The Aging Skeleton

The Aging Skeleton

Edited by

Clifford J. Rosen

Maine Center for Osteoporosis Research & Education
St. Joseph Hospital
Bangor, Maine

Julie Glowacki

Department of Orthopedic Surgery
Brigham and Women's Hospital and Massachusetts General Hospital
Harvard Medical School and Harvard School of Dental Medicine
Boston, Massachusetts

John P. Bilezikian

Department of Medicine
Division of Endocrinology
College of Physicians & Surgeons
Columbia University
New York, New York

Academic Press

San Diego New York Boston London
Sydney Tokyo Toronto

This book is printed on acid-free paper. ∞

Academic Press
a division of Harcourt Brace & Company
525 B Street, Suite 1900, San Diego, California 92101-4495, USA
http://www.apnet.com

Academic Press
24-28 Oval Road, London NW1 7DX, UK
http://www.hbuk.co.uk/ap/

Library of Congress Catalog Card Number: 98-89311

International Standard Book Number: 0-12-098655-8

PRINTED IN THE UNITED STATES OF AMERICA
99 00 01 02 03 04 QW 9 8 7 6 5 4 3 2 1

Contents

Contributors

John J. B. Anderson
Department of Nutrition, Schools of Public Health and Medicine, University of North Carolina, Chapel Hill, North Carolina 21599

Merredith August
Department of Oral and Maxillofacial Surgery, Massachusetts General Hospital, Boston, Massachusetts 02114

Daniel T. Baran
Department of Orthopedics and Physical Rehabilitation, University of Massachusetts Medical Center, Worcester, Massachusetts 01655

David J. Baylink
Departments of Medicine and Biochemistry, Jerry L. Pettis VA Medical Center, Loma Linda, California 92357

Belinda Beck
Geriatrics Research, Education and Clinical Center, Veterans Affairs Medical Center, Palo Alto; and Department of Medicine, Stanford University, Stanford, California 94304

Norman H. Bell
Department of Pediatrics, Medicine and Pharmacology, Medical University of South Carolina and Department of Veterans Affairs Medical Center, Charleston, South Carolina 29401

Paolo Bianco
Department of Experimental Medicine, University of Aquila, L'Aquila, Italy

John P. Bilezikian
Division of Endocrinology, Columbia University College of Physicians and Surgeons, New York, New York

Jean-Philippe Bonjour
Department of Internal Medicine, World Health Organization Collaborating Center for Osteoporosis and Bone Diseases, University Hospital, Geneva, Switzerland

Mary L. Bouxsein
Orthopedic Biomechanics Laboratory, Beth Israel Deaconess Medical Center and Harvard Medical School, Boston, Massachusetts 02215

David B. Burr
Departments of Anatomy and Orthopedic Surgery, Indiana University School of Medicine, Indianapolis, Indiana 46202

Dennis R. Carter
Biomechanical Engineering Division, Stanford University, Stanford, California 94305; and Rehabilitation R&D Center, Department of Veterans Affairs, Palo Alto, California 94304

Juliet Compston
School of Clinical Medicine, University of Cambridge, Cambridge, United Kingdom

Felicia Cosman
Clinical Research Center, Helen Hayes Hospital, West Haverstraw, New York

Deborah Cardamone Cusatis
Department of Health Evaluation Sciences, Hershey Medical Center, Penn State College of Medicine and University Hospitals, Hershey, Pennsylvania 17033

Leah Rae Donahue
The Jackson Laboratory, Bar Harbor, Maine

Thomas A. Einhorn
Department of Orthopedic Surgery, Boston University School of Medicine, Boston, Massachusetts 02118

Murray J. Favus
Bone Program, University of Chicago Pritzker School of Medicine, Chicago, Illinois 60637

Kathleen Forti-Gallant
Pain Program, Penobscot Pain Management, Bangor, Maine 04402

L. J. Fraher
Department of Medicine and the Lawson Research Institute, St. Joseph's Health Centre, and the Univer-

sity of Western Ontario, London, Ontario, Canada N6A 4V2

F. Michael Gloth
Department of Geriatrics, Union Memorial Hospital and Johns Hopkins University School of Medicine, Baltimore, Maryland 21218

Julie Glowacki
Skeletal Biology Laboratory, Brigham and Women's Hospital and Massachusetts General Hospital, Boston, Massachusetts

Deborah T. Gold
Department of Psychiatry and Behavioral Sciences; Center for the Study of Aging and Human Development; and Department of Sociology, Duke University, Durham, North Carolina 27708

Caren M. Gundberg
Department of Orthopedics and Rehabilitation, Yale University School of Medicine, New Haven, Connecticut 06520

Robert P. Heaney
Creighton University, Omaha, Nebraska 68131

A. B. Hodsman
Department of Medicine and the Lawson Research Institute, St. Joseph's Health Centre, and the University of Western Ontario, London, Ontario, Canada N6A 4V2

Mark C. Horowitz
Department of Orthopedics and Rehabilitation, Yale University School of Medicine, New Haven, Connecticut 06510

Leonard B. Kaban
Department of Oral and Maxillofacial Surgery, Massachusetts General Hospital, Boston, Massachusetts 02114

Dike N. Kalu
Department of Physiology, University of Texas Health Science Center, San Antonio, Texas 78284

L. Lyndon Key
Department of Pediatrics, Medicine and Pharmacology, Medical University of South Carolina and Department of Veterans Affairs Medical Center, Charleston, South Carolina 29401

Douglas P. Kiel
Harvard Medical School Division on Aging and Hebrew Rehabilitation Center for Aged Research and Training Institute, Boston Massachusetts 02131

Peter Lakatos
Department of Medicine, Semmelweis University Medical School, Budapest, Hungary

K.-H. William Lau
Departments of Medicine and Biochemistry, Jerry L. Pettis Memorial VA Medical Center, Loma Linda, California 92357

Meryl S. LeBoff
Brigham and Women's Hospital, Harvard Medical School, Boston, Massachusetts 02115

Peter Leong
Pain Program, Penobscot Pain Management, Bangor, Maine 04402

Robert Lindsay
Clinical Research Center, Helen Hayes Hospital, West Haverstraw, New York

Loren G. Lipson
Division of Geriatric Medicine, Department of Medicine, University of Southern California School of Medicine, Los Angeles, California

Tom Lloyd
Department of Health Evaluation Sciences, Hershey Medical Center, Penn State College of Medicine and University Hospitals, Hershey, Pennsylvania 17033

Kenneth W. Lyles
Duke University Medical Center, Durham, North Carolina; and GRECC, VA Medical Center, Durham, North Carolina 27705

Robert Marcus
Geriatrics Research, Education and Clinical Center, Veterans Affairs Medical Center, Palo Alto, and Department of Medicine, Stanford University, Stanford, California 94304

Carlos A. Mautalen
Clinical Hospital, University of Buenos Aires, Buenos Aires, Argentina

Jeffrey D. Moffett
Department of Orthopedic Surgery, Boston University School of Medicine, Boston, Massachusetts 02118

Subburaman Mohan
Jerry L. Pettis VA Medical Center, Loma Linda University, Loma Linda, California 92357

Douglas B. Muchmore
Lilly Research Laboratories, Eli Lilly and Company, Indianapolis, Indiana 46285

Dorothy A. Nelson
Department of Anthropology and Department of Internal Medicine, Wayne State University School of Medicine, Detroit, Michigan 48201

Michael C. Nevitt
Department of Epidemiology and Biostatistics, University of California, San Francisco, California 94105

Beatriz Oliveri
Clinical Hospital, University of Buenos Aires, Buenos Aires, Argentina

Eric Orwoll
Oregon Health Sciences University, Endocrinology and Metabolism, Portland VA Medical Center, Portland, Oregon 97207

Sacrates E. Papapoulos
Department of Endocrinology and Metabolic Diseases, Leiden University Medical Center, The Netherlands

R. L. Prince
University Department of Medicine, University of Western Australia and Department of Endocrinology & Diabetes, Sir Charles Gairdner Hospital, Nedlands, Western Australia 6009

Lawrence G. Raisz
Department of Endocrinology, University of Connecticut Health Center, Farmington, Connecticut

René Rizzoli
Department of Internal Medicine, World Health Organization Collaborating Center for Osteoporosis and Bone Diseases, University Hospital, Geneva, Switzerland

Pamela Gehron Robey
National Institute of Dental Research, National Institutes of Health, Bethesda, Maryland 20892

Simon P. Robins
Rowett Research Institute, Bucksburn University, Aberdeen, Scotland

Clifford J. Rosen
Maine Center for Osteoporosis Research, Bangor, Maine 04401

Philip D. Ross
Scientific Publications Group, Merck & Co., Inc., Rahway, New Jersey

Clinton Rubin
Musculo-Skeletal Research Laboratory, Program in Biomedical Engineering, State University of New York–Stony Brook, Stony Brook, New York 11794

Harry Rubin
Department of Molecular and Cell Biology and Virus Laboratory, University of California, Berkeley, California 94720

Janet Rubin
Department of Medicine, Emory University School of Medicine and Veterans Affairs Medical Center, Atlanta, Georgia 30033

Arthur Santora
Scientific Publications Group, Merck & Co., Inc., Rahway, New Jersey

Debra H. Schussheim
Department of Medicine, College of Physicians and Surgeons, Columbia University, New York, New York 10032

Ego Seeman
Austin and Repatriation Medical Centre, University of Melbourne, Melbourne, Australia

Markus J. Seibel
Department of Medicine, College of Physicians and Surgeons, University of Heidelberg Medical School, Heidelberg, Germany

Sherry Sherman
Clinical Endocrinology and Osteoporosis Research, National Institute on Aging, National Institutes of Health, Bethesda, Maryland 20892

Shonni J. Silverberg
Department of Medicine, Columbia University, New York, New York 10032

Mehrsheed Sinaki
Physical Medicine and Rehabilitation, Mayo Clinic, Rochester, Minnesota 55905

Ethel S. Siris
Department of Medicine, College of Physicians and Surgeons, Columbia University, New York, New York, and Toni Stabile Center for the Prevention and Treatment of Osteoporosis, Columbia-Presbyterian Medical Center, New York, New York 10032

Paula H. Stern
Department of Molecular Pharmacology and Biological Chemistry, Northwestern University Medical School, Chicago, Illinois

John L. Stock
The Medical Center of Central Massachusetts, University of Massachusetts Memorial Health Care, Worcester, Massachusetts

Thomas S. Thornhill
Department of Orthopedic Surgery, Brigham and Women's Hospital, Boston, Massachusetts

Charles H. Turner
Department of Orthopaedic Surgery and Mechanical Engineering, Biomechanics and Biomaterials Research Center, Indiana University School of Medicine, Indianapolis, Indiana 46202

Marjolein C. H. van der Meulen
Department of Mechanical and Aerospace Engineering, Cornell University, Ithaca, New York 14853

Marie Luz Villa
Department of Medicine, University of Washington School of Medicine, Mercer Island, Washington 98040

Michelle P. Warren
Department of Obstetrics and Gynecology, College of Physicians and Surgeons, Columbia University, New York, New York 10032

Richard C. Wasnich
Hawaii Osteoporosis Center, Honolulu, Hawaii 96814

P. H. Watson
Department of Medicine and the Lawson Research Institute, St. Joseph's Health Centre, and the Univer-

sity of Western Ontario, London, Ontario, Canada N6A 4V2

Catherine E. Waud
The Medical Center of Central Massachusetts, University of Massachusetts Memorial Health Care, Worcester, Massachusetts

Jonathan M. Weiner
Division of Geriatric Medicine, Department of Medicine, University of Southern California School of Medicine, Los Angeles, California 90033

Mark L. Weiss
Department of Anthropology and Department of Internal Medicine, Wayne State University, Detroit, Michigan 48201

Mitchell J. Winemaker
Brigham and Women's Hospital, Harvard Medical School, Boston, Massachusetts 02115

A. John Yates
Scientific Publications Group, Merck & Co., Inc., Rahway, New Jersey

Foreword

This remarkably substantive textbook provides a clear testament to how much new knowledge has been gained over the past 15 years on the causes and treatments of osteoporosis and other bone diseases of the elderly. These advances have all come about by a converging development of expanding activities by several diverse, but complementary, organizational forces that support research: (1) scientific societies; (2) governmental agencies supporting biomedical research; (3) the pharmaceutical and biotechnology industries; and (4) new and vital voluntary health agencies. A generation ago, it was largely held that osteoporosis was, for the most part, the inevitable consequence of aging. Much excellent research on calcium metabolism had pointed to an imbalance. That osteoporosis was largely a disease of elderly women was ascribed to the menopause with its attendant estrogen loss.

It all started in the late 1970s. The "bone doctors" in the Endocrine Society formed their own new scientific association, the American Society for Bone and Mineral Research (ASBMR), recruiting relevant basic and clinical scientists to join them in their work. The growth of the ASBMR has been nothing less than spectacular, with even more abstracts of higher quality competing for presentation at annual scientific meetings, and the creation and success of its *Journal of Bone and Mineral Research.* Even more recently in the 1990s, the International Society for Clinical Densitometry was useful with similarly spectacular growth.

Several initiatives on bone biology and its diseases were launched by the National Institutes of Health (NIH). The NIDDK, NIAMD, and NIDR had been supporting excellent intramural programs of research on bone and bone diseases. In the 1980s other institutes developed new programs targeted to bone research. The new NIAMS (I was its first director) established a new extramural program on bone biology and bone diseases with superb new leadership and became the fastest growing extramural research program in the Institute. The National Institute of Aging (NIA) also formed new programs (e.g., on menopause, frailty, basic biology), as did other Institutes. In 1993, a Federal Working Group on Bone Diseases was formed, with 15 different agencies participating in information exchange and forging collaborative activities. One landmark was the 1984 NIH Consensus Development Conference on Osteoporosis, chaired with great expertise by Dr. William A. Peck; it was a broad-ranging conference that informed both the public and professionals on the importance of hormonal replacement therapy and sufficient calcium intake to combat bone loss and recommended many new directions for research. The NIH investment in research on bone and osteoporosis has grown sharply since that time. Important research advances have been achieved; most are very well documented in this text on the aging skeleton. Moreover, public interest has risen greatly. For example, as a result of the NIH Conference on Optimal Calcium Intake in 1994, so ably chaired by Dr. John Bilezikian, the elderly have responded by increasing their intake of both calcium and vitamin D.

The major contributions of the pharmaceutical industry to the prevention and treatment of osteoporosis deserve emphasis. This excellent textbook documents the research advances that have been made. To mention a few, let us note briefly the development of calcitonin, both by injection and by nasal spray, of bisphosphonates, and of estrogen analogues.

Major contributions have also been made by the biotechnology industry in terms of accurate and precise measures of bone density by dual energy X-ray absorptiometry (DXA) and ultrasound, and new useful biochemical measurements of bone turnover. Appropriately, an entire section of this textbook is devoted to the topic of quantifying the amount and dynamics of bone loss.

In addition, organizations were created to educate the public and professionals about the issues and new developments and to arouse public interest in supporting research on osteoporosis and other bone diseases. These organizations include The National Osteoporosis Foundation, The Paget's Disease Foundation, The Osteoporosis Imperfecta Foundation, and others. Older organizations such as The National Dairy Council renewed its efforts to educate the public in skeletal health. As a result of their dedication and drive, public interest and the number of publications in the various media in this field have soared.

This textbook has been organized in a very effective manner. In the first section, aging is discussed both generally and in terms of the aging skeleton, with separate chapters on cellular, animal, and human models. In the second section, the important concepts of achieving peak bone mass by the end of the third human decade are discussed in detail, with individual chapters on racial, genetic, nutritional, hormonal, and mechanical determinants of peak bone mass. The importance of making every effort to maintain bone mass after 30 years of age is introduced. The many different mechanisms that participate in age-related bone loss are discussed individually in the chapters contained in Section III. In addition to novel perspectives on the "standard topics" of sex steroids, parathyroid hormones, and nutrition, other chapters describe recent interest in cytokines, prostaglandins, growth hormones, and pharmacologic agents. Section IV describes several new methods that have been developed to measure quantitatively, often with great precision, bone mass. Perhaps primary among these has been the development and clinical application of bone densitometry with new technologies such as DXA and ultrasound. Bone densitometry now provides major, essential guideposts to the treatment and prevention of osteoporosis and other bone diseases in our senior citizens. A testament to the importance of these new methods is the creation of a new scientific publication, *The Journal of Clinical Densitometry,* edited by Dr. Clifford J. Rosen.

The final two sections cover the consequences to the patient of bone loss (fractures) and the many methods of treating (and preventing) bone loss and osteoporosis. The discussion of fractures is thorough, including a definition of frailty fractures (more challenging than one might expect); fractures at different anatomic sites; effects of fractures on quality of life; and management issues with respect to orthopedics, pain, and nutrition. Section VI, on therapeutics, is exceptionally comprehensive, reflecting the many scientific advances that have been accomplished in this field in recent years. The rationales for calcium supplementation and vitamin D are discussed individually, as are the important benefits of estrogen replacement. There are excellent chapters on bisphosphonates, calcitonin, and the "paradoxical" efficacy of parathyroid hormone treatment. Promising yet controversial therapeutic approaches—fluorides, androgens, and growth hormones and growth-factors—are also covered individually. Also discussed are the prevention of falls and the impacts of different types of physical activity on bone and bone loss. As a result of the many recent advances in treatment as described in the text, physicians now have at hand a strong armamentarium of agents with which to prevent, and with some agents to reverse, the bone loss of the aging skeleton.

And last, the editors of this textbook deserve to be congratulated on their success in recruiting such a high caliber of contributing authors (authorities) for this volume. They are virtually all national and international leaders, constituting a "Who's Who" in bone and mineral research and related topics.

LAWRENCE E. SHULMAN, M.D., PH.D.

BETHESDA, MARYLAND

Preface

Our understanding of the basic and clinical aspects of bone biology has advanced remarkably in the past decade. In part this advance has been driven by an astonishing increase in the prevalence of osteoporosis due to the "graying" of the world's population, as well as by a heightened awareness of the disease. Equally important, the medical, social, and economic impact of osteoporotic fractures has finally been confirmed. Although it is likely that osteoporosis has existed for centuries, we are now entering a new millennium not only with the hope of effectively managing the consequences of this disease but also with the promise of its potential eradication. This book summarizes and organizes our progress in defining the complex and multifactorial events that contribute to age-related bone disease. In addition, a third of this text is devoted to a comprehensive therapeutic approach for clinicians faced with the unique problems that elderly osteoporotic individuals face on a daily basis.

In retrospect, it is easy to see how this book was born. Yet, a decade ago it would have been inconceivable even to propose a comprehensive treatise about the aging skeleton. Although low bone mass and increased skeletal fragility characterized the aging process, little else was clear. A mere 10 years ago, many clinicians and most scientists viewed osteoporosis as a normal consequence of aging rather than as a disorder with distinct pathophysiological features. There were no therapeutic paradigms for those who had sustained disabling spine and hip fractures. Worse, few older women were ever considered for treatment. Preventive strategies in this age group were not even on the "radar screen." Also, efforts to discern pathogenic pathways on a molecular or cellular level were embryonic. Moreover, little was known about the physiology of skeletal remodeling in the elderly. Clearly, times have changed. In fact, large longitudinal and cross-sectional studies of the elderly, along with newer tools to define bone remodeling, have pointed the way to a clearer understanding of the disease for all individuals. Thus, it is entirely fitting that we commit an entire textbook to delineating the mechanisms and consequences of skeletal aging.

This book is divided into six sections. Together they represent an integration of fundamental biology, epidemiology, and clinical medicine. This alignment matches the perspectives and expertise of the editors, who felt that a comprehensive review of the aging skeleton mandated this approach. In the first section, chapters focus on the general aspects of aging in higher organisms and the application of specific models of senescence to skeletal determinants such as calcium balance and remodeling. Use of *in vitro* and *in vivo* systems, with their strengths and limitations, provides an important backdrop for the next sections and introduces the reader to the rest of the book.

Bone mass is determined by the balance between peak acquisition during adolescence and maintenance throughout adult life. In the second and third sections, nutritional, heritable, environmental, mechanical, and hormonal influences are examined with respect to acquisition, maintenance, and loss of bone mass. Particular attention is given to cellular and tissue responses in the aging skeleton to perturbations of various hormones, growth factors, and cytokines. These sections are followed by an in-depth presentation of quantifiable measures of bone loss, including bone mineral density, histomorphometry, biochemical markers of bone turnover, and biomechanical determinants. In the fifth section, the biomechanical aspects of fractures and their socioeconomic and medical consequences are delineated. In the final section, a wide range of therapeutic interventions from fall prevention, to dietary recommendations, to pharmacological treatments are considered in depth. For each section, expert clinicians and scientists were selected on the basis of their investigative areas, their contributions to our current understanding of osteoporosis, and their "fit" within the overall perspective of the book. For each chapter individual themes are stressed, but all are written in a manner that is consistent with the principles and practices of both geriatric and skeletal medicine.

This textbook brings together experts in the field of bone biology and medicine to define the "aging" skeleton and to determine its implications for aging individuals. Ultimately, we hope this book will be used by students, basic and clinical scientists, geriatricians, orthopedic and oral surgeons, internists, endocrinologists, rheumatologists, gynecologists, and primary care physicians as they continue their quest for solutions to the enigmas that surround the aging process in bone. We hope that the multidisciplinary themes that emerge will stimulate further attempts to ameliorate and ultimately to prevent osteoporosis.

CLIFFORD J. ROSEN

JULIE GLOWACKI

JOHN P. BILEZIKIAN

Part I

General Aspects and Models of Aging

CHAPTER 1

Aging through the Ages

DOROTHY A. NELSON Department of Internal Medicine, Wayne State University School of Medicine, and Department of Anthropology, Wayne State University, Detroit, Michigan 48201

MARK L. WEISS Department of Anthropology, Wayne State University, Detroit, Michigan 48201

The increasing longevity of modern populations explains much of the alarming increase in the rate of osteoporotic fractures. In many respects, osteoporosis, defined as low bone mass and an increased risk of fracture, can be considered to be a consequence of age-related degenerative effects on the skeleton and other organ systems. It is not clear whether age-related changes are genetically determined (programmed) from birth or whether they result from the lifelong accumulation of structural and functional errors at the cellular level. In either case, the modification of developmental changes over the life span, such that peak bone mass can be maximized or osteoporosis avoided, should be relatively difficult.

Studies of past populations indicate that low bone mass was not a problem in human populations until relatively recently in evolutionary terms. Diseases of aging, including osteoporosis, that we see today are the manifestation of millions of years of genetic and cultural change and adaption. It is difficult to explain the adaptive value of an increased life expectancy when many of the consequences of aging would seem to be maladaptive for the population as well as the individual. This is particularly true because natural selection, the primary force responsible for adaptation, presumably cannot affect biological characteristics that occur after the age of reproduction since it acts through differential reproductive success. Thus, increasing longevity and a rising prevalence of debilitating conditions in the elderly are difficult to explain with traditional evolutionary models of adaptation. It would appear that unless the genetics of bone biology underlying low bone mass with fragility fractures in the elderly can be modified, the prevalence of osteoporosis and its public health costs may unavoidably increase as human life expectancy lengthens.

INTRODUCTION

Members of industrialized societies today look for ward to a long life expectancy. However, this is not true of many other human populations, both past and present, where an individual's lifetime may be relatively short. The increase in human longevity is a benefit of relatively recent improvements in health and nutrition, but it does come with costs. Degenerative changes and age-related diseases or conditions, associated with varying levels of morbidity and public health costs, have become more prevalent in modern society. In many respects, osteoporosis can be considered to be a consequence of age-related degenerative effects on the skeleton and other organ systems. There are, of course, well-documented factors other than aging that can contribute to an individual's risk of osteoporosis (e.g., diseases, drug exposures), but the increasing longevity of human populations explains much of the alarming increase in the rate of osteoporotic fractures.

As Stanley Garn reported in his classic study [1], bone loss after middle age is a universal phenomenon in the human species, an observation that has been corroborated by numerous studies since then. This phenomenon appears to extend to nonhuman primates as well [2,3], suggesting that human ancestors might have faced the problem of osteoporosis if they had had longer life spans. However, studies of past populations indicate that low bone mass was not a problem in human populations until the transition from gathering–hunting to agriculture some 10–12,000 years ago [4]. Figure 1 depicts 200 million years of mammalian evolution on a 12-h clock in order to put into perspective how recently hominids (i.e., human ancestors) appeared and food production began in evolutionary time. Some evidence suggests that despite apparent bone loss in some prehistoric groups, bone quality may have been preserved, reducing the likelihood of fragility fractures that are now recognized as osteoporosis (see later) [5]. It is unclear whether the occurrence of low bone mass in such populations was due to longevity in some individuals or groups, to environmental factors, or to both, but osteoporosis per se does not appear to have been a major problem until recently.

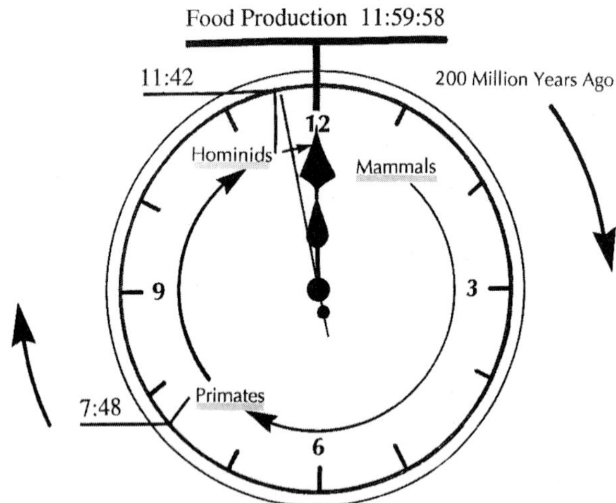

FIGURE 1 Representation of 200 million years of mammalian evolution on a 12-hr clock analog, with emphasis on recent appearance of earliest humans (hominids) and food production. From Nelson [32], copyright by European Foundation for Osteoporosis and the National Osteoporosis Foundation.

This chapter offers an anthropological perspective on aging in relation to bone health and osteoporosis. It explores some of the biocultural correlates of aging and increased longevity and their relationship to osteoporosis in an evolutionary context.

EVOLUTIONARY FORCES AND AGING

Evolution and Genetics

The primary forces of evolution are mutation and natural selection. Mutations are random alterations in the structure of genes and are the ultimate source of new genes. However, it is unlikely that a single mutation or set of mutations has resulted in the universality of age-related bone loss. Natural selection works via the differential reproductive success of the alternative genotypes to which mutation gives rise. As such it is an ordering force that increases the frequency of beneficial mutations while decreasing the frequency of deleterious ones. Benefit and detriment are relative terms and it is important to keep in mind that judging these qualities is dependent on many variables, including the species' genetic background and its ecological situation. The genetic background is determined, in part, by the effects of past evolutionary processes on other genetic traits. Viewed this way we can see that the current genetic structure of a species sets boundaries and channels of change for future possibilities. A species' history delimits a range of possibilities for future change. Adding to the complexity is the need for the coordination of gene actions affecting organisms at different times in their life cycles.

Advanced molecular and statistical techniques have allowed the identification of a number of structural candidate genes that may be involved in the etiology of osteoporosis [6–9]. However, diseases of aging, such as osteoporosis, may be influenced by regulatory loci operating at another level. Over the past several decades, molecular geneticists have elucidated several classes of genes that act as regulators of gene function; determining the timing of gene action, the polarity of the embryo, and other developmental phenomena [10,11]. Although a discussion of developmental pathways is beyond the scope of this chapter, it is important to realize that the genotype guides the development of an organism down a series of channels so as to establish the basic body plan of the individual. The body segmentation, for instance, that is seen in animals from fruit flies to humans, is affected by homeotic genes that have been highly conserved over enormous spans of evolution. The evolutionary conservation of the DNA sequence and number of these homeotic genes is a clear indication of their importance in proper development. The patterning of bone deposition and remodeling throughout the life cycle is also a fundamental developmental process. This developmental path is almost certainly affected by factors other than allelic variation for one or another protein. To the degree that the gain and loss of bone during an individual's lifetime reflects an evolved pattern of developmental rather than variation in the form of a few proteins, modification of this pattern such that peak bone mass can be maximized or osteoporosis avoided should be relatively difficult.

Aging in an Adaptive Framework

Universally encountered biological phenomena, such as age-related bone loss, have traditionally been viewed by physical anthropologists as having adaptive value, if not now, then in past populations living under difficult circumstances. In order to understand this perspective, one must appreciate the time depth over which evolution has occurred in the human species, as well as the complexity of human development over the life cycle of individuals. Both ontogeny and phylogeny are the result of interactions of genetic potential and environmental influences. These complex interrelationships have been acting on human biology over a tremendously long period, beginning with the first humans some 5 million years ago and extending back through the evolution of our primate ancestors 70 million years ago and beyond. Thus, the human biological phenomena seen today, including aging in general and the disease osteoporosis in particular, are the current manifestation of millions of years of genetic change and adaptation to different environments. Further layers of complexity are added by the behavioral and cultural capabilities of our species.

An evolutionary perspective on aging raises an interesting conundrum: if selection operates by differential reproduction of genotypes, then biological characteristics that occur after the age of reproduction cannot be easily explained. Figure 2 illustrates that the effectiveness of natural selection declines over the course of the reproductive period and varies inversely with cumulative reproductive success. How can selection operate on characteristics that evidence themselves after the reproductive years? For that matter, why do people survive beyond their reproductive years at all, especially as many of the results of aging would seem to be maladaptive for the individual?

One explanation of human longevity that has been proposed relates to the particularly human ability to provide care for the young. Hawkes *et al.* [12] propose that older members of a population, and grandmothers in particular, make important contributions to the survival and reproductive success of their lineal descendants. This model has no obvious solution to the osteoporosis puzzle, as osteoporosis as a debilitating condition should reduce one's ability to help younger generations. One could even postulate that it would be maladaptive for a population to have to take care of its elderly if resources are limited, thus making a shortened life span advantageous to the group. In this context, increasing longevity and a rising prevalence of debilitating conditions in the elderly are difficult to explain with traditional evolutionary models of adaptation. A solution to the puzzle may rest on the realization that it is only recently in evolutionary terms that people survived past middle age in appreciable numbers; there has been little time for the evolutionary impact or significance of increased longevity to become evident.

GENETICS AND LONGEVITY

While it is difficult to explain in evolutionary perspective the aging processes that occur after reproductive potential ends (menopause in women) or markedly decreases (in older men, see Fig. 3), several theoretical models have been considered (see review in Turner and Weiss [13]). The details of these are beyond the scope of this chapter, but the two major categories can be briefly described. One is a model of programmed aging that ascribes aging to phenomena built into the cells' genetic information and relies on adaptive models that require natural selection [13–16]. Alternatively, stochastic models attribute aging to the accumulation of random errors in the structure and function of cellular mechanisms, explaining senescence as the decay of homeostasis [13,17,18]. The "program" view holds that senescence is the final stage in growth and development that begins at conception [13]. As cells divide, preprogrammed genetic switches (regulatory genes) are tuned on and off. The constancy of patterns in growth and development within a species provides strong evidence for genetic programming of the life cycle [19] and, specifically, the process of aging. These may work primarily through hormonal, changes that are genetically programmed, such as menopause in human females. The stochastic models of aging focus on the accumulation of errors with age, including the "free radical theory,"

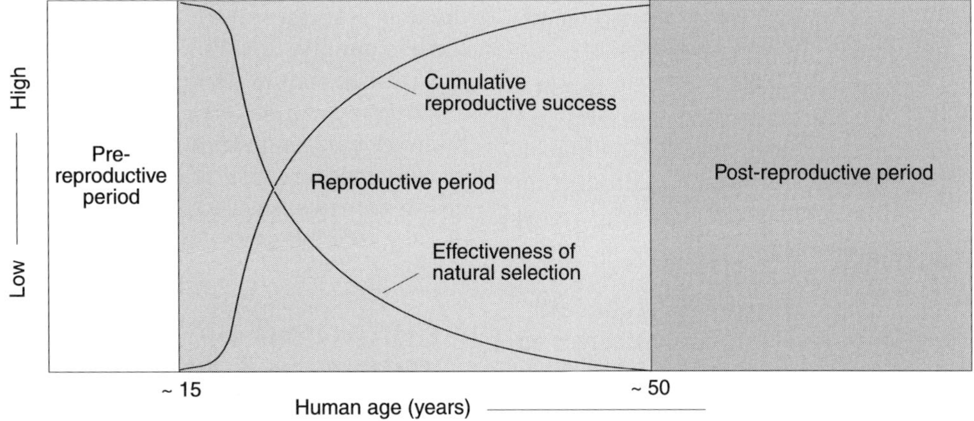

FIGURE 2 Decline in effectiveness of natural selection as reproductive success is reached over the course of an individual's reproductive period. Increasing human longevity extends the postreproductive period when natural selection has little effect. From Olshansky *et al.* [30].

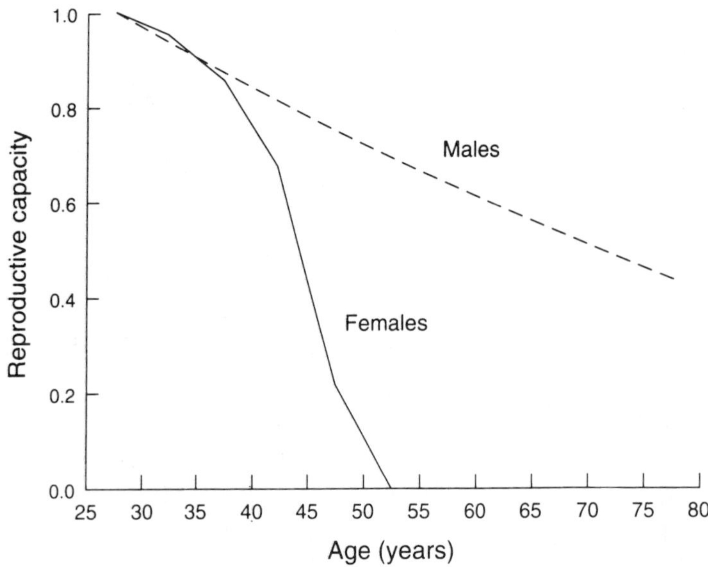

FIGURE 3 Reproductive senescence in men and women after ages 25–29 years. From Wood *et al.* [20], with permission of Oxford University Press, Inc.

decreased DNA repair, somatic mutations, and others [13,17,18]. These ideas are probably not mutually exclusive, leading us to a picture of complex interactions, at the cellular and molecular levels, between genes and environmental factors that are especially difficult to understand in human populations [13]. At present it would appear that the genetic predisposition for longevity is dependent less on genes for a long life than on *not* having genes for conditions that might cause a shorter life span [13]. In summary, aging appears to involve a "multitude of different, poorly coordinated senescent processes" rather than a single underlying process [20].

PRIMATES

Expansion of the life span past the end of the reproductive years is uncommon among nonhuman primates (see Fig. 4), and has only occurred relatively recently among humans [21]. Studies suggest that few primates living in the wild exhibit a menopause [22], although there may be an age-related decrease in reproduction in some but not all older animals. In contrast, women in industrialized society can expect to spend at least a third of their lives after menopause.

Data from observations of primates in nature compared with observations in zoo populations may shed some light on the important role of environmental factors in aging and in the expression of age-related disease [23]. Captive animals may approach or even reach their species' potential for longevity, or maximum life span [23]. Some animals live long enough to exhibit diseases of aging similar to those seen in older people. Such spontaneously occurring diseases seen in captive primates include degenerative joint disease, rheumatoid arthritis, atherosclerosis, diabetes mellitus, and osteoporosis [3]. Although it could be argued that captive animals live in artificial circumstances, they are somewhat comparable to some modern human populations who have abundant food, shelter, and medical care—in a sense, they are relying on culture to remove some of the environmental stressors experienced by animals in the wild or, by analogy, experienced by traditional peoples. Thus, in nature, primates including humans probably do not reach their maximal life span; under artificial conditions (captivity for nonhuman primates) or technologically and culturally complex conditions (people in developed countries), the maximal species life span is more often reached. If the socioeconomic burden of diseases associated with aging can be "absorbed" by the community, then they will become more prevalent. This burden may, at some point, cross a critical threshold and become a drain on resources. In nature, this is most often the case, and elderly individuals are not sustained; in contemporary life, it is recognized that the public health burden of such age-related diseases as osteoporosis may soon become a crisis.

CHANGING DEMOGRAPHICS THROUGH THE AGES

Prehistoric and Nonindustrialized Societies

In prehistoric populations, and in hunter–gatherers (until very recently), life expectancy was much shorter

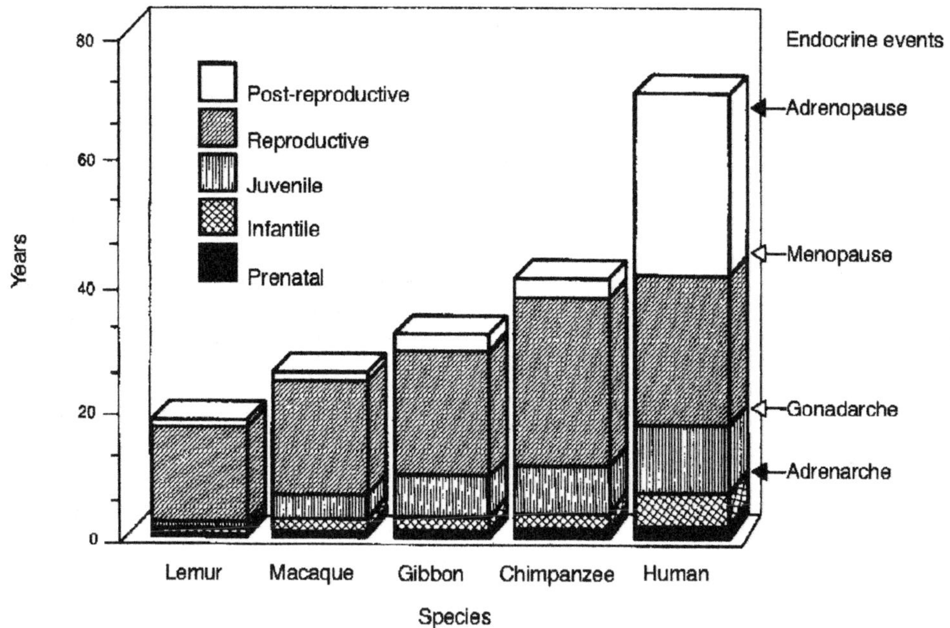

FIGURE 4 Longevity in selected primates compared with human, with duration of major life periods including postreproductive stage. From Katz *et al.* [21] with permission of Oxford University Press, Inc.

than in today's populations. However, age-related bone loss has been documented in some prehistoric populations [4,5]. In contrast with modern populations, it rarely results in osteoporosis (fractures) and its sequelae, in part because not many individuals live long enough to be affected. Furthermore, some evidence suggests that bone quality may have been maintained better in past populations than in modern populations experiencing low bone mass after midadulthood [5].

It is believed that such factors as a high infant and childhood mortality rate and a high incidence of injury deaths contributed to the lower life expectancy among prehistoric, technologically simple societies relying on gathering and hunting wild foods. Such was the case for all of humankind until the advent of agriculture some 10–12,000 years ago. Figure 1 puts into perspective this long period of human prehistory before food production. In early agricultural societies, infectious disease became a significant cause of death, which in turn limited life expectancy. Such conditions existed partly because of larger population sizes, increased sedentism and interpersonal contact, the accumulation of garbage and contaminants, and the introduction of domesticated animals. Poor nutrition was often an associated problem. Interestingly, studies of prehistoric populations have found a lower bone mass among transitional agriculturalists compared with hunter–gatherers [4,24]. Although this has been attributed in part to nutritional deficiency, particularly of calcium, it was almost certainly a combination of poor nutrition in general, periods of starvation, disease, and other stresses.

Urban Populations and Industrialized Societies

Farther along the continuum of socioeconomic complexity is the urbanization of populations, leading to the current classification of societies into preindustrial and industrial. As was seen with the transition to agriculture, this new phase was associated with new health problems, such as epidemics (e.g., the Black Death in Europe) and crime. Today's major health problems of industrialization are noninfectious diseases such as cardiovascular diseases, cancers, diabetes, and osteoporosis, which are somewhat offset by overall reductions in mortality, including infant mortality. According to this model of "epidemiologic transition" [25], the primary cause of death following the change from infectious disease is the increase in degenerative noninfectious diseases. This is associated with a longer life expectancy at birth, but not a longer life span (the limit of human life). Osteoporosis fits neatly into this model of urbanization and transition, as it appears that the more economically developed nations also have the highest evidence of osteoporotic fracture [26,27].

LOW BONE MASS IN PAST POPULATIONS

Measures of bone mass and bone quality in past populations include cortical thickness, cortical area, bone mineral content, and histomorphometry. Such studies of skeletal remains are limited by the relative imprecision with which covariates such as age and sex can be ascribed to individual skeletons. There is also some degree of error inherent in reconstructing lifeways, including dietary adaptations and physical activity types and levels. Furthermore, bone can be modified by its burial environment. With these caveats in mind, current knowledge of bone quantity and bone quality can be summarized from studies of skeletal collections from three main geographic areas: Sudanese Nubia (approximately 350 B.C. to 1450 A.D.), eastern and southwestern North America (from 2000 B.C. to the contact period), and the Arctic (from approximately 700 B.C.). There are a few additional studies from Europe and the near East. Full references to these studies can be found in Pfeiffer and Lazenby [4].

These investigations have reported that some groups appear to have low bone mass in comparison to other groups (either prehistoric and modern) that appear to have "normal" bone mass and better overall health indicators. Those studies that found a relatively low bone mass implicate such factors as chronic malnutrition associated with the origin and intensification of agriculture (North American and Nubia) or a heavy reliance on animal protein in the diet (Arctic). For example, one study reported that hunter-gatherers from 6000 years ago in what is now Illinois had thicker cortices, higher bone mineral content, and better maintenance of bone in late adulthood than maize agriculturalists from the same region, several millennia later [24]. Many investigators have suggested that the *transition* to agriculture is characterized by increases in morbidity and mortality and created health problems that are manifest in the skeleton [4]. In summary, low bone mass has been found in past populations from a variety of geographic regions, not just among the ancestors of groups currently considered to have the highest risk of osteoporosis [4], suggesting that environmental and/or cultural factors were significant contributors. Genetic differences between populations are unlikely to be the explanation for differences in bone mass, given that many of the comparative studies involved populations that were not very distant in space or time (and thus in genetics). Old age is seldom invoked as a cause of low bone mass, as life expectancy was short. Nutritional models are most commonly used, with or without a physical activity (biomechanical) component. For example, Ruff *et al.* have suggested that agriculturalists were less physically active than hunter gatherers [28], although the types and intensity of physical activity were almost a certainly a factor [29].

A recent review of paleopathological studies of bone loss suggests that despite a low bone mass in some past populations, there is little evidence of osteoporotic fracture [5]. The authors report that bone quality may have been protected, thereby reducing the likelihood of fractures due to bone fragility. One explanation is that there was some type of compensatory mechanism affecting bone architecture that may have been affected by physical activity levels [5]. These were almost certainly higher than those of modern populations, were probably high in both sexes, and were probably maintained at a relatively high level throughout the life span.

ALTERING THE HUMAN LIFE SPAN

It has been assumed that there is a "law of mortality" that is inevitable and which postulates that individuals have a decreased ability to withstand destruction after the age of sexual maturity, especially in older age. This was first voiced by the British actuary, Benjamin Gompertz, in the early 19th century. This has been expanded into a universal law of mortality that applies to all species [30], despite species differences in longevity. Olshansky *et al.* [30] described an "intrinsic mortality signature" that they believe to be characteristic of a species. However, it is possible that senescence can be modified through direct manipulation of genes or indirectly by controlling the products of gene expression [30]. For example, Banks and Fossel [31] suggested that an *in vitro* alteration of telomeres may affect cellular senescence and, if applied to humans, might ultimately alter the human life span. As always, one can expect a tradeoff for modifying a natural process (i.e., senescence), perhaps in the form of an increased prevalence of external causes of degeneration or death [30] and certainly in terms of social and economic costs. Unless the genetics of bone biology and/or other mechanisms underlying bone loss and neuromuscular degeneration can be modified, osteoporotic fracture may well be one of those diseases whose prevalence, and public health burden, will unavoidably increase as we lengthen human life expectancy.

References

1. Garn, S. M., "The Earlier Gain and the Later Loss of Cortical Bone in Nutritional Perspective." Charles C. Thomas, Springfield.
2. Burr. D. B. The relationships among physical, geometrical and mechanical properties of bone, with a note on the properties of nonhuman primate bone. *Yearbook Phys. Anthropol.* **23,** 109 (1980).
3. Sumner, D. R., Morbeck, M. E., and Lobick J. J. Apparent age-related bone loss among adult female Gombe chimpanzees. *Am. J. Phys. Anthropol.* **79,** 25–234 (1989).
4. Pfeiffer, S. K., and Lazenby R. A. Low bone mass in past and present aboriginal populations. *In* "Advances in Nutritional Re-

search" (H. H. Draper, ed.), Vol. 9, pp. 35–51. Plenum Press, New York, 1994.
5. Agarwal, S. C., and Grynpas, M. D. Bone quantity and quality in past populations. *Anat. Rec.* **246,** 423–432 (1996).
6. Morrison, N. A., Qi, J. C., Tokita, A., Kelly, P. J., Crofts, L., Nguyen, T. V., Sambrook, P. N., and Eisman, J. A. Prediction of bone density from vitamin D receptor alleles. *Nature* **207,** 284–287 (1994).
7. Kobayashi, S., Inoue, S., Hosel, T., Ouchi, Y., Shinaki, M., and Orimo, H. Association of bone mineral density with polymorphism of the estrogen receptor gene. *J. Bone Miner. Res.* **11,** 306–311 (1996).
8. Murray, R. E., McGuigan, F., Grant, S. F. A., Reid, D. M., and Ralston, S. H. Polymorphisms of the interleukin-6 gene are associated with bone mineral density. *Bone* **21,** 89–92 (1997).
9. Uitterlinden, A. G., Burger, H., Huang, Q, Yue, F., McGuigan, F. E. A., Hofman, A., van Leeuwen, J. P. T. M., Pols, H. A. P., and Ralston, S. H. Relation of alleles of the collagen Type Iα1 gene to bone density and the risk of osteoporotic fractures in postmenopausal women. *N. Engl. J. Med.* **338,** 1016–1021 (1998).
10. Nusslein-Volhard, C., and Wieschaus, E. Mutations affecting segment number and polarity in *Drosophila. Nature* **287,** 795–801 (1980).
11. Wieschaus, E. Embryonic transcription and the control of developmental pathways. *Genetics* **142,** 5–10 (1996).
12. Hawkes, K., O'Connell J. F., and Blurton-Jones, N. G. Hadza women's time allocation, offspring provisioning, and the evolution of long postmenopausal life spans. *Curr. Anthropol.* **38,** 551–577 (1997).
13. Turner, T. R., and Weiss, M. L. The genetics of longevity in humans. *In* "Biological Anthropology and Aging" (D. E. Crews and R. M. Garruto, eds.), pp. 76–100. Oxford Univ. Press, New York, 1994.
14. Hayflick, L. The limited *in vitro* lifetime of human diploid cell strains. *Exp. Cell Res.* **37,** 614–636 (1965).
15. Goldstein, S. Replicative senescence: the human fibroblast comes of age. *Science* **249,** 1129–1133 (1990).
16. Smith, J. R., (1990). DNA synthesis inhibitors in cellular senescence. *J. Geron. Bio. Sci.* **45,** B32–B35 (1990).
17. Harman, D. Free radical theory of aging: consequences of mitochondrial aging. *Age* **6,** 86–94 (1983).
18. Saul, R. L., Gee P., and Ames B. N. Free radicals, DNA damage, and aging. *In* "Modern Biological Theories of Aging" (H. R. Warner, R. N. Butler, R. L. Sprott, and E. L. Schneider, eds.), pp. 113–129. Raven Press, New York, 1987.
19. Kirkwood, J. L. Evolution and aging. *Genome* **31,** 398–405 (1989).
20. Wood, J. W., Weeks, S. C., Bentley, G. R., and Weiss, K. M. Human population biology and the evolution of aging. *In* "Biological Anthropology and Aging" (D. E. Crews and R. M. Garruto, eds.), pp. 19–75. Oxford Univ. Press, New York, 1994.
21. Katz, S. H., and Armstrong, D. F. Cousin marriage and the x-chromosome: evolution of longevity and language. *In* "Biological Anthropology and Aging" (D. E. Crews and R. M. Garruto, eds.), pp. 101–123. Oxford Univ. Press, New York, 1994.
22. Pavelka, M. S. M., and Fedigan, L. M. Menopause: a comparative life history perspective. *Yearbook Phys. Anthropol.* **34,** 13–38 (1991).
23. DeRousseau, C. J. Primate gerontology: an emerging discipline. *In* "Biological Anthropology and Aging" (D. E. Crews and R. M. Garruto, eds.), pp. 127–153. Oxford Univ. Press, New York, 1994.
24. Nelson, D. A. Bone density in three archaeological populations. *Am. J. Phys. Anthropol.* **63,** 198 (1984).
25. Omran, A. R. The epidemiologic transition: a theory of the epidemiology of population change. *Milbank Mem. Fund Quart* **49,** 509–538 (1971).
26. Parfitt, A. M. Idiosyncratic comments on the state of knowledge in osteoporosis, with particular emphasis on its limitations. *In* "Osteoporosis 1990" (C. Christiansen and K. Overgaard, eds.), Vol. 3, pp. 1845–1851. Osteopress ApS, Copenhagen, 1990.
27. Melton, L. J., III, and Cooper, C. Epidemiology. *In* "Osteoporosis" (J. C. Stevenson and R. Lindsay, eds.), pp. 65–84. Chapman & Hall, New York, 1998.
28. Ruff, C. B., Larsen, C. S., Hayes, W. C. Structural changes in the femur with the transition to agriculture on the Georgia coast. *Am. J. Phys. Anthropol.* **64,** 125–136 (1984).
29. Bridges, P. S. Bone cortical area in the evaluation of nutrition and activity levels. *Am. J. Hum. Biol.* **1,** 785 (1989).
30. Olshansky, S. J., Carnes, B. A., and Grahn, D. Confronting the boundaries of human longevity. *Am. Sci.* **86,** 52–61.
31. Banks, D. A., and Fossel M. Telomeres, cancer, and aging. *JAMA* **278,** 1345–1348 (1997).
32. Nelson, D. A. An anthropological perspective on optimizing calcium consumption for the prevention of osteoporosis. *Osteopor. Int.* **6,** 325–328 (1996).

CHAPTER 2

Human Aging at the Millennium

SHERRY SHERMAN Clinical Endocrinology and Osteoporosis Research, National Institute on Aging, National Institutes of Health, Bethesda, Maryland 20892

As we move into the third millennium, the field of biomedical research is positioned to capitalize on unprecedented advances in medicine, technology, and public health. Dramatic increases in life expectancy—25 years in the last century—have led to burgeoning numbers of older and oldest Americans as well as a profound increase in their ratio of the total population. With these monumental changes come economic, social, cultural, and medical uncertainties about the costs of enhanced life expectancy and our ability to maintain the quality of life into the very late years.

It is in the broad context of aging processes that skeletal aging must be considered. The aging of the skeleton and the associated problem of fractures in the elderly should be viewed not in isolation but against the backdrop of the aging processes per se and multifaceted issues such as comorbidity, functional limitations, and frailty. All of these elements must ultimately be considered in the still larger context of anticipated population growth, long-term care needs and their costs, and the objective of ensuring that scientific and medical advances benefit the broadest base of the U.S. population, especially its various special populations.

AGING IS HIGHLY VARIABLE

Increasingly sophisticated research in aging since the mid-1970s has led us to discard the concept of aging as an inevitable, inexorable, unified progression toward debility and infirmity before death. Now, aging is appreciated as the heterogeneous product of a genetic disposition being revealed under variable environmental, behavioral, psychosocial, and economic conditions, many of which are amenable to profound change [1].

The life span, rate(s) of aging, and predisposition to diseases are determined by genetic (or intrinsic) factors acting in concert with environmental (or extrinsic) factors. On average, aging is associated with progressive structural, functional, and metabolic alterations in a variety of tissues and systems. Many of these age-related alterations have been implicated in subsequent impairments in physiological, physical, psychosocial, and cognitive functioning. Central goals in clinical aging research have been to (1) identify the role of age-related changes in biological, social, and behavioral domains in the development of the diseases and disorders of old age, and (2) develop strategies to prevent or reduce morbidity and disability in the elderly. To address the first goal, investigators have long recognized the need to differentiate those changes that are due to "normal" aging from those pathological changes that result from disease [2]. Because "normal aging" represents those non pathological changes or "losses" that occur on "average," a more informative and useful distinction is that between "successful" versus "usual" aging [1]. This distinction is useful in evaluating potential risk factors and in developing preventive intervention studies.

The variability inherent in human aging has been a mixed blessing in aging research. There is no shortage of biological parameters, which change with age and which have potential use as biomarkers in independently and accurately estimating chronologic age. However, considerable variability between individuals within a given biological system in the inception and/or rates of change has frustrated attempts to identify and validate biomarkers [3]. Aging research has also benefited by the ample variability of aging organisms. The broad successes of research aimed at identifying and quantifying the variability contributed by environmental (or extrinsic factors) to aging or disease processes have fueled efforts to find and exploit modifiable risk factors in the conquest of disease and in the extension of active life expectancy. Appreciation of the substantial heterogeneity between individuals and groups has fostered the search for alternative explanations for health and disease. The desire to understand why some individuals age well and appear to escape many of the common chronic diseases of aging has been a motivating force in identifying and employing proactive strategies to replace "normal" or "usual" aging with "successful" aging [2]. Such efforts are successfully challenging stereotypes about the inevitability of decline in old age by generating effective strategies that can maintain or enhance physical functioning and well-being.

AGING AND BODY COMPOSITION

Profound changes in body composition occur with aging. For reasons that are incompletely understood, aging human beings lose bone [4] and muscle mass but increase their fat mass [5,6]. These changes and their associated structural and metabolic sequelae have been implicated in the development of frailty, morbidity, and disability in old age.

Bone mineral density stabilizes after the attainment of peak bone mass and begins to decline sometime between the fourth and the fifth decades. The progressive loss of bone mass with aging results in decrements in bone strength and increases the risk of osteoporosis and fractures. Hip fractures, perhaps the most devastating of fractures, accounted for nearly 281,000 hospital discharges in 1994 [7]. The sequelae of hip fractures—increased morbidity, potential permanent loss of ambulation and independence, and the need for long-term nursing home care—pose a serious public health problem [4].

Age-related bone loss, which is etiologically heterogeneous, differs by skeletal site with respect to the time of onset and rates of bone loss [4]. Rates of bone loss and the propensity to fracture are influenced by a host of factors, including gender, genetic and racial/ethnic background, estrogen and medication status, dietary intakes of calcium and vitamin D and other nutrients, levels of physical activity, body weight, and weight changes. In addition to trauma, bone mineral density, and other skeletal factors, the risk of hip fractures is influenced by nonskeletal factors such as the risk of falls, the ability to rise from a chair without using one's arms (which reflects balance and muscle strength), and visual acuity [8].

Sarcopenia, defined as a condition of reduced muscle mass, is a well-known consequence of aging and occurs in parallel with reductions in muscle strength and, to some extent, muscle quality [5]. Importantly, decreased muscle mass and strength can impair physical performance in the elderly and are associated with an increased risk of physical frailty, declines in functional capacity, impaired mobility, and falls [9]. The increased risk of falls associated with reduced lower extremity strength also reflects impairments in gait and balance and other aspects of physical performance [10]. Fortunately, strength training exercises can be effective in improving physical performance by reversing deficits in muscle mass and strength, indicating that the decline in muscle strength is modifiable and not an inexorable consequence of aging [9].

PHYSIOLOGICAL AND FUNCTIONAL CHANGES

Functional Reserve

Aging is associated with progressive reductions in functional reserve, which is the ability to successfully respond or adapt to physiologic and physical perturbations or stresses [11]. Within the cardiovascular system, decrements in maximal heart rate and maximal aerobic capacity signal potential compromises in cardiac functional reserve capacity. Additionally, structural changes, such as increases in aortic and large artery wall thickness and vascular stiffness, are associated with elevations in arterial systolic pressure and impedance in left ventricular ejection, which, in turn, lead to progressive left ventricular hypertrophy. A modifier of cardiovascular function, physical activity increases maximal oxygen uptake and maximal work capacity. However, even though physically fit individuals have higher maximal aerobic capacity, values for this parameter decline with age at rates that approximate those in their sedentary counterparts. Compensatory changes such as increased stroke volume may occur to facilitate increases in cardiac output in response to exertion [12].

Cardiovascular diseases, the leading cause of mortality in the United States, are responsible for the deaths of 50% of persons over the age of 65. Cardiovascular diseases or conditions associated with aging include hypertension, stroke, peripheral vascular disease, ischemic heart disease, cardiac arrhythmias, atrial fibrillation, and heart failure. High blood pressure (defined as a systolic blood pressure of 140 mm Hg or higher and/or a diastolic blood pressure of 90 mm Hg or higher) is very common in older adults. The most common form of high blood pressure in older persons is isolated systolic hypertension (defined as a systolic blood pressure of 140 mm Hg or higher and a diastolic pressure less than 90 mm Hg).

High blood pressure places older persons at significantly greater risk for stroke and heart disease [13].

Changes in the Immune System

Declines in immune function with aging portend an increasing incidence of infections and associated morbidity and mortality in old age as well as an increased risk of malignancies. Furthermore, in older individuals, preventive strategies, such as immunizations against influenza and other infectious agents, produce less effective responses than those produced in younger people [14]. More specifically, declines in protective immune responses reflect compromises in (1) the production of high-affinity antibodies, (2) the production of long-lasting memory immune responses after vaccination, and (3) the expression of delayed-type hypersensitivity reactions in response to antigens. Like other physiological responses, many aspects of immune function can also be influenced by extrinsic factors such as diet, physical activity, and morbidity [15].

Changes in the Endocrine System

Some of the most commonly cited age-related endocrine changes are those involved in (1) the regulation of glucose metabolism by insulin, (2) the growth hormone (GH)/insulin-like growth factor I (IGF-I) axis, (3) the secretion of parathyroid hormone, and (4), in women, the striking reduction in ovarian hormones following menopause.

Glucose Metabolism

Increases in (1) 2-hr blood glucose levels after a glucose challenge, (2) peripheral insulin resistance, and (3) higher postprandial insulin levels are associated with aging in humans [16]. However, because many older individuals exhibit responses that are comparable to those who are much younger, the assessment of extrinsic factors that can significantly affect glucose metabolism, such as diet, physical activity, and abdominal adiposity, is critical for accurate interpretation.

Growth Hormone Axis and the Somatopause

Alterations in the pulsatile characteristics of the GH and declines in spontaneous and stimulated secretion of GH, which are often accompanied by decreases in circulating levels of IGF-I, appear to be common accompaniments of aging [17] and have been termed the "somatopause" [16]. Because age-related changes, such as declining bone and muscle mass and increasing adiposity, seem to occur at the same time, these somatic changes have been attributed to changes in the GH/IGF-I axis. Not surprisingly, intense interest has focused on the potential benefits to be realized through successful paradigms designed to replenish GH and/or IGF-I. Administration of GH to healthy elderly men has achieved reductions in adiposity and increases in lean body mass and strength [18]. However, until evidence of clinically significant improvements in muscle strength, physical performance, or other functional parameters is forthcoming and concerns over adverse metabolic effects are resolved [19], the use of GH/IGF-I as an anti-aging strategy in the prevention of frailty is unwise and potentially dangerous.

Menopause

The most profound and universal alterations(s) in the aging endocrine system occurs in women and is due to menopause. The average age at which menopause occurs worldwide ranges from 45 to 55 years. The term *natural menopause* is defined by the World Health Organization as the permanent cessation of menstruation resulting from the loss of ovarian follicular activity [20]. Although the complete exhaustion of ovarian follicular reserves invariably leads to menopause, there is controversy over the relative roles played by the ovary versus the hypothalamic–pituitary unit in the transition from the pre- to postmenopausal state [21]. The postmenopausal years are characterized by a state of permanent hypergonadotropic, hypoestrogenic amenorrhea. The years leading up to menopause appear to be characterized by highly variable and unpredictable endocrine patterns, symptomatology, menstrual bleeding anomalies, and other gynecologic events. Recent findings suggest that the menopause transition, which can begin in the early forties, is a discontinuous process with varying type of ovulatory and anovulatory ovarian activity. Rather than a gradual decline in estrogen levels from the midthirties, culminating in a final menstrual period and menopause, evidence suggests that one variation of altered ovarian activity during the perimenopausal transition can be characterized by a cycle(s) of hyperestrogenism, hypergonadotropism, and diminished luteal phase progesterone secretion [22].

The public health significance of menopause extends far beyond the termination of menstrual cycle and reproductive function. Because of the known role of estrogen in the maintenance of bone mass and the prevention of fractures and in preserving a cardioprotective lipid profile, menopause and reduced levels of estrogen can have profound implications for subsequent health, morbidity, and even longevity in aging women. Not surprisingly, the role of estrogen in the prevention and/or treatment of osteoporosis, cardiovascular disease, Alzheimer's disease, and other disorders of aging, is currently the subject of numerous basic and clinical research studies, as well as large-scale clinical trials, such as the NIH Women's Health Initiative (WHI).

Andropause

Somewhat subtler is the reduction in total and free testosterone in aging men. Although representative data on the prevalence of this condition in the United States are lacking, overt hypogonadism in men, in contrast to women, is considerably less common and is not considered to be a normal concomitant of the aging processes [23,24]. Studies in hypogonadal men suggest that the administration of testosterone can increase the synthesis of skeletal muscle proteins and muscle mass [25] as well as muscle strength [26]. Testosterone, in suprapharmacologic doses, can also increase muscle mass and strength in eugonadal men and does so in an additive fashion with strength training exercises when these two modalities are combined [27].

Despite these observations, the lack of definitive findings from long-term, randomized controlled trials and concerns over side effects (elevated hematocrit, prostate enlargement, and the potential for malignancy) do not support the recommendation of testosterone as a strategy to prevent or treat frailty in older men [26]. The role of circulating testosterone levels in maintaining bone and muscle mass in old age is uncertain and remains a subject of intense research interest. Drawing on recent evidence that estrogen may be at least as, if not more, important than testosterone in the maintenance of bone mass, a recently proposed model for osteoporosis in elderly men hypothesizes that low levels of bioavailable testosterone may contribute to bone loss by compromising the amount of testosterone substrate available for estrogen production [28].

Adrenopause

Adrenopause is a term used to signify age-associated reductions in the levels of dehydroepiandrosterone (DHEA) and its sulfate (DHEAS). The common presursor for androgens and estrogens, DHEA has been called a "multifunctional steroid hormone" [29]. The rationale for the potential significance of age-related declines in DHEA(S) levels in the morbidity of old age is identical to that for growth hormone, i.e., DHEA(S) concentrations fall with age coincident with reductions in bone and lean body mass and increases in adiposity. Because higher DHEA(S) levels have also been associated with a modestly reduced risk of mortality from cardiovascular disease in men [30], there is great interest in evaluating the "antiaging" potential of DHEA(S) and its roles in promoting a sense of well-being and preventing obesity, diabetes mellitus, cancer, and heart disease.

Two small, randomized placebo-controlled trials in humans found that increasing DHEA(S) to levels comparable to those found in young adults can raise IGF-I levels and benefit men and women by (1) enhancing perceived physical and psychological well-being [31] and (2) increasing lean body mass [29]. However, it was found that only men realized significant reductions in body fat and gains in muscle strength and that other parameters, such as insulin sensitivity, were unaffected. Furthermore, while a recent uncontrolled study has reported that DHEA can increase femoral bone mass and stimulate the maturation of the vaginal epithelium while maintaining an atrophic endometrium [32], other studies suggest that DHEA offers no clinically significant benefit in enhancing immune responses [33] or psychological or cognitive performance [34]. Consequently, the significance of DHEA as an agent to improve or preserve health and physical functioning in old age remains unclear. Importantly, the rise in circulating androgen and IGF-I levels stimulated by DHEA in some regimens is of concern with respect to the potential risks of ovarian, prostate, and other cancers [16]. Until objective findings can support a clinically meaningful role for DHEA in the maintenance of health and well-being, the use of this agent as an antiaging remedy or preventive cannot be supported.

Parathyroid Hormone

Parathyroid hormone (PTH) is a key component in the regulation of calcium and phosphorus homeostasis and in the maintenance of bone mass. Endogenous PTH, which increases 35% across the adult age span in men and women [35] and correlates with elevated indices of bone resorption, is strongly implicated as a mediator of bone loss in older men and women [28]. In women, ovarian hormone status may independently modulate the sensitivity of bone to PTH, with menopause and reduced or deficient estrogen levels leading to accelerated bone loss via a permissive effect on PTH-stimulated bone resorption [28]. A substantial role for vitamin D status and calcium nutrition, alone, or in combination, as potential determinants of PTH levels has been indicated in observational [35] and intervention studies [36,37]. Importantly, reductions in PTH levels concomitant with reductions in bone loss have been accomplished with interventions using calcium [36] and calcium and vitamin D supplements [37]. In the latter study, calcium and vitamin D supplements not only stabilized bone mass, but led to a significant reduction in fractures [37].

These are but a few of an enormous number of physical, physiologic, and structural parameters that have been studied and which show changes with age. The topics and parameters discussed earlier were selected because of the potential importance of compromises in these parameters on subsequent morbidity and frailty and also because many of these parameters are modifiable and lend themselves to successful aging paradigms. Importantly, the ability to modify factors contributing to age-related disorders and diseases and their subsequent downward course of debility in the elderly has profound implications with respect to how we view aging and its true inexorable consequences.

PREVENTING FRAILTY AND PROMOTING SUCCESSFUL AGING

At the opposite end of the spectrum of successful or healthy human aging is physical frailty, which connotes a constellation of impairments underlying seriously reduced physical and cognitive functioning and an enhanced susceptibility to injuries and acute illness. Impairments in physical functioning, which can result from deficits in strength, speed, endurance balance, and mobility, can compromise an individual's ability to perform daily activities of living [11,38]. Importantly, because many of these deficits increase the propensity to fall [10], frailty is a major contributor to hip fractures and other injurious events, which can, in turn, produce devastating disabilities that require long-term care. Indeed, the demonstration by Nevitt and Cummings [39] that the type of fall is a major determinant of the type of fracture underscores the idea that falls and frailty are likely to be at least as important in the etiology of hip fractures as is bone density, strength, and other skeletal factors.

Compromised physical functioning can reflect a variety of deficits in cardiovascular performance, muscle function, bone strength, joint mobility, and control of gait and posture. These deficits and concomitant disabilities may be the sequelae of disorders of old age such as cardiovascular and peripheral vascular disease, osteoarthritis, hip fracture, diabetes, stroke, chronic obstructive pulmonary disease, visual and hearing impairments, and cognitive dysfunction [40]. As can be seen from Table I, over half the older population is afflicted with arthritis, whereas one-third has heart disease and/or hypertension. Twenty-eight percent of the older population has problems hearing, whereas over 16% have visual problems (such as cataracts) or skeletal deformities and impairments. Importantly, the prevalence of these conditions increases after age 75.

TABLE I Prevalence of Selected Reported Chronic Conditions per 1000 Persons 65 Years and Older in the United States in 1994[a]

Condition	65 years and over		
	Total	65–74 years	≥75 years
Arthritis	501.5	476.9	536.6
Hypertension	364.0	347.2	388.0
Hearing impairment	286.4	234.6	360.4
Heart disease	324.9	281.2	387.3
Deformity or orthopedic impairment	165.6	154.1	182.1
Cataracts	166.2	113.0	242.4
Chronic sinusitis	151.1	150.1	152.5
Diabetes	101.2	101.6	100.8
Tinnitus	90.1	90.1	90.0
Visual impairment	82.2	61.5	111.8

[a] From Adams and Marano [48].

POPULATION AGING

The U.S. population is aging very rapidly, with baby boomers (those born between 1946 and 1964) leading the way. Since the turn of the century, when life expectancy at birth was only 47 years, the United States has experienced spectacular increases in life expectancy, which now stands at 73 and 79 years at birth for men and women, respectively [41]. Also of note have been the gains in life expectancy at age 65, from 11.9 to 17.4 more years [42], which will herald increasing numbers of those over 85, the "oldest old" in the next millennium. Thus, the older population will become even older in the next 30 years and will comprise a much larger proportion of the U.S. population, as the large increases in life expectancy that have been realized over the last century combine with the lower birth rates that followed the birth of baby boomers.

Baby boomers will begin turning 65 in 2011 and continue to reach this milestone until the year 2030. Between now and the year 2030, as the baby boom becomes the grandparent boom, the numbers of those over 65 will double from 35 to 70 million. Most importantly, the proportion of those over 65 will rise from 12.8 to 20%, or from one in eight to one in every five Americans. Those over 85, the fastest growing segment of the population, will double in size between now and 2030 (4.3 to 8.8 million) and double again to 18.9 million between 2030 and 2050 [42].

Although the current older population is overwhelmingly white and non-hispanic, the population over 65 is becoming more racially diverse as it begins to reflect changes in the total U.S. population. In 1990, the number of elderly Hispanics was 1.1 million, less than half the size of the 2.5 million older black population and only 3.5% of the total older U.S. population. However, this rapidly growing group is expected, by 2030, to increase nearly sevenfold to 7.6 million to outnumber the expected 6.8 million older black Americans and to comprise over 10% of the total U.S. population over age 65 [42].

The "graying" of the population and its increasing ethnic diversity in the next half century will generate significant social and economic challenges in promoting healthy, successful aging. The burgeoning of the older population and the oldest old, who have the highest per capita costs for medical services, will place larger numbers of individuals at risk for disease and disability, amplify the demand for health care services, and exacerbate the fiscal burdens confronting the health care system. In anticipating these challenges, a critical need exists for the development of new cost-effective strategies aimed at maintaining quality of life and productivity in old age.

The news is encouraging. Advances in sciences, medicine, and technology are already preserving structure and function in physiological systems and enhancing human performance. Advances in molecular genetics are beginning to unravel the secrets of longevity and cellular senescence. Compromises in physical functioning in the aging population are being reversed or ameliorated as individuals with painful osteoarthritic knees and hips become the beneficiaries of hip and knee replacement surgery. Cataract surgery can rectify major deficits in vision. Vascular reperfusion strategies and programs of life-style modifications can reduce the risks of heart disease disability and death. Because the prevalence of disability has declined from 24.9% to 21.3%, there are at least 1.4 million fewer disabled older persons in the United States today than would have been predicted using 1982 disability rates [43].

Many prevention strategies appear on the surface to be modest life-style modifications. However, these modifications can profoundly alter our thinking about aging, its stereotypes, and the inevitability of diseases such as osteoporosis. For example, the success of research testing inexpensive, low-burden strategies, such as calcium and vitamin D supplementation, demonstrates that simple life-style modifications can reduce bone loss in older men and women and even reduce the risk of fractures [37]. Another strategy, estrogen supplementation, is well known for is high efficacy in preserving bone mass in postmenopausal women [44]. As other therapeutic agents are shown to be not only effective in reducing bone loss and preventing fractures, but highly acceptable for incorporation into daily routines, beliefs that bone loss and osteoporosis are the inexorable consequence of aging may need to be substantially revised.

Major inroads are being made into combating frailty and disability. Progressive resistance exercise training in nursing home residents can increase muscle mass and strength and, importantly, improve physical performance measures such as gait speed and the ability to climb stairs [9]. Even in very frail patients, physical therapy programs containing range of motion, strength, balance, and mobility exercises can significantly increase mobility and reduce the dependence on assisted devices, such as wheelchairs [45].

Modifiable risk factors can play a role in paradigms to prevent disability. This potential is apparent from findings from a very recent long-term follow-up study that demonstrated that middle-aged and older adults with better health habits with respect to physical exercise, body mass index, and smoking could postpone the onset of disability by more than 5 years. Thus the ability to survive longer, enjoy more disability-free years, and experience the compression of morbidity into fewer years at the very end of life can be influenced profoundly by life-style modifications [46].

Life-style modifications also have the potential to reduce the risk of death from chronic diseases associated with aging. In a study of major extrinsic factors believed to contribute to death, it was estimated that over half of all the deaths in the United States that occurred in 1990 were associated with modifiable risk factors and could therefore have been prevented or perhaps at least delayed [47]. The leading cause of death in individuals of all ages is heart disease, which was responsible for 33.5% of the 2.15 million deaths occurring in 1990. Malignant neoplasms and cerebrovascular diseases caused 505,000 (23.5%) and 144,000 (6.7%) of all deaths, respectively, so that these three causes accounted for nearly two-thirds of all deaths. The five most substantial contributors to mortality were determined to be tobacco (an estimated 400,000 deaths), diet and activity patterns (300,000), alcohol (100,000), and microbial agents (90,000). The previous two studies suggest that successful prevention or delay of the chronic conditions and diseases of aging through the exploitation of modifiable risk factors could make a substantial difference in the numbers of older individuals surviving and experiencing healthy, disability-free survival.

Research in aging is a relatively young field, but it is quickly becoming a most sophisticated one, and it is happening none too soon. With our aging population poised to grow to enormous numbers, successful research in aging is the key to ensure that the extra years of life will be healthy, productive, and economically sound.

References

1. Rowe, J. W., and Kahn, R. L. Human Aging: usual and successful. *Science* **237,** 143–149 (1987).
2. Shock, N. W., Greulich, R. C., Andres, R., Arenberg, D., Costa, P. T., Jr., Lakatta, E. G., and Tobin, J. D. *In* "Normal Human Aging: the Baltimore Longitudinal Study of Aging," pp. 1–4. NIH

Publication No. 84-2450, U.S. Department of Health and Human Services, U.S. Government Printing Office, Washington, DC, 1984.

3. Baker, G. T., III, and Martin, G. R. Molecular and biologic factors in aging: the origins, causes and prevention of senescence. *In* "Geriatric Medicine" (C. K. Cassel, H. J. Cohen, E. B. Larson, D. E. Meier, N. M. Resnick, L. Z. Rubenstein, and L. B. Sorenson, eds.), 3rd Ed., pp. 3–28, Springer-Verlag, New York, 1997.
4. Riggs, B. L., and Melton, L. J., III. Involutional osteoporosis. *N. Engl. J. Med.* **314,** 1676–1686 (1986).
5. Evans, W. J. What is sarcopenia? *J. Gerontol.* **50A,** 5–8 (1995).
6. Kohrt, W. M., and Holloszy, J. O. Loss of skeletal muscle mass with aging: effect on glucose tolerance. *J. Gerontol.* **50A,** 68–72. (1995).
7. Looker, A. C., Orwoll, E. S., Johnston, C. C., Jr., Lindsay, R. L., Wahner, H. W., Dunn, W. L., Calvo, M. S., Harris, T. B., and Heyse, S. P. Prevalence of low femoral bone density in older U.S. adults from NHANES III. *J. Bone Miner. Res.* **12,** 1761–1768 (1997).
8. Cummings, S. R., Nevitt, M. C., Browner, W. S., Stone, K., Fox, K. M., Ensrud, K. E., Cauley, J., Black, D., and Vogt, T. M. Risk factors for hip fracture in white women. *N. Engl. J. Med.* **332,** 767–773 (1995).
9. Fiatarone, M. A., O'Neill, E. F., Ryan, N. D., Clements, K. M., Solares, G. R., Nelson, M. E., Roberts, S. B., Kehayias, J. J., Lipsitz, L. A., and Evans, W. J. Exercise training and nutritional supplementation for physical frailty in very elderly people. *JAMA* **330,** 1769–1775 (1994).
10. Wolfson, L., Judge, J., Whipple, R., and King, M. Strength is a major factor in balance, gait, and the occurrence of falls. *J. Gerontol.* **50A,** 64–67 (1995).
11. Pendergast, D. R., Fisher, N. M., and Calkins, E. Cardiovascular, neuromuscular, and metabolic alterations with age leading to frailty. *J. Gerontol.* **48,** 61–67 (1993).
12. Wenger, N. K. Cardiovascular disease. *In* "Geriatric Medicine" (C. K. Cassel, H. J. Cohen, E. B., Larson, D. E. Meier, N. M. Resnick, L. Z. Rubenstein, and L. B. Sorensen, eds.), 3rd Ed., p. 357. Springer-Verlag, New York, 1997.
13. The Sixth Report of the Joint National Committee on Prevention, Detection, Evaluation, and Treatment of High Blood Pressure, *Arch. Intern. Med.* **157,** 2413–2446 (1997).
14. Burns, E., and Goodwin, J. S. Changes in immunologic function. *In* "Geriatric Medicine" (C. K. Cassel, H. J. Cohen, E. B. Larson, D. E. Meier, N. M. Resnick, L. Z. Rubenstein, and L. B. Sorensen, eds.), 3rd Ed., p. 585. Springer-Verlag, New York, 1997.
15. Miller, R. A. The aging immune system: primer and prospectus. *Science* **273,** 70–74 (1996).
16. Lamberts, S. W. J., van den Beld, A. W., and van der Lely, A. J. The endocrinology of aging. *Science* **278,** 419–424 (1997).
17. Corpas, E., Harman, S. M., and Blackman, M. Human growth hormone and human aging. *Endocr. Rev.* **14,** 20–39 (1993).
18. Rudman, D., Feller, A. G., Nagraj, H. S., Gergans, G. A., Lalitha, P. Y., Goldberg, A. F., Schlenker, R. A., Cohn, L., Rudman, I. W., and Mattson, D. E. Effects of human growth hormone in men over 60 years of age. *N. Engl. J. Med.* **323,** 1–6 (1990).
19. Papadakis, M. A., Grady, D., Black, D., Tierney, M. J., Gooding, G. A. W., Schambelan, M., and Grunfeld, C. Growth hormone replacement in healthy older men improves body composition but not functional ability. *Ann. Intern. Med.* **124,** 708–716 (1996).
20. WHO Scientific Group on Research on the Menopause in the 1990s, "Research on the Menopause: Report of a WHO Scientific Group." WHO technical report series, Geneva, Switzerland, 1994.
21. Wise, P. M., Krajnak, K. M., and Kashon, M. L. Menopause: the aging of multiple pacemakers. *Science* **273,** 67–70 (1996).
22. Santoro, N., Brown, J. R., Adel, T., and Skurnick, J. H. Characterization of reproductive hormonal dynamics in the perimenopause. *J. Clin. Endocrinol. Metab.* **81,** 1495–1501 (1996).
23. Tenover, J. S. Androgen administration to aging men. *Endocrinol. Metab. Clin. North Am.* **23,** 877–892 (1994).
24. Harman, S. M., and Tsitouras, P. D. Reproductive hormones in aging men. I. Measurement of sex steroids, basal luteinizing hormone and Leydig cell response to human chorionic gonadotropin. *J. Clin. Endocrinol. Metab.* **51,** 35–40 (1980).
25. Brodsky, I. G., Balagopal, P., and Nair, K. S. Effects of testosterone replacement on muscle mass and muscle protein synthesis in hypogonadal men—a clinical research center study. *J. Clin. Endocrinol. Metab.* **81,** 3469–3475 (1996).
26. Sih, R., Morley, J. E., Kaiser, F. E., Perry, H. M., III, Patrick, P., and Ross, C. Testosterone replacement in older hypogonadal men: a 12-month randomized controlled trial. *J. Clin. Endocrinol. Metab.* **82,** 1661–1667 (1997).
27. Bhasin, S., Storer, T. W., Berman, N., Callegari, C., Clevenger, B., Phillips, J., Bunnell, T. J. Tricker, R., Shirazi, A., and Casaburi, R. The effects of supraphysiologic doses of testosterone on muscle size and strength in normal men. *N. Engl. J. Med.* **335,** 1–7 (1996).
28. Riggs, B. L., Khosla, S., and Melton, L. J., III. A unitary model for involutional osteoporosis. Estrogen deficiency causes both type I and type II osteoporosis in postmenopausal women and contributes to bone loss in aging men. *J. Bone Miner Res.* **13,** 763–773 (1998).
29. Yen, S. S. C., Morales, A. J., and Khorram, O. Replacement of DHEA in aging men and women. Potential remedial effects. *Ann. N.Y. Acad. Sci.* **774,** 128–142 (1995).
30. Barrett-Connor, E., and Goodman-Gruen, D. The epidemiology of DHEAS and cardiovascular disease. *Ann. N.Y. Acad. Sci.* **774,** 259–270 (1995).
31. Morales, A. J., Nolan, J. J., Nelson, J. C., and Yen, S. S. C. Effects of replacement dose of dehydroepiandrosterone in men and women of advancing age. *J. Clin. Endocrinol. Metab.* **78,** 1360–1367 (1994).
32. Labrie, F., Diamond, P., Cusan, L., Gomez, J.-L., Bélanger, A., and Candas, B. Effect of 12-month dehydroepiandrosterone replacement therapy on bone, vagina, and endometrium in postmenopausal women. *J. Clin. Endocrinol. Metab.* **82,** 3498–3505 (1997).
33. Danenberg, H. D., Ben-Yehuda, A., Zakay-Rones, Z., Gross, D. J., and Friedman, G. Dehydroepiandrosterone treatment is not beneficial to the immune response to influenza in elderly subjects. *J. Clin. Endocrinol. Metab.* **82,** 2911–2914 (1997).
34. Wolf, O. T., Neumann, O., Hellhammer, D. H., Geiben, A. C., Strasburger, C. J., Dressendörfer, R. A., Pirke, K.-M., and Kirschbaum, C. Effects of a two week physiological dehydroepiandrosterone substitution on cognitive performance and well-being in healthy elderly women and men. *J. Clin. Endocrinol. Metab.* **82,** 2363–2367 (1997).
35. Sherman, S. S., Hollis, B. W., and Tobin, J. D. Vitamin D status and related parameters in a healthy population: the effects of age, sex, and season. *J. Clin. Endocrinol. Metab.* **71,** 405–413 (1990).
36. Riggs, B. L., O'Fallon, W. M., Muhs, J., O'Connor, M. K., Kumar, R., and Melton, L. J. III. Long-term effects of calcium supplementation on serum parathyroid hormone level, bone turnover, and bone loss in elderly women. *J. Bone Miner. Res.* **13,** 168–174 (1998).
37. Dawson-Hughes, B., Harris, S. S., Krall, E. A., and Dallal, G. E. Effect of calcium and vitamin D supplementation on bone density in men and women 65 years of age or older. *N. Engl. J. Med.* **337,** 670–676 (1997).

38. Schultz, A. B. Muscle function and mobility biomechanics in the elderly: an overview of some recent research. *J. Gerontol.* **48,** 60–63 (1993).
39. Nevitt, M. C., and Cummings, S. R. Type of fall and risk of hip and wrist fractures: the study of osteoporotic fractures. *J. Am. Geriatr. Soc.* **41,** 1226–1234 (1993).
40. Fried, L. P., and Guralnik, J. M. Disability in older adults: evidence regarding significance, etiology, and risk. *J. Am. Geriatr. Soc.* **45,** 92–100 (1997).
41. Ventura, S. J., Peters, K. D., Martin J. A., and Maurer, J. D., "Births and Deaths: United States, 1996." Monthly Vital Statistics Report **46,** No. 1(S) 2, Table D, p. 5. U.S. Dept. of Health and Human Services, Hyattsville, MD, 1997.
42. Hobbs, F. B., and Damon, B. L. Chapter 2. Numerical Growth. *In* "65+ in the United States." Current Population Reports, Special Studies, **P23-190,** pp. 2-1 to 2-27. U.S. Bureau of the Census, U.S. Government Printing Office, Washington, DC, 1996.
43. Manton, K. G., Corder, L., and Stallard, E. Chronic diability trends in the elderly United States populations: 1982–1994. *Proc. Natl. Acad. Sci. USA* **94,** 2593–2598 (1997).
44. The Writing Group for the PEPI. Effects of hormone therapy on bone mineral density: results from the postmenopausal estrogen/progestin interventions (PEPI) trial. *JAMA* **276,** 1389–1396 (1996).
45. Mulrow, C. D., Gerety, M. B., Kanten, D., Cornell, J. E., DeNino, L. A., Chiodo, L., Aguilar, C., O'Neil, M. B., Rosenberg, J., and Solis, R. M. A randomized trial of physical rehabilitation for very frail nursing home residents. *JAMA* **271,** 519–524 (1994).
46. Vita, A. J., Terry, R. B., Hubert, H. B., and Fries, J. F. Aging, health risks and cumulative disability. *N. Engl. J. Med.* **338,** 1035–1041 (1998).
47. McGinnis, J. M., and Foege, W. H. Actual causes of death in the United States. *JAMA* **270,** 2207–2212 (1993).
48. Adams, P. F., and Marano, M. A. *Vital Health Stat.* **10**(193). 81–82 (1994).

Aging and Calcium Balance

ROBERT P. HEANEY Creighton University, Omaha, Nebraska 68131

INTRODUCTION

Definition

Calcium balance is the difference between the amount of calcium an organism ingests every day and how much it loses, principally through measured excreta, but also through nonmeasured routes such as shed hair, skin, nails, sweat, and other body secretions. Calcium balance is normally positive during growth, when an individual is amassing tissue. Theoretically it should be zero in full maturity, and often it will be negative during involution, when tissue mass is declining.

While calcium is a constituent of all tissues, more than 99% of body calcium is found in bone and teeth. Thus, the total body calcium balance overwhelmingly reflects skeletal tissue balance. Positive calcium balance means the body is adding bone, either as primary growth or repair of prior deficits; zero balance reflects bone equilibrium; and negative balance reflects bone loss. This much is straightforward. Difficulty arises both in measuring balance and in interpreting what is measured.

Measurement of Balance

Typically, calcium balance has been measured by placing individuals or animals on a constant diet under tightly controlled, inpatient conditions, collecting all excreta, and chemically analyzing both input and output for calcium. In humans the balance period must be at least 8 days in length, and preferably twice that long. The method, which has been the classic approach of nutrition research during most of the 20th century, is expensive and time-consuming. Because the method ignores dermal loss, it produces results systematically biased toward positive balance. It is also inherently imprecise, a problem that becomes worse for poorly absorbed nutrients such as calcium. This is because fecal calcium will almost always be nearly as large as dietary intake, because food residue flow through the colon is turbulent, and because methods for relating fecal pools to defined intake periods are weak [1]. The fecal transit problem can be effectively bypassed by using isotopic calcium tracers to measure actual *absorbed* calcium, with a substantial improvement in precision [1]. The other shortcomings can be partially offset by extending the duration of the balance study, by large sample sizes, and by comparing different test conditions within subject. Unfortunately, these stratagems themselves often create other problems.

As a result of these difficulties, few calcium balance studies are performed today. Instead, balance is estimated from a long-term change in total body bone mineral, using dual energy X-ray absorptiometry (DXA), either regionally or for the total skeleton. This method catches dermal loss and is applicable to free-living individuals on uncontrolled diets. Mass balances and DXA produce equivalent and interconvertible results. Balance is a *rate* (i.e., mass units per day), and DXA differences are the *integral* of that rate (i.e., mass units) over the time between measurements. However, despite the quite good accuracy and sensitivity of DXA, skeletal changes that are physiologically important are usually small relative to baseline values and correspondingly hard to detect over reasonable time periods. Typical changes in bone balance, even extending over many months, will usually be less than the sensitivity of the method: Accordingly, paired DXA measurements usually need to be spaced 1 or more years apart, so the method is not suitable for studying short-term change in individuals. Nevertheless, as with classical balances, this sensitivity tissue can be addressed by studying large numbers of subjects. In both situations, precision improves with the square root of the sample size.

Table I Comparative Precision for Three Balance Methods

Method	95% confidence interval of estimate[a]
Classical mass balance[b]	±110 mg/day
Ca tracer augmented mass balance[b]	±29 mg/day
Total body bone mineral by DXA[c]	±78 mg/day

[a] For zero balance in a single individual with a Ca intake of 800 mg/day.
[b] See Heaney [1] for assumptions.
[c] Assuming 1% long-term measurement precision.

Table I compares the sensitivity of the available methods, expressing sensitivity as the upper and lower boundaries for the 95% confidence interval around a measured value of zero balance in a single subject, employing an 8-day mass balance, a 1-year DXA intermeasurement interval, and fairly optimistic estimates for analytical error, both for mass balance components [1] and for long-term DXA precision. As can be seen, the tracer-augmented mass balance is the most sensitive, followed by DXA and classical mass balance. By either of the last two methods, a zero balance measurement in a single individual is equally compatible with either biologically significant bone loss or fairly impressive bone gain.

Interpretation of Balance Results

A second difficulty arises in interpreting the results of balance measurements. The fact of age-related bone loss is well documented. Inescapably, bone loss means negative calcium balance, theoretically detectable either by mass balance methods or by DXA, but what cannot be so clearly concluded is *why* the balance is negative. Is the bone undergoing atrophy, pumping its minerals out of the body and thus producing a measurable excess of excreted calcium over ingested calcium; is the excessive loss the primary event, with the body's regulatory systems tearing down bone so as to access its calcium, thereby maintaining extracellular fluid [Ca^{2+}], or are both processes happening, the second superimposed on the first?

Ever since the late 1940s there has not been a scientific consensus on the answer to this question. However, with the publication of a large number of clinical trials and key physiological studies since 1990, it is now quite certain that, for most people 65 years of age or older, both processes are going on, usually at the same time. Before dissecting them apart and exploring their implications, it will be worth reviewing the notion of a calcium requirement, how the calcium economy operates at intakes above and below the requirement, and what is known of how the components of the calcium regulatory system change with age.

THE CALCIUM REQUIREMENT

Calcium: A Plateau Nutrient

Calcium is a threshold, or plateau nutrient, a concept that is illustrated in Fig. 1. What is meant by this term is that when one graphs bony response against calcium intake, starting from clearly deficient levels, response rises as a function of intake up to some point (the thresh-

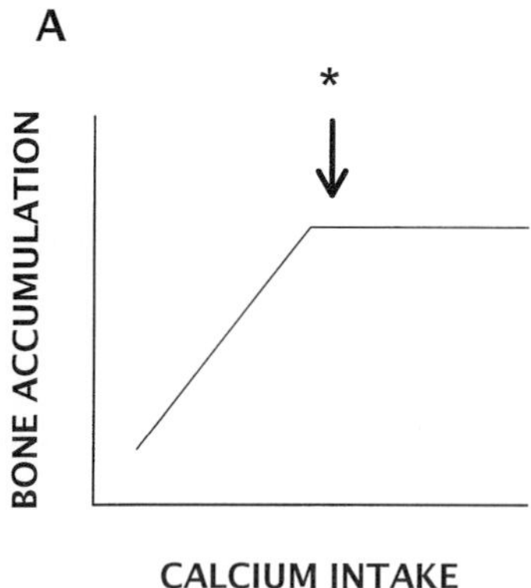

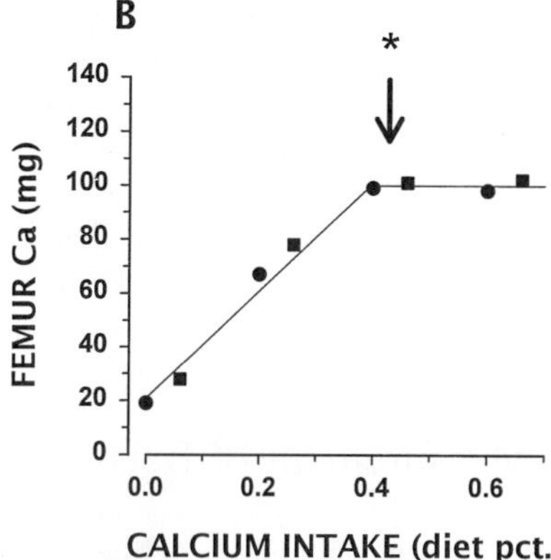

Figure 1 Threshold behavior of calcium intake. (A) Theoretical relationship of bone accumulation to intake. Below a certain value—the threshold—bone accumulation is a linear function of intake (the ascending line); in other words, the amount of bone that can be accumulated is limited by the amount of calcium ingested. Above the threshold (the horizontal line), bone accumulation is limited by other factors and is no longer related to calcium intake. (B) Actual data from two experiments in growing rats showing how bone accumulation does, in fact, exhibit a threshold pattern. Asterisks represent minimum requirement. Redrawn from data in Forbes *et al.* [2]. Copyright Robert P. Heaney, 1992. Reproduced with permission.

old), above which response plateaus. This behavior is most straightforwardly brought out during growth (as in Fig. 1B), when the amount of bone that can be amassed is strictly limited by intake. But, when calcium intake is high enough to supply the demands of the genetic program, as modified by mechanical loading, these latter factors become controlling and calcium intake no longer exerts an effect. Additional calcium will make no more bone.

The same basic relationship holds for all life stages, even when bone may be undergoing some degree of involution. The threshold concept is generalized to all life situations in Fig. 2A, which shows schematically what the intake/retention curves look like during growth, maturity, and involution. In brief, the plateau occurs at a positive value during growth, at zero retention in the mature individual, and sometimes at a negative value in the elderly. Available evidence suggests that the plateau during involution is at a negative value in the first 3–5 years after menopause, rises to zero for the next 10–15 years, and then becomes increasingly negative with age in the old elderly.

In Fig. 2B, which shows only the involutional curve, there are two points located along the curve: one below (B) and one above (A) the threshold. At *A,* calcium retention is negative for reasons intrinsic to the skeleton, whereas at *B,* involutional effects are compounded by inadequate intake, which makes the balance more negative than it needs to be. Point *B* (or below) is probably where most older adults in the industrialized nations would be situated today. The goal of calcium nutrition in this life stage is to move them to point *A,* thereby making certain that insufficient calcium intake is not aggravating any underlying bone loss.

Functional Indicator of Nutritional Adequacy

The functional indicator of nutritional adequacy for such a threshold nutrient is termed "maximal retention" and can be located in Figs. 1A and 2A at the asterisks above the curves. The intake corresponding to this point represents the requirement. Calcium retention in this sense is "maximal" only in that further intake of calcium will produce no further retention. (This is in contrast to treatment with hormones or drugs, which can clearly lead to further calcium retention). This approach was used by the Food and Nutrition Board of the National Academy of Sciences for the first time in its development of recommended intakes for calcium in 1997 [3].

Calcium is a unique nutrient in another respect. Most other nutrients, when ingested above the optimal intake level, continue to increase their body reserves, often to the point of producing toxicity (e.g., fat and fat-soluble vitamins), but because the calcium reserve is in the form of bone tissue, and bone tissue mass is regulated by cellular processes, any calcium intake in excess of *skeletal* need is simply excreted. The fact that the body cannot store bone above the level of current need is what creates the plateau. This fact also explains why the calcium requirement remains high throughout life.

The action of calcium supplementation in this regard is well illustrated by a study of Reid *et al.* [4] in post-

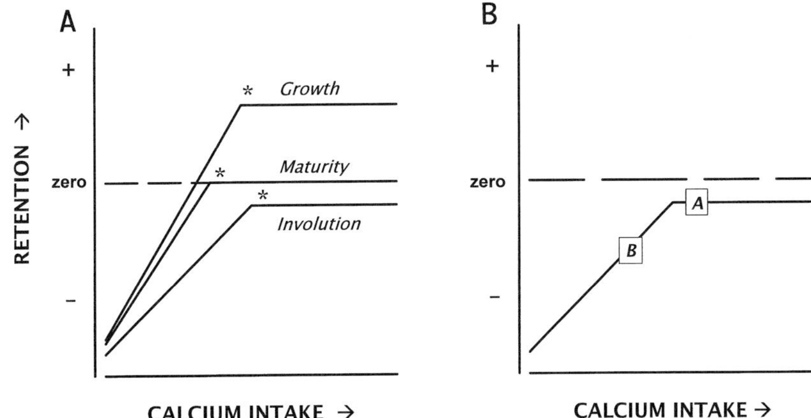

FIGURE 2 (A). Schematic Calcium intake and retention curves for three life stages. Retention is greater than zero during growth, zero at maturity, and may be negative during involution. Asterisks represent minimum requirement. (B). The involution curve only. Point B designates an intake below the maximal calcium retention threshold, whereas point A designates an intake above the threshold. Copyright Robert P. Heaney, 1998. Reproduced with permission.

menopausal women. Initially, Bone Mineral Density (BMD) in a calcium-supplemented group rose above the starting value, i.e., there was apparent bone gain; but this reflected the expected remodeling transient. Data for year 2 and beyond showed continuing bone loss, despite the high calcium intake. However, the calcium-supplemented group was losing significantly less rapidly than the placebo-treated controls [5]. The study was not dose ranging, but, for the sake of illustration, if one assumes that the intake achieved in the calcium-supplemented subjects was above the threshold of Fig. 2B, then the continuing bone loss reflects nonnutritional factors. Thus the calcium-supplemented individuals in the Reid study can be said to have been at point *A* in Fig. 2B and the placebo-treated at point *B*.

Optimal Calcium Intake

If the requirement is defined in terms of the concepts set forth in Fig. 2, then the average requirement for a population is given by the mean of the intakes at which the individuals reach the plateau or threshold value. Current best estimates for this average calcium requirement are in the range of 1000 mg/day for mature adults, rising with age to 1200–1400 mg/day by age 75 [3,6]. These are *average* figures. Assuming a population coefficient of variation for the distribution of requirements around the mean on the order of 10%, the corresponding best intimate of a recommended daily allowance would be 1200 mg/day for mature adults, rising to 1400–1600 mg/day for the elderly.

THE CALCIUM ECONOMY

The Skeleton in Vertebrate Evolution

During the marine phase of vertebrate evolution, the bony skeleton evolved as a reserve for the scarce nutrient, phosphorus, which was virtually absent from sea water. When vertebrates crawled out of the supporting aquatic environment, the skeleton acquired both a second homeostatic and a mechanical function, serving as both a reservoir and a sink for calcium, in addition to its newly essential structural role. Whereas the diets of early terrestrial vertebrates were calcium rich, food intake was episodic, and means had to be developed to maintain the constancy of extracellular fluid calcium ion concentration (ECF [Ca^{2+}]) in the face of widely varying inputs. (In a marine environment this could be accomplished by controlling calcium flux across the gill membranes.) The result is the well-known parathyroid hormone (PTH)–calcitriol regulatory loop preventing hypocalcemia and the calcitonin loop preventing hypercalcemia. The former is of greater relevance in the context of this chapter.

Paleolithic Calcium Intake

As far as can be discerned, calcium was a surfeit nutrient in the environment in which hominids evolved [7]. It is probably a consequence of this dietary abundance that intestinal calcium absorption is inefficient, renal conservation of calcium weak, and dermal calcium losses unregulated. Gross intestinal absorption in adults, at prevailing intakes, averages about 30%; because substantial quantities of calcium enter the digestive tract with gastrointestinal secretions, net absorption is generally in the range of 10 to 20% [8,9]. Additionally, many dietary components interfere with renal calcium conservation, notably sodium, acid load, and sulfur-containing amino acids. These agencies create a floor below which urinary calcium cannot be reduced, despite the effects of PTH on renal tubular calcium reabsorption. Finally, resting dermal losses (i.e., without sweating) may be in the range of 60 mg/day [10], and sweating can cause losses 5–10× that large [11]. The net result of these excretory forces is that obligatory calcium losses in sedentary adults on typical diets are generally in the range of 160–240 mg/day.

With a diet like that of our paleolithic ancestors (i.e., a calcium density of ~70 mg/100 kCal), a low absorption efficiency would be quite sufficient to offset regular obligatory losses and to adapt to day-to-day variability in intake and excretion (see later). However, despite upregulation of intestinal calcium absorption efficiency on low intakes, adaptation may not be so easily accomplished on contemporary diets. An overview of the control system will make clear why that is so. Two distinct feedback loops are involved. One is the loop regulating bone remodeling and the other is the loop maintaining ECF [Ca^{2+}].

Overlapping Control Loops

Briefly, bone is constantly being remodeled, a process that begins first with activation at a local site, followed by osteoclastic erosion into the bony surface, and later by osteoblastic in-filling of the resulting cavity. Two features of this remodeling scheme are important in our context. First, although PTH is secreted in response to demands of the ECF [Ca^{2+}], the hormone is also the principal determinant of the bone remodeling activation threshold, and hence of the amount of remodeling in the total skeleton. (PTH also stimulates existing osteoclasts to resorb bone more avidly.) Second, remodeling at each site is asynchronous (resorption first, formation later). This means that while, under steady-state conditions, resorption at one site will be matched by formation at another, a change in remodeling increases or decreases osteoclastic resorption without a corresponding effect on mineralization of forming bone at sites activated previously. Thus, an increase in PTH makes surplus calcium available immediately, as acutely more bone is being resorbed than is currently being formed. Later, of course, when formation begins at the newly activated sites, there will be a demand to repay the loan of the previous "surplus" calcium. This phase lag between resorption and formation, which is normally of several weeks' duration, is admirably suited to mammalian calcium ion homeostasis. Generally the diet, rich in calcium, supplies the animal's needs, but in periods of fasting or famine, when food is scarce or unavailable, the internal calcium reserves are tapped. Later, when food sources are plentiful again, the loan is automatically repaid from the diet.

A unique feature of the ECF [Ca^{2+}] control loop is that PTH acts not just on bone, but on the gastrointestinal tract and the kidney as well. PTH is a principal regulator of the renal 1-α-hydroxylase, which converts 25-hydroxyvitamin D to 1,25-dihydroxyvitamin D, the hormonally most potent form of vitamin D, which in turn acts on the gastrointestinal tract to increase the extraction of calcium from ingested food. PTH also acts on the kidney to increase renal tubular calcium reabsorption, thereby decreasing renal excretory losses. However, slowing losses does not, of itself, compensate for a deficiency; it just slows or halts its progression. Thus it is the gastrointestinal tract and the bone that must provide the calcium needed to compensate for increased losses or reduced intake. The three effector organs (gastrointestinal tract, kidney, bone) are linked only by the common level of circulating PTH, which bathes and influences them all.

Quantitative Operation of the System

So much is generally recognized. What is less well characterized, and often ignored, are the *quantitative* workings of the system. It is commonly, if erroneously, assumed that because intestinal calcium absorption efficiency is low, upregulation will fully compensate for declines in intake (or increases in excretory loss). Examples include a calcium challenge, such as antler building in deer each spring, or human consumption of a low calcium diet. Under these circumstances, ECF [Ca^{2+}] tends to fall, as losses are not fully replaced from absorbed food calcium. The result is an increase in PTH secretion, which activates more bone resorption, increases renal conservation, and increases calcium absorption efficiency. The net effect with respect to total bone mass depends on the relative responsiveness of the three effector organs and on their capacity to provide the needed extra calcium [12]. Sensitivity of the effectors is genetically and hormonally determined, whereas the *capacity* to respond is largely determined by unregulated factors outside the control loop, such as the calcium content of the diet and coingestion of nutrients that force obligatory loss.

As PTH rises, extra calcium enters the ECF from newly activated bone remodeling loci, as well as from increased intestinal absorption via the direct action of PTH to facilitate 1,25-dihydroxyvitamin D synthesis. Excretory losses are reduced by better renal conservation. If, for some reason, the bony response is blunted, PTH continues to rise, forcing more intestinal absorption and better renal conservation. Conversely, if bone is highly responsive to PTH, the hormone level rises less because the needed calcium is supplied readily from the nearly limitless skeletal reserves. As a result, less improvement in external calcium utilization ensues. Similarly, if the gastrointestinal tract is unresponsive or the diet is so poor that its capacity to yield calcium is limited, then the PTH secretion rises further and bone is driven to meet the needs of the ECF [Ca^{2+}]. The two key insights here are (1) it is ECF [Ca^{2+}] that is being regulated, not bone mass, and (2) the dose–response relationships for the three effector organs are independent of one another.

Thus, American blacks (and probably African blacks as well) have a bony resorptive apparatus relatively resistant to PTH. As a result, they develop and maintain a higher bone mass than Caucasians and Asians, despite an often poor diet. As predicted from the foregoing, they exhibit higher PTH and 1,25-dihydroxyvitamin D levels [13]. In this way they utilize and conserve diet calcium more efficiently than Caucasians. The opposite situation occurs at normal menopause. Because estrogen appears to decrease bony responsiveness to PTH, estrogen loss at menopause increases the skeletal response to PTH. This is a part of the explanation for the increase in calcium requirement after menopause [3,6].

At the same time, it is useful to bear in mind that there is a huge disproportion between the body's needs for calcium and the calcium content of even a poor diet. Even at the peak of the adolescent growth spurt, bony growth could be accommodated nicely by the calcium contained in little more than a single serving of milk, if that calcium could be absorbed efficiently and fully conserved once absorbed. So, in theory at least, even calcium-poor diets could be adequate. This fact may explain why nutritional scientists had been slow to accept the life-long importance of a high calcium intake for contemporary humans. If the calcium were in the diet and the body was not fully accessing it, then—it was argued—the body did not need it.

That argument was recognized as flawed after the publication of several randomized, controlled trials,[1] showing that the body would indeed use extra calcium and improve calcium balance if the mineral were provided by high calcium intakes. Failure to retain calcium at low intakes reflected the fact that human absorption and conservation efficiencies for calcium are simply not up to the challenge of low intake, particularly when the bony reserves are so accessible. (As already pointed out, there was no evolutionary need for hominids to develop the type of absorption and excretory conservation that is needed for today's diets, when then available foods provided a surplus of calcium. Although our diets are modern, our physiologies are paleolithic.)

Age-Related Changes in Operation of the Control System

Important changes occur in the inputs and settings of this system with age. Calcium intake among U.S. women falls from early adolescence to the end of life. In National Health and Nutrition Examination Survey-II, the median calcium intake was 793 mg in early adolescence, 550 mg in the 20s, and 474 mg at menopause [15]. At the same time, absorption efficiency also falls with age. Peripubertal girls absorb calcium with about 45% greater efficiency for the same intake than do perimenopausal women [16]. In general, after age 40, absorption efficiency drops by about 0.2 absorption percentage points per year, with an added 2.2 percentage point drop across menopause [8]. A part of this decline may be due to a decrease in mucosal mass, which, in animals, is known to vary with food intake. In practical terms, if a 40-year-old woman absorbed a standard load at an efficiency of 30%, the same woman, at age 65 and deprived of estrogen, would absorb the same load at an efficiency of 22.8%, or almost a 25% worsening in absorptive performance. Vitamin D status declines with age as well [17,18], although this is a function of solar exposure and milk consumption. However, in Europe, where solar vitamin D synthesis is low for reasons of geography and climate, and milk is generally not fortified, the serum 25(OH)D concentration drops from over 100 nmol/liter (40 ng/ml) in young adults to under 50 nmol/liter (20 ng/ml) in individuals over age 70 [17,18]. Not surprisingly, serum PTH rises with age as a consequence of this aggregate of age-related changes. Twenty-four-hour integrated PTH is 70% higher in healthy 65-year-old women consuming diets containing 800 mg calcium per day than in third decade women on the same diets [19]. That this difference is due to insufficient absorptive input of calcium is shown by the fact that the discrepancy can be completely obliterated by increasing calcium intake in older women [19].

[1]See the review by Heaney [14] for a summary of these trials, as well as the more recent compilation of studies by the Food and Nutrition Board of the National Academy of Science [3].

Two Examples of System Operation

As implied in the foregoing, it is a *quantity* that is being optimized (i.e., ECF [Ca^{2+}]); this is accomplished by the algebraic sum of various *quantitative* inputs and outputs. While the operation of this, or any feedback loop, must first be sketched out qualitatively, in the final analysis it is the quantitative operation of the system that will determine what ultimately happens, in this case to the size of the calcium reserve, i.e., the mass of the skeleton. Two examples will serve to illustrate the quantitative operation of the system. One highlights the contrast between calcium handling at menarche and menopause and the second describes the response of the system to a fixed increase in obligatory loss.

MENARCHE AND MENOPAUSE

True trabecular bone density increases by about 15% across menarche [20], and about the same quantum of bone is lost across menopause [21]. Curiously, administration of estrogen to women more than 3 years postmenopausal has generally failed to reproduce the pubertal increase in BMD, and it has been customary to say, in recent years, that apart from whatever remodeling transient estrogen replacement therapy (ERT) may produce in postmenopausal women [22], its principal effect on bone is to stabilize bone mass, not to restore what had been lost. However, this conclusion was drawn without attending to the quantitative aspects of the age-related changes in the calcium economy, summarized in the foregoing. Table II assembles published data for

TABLE II Net Calcium Absorption at Menarche and Menopause

	Menarche	Menopause
Ca intake[a]	793 mg/day	474 mg/day
Ca absorption efficiency[b]	35.2%	30.5%
Endogenous fecal Ca[c]	67 mg/day	102 mg/day
Net Ca absorption	212 mg/day	42 mg/day

[a] NHANES-II median values [15].
[b] Heaney *et al.* [8] and O'Brien *et al.* [16]; values adjusted to intake.
[c] Heaney *et al.* [23].

median calcium intake and mean data for absorption efficiency and endogenous fecal calcium loss, and shows very clearly how quantitative changes in the 40 years from menarche to menopause account for the rather different performance of the two age groups. In brief (and despite an intake less than recommended), a peri-pubertal girl is able to achieve net absorption of over 200 mg of calcium from the median diet calcium content of her age cohort, whereas an early menopausal woman extracts less than one-fifth as much from hers. The drop in intake amounts to about 40%, but the drop in net absorption is 80%. As Table II shows, this is the resultant of lower intake, lower absorption efficiency, and higher digestive juice calcium losses. Given the level of obligatory losses at midlife, the absorbed quantity from prevailing diets is simply insufficient to support an estrogen-stimulated increase in BMD. As would be predicted from this understanding, higher calcium intakes lead to higher retention (see later).

RESPONSE TO ADDITIONAL LOSSES

An individual increasing his/her sodium intake by an amount equivalent to a single daily serving of a fast-food fried chicken meal experiences an increase in urinary calcium of about 40 mg/day [24]. Without compensating adjustments in input to the ECF, $[Ca^{2+}]$ drops. PTH, of course, rises, and with it, calcitriol synthesis. Published data allow rough estimation that a calcium drain of this magnitude would produce an increase in calcitriol level of about 6–7 pmol/liter [25], and dose–response data for calcitriol indicate that this stimulus would increase calcium absorption efficiency by about two to three absorption percentage points [26]. While it is commonly (and uncritically) considered that the absorptive apparatus is able to compensate both for a change in intake and for a change in excretory loss, quantitative considerations make it clear that this depends entirely on the level of calcium in the diet. A 2–3% increase in extraction from a 2000-mg diet yields 40–60 mg of extra calcium, whereas, the same absorptive increase from a 200-mg diet yields at most only 4–6 mg, and probably less.[2] Thus, on a high calcium diet, the body easily compensates for varying drains: both bone and ECF $[Ca^{2+}]$ are protected. However, on a low calcium diet, while the ECF $[Ca^{2+}]$ is protected, bone is not.

The Importance of Calcium Intake

In brief, as the body adjusts to varying demands, the portion of the demand met by bone will be determined by the level of diet calcium—the one critical component of the system that is not regulated. However, it must also be stressed that while an adequate calcium intake is a necessary condition for bone building and for adaptation to varying calcium demands, it is not by itself sufficient. Calcium alone will not stop estrogen deficiency bone loss or disuse loss (because neither is due to calcium deficiency). By the same token, however, recovery from immobilization or restoration of bone lost because of hormone deficiency will not be possible without an adequate supply of the raw materials needed to build bone substance.

This need for supplemental calcium has become increasingly clear as awareness of the essential role of calcium has grown in recent years, and increasing numbers of studies have combined calcium with other agents. Probably the earliest report of such a study, a retrospective compilation of Mayo Clinic osteoporosis treatment data [27], showed a synergistic effect on reducing vertebral fracture rate in osteoporotic women by adding calcium and vitamin D to estrogen replacement therapy and fluoride, with the greatest reduction being found with the combination of all four agents. More recently, Davis *et al.* [28] showed a substantial enhancement of the bone protective effect of ERT in postmenopausal women also given calcium. Most convincing of all, Nieves *et al.* [29], in a meta-analysis of 31 published randomized, controlled trials using ERT, segregated trials according to whether calcium was added to the ERT regimen. There was a strikingly greater, and more than additive, effect when calcium was incorporated into the regimen. Figure 3 displays data from this study.

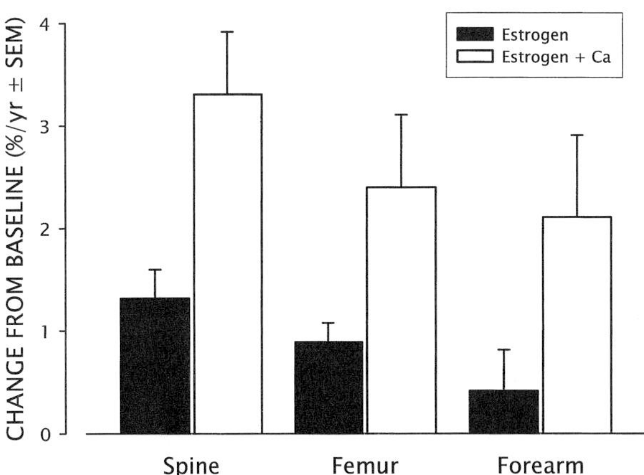

FIGURE 3 Mean skeletal response at three measurement sites to estrogen replacement therapy, with and without supplemental calcium, from 31 published randomized, controlled trials of estrogen in postmenopausal women. Calcium intake in the unsupplemented and the supplemented groups averaged 589 and 1189 mg/day, respectively. Redrawn from Nieves *et al.* [29], reproduced with permission.

[2]This is because extraction efficiency is already relatively high on low intakes and there is less calcium still unabsorbed on which the mucosa can work to extract additional calcium.

SUMMARY

Calcium balance is the resultant of several interacting forces, including nutrition, hormonal status, disuse, and general involution. Minimization of the structural impact of a negative calcium balance (i.e., a depleted skeleton) requires a multifaceted approach, including, but not limited to, an adequate calcium intake. Because calcium utilization is inefficient even during growth, and becomes more so with age, calcium intake requirements are high and rise with age. Intakes of healthy elderly persons should be in the range of 1400–1600 mg/day, and patients with osteoporosis being treated with bone active agents may need substantially more to realize the full benefit of their antiosteoporosis therapies. The goal of a high calcium intake in the elderly is both to make certain that inadequate calcium is not compounding the other negative factors influencing the aging skeleton and to support any bone-building potential that may reside in current and future antiosteoporosis therapies.

References

1. Heaney, R. P. En recherche de la difference. *Bone Miner.* **1,** 99–114 (1986).
2. Forbes, R. M., Weingartner, K. E., Parker, H. M., Bell, R. R., and Erdman, J. W., Jr. Bioavailability to rats of zinc, magnesium and calcium in casein-, egg-, and soy protein-containing diets. *J. Nutr.* **109,** 1652–1660 (1979).
3. Dietary reference intakes for calcium, magnesium, phosphorus, vitamin D, and fluoride. Food and Nutrition Board, Institute of Medicine, National Academy Press, Washington, DC, 1997.
4. Reid, I. R., Ames, R. W., Evans, M. C., Gamble, G. D., and Sharpe, S. J. Effect of calcium supplementation on bone loss in late postmenopausal women. *N. Engl. J. Med.* **328,** 460–464 (1993).
5. Reid, I. R., Ames, R. W., Evans, M. C., Gamble, G. D., and Sharpe, S. J. Long-term effects of calcium supplementation on bone loss and fractures in postmenopausal women: a randomized controlled trial. *Am. J. Med.* **98,** 331–335 (1995).
6. NIH Consensus Conference: Optimal Calcium Intake. *J. Am. Med. Assoc.* **272,** 1942–1948 (1994).
7. Eaton, B., and Nelson, D. A. Calcium in evolutionary perspective. *Am. J. Clin. Nutr.* **54,** 281S–287S (1991).
8. Heaney, R. P., Recker, R. R., Stegman, M. R., and Moy, A. J. Calcium absorption in women: relationships to calcium intake, estrogen status, and age. *J. Bone Miner. Res.* **4,** 469–475 (1989).
9. Heaney, R. P. Assessment and consistency of calcium intake. *In* "Nutritional Aspects of Osteoporosis" (P. Burckhardt and R. P. Heaney, eds.), Vol. 85, pp. 99–104. Serono. Raven Press, New York, 1991.
10. Charles, P. Metabolic bone disease evaluated by a combined calcium balance and tracer kinetic study. *Danish Med. Bull.* **36,** 463–479 (1989).
11. Klesges, R. C., Ward, K. D., Shelton, M. L., Applegate, W. B., Cantler, E. D., Palmieri, G. M. A., Harmon, K., and Davis, J. *J. Am. Med. Assoc.* **276,** 226–230 (1996).
12. Heaney, R. P. A unified concept of osteoporosis. *Am. J. Med.* **39,** 877–880 (1965).
13. Bell, N. H., Greene, A., Epstein, S., Oexmann, M. J., Shaw, S., and Shary, J. Evidence for alteration of the vitamin D-endocrine system in blacks. *J. Clin. Invest.* **76,** 470–473 (1985).
14. Heaney, R. P. Nutritional factors in osteoporosis. *Annu. Rev. Nutr.* **13,** 287–316 (1993).
15. Carroll, M. D., Abraham, S., and Dresser, C. M. *In* "Dietary Intake Source Data: United States, 1976-80, Vital and Health Statistics, Series 11-No. 231. DHHS Pub. No. (PHS) 83-1681, National Center for Health Statistics, Public Health Service, U. S. Government Printing Office, Washington, DC, 1983.
16. O'Brien, K. O., Abrams, S. A., Liang, L. K., Ellis, K. J., and Gagel, R. F. Increased efficiency of calcium absorption during short periods of inadequate calcium intake in girls. *Am. J. Clin. Nutr.* **63,** 579–583 (1996).
17. McKenna M. J., Freaney, R., Meade, A., and Muldowney, F. P. Hypovitaminosis D and elevated serum alkaline phosphatase in elderly Irish people. *Am. J. Clin. Nutr.* **41,** 101–109 (1985).
18. Francis, R. M., Peacock, M., Storer, J. H., Davies, A. E. J., Brown, W. B., and Nordin, B. E. C. Calcium malaborption in the elderly: the effect of treatment with oral 25-hydroxyvitamin D_3. *Eur. J. Clin. Invest.* **13,** 391–396 (1983).
19. McKane, W. R., Khosla, S., Egan, K. S., Robins, S. P., Burritt, M. F., and Riggs, B. L. Role of calcium intake in modulating age-related increases in parathyroid function and bone resorption. *J. Clin. Endocrinol. Metab.* **81,** 1699–1703 (1996).
20. Gilsanz, V., Gibbens, D. T., Roe, T. F., Carlson, M., Senac, M. O., Boechat, M. I., Huang, H. K., Schulz, E. E., Libanati, C. R., and Cann, C. Vertebral bone density in children: effect of puberty. *Radiology* **166,** 847–850 (1988).
21. Genant, H. K., Cann, C. E., Ettinger, B., Gordan, G. S., Kolb, F. O., Reiser, U., and Arnaud, C. D. Quantitative computed tomography for spinal mineral assessment. *In* "Osteoporosis" (C. Christiansen *et al.,* eds.), pp. 65–72. Department of Chemistry, Glostrup Hospital, Copenhagen, Denmark, 1984.
22. Heaney, R. P. The bone remodeling transient: implications for the interpretation of clinical studies of bone mass change. *J. Bone Miner. Res.* **9,** 1515–1523 (1994).
23. Heaney, R. P., and Recker, R. R. Determinants of endogenous fecal calcium in healthy women. *J. Bone Miner. Res.* **9,** 1621–1627 (1994).
24. Itoh, R., and Suyama, Y. Sodium excretion in relation to calcium and hydroxyproline excretion in a healthy Japanese population. *Am. J. Clin. Nutr.* **63,** 735–740 (1996).
25. Dawson-Hughes, B., Stern, D. T., Shipp, C. C., and Rasmussen, H. M. Effect of lowering dietary calcium intake on fractional whole body calcium retention. *J. Clin. Endocrinol. Metab.* **67,** 62–68 (1988).
26. Heaney, R. P., Barger-Lux, M. J., Dowell, M. S., Chen, T. C., and Holick, M. F. Calcium absorptive effects of vitamin D and its major metabolites. *J. Clin. Endocrinol. Metab.* **82,** 4111–4116 (1997).
27. Riggs, B. L., Seeman, E., Hodgson, S. F., Taves, D. R., and O'Fallon, W. M. Effect of the fluoride/calcium regimen on vertebral fracture occurrence in postmenopausal osteoporosis. *N. Engl. J. Med.* **306,** 446–450 (1982).
28. Davis, J. W., Ross, P. D., Johnson, N. E., and Wasnich, R. D. Estrogen and calcium supplement use among Japanese American women: effects upon bone loss when used singly and in combination. *Bone* **17,** 369–373 (1995).
29. Nieves, J. W., Komar, L., Cosman, F., and Lindsay, R. Calcium potentiates the effect of estrogen and calcitonin on bone mass: review and analysis. *Am. J. Clin. Nutr.* **67,** 18–24 (1998).

CHAPTER 4

Constraints of Experimental Paradigms Used to Model the Aging Skeleton

JANET RUBIN Department of Medicine, Emory University School of Medicine and Veterans Affairs Medical Center, Atlanta, Georgia 30033
HARRY RUBIN Department of Molecular and Cell Biology and Virus Laboratory, University of California, Berkeley, California 94720
CLINTON RUBIN Musculo-Skeletal Research Laboratory, Program in Biomedical Engineering, State University of New York, Stony Brook, New York 11794

INTRODUCTION: BONE AS A COMPLEX SYSTEM

Can these bones live?
Ezekiel

The human skeleton is a multifunctional organ that facilitates locomotion, protects internal organs, and serves as the primary reservoir of mineral. In accommodating these diverse functional, structural, and metabolic roles, the skeleton's remarkable ability to maintain relative homeostasis is achieved via poorly understood and complex control mechanisms. During the aging process, the skeleton retains its capacity for providing mineral to the organism, but the bones become fragile over time. The functional demands on the aging skeleton continue to provide a barrage of mechanical stimuli, but the skeleton becomes less able to respond appropriately, resulting ultimately in fracture. The skeleton's susceptibility to the ravages of aging thus puts the organism at great risk.

This book readily demonstrates the diversity of contributing causes of bone loss and their relationships to age-related bone loss. It is apparent that the skeletal failure that parallels the aging process arises from complex, multifactorial etiologies. Subtle changes in the conformation of the mineral constituents of the bone, attenuation of mechanotransduction to the cell, progressive sarcopenia, neurologic degeneration, altered balance of formative and resorptive activity, genetic predisposition to osteopenia, microdamage, and corrosion of the organic matrix are only a few of the many potential sources of deterioration that conspire toward structural failure. To better understand the means by which age slowly but inevitably affects the skeleton, it is essential that the interdependence of distinct etiologies be considered.

How do we appropriately study the aging process in bone? As scientists, we approach the complications of aging at many levels, from processes at the whole organism to the molecular machinery. Because we are constrained by the systems with which we study the aging skeleton, we must appreciate the limits of the information gained. While singular scientific strategies to understand the consequences of aging are important, it is essential to consider the results in the light of the interdependent nature of a complex biological system. Ultimately, our goal is to emphasize that the skeleton, particularly the aging skeleton, must be considered at many different levels.

This chapter uses some of the models employed for studying the aging process to emphasize the interdependence of diverse and distinct entities in determining the etiology of age-related bone disease. This is not meant to be an exhaustive review, but rather a vehicle to examine how overinterpretation of a specific model at one level (e.g., *in vitro* studies of osteoblasts) could oversimplify our understanding of how aging affects the whole skeleton. Beginning at the organismal level, we consider the clinical interpretation of fracture risk in aging humans; Chapters 10, 24, and 26 also include some of these issues. At the tissue level, the use of the rat as a model for age-related bone deficiency is evaluated; Chapter 5 also examines the strengths and weaknesses of whole animal models of aging. From these *in vivo* systems, we turn to *in vitro* systems, with the goal of evaluating whether an "old" cell can realistically serve as a model of aging; Chapter 7 also discusses the interpretation of cellular studies. Finally, we offer an epigenetic approach to modeling age-related changes at the level of the cell.

THE AGING HUMAN: BONE MINERAL DENSITY IS ONLY PART OF FRACTURE RISK

Youth is wasted on the young.
Somerset Maugham

Bone mineral density is the most important index of fracture risk. Data sets of bone density suggest that for each standard deviation below peak bone mass, the fracture risk increases by at least 1.5- to 2-fold [1]. A decrease in mineral density normally parallels the aging process, and this loss of bone density is estimated to account for as much as 80% of the decrease in strength in the elderly skeleton [2]. However, it is important to emphasize that these data arise from and are applicable primarily to women, particularly women past the age of menopause. What these data mean for young women, children, or men, who have been less studied and fracture less, is not yet clear. To illustrate this point, consider that a 70-year-old woman with an equivalent bone density to that of a 20 year old is subject to nearly a 10-fold increase in fracture risk [3]. This suggests that fracture risk is influenced by factors that bone mineral density cannot measure, such as the risks of falling that an older population incurs through frailty and ill-health or the reduced ability to protect the body during a fall. There are, of course, many other intrinsic skeletal components that are affected by aging. We review several that may contribute to the risk of failure in the aging skeleton.

Bone size is critical to fracture risk: less energy is required to break a small bone than a large one. Peak bone size is determined largely by genetic indices and in essence is not affected by aging [4,5]. Nevertheless, the fracture risk of a patient based on deviations from Z or T scores (variability from age matched or peak mass, respectively) does not account for the size of the women. For this reason, smaller women will have lower apparent bone mineral density and, by this criterion, may fall into a category of risk as assessed by dual energy x-ray absorptiometry (DXA), even though their skeletons are quite appropriate for functional needs. A petite woman with a T score 1.5 standard deviations below normal may in fact be at no increased risk at all. The decision to treat to prevent fracture morbidity therapy should be based on criteria that also appreciate the stature of the patient, as well as the rate of change of bone density.

Properties other than size and mass are also key contributors to the structural competence of bone. These include functional parameters such as levels of exercise and morphologic parameters such as the long bone curvature, the girth and geometry of the cross-sectional area, the trabecular organization (e.g., connectivity), and even nutritional factors such as calcium intake, which contribute to the rate of bone turnover as well as bone mass. Just as bone strength is achieved by a complex interdependence of many diverse factors, degeneration of the skeleton is a product of many interacting events. With aging, extrinsic factors such as (lack of) exercise, (lack of) nutrition, smoking, and drinking influence the microarchitecture and morphology that ultimately determine structural sufficiency.

The ultrastructural components of bone provide strength while maintaining lightness and mobility. The composite structure of bone allows it to withstand compression, as well as survive tensile strain, bending, and twisting. The inorganic phase of bone, hydroxyapatite crystals arrayed in a protein matrix, provides the compressive resistant component. Individual calcium phosphate crystals of multiple sizes are imbedded in and around the fibrils of the collagen type I lattice [6]. The organization of the crystal, and its relationship to constituents such as collagen, is influenced by external factors such as hormones, cytokines, and functional stimuli, all which are subject to change in an aging, and perhaps diseased milieu. Considering that bone is constantly remodeling, subtle defects in the collagen scaffold, or in an osteoid that does not organize or mineralize in an "optimal" manner, will eventually, albeit slowly, undermine the skeleton's ability to resist load bearing.

Hydroxyapatite, as effective as it may be in resisting compressive loads, has very poor structural properties when subjected to tensile loads. As in concrete, a material that excels at resisting compression but is poor in resisting tension, tensile elements (e.g., steel rods known as reinforcing bar) are added to create a composite material that can cope with complex loading environments. In the case of bone, tensile strength arises from collagen fibrils organized into lamellae. Lamellae vary in thickness, and the collagen orientation between adjacent plates can rotate by as much as 90°, permitting the tissue to resist forces and moments acting from several different directions, much like the added strength of plywood provided by distinct orientation of each layer of the composite [7]. While this ultrastructural organization is, to a certain extent, defined by the genome, the functional environment contributes to the distribution of lamellae as well as the osteons that house them [8]. Given that more than 80% of functionally engendered strains (deformation) are due to bending (and thus a high percentage of strain is tensile), the structural quality of the bone "organ" may ultimately be determined by the quality of the collagen and the organization of the microarchitecture (e.g., circumferential lamellae, primary and/or secondary osteons). While studies such as DEXA or CT scanning fail to monitor the organic constituents of the bone, studies have shown that collagen itself deteriorates with age and undoubtedly contributes to the declining material properties of the skeleton [9].

Alterations in *either* the organic (e.g., collagen) or the inorganic (e.g., hydroxyapatite) matrix components can bring about changes in the bone strength. Mutations in the collagen gene give rise to several genetic skeletal problems, some of which increase fracture risk. In osteogenesis imperfecta (OI), mutations in the primary structure of type I procollagen lead to brittle and easily fractured bones [10,11]. The origin of the fragility of OI bone is not completely understood, but points to microarchitectural changes. This disease has been studied using several mouse models, including the osteogenesis imperfecta mouse model (*oim*), which produces only collagen a1. The bone crystals in the absence of collagen a2 appear to be thinner and possibly disoriented [12]. Another disorder of collagen resulting in excessively fragile bone is fibrogenesis imperfecta ossium [13], a rare disorder where the skeleton is replaced by disorganized collagen-deficient tissue. The natural history of this disease reveals a progressive replacement of bone by abnormal collagen with randomly orientated fibrils of varying thickness. Calcification of the collagen is greatly delayed, implying that the highly organized morphology of the collagen substrate is important not only for strength, but for biomineralization. It is possible that aging affects collagen production or its mineralization.

Several clinical findings emphasize that the microarchitecture of bone is also a critical determinant of fracture risk. For example, volumetrically, the amount of mineral contained in each unit of bone is similar when comparing black to white women [14]. However, white women fracture at twice the rate of black women [15]. To a certain extent, the reduced fracture incidence is influenced by the proportionately larger bone size found in black women [16,17] and because black women may have a greater cortical thickness [18]. It has been suggested that black women have thick trabeculae, presenting less surface area to be remodeled, thus preserving continuity [17]. Studies from Weinstein and Bell [19] concur that black adults have lower bone turnover, which may also contribute to the lower fracture rate measured in blacks. Together, these data suggest that concentrating on areal bone density does not necessarily inform us completely of the etiology of fracture risk. No place is this better demonstrated than in the subtle increases in areal bone mineral density that accompany the use of alendronate, changes that cannot fully explain the precipitous drop in fracture risk; bone structure is enjoying some benefit of treatment that is not being quantified by DXA [20]. What is clear is that we must consider parameters beyond bone density that contribute to bone quality such as turnover, connectivity, organic constituents, ultrastructural integrity, and organization. With an improved understanding of what provides the skeleton with its structural success, we may be able to identify which parameters become dysfunctional in the aging human.

THE AGING RAT: USING ANIMAL MODELS TO STUDY AGING IN HUMANS

That man with all his noble qualities . . . still bears in his bodily frame the indelible stamp of his lowly origin.

C. Darwin (final words)

Consider the evolution of vertebrates. First signs of life popped up on our planet around 4 billion years ago. The first known vertebrates, armored jawless fishes called Agnathans, did not appear for another 3.5 billion years, 480 million years ago during the Ordovician period [21]. Hominids have existed for only 3.2 million years. Humans "anatomically similar" to current residents appeared only 100,000 years ago. Of all the animals running, floating, flying, or swimming around, less than 3% are vertebrates. There is a perplexing degree of homology between the genome of the human and chimpanzee (99%), a high degree of homology between human and rat (93%), and a humbling degree of similarity to the fruit fly (75%), suggesting strong, intricate ties among essentially all Animalia. Given the high degree of genomic homology across mammals and the relatively brief time with which we humans have been around, it seems reasonable that animal models of human bone disease would provide valuable insight into the pathogenesis and etiology of the aging skeleton. To a certain extent that is true, but it is essential to approach these models with a strong sense of their limitations.

The great majority of *in vivo* protocols used to study the aging process in general, and the aging skeleton in particular, focus on *Rattus novegicus,* the laboratory rat. As important as the rat may be as a tool for the study of aging, it must be emphasized that the rat skeleton is unusual in that growth may slow following a few months, but never actually ceases [22,23]. Indeed, bone loss does not occur until an exogenous distress is imposed, such as estrogen or androgen deficiency. Interpretation of the roles of insulin-like growth factor I (IGF-I) or other bone formative agents (e.g., exercise) in influencing the aging rat skeleton then are complicated by the need to extrapolate from a model of slowed growth to the human condition of rapid decline. Circumspection is, of course, essential in any case of using an animal to model a human disease. The complexities inherent in the aging process, a natural condition of deterioration rather than a disease per se, may be difficult to study through experimental perturbations of growth in the rat.

The 1994 U.S. FDA guidelines for preclinical and clinical evaluation of agents used in the treatment or prevention of postmenopausal osteoporosis suggest that the ovariectomized rat be used as the primary model system for preclinical investigations [24]. Because rats are readily available and because ovariectomized rats consistently and predictably lose bone at specific sites of the skeleton, many laboratories find them useful. As convenient as the model may be, it is critical to consider whether the "aging" rat skeleton is a realistic appraisal of the aging human.

For example, it is unclear whether effects of growth hormone or IGF-I on rats can be extrapolated to clinical use [25]. Somatomedin C, or IGF-I, has pleiotropic effects in bone. It was first discovered as the sulfation factor released from the liver after administration of the growth hormone and it was shown to stimulate bone growth [26]. It is important to note that growth hormone alone fails to initiate growth, as it requires the presence of IGF-I. In the absence of IGF-I, a condition caused by resistance to growth hormone as described in multiple pediatric syndromes, children fail to grow [27,28]. Because of the direct association of IGF-I with growth, it seems reasonable that IGF-I, in isolation, might be able to induce bone formation in animals and bone cell cultures [29,30].

Whereas clinical applications of IGF-I focus on the treatment of growth disorders, it was proposed that a deficiency of this hormone may underlie the inability of bone formation to compensate for the increased resorption present in aging individuals [31]. In support of this hypothesis, a subset of older men was found to have IGF-I levels in the lower quartile [32]. To directly test whether the skeletal consequences of IGF-I deficiency can be treated, Wakisaka and colleagues [33] locally infused IGF-I into the femurs of old rats. The results were certainly compelling in that procollagen, osteopontin, alkaline phosphatase, and osteocalcin increased significantly [33]. Further, the increase in the bone formation rate was paralleled by a decrease in eroded surface and osteoclast surface, leading the authors to conclude that local administration of IGF-I improves trabecular bone status.

A more comprehensive understanding of the effect of stimulating the IGF-I/growth hormone axis in rats can be found in a study by Oxlund and colleagues [34]. Twenty-one-month-old rats were injected with growth hormone, thus causing substantial increases in IGF-I. As suspected, this intervention caused a brisk increase in femoral bone formation associated with improved breaking load and stiffness of the femur. Mild exercise along with IGF-I stimulated a synergistic increase in bone formation accompanied by yet further advances in strength parameters. On initial inspection, these data appear to support the case for a role for IGF-I in the treatment of bone disease. However, on closer examination, it becomes clear that IGF-I treated bones grew in both length and breadth and that the increase in strength was due to the greater size of bones in the hormonally manipulated animals rather than an increase in formation in the sense of remodeling. Thus, while IGF-I is an effective means to stimulate the growth plate of rats, it remains problematic to extrapolate data shown to cause bone growth in an animal that can continue to grow to a human skeleton that long ago lost that capacity.

The rat model has been used frequently to herald salutary therapeutics in the aging human skeleton. Parathyroid hormone stimulates bone formation in aged ovariectomized rats [35,36], as does basic fibroblast growth factor [37]. It is not clear whether this is true for nongrowing animals. Studies assessing alternate compounds, such as androgen, in "maintaining" the mass of the rat skeleton [38,39] may instead be reestablishing a faster rate of bone growth, and thus increases in bone density arise from an overall increase in bone size. Even in presumably straightforward situations that evaluate the potential of mechanical stimuli to differentially influence gene expression (e.g., the quest for the "mechanogene"), investigators using the rat are faced with the task of discriminating those genes that are involved in normal growth patterns versus bone modeling as caused by mechanical loading; ironically, the very gene that is being sought may be masked as it may also be involved in growth [40] or wound healing [41].

Growth in any animal is, indeed, a polygenic phenomenon, creating many problems for analysis. Thus, when considering manipulations of aged rats that induce changes in bone density or strength, it is essential to take into account that rats are continuously growing and that the aging rat skeleton might better be described as one in which growth is altered by changes in the hormonal environment. While the rat may be an effective initial screening tool to identify anabolic agents, we must accept the limitations in extrapolating perturbations of bone growth to the slow, progressive degeneration of bone morphology.

WHAT IS AN AGING CELL?

You will recognize, my boy, the first sign of old age: it is when you go out into the streets of London and realize for the first time how young the policemen look.

Sir Seymour Hicks

The skeleton can be examined on many hierarchical levels. Few would disagree that cell function underlies the creation of these levels, as each requires active biological processes to arrange the bone structure and respond to signals to form and remodel the mineralized environment. Considering that aging represents the villainous deorchestration of this complex, interdependent process, it would make sense to conclude that the study of the etiology of aging requires experiments with aging cells. However, a multitude of problems arise in first defining what an "old cell" actually is and whether the imposed limitations of the culture dish will obfuscate understanding of cell function within a degenerating physiologic system.

Perhaps the first set of problems involves the choice of which cell to study. Because osteoblasts are predominantly responsible for forming bone, this would appear a reasonable place to start. Indeed, evidence shows that a reduced osteoprogenitor pool is present in aged humans [42]. Further, bone from older individuals differs from that from younger ones [43]. An optimistic plan to address insufficient bone formation in the elderly might be to transplant osteoprogenitor cells from a young donor into an old individual. In concert with the age-induced attenuation of osteoblast activity, bone resorption outpaces bone formation, raising the issue that part of the problems facing the aging skeleton involves the proliferation of too many osteoclasts from the marrow progenitor pool. Is it the cells themselves that fail? Alternately, the controls on cell recruitment—osteoprogenitor or osteoclast—may fail with age.

Considering the nature of the bone loss, progressive over decades, and the very small percentage of cells residing in the bone that are osteoblasts or osteoclasts, the failure that coincides with aging may, in reality, be caused by the activity (or inactivity) of another cell. Perhaps *neither* bone forming nor resorbing cells are deficient: the cell that may control the response of these other cells may, in fact, be the bone osteocyte. The osteocyte is poised in the calcified matrix, tightly interconnected to neighboring osteocytes and bone lining cells, and is well positioned and designed to respond to mechanical and hormonal signals [44]. Unfortunately, the osteocyte, fixed in phenotype by sealing within the bone, is difficult to harvest and difficult to culture. Even those investigators who have successfully cultured these recalcitrant cells [45] must consider if denying them their matrix environment in reality denies them of their functional phenotype. In any case, the study of aging by examining specific cell types must be circumspect, as the very selection of the cell to be studied will divulge different sets of information. While the *in vitro* results may be very exciting, extrapolation of results derived from the unique environment of the incubator to the unique environment of the organism must be performed with caution.

Perhaps as difficult a problem as selection of the critical cell type is the selection of an appropriate *in vitro* model with which to study the cellular process of aging. Two paradigms to model the aging cell have been used most frequently in the literature. The first is to allow cells to continuously divide, eventually reaching a point of suspected senescence in the laboratory dish, and to identify the changes that overcome that cell population during these late divisions. The second is to harvest cells from aged animals and to compare how these cells respond differently in culture from those harvested from young animals. It is important to consider the attributes and limitations of each of these approaches.

No normal diploid human cells have been shown to proliferate indefinitely *in vitro*. This observation gave rise to the theory that normal cells have a fixed limit in replicative capacity [46]. The critical question is whether this *in vitro* process can be compared with that occurring in the organism. There are many differences, the most overreaching one being that calculations of the numbers of cell replications within the organism suggest that their capacity to divide is not fixed and depends rather on the needs of the self-renewing organs. For certain tissues and organs, the continued natural replication far exceeds the *in vitro* boundaries as assigned by the "Hayflick limit," i.e., that there is a fixed limit of replication within a two-dimensional culture dish [47]. This inconsistency begs the question of what we can learn from cells removed from their spatially, chemically, and temporally information-rich environment to an artificial monolayer culture, bathed in medium rich with growth stimuli—a radical change which may, in itself, mask any accrued signals that incriminate a particular host environment. While we must accept that *in vitro* cell cultures are a critical avenue to uncovering mechanisms of events, we must also realize that the culture dish is a poor substitute for aging. In essence, the subtle shifts in biological processes that arise from environmental information encoded over many years will probably not be approachable by cells senescing in the laboratory environment.

Perhaps a level of cell senescence could be assigned to osteoprogenitor cells according to the donor age. Several studies have suggested that older individuals can supply less osteoprogenitor cells [42,48–50], and marrow replicative capacity (i.e., supply of bone stem cells) is held to decrease with age [51]. Osteoprogenitor cells harvested from an old animal might behave differently when compared to those from a newborn because of subtle acquired damage in the genetic apparatus. Alternatively, the cells may respond differently because of faulty programming delivered by the aged environment, magnified by the onset of age-related diseases. To illustrate this point, an experiment involving harvesting osteoprogenitor cells from weight bearing versus skeletally unloaded rats was performed. Five days of hindlimb elevation led to significant decrements in the proliferative capacity and functional parameters of bone marrow stromal cells [52]. This work suggested that these cells were able to retain a memory of their donor environment. Along the same lines, i.e., the ability of the donor environment to program cells, systemic administration of the bone anabolic agent prostaglandin E_2 leads to an increased osteogenic capacity of harvested bone marrow cells [53]. Because disease states are more common in the elderly, the presence of disease, rather than age itself, might account for various reports of an inverse correlation between donor age and population doublings *in vitro* [47]. With regard to bone, this question may be answered by taking old osteoprogenitor cells, tagged with regard to identity, and transplanting to a young animal or transplanting young cells to an old environment. In this way the contribution of the environment—the hormones, cytokines, and structural environment present in the aged individual—can be assessed.

It will also be important to separate the ability of aged cells to proliferate (e.g., refreshing bone forming units) from the ability of these cells to function properly. At this time, research has focused on capturing an osteoprogenitor supply characterized by the ability to function phenotypically as osteoblasts while continuously proliferating. It is, however, not a certainty that osteoprogenitor cells with robust proliferative capacity will function appropriately. One experiment suggesting that aged bone may be deficient in response to mechanical stimuli was performed using rat alveolar bone. Mechanically stressed rat alveolar bone showed that the bone formation activity of osteoblasts declined with age, despite no evidence of difference in number of these cells [54]. These issues with regard to aged bone cells remain to be solved.

AN ALTERNATIVE APPROACH TO CELLULAR AGING

Thus the whirligig of time brings in his revenges.
Shakespeare (*Twelfth Night*)

The aging field, which was at one time itself almost moribund, was revitalized by the claim that cells had a genetically fixed limit to the number of replications they could undergo, the so-called Hayflick limit [55,56]. This conclusion was in fact an interpretation of the evidence that human fetal fibroblasts explanted to cell culture could not be carried beyond 50 divisions. There are many reasons to question whether this limit on proliferation arises from genetic machinery; an equally reasonable interpretation would conclude that the Hayflick limit reflects the cumulative damage resulting from the failure of the cells to adapt to the radically foreign environment of cell culture [47,57].

This is not the place to recount the multifaceted case against the genetically fixed limit on replicative life span, but it is instructive to consider why it had such a profound impact on the field of aging. For one thing, the idea of a fixed replicative life span for all animal cells was a broad generalization that had an appealing simplicity. For another, it was based on an (almost) invariably reproducible experiment of cell culture, thus calling out for biological and biochemical correlation. The mass of such correlations collected since the late 1960s has yielded much information that indeed has some validity for understanding long-range cellular changes that accompany aging. The problem with these explanted cells, however, is that their replicative capacity starts going downhill as soon as they are plated in culture. The encroaching limit could, in fact, be an indicator of the inability of the cell to cope with the new environment rather than reflecting a genetically fixed limit on replication.

In seeking a generalizable *in vitro* model system, it would make sense to use cells that are fully adapted to growth in culture just as our own cells are fully adapted to function within organs. There are many such established cell lines fully adapted to life in the laboratory dish, and some even mirror the growth regulatory properties of normal cells without the decline in function that inevitably occurs with freshly explanted cells (primary cultures). Some general findings about cell behavior have already been made with such cells that should have significance in the process of cellular aging. First and foremost of these is that when cells are subject to an extended period of physiological stress, such as crowding or cytotoxic treatment, some cells may die, but a larger fraction of survivors will incur heritable damage such that they and all their descendants grow at a slower rate than the original population [58,59]. The connection with cellular aging is that cells in various organs in experimental animals multiply more slowly in the aged animal. Thus, a general property of aging cells can be modeled in cell culture.

Second, somatic cell genetics reveals that deletions of large chunks of genetic material (multiallelic deletions) are associated with a reduction in growth rate. In contrast, local mutations do not affect growth [60–63]. Multiallelic deletions, in fact, accumulate in somatic cells with age [64]. Hence, culture manipulations that generate multiallelic deletions may model the aging process.

There are also epigenetic effects in aging that require the presence of multicellular populations and may be difficult to reproduce in culture. An example concerns the inactivation of the X chromosome in cells of female mammals. In the livers of young mice, only about 1 cell in 2000 has two active X chromosomes [65]. In old female mice, however, control of X inactivation is relaxed such that about 1 cell in 40 has two active X chromosomes. While this is no doubt a product of changes at the level of the cell, those effects are multiplied in multicellular aggregates where regulatory controls are gradually weakened by aging.

The relevance of such observations is that general findings made with cells in culture or in the animal can be cautiously related to one another and eventually applied to specific tissues. This can be illustrated with an example with relevance to aging from the field of neoplastic transformation and its relation to cancer. If murine NIH/3T3 cells are kept under long-term growth constraints (crowding or limited availability of growth factors), neoplastically transformed cells appear [66,67]. Transformation is recognized by the formation of multilayered, disordered layers of cells in culture and an ability to produce tumors in immunologically deficient mice with these cells. At high densities, recapitulating a more normal environment, these transformed cells multiply rapidly. At low population densities, paradoxically, the cells grow at a lower rate than their progenitors and continue to do so indefinitely [68]. The heritability of the altered growth regulation is therefore an indication of genetic damage to the cells. Somatic cell genetics has shown that mutations that result in slowed growth are almost invariably large-scale deletions of DNA or rearrangements of DNA (see earlier discussion). The former are the most common lesion found in solid epithelial cancers and the latter are common in leukemias [69]. Multiallelic deletions are also ubiquitous in the cells of aging mice [64]. The situation is analogous to the situation in the aging organism, where large genetic changes appear in many more cells than undergo transformation, but those changes are a prerequisite for transformation and ultimately to cancer [64]. So a set of correlations exists among neoplastic transformation, deletions, human cancer, and aging, from the culture dish to the animal.

Cell culture does offer the versatility to bring out all the relations described here and specialized aspects that may be applicable to studying aging of the skeleton. Questions that will be pertinent to the skeleton include determining to what extent deletions and genetic rearrangements are found in aging bone. We will want to know whether constraints on growth and metabolism in skeletal tissue create genetic mutations analogous to aging bone cells. In the end, we may be able to answer whether these alterations can be related to loss of function and increased fragility of bone with age.

SUMMARY

There are so few who can grow old with a good grace.

Sir Richard Steele

In conclusion, even with all these data, reports, and hypotheses, we still ask what determines the increased risk of hip fracture in a 70 year old in relation to a 20 year old who has the same bone density. We believe the answer will arise out of studies that consider the entire musculoskeletal system (and beyond) rather than attribute age-related complications to any specific etiology in isolation. The 70 year old must contend with decreased agility in response to falling, predisposing him/her to hip fracture. Further, aged bone may not respond to the loading environment appropriately. The improved moment of inertia that comes from periosteal expansion in the aging process may be composed of poor mineral, organic components, or both. The etiology of osteopenia has even been proposed to arise not from the failings of the bone tissue, but as an appropriate adaptation to the degeneration of muscle, i.e., osteopenia follows sarcopenia [70].

Moving from the organismal to the tissue level, aged bone may have a decreased ability to repair damage, it may accumulate microdamage and thus disrupt intercellular communication, or it may have a depressed (or opposite) response to pharmaceutical treatments developed in young animals. We must be cautious in presuming that growing animals will respond analogously to humans, both in terms of age and aging physiology. We must even ask the question if animals used in laboratory research do indeed age over their short life spans.

Moving to the next level of complexity, the cell, it is important to argue that investigations of age-related deficits in cellular functions consider all the cells involved in bone remodeling. Concurrently, we must ask if these cells adequately represent their counterparts in the temporal–spatial biochemical–biophysical milieau of bone. Because the usual two-dimensional *in vitro* culture environment imposes radical changes in the collected cells, interpretation may be possible if genetic defects are present or if the cells retain adequate memory of their donor environment. Both these provisos require assumptions that may be difficult to analyze when moving from the level of the gene to the cell, to the organ, and then to the aging animal. Perhaps the most powerful techniques for studying cell function will involve the transplantation of young cells into the aged animal and vice versa. In this way the attributes of the intrinsic cellular machinery can be compared to changes in the host environment.

In interpreting studies of human and animal models of disease, an awareness of the hierarchy of bone must be used to arrive at a comprehensive understanding of what aging means for the skeleton. Obviously, this is a daunting task. It is essentially impossible for a single investigator or team to successfully tackle the complex interactions of a complex interdependent system such as the skeleton. Nor do we wish to imply that everyone should abandon their patch clamps, thermocyclers, cell cultures, DXA measurements, or turkey ulnae. Their contributions are critical to the science which we, as a discipline and a society, require to move forward. However we approach these important issues, it remains essential that we appreciate the intricate interdependence of countless distinct elements that all contribute toward the achievement of a successful skeleton, just as we must appreciate how many distinct elements conspire to the degeneration of the aging skeleton.

References

1. Melton, L. J., Atkinson, K. J., OFallon, W. M., Wahner, H. W., and Riggs, B. L. Long term fracture prediction by bone mineral assessed at different skeletal sites. *J. Bone Miner. Res.* **8,** 1227–1233 (1993).
2. Singer, K., Edmonston, S., Day, R., Breidahl, P., and Price, R. Prediction of thoracic and lumbar vertebral body compressive strength: correlations with bone mineral density and vertebral region. *Bone* **17,** 167–174 (1995).
3. Burr, D. B., Forwood, M. R., Fyhrie, D. P., Martin, R. B., Schaffler, M. B., and Turner, C. H. Bone microdamage and skeletal fragility in osteoporotic and stress fractures. *J. Bone Miner. Res.* **12,** 6–15 (1997).
4. Christian, J. C., Yu, P., Slemenda, C. W., and Johnston, C. C. Heritability of bone mass. *Am. J. Hum. Genet.* **44,** 429–433 (1989).
5. Pocock, N. A., Eisman, J. A., Hopper, J. L., Yeates, M. G., Sambrook, P. N., and Eberl, S. Genetic determinants of bone mass in adults. *J. Clin. Invest.* **80,** 706–710 (1987).
6. Weiner, S., and Traub, W. Bone structure: from angstroms to microns. *FASEB J.* **6,** 879–885 (1992).
7. Alexander, M. "Bones: The Unity of Form and Function." Macmillan, New York, 1994.
8. Skedros, J. G., Mason, M. W., Nelson, M. C., and Bloebaum, R. D. Evidence of structural and material adaptation to specific strain features in cortical bone. *Anat. Rec.* **246,** 47–63 (1996).
9. Oxlund, H., Mosekilde, L., and Ortoft, G. Reduced concentration of collagen reducible cross links in human trabecular bone with respect to age and osteoporosis. *Bone* **19,** 479–484 (1996).
10. Prockop, D. J., and Kivirikko, K. I. Heritable diseases of collagen. *N. Engl. J. Med.* **311,** 376–386 (1984).
11. Prockop, K. J. Mutations that alter the primary structure of type I collagen. *J. Biol. Chem.* **265,** 15349–15352.
12. Misof, K., Landis, W. J., Klaushofer, K., and Frati, P. Collagen from the osteogenesis imperfecta mouse model (oim) shows reduced resistance against tensile stress. *J. Clin. Invest.* **100,** 40–45 (1997).
13. Carr, A. J., Smith, R., Athanasou, N., and Woods, C. G. Fibrogenesis imperfecta ossium. *J. Bone Jt. Surg. Br. J.* **77,** 820–829 (1995).
14. Seeman, E. From density to structure: Growing up and growing old on the surfaces of bone. *J. Bone Miner. Res.* **12,** 509–521 (1997).
15. Patel, D. N., Pettifor, J. M., Becker, P. J., Grieve, C., Leschner, K. The effect of ethnic group on appendicular bone mass in children. *J. Bone Miner. Res.* **7,** 263–272 (1992).
16. Han, Z. H., Palnitkar, S., Sudhaker Rao, D., Nelson, D., and Parfitt, A. M. Effect of ethnicity and age or menopause on the structure and geometry of iliac bone. *J. Bone Miner. Res.* **11,** 1967–1975 (1996).
17. Han, Z. H., Palnitkar, S., Sudhaker Rao, D., Nelson, D., and Parfitt, A. M. Effects of ethnicity and age or menopause on the remodeling and turnover of iliac bone: implications for mechanisms of bone loss. *J. Bone Miner. Res.* **12,** 498–508 (1997).
18. Garn, S. N., and Clark, D. C. Nutrition, growth, development, and maturation: findings from the ten state nutrition survey of 1968-1979. *Pediatrics* **56,** 306–319 (1975).
19. Weinstein, R. S., and Bell, N. H. Diminished rates of bone formation in normal black adults. *N. Engl. J. Med.* **319,** 1698–1701 (1988).
20. Ensrud, K. E., Black, D. M., Palermo, L., Bauer, D. C., Barrett-Connor, E., Quandt, S. A., Thompson, D. E., and Karpf, D. B. Treatment with alendronate prevents fractures in women at highest risk: results from the Fracture Intervention Trial. *Arch. Intern. Med.* **157**(22), 2617–2624 (1997).
21. Long, J. "The Rise of the Fishes." John Hopkins Press, Baltimore, MD, 1995.

22. Riesenfeld, A. Age changes of bone size and mass in two strains of senescent rats. *Acta Anat.* **109,** 63–69 (1981).
23. Baron, R., Tross, R., and Vignery, A. Evidence of sequential remodeling in rat trabecular bone: morphology, dynamic histomorphometry, and changes during skeletal maturation. *Anat. Rec.* **208,** 137–145 (1984).
24. "Guidelines for Preclinical and Clinical Evaluation of Agents Used in the Prevention or Treatment of Postmenopausal Osteoporosis." Food and Drug Administration, April 1994.
25. Inzucchi, S. E. Growth hormone in adults: indications and implications. *Hosp. Pract.* Jan **15,** 79–96 (1997).
26. Daughaday, W. H., Herington, A. C., and Phillips, L. S. The regulation of growth by endocrines. *Annu. Rev. Physiol.* **37,** 211 (1975).
27. Rosenbloom, A. L., Aguirre, J. H., Rosenfeld, R. G., and Fielder, P. J. The little women of Loja—GH-receptor deficiency in an inbred population of southern Ecuador. *N. Engl. J. Med.* **323,** 1367-1374 (1990).
28. Laron, Z., Pertzelan, A., and Mannheimer, S. Genetic pituitary dwarfism with high serum concentration of growth hormone—a new inborn error of metabolism? *Isr. J. Med. Sci.* **2,** 152–155 (1966).
29. Hock, J. M., Centrella M., and Canalis, E. IGF has independent effects on bone matrix formation and cell replication. *Endocrinology,* **122,** 254–260 (1998).
30. McCarthy, T. L., Centrella, M., and Canalis, E. Regulatory effects of IGF 1 and 2 on bone collagen synthesis in rat calvarial cultures. *Endocrinology* **124,** 301–309 (1989).
31. Liang, C. T., Barnes, J., Seedor, H., Quartuccio, H. A., Bolander, M., Jeffery, J. J., and Rodan, G. A. Impaired bone activity in aged rats: alterations at the cellular and molecular levels. *Bone* **13,** 435–441 (1992).
32. Rudman, D., Feller, A. G., Nagraj, H. S., Gergans, G. A., Lalitha, P. Y., Goldberg, A. F., Schlenker, R. A., Cohn, L., Rudman, I. W., and Mattson, D. E. Effects of human growth hormone in men over 60 years old. *N. Eng. J. Med.* **323,** 1–6, (1990).
33. Wakisaka, A., Tanaka, H., Barnes, J., and Liang, C. T. Effect of locally infused IGF-I on femoral gene expression and bone turnover activity in old rats. *J. Bone Miner. Res.* **13**(1), 13–19 (1998).
34. Oxlund, H., Andersen, N. B., Ortoft, G., Orsov, H., and Andreassen, T. T. Growth hormone and mild exercise in combination markedly enhance cortical bone formation and strength in old rats. *Endocrinology* **139,**(4), 1899–1904 (1998).
35. Miller, S. C., Hunziker, J., Mecham, M., and Wronski, T. J. Intermittent PTH administration stimulates bone formation in the mandibles of aged ovariectomized rats. *J. Dent. Res.* **76**(8), 1471–1476 (1997).
36. Sato, M., Zeng, G. Q., and Turner, C. H. Biosynthetic human PTH effects on bone quality in aged ovariectomized rats. *Endocrinology* **138**(10), 4330–4337 (1997).
37. Nakamura, K., Kurokawa, T., Aoyama, I., Hanada, Tamura, M., and Kawaguchi, H. Stimulation of bone formation by intraosseous injection of basic fibroblast growth factor in ovariectomized rats. *Int. Orthop.* **22**(1), 49–54 (1998).
38. Vanderscheuren, D. Androgens and their role in skeletal homeostasis. *Horm. Res.* **46**(2), 95–98 (1996).
39. Lea, C. K., and Flanagan, A. M. Physiological plasma levels of androgens reduce bone loss in the ovariectomized rat. *Am. J. Physiol.* **274**(2 pt 1), E328–E335 (1998).
40. Mason, D., Suva, L., Genever, P., Patton, A., Seuckle, S., Hillam, R., and Skerry, T. Mechanically regulated expression of a neural glutamate transporter in bone: a role for excitatory amino acids as osteotropic agents. *Bone* **20,** 199–205 (1997).
41. Miles, R., Turner, C., Santerre, R., Tu, Y., McClelland, P., Argot, J., DeHoff, B., Mundy, C., Rosteck, P., Bidwell, J., Sluka, J., Hock, J., and Onyia, J. Analysis of differential gene expression in rattibia after an osteogenic stimulus *in vivo:* Mechanical loading regulates osteopontin and myeloperoxidase. *J. Cell Biochem.* **68,** 355–365 (1998).
42. Sutherland, M. S., Rao, L. G., Muzaffar, S. A., Wylie, J. N., Wong, M. M., McBroom, R. J., Murray, T. M. Age-dependent expression of osteoblastic phenotypic markers in normal human osteoblasts cultured long-term in the presence of dexamethasone. *Osteop. Int.* **5**(5), 335–343 (1995).
43. Nyssen-Behets, C., Delaere, O., Duchesne, P. Y., and Dhem, A. Aging effect on inductive capacity of human demineralized bone matrix. *Arch. Orthop. Trauma Surg.* **115**(6), 303–306 (1996).
44. Rubin, J., and Rubin, C. Osteoblasts, osteocytes, and osteoclasts. *In* "Current Opinion in Orthopaedics" (W. R. J. Rennie and J. H. Herndon, eds.), Vol. 8, pp. 34–42.
45. Aarden, E. M., Wassenaar, A. M., Alblas, M. J., and Nijweide, P. J. Immunocytochemical demonstration of extracellular matrix proteins in isolated osteocytes. *Histochem. Cell Biol.* **106**(5), 495–501 (1996).
46. Hayflick, L. Aging, longevity and immortality. *Exp. Gerontol.* **27,** 363–368 (1992).
47. Rubin, H. Cell aging *in vivo* and *in vitro. Mech. Ageing Dev.* **98,** 1–35 (1997).
48. Becerra, J., Andrades, J. A., Ertl, D. C., Sorgente, N., and Nimni, M. E. Demineralized bone matrix mediates differentiation of bone marrow stromal cells *in vitro:* effect of age of cell donor. *J. Bone Miner. Res.* **11**(11), 1703–1714 (1996).
49. Tanaka, H., and Liang, C. T. Mitogenic activity but not phenotype expression of rat osteoprogenitor cells in response to IGF-I is impaired in aged rats. *Mech. Ageing Dev.* **92**(1), 1–10 (1996).
50. Inoue, K., Ohgushi, H., Yoshikawa, T., Okumura, M., Sempuku, T., Tamai, S., and Dohi, Y. The effect of aging on bone formation in porous hydroxyapatite: biochemical and histological analysis. *J. Bone Miner. Res.* **12**(6), 989–994 (1997).
51. Morrison, S. J., Uchida, N., and Weissman, I. L. The biology of hematopoietic stem cells. *Annu. Rev. Cell Dev. Biol.* **11,** 35–71 (1995).
52. Kostenuik, P. J., Halloran, B. P., Morey-Holton, E. R., and Bikle, D. D. Skeletal unloading inhibits the *in vitro* proliferation and differentiation of ratosteoprogenitor cells. *Am. J. Physiol.* **273**(6 Pt 1), E1133–E1139 (1997).
53. Weinreb, M., Suponitzky, I., and Keila, S. Systemic administration of an anabolic dose of PGE2 in young rats increases the osteogenic capacity of bone marrow. *Bone* **20**(6), 521–526 (1997).
54. Kabasawa, M., Ejiri, S., Hanada, K, and Ozawa, H. Effect of age on physiologic and mechanically stressed rat alveolar bone: a cytologic and histochemical study. *Int. J. Adult Orthodon. Orthognath. Surg.* **11**(4), 313–327 (1996).
55. Hayflick, L., and Moorhead, P. The serial cultivation of human diploid cell strains. *Exp. Cell Res.* **25,** 585–621 (1961).
56. Hayflick, L. The limited *in vitro* lifetime of human diploid cell strains. *Exp. Cell Res.* **37,** 614–636 (1965).
57. Rubin, H. Telomerase and cellular lifespan: End of the debate? *Nature Biotechnol.* **16,** 396–397 (1998).
58. Rubin, H., Yao, A., and Chow, M. Heritable, population-wide damage to cells as the driving force of neoplastic transformation. *Proc. Natl. Acad. Sci. U.S.A.* **92,** 4843–4847 (1995).
59. Chow, M., and Rubin, H. Ubiquitous, heritable damage in cell populations that survive treatment with methotrexate. *Proc. Natl. Acad. Sci. U.S.A.* **94,** 8773–8778 (1997).

60. Hozier, J., Sawyer, J., Clive, D., and Moore, M. Chromosome 11 aberrations in small colony L5178Y TK-/-mutants early in their clonal history. *Mutat. Res.* **147,** 237–242 (1985).
61. Applegate, M. L., Moore, M. M., Broder, C. B., Burrell, A., Juhn, G., Kasweck, K. L., Lin, P. F., Wadhams, A., and Hozier, J. L. Molecular dissection of mutations at the heterozygous thymidine kinase locus in mouse lymphoma cells. *Proc. Natl. Acad. Sci. U.S.A.* **87,** 51–55 (1990).
62. Xia, F., Amundson, S. A., Nickoloff, J. A., and Liber, H. L. Different capacities for recombination in closely related human lymphoblastoid cell lines with different mutational responses to x irradiation. *Mol. Cell. Biol.* **14,** 5850–5857 (1994).
63. Evans, H. H. The prevalence of multilocus lesions in radiation-induced mutants. *Radiat. Res.* **137,** 131–144 (1994).
64. Vijg, J., Martijn, E. T., Martus, H. J., and Boerrigter, M. Transgenic mouse models for studying mutations *in vivo:* applications in aging research. *Mech. Ageing Dev.* **99,** 257–271 (1997).
65. Wareham, K. A., Lyon, M. F., Glenister, P. H., and Williams, E. D. Age related reactivation of an X-linked gene. *Nature* **327,** 725–727 (1987).
66. Rubin, H., and Xu, K. Evidence for the progressive and adaptive nature of spontaneous transformation in the NIH 3T3 cell line. *Proc. Natl. Acad. Sci. U.S.A.* **86,** 1860–1864 (1989).
67. Yao, A., Rubin, A. L., and Rubin, H. Progressive state selection of cells in low serum promotes high density growth and neoplastic transformation in NIH 3T3 cells. *Cancer Res.* **50,** 5171–5176 (1990).
68. Chow, M., and Rubin, H. Irreversibility of cellular aging and neoplastic transformation: A clonal analysis. *Proc. Natl. Acad. Sci. U.S.A.* **93,** 9793–9798 (1996).
69. Rodriguez, E., Sreekanitaiah, C., and Chaganti, R. S. K. Genetic changes in epithelial solid neoplasia. *Cancer Res.* **54,** 3398–3406 (1994).
70. Huang, R., McLeod, K., and Rubin, C. Changes in the dynamics of muscle contraction as a function of age; A contributing factor to the etiology of osteoporosis? *J. Gerontol.,* in press.

CHAPTER 5

Animal Models of the Aging Skeleton

DIKE N. KALU Department of Physiology, University of Texas Health Science Center at San Antonio, San Antonio, Texas 78284

CHARACTERISTICS OF HUMAN SKELETAL AGING

Animals models of the aging skeleton should closely resemble those of human skeletal aging. Therefore, in order to determine what an animal model of human skeletal aging should accomplish, it is first necessary to briefly describe the characteristics of the human model.

Changes in Bone Mass with Aging

The skeleton of humans undergoes predictable age related changes in bone mass [1] (Fig. 1A). The first two decades of life are characterized by rapid bone growth, followed by the attainment of peak bone mass between 20 and 30 years of age. Bone mass remains at this peak level for a relatively brief period and is then followed by a gradual but progressive loss of bone. This age-related bone loss occurs in all individuals in both males and females. However, there is sexual dimorphism in the process. Females achieve a lower peak bone mass than males, and a period of rapid bone loss that lasts for about 10 years following menopause is superimposed on the age-related bone loss that occurs in all individuals. Age-related bone loss results from an imbalance in the remodeling of bone.

Bone Remodeling

Bone is continuously remodeled throughout life. Bone remodeling is the breakdown and reformation of bone involving an initiating resorption phase and subsequent formation phase, with a reversal phase occurring between resorption and formation [2,3] (Fig. 1B). Remodeling is initiated by the appearance of osteoclasts in bone at the sites to be remodeled, such as the cortical endosteal and trabecular endosteal surfaces. The osteoclasts resorb a quantum of bone and then disappear. After a brief period, the cavity formed by osteoclasts is lined by osteoblasts, which then refill the cavity with new bone. Newly formed resorption cavities and those in the process of being refilled with bone are termed bone multicellular units (BMUs). When the refilling process is completed, the resultant new bone is called a bone structural unit (BSU), Haversian system, or osteon. Bone remodeling prevents or removes areas of fatigue and microdamage within bone and thereby maintains the mechanical competence of bone by renewing its components. Bone remodeling determines the amount of bone present at any time. In young adults, the coupling of bone formation to resorption is balanced; there is no net loss of bone, and bone mass is stable. With aging there is a remodeling imbalance and less bone is formed than is resorbed. An ideal animal model of skeletal aging should demonstrate predictable changes in bone mass with aging and a remodeling imbalance that results in age-related bone loss.

Osteoporosis

Osteoporosis is a disease characterized by low bone mass, microarchitechtural deterioration of bone, enhanced bone fragility, and increased fracture risk. The disease is classified as primary or secondary. Secondary osteoporosis is usually associated with a recognizable disease or medical therapy and accounts for about 10% of osteoporotic conditions. It will not be considered here. Our main focus is primary osteoporosis, which is associated mainly with aging. Two forms have been

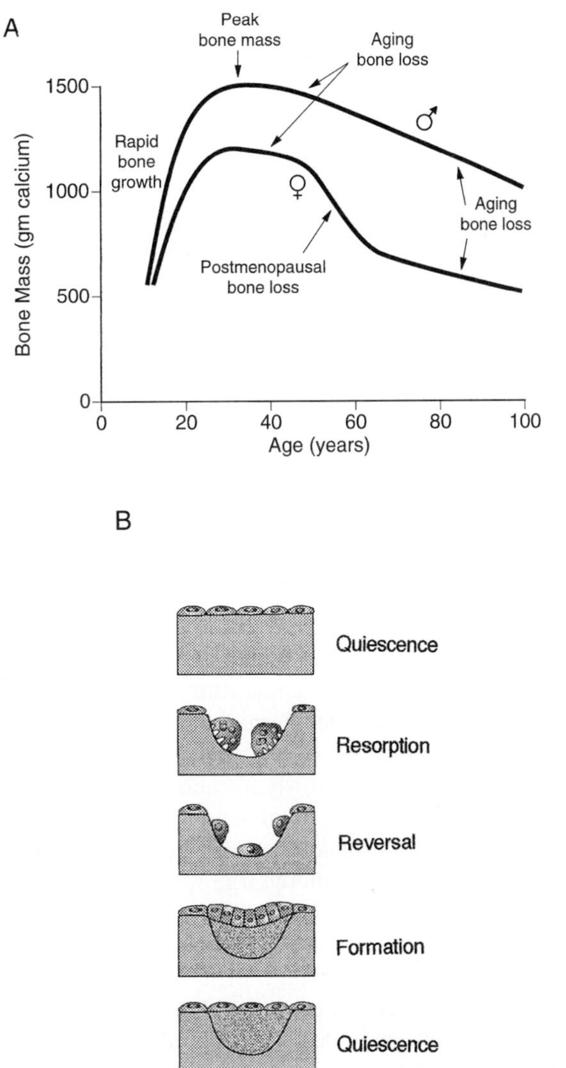

FIGURE 1 (A) Changes in bone mass with aging in men and women. Modified from Kassem *et al.* [1]. (B) Remodeling sequence in normal adult bone. Modified with permission from Parfitt [3].

described: type 1 and type 2 osteoporosis [1]. Accelerated bone loss following menopause and low peak bone mass are important risk factors for postmenopausal or type 1 osteoporosis. The latter is characterized by an accelerated loss of cancellous (trabecular) bone, which ranges from thinning to complete removal of trabecular plates by osteoclasts, thereby disrupting the trabecular lattice network and connectivity. Loss of cortical (compact) bone also occurs but is less marked and is characterized by accelerated endocortical resorption, increased intracortical porosity, expanded marrow space, and thin cortices. The primary defect in type 1 osteoporosis is excessive bone resorption, whereas in type 2 or senile osteoporosis, the imbalance in bone remodeling is attributed mainly to decreased bone formation with aging [1]. Although fractures are the hallmark of osteoporosis in humans, in terms of developing an animal model, it is of much greater significance that the pathophysiological alterations that lead to bone loss are the same in humans as in the animal model, even if bone loss in the animal model does not result in fractures [4].

THE ANIMAL MODEL PARADOX

An animal model of human aging skeleton can be defined as a living animal in which spontaneous or induced bone loss can be studied and in which the characteristics of the bone loss and its sequalae resemble those found in humans in one or more respects [4]. One of the difficulties in establishing an animal model is that the characteristics and pathogenesis of the disease for which an animal model is being proposed are often not completely known at the time the model is sought. If a disease or condition is not fully understood, how can one design a good animal model of the disease? This is the *animal model paradox.* However, according to our definition, the characteristics of an animal model of the aging skeleton need not be an exact replica of the human condition in order for the model to be useful for studying aspects of aging bone loss. An animal model should be based on the available information and should be modified and updated as new information on the disease or the model evolves. Even then an exact replica of the disease may never be found.

CHARACTERISTICS OF A GOOD ANIMAL MODEL

Good animal models share at least four characteristics: convenience, relevance, predictability, and appropriateness [4–6]. Convenience refers to ease, and for a long time it was the main criterion for choosing an animal model. However, convenience should not be the predominating factor in the choice of a model, as individuals, with adequate training and experience, can become adept with a model that at first seemed formidable. Relevance refers to the comparability of a phenomenon being studied in an animal to that seen in the human. Predictability refers to the capability of the model to foretell the anticipated outcome. Appropriateness refers to the complex of other factors such as availability, cost, facilities required, and environmental considerations that make a given species best for studying a particular phenomenon. Good animal models of skeletal aging will meet these criteria.

WHY ANIMAL MODELS OF THE AGING SKELETON ARE REQUIRED

Osteoporosis is a common disease of the aging skeleton and all individuals are potential candidates for osteoporosis if they live long enough, as bone loss with aging is a universal occurrence. The underlying reasons for age-related bone loss are only partially understood and strategies for managing osteoporosis are still evolving. A good animal model should be capable of bridging information deficits and providing new insights about the disease it models. The development and application of appropriate animal models of human bone loss are legitimate components of the quest to understood, manage, and possibly even prevent the occurrence of osteoporosis in the future.

CANDIDATE ANIMAL MODELS OF AGING BONE LOSS

Several animal species are candidate models for human aging bone loss. These include rats, mice, dogs, minipigs, sheep, ferrets, and nonhuman primates. The rat model has been studied more extensively than all the other candidate models combined by a large margin. For this reason the rat model will be discussed first and in some depth as the prototypic model of human skeletal aging. Some of the issues to be discussed relate not only to the rat model but also to other species that will be considered subsequently. Additional information on the rat model can be found in several reviews [4,7–11].

Rats

The ovariectomized rat model is the most widely used animal model of aging bone loss because it fulfills the four desired characteristics: convenience, relevance, predictability, and appropriateness. Rats are familiar and common laboratory animals; Studies with rats can be carried out easily under the standardized conditions of the laboratory; They are relatively inexpensive, and bone changes can be induced in a short time. Even though the rat is the most commonly studied model of bone loss, resistance and negative mind-set about the unsuitability of the rat skeleton for studying issues concerning human osteoporoses are a historical truth [8]. Some appreciation of the nature of this resistance is important as the issues involved apply also in varying degrees to other potential animal models of human bone loss. These issues will be discussed only briefly.

OSTEOPOROSIS IS A COMMON DISEASE

A notable impediment to the development of the rat model has nothing to do with the appropriateness of the rat as a model of skeletal aging. Rather it has to do with the fact that osteoporosis is not rare [12]. About 20 million people are afflicted with the disease in the United States alone, and the millions of people that reach menopausal age annually provide a ready pool of subjects for studying osteoporosis. Since the best study of man is man, there was no real pressure to seek an animal model for the disease with so many human equivalents. However, it is clear that as a result of ethical and other constraints, sole reliance on human subjects for studying osteoporosis limits the ability to test new hypotheses and to evaluate new potential therapies for the disease.

EXPLOSION IN BONE RESEARCH BYPASSED ANIMAL MODELS

The seventies and eighties witnessed a tremendous explosion in basic research on bone that was dominated by *in vitro* bone studies in tissue culture. These studies have greatly advanced and enriched our basic understanding of bone and of the role of local factors in the regulation of bone metabolism [13]. In the process, *in vivo* bone research and animal models were bypassed. It was believed that such *in vivo* animal studies are incapable of yielding information that is relevant to human bone loss [8]. We now know that this view is a misconception. Misconceptions about the rat as a model for human bone loss retarded research in this area by at least two decades.

RATS AND CONTINUED GROWTH THROUGHOUT LIFE

An often heard criticism of the rat model of skeletal aging is that the rat is continuously growing and is, therefore, unsuitable as a model of human bone loss that starts after the attainment of skeletal maturity. There is no doubt that laboratory rats fed *ad libitum* continue to increase their body weight for a substantial part of their life span (Fig. 2). Because most earlier studies on rats were carried out on young growing animals, this led to the notion that the rat skeleton is also growing continuously and rapidly throughout life. This is not the case (Fig. 2) [14,15]. In 1982, Yu *et al.* [16] reported that the increase in body weight after adulthood in F344 rats is due more to increased adiposity than to an increase in lean body mass just as in humans and that at advanced age rats lose both lean body mass and adiposity. Twenty-five years earlier, Berg and Harmison [17] reported that in both male and female Sprague–Dawley rats, linear growth of the tibia was rapid until about 170 days and then declined, and in old animals there was no longer evidence of osteogenesis in the epiphyseal growth plate,

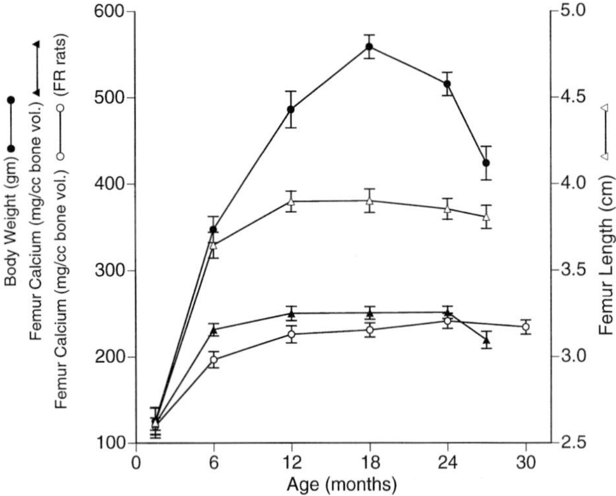

FIGURE 2 Changes in body weight, bone length, and bone calcium content with age in F344 male rats fed *ad libitum.* Note that rats do not continue to grow indefinitely and that the body weight continued to increase when bone calcium had stabilized. Animals that were food restricted (FR) to 60% of the *ad libitum* food intake had lower bone calcium and did not experience terminal bone loss. Modified from Kalu *et al.* [14]; © The Endocrine Society.

indicating that linear bone growth had stopped. In every instance where rats have been studied carefully over a prolonged period, linear bone growth has been reported to slow down considerably and even stop at advanced age [14,15,17,18]. The onset of the slowing down, the time of stoppage of linear growth as a result of the closure of the epiphyses, and the peak bone mass attained vary with the strain of rats and is modulated by gender and environmental factors such as diet (Fig. 2).

RATS AND BONE LOSS WITH AGING

Another common criticism of the rat model is that rats do not normally experience a progressive age-related decline in bone mass that is analogous to the bone loss that occurs with aging following the attainment of peak bone mass in humans (Figs. 1 and 2). However, at advanced age, rats fed *ad libitum* experience terminal bone loss (Fig. 2) [14,19] that is more likely related to disease that is common in aging rats. The apparent stability of the rat skeleton can be used to advantage in the development of specific models of bone loss [15]. For instance, during the period of skeletal stability in rats, any bone loss that results from a manipulation such as low dietary calcium, hormone therapy, hormone deficiency, or mechanical challenge can be attributed solely to that manipulation uncomplicated by normal aging bone loss of uncertain etiology as occurs in humans. Nonetheless, it is not absolutely true that apart from terminal bone loss, rats do not lose bone with aging if one considers the cancellous and cortical components of the skeleton separately. Loss of cancellous bone in the appendicular skeleton occurs with aging in rats [20], but cortical bone is more resistant to loss with aging. Because the cancellous component of long bones is small, demonstration of the age-related loss of cancellous bone in rats requires the application of sensitive bone measurement techniques such as bone histomorphometry [20]. The age-related loss of cancellous bone, which occurs in rats as in humans, appears to be independent of ovarian hormone status and has, so far, received little attention.

BONE REMODELING IN THE RAT

Perhaps the most serious indictment of the rat as an inappropriate model of human bone loss is the misconception that the mature rat skeleton does not remodel as human skeletons do. Because age-related bone loss in humans is due to a remodeling imbalance in which less bone is formed than is resorbed, it has been argued that an animal whose skeleton does not remodel cannot be an appropriate model of human bone loss. Contrary to common perception, even old literature indicates that the rat skeleton undergoes remodeling in a similar manner as human skeleton, involving the activation, resorption, and formation phases of a typical BMU [21]. More recently, bone remodeling was demonstrated elegantly in a study of tibial and vertebral cancellous and endocortical bones in rats of different ages using a combination of *in vivo* fluorochrome labeling with cement line staining. Remodeling was observed to increase with age and by 12 months remodeling accounted for over 90% of turnover activity in vertebral cancellous bone and 66% of turnover activity in proximal tibial metaphysis with similar trends of increased remodeling activity with age in tibial and vertebral endocortical sites [22]. Rat bones do remodel.

LATENT REMODELING CAPACITY OF RAT CORTICAL BONE

The paucity of Haversian systems in cortical bone in rats contributed to the notion that rats have a nonremodeling skeleton. However, whereas most young adult rats (<8 months) lack cortical Haversian systems, intracortical remodeling can be found in older rats [23,24]. Even in young adult rats, an appropriate stimulus such as PGE-2 therapy [24] and low dietary calcium [23] can activate intracortical remodeling, creating a porous cortex with concentric lamellae that have the characteristics of Haversian systems present in the adult human skeleton. Thus, cortical bone in the rat has latent remodeling capacity [4]. Therefore, it is likely that the same basic mechanisms of bone remodeling exist in rats and humans and that the same remodeling defects that cause age-related bone loss in humans underlie bone loss in rat models of skeletal aging. However, in view of the dearth of intracortical remodeling in the rat, rats are not ideal for investigating issues where BMUs are the primary focus. For such studies, animal models whose bones normally have numerous Haversian systems are more appropriate, as discussed later.

The Ovariectomized Rat Model of Postmenopausal Bone Loss

The most common expression of skeletal aging is the bone loss that occurs in women following menopause. Having placed in context some of the common questions and misconceptions about the rat skeleton, we will now examine the rat model of postmenopausal bone loss. Rats have a 4-day estrous cycle in which an increase in estrogen levels occurs once every 4 days. Rats do not have a natural menopause analogous to that of women, but they can be ovariectomized to make them estrogen deficient, thus simulating menopause. Saville [25] is usually credited with pioneering the development of the ovariectomized rat model of human postmenopausal bone loss. He castrated female rats at 21 days of age and observed that, with time, the ovariectomized rats had less bone calcium per unit volume of bone than control animals. This basic finding has been confirmed repeatedly by numerous investigators in young and old rats using a variety of techniques to measure bone mass and its indices [4,7]. It should, however, be noted that Saville's study did not strictly demonstrate bone loss as lower bone mass in his rapidly growing young ovariectomized animals could have been due mainly to decreased bone accretion relative to controls. Such relative osteopenia in young growing ovariectomized animals does not accurately model postmenopausal bone loss that occurs after the attainment of skeletal maturity. It is in the use of rats that are still growing that the ovariectomized rat model is most often misused if appropriate controls are not included. It is only when the final bone mass of ovariectomized rats is also lower than that of the baseline control that true bone loss has occurred [4]. These problems are avoided if aged animals with stable bone mass are used to model postmenopausal bone loss.

The Aged Rat Model

The use of aged rats to model postmenopausal bone loss ensures that bone loss following ovariectomy is not complicated by the continued bone growth that occurs in young growing animals. To establish an aged ovariectomized rat model, it is first necessary to characterize the bone growth pattern of female rats to establish the time of skeletal maturity and to determine the appropriate age at which to ovariectomize rats. In such a study using female Wistar rats, it was observed that as in male F344 rats (Fig. 2), bone growth was highest from 1 to 3 months of age, slowed between 3 and 6 months, and by 12 months all bone parameters measured had reached plateau levels, with no further significant change up to 24 months of age [15]. From these considerations, 12 months was chosen as the age at which to base the aged rat model. However, the age when rat bone parameters achieve stable levels is influenced by diet, strain of rat, and environmental conditions and has to be established for each strain of rat. What is significant about the aged rat model is that the rats are at an age when bone mass has stabilized, and the epiphyses have practically fused with little or no continued linear bone growth. Therefore, the aged rat model is dubbed "aged" not because the rats are senescent, but rather because their skeletal characteristics have stabilized at a level close to that of aged rats. The aged rat model ensures that skeletal changes observed following ovariectomy are due primarily to ovarian hormone deficiency, uncomplicated by continued rapid bone growth as occurs in younger animals or by senile bone loss and disease that can occur later in the life of the rat [15]. In the aged rat model, the animals are usually sacrificed several months after ovariectomy to permit significant loss of bone, especially if cortical bone loss is also required.

In some studies, rats have been ovariectomized at 24 months of age to examine the skeletal effects of ovarian deficiency. A beginning age of 24 months for ovariectomy studies is too old; it is analogous to studying the early effects ovarian hormone deficiency on bone in an 80-year-old woman. Also, aged rats are prone to tumors and diseases such as chronic nephropathy that can alter bone metabolism and confound the effects of experimental manipulations on bone. Some have argued that not enough cancellous bone remains in aged rats to make the aged rat model useful for skeletal studies. This problem can occur in retired breeders in which cancellous bone is depleted as a result of repeated breeding [26]. Aged virgin female rats still have substantial amounts of cancellous bone in their proximal tibia, distal femur, and vertebral bodies and should be used instead of retired breeders.

The Mature Rat Model

Although the aged rat model has many of the characteristics to look for in an animal model of postmenopausal bone loss and is the preferred model, aged rats are expensive, their availability is limited, and a long period elapses before the effects of ovariectomy on their bones are manifest [4]. In constrast, younger rats (approximately 3 months old) are more readily available, they are not very expensive, the effects of ovariectomy on their skeleton are manifest in a few weeks, and the characteristics of the bone loss are similar to those of the aged rat model [4,7,15,20]. These attributes account for the widespread use of younger rats for studying bone loss due to ovarian hormone deficiency. The author has designated models based on rats aged about 3 months as the "mature rat model" to differentiate them from the "aged rat model" of postmenopausal bone loss [4]. The term "mature" is used loosely to emphasize that these rats are reproductively mature and capable of responding appropriately to sex hormone deficiency and its sequalae following ovariectomy. In a typical experiment with the mature rat model, 90-day-old Sprague–Dawley rats are ovariectomized or sham operated and are sacrificed 1 or more months later depending on the nature of the study. A typical finding is that the ovariectomized animals quickly lose cancellous bone at the proximal tibial and distal femoral metaphyses. This is associated with an increase in osteoclast and osteoblast numbers, which is consistent with bone resorption exceeding bone formation as in the aged rat model [4,7,15,20]. It is now generally considered that the characteristics of the bone loss due to ovariectomy in the mature and aged rat models share sufficient similarities with those of early postmenopausal bone loss to make them appropriate for studying problems related to this condition [4,7,15,20].

Rat Model Based on Treatment with LHRH Agonist

A family of luteinizing hormone-releasing hormone (LHRH) agonists are used clinically to suppress endogenous gonadotropin secretion. This results in inhibition of ovulation and follicular activity. Patients treated with LHRH agonists have low estrogen levels and are at risk of accelerated loss of bone as in postmenopausal women [27]. As a result of the hypogonadism associated with LHRH agonist therapy, treatment of rats with LHRH agonists has been explored as an alternative way to induce estrogen deficiency osteopenia without surgical intervention to remove the ovaries. Such studies have been found to be just as effective as surgical ovariectomy in lowering blood estrogen levels and inducing osteopenia in rats [28]. Because the withdrawal of LHRH agonist therapy restores normal hypothalamic–pituitary function and reverses the bone loss, this model can give insights on ovarian hormone deficiency osteopenia that cannot be obtained from irreversible surgical castration. The model is of interest and merits more attention.

Applications of the Ovariectomized Rat Model

The ovariectomized rat model has been used mainly for two types of studies: (1) to explore the pathogenesis of post menopausal bone loss and (2) for the preclinical testing of potential therapies for osteoporosis.

Pathogenesis of Postmenopausal Bone Loss

Until recently, studies on the interaction of sex hormone deficiency with calcium-regulating hormones and the regulation of calcium homeostasis dominated the search for the humoral etiology of postmenopausal bone loss, but the nature of the roles of calcium-regulating hormones, if any, remains uncertain [29,30]. The inconclusive findings may relate, in part, to the heterogeneity of human populations and to the difficulty in standardizing human studies. For this reason the ovariectomized rat model, in the rigorously controlled environment of the laboratory, is ideal for seeking the role of calcium-regulating hormones in the etiology of estrogen deficiency bone loss. Changes in the levels of these hormones following ovariectomy have been investigated in studies using the aged rat model [15,31]. It was observed that although bone loss, with the characteristics of postmenopausal bone loss, occurred in ovariectomized rats, changes in the levels of calcium-regulating hormones could not account for the bone loss [15,31]. Subsequently, the ovariectomized rat model has been used to examine newer hypotheses of postmenopausal bone loss. According to one hypothesis, ovarian hormone deficiency following menopause enhances the expansion of a pool of marrow-derived progenitor cells that differentiate to osteoclasts that enhance bone resorption and increase bone loss [32,33]. The hypothesis was first tested in ovariectomized mice where the technique for examining marrow-derived osteoclast progenitors had been well worked out. It was observed that in comparison to sham-operated control mice, ovariectomy caused a fourfold increase in osteoclast-like cells in *ex vivo* cultures of bone marrow cells [32]. In a subsequent study in ovariectomized rats, a similar increase in marrow-derived osteoclast-like cells was accompanied by increased trabecular osteoclasts and decreased cancellous bone. The changes were reversed by estrogen therapy, giving credence to the new hypothesis [33] (Fig. 3). These studies illustrate how *in vivo* studies on ovariectomized rodent models can be combined with *in vitro* studies to explore new hypotheses about aging bone loss that are not easy to investigate directly in humans due, in this case, to the difficulty in obtaining human bone marrow routinely from ovariectomized women.

Preclinical Testing of Drugs for Osteoporosis Therapy

It is in the area of preclinical testing of potential drugs for osteoporosis therapy that the ovariectomized rat bone loss model has received the most attention. There are two main approaches to osteoporosis therapy by pharmacological intervention: preventive therapy to

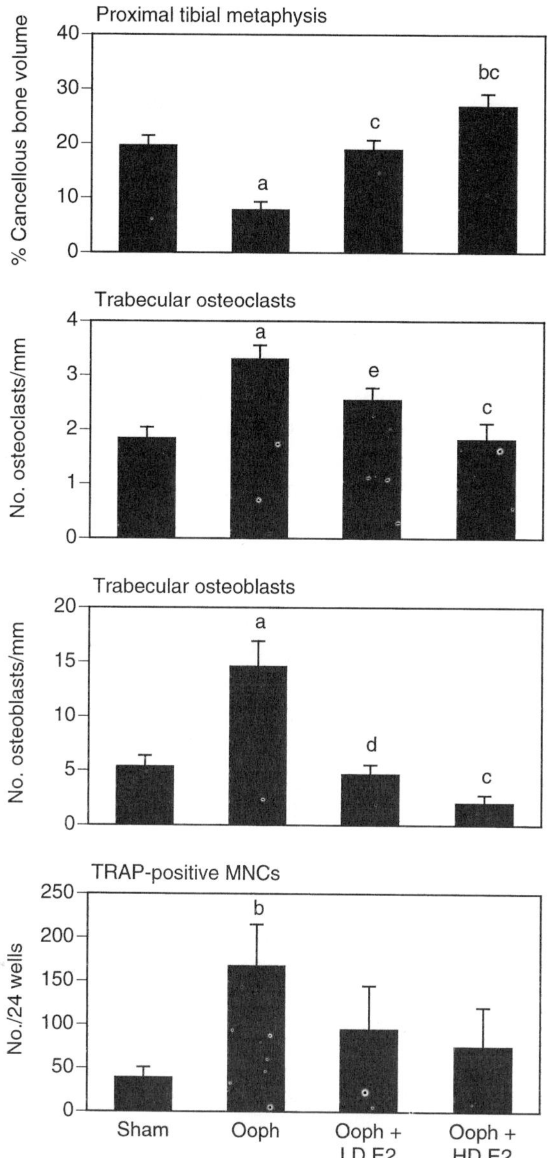

FIGURE 3 Effects of ovariectomy (oophorectomy, Ooph) and 17β-estradiol (E_2) on cancellous bone volume, trabecular osteoclast, and osteoblasts at the proximal tibial metaphysis and on *ex vivo* formation of TRAP-positive multinucleated cells (MNCs) from mononuclear marrow cells in culture. LD, low dose (20 ng E_2/100 g body wt/day); HD, high dose (500 ng E_2/100 g body wt/day). Rats were sacrificed after 35 days. Data are means ± SE. $^a p < 0.001$, vs sham; $^b p < 0.05$, vs sham; $^c p < 0.001$, vs Ooph; $^d p < 0.01$, vs Ooph; $^e p < 0.05$, vs Ooph. Modified from Kalu *et al.* [33], with permission from Elsevier Science.

arrest the progression of the bone loss and restorative therapy to rebuild bone in established osteoporosis (Fig. 4). The former has been investigated extensively using the ovariectomized rat model.

Preventive Therapy to Arrest the Progression of Bone Loss In the ovariectomized rat model, ovarian hormone deficiency results in marked cancellous osteopenia that is evident as early as 2 weeks following ovariectomy [20,34]. The model is therefore ideal for studying potential antiresorptive drugs for preventing the initiation or progression of cancellous bone loss. Such antiresorptive drugs act by decreasing bone remodeling and include estrogens, estrogen agonist–antagonists, bisphosphonates, and calcitonin. These drugs exert similar effects on bone loss in humans as in the mature and aged ovariectomzied rat bone loss models [4,7]. The proximal tibia and distal femur are favorite sites for bone loss studies in the rat model, in part, because they contain substantial cancellous bone, and they lose this bone at a fast rate, thereby permitting a study to be completed in a short period of time. However, even the vertebral bodies and the neck of the femur of rats lose significant amounts of cancellous bone following ovariectomy and should always be included in evaluation of therapeutic agents because they are important sites of bone loss and fracture in humans. Preventive drug therapy is usually begun immediately following ovariectomy; if started later, additional appropriate controls should be included. It has been emphasized previously, and rightly so, that histomorphometric cancellous bone measurements should be made in the secondary spongiosa [35]. This should not exclude the concomitant exploration of whether the therapy under investigation also affects the primary spongiosa if the mature rat model with still-open epiphyses is used. Anabolic agents for bone which act primarily to stimulate bone formation, have also been evaluated for their efficacy as preventive therapy. Care should be exercised when anabolic agents are studied because such drugs may also increase growth plate activity in the mature rat model or reactivate the growth plate if it is not completely fused in aged rats. Increased growth plate activity can increase cancellous bone volume and confound the interpretation of findings derived from drug therapy.

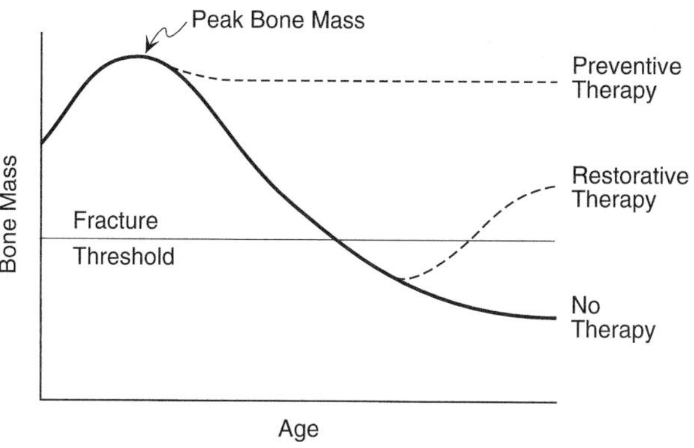

FIGURE 4 Schematic illustration of the two types of therapies that can be investigated using the ovariectomized rat bone loss model.

Restorative Therapy to Rebuild Bone in Established Osteoporosis Studies in which the intent is to rebuild bone after bone loss is established should use the aged rat model to minimize problems related to continued linear bone growth and its stimulation. Before initiating drug therapy in restorative studies, significant bone loss should have occurred and bone mass reestablished at a lower level following ovariectomy. In a typical restorative experiment to examine whether a new drug can rebuild lost bone, at least seven groups of rats should be studied: group 1, baseline control; group 2, sham-operated control; group 3, ovariectomized (ovx); group 4, sham; group 5, ovx; group 6, ovx + low dose drug; and group 7, ovx + high-dose drug. Group 1 should be killed at the beginning of the study; groups 2 and 3 should be killed after about 3 months to establish that bone loss had occurred before initiating therapy in groups 4 to 7. Groups 4 to 7 should receive drug and solvent vehicle therapies as appropriate from the beginning of the fourth month following surgery. The length of drug therapy depends on the anticipated potency of the drug being tested. If it is planned to sacrifice rats at timed intervals following the initiation of drug therapy, additional groups of rats will be required. The attributes of a good restorative protocol include the following: Bone mass or its indices in groups 1, 2, and 4 should not differ significantly, indicating that bone mass had reached stable levels when the study was initiated. If the rats were still growing during the experimental period, as determined by comparison of the bone mass of groups 1, 2, and 4, this should be taken into account in the interpretation of results. Studies that do not include group 1 lack rigor, and studies that lack groups 2 and 3 cannot claim to be studying the restoration of bone mass because it would be uncertain whether bone loss had occurred and by how much before the initiation of drug therapy. An ideal protocol is a longitudinal study in which each animal serves as its own control and several measurements are made at timed intervals in the course of the study. However, only investigators with access to densitometric instruments can do longitudinal studies. In restorative studies, it is not absolutely necessary that bone mass completely stabilizes at a new lower level before drug therapy is initiated as there may not be enough cancellous bone remaining to serve as a template for restoring bone mass. However, for bone restoration to have occurred, bone mass following drug therapy should not only be higher than that of the terminal ovariectomized controls (group 5), it should also be higher than the level at the time therapy was initiated (group 3). Drug therapy experiments to increase cancellous bone volume should also determine the effects of therapy on growth plate activity. If the drug being studied is known to have the potential to alter growth plate activity, the mature rat model (3 month old) is inappropriate and should not be used. If the drug reactivates residual linear growth in the aged rat model, linear growth rate should be determined for each bone and cancellous bone measurement made at age-equivalent areas for all bones [35–37].

Cortical Bone in Restorative Therapy The protocol just outlined is suitable for studying the restoration of cancellous bone that is lost rapidly following ovariectomy. The protocol is also applicable to cortical bone, but a longer time may be required to first establish cortical osteopenia, which occurs at a slower rate following ovariectomy. The rat model can provide only limited information on cortical osteopenia because of its lack of significant intracortical remodeling, which is prevalent in the human skeleton. However, ovariectomized rats can model the increased endocortical remodeling imbalance that thins cortical bone and increases marrow area in the diaphysis of long bones following menopause [38,39]. In a restorative therapy study using the aged rat model [40], it was observed that ovariectomy caused a significant increase in tibial diaphyseal marrow area ($p < 0.0001$) and a significant decrease in the percentage cortical bone area ($p < 0.0001$) by 3 months. Growth hormone therapy started at 4 months following ovariectomy reversed the decrease in cortical bone with no significant effect on marrow area. In addition, GH increased the periosteal mineral apposition rate and the bone formation rate measured by fluorochrome labeling. These findings indicate that GH can rebuild cortical bone following loss due to ovariectomy in aged rats and that it mediates its effect not by replacing bone lost from the endocortical surface, but by stimulating periosteal expansion of cortical bone as a result of an enhanced formation of new bone. Cortical bone measurements are usually made on sections prepared from just above the tibio–fibula junction and ground for static and dynamic histomorphometry [41]. The junctional sampling site is superior to measurements made at the middiaphysis of long bones because if a drug modulates linear bone growth, the middiaphysis of the control and drug-treated animals may not necessarily be equivalent in age.

Bone Measurements

The bone measurements that should be made in studies based on the rat bone loss model depend, in part, on the questions being addressed and the techniques that are available to the investigator. However, the animal model bone research field is now at a stage where bone histomorphometry involving static and dynamic measurements has emerged as the gold standard. The ASBMR histomorphometric nomenclature should be used [42]. Other simple bone measurements such as anthropometric measures of length, weight, volume, and density can yield valuable information but are not sufficient by themselves. Biochemical markers of bone turnover in blood and urine should be measured; some kits are now available commercially for the murine species. Molecular mechanisms involving the expression of mRNAs for bone matrix proteins and growth factors should be explored if the capability exists [43,44]. Other factors affecting bone mass, such as the disposition of dietary calcium, should not be ignored. Because estrogen increases the absorption of calcium [45,46] and estrogen receptors are present in intestinal cells [47,48], the investigation of factors that affect bone such as estrogen agonist/antagonists should also explore their effects on calcium absorption.

Measurement of Mechanical Properties of Bone

In humans the hallmark of osteoporosis is an increase in the fracture rate due to decreased bone strength. Because the induction of osteopenia in rats does not usually result in fractures, in animal model studies of bone loss and its modulation, mechanical properties of bone are determined as a measure of the potential of therapeutic agents to decrease or prevent osteoporotic fractures. Mechanical testing should be carried out on, at least, vertebral bodies, long bones (femur or tibia), and the femoral neck [49]. The vertebral bodies and femoral neck are selected because they are clinically important sites of frequent fractures in humans. Like human vertebral bodies, those of rats contain both cancellous and cortical bone that is covered by periosteal tissue. Femoral neck sites are also composed of both cortical and cancellous bone; in rats they are load bearing just as they are in humans but the loading patterns are different. Although osteoporotic fractures do not usually occur in the diaphysis of long bones in humans, testing the long bones of rats is important for at least three reasons [49]: (1) Rat long bones, like human long bones, are covered by periosteal tissue and can therefore give information on whether a therapy can potentially stimulate subperiosteal bone apposition in human bones. (2) Data obtained from diaphysial bone will give additional information on the quality of bone following the addition of new cortical bone. (3) Because diaphyses are composed of essentially pure cortical bone, their mechanical properties would likely indicate whether "cortical steal" occurred drug therapy, especially with anabolic hormones. "Cortical steal" is the presumed mobilization of calcium from cortical bone for redeposition in cancellous bone.

FDA Guidelines

In 1994 the United States Federal Drug Administration published its guidelines for the evaluation of drugs used for the treatment of osteoporosis [50]. The guidelines stipulated that preclinical studies of bone quality (mass, architecture, and strength) should be performed in two species, one of which must be the ovariectomized rat. The recognition by the FDA of the ovariectomized rat as an appropriate model for investigating issues relevant to human postmenopausal bone loss gave a tremendous boost to studies using the model. However, there are problems with some of the recommendations of the guidelines for the use of the ovariectomized rat model with regard to the duration of ovariectomy, end point measurements, and the characterization of the rat as a nonremodeling species, thereby perpetuating the notion that rat bones do not remodel. Some of these problems have been discussed [51]. Because no single animal species duplicates all the characteristics of human osteoporosis, the guidelines also recommended that the evaluation of drugs for osteoporosis therapy should include a second study on a large animal model with a remodeling skeleton.

OTHER ANIMAL MODELS OF BONE LOSS

Because the rat is used so widely as a model of postmenopausal bone loss one may ask why other models are necessary. There are several reasons for requiring other animal models of aging bone loss. First, it has already been mentioned that rats have low levels of Haversian remodeling, which make them not ideal for answering questions related specifically to Haversian remodeling parameters, such as the mean wall thickness of BMUs [52]. Second, while the ovariectomized rat successfully models accelerated bone loss due to menopause, there are, as yet, no generally accepted models for normal age-related bone loss that occurs with aging in all individuals, and predisposes to senile or type 2 osteoporosis. Third, models of bone loss in males have received very little attention. These are serious deficits because with the continuing increase in the longevity of human populations, all individuals are potential candidates for osteoporosis. The species that are being explored to complement the rat model include mice, dogs, sheep, minipigs, ferrets, and nonhuman primates. Because none has received the magnitude of attention that has been given to the rat and because of the constraints of space, each will receive only a brief moment. The interested reader is referred to other publications on the subject [9–11,52].

Mice

The mouse has a long history of being used in studies of age-related bone loss and has some important attributes in this regard. The growth plate has been reported to fuse early, at about 3–4 months of age; peak bone density is reached within 6 months; senescent bone changes begin around 1 year of age; and osteopenia increases with advancing age [9]. The age-related bone loss occurs in both cancellous and cortical bone and is believed to be similar to age-related osteoporosis in humans. There are, however, significant strain and gender differences in bone changes with age in mice. Although the epiphyses are reported to fuse early (3–4 months of age), linear bone growth in some strains is still evident between 8 and 12 months of age [53]. The bone loss that occurs commonly with aging in mice is accentuated in the SAM-P/6 mice whose bone density peaks at about 4 months and subsequently falls progressively with age in both long bones and vertebral bodies [54,55]. Fractures occur spontaneously in this strain, making it a useful model of fragility fracture as well [54,55]. This strain is currently being exploited to seek the etiologic mechanisms that underlie age-related bone loss that leads to type 2 osteoporosis.

The mouse has also been used as a model of accelerated bone loss due to ovarian hormone deficiency as occurs following menopause. As in rats, mice experience a rapid loss of cancellous bone following ovariectomy and estrogen therapy prevents the bone loss [56]. However, estrogen therapy in mice prevents bone loss mainly by stimulating bone formation in contrast to inhibiting resorption as in the ovariectomized rat, which is believed to model the human condition better [56]. Compared to rats, the mouse is small, making mouse bones difficult to handle, and, like rats, mice lack substantial intracortial remodeling. Because of these considerations, it is difficult to make a case for the ovariectomized mouse as an alternative small animal model of postmenopausal bone loss, especially as the rat model, with its convenient bone size, is so well characterized and established. However, the mouse is a potentially useful model for studying the mechanism of the bone anabolic effects of estrogen, which some believe also occurs in rats [57,58] and humans but is only easy to demonstrate in mice [56]. The mouse also has the potential of being a convenient model for evaluating new bone anabolic therapies where estrogen deficiency is not a primary consideration, in which case its small size will be advantageous when new drugs are available only in small amounts.

Another area in which the mouse is being increasingly used in studying aspects of skeletal aging is in the investigation of the genetic basis of peak bone mass [53]. Peak bone mass and the subsequent rate of bone loss are considered to be among the most important determinants of an individual's likelihood to develop osteoporosis due to age-related bone loss. The study of identical twins has yielded much useful information on the genetic basis of population variations in peak bone density. In the human population, dizygotic and monozygotic twin pairs are not very common. In contrast, inbred strains of mice offer an unlimited supply of mice that are genetically identical within strain but genetically different between strains. In mice, bone density varies over a wide range and differs between strains. The differences in bone density between inbred strains of mice that are raised under identical conditions demonstrate genetic regulation of bone density. Therefore, appropriate studies of inbred strains of mice with different bone densities could be used to identify genes that determine peak bone mass and their biological functions [53]. These types of studies are in progress in various laboratories.

LARGE NONRODENT ANIMAL MODELS OF AGING BONE LOSS

Large nonrodent animal species have been studied almost exclusively as models for the investigation of osteoporosis therapies in bone remodeling species with well-established Haversian systems. The stipulation by the United States FDA [50] that the preclinical testing of drugs should include the evaluation of the drug in one of these species has increased interest in the evaluation of the appropriateness of large nonrodent animal species as models of human skeletal bone loss. The following is a brief description of models based on dogs, sheep, minipigs, ferrets, and nonhuman primates. Additional information on these species can be found in other reviews [9–11,52].

Dogs

The dog skeleton shares many characteristics with human skeleton. As in humans, the dog skeleton remodels and has well-developed Haversian system; its epiphyses fuse following maturity; it has similar proportions of cancellous and cortical bone as humans; and it loses bone with aging. The female beagle dog has been evaluated extensively as a model of postmenopausal bone loss. However, reports on the nature of the skeletal response of the dog skeleton to ovarian hormone deficiency are conflicting. One group typically finds that ovarian hormone deficiency in dogs results in a decreased cancellous bone mass, a decreased trabecular mean wall thickness, an increased osteoblast number, and a decreased bone formation rate per osteoblast, with no change in bone resorption parameters [59]. The investigators concluded that the etiologic factor for bone loss following estrogen deficiency in beagle dogs is decreased bone formation due to osteoblastic insufficiency [59]. In contrast, other reports indicate that bone turnover and indices of bone formation and resorption increase following ovariectomy, but with a transient or no significant loss of bone [60]. These conflicting findings have made the ovariectomized dog a controversial model of ovarian hormone deficiency bone loss. The reasons for the conflicts are uncertain but may relate, in part, to the low estrous cycle of dogs [61]. The dog is a seasonal breeder and cycles only once or twice per year, unlike humans with a 28-day cycle and rats, which have 4- to 5-day cycles. In order words, a peak increase in estrogen occurs only once or twice per year in the dog, once every 28 days in humans, and once every 4–5 days in rats. If the frequency of peak estrogen levels in different species mirrors the proportion of time the skeleton is dominated by estrogen, it will explain why the dog skeleton appears not to be a sensitive and predictable model of estrogen deficiency bone loss. However, with its rich Harvesian system, the dog skeleton should be a useful model for the evaluation of Haversian remodeling parameters in studies where estrogen status is not an important factor [10].

Sheep

The female sheep (ewe) is a large remodeling animal that has potential for the assessment of osteoporosis therapies. The attraction of the sheep is that aged animals are in large supply; they are docile with simple husbandry needs, and they are easy to work with [62]. Although young sheep have a plexiform cortical bone type, older ($\geq$ 7 months) sheep remodel their skeleton and have well-developed Haversian systems [62,63]. The sheep is useful for investigating the *in vivo* effects of potential osteoporosis therapies on bone in an intact remodeling species. There is also considerable interest in using the ovariectomized sheep as a model of postmenopausal bone loss, but this has been the subject of only a few studies. Typically, in sheep, ovariectomy increases bone turnover and reduces bone mineral density, and a further loss of bone due to ovariectomy is prevented by estrogen therapy [62,63]. Although these findings are analogous to humans, studies with the ovariectomized sheep should be undertaken with caution because these animals have skeletal characteristics that confound their use as a model of postmenopausal bone loss [62–66]. Their skeleton undergoes seasonal variations in bone loss and bone mass; bone formation rates are severely depressed in the winter months and animals can spontaneously lose and regain bone during an experimental period; biomechanical parameters correlate with BMD at the femur but not at vertebral sites due probably to unusually large vertebral arches; all bones do not respond consistently and similarly to changes in BMD following ovariectomy; and estrogen therapy may increase BMD for reasons that are not clear [62–66]. These difficulties associated with the sheep skeleton indicate that in order to make the ovariectomized sheep a useful large remodeling model of postmenopausal bone loss suitable for assessing osteoporotic therapies, investigators working on the sheep need to characterize rigorously their model with respect to strain, season, diet, bones, and skeletal sampling sites, length of ovarian hormone deficiency, and appropriate controls to ensure that observations made following ovariectomy and/or therapy meet the criteria of predictability.

Pigs

Pigs have skeletal characteristics that make them potentially good large animal model for skeletal research [67], but they have not been studied extensively. Similar to humans, pigs have a continuous estrous cycle about 20 days long; they reach puberty early (within 6 months); they have cortical and cancellous bone with a well-developed Haversian system and BMU-based bone remodeling. The attractiveness of the pig model is enhanced by the availability of miniature pigs. Miniature laboratory pigs are of modest size and are available commercially. They weigh only about 50 kg in contast to mature farm pigs, which weight about 150 kg. Mechanical competence studies on minipigs treated with fluoride indicate that this model can yield results predictive of the skeletal response of humans [67]. They also respond appropriately to ovariectomy, but an optimum loss of bone due to ovariectomy required a mild restriction of dietary calcium. Compared to humans, pigs have a much higher bone mass, a denser trabecular network, and a different loading pattern of the skeleton, but these disadvantages are common to other large animal models to varying extents [67].

Ferrets

Ferrets have been studied even less well than pigs with respect to skeletal aging. Nonetheless they are attractive for modeling human bone loss because they are small, easily available animals with well-developed BMU-based remodeling in both cortical and trabecular bone. They have a short life span of 3–4 years. At 7 months of age, when the epiphyses fuse, the approximate weights of males and females are 1800 and 600 g, respectively. Females lose bone following ovariectomy as in humans [68]. However, their bone mass is influenced negatively by a decreased exposure to light and unbred females are prone to aplastic anemia due to prolonged estrus. With their BMU-based remodeling, ferrets and miniature pigs deserve further exploration as models for skeletal studies.

Nonhuman Primates

Nonhuman primates offer a model of bone aging with characteristics that, compared to other models, are closest to those of humans. As in humans, nonhuman primates have BMU-based remodeling; the length of their menstrual cycle is similar to that of humans; they exhibit irregular cycles with aging; some assume erect posture with similar bone loading patterns as humans; and they lose bone mass at an advanced age and with immobilization as in humans. These shared characteristics with humans make primates very attractive for studies of human skeletal aging. Most of such studies have so far focused on primates as models of ovarian hormone deficiency bone loss [69–71]. Despite similarities in the hormonal profile of women and female nonhuman primates, "menopause" occurs chronologically much later in nonhuman primates. Even with their shorter life span compared to humans, reliance on natural menopause will greatly limit the use of nonhuman primates for bone aging studies. Like other species, nonhuman primates have to be ovariectomized to induce ovarian hormone deficiency and postmenopausal-type bone loss. Several studies indicate that ovarian hormone deficiency due to surgical ovariectomy or chemical castration does, indeed, cause bone loss in nonhuman primates as in humans. In one study of female rhesus monkeys (*Macaca mulata*), GnRH agonist therapy caused an amenorrheic anovulatory condition, decreased estrogen levels, and increased serum osteocalcin levels, an index of bone turnover [69]. In addition, BMD of the humerus and caudal vertebrae was reduced by 2 months but returned to pretreatment levels 5 months following the cessation of GnRH therapy. In this study there were only three animals, which also served as their own controls. A recent and more extensive study carried out with surgically ovariectomized animals yielded results that are also in line with findings in postmenopausal women [71]. Eighteen cynomolgus monkeys were surgically ovariectomized and 19 were sham operated. For much of the experimental period the animals were fed a low calcium diet (0.14% Ca) that provided a calcium intake that was similar to that of postmenopausal women. Ovariectomy increased bone turnover, accelerated bone loss, reduced bone mass below baseline, and lowered vertebral and femoral bone strength [71]. These findings further support the appropriateness of the ovariectomized nonhuman primate as a model of postmenopausal bone loss. The finding of absolute bone loss following ovariectomy in this study is of note in view of previous reports of relative bone loss due, in part, to failure to gain bone in ovariectomized primates [70].

Although the ovariectomized nonhuman primate best models postmenopausal bone loss in comparison to other species, studies with nonhuman primates are restricted to only a few dedicated centers. In addition to the special facilities that are required and the large expense involved in such studies, additional issues to consider in the use of nonhuman primates for skeletal studies have been emphasized [71]: Group housing of primates, although desirable, produces extreme stress, infighting, weight loss, and mobidity, all of which can have an impact on bone, and even increased mortality. Large variance occurs in bone parameters in primate studies, which calls for large numbers of animals in order to achieve adequate statistical power. A sample size of 19 to 25 has been suggested, which translates to about 100 animals to test one osteoporosis drug at two dose levels in preventive therapy (sham, 25; ovx, 25; ovx + low dose drug, 25; ovx + high dose drug, 25). This is a large number of nonhuman primates, especially for a species that is not easily available. The importance of using aged primates whose bone mass has stabilized at its peak level before ovariectomy has also been emphasized [71]. Unlike laboratory-reared monkeys, aged monkeys captured from the wild may resume bone accretion when maintained on a laboratory diet, with its higher calcium content. Such animals should be allowed to first achieve a stable bone mass before initiating ovariectomy to minimize complications from resumed bone accretion. Therefore, nonhuman primate models, despite their close genetic proximity to humans, require rigorous standardization with respect to housing, dietary calcium intake, age at ovariectomy, length of time following ovariectomy, and length of acclimatization to laboratory diets if captured in the wild.

SUMMARY

Only a few years ago a book on human skeletal aging would most certainly not include a chapter on animals models of human skeletal aging. The fact that such chapters are now becoming standard features of esteemed books on bone and osteoporosis [10,52] is evidence that animal model study has come of age and will finally assume its rightful position as a legitimate component of the armamentarium for investigating issues relevant to human age-related bone loss. In the past, studies with animal models of age-related bone loss appeared to emphasize studies with a predictable outcome because of their similarities to studies that have been done in humans. This was an inevitable part of the process of validating and legitimizing the relevance of these *in vivo* animal studies. Most such studies have been in the area of testing new drugs for osteoporosis therapies in the ovariectomized rat model, and these studies have been very successful. However, *in vivo* animal bone research should not be restricted to the investigation of osteoporosis therapies in ovariectomized animal models. *In vivo* bone studies can be employed usefully for evaluating diverse questions relevant to human bone physiology and disorders and should be recognized as powerful and appropriate tools for research on bone from the growing period through maturation to aging and senescence.

Acknowledgments

This study was supported in part by a grant from NIH AG13309 and a University Grant Program for Osteoporosis from Procter and Gamble pharmaceuticals. I thank Dr. Jameela Banu for her help in the preparation of this manuscript.

References

1. Kassem, M., Melton, L. J., and Riggs, B. L. The TypeI/Type II mode for involutional osteoporosis. *In* "Osteoporosis" (R. Marcus, D. Feldman, and J. Kelsay, eds.), pp. 691–702. Academic Press, New York, 1996.
2. Frost, H. M. Tetracycline based histologic analysis of bone remodeling. *Calif. Tissue Res.* **3,** 211–237 (1969).
3. Parfitt, A. M. Bone remodeling: Relationship to the amount and structure of bone, and the pathogenesis and prevention of fractures. *In* "Osteoporosis: Etiology, Diagnosis and Management" (B. L. Riggs, and L. J. Melton III, eds.), pp. 45–93. Raven Press, New York, 1988.
4. Kalu, D. N. The ovariectomized rat model of postmenopausal bone loss. *Bone Miner.* **15,** 175–192 (1991).
5. "Introduction: Mammalian Models of Research on Aging," pp. 1–6. National Academy Press, Washington DC, 1981.
6. Frenkel, J. K. Introduction: Choice of animal models for the study of disease process in man. *Fed. Proc.* **28,** 160–161 (1969).
7. Wronski, T. J., and Yen, C. F. The ovariectomized rat as an animal model for postmenopausal bone loss. *Cells Mater.* **1**(Suppl.), 69–74 (1991).
8. Frost, H. M., and Jee, W. S. S. On the rat model of human osteoporoses. *Bone Miner.* **18,** 227–236 (1992).
9. Ornoy, A., and Katzburg, S. Osteoporosis: Animal models for the human disease. *In* "Animal Models of Human Related Calcium Metabolic Disorders" (A. Ornoy, eds.), pp. 105–126. CRC Press, New York, 1995.
10. Kimmel, D. B. Animal models for *in vivo* experimentation in osteoporosis research. *In* "Osteoporosis" (R. Marcus, D. Feldman, and J. Kelsy eds.), pp. 671–690. Academic Press, New York, 1996.
11. Jee, W. S. S. Proceedings of the International Conference on Animal Models in the Prevention and Treatment of Osteopenia. *Bone* **4**(Suppl.), 113S-466S (1995).
12. Osteoporosis: Consensus Conference. *J. Am. Med. Assoc.* **252,** 799-802 (1984).
13. Favus, M. J., ed. "Primer on the Metabolic Bone Diseases and Disorders of Mineral Metabolism," 3rd ed. Lippincott-Raven, New York, 1996.
14. Kalu, D. N., Hardin, R. H., Cockerham, R., and Yu, B. P. Aging and dietary modulation of rat skeleton and parathyroid hormone. *Endocrinology* **115,** 1239–1247 (1984).
15. Kalu, D. N., Liu, C. C., Hardin, R. R., and Hollis, B. W. The aged rat model of ovarian hormone deficiency bone loss. *Endocrinology* **124,** 7–16 (1989).
16. Yu, B. P., Masoro, E. J., Murata, I., Bertrand, H. A., and Lynd, F. T. Life span study of SPF Fischer 344 male rats fed ad libitum or restricted diets: longevity, growth, lean body mass and disease. *J. Gerontol.* **37,** 130–141 (1982).
17. Berg, B. N., and Harmison, C. R. Growth, disease and aging in the rat. *J. Gerentol.* **12,** 370–377 (1957).
18. Mori, S., Jee, W. S. S., Li, X. J., Chan, S., and Kimmel, B. D. Effects of prostaglandin E_2 on the production of new cancellous bone in the axial skeleton of ovariectomized rats. *Bone* **11,** 103–113 (1990).
19. Kalu, D. N., Masoro, E. J., Yu, B. P., Hardin, R. R., and Hollis, B. W. Modulation of age related hyperparathyroidism and senile bone loss in Fischer rats by soy protein and food restriction. *Endocrinology* **122,** 1847–1854 (1988).
20. Wronski, T. J., Dann, L. M., Scott, K. S., and Cintron, M. Long term effects of ovariectomy and aging on the rat skeleton. *Calcif. Tissue Int.* **45,** 360–366 (1989).
21. Baron, R., Tross, R., and Vignery, A. Evidence of sequential remodeling in rat trabecular bone: morphology, dynamic histomorphometry, and changes during skeletal maturation. *Anat. Rec.* **208,** 137–145 (1984).
22. Erben, R. G. Trabecular and endocortical bone surfaces in the rat: modeling or remodeling? *Anat. Rec.* **246,** 39–46 (1996).
23. Ruth, E. B. Bone studies II: an experimental study of the Haversian-type vascular channels. *Am. J. Anat.* **93,** 429–455 (1953).
24. Jee, W. S. S., Mori, S., Li X. J., and Chan, S. Prostaglandin E_2 enhances cortical bone mass and activates intracortical bone remodeling in intact and ovariectomized female rats. *Bone* **11,** 253–266 (1990).
25. Saville, P. D. Changes in skeletal mass and fragility with castration in the rat: a model of osteoporosis. *J. Am. Geriat. Soc.* **17,** 155–166 (1969).
26. Binkley, N., and Kimmel, D. B. Effect of age and parity on skeletal response to ovariectomy in rats. *J. Bone Miner. Res.* **9**(Suppl. 1), S197 (1994).
27. Devogelear, J.-P. DeDeuxaisnes, C. N., Donnez, J., and Thomas, K. LHRH analogues and bone loss. *Lancet* **1,** 1498 (1987).
28. Goulding, A., and Gold, E. A new way to induce estrogen deficiency osteopenia in the rat: Comparison of the effects of surgical ovariectomy and administration of LHRH agonist buserelin on bone resorption and composition. *J. Endocrinol.* **121,** 293–298 (1989).
29. Kalu, D. N. Bone. *In* "Handbook of Aging" (E. J., Masoro, ed.), pp. 395–411. Oxford Univ. Press, New York, 1995.
30. Morris, H. A., O'Loughlin, P. D., Mason, R. A., and Schulz, S. R. The effect of oophorectomy on calcium homeostasis. *Bone* **17**(Suppl.), 169S–174S (1995).
31. Kalu, D. N., and Hardin, R. R. Evaluation of the role of calcitonin deficiency in ovariectomy induced osteopenia. *Life Sci.* **34,** 2393–2398 (1984).

32. Kalu, D. N. Proliferation of trap positive multinucleate cells in ovariectomized mice. *Proc. Soc. Exp. Biol. Med.* **195,** 70–74 (1990).
33. Kalu, D. N., Salerno, E., Liu, C. C., Ferraro, F., Arjmandi, B. H., and Salih, M. A. Ovariectomy-induced bone loss and the hematopoietic system. *Bone Miner.* **23,** 145-161 (1993).
34. Gasser, J. A. Assessing bone quality by pQCT. *Bone* **17**(Suppl.), 145S–154S (1995).
35. Kimmel, B. D., and Jee, W. S. S. A quantitative histologic analysis of the growing long bones metaphysis. *Calcif. Tissue Int.* **32,** 113-122 (1980).
36. Yeh, J. K., Chen, M.-M., and Aloia, J. F. Skeletal alterations in hypophysectomized rats: I. A histomorphometric study on tibial cancellous bone. *Anat. Rec.* **241,** 505–512 (1995).
37. Jee, W. S. S., Inoue, J., Jee, K. W., and Haba, T. Histomorphometric assay of the growing long bone. *In* "Handbook of One Morphology" (H. Takahashi, ed.), pp. 101–122. Nishimura Niigata City, Japan, 1983.
38. Garn, S. M. Bone loss and aging. *In* "The Physiology and Pathology of Human Aging" (R. Goldman and M. Rockstein, eds.), pp. 39–57. Academic Press, New York, 1975.
39. Kalu, D. N., Hardin, R. R., and Cockerham, R. Evaluation of the pathogenesis of skeletal changes in ovariectomized rats. *Endocrinology* **115,** 507–512 (1984).
40. Orhii, P. B., Norland, K. A., and Kalu, D. N. Growth hormone therapy restores cortical bone following loss due to ovariectomy in aged rats. *J. Bone Miner. Res.* **12**(Suppl. 1), T555 (1997).
41. Jee, W. S. S., Mori, S., Li X. J., and Chan, S. Prostaglandin E_2 enhances cortical bone mass and activates intracortical bone remodeling in intact and ovariectomized female rats. *Bone* **11,** 253–266 (1990).
42. Parfitt, A. M., Drezner, M. K., Glorieux, F. H., Kanis, J. A., *et al.* Bone histomorphometry: standardization of nomenclature, symbols and units. *J. Bone Miner. Res.* **2,** 595–610 (1987).
43. Salih, M. A., Lui, C. C., Arjmandi, B. H., and Kalu, D. N. Estrogen modulates the mRNA levels for cancellous bone proteins of ovariectomized rats. *Bone Miner.* **23,** 285–299 (1993).
44. Westerlend, K. C., Wronski, T. J., Evans, G. L., and Turner, R. T. The effect of longterm ovarian hormone deficiency on transforming growth factor-beta and bone matrix mRNA expression in rat femora. *Biochem. Biophys. Res. Commun.* **200,** 283–289 (1994).
45. Caniggia, A., Gennasi, C., Borella, G., Benant, M., *et al.* Intestinal absorption of calcium-47 after treatment with oral estrogen and gestagen in senile osteoporosis. *Br. Med. J.* **4,** 30–32 (1970).
46. Arjmandi, B. H., Hollis, B. W., and Kalu, D. N. *In vivo* effect of 17 beta-estradiol on intestinal calcium absorption in rats. *Bone Miner.* **26,** 181–189 (1994).
47. Arjmandi, B. H., Salih, M. A., Herbert, D. C., Sims, S. H., and Kalu, D. N. Evidence for estrogen receptor-linked calcium transport in the intestine. *Bone Miner.* **21,** 63–74 (1993).
48. Salih, M. A., Sims, S. H., and Kalu, D. N, Putative intestinal estrogen receptor: evidence for regional differences. *Mol. Cell. Endocrinol.* **121,** 47–55 (1996).
49. Mosekilde, L. Osteoporosis—mechanisms and models. *In* "Anabolic Treatments for Osteoporosis" (J. F. Whitfield and P. Morley, eds.), pp. 31–58. CRC Press, New York, 1998.
50. Guidelines for Preclinical and Clinical Evaluation of Agents Used for the Prevention or Treatment of Postmenopausal Osteoporosis, Division of Metabolism and Endocrine Drug Products, Food and Drug Administration, 1994.
51. Thompson, D. D., Simmons, H. A., Pirie, C. M., and Ke, H. Z. FDA guidelines and animal models for osteoporosis. *Bone* **17**(Suppl.), 125S–133S (1995).
52. Geddes, A. D. Animal models of bone disease. *In* "Principles of Bone Biology" (J. P., Bilezikian, L. G., Raisz, and G. A. Rodan, eds.), pp. 1343–1354. Academic Press, New York, 1996.
53. Beamer, W. G., Donahue, L. R. Rosen, C. J., and Baylink, D. J. Genetic variability in adult bone density among inbred strains of mice. *Bone* **18,** 397–403 (1996).
54. Takeda, T., Hosokawa, M., and Higuchi, K. Senescence-accelerated mouse (SAM). A novel murine model of accelerated senescence. *J. Am. Ger. Soc.* **37,** 911–919 (1991).
55. Matsushita, M., Tsuboyama, T., Kasai, R., *et al.* Age related changes in bone mass in the senescent accelerated mouse: SAM-R/3 and SAM-P/6 as new murine models for senile osteoporosis. *Am. J. Pathol.* **125,** 276–283 (1986).
56. Bain, S. D., Bailey, M. C., Celino, D. L., Lantry, M. M., and Edwards, M. W. High dose estrogen inhibits bone resorption and stimulates bone formation in the ovariectomized mouse. *J. Bone Miner. Res.* **8,** 435–442 (1993).
57. Chow, J. W., Lean J. M., and Chambers, T. J. 17 beta-estradiol stimulates cancellous bone formation in female rats. *Endocrinology* **130,** 3025–3032 (1992).
58. Takano-Yamamoto, T., and Rodan, G. A. Direct effects of 17 beta-estradiol on trabecular bone in ovariectomized rats. *Proc. Natl. Acad. Sci. U.S.A.* **87,** 2172–2176 (1990).
59. Malluche, H. H., Fargere, M.-C., Kush, M., and Friedler, R. Osteoblast insufficiency is responsible for maintenance of osteopenia after loss of ovarian function in experimental beagle dogs. *Endocrinology* **119,** 2649-2654 (1986).
60. Boyce, R. W., Franks, A. F., Jankowsky, M. C., Orcutt, C. M., *et al.* Sequential histomorphometric changes in cancellous bone from ovariohysterectomized dogs. *J. Bone Miner. Res.* **5,** 947–953 (1990).
61. Miller, S. C., Bowman, B. M., and Jee, W. S. S. Available animal models of osteopenia—small and large. *Bone* **17**(Suppl.), 117S–123S (1995).
62. Newman, E., Turner, A. S., and Wark, J. D. The potential of sheep for the study of osteopenia: current status and comparison with other animal models. *Bone* **16**(Suppl.), 277S–284S (1995).
63. Hornby, S. B., Ford, S. L., Mase, C. A., and Evans, G. P. Skeletal changes in the ovariectomized ewe and subsequent response to tretment with 17 beta-estradiol. *Bone* **17**(Suppl.), 387S–394S (1995).
64. Turner, A. S., Mellinekrodt, C. H., Alvis, M. R., and Bryant, H. V. Dose response effects of estradiol implants on bone mineral density in ovariectomized ewes. *Bone* **17**(Suppl.), 421S–427S (1995).
65. Turner, A. S., Alvis, M., Myers, W., Stevens, M. L., and Lundy, M. W. Changes in bone mineral density and bone specific alkaline phosphatase in ovariectomized ewes. *Bone* **17**(Suppl.), 395S–402S (1995).
66. Deloffre, P., Hans, D., Rumelhart, C., Mitton, D., Tsouderos, Y., and Meunier, P. J. Comparison between bone density and bone strength in glucocorticoid-treated ewe. *Bone* **17**(Suppl.), 409S–414S (1995).
67. Mosekilde, L., Weisbrode, S. E., Safron, J. A., Stills, H. F., *et al.* Evaluation of the skeletal effects of combined mild dietary calcium restriction and ovariectomy in Sinclair S-1 minipigs: A pilot study. *J. Bone Miner. Res.,* **8,** 1311–1321 (1993).
68. Mackey, M. S., Stevens, M. L., Ebert, D. C., Tressler, D. L., Combs, K. S., Lowry, C. K., Smith, P. N., and McOsker, J. E. The ferret as a small animal model with BMU-based remodeling for skeletal research. *Bone* **17**(Suppl.), 191S-196S (1995).
69. Mann, D. R., Gould, K. G., and Collins, D. C. A potential primate model for bone loss resulting from medical oophorectomy or menopause. *J. Clin. Endocrinol. Metab.* **71,** 105-110 (1990).
70. Thompson, D. D., Seedor, J. G., Quartuccio, H., Solomon, H., *et al.* The bisphosphonate, alendronate, prevents bone loss in ovariectomized baboons. *J. Bone Miner. Res.* **7,** 951–960 (1992).
71. Jerome, C. P., Turner, C. H., and Lees, C. J. Decreased bone mass and strength in ovariectomized Cynomolgus monkeys (*Macaca fascicularis*). *Calcif. Tissue Int.* **60,** 265–270 (1997).

CHAPTER 6

Human Diseases as Models of Accelerated Aging

JONATHAN M. WEINER AND LOREN G. LIPSON
Division of Geriatric Medicine, Department of Medicine, University of Southern California School of Medicine, Los Angeles, California 90033

THE AGING IMPERATIVE

The United States population is aging more rapidly than ever. This phenomenom is worldwide and will continue into the foreseeable future. Many disease states have been categorized as states of accelerated aging. The purpose of this chapter is to use these disease states to understand better the mechanism of aging. Three diseases will be discussed: one common and two uncommon. Answering questions of why and how we age could lead to new preventive approaches to this phenomenon.

Why has 65 been considered to be the benchmark of the elderly? At the end of the 19th century, Otto von Bismark told the Prussian people that if they worked hard, they would be rewarded at the age of 65 with a pension. Suffice it to say, at that time the average life span was 47 years and soldiers in the army did not usually live beyond 30 years. Bismark was popular with the government because he gave virtually no pensions. In the 1930s when the United States social security system was founded, planners looked to this precedent and picked the age of 65, an age reached by relatively few in the population. Time, however, has proved that former fact to be fiction. On average, we now live to the age of 77. The 20th century has been witness to an unprecedented 30-year gain in longevity.

According to the United States Census Bureau, in the year 1900, 3.1 million Americans were over the age of 65, only 4% of the population. In the year 1994, 33.2 million people were over the age of 65, 12.5% of the population [1]. Because of these trends, it is inevitable that society will have to face new challenges, both foreseeable and not, over the next 50 years. Aging per se is therefore becoming a biological event for which we need greater understanding.

THE MECHANISM OF AGING

Physiology of Aging

Medical advances have played a major role in the aging of our population. As noted in Table I [2], the predominant cause of death in the elderly is cardiovascular disease. The second most common cause is malignancy. In 1991 "seven in ten deaths [in the] elderly could be attributed to either heart disease, cancer, or stroke" [1]. The particular statistics, however, show that among these organ systems, morbidity and mortality for a given illness have decreased. One example of this was the Scandinavian Simvastatin Survival Study, which showed that one antilipid agent could decrease the mortality rate in patients who suffered from cardiovascular disease and hypercholesterolism [3]. Similar advances have been shown in stroke prevention, malignancy screening, and diabetic management.

The aging human body undergoes many physiologic changes. Functions of all organ systems are irreversibly altered. It appears that organ dysfunction results from two pathways. There is a slow dysfunction related to an independent biological clock, and a second dysfunction that relates specifically to organic disease. The cardiac

TABLE I Death Rates per 100,000 Population and Percentages for the 10 Leading Causes of Death among Persons 65 and Older: 1970, 1978, and 1986 (by Rank Order and Age for 1986)[a]

Cause of death ICD code[b]	1970	1978	1986 death rate: 65 and older	1986 death rate: 65–74	1986 death rate: 75–84	1986 death rate: 85 and older	Percentage of deaths 65 and older
All causes	5892.1	5293.5	5102.0	2801.4	6348.2	15398.9	100.0
Diseases of heart	2683.3	2331.1	2122.2	1043.0	2637.5	7178.7	41.6
Malignant neoplasms including neoplasms of lympnatic and hematopotetic tissues	923.4	1002.4	1056.6	847.0	1287.3	1612.0	20.7
Cerebrovascular diseases	847.5	622.0	443.5	164.1	573.8	1762.6	8.7
Chronic obstructive pulmonary diseases and allied conditions	102.2	66.1	214.8	149.2	295.0	362.9	4.2
Pneumonia and influenza	200.4	193.2	208.5	58.6	242.8	1032.1	4.1
Diabetes mellitus	131.4	101.3	93.4	59.2	121.9	213.9	1.8
Accidents and adverse effects	135.9	100.3	86.2	49.0	106.3	252.2	1.7
All other accidents and adverse effects	99.7	75.8	64.2	31.2	77.5	226.9	1.3
Motor vehicle accidents	36.2	24.5	22.0	17.9	28.8	25.3	0.4
Atherosclerosis	149.7	115.0	73.9	16.0	74.8	232.6	1.5
Nephritis, nephrotic syndrome, and nephrosis	23.7	25.6	61.2	26.8	79.4	216.3	1.2
Septicemia	7.5	19.5	50.8	22.6	64.6	181.9	1.0
All other causes residual	637.5	700.6	691.8	365.9	929.4	2153.7	11.7

[a] Source: National Center for Health Statistics. Vital Statistics of the United States. 2, 1970 and 1978: 1986, unpublished tabulations.
[b] International Classification of Diseases, ninth revision. 1980.

and dermatological systems are excellent examples of these two mechanisms at play. Heart rate in the sitting position decreases with age [4]. Collagenous and elastic tissue increases with increased age around the conduction system, thus causing increases in atypical beats and a predisposition to arrhythmias [5]. In addition, there are also changes in preload, contractile state, and coronary blood flow [6]. Cutaneous aging results in reductions in the skin's ability to heal and to protect. In addition, it is more difficult for the skin to control temperature. Finally, changes in hair and tensile strength result in cosmetic changes, which are the most apparent marker of aging [7,8]. Figure 1 [9] shows that renal function, pulmonary function, and basal metabolic rate also decline with aging.

Theories of Aging

THE ERROR THEORY OF AGING

Many theories have been advanced to explain why we age. As is true for most issues about which many explanations are proposed, no one concept is likely to account solely for the aging process. Rather, a combination of the following theories together help to answer the question "why do we age?"

Orgel proposed the "error theory" in 1963. The theory was based on the genetic code. As transcription takes place and proteins are made, small errors inevitably take place from time to time. In a perfectly monitored cellular system, if tRNA produces an incorrect amino acid sequence, for example, corrections are made. If not properly corrected, the resulting protein would be slightly altered with resultant small changes in function. If this protein aids in the production of other proteins, the abnormal protein can lead to other errors. Moreover, as a cell ages, the chances of error increase; the abnormal proteins will eventually result in more lasting alterations in intracellular and extracellular functions associated with the abnormal proteins. This may even cause cell death [10,11]. The error theory has met with some difficulties. Aging cells do not contain erroneous proteins, and if erroneous proteins are introduced into a cell, the cell does not age prematurely. Other theories on aging are built around the genetic code. Von Hahn suggested that errors at the DNA level might cause aging in a way similar to the "error theory" [12]. Unfortunately, it is difficult to evaluate how putative DNA errors would translate into cellular errors. This theory remains untested.

THE FREE RADICAL THEORY OF AGING

A second concept is widely known as the "free radical theory." In order to understand the theory as origi-

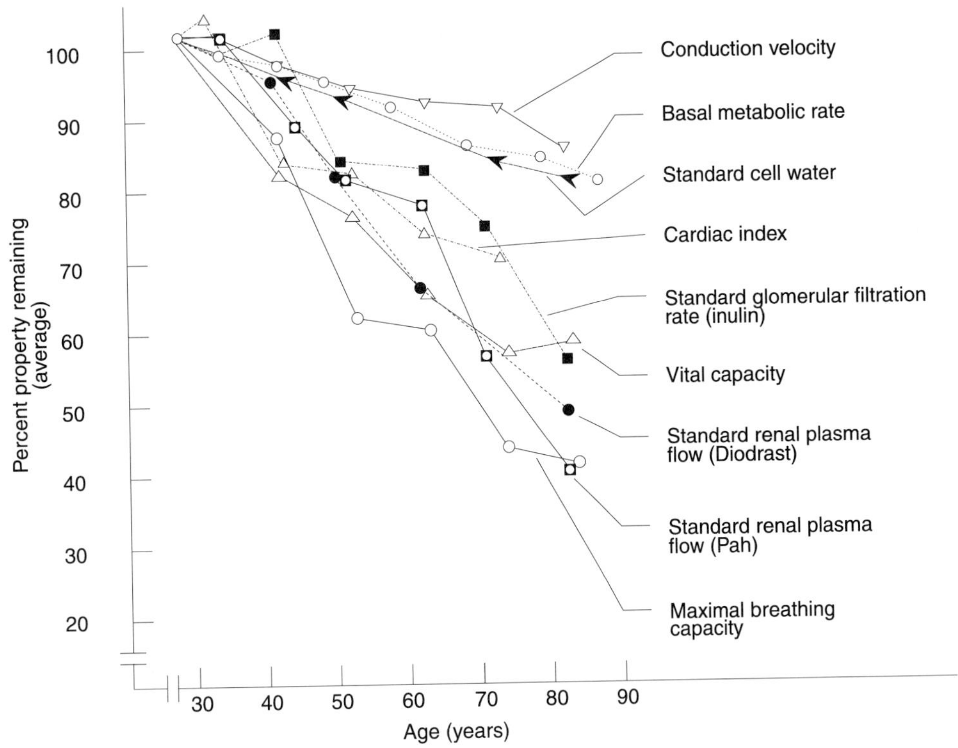

Figure 1 Average age differences in physiological functions among normal male subjects aged 30–90 years.

nally postulated by Harman in 1956 [13], free radical reactions must first be understood. During a chemical reaction, there may be a transient presence of a highly reactive intermediate with an unpaired electron [14]. This intermediate is called a free radical. Free radicals originate mainly from oxidation and can accumulate over time. With the accumulation of free radicals, cellular function decreases and cell death eventually follows. Collagen and elastin are two major tissue proteins affected by free radical formation during aging. Studies involving the addition of antioxidants either to animals or to cells in culture would test this idea by preventing the accumulation of free radicals. Such studies have not been associated with reductions in mortality [15].

The Hayflick Model of Aging

Hayflick's observations led to a third theory of aging. Hayflick observed that human diploid fibroblasts would double only a finite number of times. Despite an ability of the remaining cells to continue to survive for several months, they will not continue to divide beyond approximately 50 doublings [16]. It was and is still believed that if the reason for this doubling cessation is understood, scientist will be able to know why we age. Later research by Hayflick and others has continued to support this finding. Chapter 7 of this volume includes a discussion of the telomere explanation for the finite replication capacity of normal cells. Experiments between hybrids of elderly human diploid fibroblasts and immortalized cell lines still showed a finite division potential [17]. The manipulation of DNA synthesis and mitogenic growth was successful in altering this finite potential, but no true mechanism was identified [17]. Furthermore, many cells do not depend on their function or survival on the capacity to divide so it is hard to imagine that this theory would accommodate many examples of cellular aging.

DISEASES THAT CAN ACCELERATE THE AGING PROCESS

Diabetes Mellitus

Diabetes mellitus is an organic disease characterized by defects in insulin production and glucose utilization. It is associated over time with cardiovascular, neuropathic, renal, and atherosclerotic complications. This disease helps illustrate some principles of aging. The clinical manifestations of diabetes parallel the many comorbid conditions found in aging individuals. Inde-

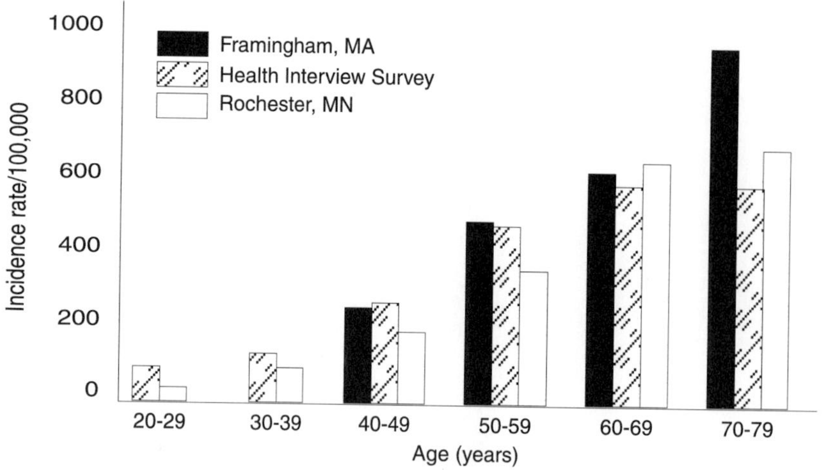

FIGURE 2 Annual incidence of noninsulin-dependent diabetes mellitus in three surveys.

pendent of age, the illness itself appears to accelerate the aging process in affected individuals.

Aging in general is associated with a decline in glucose tolerance. Studies show a 1-mg/dl increase in fasting plasma glucose accompanied by a 9- to 10-mg/dl increase in the oral glucose tolerance test (OGTT) per decade of life [18]. Type 2 diabetes is found in 3–5% of persons between the third and fifth decade of life. This incidence increases to 10% by age 60 and can reach 16–20% by age 80 [19] Figure 2 [20] represents consistent findings from the Framingham, Health Interview and the Rochester studies. Table II [18] depicts OGTT results in the National Health and Nutrition Examination Survey II (1976–1980). It is clear that abnormalities of glucose metabolism increase with age. The elderly patient develops decreased insulin secretion from the pancreatic β cells. Furthermore, insulin that is secreted has a reduced effect on the muscle uptake of glucose. Finally, the liver in the elderly may produce excess amounts of glucose. The combination of these three impairments leads to the state of hyperglycemia. Table III [19] lists the factors responsible for development of type 2 diabetes in the elderly and hyperglycemia of aging.

Elderly patients with diabetes have higher mortality and morbidity rates. This disease state slows wound healing and accelerates cataracts, microaneuryusms, neurologic dysfunction, and large and small vessel atherosclerosis. The ramifications of elderly patients developing peripheral neuropathy and increasing their risk of lower extremity cellulitis infection are compounded by poor wound healing and microvascular disease. In addition, immobility and a predisposition to obesity compounds potential difficulties and will increase the risk of cardiovascular disease.

The elderly have an increased prevalence of hyperglycemia and its resulting morbidity and mortality. Dia-

TABLE II OGTT Results in the National Health and Nutrition Examination Survey II (1976–1980)

	Age in years			
	20–44	45–54	55–64	65–74
1. Diabetes known prior to testing	1.1%	4.3%	6.6%	9.3%
2. Diabetes revealed through testing	1.0%	4.4%	6.5%	8.6%
Total prevalence of diabetes	2.1%	8.7%	13.1%	17.9%
3. Impaired glucose tolerance	6.5%	14.9%	15.2%	22.9%
Total diabetes and impaired glucose tolerance	8.6%	23.6%	28.3%	40.8%

TABLE III Factors Responsible for Development of Type 2 Diabetes in the Elderly and Hyperglycemia of Aging

Type 2 diabetes in the elderly	Hyperglycemia of aging
Altered pancreatic islet function Insulin Glucagon Somatostatin	Decreased insulin biosynthesis and/or secretion
	Alterations in insulin action Receptor Postreceptor of intracellular
Insulin resistance Receptor binding Postreceptor defects	Decreased peripheral glucose utilization
	Changes in body composition
	Changes in diet
	Decreased physical activity

betes mellitus itself, however, appears to accelerate the aging process independently. Collagen, fibroblasts, capillary basement membranes, and atherogenesis appear to show changes in diabetics similar to those in natural aging. These changes are described in Table IV [21]. Collagen fiber polymerization and cross-linking increase with age despite decreased amounts of connective tissue collagen [22]. Collagen in the elderly consequently becomes more resistant to turnover. An accurate prediction of chronological age can actually be made by measuring the time it takes to digest a known quantity of collagen by collagenase. In type I diabetics, who have had diabetes mellitus for many years, collagen digestion test results indicate an age that is more than twice their actual chronological age. As human beings age, skin fibroblasts cannot be maintained in culture after a specific chronological time. As mentioned earlier, this was a major identifiable principle of cellular aging. When young skin fibroblasts from diabetics were grown in culture with aged skin fibroblasts from non-diabetics, the viability was the same. This once again suggested that although the diabetic fibroblasts came from individuals of younger chronological age, they behaved like cells from aged nondiabetics [23].

Even when controlled, diabetes is associated with changes in extracellular matrix components, including the degree of glycosylation of proteins. Capillary basement membranes can become thickened, a process of aging that is accelerated in diabetics [24]. A last example of premature aging in the diabetic is seen in smooth muscle and endothelial cells that show early changes of accelerated atherogenesis and atherosclerosis [25].

Premature aging in diabetics can be seen in other organ systems. Diabetics develop microvascular disease that results in arteriolar and precapillary reductions in blood flow. Until recent years, peripheral neuropathy was thought to be *pathonogmonic* for diabetes and a few relatively rare neurologic conditions. Malfunction of the autonomic nervous system and the sensory nervous system is a common result of long-standing, poorly controlled diabetes. Patients with diabetes develop difficulty with gastroperesis, orthostatic hypotension, and sexual dysfunction. They also develop sensory loss to fine touch and vibration in the stocking-glove distribution. These physiologic changes occur as part of the aging process and are evidenced by the growing number of older nondiabetic individuals with autonomic and peripheral neuropathies, but in diabetics, these changes occur earlier. A 65 year old with diabetes for 15 years may show signs of neuropathy seen typically in an 85 year old without diabetes. Another example is precapillary blood flow. Diabetics ranging from age 19 to 72 were compared with age- and gender-matched controls. Reaction time and flow rate were impaired in the entire diabetic population but in the control group, impairment was evident only as a function of age. Again, diabetes appears to mimic many physiologic elements of aging [26].

TABLE IV Diabetes Mellitus as a State of Accelerated Aging

Cell or organelle studied	Consequence on aging
Collagen	Abnormal formation; increased polymerization and aging
Fibroblast cell culture	Decreased replication and culture viability
Capillary basement membrane	Increased rate of age-related thickening
Arterial smooth muscle endothelial cells	Increased age effects on lipid metabolism

Progerioid Syndromes

Although aging influences the onset of diabetes and diabetes causes premature aging, other conditions are marked by premature aging. Hutchinson–Gilford syndrome, Werner's syndrome, acrogeria, ataxia telangiectasia, Cockayne's syndrome, Down's syndrome, familial cervical liposysplasia, Seip syndrome, and familial hypercholeterolemia are all inherited syndromes associated with premature aging. Identifying criteria for these progeroid syndromes can be found in Table V [28]. This chapter focuses on Hutchinson–Gilford syndrome and Werner's syndrome.

HUTCHINSON–GUILFORD

Hutchinson–Guilford [27] (progeria) is an inherited disorder thought to be sporadic and autosomal dominant in as much as it has a low frequency of recurrence in families and there is an absence of consanguinity. Some sources have labeled the disease pattern as autosomal recessive, but others disagree [28]. The unusual penetrance pattern may be the result of a germ line mutation. Jonathan Hutchinson initially described the illness in 1886. He described a 3.5-year-old boy who had the appearance of an old man [29]. Hastings Gilford had a similar case and termed the illness "progeria," taken from the Greek word for old age, "geras" [30]. Currently the illness affects 1 in 8 million infants [31]. The ratio of male to female is 1.5 : 1. Ninety-five percent of affected infants are Caucasian [31]. Infants with progeria appear to be normal at birth. The diagnosis is often made within the first year of life, when the infant develops at a profoundly retarded rate. There is little hair and subcutaneous fat over the scalp. They have

TABLE V Selected Major Criteria for the Identification of Genetic Progerioid Syndromes of Humans

Criteria	Syndrome	
	Unimodal	Segmental
Increased susceptibility to one or more types of neoplasms of relevance to aging	Polyposis, intestinal, type III	Ataxia telangiectasia
Increased frequencies of nonconstitutional chromosomal aberrations	Porokeratosis of Mibelli	Werner's
Dementia and/or relevant degenerative neuropathology	Alzheimer's disease of brain	Down's
Premature graying or loss of hair	White hair, prematurely	Progeria
Amyloid depositions	Amyloid, type III (cardiac form)	Down's
Increased depositions of lipofuscin pigments	Neuronal ceroid lipofuscinosis (Parry type)	?Cockayne's
Diabetes mellitus	Diabetes mellitus, autosomal dominant (mild juvenile form)	Seip's
Disorder of lipid metabolism	Familial hypercholesterolemia	Cervical lipodysplasia, familial
Hypogonadism	Kallmann's syndrome	Myotonic dystrophy
Autoimmunity	Thyroid autoantibodies	Down's
Hypertension	Hypertension, essential	Turner's
Degenerative vascular disease	Amyloidosis, cerebral, arterial	Werner's
Osteoporosis	Osteoporosis, juvenile	Klinefelter's
Cataracts	Cataract, nuclear total	Werner's
Regional fibrosis	Antitrypsin deficiency of plasma with chronic obstructive pulmonary disease	Werner's
Variations in amounts and/or distributions of adipose tissue	Adiposis dolorosa	Progeria

normal to above normal intelligence. Sexual maturation is usually delayed. The most common clinical features are sclerodermoid changes over the lower abdomen, flanks, and upper thighs. It is also common for progerioid infants to have loose skin wrinkled over the phalanges. The appearance is similar to that of an elderly man or woman. They are described to have a "horse riding" stance due to a coxa valga. This also results in a shuffling, wide-based gait. The average age of death is 12–13 years [31], with a range of 7 to 27 years. Paralleling death in aging individuals, 80% of patients with progeria die of myocardial infarction or congestive heart failure [27].

The cause of premature aging associated with progeria is unknown. One finding is an increased level of urinary hyaluronic acid. The excretion of hyaluronic acid is 7 to 14 times the normal level [27]. Hyaluronic acid acts as an antiangiogenesis factor. Its metabolites act to stimulate angiogenesis. Based on this proposed mechanism, alterations in the metabolism of hyaluronic acid would have a dramatic impact on development and growth. In normal adults, hyaluronic acid excretion increases with age. Also described is a consistent increase in the glycoprotein, gp200, in skin fibroblasts of patients with progeria. This alteration in glycosylation likely plays a role in the precocious senility. Patients with progeria also display elevations in growth hormone levels and basal metabolic rate (BMR). Abdenur *et al.* [32] attempted to treat these infants with a nutritional and growth hormone treatment. With the hypothesis that the failure to thrive was a result of the increased BMR, the investigators believed that by maintaining the higher nutritional demands, disease progression may be slowed. They did indeed accomplish these goals. Patients developed increased levels of growth factors and decreased BMR. The progression of atherosclerotic disease and thus aging, however, was not prevented.

WERNER'S SYNDROME

Another disease in which hyaluronic acid is elevated is Werner's syndrome. Werner's syndrome, also known as adult progeria, is now known to be a recessive genetic disorder caused by the mutations in the DNA helicase gene (WRN) [33]. The gene has been mapped to chromosome 8 (8p12) [34]. In 1904, a German ophthalmologist described four siblings with sclerodermoid skin and bilateral cataracts [35]. The earliest symptoms may appear during the second decade with the premature graying of hair. Voice pitch is altered to a high squeak. By the third decade, patients may develop visual disturbances. Patients will also at this time develop skin atrophy and loss of subcutaneous fat of the limbs, predisposing them to leg ulcers. As the fourth decade approaches, osteoporosis and diabetes mellitus begin to appear. Fertility is affected due to severe hyalinization of the seminiferous tubules in males and loss of primary follicles in the ovaries of females. Finally, as is the case with normal physiologic aging, there are many case reports of malignancies not usually found in this age group, which appears to be further evidence of accelerated aging. Death occurs on average at the end of the fourth decade or in the fifth decade. Werner's patients usually die with diagnoses of cataracts, osteoporosis, diabetes, cancer, and atherosclerosis. As is the case in progeria, the leading cause of death is cardiovascular disease [36].

Werner's syndrome is also associated with an elevation of urinary excretion of hyaluronic acid [27]. As is the case in progeria, it is difficult to pinpoint the exact cause of aging in these patients. In addition to abnormalities of hyaluronic acid metabolism, the gene WRN appears to be involved in DNA helicase production [29]. The DNA helicase is a vital enzyme for DNA transcription repair. Thus, DNA may become unwound or wound incorrectly. Other findings in Werner's suggest an aging mechanism overlapping with diabetes. Fibroblasts from the skin of patients with Werner's syndrome grow poorly in culture and show less response than controls to platelet-derived growth factor [37]. Fibroblasts from acral sclerodermoid skin similarly showed a delay of collagenase activity. The same group also designed a study in which fibroblasts from normal donors were placed into serum of Werner's syndrome patients. The result was stimulation of collagen synthesis and inhibition of collagenase in the previously normal fibroblasts [38]. In addition to collagen disregulation, another finding showed that hydroxyproline was increased in biopsies of sclerodermoid skin. This is believed to be the result of replacement of adipose tissue with connective tissue [39].

SUMMARY

Aging appears to be an ongoing imperative of life. Using the principles of aging and certain pathophysiologic illness displaying accelerated aging, we can continue to look for clues. In diabetes mellitus, progeria, and Werner's syndrome, fibroblast function is altered in a pattern similar to aging. In addition, all three patient groups suffer morbidity and mortality from cardiovascular illness similar to the general aging population. More research and observation are needed to understand more completely the mechanism of aging.

References

1. United States Census Bureau, May 12, 1997.
2. Schneider, E. L., and Rowe, J. W., "Handbook of the Biology of Aging," 3rd Ed. p. 11. Academic Press, New York, 1990.
3. Scandinavian Simvastatin Survival Study Group. Randomized trial of cholesterol lowering in 4444 patients with coronary heart disease: the Scandinavian Simvastain Survival Study (4S). *Lancet* **344,** 1383–1389 (1994).
4. Jose, A. D. Effect of combined sympathetic and parasympathetic blockade on heart rate and cardiac function in man. *Am. J. Cardiol.* **18,** 476 (1966).
5. Fleg, J. L., and Kennedy, H. L. Cardiac arrythmias in healthy elderly population: Detection by 24 hour ambulatory electrocardiography. *Chest* **81,** 302 (1982).
6. Lakatta, E. G. Determinants of cardiovascular performance: Modification due to aging. *J. Chronic Dis.* **36,** 15 (1993).
7. Lavker, R. M., and Sun, T. T. Heterogeneity in epidermal basal keratinocytes: Morphological and functional correlations. *Science* **215,** 1239 (1982).
8. Lavker, R. M., *et al.* Morphology of aged skin. *Clin. Geriatr. Med.* **5,** 53 (1989).
9. Shock, N. W. *In* "Proceedings of Seminars" (F. C. Jeffers, ed.), pp. 123–140. Center for the Study of Aging and Human Development, Duke University, Durham, NC, 1962.
10. Orgel, L. E. Aging of clones of mammalian cells. *Nature* **243,** 441–445 (1963).
11. Orgel, L. E. The maintenance of the accuracy of protein synthesis and its relevance to aging. *Proc. Natl. Acad. Sci. USA* **49,** 517–521 (1963).
12. Von Hahn, H. P. The regulation of protein synthesis in the aging cell. *Exp. Gerontol.* **5,** 323–334 (1970).
13. Harman, D. A theory based on free radical and radiation chemistry. *J. Gerontol.* **11,** 298–300 (1956).
14. Nohebel, D. C., and Walton, J. C. "Free Radical Chemistry." University Press, Cambidge, MA, 1974.
15. Cutler, R. G. Antioxidants and longevity of mammalian species. *In* "Molecular Biology of Aging" (A. D. Woodhead, A. D. Blackett, and A. Hollaender, eds.), pp. 15–73. Penum Press, New York, 1985.
16. Hayflick, L., and Moorhead, P. S. The serial cultivation of human diploid cell strains. *Exp. Cell Res.* **25,** 585 (1961).
17. Stein, G. H., Namba, M., and Corsaro, C. M. Relationship of finite proliferative life span, senescence, and quiescence in human cells. *J. Cell Physiol.* **122,** 343–349 (1985).
18. Shimokata, H., *et al.* Age as independent determinant of glucose tolerance. *Diabetes* **40,** 44 (1991).
19. Lipson, L. G. Diabetes in the elderly: diagnosis, pathogenesis, and theory. *Am. J. Med.* **80**(5a), 10–21 (1986).
20. Wilson, P. W. F., Anderson, K. M., and Kannel, W. Epidemiology of diabetes mellitus in the elderly. The Framingham Study. *Am. J. Med.* **80**(5a), 3–9 (1986).
21. Lipson, L. G., "Diabetes Mellitus in the Elderly: Special Problems, Special Approaches," pp. 1–16. Co Medica, New York, 1985.
22. Hamlin, C. R., Kohn, R. R., and Luschin, J. H. Apparent accelerated aging of human collagen in diabetes mellitus. *Diabetes.* **24,** 902–904 (1975).
23. Goldstein, S., Moerman, E. J., Soeldner, J. S., *et al.* Diabetes mellitus and genetic prediabetes: decreased replicative capacity of cultured skin fibroblasts. *J. Clin. Invest.* **63,** 358–370 (1979).
24. Kilo, C., Vogler, N., and Williamson, J. R. Muscle capillary basement membrane changes related to aging and to diabetes mellitus. *Diabetes* **21,** 881–905 (1972).

25. Bierman, E. L. Atherosclerosis and aging. *Fed. Proc.* **37,** 2832–2836 (1978).
26. Stansberry, K. B., *et al.* Impairment of peripheral blood flow response in diabetes resembles an enhanced aging effect. *Diabetes Care* **20**(11), 1711–1716 (1997).
27. Brown, W. T. Progeria: A human disease model of accelerated aging. *Am. J. Clin. Nutr.* **55,** 1222S (1992).
28. Martin, G. M., and Turker, M. S. Genetics of human disease, longevity and aging. *In* "Principles of Geriatric Medicine and Geronotology" (W. R. Hazzard, E. L. Bierman, J. P. Blass, W. H. Ettinger, and J. B. Halter, eds.), 3rd ed. pp. 19–35. McGraw-Hill, New York, 1994.
29. Hutchinson, J. Congenital absence of hair and mammary glands with atrophic condition of the skin and its appendages in a boy whose mother had been almost totally bald from alopecia areata from the age of six. *Medicochir Trans.* **69,** 473–477 (1886).
30. Guilford, H. Progeria: A form of senilism. *Practitioner* **73,** 188–217 (1904).
31. DeBusk, F. L. The Hutchinsoin–Gilford progeria syndrome. *J. Pediatr.* **90,** 697–724 (1972).
32. Abdenur, J. E., *et al.* Response to nutritional and growth hormone treatment in progeria. *Metab. Clin. Exp.* **46**(8), 851–856 (1997).
33. Gray, M. D., *et al.* The Werner syndrome protein is a DNA helicase. *Nature Genet,* **17**(1), 100–103 (1997).
34. Goto, M., *et al.* Genetic linkage of Werner's syndrome to five markers on chromosome 8. *Nature* **355,** 735 (1992).
35. Werner, O., "Uber Katarakt in Verbindung mt Sklerodermie." Doctoral dissertation, Kiel University, 1904.
36. Salk, D., *et al.,* "Werner's Syndrome and Human Aging." Plenum Press, New York, 1985.
37. Bauer, E. A., Silverman, N., Busiek, D. F., *et al.* Diminished response of Werner's syndrome fibroblasts to growth factors PDGF and FGF. *Science* **234,** 1240–1243 (1986).
38. Bauer, E. A., Uitto, J., Tan, E. M., *et al.* Werner's syndrome: Evidence for preferential regional expression of a generalized mesenchymal cell defect. *Arch. Dermatol.* **124,** 90–101 (1988).
39. Salk, D. Werner's syndrome: A review of recent research with analysis of connective tissue metabolism, growth control of cultured cells, and chromosomal aberrations. *Hum. Genet.* **62,** 1–15 (1982).

CHAPTER 7

Cellular Models of Human Aging

JULIE GLOWACKI Orthopedic Research, Brigham and Women's Hospital, Harvard Medical School; and Skeletal Biology Research Center, Massachusetts General Hospital, Harvard School of Dental Medicine, Boston, Massachusetts 02115

INTRODUCTION

There are many compatible and incompatible theories to explain age-related increases in disease and mortality. Finding age-related loss of function in many organ systems suggests either a single control point within an organism or innate common changes that occur throughout diverse tissue and organ types. There are two major types of aging theories, those that involve the accumulation of damage and those that have a genetic basis (Table I). Some theories have been derived from theoretical considerations and some from experimental data. Different models can be used to describe the theories or to test predictions based on the theories. Mathematical models of stochastic and deterministic influences on aging have been developed from data ranging in type from population statistics to locations of frequent somatic mutations in DNA. Molecular models of causes or effects of aging include postsynthetic changes in extracellular molecules such as collagen and elastin and in intracellular molecules such as DNA and enzymes. *Drosophila,* yeast, fungi, and the nematode *Caenorhabditis elegans* have provided detailed information about genetics and inheritance patterns for longevity. Animal models have been useful in testing theories about caloric restriction and genetic features that result in accelerated senescence. Precious colonies of aged rats and mice, either on standard chow or calorie restriction, are available from the National Institutes of Health and are widely used for experimentation.

Cellular models of human aging rely mainly on methods of cell biology and biochemistry. Cultivation of tissue and cells was developed at the beginning of this century. The challenge at that time was to develop growth media and conditions that were favorable for distinct cells types. Many investigators in the 1950s and 1960s formulated media that could be used for different types of cells and tissues, many of which are used today, retaining the scientists' names (Puck, Dulbecco, Eagle, Moscona, Ham). Since then, many of the obstacles to consistent and convenient cell and tissue culture have been removed, not the least of which is the commercial availability of media, sera, and culture vessels. Early progress on cultivating human cells concerned malignant tissues and highly proliferative tissues, such as spleen and bone marrow. Cellular models of human aging depended on suitable techniques for the *in vitro* growth of normal cells and tissues.

Although there are many differences between cultured cells and their counterparts *in vivo,* in part stemming from their dissociation from the three-dimensional array of tissues, research on mechanisms of cellular aging has been highly productive in developing and testing various theories. Three major approaches have been used in cytogerontology [1]. One is to follow cell cultures from normal donors through subcultivation *in vitro.* Comparisons of molecular or cellular features are made between cells from early and late passages. The second is to compare *in vitro* features of early passage cells from old and young individuals. The third is to compare cells obtained from individuals with accelerated aging syndromes, such as progeria or Werner syndrome, with cells from age-matched normal donors.

REPLICATIVE SENESCENCE

Aging *in Vitro*

Cells taken from an organism are called primary cells and will multiply in culture vessels. Upon reaching con-

TABLE I Mechanisms of Cellular Aging: Major Theories

Replicative senescence
Dimished proliferation
Dimished repair
Diminished differentiated function
Resistance to mutagenesis
Genomic damage, instability
Methylation patterns
Oxidation, glycosylation, conjugation, cross-links
Premutagenic changes
Mitochondrial DNA damage
Oxidation
Deletions, duplications, point mutations
Gene expression
Transcription factors
Modifications of cellular proteins
Stress response proteins
Heat shock proteins
Modifications in extracellular matrix proteins
Increased carbonyl content
Oxidation of amino acid residues
Increased glycation and glycosylation
Protein degradation

fluence, the primary culture can be subcultured into two new vessels; this process can be repeated at intervals, with the cells retaining many characteristics of the starting tissue. Alexis Carrel, one of the early investigators impressed with this process, proposed that somatic cells had an infinite life span *in vitro* [2]. It is now generally accepted that this is not the case. Fresh cells grow rapidly for a finite period, then their growth rate progressively declines. After several months, the cells stop growing and eventually they degenerate and die. Hayflick and Moorhead described the three phases of cell growth, decline, and senescence (Fig. 1) and showed that for cultured human fibroblasts, senescence takes place after some 50 generations when approximately 10^{22} cells have been produced from each primary cell [3,4]. It was clearly shown that it was not chronological time or metabolic history that was associated with senescence, but the finite number of cell divisions. Cells isolated from individuals of different age would therefore be expected to proliferate to different extents. Human embryonic cells will grow for some 50 generations and cells from adult tissue enter senescence after 20 generations. Although it may be overly simplistic to extrapolate the behavior of cells *in vitro* to mechanisms of *in vivo* aging and although the artificial nature of culture conditions is likely to introduce artifacts in cell behavior, finding more replicative capacity for cells from younger than older subjects is consistent with the Hayflick theory. Studies with cells from patients with Werner syndrome, progeria, or other conditions of accelerated aging or age-related disorders also support the relevance of proliferative capacity to *in vivo* aging.

The Cell Cycle

A strict sequence of events leads to the duplication of cells, called the cell cycle. DNA synthesis and cell division are the two most obvious events. Appreciation of the events in the cell cycle and in the stringent regulation of a cell's progression through the cycle is fundamental to understanding the significance of changes detected in senescent cells.

DNA synthesis occurs in S phase, beginning slowly, reaching a maximum, and decelerating until DNA synthesis is complete, in 6 to 7 hr for mammalian cells. DNA replication is paralleled by histone gene expression, producing the basic chromosomal proteins necessary for packaging newly replicated DNA into chromosomes. After a short period, G2, usually 2 to 3 hr, the first evidence of mitosis is detectable in cell culture.

Mitosis of cells in culture is heralded by the rounding of the cell in early prophase. In this phase, chromosomes condense and the nuclear membrane disappears. In metaphase, the condensed chromosomes are massed in the center of the cell, which is only loosely attached to the dish. The centrioles migrate to opposite poles of the cell and the mitotic spindle is formed, joining the cell membrane through the centrioles to the centromere of each chromosome. At anaphase, the two sets of chromosomes move to opposite poles and at telophase, they decondense while the cell membrane encloses each new daughter cell. As the cells flatten, the nuclear membranes and nucleoli reform. Mitosis requires 1 hr for mammalian cells. After mitosis, the cells enter the G1 phase, the duration of which accounts for variations in cycle time for different cell types, from unmeasurable for some cells to longer than 20 hr for others. In G1, cells retain enzymes required for the next round of DNA synthesis. Cells that have lost these enzymes are not prepared for DNA synthesis and enter into a quiescent phase, G0. Addition of a stimulus can return the cells to G1. Nonreplicating, terminally differentiated cells are generally arrested in the G0 stage.

Intracellular Inhibitors of Growth

In brief, different types of factors regulate the different phases of the cycle. Upon stimulation to proliferate, the fos/jun-related early response genes activate the genes needed for DNA biosynthesis [5]. Cyclin-related

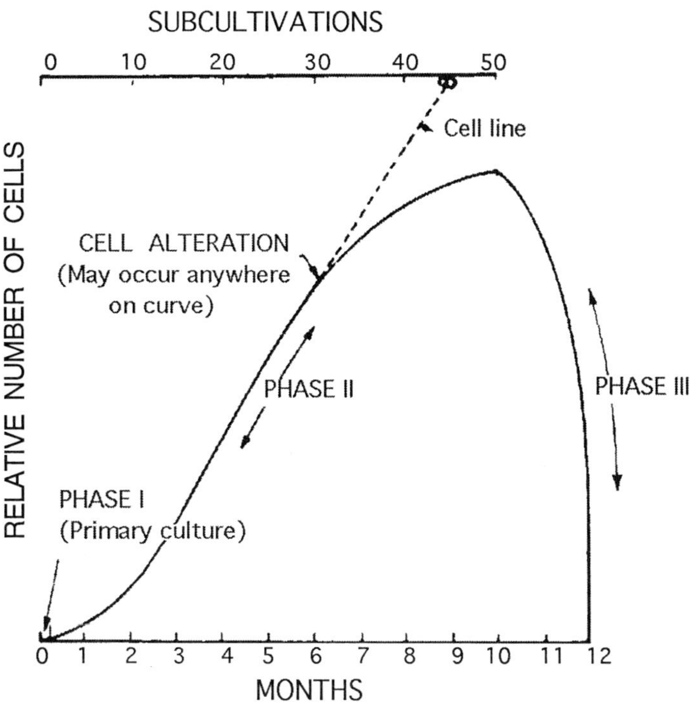

FIGURE 1 Representation of the change in relative numbers of normal somatic cells after phase I, the primary culture during which they form a confluent monolayer. Cells in phase II expand as cell strains but enter phase III with declining growth, senescence, and a finite life span unless an alteration transforms them into a cell line with an infinite life span. Reproduced with permission from Hayflick and Moorhead [3].

proteins control cycle progression by activating kinases that phosphorylate transcription factors that, in turn, regulate genes of proliferation [6]. The proliferation of normal cells is thought to be regulated by growth-promoting protooncogenes counterbalanced by growth-constraining tumor suppresser genes. The most thoroughly investigated tumor suppresser genes are RB1 (the retinoblastoma tumor suppresser protein) and p53. Inactivation of these genes can be achieved by a protein called large T antigen, which is encoded by the transforming gene of SV40. Thus the oncoprotein of SV40 neutralizes the two major proteins that exert a negative control on cell growth, resulting in the immortalization of the target cell. The same phenomenon occurs with human papilloma virus type 16 and with adenovirus type 5. Cell transformation by inactivation of RB1 and p53 can also be achieved by point mutations and deletions in somatic cells, a mechanism documented in many human cancers. Evidence suggests that p53 is involved in a DNA damage response pathway that is activated on formation of dicentric chromosomes when telomeres are lost. Activation of p53 produces a block in the G1 phase that is manifest as senescence [7].

Understanding of the roles of protooncogenes and the cyclins in growth, differentiation, and cancer sets the stage for characterization of cellular senescence. Because senescent cells appear to be blocked in the G1 phase and cannot enter S phase, comparisons have been made between the responses of young and old quiescent fibroblasts to serum stimulation. Of the genes that are altered in senescent cells, there are several candidate causal genes [8,9]. At this time, evidence indicates that the immediate causes of the failure of senescent cells to proliferate are the repression of growth regulators and overexpression of the growth inhibitors. Replicative senescence has been attributed to the repression of three key transcription regulators (c-fos, Id, and E2F), the overexpression of a cdk inhibitor, and to the constitutive expression of the growth inhibitors p53 and RB1, most likely mediated by the repression of mdm2 and ensuing overexpression of p21. Any one of these would be sufficient to inhibit proliferation, but unsuccessful attempts to reactivate proliferation by providing cells with c-fos, Id, E2F, and mdm2 [10] support the view that over- or constitutive expression of growth inhibitors (tumor suppressor genes) may have central importance in aging (Fig. 2). There are conflicting data about changes in p53 levels, perhaps explained because expression depends on exposure to mitogens. With *in vitro* senescence, there is an increase in p53 protein and in mRNA when the

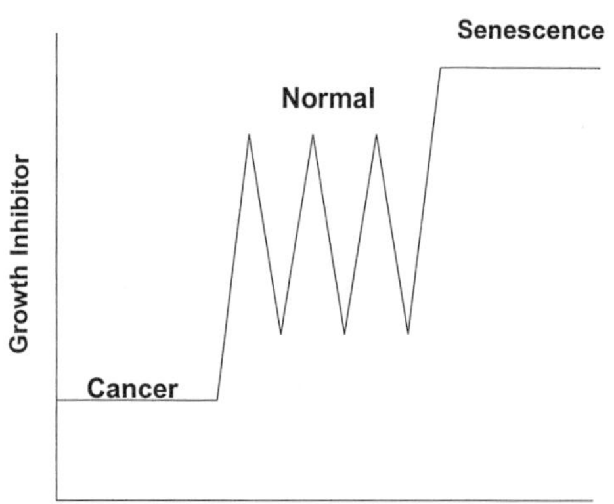

FIGURE 2 Relative level of activity of cell growth inhibitors (tumor suppressor genes, e.g., p21, p53 or RB) in cancer, normal growth, and senescence. In normal cells, growth inhibitors are downregulated when quiescent cells are exposed to a mitogen. Many cancers are characterized by neutralization of these inhibitors. Senescence may be explained by constitutive expression of these inhibitors.

latter is expressed on a per cell basis, but not always on the basis of total RNA [11]. Even when p53 mRNA per total RNA was reported to be similar in early and late passage cells, its DNA-binding activity and transcriptional activity were increased in the senescent cells [12]. Use of stable p53 reporter constructs demonstrated an inverse relationship between p53 expression and DNA synthesis in cultured cells [13]. Overexpression of a p53 transgene resulted in the arrest of the cell cycle and induction of the senescent phenotype [14]. To the converse, microinjection of monoclonal antibodies to p53 induced senescent cells to reenter S phase, undergo mitosis, and result in increased cell numbers [15]. Evidence for both p53 and RB involvement in cellular senescence came from transfections of cells with wild-type SV40 T antigen or a mutant form lacking either the p53- or the RB-binding domains [16]. Human fibroblasts immortalized with the wild-type transgene became senescent upon deinduction of T antigen, but only if the p53- and RB-binding domains were intact.

Until recently, there was no clear understanding of the mechanism by which a cell's ability to divide was diminished with aging. As discussed later, telomeres play a central role in proliferative capacity. Evidence suggests that p53 is activated as a result of telomere shortening to a critical length. Other data shed some light on the relationship between senescence and apoptosis, or programmed cell death. It was shown that expression of p53 induces apoptosis in a myeloid leukemic cell line [17]. Such information supports the view that genes that promote cellular senescence do so, in part, by leading to the death of certain cell types rather than to transformation or the risk of transformation, in light of increased cell damage.

Other data indicate additional mechanisms that can be linked to cellular senescence. Inactivation of the G2 checkpoint in fibroblasts expressing the E6 oncoprotein was coincident with telomere erosion and chromosomal abnormalities [18]. Inactivation of p21 (an inhibitor of cyclin-dependent kinase) averted senescence in normal fibroblasts [19].

There are those who speculate that replicative senescence is a fundamental mechanism, at least in mammals, for suppressing the consequences of life: chromosomal change, malignant mutations, and mitochondrial damage [20]. Replicative senescence may have evolved to curtail tumorigenesis, but may also have the unselected effect of contributing to age-related pathologies, including cancer [21].

TELOMERE LENGTH

Recent information on telomeres in cancer and in aging shed mechanistic light on the phenomenon of replicative senescence. Human telomeres consist of repeats of the sequence TTAGGG at the ends of chromosomes. They serve to protect chromosomal ends from degradation and fusion with other chromosomes. They are required by DNA polymerase to initiate 5′-to-3′ DNA replication, which occurs on one strand of DNA as a discontinuous process and produces separate segments called Okazaki fragments (Fig. 3a). Degradation of the RNA primers in the lagging strand is followed by ligation of the fragments, but the 3′ end of the parental strand is left incompletely copied (Fig. 3b) [22–25]. Telomere length is about 15 kbp in germline cells, but is significantly shorter in most human somatic tissues. With each cell division *in vitro,* human telomeres shorten by 50 to 100 bp. This shortening is linked to decreased replicative capacity of cells. When several kilobase pairs are lost, cells stop dividing and senesce. The telomere hypothesis of cellular aging proposes that cells become senescent when a threshold telomere length is reached [26]. Somatic cells show a loss of the terminal restriction fragments, determined by the size of the sequences that hybridize to a $(CCCTAA)_3$ probe (Fig. 4). When the end is lost or reaches a critical length in one telomere, a checkpoint is reached, the Hayflick limit, and the cell can no longer divide. At cell crisis, gross chromosomal aberrations are evident. The telomere hypothesis is upheld by measures of telomere length in cells obtained from young and old subjects, resulting in an estimate of loss of telomere length by 15 bp/year *in vivo.* In contrast to normal senescent cells, certain stem cells or germline cells maintain telomere length by telomerase activity and have a greater proliferative capacity, i.e., a longer life span, than somatic cells. Furthermore, many

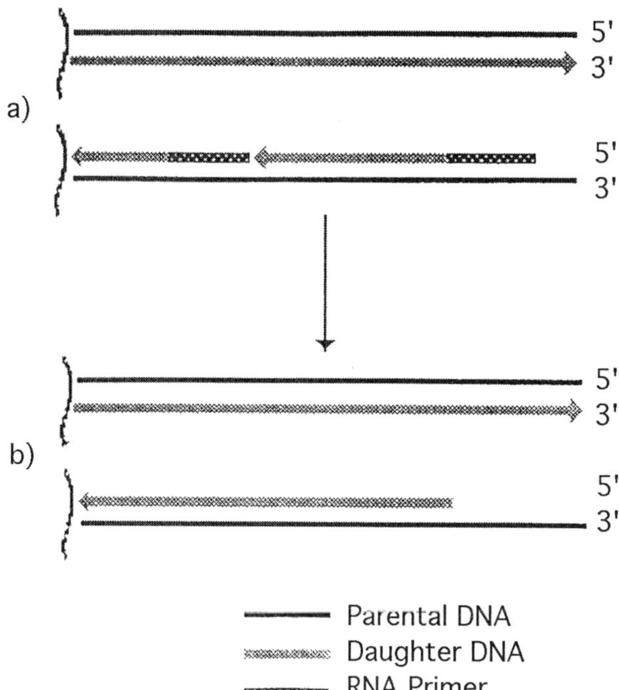

FIGURE 3 The end replication problem. (a) In DNA replication, the 3′-5′ parental strand is copied in a continuous manner by DNA polymerase, but the 5′-3′ strand is copied discontinuously as Okazaki fragments with labile RNA primers. (b) After removal of the RNA primers, filling of the gaps, and ligation of the fragments, the 3′ end of the parental strand is incompletely copied with shortening after each round of DNA replication. Reprinted from Harley [26], with permission from Elsevier Science.

transformed or immortalized cells are characterized by the maintenance of telomere length, either by the activation of telomerase or by an alternative mechanism. Telomerase is a ribonucleoprotein polymerase that specifically catalyzes the extension of the 3′ ends of the parent DNA [27,28].

Although many factors influence the regulation of telomere length in different organisms, such as DNA replication enzymes, telomerase, telomere-binding proteins, telomere-capping proteins, and repressors of telomerase [29], in human cells telomere length is not maintained with cell division and telomerase is not active in normal tissues to mediate the elongation of shortened telomeres. Not all cells in an individual have the same replicative history. Studies in vascular tissue reveal differences in telomere length in different anatomical sites. Endothelial cells from iliac arteries showed a greater rate of telomere shortening than endotheliocytes from iliac veins [24]. Those data are consistent with higher hemodynamic stress and greater cell turnover in arteries. A large body of indirect evidence suggests a causal relationship between telomere loss and replicative senescence [26,30–33]. In general, species with long life spans have somatic cells with longer replicative potential *in vitro.*

There are two studies that provide direct evidence supporting the hypothesis that telomere length determines the proliferative capacity of human cells. In a study in which mortal cells were fused with an immortal line in which telomeres were elongated, it was found that the resulting hybrid had a longer life span than hybrids in which telomeres were not elongated [34]. The telomere hypothesis recently gained weighty evidence in its support. Human cells that were transfected to express the reverse transcriptase subunit of telomerase displayed elongation of telomeres and spectacular continuation of proliferation [35]. They did not appear to be malignant; rather those cells maintained the normal karyotype and morphology through many generations. The ultimate test will be whether the introduction of telomerase in somatic cells will maintain telomere length and extend the cell's life span without introducing genomic instability, loss of contact inhibition, and anchorage independence that characterize transformed cancer cells.

It had been thought that telomere shortening is a tumor-suppressing mechanism, but that does not appear to be the case for all species. Studies with telomerase knockout mice showed that their cells, which did display accelerated senescence, were in fact capable of malignant transformation [36]. Clearly, many mechanisms can lead to malignant changes in cells and there are many ways in which senescence and cancer are uncoupled. Unfortunately, though, mouse cells are not good models for evaluating the role of telomeric decline in senescence because the mouse does not have stringent repression of telomerase in somatic tissues and the mouse has telomeres three times longer than human's; nevertheless, murine cells do not live longer *in vitro* [37].

There is great interest in the precise mechanisms whereby telomere shortening leads to a senescent phenotype [21]. As mentioned earlier, telomere shortening may be recognized by a "surveillance" function of p53 as a form of chromosomal damage. Data that support this hypothesis were obtained from fibroblasts of subjects with ataxia telangiectasia [7]. Those cells lost telomeres at an accelerated rate and the formation of dicentric chromosomes coincided with the activation of p53 protein and premature senescence.

The telomere hypothesis may be shown to be oversimplified as more is learned about participating and alternate mechanisms of cellular aging. On the one hand, one group of scientists is attempting to "treat" senescence by upregulating telomerase; on the other hand, other investigators are attempting to treat cancer by inhibiting telomerase. The delicate control of cell division is balanced by many factors to allow cells to

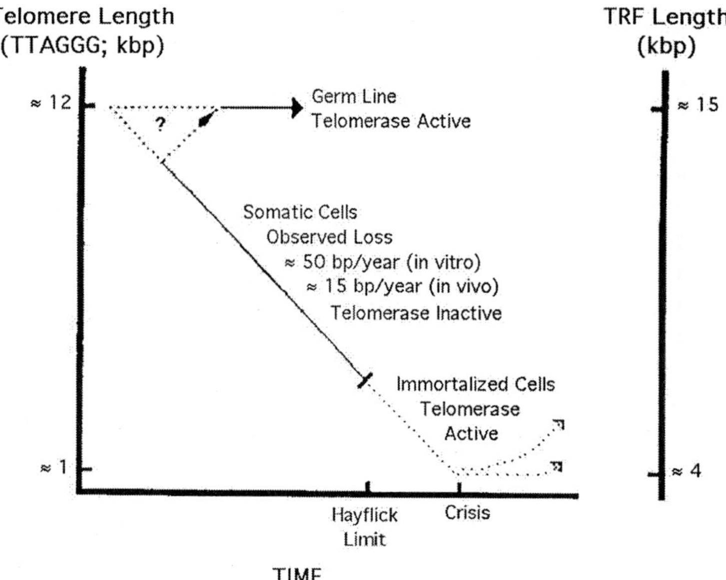

FIGURE 4 The telomere hypothesis for human cell aging and transformation. Telomere length [or length of genomic DNA that hybridizes to a $(CCCTAA)_3$ probe] and TRF (or terminal restriction fragment) are maintained in germline cells or cells with activated telomerase. Otherwise, as in human fibroblasts, telomeres shorten by 50 bp/doubling *in vitro* or by 15 bp/year *in vivo*. Reprinted from Harley [26], with permission from Elsevier Science.

grow within limits. The linkage of telomere shortening to constitutive expression of growth inhibitors (tumor suppresser genes) provides a satisfying unifying hypothesis for future investigations.

GENE EXPRESSION

Somatic Chromosomal Mutations

Aging can be explained in part as a stochastic process of molecular damage. This is described as a somatic mutation theory, according to which generalized deterioration of the genome throughout an organism or specific damage to vulnerable domains results in loss of function or senescence. This theory is usually associated with Szilard [38]. Spontaneous chromosomal rearrangements occur more commonly in cells from older than younger individuals. Peripheral blood lymphocytes have become a model for studying chromosomal aberrations in humans; they show between two- and ninefold increases in gross rearrangements with age [39].

At a higher level of analysis, somatic mutations can be measured in selectable genes, e.g., hypoxanthine–guanine phosphoribosyltransferase (HPRT). Mutation frequency of HPRT was reported 0.6×10^{-6} in newborns and 16×10^{-6} in the aged [40]. The functional significance of somatic mutations is unclear. Among known human disease loci, there are certain features that render those sites prone to mutations, e.g., the presence of highly mutable CpG sites, the degree of sequence repeats, or aspects of regional genomic architecture [41]. Such hot spots may provide a physical link between the concepts of stochastic and programmed processes in senescence.

The free radical theory of aging is based on the nature of free radical reactions and their ubiquitous presence in living systems, being generated from enzymatic and, to a lesser extent, nonenzymatic reactions. The former include reactions in the respiratory chain. Reactive oxygen species (ROS) can interact with intracellular nucleic acids, proteins, and lipids. ROS are the best known factors that can cause molecular alterations in living systems. Efficient repair systems are needed to remove such by-products from tissues. Various age-associated biochemical changes in DNA have been identified (reviewed in Ref. 42), including oxidation products, conjugates of DNA nucleotides with genotoxic malondialdehyde (the major product of lipid peroxidation), bulky covalent I-compounds (some of which are linked to diet but are paradoxically increased with calorie restriction), glycosylation, protein–DNA cross-links, and alterations in methylation patterns.

Somatic Mutations in Mitochondrial DNA

Mutations in mitochondrial DNA (mtDNA) may also account for senescence-related cellular changes.

Mitochondria are semiautonomous cell organelles. The majority of mitochondrial proteins are encoded in nuclear DNA, synthesized in the cytoplasm, and imported into mitochondria. mtDNA is 16.6 kb in length and encodes 13 proteins of respiration and 22 tRNAs and 2 rRNAs. It is particularly vulnerable to damage, with up to a 100-fold greater mutation rate than nuclear DNA; mtDNA is naked, lacking histones, and there is little DNA repair capacity in mitochondria. Mitochondrial DNA is inherited via the oocyte cytoplasm and is thus of maternal origin. A number of specific myopathies, duplications, deletions, or point neuropathies, and encephalomyopathies are due to specific mtDNA mutations, either inherited as such or acquired during embryogenesis [43]. With aging, there is an increase in the number of large deletions [44]. Although deletions in mtDNA increase with aging up to 10,000-fold, they represent only 0.1% of the total mtDNA in that tissue. The mutant mtDNA appears to be distributed in a mosaic manner, however, with some cells completely energy deficient, as determined by histochemical staining for cytochrome c oxidase [45]. The accumulation of bioenergitically defective cells may reach a threshold for diminished organ function.

The damage to mtDNA may be due to free radicals that are generated within the organelle. Oxidative damage to mtDNA is reported to be 10 times the level for nuclear DNA for the same tissue [46]. Evidence from studies of mtDNA in particular has resulted in a blending of somatic mutation and free radical theories of aging. Accumulation of damage may account for age-related decreases in bioenergetic functions of tissues. Cells of the central nervous system, cardiac muscle, skeletal muscle, and liver would be especially vulnerable to this degeneration. Thus the mtDNA theory of aging addresses generalized aspects of aging as well as age-associated diseases of specific organ systems.

Regulation of Gene Expression

Analyses of cells as they become senescent indicate an array of changes in gene expression, including the repression of growth stimulatory genes, overexpression of growth inhibitory genes, and interference with downstream pathways. Molecular analyses have identified many changes in gene expression and activity during cellular aging, but the question is always which changes could be causal and which result from senescence. Aging alters the level of constitutive gene expression and gene regulation by hormonal or cytokine factors. Some age-associated changes have been shown as alterations in rates of transcription, in pools of mRNA, and steady-state levels of proteins.

Comparison of cDNA libraries from senescent and normal fibroblasts shows differential expression of known and unknown genes [47]. One of the genes upregulated in late passage fibroblasts was identified as IGFBP-3 [48]. In addition, novel genes have been discovered by subtractive enrichment of a cDNA library from a subject with Werner syndrome of premature aging [49]. One of these, S1-5, which contains EGF-like consensus sequences, was overexpressed in late passage normal cells and was induced by the growth arrest of early passage cells [50]. This experimental approach also led to the discovery that there are reduced functional integrin–fibronectin receptors ($\alpha_5\beta_1$) on senescent fibroblasts [51]. A number of the other genes that are overexpressed in late passage fibroblasts have been identified, including a calcium-binding smooth muscle protein [52], a lysyl oxidase-like protein involved in cell adhesion [53], a calcium-binding protein involved in cell membrane currents [54], plasminogen activator inhibitor-1 (PAI-1) [55], and osteonectin [55]. There are some data showing that some of these genes are coordinately upregulated due to an increase in the stability of mRNA, but others also show increased rates of transcription [55].

Similar differential screening and subtractive hybridization techniques with rat embryo fibroblast cell lines that were conditionally immortalized with SV40 T antigen resulted in cloning of eight senescence-induced genes and one senescence-repressed gene [56]. Three of those genes encode for extracellular matrix proteins (α1-procollagen, osteonectin, and fibronectin); some of the others are involved in calcium-dependent signal transduction pathways. Those genes were also found to be overexpressed in human osteoblasts and in normal rat fibroblasts that were undergoing senescence *in vitro*. Information is needed whether such changes are separate effects of aging or multiple consequences of a single cause.

Stress response genes provide a valuable example of age-associated changes in cellular reactions to various stresses in eliciting protective and reparative processes [57]. Common experimental tools for revealing age-related changes include exposure to stimuli such as bacterial endotoxin or lipopolysaccharide, oxidative radicals, phorbol esters, heavy metals, hyperthermia, or ultraviolet radiation. There is sufficient similarity in a cell's response to those diverse stimuli to generalize about mechanisms that are altered with aging. Aging alters NF-κB, Ap-1 (fos, jun), heat shock factors, CCAAT/enhancer binding protein (C/EBPs), and the glucocorticoid receptor, each of which is involved in a cell's response to stresses. There is a large literature on the effects of aging to suppress the many signal pathways and the cascades of downstream events that are mediated through those stress response genes. It has been proposed that these transcriptional activities are linked to signal transduction and/or redox pathways [57]. Thus it may be possible to merge the free radical theory to specific gene expression.

FUNCTIONAL SENESCENCE *IN VITRO*

General

Many observational and associational studies have provided a catalog of changes that cells undergo with aging. Skin fibroblasts have been a useful model for functional senescence. Human skin imparts visible information about our age: with aging, skin becomes thinner, looses elasticity, and develops wrinkling. These tissue changes reflect the accumulation of old matrix and the decreased renewal of old with new. At the level of the cell, phenotypic signs of aging depend on the cell type, but for the commonly studied cells, fibroblasts and endothelial cells, they are increased cell size, increased accumulation of lysosomes, and generalized decreased rates of protein synthesis and degradation.

Late passage fibroblasts show increased levels of proteins encoded by overexpressed genes, of which IGFBP-3 has greatest interest. Both the absolute amount of IGFBP-3 protein and the molar ratio of IGFBP-3/IGF-II were higher in senescent cells, but it is not clear whether IGFBP-3 plays an adaptive or causal role in senescence [58]. In addition, fetal cells secreted the lowest levels of IGFBP-3, and postnatal cells showed a strong positive correlation between donor age and accumulation of IGFBP-3 in conditioned medium [59]. It is likely that IGF and its binding proteins are involved in cellular senescence. Transfection of full-length IGFBP-3 cDNA into fibroblasts reduced colony formation and exogenous IGFBP-3 inhibited IGF-I-stimulation of DNA synthesis in early passage cells [60].

Senescence-associated β-galactosidase (SA-β-Gal) has been used to identify and enumerate senescent human cells. It is active at pH 6.0 and is readily distinguished from the lysosomal enzyme, which is active at pH 4.0. It is not proposed to be a cause of cellular aging, but it is a change that invariably accompanies cellular aging both *in vivo* and *in vitro* [61]. A variety of cultures, including human fibroblasts, keratinocytes, endothelial cells, and mammary epithelial cells, show more SA-β-Gal-positive cells with passage number. Terminally differentiated cells and serum-deprived quiescent cells did not express the marker; thus its appearance was restricted to senescence. In addition, in both dermis and epidermis, SA-β-Gal-positive cells were found to be more abundant in older than younger subjects [10]. These findings support the view that senescent cells do accumulate in aged tissue. It will be important to determine whether the marker is linked to processes that are altered with aging, like wound repair. Even if the accumulation of such cells does not contribute to tissue or organ age-associated pathology, more information about the distribution of this marker in skeletal and other tissues would be useful. Development of other gene or functional markers will be needed for progress with cellular models of human aging.

Age-associated posttranslational changes in proteins include general biochemical alterations that may be conformational or covalent. Modifications can be detected by measurements of specific enzyme activity, thermal stability, extent of carbonyl modifications, oxidation of amino acids residues, glycation, glycoxidation, and conjugation with lipid oxidation products such as malondialdehyde. Some of the age-related modifications of cellular phosphoproteins may be due to autophosphorylation or activation of new isozyme genes [62]. Of particular interest are the advanced glycosylation end products (giving the abbreviation AGEs) that are formed by multiple pathways, are increased with aging, and are implicated in Alzheimer's, diabetes, and certain eye disorders (reviewed in Ref. 63). Cellular and tissue accumulation of damaged proteins is dependent on the concentration of ROS, inhibitors of oxidation, and the rate of degradation of oxidized proteins. Although it is appreciated that there is an age-dependent loss of neutral protease activity [64], it is likely due to a combination of mechanisms including gene expression, rate of enzyme synthesis, posttranslational modifications, inhibition by other proteins, and by oxidation itself. A large number of factors are involved in determining the accumulation of modified proteins with age. The level of protein damage may be the net effect of a vast number of age-related changes that are ultimately manifested by this measure. The free radical theory of aging holds that proteins, as well as DNA, show age-associated accumulation of damage that leads to specific "free radical diseases." Atherosclerotic lesions can be initiated and enhanced by irritants like those formed by the oxidation of lipoproteins or oxidative polymerization. Support for the importance of the antioxidant defense mechanism is indicated by the increased life span of *Drosophila* that overexpress antioxidant enzymes. The free radical theory gives rise to the idea that aging or its effects can be inhibited by antioxidant therapies. Amyloidosis and immune deficiency of age have both been inhibited in animals with antioxidant therapy [42]. Controlled clinical evaluation is needed to show whether the human life span can be prolonged by diets and supplements designed to minimize free radical reactions.

In sum, studies with model cell systems indicate that aging is associated with an overall decline in protein synthesis and turnover and an accumulation of damaged molecules. Both increases and decreases are found in the levels of specific proteins; such variations may be due to particular mechanisms of gene regulation or may reflect the generalized loss of control of gene expression [65,66].

Bone Cells

It is possible to isolate and cultivate cells from human bone with phenotypic features of osteoblasts or osteocytes [67,68]. Alkaline phosphatase activity and gene expression, synthesis of collagen type I, and expression of bone sialoprotein and osteocalcin are standard markers of bone cell activity. Human osteoblasts showed the same age-dependent decrease in growth rate as did dermal fibroblasts from the same normal subjects [69]. A study of 87 subjects aged 2 to 88 years showed no age difference in cell growth or in total protein, alkaline phosphatase, and osteocalcin synthesis, but did report an age-dependent decrease in the numbers of cells at confluence [70]. A more recent investigation showed that mitogenic responses of human trabecular osteoblasts showed an age-dependent decline in response to various agents, including parathyroid hormone (PTH), growth hormone, calcitonin, transforming growth factor β, IGF-I, and platelet-derived growth factor [71]. Alkaline phosphatase activity was reported to not differ with age or gender, but osteocalcin was lower in cells from women than from men and also showed a significant decrease with the age of the donor [72]. A recent investigation of endosteal bone cells found that cell growth and protein production were impaired in cultures from men over the age of 50 years and that production of osteocalcin upon treatment with 1,25-dihydroxyvitamin D_3 was significantly depressed in older donors (>50 years of age) [73]. A comparison of human osteoblasts showed lower cyclic AMP responses to PTH by cells from older than from younger subjects and by cells from osteoporotic subjects than from controls [74]. This indicates that analysis of risk factors for osteoporosis may be advisable for studies with bone cells from older subjects. Further, as in many studies of human cell types, it is likely that culture conditions are important in integrating information from different reports. Clearly, more information is needed from studies with isolated osteoblasts from young and old individuals.

The osteogenic potential of bone marrow was demonstrated by classic work of Friedenstein *et al.* [75] and Ashton *et al.* [76]. Age-related histological changes in marrow from red to white, to fatty, and to gelatinous are associated with diminished bone mass [77]. Changes in the relative functional activities of marrow-derived, bone-forming osteoblasts and bone-resorbing osteoclasts could account for differences in skeletal metabolism with aging. Some literature exists in support of this hypothesis, mainly from animal studies. Age-related defects have been shown in the number and proliferative potential of mouse and rat stromal cells and an associated increase was observed in the osteoclast progenitor pool in those animals [78–84]. Human bone marrow cells have been examined for osteogenic potential *in vitro* [85–87], but there is little direct information on the molecular effects of age. An examination of 28 samples of marrow from men between 37 and 80 years of age showed an age-related decline in differentiation of osteoblasts in 3D culture ($r = -0.48$, $p < 0.01$) [88]. This is consistent with the hypothesis that with age, human bone marrow cells have reduced potential for osteoblastogenesis (Fig. 5). More information is needed to determine whether this is due to a loss of progenitor or precursor cells, to diminished capacity to function as osteoblasts, to alterations in the environment to promote adipogenesis, to increased potential to support osteoclastogenesis, or to all of these and other possibilities. Such information is needed before rational schemes for intervention can be contemplated.

Several studies with human bone marrow cells suggest that donor age influences a number of properties that may be involved in skeletal metabolism. For example, human marrow cells secrete IGF-I, IGF-binding proteins, and IGFBP-3 protease, with IGFBP-3 showing an increase with age [89]. That increase was similar to that previously found for human skin fibroblasts [58]. There is some information about the effects of age on osteoclastogenesis in cultured human marrow. There is

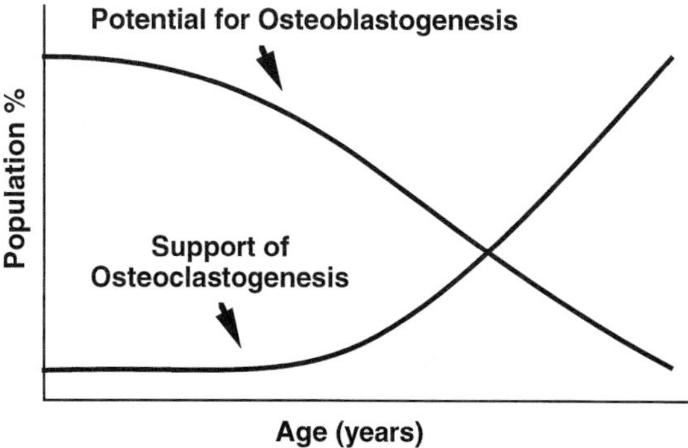

FIGURE 5 Hypothesis on the role of bone marrow in skeletal aging. With age, the number of stromal cells with the capacity to differentiate to osteoblasts may decrease. This may be linked to an increased capacity of stromal cells to support differentiation of osteoclasts from hematopoietic cells. Both of these changes could contribute to loss of bone mass with age.

an increase in the number of osteoclast-like cells generated *in vitro* [90] and an increase in constitutive secretion of interleukins-6 and -11, both of which stimulate osteoclast differentiation [91]. These data are consistent with the hypotheses presented in Figure 5. Thus, it appears that marrow cell cultures may be useful in the analysis of age-related changes in the roles of marrow cells and products in skeletal metabolism.

Tissues That Produce Sex Steroids

There have been cell culture studies of ovaries and testes from aging humans, but most of it concerns development of eggs and sperm. Data are available that indicate that there is a primary impairment of testosterone synthesis from progesterone and pregnenolone in cells from elderly men [92–94].

The adrenal gland can be linked to skeletal senescence because of the adrenopause (see Chapter 15) and the gradual decline of serum dehydroepiandrosterone (DHEA) and its sulfated form (DHEAS). DHEA(S) has been shown to influence serum IGF-I levels in humans [95]. Cell culture techniques may become important for our understanding of the effects of age on adrenal cortex function. Plasma DHEA(S) levels reflect synthesis by the adrenal cortex. The cortex is composed of three morphological zones: the outer zona glomerulosa, the middle zona fasciculata, and the inner zona reticularis. The glomerulosa is the site of aldosterone synthesis, the fasciculata is the source of glucocorticoids, and the reticularis is the zone responsible for the synthesis of DHEA(S). There are some indications that the fasciculata may also synthesize DHEA, but there is no information about its contribution during growth and aging. Unlike basal plasma cortisol concentration and its stimulation by adrenocorticotropic hormone (ACTH), both of which are maintained in aging, DHEA(S) declines after young adulthood to very low or negligible levels after age 70 (reviewed in Chapter 15). Although the ratio of DHEA(S) to cortisol biosynthesis varies widely in human health and disease, each is under regulatory control by ACTH [96]. Analysis of steroid synthesis by cultured fetal human adrenocortical cells from the reticularis shows that the major intermediates of DHEA, 17α-hydroxypregnenolone and 17α-hydroxyprogesterone, are the same intermediates used in the fasciculata for the synthesis of cortisol. In the adrenal there are multiple points of enzymatic competition for intermediate substrates, with the key determining enzyme being 3β-hydroxysteroid dehydrogenase (3β-HSD). Measures of the level of mRNA, protein, and activity of 3β-HSD indicate its abundance outside the reticularis; if this enzyme is inhibited, even the fasciculata will synthesize DHEA. Hornsby and Aldern [97] proposed that adrenarche may be viewed as tissue remodeling of the adrenal, resulting in the increased production of DHEA, and that, by analogy, the adrenopause may reflect a decrease in the number of functional reticularis cells. Tests of this hypothesis require greater understanding of the regulation of adrenal enzymes and availability of human tissue.

CELLULAR AGING IN PROGERIA AND WERNER SYNDROMES

Diseases of accelerated aging are rare and may be poor models for normal aging (see Chapter 6). Progeria syndrome (Hutchinson–Gilford syndrome) has a clinical picture different from the process of normal aging. Subtle indicators of disease may be present within the first year of life. Early manifestations imply fundamental deficiencies in growth: skeletal hypoplasia and dysplasia, marked delay in ossification of fontanels, delayed eruption of dentition, and hypoplasia of hair follicles and nails. Later abnormalities suggest premature aging: relentless arterial atheromatosis, left ventricular hypertrophy, thinning of skin, and loss of subcutaneous fat. Although the syndrome is more complex than natural aging, prudent use of progeric cells can provide a reference for cellular studies of normal senescence. Werner syndrome is an autosomal recessive disorder, characterized by the premature onset and accelerated rate of geriatric disorders such as atherosclerosis, diabetes mellitus, osteoporosis, cataracts, and various neoplasms. It is usually not diagnosed until young adult life. Cockayne syndrome, acrogeria, and metageria have been described with senile-like appearance, but are not well characterized.

Cellular and DNA replicative potentials have been shown to be reduced in cells from unrelated patients with Werner syndrome and in a progeric strain called CRL 1277 [98].

Analyses of cells from subjects with Werner syndrome showed greater shortening of telomeres [99]. Those cells also showed other features indicative of premature cellular aging, such as elevated rates of nonhomologous recombination and decreased repair of DNA; all three of these abnormalities were suggestive of fundamental alterations in DNA.

The Werner syndrome gene has been cloned and encodes for a protein that is a member of the RecQ family of DNA helicases and that catalyzes DNA unwinding [100]. Several helicase gene mutations have been discovered, especially in a Japanese series [101].

A number of abnormalities have been found in the functional capacity of skin fibroblasts from Werner syndrome patients, including an increased synthesis of collagen and a decreased synthesis of collagenase [102], an increased synthesis of hyaluronan [103], a greater synthesis of fibronectin [104], and alterations in cell surface glycosaminoglycans [105]. In addition, Werner fibroblasts also show diminished mitogenic and regulatory responses to platelet-derived growth factor (PDGF) and fibroblast growth factor (FGF) [106]. Differential screening of cDNA expression libraries indicated that a number of genes are overexpressed in Werner syndrome compared to normal fibroblasts [107,108]. Of the nine known and nine unknown genes, at least five were also overexpressed in late passage normal fibroblasts and may be specific for senescence not for Werner syndrome. Those include insulin-like growth factor I-binding protein 3 (IGFBP-3), α 1 (I) procollagen, fibronectin, WS3-10, and WS9-14. Expression of many of these genes is greater in late passage than early passage normal fibroblasts.

SUMMARY

Is aging fundamentally a stochastic or programmed event? Human aging is a complex process likely to involve multiple mechanisms of damaging changes. It is likely that several mechanisms contribute to cellular senescence. Evidence presented here shows how readily the various aging theories can be merged. A unified theory would hold that aging results from the combined effects of damage to vulnerable regulatory genes linked to the shortening of telomeres. Oxidative damage to nuclear DNA, including base alterations, single-strand breaks, sister chromatid exchanges, and DNA–protein cross-links, is termed oxygen toxicity or the oxygen paradox, a fundamental risk in aerobic life forms. Impairment of repair mechanisms may also be attributed to oxygen toxicity, but at the level of mitochondrial DNA, peroxidation of membrane lipids, and protein cross-links.

Research in aging and in cancer provides us with the two-stage model of cellular senescence. The first stage is mediated by cellular proteins in the p53, p21, or p16/RB pathways. Mortality is dodged by tumor virus proteins that bind to and inactivate these tumor suppressers. The second independent stage is linked to critical telomere shortening. At this point, mortality can be evaded by expression or activation of telomerase.

Progress in understanding aging of the skin may have some implications for skeletal aging. Unlike some organs that contain postmitotic cells, e.g., nerve, muscle, and fat, the epithelial and stromal cells of the skin are mitotically competent, although they cannot divide indefinitely. Replicative senescence is generally viewed as a tumor suppressor mechanism but can in fact contribute to the rise in skin cancer that occurs with age. A possible explanation offered by Campisi is that the accumulation of senescent keratinocytes and fibroblasts compromises skin function but also changes critical elements of the microenvironment, like growth factors and inflammatory cytokines [109]. This fascinating idea suggests that mechanisms that have evolved to protect an organism from cataclysmic harm can contribute to compromised viability over time.

Scientists have been fascinated by the biology of aging since it was appreciated that there is a process of senescence that could be dissociated from specific diseases. There is continuous development of research tools to formulate and test hypotheses about causes and prevention. Although extrapolation from *in vitro* data to *in vivo* mechanisms of aging are to be made cautiously and although animal cell models may have limited value for human physiology, cellular models have inspired testing of the theory of replicative senescence and new ideas about telomere shortening with the status of cells *in vivo*. Progress in biogerontology has been made on multiple fronts, but with little integration among those investigating mammalian aging and those working on yeast, nematodes, and *Drosophila,* where longevity genes have been catalogued and where associations have been made with functional norms [110]. Clues for human counterparts to longevity genes may be obtained from work on senescence genes in other species. However, there is discouraging evidence that certain experimental models, such as mice, may have very limited relevance for human aging.

A major question is whether the study of *in vitro* cellular aging can help to elucidate the processes of aging *in vivo*. It is clear that the growth capacity of a variety of human cell types decreases with increasing donor age. Serial passaging of cells mimics many of the differences seen between cells from young and old people. There is strong evidence that telomere length is a cause of replicative senescence and that it may be a useful correlate for examining age-associated processes. Recent molecular analyses show numerous changes in gene expression that occur as cells age. Fibroblasts have been very useful as a model system, but other cell types, especially osteoblasts and marrow progenitors of osteoblasts and osteoclasts, are needed to define the relationship between replicative and functional senescence.

Acknowledgments

Pam Oborne is gratefully appreciated for her skillful assistance in the preparation of this chapter. Karen Aneshansley was very helpful with the figures. Support was provided in part by NIH Grants AG12271 and AG13519.

References

1. Hayflick, L. The cell biology of aging. *Clin. Geriatr. Med.* **1,** 15–27 (1985).
2. Carrel, A. On the permanent life of tissues outside the organism. *J. Exp. Med.* **15,** 516–528 (1912).
3. Hayflick, L., and Moorhead, P. S. The serial cultivation of human diploid cell strains. *Exp. Cell Res.* **25,** 585–621 (1961).
4. Hayflick, L. Mortality and immortality at the cellular level. A review. *Biochemistry (Moscow)* **62,** 1180–1190 (1997).
5. Johnson, L. F. G1 events and the regulation of genes for S-phase enzymes. *Curr. Opin. Cell Biol.* **4,** 149–154 (1992).
6. MacLachlan, T. K., Sang, N., and Giordano, A. Cyclins, cyclin-dependent kinases and cdk inhibitors: Implications in cell cycle control and cancer. *Crit. Rev. Eukaryot. Gene Exp.* **5,** 127–156 (1995).
7. Vaziri, H., Werst, M. D., Allsopp, R. C., Davison, T. S., Wu, Y. S., Arrowsmith, C. H., Poirier, G. G., and Benchimol, S. ATM-dependent telomere loss in aging human diploid fibroblasts and DNA damage lead to the posttranslational activation of p53 protein involving poly(ADP-ribose)polymerase. *EMBO. J.* **16,** 6018–6033 (1997).
8. Smith, J. R., and Pereira-Smith, O. M. Replicative senescence: Implications for *in vivo* aging and tumor suppression. *Science* **273,** 63–67 (1996).
9. Monti, D., Grassilli, E., Troiano, L., Cossarizza, S. A., Salvioli, S., Barbieri, D., Agnesini, C., Bettuzzi, S., Ingletti, M. C., Corti, A., and Franceschi, C. Senescence, immortalization, and apoptosis: An intriguing relationship. *Ann. N.Y. Acad. Sci.* **673,** 70–82 (1992).
10. Campisi, J., Dimri, G., and Hara, E. Control of replicative senescence. *In* "The Biology of Aging" (E. L. Schneider and J. W. Row, eds.), 4th ed., pp. 121–149. Academic Press, San Diego, 1996.
11. Kulju, K. S., and Lehman, J. M. Increased p53 protein associated with aging in human diploid fibroblasts. *Exp. Cell Res.* **217,** 336–345 (1995).
12. Atadja, P., Wong, H., Garkavtsev, I., Veillette, C., and Riabowol, K. Increased activity of p54 in senescing fibroblasts. *Proc. Natl. Acad. Sci. USA* **92,** 8348–8352 (1995).
13. Gire, V., and Wynford-Thomas, D. Reinitiation of DNA synthesis and cell division in senescent human fibroblasts by microinjection of anti-p53 antibodies. *Mol. Cell Biol.* **18,** 1611–1621 (1998).
14. Sugrue, M. M., Shin, D. Y., Lee, S. W., and Aaronson, S. A. Wild-type p53 triggers a rapid senescence program in human tumor cells lacking functional p53. *Proc. Natl. Acad. Sci. USA* **94,** 9648–9653 (1997).
15. Bond, J., Haughton, M., Blaydes, J., Gire, V., Wynford-Thomas, D., and Wyllie, F. Evidence that transcriptional activation by p53 plays a direct role in the induction of cellular senescence. *Oncogene* **13,** 2097–2104 (1996).
16. Shay, J. W., Pereira-Smith, O. M., and Wright, W. E. A role for both RB and p53 in the regulation of human cellular senescence. *Exp. Cell Res.* **196,** 33–39 (1991).
17. Yonish-Rouache, E., Resnitzky, D., Lotem, J., Sachs, L., Kimchi, A., and Oren, M. Wild-type p53 induces apoptosis of myeloid leukaemic cells that is inhibited by interleukin-6. *Nature* **352,** 345–347 (1991).
18. Filatov, L., Hurt, J., Byrd, L., Golubovskaya, V., and Kaufmann, W. Inactivation of G2 checkpoint function and telomere erosion may destabilize chromosomes in human fibroblasts expressing HPV16 E6 oncoprotein. *Proc. Annu. Meet. Am. Assoc. Cancer Res.* **38,** A2405 (1997).
19. Brown, J. P., Wei, W., and Sedivy, J. M. Bypass of senescence after disruption of p21 CIP1/WAF1 gene in normal diploid human fibroblasts. *Science* **277,** 831–834 (1997).
20. Wynford-Thomas, D. Telomeres, p53 and cellular senescence. *Oncol. Res.* **8,** 387–398 (1996).
21. Campisi, J. The biology of replicative senescence. *Eur. J. Cancer* **33,** 703–709 (1997).
22. Allsopp, R. C., Chang, E., Kashefi-Aazam, M., Rogaev, E. I., Piatyszek, M. A., Shay, J. W., and Harley, C. B. Telomere shortening is associated with cell division *in vitro* and *in vivo*. *Exp. Cell Res.* **220,** 194–200 (1995).
23. Allsopp, R. C., and Harley, C. B. Evidence for a critical telomere length in senescent human fibroblasts. *Exp. Cell Res.* **219,** 130–136 (1995).
24. Chang, E., and Harley, C. B. Telomere length and replicative aging in human vascular tissues. *Proc. Natl. Acad. Sci. USA* **92,** 11190–11194 (1995).
25. Notaro, R., Cimmino, A., Tabarini, D., Rotoli, B., and Luzzatto, L. *In vivo* telomere dynamics of human hematopoietic stem cells. *Proc. Natl. Acad. Sci. USA* **94,** 13782–13785 (1997).
26. Harley, C. B. Telomere loss: Mitotic clock or genetic time bomb? *Mutat. Res.* **256,** 271–282 (1991).
27. Greider, C. W. Telomere length regulation. *Annu. Rev. Biochem.* **65,** 337–365 (1996).
28. Dahse, R., Fiedler, W., and Ernst, G. Telomeres and telomerase: Biological and clinical importance. *Clin. Chem.* **43,** 708–714 (1997).
29. Oshimura, M., and Barrett, J. C. Multiple pathways to cellular senescence: Role of telomerase repressors. *Eur. J. Cancer* **33,** 710–715 (1997).
30. Levy, M. Z., Allsopp, R. C., Futcher, A. B., Greider, C. W., and Harley, C. B. Telomere end-replication problem and cell aging. *J. Mol. Biol.* **225,** 951–960 (1992).
31. Arino, O., Kimmel, M., and Webb, G. F. Mathematical modeling of the loss of telomere sequences. *J. Theor. Biol.* **177,** 45–57 (1995).
32. Counter, C. M. The roles of telomeres and telomerase in cell life span. *Mutat. Res.* **366,** 45–63 (1996).
33. Morin, G. B. Telomere control of replicative lifespan. *Exp. Gerontol.* **32,** 375–382 (1997).
34. Wright, W. E., Brasiskyte, D., Piatyszek, M. A., and Shay, J. W. Experimental elongation of telomeres extends the lifespan of immortal x normal cell hybrids. *EMBO J.* **15,** 1734–1741 (1996).
35. Bodnar, A. G., Ouellette, M., Frolkis, M., Holt, S. E., Shiu, C. P., Morin, G. B., Harley, C. B., Shay, J. W., Lichtsteiner, S., and Wright, W. E. Extension of life-span by introduction of telomerase into normal human cells. *Science* **279,** 349–352 (1998).
36. Blasco, M. A., Lee, H. W., Hande, M. P., Samper, E., Lansdorp, P. M., DePinho, R. A., and Greider, C. W. Telomere shortening and tumor formation by mouse cells lacking telomerase RNA. *Cell* **91,** 25–34 (1997).
37. Kipling, D., and Cooke, H. J. Hypervariable ultra-long telomeres in mice. *Nature* **347,** 400–402 (1990).
38. Szilard, L. On the nature of the aging process. *Proc. Natl. Acad. Sci. USA* **71,** 1124–1135 (1959).
39. Prieur, M., Achkar, W. A., Aurias, A., Coutirier, J., Dutrillaux, A. M., Dutrillaux, B., Flury-Herard, A., Gerbault, M., Seureau, T., Hoffschir, F., Lamoliatte, E., LeFrancois, D., Lombard, M., Muleris, M., Ricoul, M., and Sabatier, L. Acquired chromosome rearrangements in human lymphocytes: Effect of aging. *Hum. Genet.* **79,** 147–150 (1988).

40. Carrano, A. V. Summary of the workshop on mammalian *in vivo* somatic mutation. *Genome* **31,** 458–459 (1989).
41. Cooper, D. N., and Krawezak, M. The mutational spectrum of single base-pair substitutions causing human genetic disease: Patterns and predictions. *Hum. Genet.* **85,** 55–74 (1990).
42. Randerath, K., Randerath, E., and Filburn, C. Genomic and mitochondrial DNA alterations with aging. *In* "The Biology of Aging" (E. L. Schneider and J. W. Row, eds.), 4th Ed. pp. 198–214. Academic Press, San Diego, 1996.
43. Shoffner, J. M., and Wallace, D. C. Oxidative phosphorylation diseases: Disorders of two genomes. *Adv. Hum. Genet.* **19,** 267–330 (1990).
44. Cortopassi, G. A., Shibata, D., Soong, N. W., and Arnheim, N. A pattern of accumulation of a somatic deletion of mitochondrial DNA in aging tissues. *Proc. Natl. Acad. Sci. USA* **89,** 7370–7374 (1992).
45. Muller-Hocker, J. Cytochrome-c-oxidase deficient cardiomyocytes in the human heart—an age-related phenomenon: A histochemical ultracytochemical study. *Am. J. Pathol.* **134,** 1167–1173 (1989).
46. Richter, C., Park, J. W., and Ames, B. N. Normal oxidative damage to mitochondrial and nuclear DNA is extensive. *Proc. Natl. Acad. Sci. USA* **85,** 6465–6467 (1988).
47. Goldstein, S., Niewiarowski, S., and Singal, D. P. Pathological implications of cell aging *in vitro. Fed. Proc.* **34,** 56–63 (1975).
48. Goldstein, S., Murano, S., Benes, H., Moerman, E. J., Jones, R. A., Thweatt, R., Shmookler Reis, R. J., and Howard, B. H. Studies on the molecular–genetic basis of replicative senescence in Werner syndrome and normal fibroblasts. *Exp. Gerontol.* **24,** 461–468 (1989).
49. Lecka-Czernik, B., Moerman, E. J., Jones, R. A., and Goldstein, S. Identification of gene sequences overexpressed in senescent and Werner syndrome human fibroblasts. *Exp. Gerontol.* **31,** 159–174 (1996).
50. Lecka-Czernik, B., Lumpkin, C. K., Jr., and Goldstein, S. An overexpressed gene transcript in senescent and quiescent human fibroblasts encoding a novel protein in the epidermal growth factor-like repeat family stimulates DNA synthesis. *Mol. Cell Biol.* **15,** 120–128 (1995).
51. Hu, Q., Moerman, E. J., and Goldstein, S. Altered expression and regulation of the alpha5beta1 integrin-fibronectin receptor lead to reduced amounts of functional alpha5beta1 heterodimer on the plasma membrane of senescent human diploid fibroblasts. *Exp. Cell Res.* **224,** 251–263 (1996).
52. Thweatt, R., Lumpkin, C. K. Jr., and Goldstein, S. A novel gene encoding a smooth muscle protein is overexpressed in senescent human fibroblasts. *Biochem. Biophys. Res. Commun.* **187,** 1–7 (1992).
53. Saito, H., Papaconstantinou, J., Sato, H., and Goldstein, S. Regulation of a novel gene encoding a lysyl oxidase-related protein in cellular adhesion and senescence. *J. Biol. Chem.* **272,** 8157–8160 (1997).
54. Liu, S., Thweatt, R., Lumpkin, C. K. Jr., and Goldstein, S. Suppression of calcium-dependent membrane currents in human fibroblasts by replicative senescence and forced expression of a gene sequence encoding a putative calcium-binding protein. *Proc. Natl. Acad. Sci. USA* **91,** 2186–2190 (1994).
55. Wang, S., Moerman, E. J., Jones, R. A., Thweatt, R., and Goldstein, S. Characterization of IGFBP-3, PAI-1 and SPARC mRNA expression in senescent fibroblasts. *Mech. Aging Dev.* **92,** 121–132 (1996).
56. Gonos, E. S., Derventzi, A., Kveiborg, M., Agiostratidou, G., Kassem, M., Clark, B. F., Jat, P. S., and Rattan, S. I. Cloning and identification of genes that associate with mammalian replecative senescence. *Exp. Cell Res.* **240,** 66–74 (1998).
57. Papaconstantinou, J., Reisner, P. D., Liu, L., and Kuninger, D. T. Mechanisms of altered gene expression with aging. *In* "The Biology of Aging" (E. L. Schneider and J. W. Row, eds.), 4th Ed. pp. 150–183. Academic Press, San Diego, 1996.
58. Goldstein, S., Moerman, E. J., Jones, R. A., and Baxter, R. C. Insulin-like growth factor binding protein 3 accumulates to high levels in culture medium of senescent and quiescent human fibroblasts. *Proc. Natl. Acad. Sci. USA* **88,** 9680–9684 (1991).
59. Goldstein, S., Moerman, E. J., Jones, R. A., and Baxter, R. C. Accumulation of insulin-like growth factor binding protein-3 in conditioned medium of human fibroblasts increases with chronologic age of donor and senescence *in vitro. J. Cell Physiol.* **156,** 294–302 (1993).
60. Moerman, E. J., Thweatt, R., Moerman, A. M., Jones, R. A., and Goldstein, S. Insulin-like growth factor binding protein-3 is overexpressed in senescent and quiescent human fibroblasts. *Exp. Gerontol.* **28,** 361–370 (1993).
61. Dimri, G. P., Lee, X., Basile, G., Acosta, M., Scott, G., Roskelley, C., Medrano, E. E., Linskens, M., Rubelj, I., Pereira-Smith, O., *et al.* A biomarker that identifies senescent human cells in culture and in aging skin *in vivo. Proc. Natl. Acad. Sci. USA* **92,** 9363–9367 (1995).
62. Kahn, A., Meienhofer, M. C., Guillouzo, A., Cottreau, D., Baffet, G., Henry, J., and Dreyfus, J. C. Modifications of phosphoproteins and protein kinases occurring with *in vitro* aging of cultured human cells. *Gerontology* **28,** 360–370 (1982).
63. Levine, R. L., and Stadtman, E. R. Protein modifications with aging. *In* "The Biology of Aging" (E. L. Schneider and J. W. Row, eds.), 4th ed., pp. 184–197. Academic Press, San Diego, 1996.
64. Starke-Reed, P. E., and Oliver, C. N. Protein oxidation and proteolysis during aging and oxidative strews. *Arch. Biochem. Biophys.* **275,** 559–567 (1989).
65. Chen J. J., Brot, N., and Weissbach, H. RNA and protein synthesis in cultured human fibroblasts derived from donors or various ages. *Mech. Aging Dev.* **13,** 285–295 (1980).
66. Dimri, G. P., Testori, A., Acosta, M., and Campisi, J. Replication senescence: Aging and growth-regulatory transcription factors. *Biol. Sig.* **5,** 154–162 (1996).
67. Beresford, J. N., Fedarko, N. S., Fisher, L. W., Midura, R. J. Yanagoshita, M., Termine, J. D., and Robey, P. G. Analysis of the proteoglycans synthesized by human bone cells *in vitro. J. Biol. Chem.* **262,** 17164–17172 (1987).
68. Chaudhary, L. R., Spelsberg, T. C., and Riggs, B. L. Production of various cytokines by normal human osteoblast-like cells in response to interleukin-1 beta-estradiol. *Endocrinology* **130,** 2528–2534 (1992).
69. Fedarko, N. S., D'Avis, P., Frazier, C. R., Burrill, M. J., Fergusson, V., Tayback, M., Sponseller, P. D., and Shapio, J. R. Cell proliferation of human fibroblasts and osteoblasts in osteogenesis imperfecta: Influence of age. *J. Bone Miner. Res.* **10,** 1705–1712 (1995).
70. Evans, C. E., Galasko, C. S., and Ward, C. Effect of donor age on the growth *in vitro* of cells obtained from human trabecular bone. *J. Orthop. Res.* **8,** 234–237 (1990).
71. Pfeilschifter, J., Diel, I., Pilz, U., Brunotte, K., Naumann, A., and Ziegler, R. Mitogenic responsiveness of human bone cells *in vitro* to hormones and growth factors decreases with age. *J. Bone Miner. Res.* **8,** 707–717 (1993).
72. Chavassieux, P. M., Chenu, C., Valentin-Opran, A., Merle, B., Delmas, P. D., Hartman D. J., Saez, S., and Meunier, P. J.

Influence of experimental conditions on osteoblasy activity in human primary bone cell cultures. *J. Bone Min. Res.* **5,** 337–343 (1990).

73. Battmann, A., Battmann, A., Jundt, G., and Schulz, A. Endosteal human bone cells (EBC) show age-related activity *in vitro. Exp. Clin. Endocrinol Diabetes* **105,** 98–102 (1997).

74. Wong, M. M., Rao, L. G., Ly, H., Hamilton, L., Ish-Shalom, S., Sturtridge, W., Tong, J., McBroom, R., Josse, R. G., and Murray, T. M. *In vitro* study of osteoblastic cells from patients with idiopathic osteoporosis and comparison with cells from non-osteoporotic controls. *Osteoporosis Int.* **4,** 21–31 (1994).

75. Friedenstein, A. J., Latzinik, N. W., Grosheva, A. G., and Gorskaya, U. F. Marrow microenvironment transfer by heterotopic transplantation of freshly isolated and cultured cells in porous sponges. *Exp. Hematol.* **10,** 217–227 (1982).

76. Ashton, B. A., Allen, T. D., Howlett, C. R., Eaglesom, C. C., Hattori, A., and Owen, M. Formation of bone and cartilage by marrow stromal cells in diffusion chambers *in vivo. Clin. Orthop.* **151,** 294–307 (1980).

77. Meunier, P., Aaron, J., Edouard, C., and Vignon, G. Osteoporosis and the replacement of cell populations of the marrow by adipose tissue. A quantitative study of 84 iliac bone biopsies. *Clin. Orthop.* **80,** 147–154 (1971).

78. Kahn, A., Gibbons, R., Perkins, S., and Gazit, D. Age-related bone loss. A hypothesis and initial assessment in mice. *Clin. Orthop.* **313,** 69–75 (1995).

79. Bergman, R. J., Gazit, D, Kahn, A. J., Gruber, H., McDougall, S., and Hahn, T. J. Age-related changes in osteogenic stem cells in mice. *J. Bone Miner. Res.* **11,** 568–577 (1996).

80. Perkins, S. L., Gibbons, R., Kling, S., and Kahn, A. J. Age-related bone loss in mice is associated with an increased osteoclast progenitor pool. *Bone* **15,** 65–72 (1994).

81. Kahn, A., Meienhofer, M. C., Guillouzo, A., Cottreau, D., Baffet, G., Henry, J., and Dreyfus, J. C. Modifications of phosphoproteins and protein kinases occurring with *in vitro* aging of cultured human cells. *Gerontology* **28,** 360–370 (1982).

82. Kahn, A., Gibbons, R., Perkins, S., and Gazit, D. Age-related bone loss. A hypothesis and initial assessment in mice. *Clin. Orthop.* **313,** 69–75 (1995).

83. Frenkel, B., Capparelli, C., Van Auken, M., Baran, D., Bryan, J., Stein, J. L., Stein, G. S., and Lian, J. B. Activity of the osteocalcin promoter in skeletal sites of transgenic mice and during osteoblast differentiation in bone marrow-derived stromal cell cultures: effects of age and sex. *Endocrinology* **138,** 2109–2116 (1997).

84. Roholl, P., Blauw, E., Zurcher, C., Dormans, J., and Theuns, H. Evidence for a diminished maturation of pre-osteoblasts into osteoblasts during aging in rats: An ultrastructural analysis. *J. Bone Min. Res.* **9,** 355–366 (1994).

85. Long, M. W., Williams, J. L., and Mann, K. G. Expression of human bone-related proteins in the hematopoietic microenvironment. *J. Clin. Invest.* **86,** 1387–1395 (1990).

86. Vilamitjana-Amedee, J., Bareille, R., Rouais, F., Caplan, A. I., and Harmand, M. F. Human bone marrow cells express an osteoblastic phenotype in culture. *In Vitro Cell Dev. Biol. Anim.* **29A,** 699–707 (1993).

87. Cheng, S. L., Yang, J. W., Rifas, L., Zhang, S., and Avioli, L. Differentiation of human bone marrow osteogenic stromal cells *in vitro:* Induction of the osteoblast phenotype by dexamethasone. *Endocrinology* **134,** 277–286 (1994).

88. Mueller, S. M., Mizuno, S., and Glowacki, J. The effect of age on the osteogenic potential of human bone marrow cells cultured in three-dimensional collagen sponges. *Bone* **23,** S536 (1998).

89. Rosen, C. J., Verault, D., Steffens, C., Cheleuitte, D., and Glowacki, J. Effects of age and estrogen status on the skeletal IGF regulatory system: Studies with human marrow. *Endocrine* **7,** 77–80 (1997).

90. Glowacki, J. Effect of age on human marrow. *Calcif. Tissue Int.* **56S,** 50–51 (1995).

91. Cheleuitte, D., Mizuno, S., and Glowacki, J. *In vitro* secretion of cytokines of human bone marrow: Effects of age and estrogen status. *J. Clin. Endocr. Metab.* **83,** 2043–2051 (1998).

92. Hammar, M. Impaired *in vitro* testicular endocrine function in elderly men. *Andrologia* **17,** 444–449 (1985).

93. Hammar, M., Petersson, F., and Berg, A. A. *In vitro* conversion of progesterone in the human testis at different ages, pathophysiological conditions, and during treatment with estrogens or gonadotrophic hormones. *Arch. Androl.* **14,** 143–149 (1985).

94. Hammar, M., Ahlstrand, C., Berg, A. A., and Lackgren, G. *In vitro* conversion of 3H-pregnenolone by human testicular tissue from fetal age to senescence. *Arch. Androl.* **13,** 203–212 (1984).

95. Morales, A. J., Nolan, J. J., Nelson, J. C., and Yen, S. S. C. Effects of replacement dose of dehydroepiandrosterone in men and women of advancing age. *J. Clin. Endocrinol. Metab.* **78,** 1360–1367 (1994).

96. Hornsby, P. J. Biosynthesis of DHEAS by the human adrenal cortex and its age-related decline. *Ann. N.Y. Acad. Sci.* **774,** 29–46 (1995).

97. Hornsby, P. J., and Aldern, K. A. Steroidogenic enzyme activities in cultured human definitive zone adrenocortical cells: Comparison with bovine adrenocortical cells and resultant differences in adrenal androgen synthesis. *J. Clin. Endocrinol. Metab.* **58,** 121–130 (1984).

98. Fujiwara, Y., Kano, Y., Ichihashi, M., Nakao, Y., and Matsumura, T. Abnormal fibroblast aging and DNA replication in the Werner syndrome. *Adv. Exp. Med. Biol.* **190,** 459–477 (1985).

99. Yu, C. E., Oshima, J., Fu, Y. H., Wijsman, E. M., Hisama, F., Alisch, R., Matthews, S., Nakura, J., Miki, T., Ouais, S., Martin, G. M., and Mulligan, J. Positional cloning of the Werner's syndrome gene. *Science* **272,** 258–262 (1996).

100. Gray, M. D., Shen, J. C., Kamath-Loeb, A. S., Blank, A., Sopher, B. L., Martin, G. M., Oshima, J., and Loeb, L. A. The Werner syndrome protein is a DNA helicase. *Nat. Genet.* **17,** 100–103 (1997).

101. Matsumoto, T., Imamura, O., Yamabe, Y., Kuromitsu, J., Tokutake, Y., Shimamoto, A., Suzuki, N., Satoh, M., Kitao, S., Ichikawa, K., Kataoka, H., Sugawara, K., Thomas, W., Mason, B., Tsuchihashi, Z., Drayna, D., Sugawara, M., Sugimoto, M., Furuchi, Y., and Goto, M. Mutation and haplotype analyses of the Werner's syndrome gene based on its genetic structure: Genetic epidemiology in the Japanese population. *Hum. Genet.* **100,** 123–130 (1997).

102. Bauer, E. A., Uitto, J., Tan, E. M., and Holbrook, K. A. Werner's syndrome. Evidence for preferential regional expression of a generalized mesenchymal cell defect. *Arch. Dermatol.* **124,** 90–101 (1988).

103. Nakamura, T., Takagaki, K., Kubo, K., Saito, T., Endo, M., Mori, S., Morisaki, N., Saito, Y., and Yoshida, S. Hyaluronate synthesized by cultured skin fibroblasts derived from patients with Werner's syndrome. *Biochim. Biophys. Acta* **1139,** 84–90 (1992).

104. Rasoamanantena, P., Thweatt, R., Labat-Robert, J., and Goldstein, S. Altered regulation of fibronectin gene expression in Werner syndrome fibroblasts. *Exp. Cell. Res.* **213,** 121–127 (1994).

105. Mitsui, Y., Yamamoto, K., Yamamoto, M., and Matuoka, K. Cell surface changes in senescent and Werner's syndrome fibroblasts:

their role in cell proliferation. *Adv. Exp. Med. Biol.* **190,** 567–585 (1985).

106. Bauer, E. A., Silverman, N., Busiek, D. F., Kronberger, A., and Deuel, T. F. Diminished response of Werner's syndrome fibroblasts to growth factors PDGF and FGF. *Science* **234,** 1240–1243 (1986).
107. Lecka-Czernik, B., Moerman, E. L., Jones, R. A., and Goldstein, S. Identification of gene sequences overexpressed in senescent and Werner syndrome human fibroblasts. *Exp. Gerontol.* **31,** 159–174 (1996).
108. Murano, S., Thweatt, R., Shmookler Reis, R. J., Jones, R. A., Moerman, E. J., and Goldstein, S. Diverse gene sequences are overexpressed in Werner syndrome fibroblasts undergoing premature replicative senescence. *Cell. Biol.* **11,** 3905–3914 (1991).
109. Campisi, J. The role of cellular senescence in skin aging. *J. Investig. Dermatol. Symp. Proc.* **3,** 1–5 (1998).
110. Jazwinski, S. M. Longevity, genes, and aging. *Science* **273,** 54–59 (1996).

Part II

Determinants of Peak Bone Mass; Maintenance of Peak Bone Mass

CHAPTER 8

Genetic Determinants of the Population Variance in Bone Mineral Density

EGO SEEMAN Austin and Repatriation Medical Centre, University of Melbourne, Melbourne, Australia

THE QUESTION

The relevant end point in studying the pathogenesis of bone fragility is fracture. Are there genetic and environmental factors that explain why fractures occur more often in older than in younger persons, more often in some communities than in others, and more often in women than in men? As fractures are uncommon annual events in an individual, it is difficult to detect a truly existing association between fractures and a genetic marker or an environmental exposure. Thus, the low annual incidence of fractures virtually precludes the use of this end point as a means of identifying the causes of bone fragility in an individual or population.

Areal bone mineral density (BMD) is a surrogate measure of the breaking strength of bone *in vitro* and of fracture risk *in vivo*. Thus, the questions become (1) are there genetic and environmental factors that partly explain why areal BMD is lower in patients with fractures than in age-matched controls and (2) are there genetic and environmental factors that explain why areal BMD is lower in women than in men and lower in whites than in blacks (and therefore may account for gender and racial differences in fracture rates)? What genetic and environmental factors explain the variance in areal BMD in a healthy premenopausal population, therefore explaining why some individuals have higher areal BMD while others have lower areal BMD? What are the genetic and environmental factors that account for the variance in bone loss during aging?

Patients with fractures have reduced areal BMD relative to age-matched controls. This deficit may be due to the attainment of a low peak areal BMD, excessive bone loss, or both. As the areal BMD measurement does not completely adjust for bone size, the lower areal BMD may also be due to patients with fractures having smaller bones than controls [1,2]. Smaller bone size in patients with fractures may be due to the attainment of a smaller skeleton during growth or to the failure of periosteal expansion during aging. The lower bone mass in the (smaller) bone—the lower volumetric BMD—may be due to reduced mineral accrual within the periosteal envelope of the smaller bone during growth, excessive bone loss during aging, or both.

Thus, insight into the genetic and environmental factors contributing to "osteoporosis"—areal BMD reduced by 2.5 standardized deviations or more below the young adult normal mean—requires the systematic study of (i) the growth in size of the skeleton, i.e., periosteal growth, (ii) the mineral accrual that occurs within the confines of a regions periosteal envelope, i.e., the mechanisms responsible for the formation of cortical thickness: endocortical expansion before and during puberty and endocortical contraction in late puberty, (iii) the mechanisms responsible for increasing trabecular number and thickness, (iv) the mineralization of matrix that forms the true (material) density of bone, (v) age-related periosteal expansion, and (vi) age-related cortical and trabecular bone loss. The same questions arise when comparing genders and races. What are the genetic and environmental factors that account for any differences in the bone size, mass, and volumetric BMD between genders and races that may explain gender and racial differences in fracture rates?

IS "BMD" A SUITABLE PHENOTYPIC END POINT?

Areal BMD is a surrogate of the breaking strength of bone and is a sensitive predictor for fracture. However, areal BMD may not be the correct phenotypic end point when questions are asked about genetic and environmental factors responsible for bone fragility because areal BMD is not a specific, unambiguous structure with identifiable physiological control mechanisms. It is a summation of periosteal and endosteal (endocortical, intracortical, trabecular) surface modeling and remodeling. Periosteal expansion and remodeling determine external bone size, and are independent predictors of bone strength. Endocortical expansion is less than periosteal expansion before puberty (otherwise cortical width would not increase as the external size of the bone increases). The endocortical surface then contracts at puberty in females, probably less in males, and to a different degree from bone to bone. Of final cortical thickness, 75% is due to periosteal expansion whereas 25% is due to endocortical contraction at the metacarpals, but at the femur 95% of midshaft femur is due to periosteal expansion with little contribution from endocortical contraction [3]. The *relative* behavior of these two surfaces establishs cortical thickness. Thus, even cortical thickness is not a single entity; it is the net result of the modeling and remodeling on these two surfaces. The surfaces behave differently because they are regulated differently. Cortical thickness is the net result of the actions of the differing regulators on the absolute *and relative* growth of these two surfaces.

Just as areal BMD and cortical thickness are the net result of differing regulatory processes, volumetric BMD may also be an unsuitable phenotype for the identification of genetic regulators of bone fragility because volumetric BMD is a function of the bone size and the regulators of bone size, and the mass contained within its periosteal envelope, and the regulators that influence each of the structural components of mass. The same deficit in volumetric BMD may be produced by entirely different mechanisms that will be obscure unless mass and size are studied separately. For example, oophorectomy in growing rats produces a larger bone than sham-operated animals but the accrual of mass is no different than sham-operated controls. The combination of a reduction in mass relative to the (larger) bone size results in reduced volumetric BMD. Orchiectomy results in a reduction in growth in mass and size, but the reduction in mass is greater than the reduction in size so that volumetric BMD is reduced. Thus, the pathogenetic mechanisms resulting in osteoporosis in the growing female and male rat are entirely different [4].

To identify the regulators of growth in the dimensions of volume and structural components of mass, it is necessary to first measure the pattern of growth of each of these skeletal surfaces describing the age-, gender-, and race-specific mean *and* population variance during growth. When these measurements are obtained, it may then be possible to determine what genetic and environmental factors account for the variance within a group specified by age, gender, and race.

RELATIVE GROWTH IN BONE MASS AND SIZE DETERMINES VOLUMETRIC BMD

Little is known about the genetic or environmental factors regulating the gain in bone mass. Both BMC and areal BMD are size-dependent expressions of "density." Both increase during growth because the bone enlarges. When size is taken into account by expressing the bone mass as a function of its size, as volumetric BMD, then this expression of density appears to be independent of age [5–7]. This is illustrated in Fig. 1 where it is shown that volumetric BMD is constant during growth. An individual with volumetric BMD at the 5th percentile in the first 5 years of life will probably have volumetric BMD at the 5th percentile in young adulthood. The same applies for individuals with volumetric BMD at the 95th percentile, i.e., volumetric BMD probably "tracks."

If volumetric BMD is independent of age, then the position of an individuals volumetric BMD relative to his/her peers in the population distribution must be determined very early, perhaps *in utero*. For volumetric BMD to be independent of age, its components—bone size and mass—must increase in proportion. If this is correct, then this growth in size and the growth in mass within its periosteal envelope must be coordinated and thus coregulated so that the enlarging bone gains an increasing bone mass within it (as cortical shell and trabeculi). The proportional changes in mass and size will vary for each individual and that proportion will determine the absolute level of volumetric BMD, i.e., the level of volumetric BMD—whether it is in the lower, middle, or upper part of the population distribution—will be determined by the *relative* growth in mass and size.

Persons with volumetric BMD in the 95th percentile must accrue more bone per unit volume of *the* bone than individuals with volumetric BMD at the 5th percentile. If the growth in mass (relative to its mean) is greater than the growth in size (relative to its mean), volumetric BMD will be in the higher part of the population distribution. If growth in mass is less than growth in size,

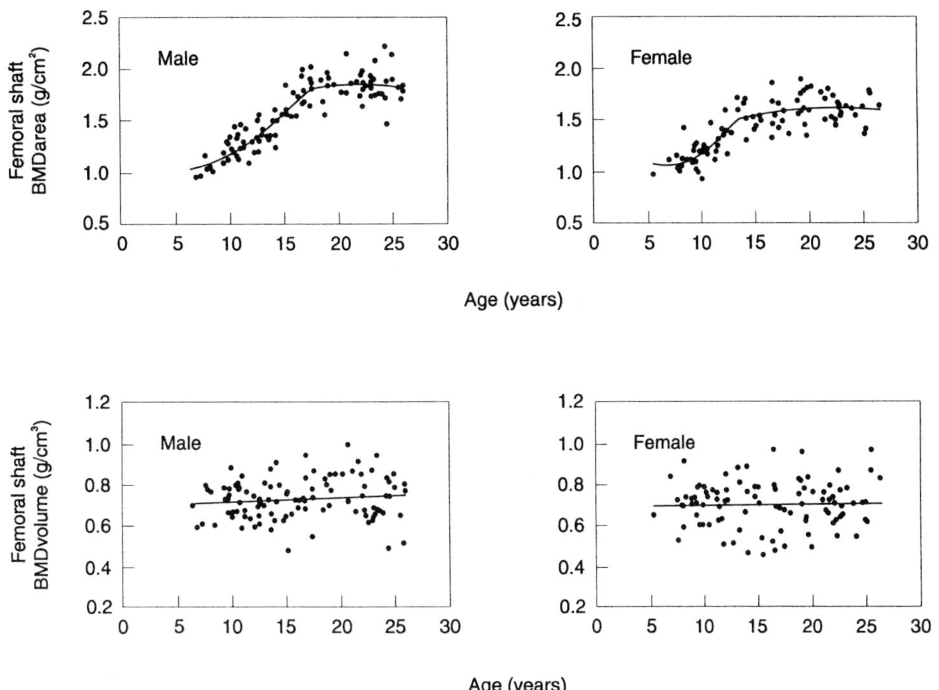

FIGURE 1 Areal bone mineral density (BMD, g/cm^2) at the femoral midshaft increases with advancing bone age in males and females whereas volumetric BMD (g/cm^3) is independent of bone age. Reproduced with permission from Lu *et al.* [5].

volumetric BMD will be in the lower part of the population distribution. If the growth in mass and size are proportional, i.e., both are in the *same* position (irrespective of the position) in the population distribution for that trait, then volumetric BMD will be in the mid-normal range (Fig. 2). Thus, volumetric BMD is not a function of the absolute increase in bone mass or size, it is a function of the *relative* growth in bone size and the mineral accrued within it.

The variance in volumetric BMD in the population may be achieved in part by the variable combinations of growth in mass and size. Identification of genetic and environmental factors regulating the growth in size, growth in mass, and their coregulation requires that the growth of each of these components of size—length, width, depth, and mass—be measured. Identification of the existence of a genetic component of variance is suggested by finding that the intrapair correlation between the same traits in monozygotic twins is higher than in dizygotic pairs. Identification of genetic factors responsible for the resemblance (covariance) between two different traits is suggested by finding that the cross-trait, cross-twin correlation is higher in monozygotic than in dizygotic pairs. As discussed in the last section of this chapter, the correlation between lean mass and areal BMD is likely to be the result of genes that coregulate the size of each of these traits [8].

The variance in bone size, like height, does not appear to increase during growth, i.e., like height, bone size may track during growth. In contrast, the variance in bone mass may increase with advancing age. The increasing scatter suggests that some individuals gain more bone for a given bone size and mass than others; these individuals may come to have the higher volumetric BMD in adulthood (Fig. 3) [3]. In morphological terms, a higher volumetric BMD may be achieved in one (or more) of four ways: increasing cortical thickness by reduced endocortical expansion relative to periosteal expansion before puberty, greater endocortical contraction during puberty, by increasing trabecular numbers that originate in the epiphyseal plate forming a primary and secondary spongiosa, by increasing trabecular thickness during puberty, or by increasing the true mineral (material) BMD of these structures [9].

It is unlikely that growth in size and mass is independent. A larger bone may need relatively less bone to maintain the same bone strength and may be able to lose more bone before fragility emerges. A bigger bone may need a *proportionally* smaller cortical thickness for biomechanical competence. Gilsanz *et al.* [10] matched 80 black females and males with 80 whites of the same gender, age, bone age, pubertal stage, height, and weight and reported that blacks had longer legs and a larger

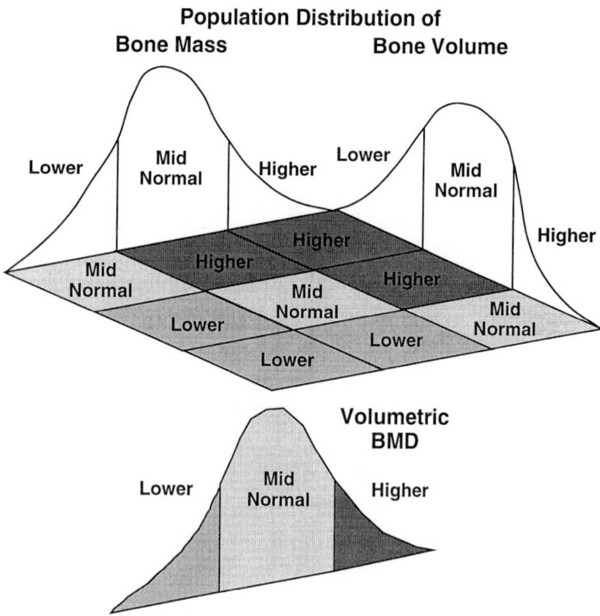

FIGURE 2 The population distribution of volumetric bone mineral density (BMD) may be the result of differing relative contributions of bone mass and size. Tertials of bone mass and bone volume and the nine possible levels of volumetric BMD resulting from combinations of these traits are shown. Midnormal volumetric BMD results when mass and size are in the same tertials in their respective trait distributions, irrespective of whether this is in the upper, middle, or lower tertial. Higher volumetric BMD results when growth in mass (relative to its population mean) is greater than the growth in size (relative to its population mean). Lower volumetric BMD results when growth in mass is less than growth in size relative to their respective trait means.

femoral midshaft cross-sectional area but no racial differences in femoral midshaft cortical thickness or its true (material) BMD. Thus, the bigger bone has a *proportionally* thinner cortex than the smaller bone of the white. Blacks had shorter trunk length and vertebral height but the same vertebral cross-sectional area. The shorter vertebral body in blacks had a higher trabecular BMD due to thicker trabeculae (not greater numbers) than whites. Thus, the smaller bone had more bone within its periosteal envelope.

POLYMORPHISMS AND GROWTH

What genetic or environmental factors confer a higher or lower volumetric BMD? This information is unavailable but important because the position of an individuals peak volumetric BMD in young adulthood determines the volumetric BMD many years later. Whether some individuals gain a greater cortical thickness by less endocortical expansion relative to periosteal expansion before puberty or greater endocortical contraction during puberty is not known. Prepubertal growth is growth hormone (GH) and insulin-like growth factor 1 (IGF-1) dependent. Pubertal growth is sex hormone dependent. GH/IGF-1 and sex steroids may affect the periosteal and endosteal surfaces, permitting cortical thickening and trabecular thickening. Whether some girls have a greater skeletal response to GH/IGF-1 is uncertain. If so, whether there may be a genetic marker such as a GH/IGF-1 or estrogen receptor (ER) polymorphism associated with a differing response to these growth factors is also unknown.

Using quantitative computed tomography, Rosen *et al.* [11] reported differences in femoral volumetric BMD of up to 50% between C3H/HeJ (C3H) and C57BL/6J (B6) mouse strains. Serum IGF-I was over 35% higher in C3H than in B6. F1 progeny had IGF-1 and femoral BMD levels intermediate between the parental strains. F2 progeny with the highest BMD had the highest IGF-1 whereas skeletal IGF-1 in calvariae, tibiae, and femora was ~30% higher in C3H than in B6 mice. The authors inferred that the difference in volumetric BMD between strains may be related to systemic and skeletal IGF-I synthesis. The morphological basis of the higher volumetric BMD in this strain may be either thicker cortices or higher true (material) BMD of the cortical bone itself (free of canals and canaliculi). It is unclear which of these mechanisms accounted for the differences in volumetric BMD in these strains. (Parenthetically, for a given external bone size, if cortical thickness increased due to endocortical apposition then the bending strength of bone may not increase, although the thicker cortices may protect from later endocortical resorption. If true BMD is increased, this may not necessarily increase bone strength.)

Sainz *et al.* [12] reported associations between VDR and femoral cortical true BMD in 100 normal prepubertal Americans of Mexican descent, aged 6.7 to 11.7 years. Care was taken to match for bone age, height, weight, body surface area, or BMI between the groups. Girls with aa and bb genotypes had a 2–3% higher femoral true (material) BMD and 8–10% higher vertebral trabecular BMD than those with AA and BB genotypes. The 23 girls with the aabb genotype had 2% higher femoral and 12% higher vertebral BMD than the 14 girls with the AABB genotype. VDR alleles were not associated with vertebral or with femoral cross-sectional areas or cortical bone area. Gunnes *et al.* [13] reported changes in areal BMD over about 4 years in 273 healthy boys and girls aged 8.2 to 16.5 years at the spine, proximal femur, radius, and whole body and forearm. No association between VDR genotype and BMD was found at any site in boys or girls before or after adjustment for calcium intake, physical activity, age, weight, or height.

Mizunuma *et al.* [14] reported the association of ER polymorphisms, lumbar BMD, and bone turnover in 173 pre- and postmenopausal women. Women with the

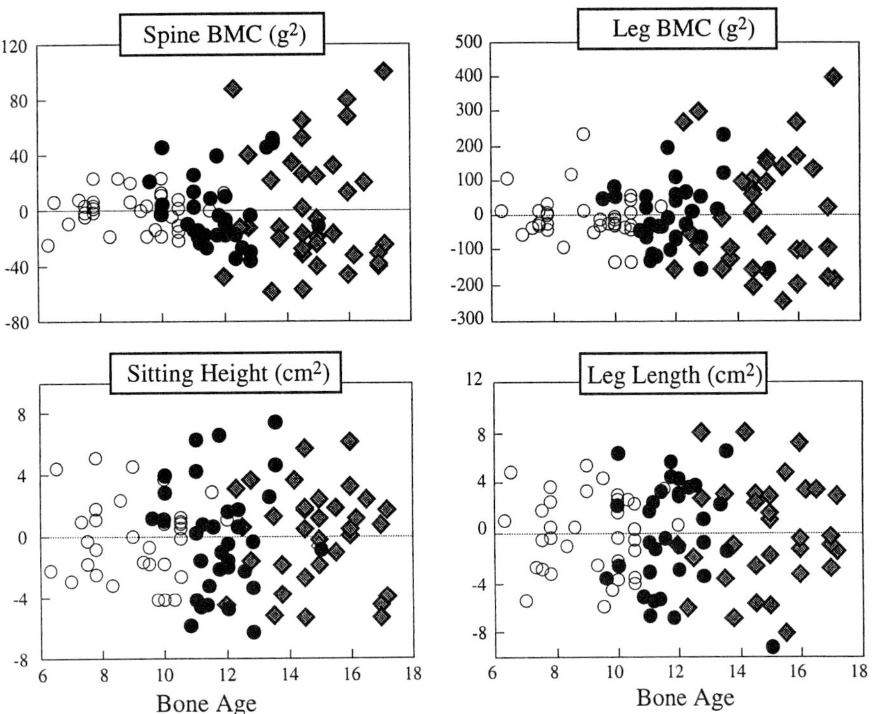

FIGURE 3 Bone age-adjusted residuals for spine and leg bone mineral content (BMC) increase with advancing age whereas bone age-adjusted residuals for sitting height and leg length do not. Prepubertal (○), peripubertal (●), and postpubertal (◆). Reproduced with permission from Bass *et al.* [3].

Xx genotype had higher BMD than those with the xx genotype. The authors suggested that the Xx genotype may be associated with a greater accretion of bone during young adulthood. There are no studies available examining the morphological basis of any higher areal BMD associated with ER genotypes. Whether the ER polymorphism predicts a greater endocortical contraction, a smaller medullary cavity, a greater cortical thickness, or a greater trabecular thickness has not been examined.

Whether VDR genotypes are associated with differences in bone size or body size is uncertain. If so, the mechanisms that may mediate differences in size (producing differences in areal BMD but not necessarily differences in volumetric BMD) are uncertain. Suarez *et al.* [15] report an association between VDR polymorphism and anthropometric data in 423 infants. Girls with the BB genotype had greater length, weight, and body surface area at 2 years than bb girls. Boys with the BB genotype had lower weight, BMI, and body surface area at 2 years than bb and Bb boys. As a result, gender-related differences were observed in Bb and bb but not BB populations. In a longitudinal analysis of 145 full-term babies, gender-related differences in length, weight, and body surface area existed in the bb infants. The significance of these observations is unclear. Keen *et al.* [16] reported an association between VDR genotypes and weight at 1 year ($F = 4.22$, $P = 0.04$) in 66 British women of mean age 65.5 years for whom detailed birth records were available. The tt group had a 7% greater weight than the TT group. However, the VDR genotype had no detectable effect on BMD at the spine or proximal femur, height, and weight in adulthood.

Trabecular volumetric BMD is determined by trabecular number, thickness, and the true material density of a trabecula. Trabecular volumetric density of the cancellous bone of the spine varies by race but not by gender [10,17,18]. Males and females of the same race have the same trabecular numbers and trabecular thickness; at peak, trabecular volumetric BMD is the same in males and females of the same race. Most histomorphometric studies have been cross-sectional with few individuals within the same decade. Thus, the structural basis of the age-specific variance in volumetric BMD within a given decade is unknown. Do women with peak volumetric trabecular BMD at the 5th percentile have fewer trabeculae or thinner trabeculae or both? What is the pathogenetic basis of these differences? Blacks have the same trabecular numbers but greater trabecular thickness than whites of the corresponding gender. Studies of the development of racial differences in trabecular thickness may provide insight into the physiological basis of the age- and gender-specific variance in volumetric peak BMD.

Harris *et al.* [19] determined the *Fok*I genotype in 72 black and 82 white premenopausal women aged 20 to 40 years. Four percent of blacks and 18% of whites were homozygous for ff, and 65 and 37% were homozygous for FF, respectively. In whites, women with the ff genotype had 4.3% lower total body BMD and 12.1% lower femoral neck BMD than FF ($P = 0.014$ and 0.001). Lumbar BMD did not differ by genotype. Adjustment for the *Fok*I genotype reduced the racial difference in femoral neck BMD by 35%. The authors suggest that the polymorphism appears to influence peak BMD and that differences in its distribution may explain racial variations in BMD. The morphological basis of these racial- and genotype-specific differences in areal BMD was not provided. In contrast, Gross *et al.* [20] reported that women with the ff genotype (15% subjects) had 12.8% lower lumbar spine BMD than the FF group. Follow-up over 2 years showed that the decrease in femoral neck BMD was greater in women with ff than with FF (−4.7 vs −0.5%, $P = 0.005$).

Arai *et al.* [21] reported a thymidine–cytosine (T-C) transition polymorphism at the translation initiation codon of the VDR gene in 239 Japanese females aged 24 to 70 years. Among 110 premenopausal women, lumbar spine BMD was 12.0% higher for mm than MM homozygotes (1.043 ± 0.025 versus 0.931 ± 0.026 g/cm^2, respectively). Cloned DNA from the ATG (M allele) variant yielded a 50-kDa protein (designated MP) whereas that from the ACG (m allele) variant yielded a 49.5-kDa protein (mP) in transfected COS-7 cells. Vitamin D-dependent activation of a luciferase reporter construct in transfected HeLa cells was increased 19.5-, 11.2-, and 15.5-fold in cells expressing, respectively, mP, MP, and both mP and MP. The extent of expression of mP was ~20% less than that of MP both *in vitro* and in transfected HeLa cells. The authors conclude that the T-C polymorphism results in synthesis of a smaller protein with increased biologic activity, which is associated with increased BMD. In contrast, Eccleshall *et al.* [22] reported that the start codon polymorphism (SCP) of the VDR gene, examined in 174 premenopausal French women aged 31 to 56 years, was unrelated to the *Bsm*I genotype, to BMD at any site, or to calcium, PTH, or vitamin D levels. NTX was 33.5% higher in ff than FF women ($P = 0.004$), indicative of a difference in bone resorption rate, but no other biochemical markers differed.

Inferences are difficult to make when results are so contradictory. The morphological basis underlying genotypic and racial differences in BMD was not defined in the study by Harris *et al.* [19] in which the femoral neck, not the lumbar spine, was lower in the ff group. In the study by Gross *et al.* [20] the lumbar spine was reduced but rates of loss were greater during follow-up at the femoral neck. Moreover, because the areal BMD measurement does not entirely adjust for bone size, there may be differences in bone size between the genotypes within a race or differences in bone size between the races that may partly account for the differences attributed to the genotype. The problem of size cannot be taken into account by statistical adjustment for size using weight, height, or body mass index because genders and races differ by body segment lengths; the size of the region being studied should be measured.

HIP AXIS LENGTH AND GENOTYPES

Hip axis length (HAL), the distance from greater trochanter to inner pelvic brim, is purported to be an independent predictor of hip fractures. HAL increases during growth to reach a peak length at 15 years [23]. Height-adjusted correlations for HAL in 176 monozygotic (MZ) pairs versus 128 dizygotic (DZ) pairs were 0.79 (95% CI 0.73, 0.84) versus 0.54 (95% CI 0.39, 0.68). About 80% of variation in HAL was attributable to additive genetic factors, which fell to 51% on adjusting for shared environmental factors. The authors suggested that about 10% of the increased risk of hip fracture associated with maternal hip fracture history may be due to genes determining HAL. In a study of adult twins, MZ correlations for areal BMD and geometry ranged between 0.36 and 0.81 and were higher than the DZ trait correlations except femoral neck [24]. Heritability was between 0.72 and 0.78 for regional areal BMD, the center of mass of the femoral neck, and the resistance of the femoral neck to forces experienced in a fall, but not for femoral neck length. Arden *et al.* [25] reported that heritability in 128 identical and 122 non-identical pairs of female twins aged 50 to 70 years was 0.62 (CI 0.22, 1.02) for HAL and was unchanged after adjustment for areal BMD, suggesting that variances for bone architecture as well as areal BMD are partly determined genetically.

Differences in HAL have been observed between genders and races and between hip fracture cases and controls. Faulkner *et al.* [26] reported that HAL was 3.4% greater in 64 hip fracture cases compared with 134 controls. For each SD increase in HAL, fracture risk increased 1.8-fold (95% CI 1.3, 2.5), and for each SD fall in BMD, fracture risk increased 2.7-fold (95% CI 1.7, 4.3). Boonen *et al.* [27] compared 105 women with spine fractures (type I or postmenopausal osteoporosis), 30 with hip fractures (type II or senile osteoporosis), and 75 controls. Femoral neck areal BMD was no different in the two osteoporotic groups, but HAL was greater in the type II group relative to the others. Women with spinal fractures were the same height as the hip fracture cases. If the hip fracture cases had been matched with women in the spinal fracture group who were shorter (but who would have been the same height had they not had spinal fracture), then the difference in HAL may have been even greater.

The 40% lower rate of hip fracture in Asian women and 50% lower hip fracture rates in black women relative to white women are inferred to be due to a greater HAL in whites. HAL was 6.7 ± 0.4 in 135 whites, 6.3 ± 0.3 in 74 Asians, and 6.4 ± 0.4 cm in 50 blacks ($P < 0.01$ for Asians and blacks compared with whites) with differences persisted after height adjustments [28]. The shorter HAL conferred an odds ratio for hip fracture of 0.53 (95% CI, 0.37 to 0.76, Asian) and of 0.68 (95% CI, 0.55 to 0.85, blacks) compared to whites. Nelson *et al.* [29] reported that 34 black and 160 white men aged 23 to 80 years had no difference in HAL. Mikhail *et al.* [30] found greater HAL and femoral neck width in 50 black compared to white premenopausal women.

In a study of 57 Japanese and 119 white women, whites had greater femoral neck BMC (3.91 vs 3.02 g), cross-sectional moment of inertia (0.99 vs 0.57 cm^4), femoral neck length (5.6 vs 4.4 cm), and femoral neck angle (130 vs 128°). The lower risk of femoral neck fracture in Japanese women was attributed to a shorter femoral neck and a smaller femoral neck angle [31]. Daniels *et al.* [32] reported that premenopausal whites had a longer femoral neck axis length than blacks (6.5 ± 0.4 vs 6.1 ± 0.4 cm). Among postmenopausal subjects, the femoral neck axis length was 6.5 ± 0.4 cm in whites and 6.0 ± 0.3 cm in blacks. Chin *et al.* [33] reported that femoral neck length in premenopausal women was 61.5 mm in 52 Chinese, 61.5 mm in 50 Indians, 66.0 mm in 71 Europeans, and 68.2 mm in 52 Polynesians. HAL in the respective groups was 98.0, 94.5, 102.3, and 106.4 mm. The Polynesians were heavier and taller than other groups, followed by the Europeans. The lower incidence of hip fracture in Asians was attributed to a shorter femoral neck length. The very low incidence of hip fracture in Polynesians could not be reconciled with the larger HAL. Reid *et al.* [34] reported a secular increase in HAL and femoral neck length between 1953 and 1990 and suggested that the increased HAL could account for much of the increase in fracture rates in the last 40 years.

The notion of a "longer" or "shorter" HAL may be a function of the size of the femur itself. Height adjustments are unlikely to be a satisfactory way of adjusting for differences in bone size because of racial differences in body segment lengths. Because women have shorter legs than men, a shorter HAL is difficult to reconcile with the higher hip fracture rates in women than in men. Asians have shorter legs than whites of comparable height. Thus the shorter HAL may reflect this difference in bone size. Finding a shorter HAL in blacks may be a conservative bias as blacks have longer legs than whites. A secular increase in HAL may occur along with a secular increase in lower body size. Whether these differences in HAL "cause" gender, racial, and secular differences in hip fractures is speculative. No randomized trials have been undertaken where a group of subjects were stratified by HAL matching by design so that important factors influencing hip fracture risk were equally represented in both groups (e.g., bone mass, size, density, age, illnesses).

ISSUES IN STUDY DESIGN THAT MAY PARTLY ACCOUNT FOR DISCREPANT ASSOCIATIONS BETWEEN BMD AND GENOTYPES

The reported associations between areal BMD in young adults or elderly persons and polymorphisms of the vitamin D receptor, estrogen receptor, and type 1 collagen genes are inconsistent and contradictory [35–38]. Reanalysis of original data reporting higher BMD in the bb genotype of the VDR gene revealed misgenotyping of DNA samples in a proportion of the twins, invalidating the reported notion that 70% of the genetic variance was attributable to VDR polymorphisms [39,40]. Many investigators report no association with VDR genotypes [41–44] whereas others report higher areal BMD in subjects with the BB genotype [45,46]. Thus, associations with higher or lower areal BMD with VDR genotypes vary from study to study. Among the studies published to date, only a small proportion of the population variance, if any, is explained by the VDR, ER, or Col I A1 genotypes [37,47]. Thus, it is reasonable to conclude that genotyping is unlikely to be a useful means of identifying individuals with higher or lower areal BMD or at higher or lower risk of fracture.

If there is an association between any of the genotypes studied and bone fragility, then the association remains undefined at this time. The reasons for this are uncertain. Perhaps the vagaries of the phenotype, areal BMD, preclude detection of any true association with a genetic marker associated with skeletal growth and aging. The role of genetic markers in skeletal growth and aging are undefined themselves. The genes and gene products that regulate the gain in any specific dimension of bone size, accrual of cortical bone, mineralization of bone, determination of trabecular number, or density that regulate activation frequency, bone formation, or resorption at the level of the basic multicellular unit or that regulate periosteal apposition during aging are unknown.

In addition, there are problems in the design of many of the studies that may contribute to the lack of reproducible data. Associations have been reported among genetic markers and more rapid gain in bone size, greater effects of calcium on bone mass during growth, greater bone loss during aging, and greater response to drug therapy. In most studies, the reported associations between genotype and the gain in bone during growth and calcium intake, the loss of bone during aging, and the greater responsiveness to treatment were detected by post hoc analyses, i.e., choices of which genotype group(s) to be compared were made based on data rather than a priori. Most analyses in the literature have compared one genotype against the other two instead of finding a linear association across three genotypes. Post hoc analysis is hypothesis generating, not hypothesis testing. In post hoc analyses the nominal P value attached to the "findings" is not meaningful given that typically a large number of other comparisons are carried out, and usually only the "significant" (i.e., $P < 0.05$) findings are reported.

An association between VDR polymorphisms and the effect of calcium supplementation on the gain in bone mass has been reported in prepubertal girls with a low intake of dietary calcium but not in girls with a high intake of calcium [48]. In 14 girls with the BB genotype, femoral and radial bone mass (but not spinal) increased greatly in response to dietary calcium supplementation than the 40 girls with the bb genotype. The latter group had a higher spontaneous gain in bone mass, which was uninfluenced by calcium supplementation.

Although these data are potentially important, unmeasured confounding factors may explain the observations because randomization to treatment or placebo is carried out without prior stratification by genotype. The hypothesis being tested in the study was whether calcium supplementation influences growth in bone mass and size. If the question concerns the influence of genotype on the response to calcium, then the groups should be first stratified by genotype and then randomized to either placebo or calcium within each genotype. To determine whether one genotype is associated with a greater gain in bone mass during growth also requires that the samples in each genotype are matched by age, bone age, and pubertal status, as well as according to whether individuals (with the same growth velocity) are on the accelerating or decelerating limb of the growth velocity curve.

Changes in growth are large and these confounders have large effects on the growth of bone mass and bone size. If any one of the confounders is overrepresented in one of the genotypes, the greater change in that genotype may be falsely attributed to the genotype. It is very difficult to match for these variables when there are several genotypes to be compared, particularly when one genotype is uncommon and so sample sizes may be small. Under these circumstances, a true association between a genotype and greater bone gain may be difficult to identify because of sample size limitations. Similarly, if the question concerns greater bone loss during aging in a given genotype, stratification by chronological age, years since menopause, and baseline BMD is needed.

BONE LOSS AND GENOTYPES

Several studies suggest an association between rates of bone loss and VDR genotypes. Krall *et al.* [49] reported that the group with the BB genotype lost bone more rapidly at the femoral neck than did bb or Bb groups. Yamagata *et al.* [50] reported that seven women with the BB genotype lost bone more rapidly during 12 months than the other two genotype groups. Ferrari *et al.* [51] reported that among 72 subjects aged around 74 years who participated in a calcium supplementation trial over 18 months that bone loss at the lumbar spine of over 0.48% per year was found in 7 of 9 subjects with the BB allele, in 15 of 37 with Bb, and in 8 of 26 with bb ($P < 0.01$). Rate of change was greater in BB subjects ($-2.3 \pm 1.0\%$ per year) than in bb ($0.7 \pm 0.7\%$ per year) and Bb subjects ($1.0 \pm 0.7\%$ per year). There were no differences in bone loss at the proximal femoral BMD between the genotype groups.

Bone loss after menopause is estrogen dependent. In the elderly, secondary hyperparathyroidism associated with calcium malabsorption may partly contribute to bone loss by increasing cortical bone remodeling. Perhaps polymorphisms of the ER gene or PTH receptor gene may be associated with activation frequency at differing stages of the aging process. Han *et al.* [17] investigated the presence of three restriction fragment length polymorphisms at the ER gene locus in 248 healthy postmenopausal Korean women aged 41 to 68 years. No relationship was present between genotypes and z score of lumbar BMD or response to HRT in terms of BMD mean decrements in biochemical markers. In contrast, Kobayashi *et al.* [52] investigated 238 postmenopausal Japanese aged 45 to 91 years. *Pvu*II (P or p) and *Xba*I (X or x) restriction fragment length polymorphisms were analyzed. z scores of BMD at lumbar spine and total body increased from homozygotes for the Px haplotype (PPxx), to heterozygotes (PPXx, Ppxx), to those lacking the Px haplotype (PPXX, PpXX, ppXx, and ppxx), leading the authors to conclude that a variation in the ER gene partly explains low BMD in postmenopausal Japanese women.

Willing *et al.* [53] examined the association between BMD and changes in BMD over 3 years in about 250 women and polymorphisms for the VDR, ER, type 1 collagen, and other genetic markers. ER polymorphisms predicted BMD but not changes in BMD. VDR polymorphisms were not associated with BMD or changes in BMD. Gene–gene interactions were reported as certain combinations of bb and (−/−) *Pvu*II had higher and BB and (−/−) *Pvu*II had lower BMD. Krall *et al.* [49] reported that 229 healthy postmenopausal women at 0.5 to 37 years postmenopause had greater rates of bone loss over 2 years in the BB group at the femoral neck, radius, and spine.

If the question is whether bone loss is more rapid in one genotype then the subjects should be stratified by genotype with prior matching by age, baseline BMD, menopausal status, body weight, and other factors that may influence the rate of loss. In some studies, cross-sectional data are used and the diminution across age is referred to as a "rate" of loss. For example, Uitterlinden *et al.* [47] reported that 526 women with the Ss genotype had 2% lower femoral neck and lumber spine BMD, whereas 58 with the ss genotype had 4% lower femoral neck and 6% lower lumbar spine BMD compared to 2294 women with the SS genotype of COLIA1. Differences were smaller (and not reported) but still significant after adjusting for the lower body weight in the ss group. The genotype explained 0.2–0.4% of the variance in BMD. Women with Ss or ss were overrepresented in the 111 women with nonverterbal fractures (RR = 1.3 95% CI 1.1,2.1). When stratified by age, the authors found no BMD differences in the 55–65 year olds according to genotype. Among the 75–80 year olds the 91 Ss had 5% lower femoral neck BMD ($P = 0.03$) and 3% lower lumbar spine BMD (NS) than the 205 SS. The 7 ss group had 12% lower at the femoral neck and 20% lower at the spine ($P = 0.04$ and 0.004, respectively). These cross-sectional data do not provide compelling evidence for more rapid bone "loss" in the ss or Ss genotype and it is difficult to conclude, as the authors do, that genotyping at this site may complement information for fracture risk gained from the BMD measurement.

VAGARIES OF THE NOTION OF BONE "LOSS"

Just as the vagaries of areal and volumetric BMD may be an impediment to understanding the causes of bone fragility, the lack of specificity in characterizing bone "loss" into its distinct morphological components is likely to be an impediment in the search for genetic and environmental factors contributing to bone "loss." Bone "loss" is not resorptive "removal" of bone, it is also failure of bone formation. Bone "loss" during aging is the net result of the amount of bone resorbed on the endosteal (intracortical, endocortical, trabecular) surfaces and the amount formed on the periosteal surface. The net amount of bone resorbed on the endosteal surfaces is a function of the imbalance between the absolute amount of bone resorbed and formed at the level of the BMU and the rate of bone remodeling (activation frequency). Thus, examining the rate of bone loss using densitometry as a phenotypic end point to identify causes of bone loss may not be useful as individuals may lose the same amount of bone by entirely different mechanisms; imbalance at the BMU may be the same but due to reduced formation in some patients and due to increased bone resorption in others. Alternatively, the imbalance at the BMU may be less but the remodeling rate may be high. Any genetic or environmental factors contributing to reduced formation, increased resorption, and activation frequency will be obscure unless the heterogeneity of bone loss between individuals and in an individual at different times of life are recognized and taken into account.

Changes on the endosteal surfaces may be obscured by periosteal apposition. An example of this process is the comparison of bone loss in men and women. Bone loss is greater in women than in men, not only because endocortical bone resorption is greater in women than in men, but also because men have greater periosteal apposition, which offsets the bone loss. Using densitometry, the "slower" bone loss in men than in women will be attributed to reduced bone resorption but it is also due to the greater periosteal bone formation. Periosteal apposition differs by region, gender, perhaps race, and perhaps according to biomechanical factors. These components of bone remodeling are not defined in terms of their age-, gender-, and menopause-specified means and variances. Little is known of the means and variances of activation frequency, endocortical, trabecular, and intracortical resorption, and periosteal apposition. Candidate genes for each of these traits are unknown.

CALCIUM ABSORPTION AND GENOTYPES

As bone loss in the elderly may be partly explained by secondary hyperparathyroidism due to calcium malabsorption, more rapid bone loss in one genotype may be the result of an association between reduced calcium absorption and one of the VDR genotypes. Gennari *et al.* [54] examined this possibility in 120 postmenopausal women aged 52 to 75 years. VDR genotypes showed no significant association with femoral neck or lumbar

BMD (although subjects with the aabbTT genotype had 13% higher lumbar BMD than AABBtt and 12% higher lumbar BMD than AaBbTt subjects). Intestinal calcium absorption, measured with SrC12, was lower in BB than in bb, in tt than in TT, and in AABBtt than in aabbTT or AaBbTt genotypes. PTH, alkaline phosphatase, and vitamin D metabolites did not differ by genotype. Zmuda *et al.* [55] studied 156 African American women aged 65 years and older and reported that fractional Ca-45 absorption was 14% lower in women with *BB* than *bb* genotype ($P = 0.08$) but no association between VDR genotypes and BMD was observed between the BMD and the VDR genotypes or bone turnover markers. In another study, women with the BB and bb genotypes had similar fractional calcium absorption on a high calcium intake. However, women with the BB genotype had a lower fractional calcium absorption and a reduced incremental rise in intestinal calcium absorption in response to calcium restriction than those with the bb genotype [56]. Kinyamu *et al.* [57] reported no differences in intestinal VDR protein concentration, calcium absorption, or serum 1,25-dihydroxyvitamin D among 92 Caucasian women aged 25 to 83 years as a group or in the 25- to 35-year or 65- to 83-year-old women. Francis *et al.* [58] reported that no association between fractional calcium absorption or BMD and VDR genotypes in 20 men aged around 60 years with vertebral crush fractures and 28 controls. Barger-Lux *et al.* [59] found no relationship between the allele and the receptor density in duodenal mucosa among 35 premenopausal women.

BIOCHEMICAL MEASUREMENTS OF BONE TURNOVER AND GENOTYPES

Garnero *et al.* [60] studied 189 healthy premenopausal women aged 31 to 57 years. No differences in bone formation (osteocalcin, bone alkaline phosphatase, PICP), bone resorption (CrossLaps, NTX), or BMD (at spine, femur, radius, whole body; measured by DXA) existed among the three VDR genotypes. These polymorphisms were concluded not to be predictive of bone turnover or BMD in these premenopausal women. Garnero *et al.* [61] also reported an analysis of VDR gene polymorphisms in 268 postmenopausal women aged 50 to 70 years. These investigators found no relation of VDR genotype and BMD at spine, hip, forearm, or whole body, with rate of bone loss or with markers of bone formation or bone resorption. There were no differences in age, years since menopause, body mass index, or dietary calcium intake that may obscure any associations. Rates of bone loss measured over 2 years were significant but did not differ among the genotypes. Analyses confined to 128 women within 10 years of menopause did not identify more rapid bone loss in any of the genotypes.

BMD RESPONSES TO INTERVENTION AND GENOTYPES

If the question concerns the detection of a greater response to treatment in a genotype then it is important to first stratify by genotype and then to randomize to placebo versus intervention. In this way, known (age, years postmenopause, dietary calcium intake, baseline BMD) *and* unknown confounders may be controlled so that any observed difference in rates of loss may be inferred to be causally related to the genotype differences. Graafmans *et al.* [62] reported the results of a 2-year study in 81 women aged about 70 years receiving placebo or vitamin D (400 IU daily). Increased BMD in the vitamin D group relative to the placebo group was 4.4% in the BB genotype ($P = 0.04$), 4.2% in the Bb genotype, and −0.3% in the bb genotype group.

The hypothesis that an intervention has a greater effect in one genotype than another has been tested by showing a treatment effect relative to placebo in one genotype but not the other. The hypothesis is tested rigorously by showing that the change (effect in treated minus effect in placebo group) is greater in one genotype than another. Without this approach, a greater effect in one genotype could have been due to confounders. Unless meticulous attention is given to matching the genotypes by these factors, ensuring sufficient numbers are available in each group to detect small but biologically important effects, then a greater effect in one genotype may reflect problems in study design rather than biological diversity.

FRACTURE RATES AND GENOTYPES

If a genotype is associated with an increased fracture risk due to an association with lower BMD or undefined factors, then the genotype should be more prevalent in fracture cases than in nonfracture cases. This has been reported by Uitterlinden *et al.* [47]. Women with Ss or ss were overrepresented in the 111 women with nonvertebral fractures (RR = 1.3 95% CI 1.1,2.1). Among the SS group, 5.4% (64 of 1194) had incident nonvertebral fractures whereas 4.6% (44 of 949) had prevalent vertebral fractures. Among the Ss group, the corresponding fracture data were 7.4% (39 of 526) and 6.7% (28 of

420), respectively; neither fracture type differed by Ss or SS genotype. Among the ss group, 13.8% (8 of 58) had incident nonvertebral fractures and 4.5% (2 of 44) had prevalent vertebral fractures. The only significant odds ratio for incident nonvertebral fractures in the ss was 2.6 (95% confidence interval 1.2, 5.9).

A true association between genotypes and areal BMD and a truly higher prevalence of a genotype in fracture cases may be missed in studies involving small sample sizes. This is a common problem in many studies of healthy individuals and in *most* studies of patients with fractures. The likelihood of finding a higher prevalence of a given genotype among fracture cases is remote given the sample sizes reported. For example, Berg *et al.* [63] detected no association between rate of bone loss and VDR genotypes among 77 of 118 participants followed since 1977. Nineteen of 49 women sustained a fracture over the 18-year study period. No difference in the fracture rate existed between the groups with different vitamin D receptor genotypes. Houston *et al.* [46] reported that among 171 pre- and postmenopausal women aged 45 to 88 years, individuals with the bb genotype had a lower BMD at lumbar spine and femoral neck than those with the BB genotype. No genotype was overrepresented among the 44 women with vertebral fracture. Riggs *et al.* [64] found that no VDR genotype was overrepresented in 43 women with osteoporosis compared to 139 controls. Frequencies of the *Bsm*I genotypes were 16% BB, 47% Bb, and 37% bb in healthy women and 22% BB, 50% Bb, and 28% bb in osteoporotic women.

CONFOUNDING

Confounding or gene–environment interaction may partly contribute to the contradictory data. Susceptibility gene–environment interactions have been proposed to account for the null or contradictory data. Gene–environment interactions may occur but are difficult to identify. Small study samples, low frequency of a susceptibility gene, and low exposure to an environmental factor may preclude the detection of this interaction. The difficulty in identifying an increased risk due to gene–environment interaction is even greater if the exposure results in an increased fracture risk through nongenomic mechanisms. These methodological limitations may result in negative results interpreted as "no effect" rather than "no detectable effect."

If the genotype effect is expressed only in the presence of a low calcium intake, then null results will occur in studies of populations in which the intake is high. The study by Ferrari *et al.* [48] in children receiving calcium supports this notion. In addition, Kiel *et al.* [65] reported no differences in BMD comparing VDR genotypes among 328 subjects aged 69 to 90 years. For subjects with a calcium intake >800 mg/day, trochanteric BMD was higher in bb than in BB groups. For those with a calcium intake <500 mg/day, radial BMD was lower in those with bb than the BB genotype. Comparison of groups with >800 and <500 mg/day showed that BMD was 7 to 12% higher at all hip and radial sites but not at the spine in subjects with the bb genotype who received the higher calcium intake. In a study of 72 adults by Ferrari *et al.* [51], the rate of change in bone mass was independent of calcium intake in BB and bb groups, but in Bb subjects there was a correlation between rate of change in lumbar spinal BMD and mean daily calcium intake (7% per g Ca per day, $r = 0.35$, $P = 0.02$).

The possible effect of body weight on the association between VDR genotypes and bone mass has been reported by Vandevyver *et al.* [66]. VDR gene polymorphism in 807 healthy Belgian postmenopausal women aged 75.5 ± 5.0 and in 84 women with osteoporosis aged around 67 years suggested that the frequencies of the genotypes did not differ in the groups. Age, weight, and height adjusted BMD at the spine and proximal femoral, and proximal radial BMD did not differ with the VDR genotype. On exclusion of women with obesity (BMI > 30 kg/m^2), femoral neck BMD was 5% higher in those with bb than BB and 5% higher in those with aa than AA ($P < 0.05$, both). The authors inferred that environmental factors may affect the detection of an association between BMD and genotype. Barger-Lux *et al.* [59] reported BMC was highest for the bb allele and lowest for the BB allele among 32 healthy premenopausal women aged around 37 years. On adjusting BMC for body weight, its association with the VDR polymorphism disappeared. It is difficult to interpret the changes in the associations before and after adjustment for body weight in these studies. It is likely that the observations were made by post hoc analyses. The test of gene–environment interaction is to demonstrate a dose–response relationship between increasing body weight and age-adjusted BMD, which differs by slope and intercept according to genotype.

THE MISLEADING NOTION OF HERITABILITY

The study of the genetic regulation of the skeletal growth and aging is impeded by the mistaken notion of heritability. The heritability of a trait is not a constant in nature that cannot be modified. If a trait has a high "heritability," this does not mean that little can be done to influence it on an individual basis. Based on twin studies, about 80% of the age-adjusted variance in areal BMD is "heritable" or "genetically determined." The view is often expressed that there is, therefore, 20% of variation "left" to modify. The implication is that environmental factors account for little variation between individuals and it is therefore difficult to alter areal BMD in an individual. The fallacy of this notion of constancy of heritability is seen readily by examining the increases in total height, sitting height, and leg length during the last 50 years [67]. Height is a heritable trait in the sense that the cross-sectional variance appears to be largely explained by genetic factors [68].

Variance is a mathematical measure of the scatter or the between-individual differences in a trait within a specific population. Variance is the sum of the squared distances of each point from the mean (variance in areal BMD having the units g^2/cm^4). Heritability is the proportion of total variance attributable to genetic factors [68,69]:

$$\text{Heritability (\%)} = 100 \times \text{genetic variance} / \text{total variance},$$

where total variance = genetic variance + environmental variance + measurement error.

The heritability of a trait has no single unique value but varies according to which factors are taken into account in specifying the mean, and in partitioning the total variance, in the specific population being studied. The heritability estimate is applicable only to the population and environment from which the sample is drawn. Heritability is not the proportion of an individual's areal BMD attributable to genetic factors. The term does not identify a percentage or a morphologically identifiable part of a trait that is genetically determined or the proportion of disease attributable to genetic factors as often stated [70]. It is incorrect to state that "80%" of areal BMD is due to genes, that a given percentage of fractures is due to genetic factors, and that a given percentage of the population having BMD below 2.5 SD is due to genetic factors. Heritability refers to possible causes of variation-variation in a trait across a particular population.

If total variance (the denominator) increases with age due to an increase in both genetic and environmental variances, but the environmental variance increased more than the genetic variance, then heritability decreases. If the total variance increases due to an increase in the environmental variance, the heritability will decrease despite genetic variance remaining unchanged. If measurement error is high, then the heritability estimate cannot be high because the error component is contained in the denominator.

The value of quantifying genetic and environmental components in absolute terms is seen when candidate genes or environmental factors are fitted to determine whether genetic or environmental factors may explain the variance. Quantifying the total variance and estimating genetic and environmental components of variance are based on principles derived by R.A. Fisher 80 years ago. Modeling can be achieved by studying correlations between twins using the classic twin model, i.e., under the assumption that MZ twin pairs share environmental factors pertinent to the trait to the same extent as DZ twin pairs [68]. If the MZ correlation exceeds the DZ correlation, the model must attribute the excess to the effect of shared genes. If the only reason why twins are correlated is because they share genes, the correlation between MZ pairs will be twice that between DZ pairs. If the DZ correlation is greater than one-half the MZ correlation, then the amount by which it is greater must be attributed by the model to the effects of environmental factors shared by twins: the common environment variance.

GENETIC AND ENVIRONMENTAL COMPONENTS OF VARIANCE IN AREAL BMD

Smith *et al.* [71] reported that the total variance in areal BMD and bone width but not height increased with advancing age and was higher in adult twins compared with juvenile twins (Fig. 4). Hopper *et al.* [72] reported that the total variance in areal BMD increased during pubertal growth and that most of the variance is attributable to unmeasured genetic factors (Fig. 5). The genetic variance in twins aged 13–17 years was less than in twins aged 10–13 years, whereas the common environmental variance was higher in the 13- to 17-year-old group. Factors responsible for the common environmental variance are unknown. The covariance, a measure of resemblance, increased in MZ twins as did the total variance, whereas the covariance of DZ twins increased during adolescence but then decreased in early adulthood. Identical twins are more likely to choose a similar life-style in adulthood so remain similar, whereas DZ twins are more likely to pursue a more independent life-style and consequently become increasingly dissimilar.

In elderly twins, Flicker *et al.* [73] reported that the genetic variance accounts for most of the total variance in areal BMD, but a common environmental component of variance was identified (Fig. 6). The absolute and relative sizes of the genetic and environmental components of variance varied from site to site. Seeman *et al.* [8] reported that the genetic variance accounted for 65% of the total variance at the femoral neck in adult twins (Fig. 7). When adjusted for age and lean mass, the ge-

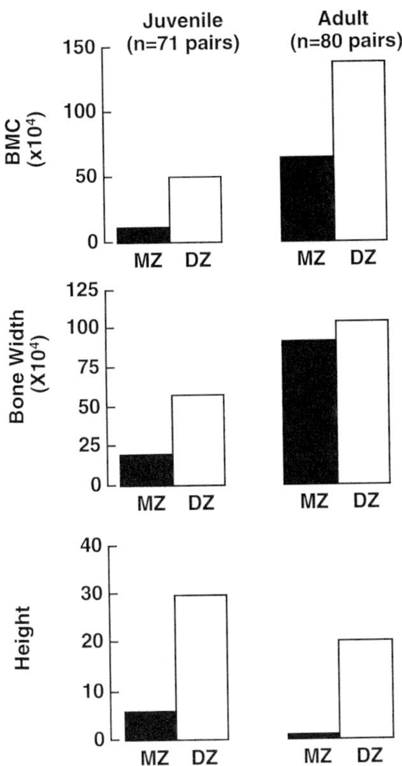

FIGURE 4 The variance with age increases in monozygotic (MZ, black bars) and dizygotic (DZ, white bars) twins for bone mass and width. Variance in height did not increase. Adapted from Smith *et al.* [71].

netic variance decreased by 16% at the femoral neck but the common environmental variance remained unchanged. At the lumbar spine, neither the genetic nor the common environmental variance changed after adjusting for age and lean mass. This is consistent with cross-sectional and within-pair analyses that showed that areal BMD is associated with lean mass, the more so at femoral sites. A reduction in variance of proximal femoral areal BMD, but not spine areal BMD, after adjusting for lean mass could suggest that exercise may be important at the former site. If this were the case, however, then the fall in variance on adjusting for lean mass should have been in the environmental component (although genetic factors may also explain variation in exercise). The observed fall in the genetic component suggests that there are genetic determinants of both areal BMD and lean mass, i.e., there are genes that influence variation in both areal BMD and lean mass.

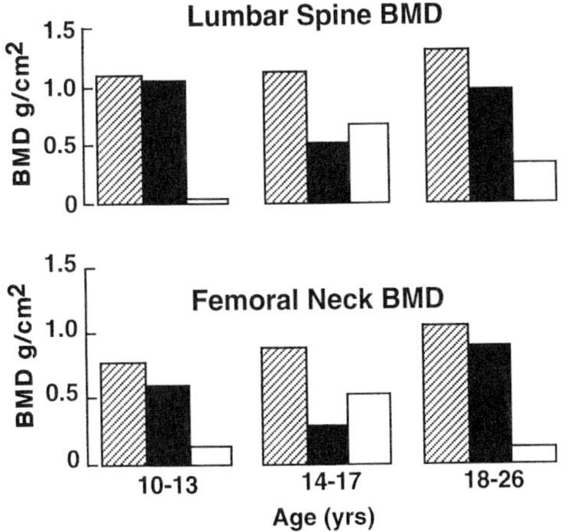

FIGURE 5 Total variance (hatched bars) in areal bone mineral density (BMD) at the lumbar spine and femoral neck is attributable largely to genetic factors (black bars). In twins aged 13–17 years, there was a significant common environmental component of variance (white bars). Adapted from Hopper *et al.* [72].

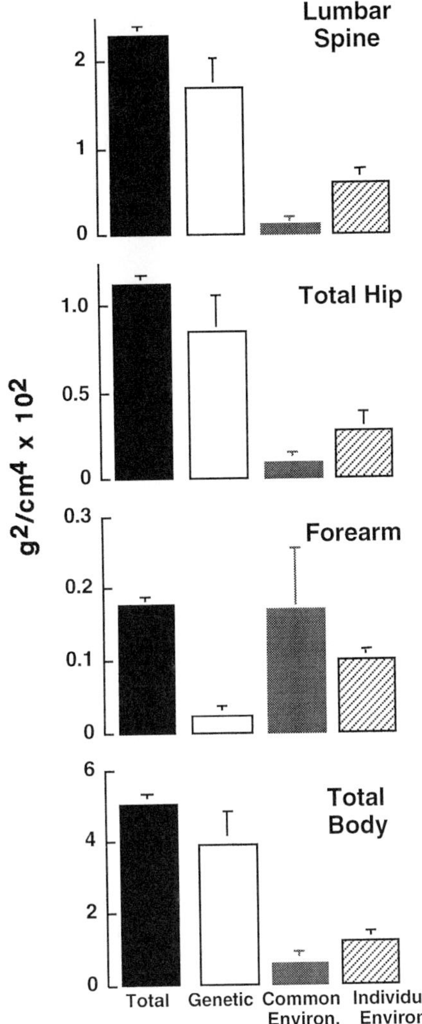

FIGURE 6 Total variance (black bars) and its components: genetic (white bars), common environmental (gray bars), and individual environmental (hatched bars). Genetic variance in elderly twins accounts for most of the total variance in areal BMD, but a large common environmental component was identified at the forearm. Adapted from Flicker *et al.* [73].

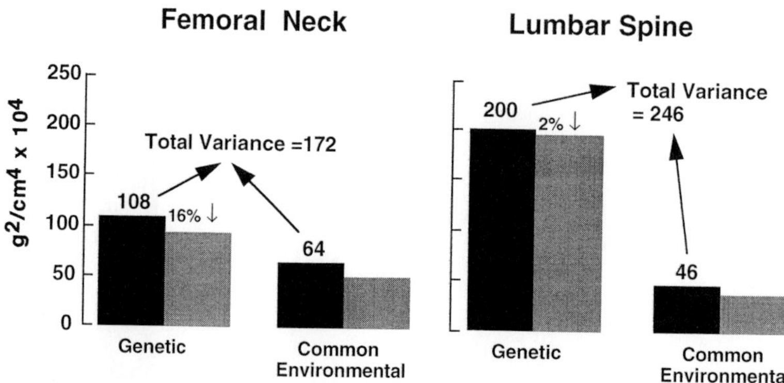

FIGURE 7 Total variance was lower at the femoral neck than at the lumbar spine. For femoral neck areal bone mineral density, the age-adjusted genetic variance (black bars) decreased by 16% after adjusting for lean mass (gray bars); the common environmental variance remained unchanged. At the lumbar spine, adjusting for lean mass reduced the genetic variance by only 2%. Adapted from Seeman *et al.* [8].

To address this, the covariance between lean mass and bone mass was examined by comparing the cross-trait correlations in an individual and between co-twins. The cross-trait correlation in self, i.e., between an individual's total body lean mass and her own femoral neck areal BMD, was about 0.25. The cross-twin, cross-trait correlation (lean mass in twin 1 versus areal BMD in twin 2) was similar to the cross trait correlation in self for the MZ twins and greater than in DZ twins (Fig. 8). When height was taken into account, the cross-trait correlations in self decreased and the cross-trait, cross-twin correlations were not different between MZ and DZ pairs, suggesting that genes regulating size are involved in genes that are common to areal BMD and lean mass [8].

In a study of 227 pairs of monozygous and 126 pairs of dizygous female twins aged 45 to 70 years, Arden and Spector [74] reported higher intraclass correlations for muscle strength and mass in monozygous than in dizygous twins (0.69 ± 0.03 vs 0.41 ± 0.07 for lean body mass, 0.49 ± 0.05 vs 0.31 ± 0.08 for grip strength, 0.44 ± 0.60 vs 0.14 ± 0.10 for leg extensor strength, after adjusting for age, height, and weight). Heritability estimates demonstrated a genetic component to lean body mass, grip strength, and leg extensor strength of 0.46, 0.30, and 0.52, respectively. However, the total additive genetic influence of BMD was reduced on adjusting for muscle variables, suggesting that there may be common genetic factors regulating muscle and bone mass. The authors also reported an independent associa-

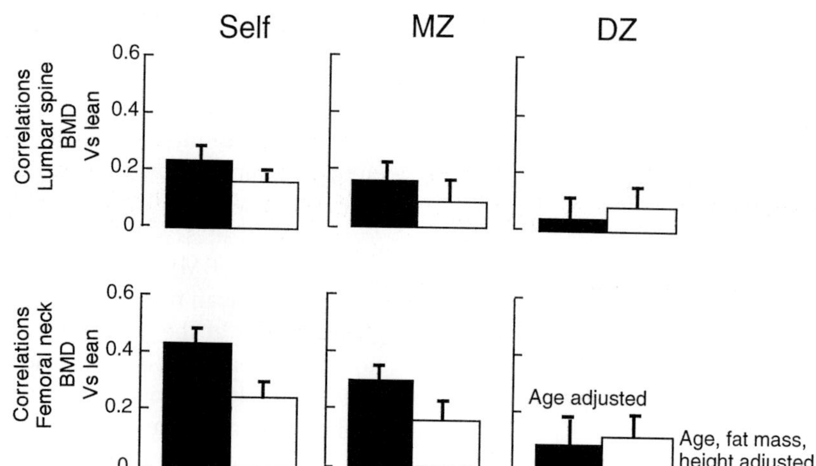

FIGURE 8 Cross-correlations in lumbar spine and femoral neck bone mineral density (BMD) with total body lean mass in an individual (Self) and BMD in one twin with lean mass in the other for MZ and DZ pairs. Adapted from Seeman *et al.* [8].

tion between muscle strength and bone mass after adjusting for lean mass.

In a study of in 57 monozygotic and 55 dizygotic female twin pairs aged 52.8 ± 13 years, Nguyen *et al.* [74] reported that intrapair differences in lean mass were associated with intrapair differences in femoral neck BMD, fat mass was associated with TBBMD, whereas both lean and fat mass were independent determinants of lumbar BMD. In contrast to the previously described studies, these investigators reported that the genetic correlation of lean mass and BMD was not significant and that the association between lean and fat mass was attributable mainly to environmental factors. The authors concluded that lean and fat mass and BMD are under strong genetic regulation, but that the associations between them are mediated largely via environmental influences. Reasons for the disparate observations are not apparent.

Guesens *et al.* [76] reported an association between muscle strength and VDR genotypes. The investigators found no association between BMD at the femoral neck, lumbar spine, and proximal forearm and VDR genotypes in 501 healthy women aged above 70 years. However, in a post hoc analysis in nonobese women, femoral neck BMD was 5% higher in women with bb than BB genotypes (z scores were -0.35 ± 0.13 for BB, -0.09 ± 0.07 for Bb, and -0.04 ± 0.09 for bb). Women with the BB genotype had 23% lower quadriceps strength than those with the bb genotype, which remained significant after adjusting for age, calcium intake, and femoral neck BMD. The reason for adjusting for BMD is not apparent. Whether there were differences in exercise activity or muscle size that may account for the muscle strength differences was not examined. After correction for quadriceps strength, no difference in femoral neck BMD was found between the VDR types in nonobese women. From these data, the authors inferred that an association exists between muscle strength and an allelic variant at the VDR locus in nonobese elderly women, which could contribute to the association between VDR polymorphism and femoral neck BMD.

SUMMARY

Heritability refers to one possible explanation of variance in a trait such as areal bone mineral density. Heritability is the proportion of the total population variance (genetic plus environmental) in areal BMD attributable to genetic factors. The term does not refer to an identifiable part of an individual's areal BMD that is inherited. The statement "80% of areal BMD is genetically determined leaving only 20% to modify" is flawed; heritability is not a constant proportion leaving 20% "due to" environmental factors that can be changed. The size of the total population variance depends on the factors chosen to describe the trait mean (such as age, gender, height, body composition). If total variance increases due to an increase in the environmental variance, without change in the genetic variance, heritability will decrease. Thus, "heritability"—a proportion—and "genetic variance"—an absolute—may give different impressions of the "strength" of genetic factors.

Areal BMD is not a specific and unambiguous morphological structure with identifiable physiological control mechanisms. It is the net result of the modeling and remodeling on the periosteal and endosteal surfaces that give the bone its mass, size, and architecture. Each surface behaves differently during growth and aging because each is regulated differently. The ambiguity of areal BMD is likely to make this an unsatisfactory phenotype for the identification of genes that contribute to the regulation of skeletal growth and aging. No gene, gene product, or gene polymorphism has been reproducibly and credibly shown to account for a given proportion of the variance in areal BMD. Data concerning candidate markers such as polymorphisms of the vitamin D receptor, estrogen receptor, and type 1 collagen genes are inconsistent, partly because of the questionable value of the phenotype being studied, the use of genetic markers of uncertain biological function, flaws in study design such as small sample sizes, failure to account for confounding, lack of stratification and/or randomization prior to intervention, reliance on statistical adjustment rather than study design, and the use of post hoc analyses to infer causation.

These flaws need to be addressed. Distinct morphological structures (trabecular number, thickness, periosteal and endocortical width, cortical thickness) should be quantified according to their age-, gender-, and race-specific means and variances. Genetic and environmental factors should be sought that explain variance in (i) periosteal expansion before puberty (forming external bone size), (ii) endocortical contraction at puberty (determining cortical thickness), (iii) trabecular number (which do not differ by race or gender) and thickness (which varies by race but not by gender), (iv) periosteal modeling during aging (offsetting bone loss), and (v) endosteal remodeling during aging (producing cortical thinning, trabecular thinning, and perforation). Expressing variance in absolute terms and fitting candidate genetic and environmental factors that may explain variance are hypothesis generating. Controlled randomized trials with prior stratification by genotype are needed to identify genotype-specific effects. The null hypothesis states that no biologically meaningful effect exists among genotypes, skeletal growth, aging, and effects of treatment. This hypothesis cannot be rejected until the studies are properly designed by stratification and control of confounding by design, rather than using statistical "adjustment."

References

1. Gilsanz, V., Loro, M. L., Roe, T. F., Sayre, J., Gilsanz, R., and Schulz, E. E. Gender differences in vertebral size in adults: biomechanical implications. *J. Clin. Invest.* **95,** 2332–2337 (1995).
2. Vega, E., Ghiringhelli, G., Mautalen, C., Valzacchi, G. R., Scaglia, H., and Zylberstein, C. Bone mineral density and bone size in men with primary osteoporosis and vertebral fractures. *Calcif. Tissue Int.* **62,** 465–469 (1998).
3. Bass, S., Pearce, G., Tabensky, A., Hendrich, E., Delmas, P. D., Seeman, E. Differing rates of skeletal maturation: Size versus mass, axial versus appendicular, periosteal versus endocortical, apparent versus true density. Antecedents of site-specific deficits in osteoporosis? Submitted.
4. Zhang, X. Z., Kalu, D. N., Erbas, B., Hopper, J. L., Seeman, E. The effect of gonadectomy on bone size, mass and volumetric density in growing rats may be gender-, site-, and growth hormone-dependent. Submitted.
5. Lu, P. W., Cowell, C. T., Lloyd-Jones, S. A., Broidy J., and Howman-Giles, R. Volumetric bone mineral density in normal subjects, aged 5–27 years. *J. Clin. Endocrinol. Metab.* **81,** 1586–1590 (1996).
6. Zamberlan, N., Radetti, G., Paganini, C., Gatti, D., Rossini, M., and Braga, V. Evaluation of cortical thickness and bone density by roentgen microdensitometry in growing males and females. *Eur. J. Pediatr.* **155,** 377–382 (1996).
7. Warner, J., Cowan, F., Dunstan, F., Evans, W., Webb, D., and Gregory, J. Measured and predicted bone mineral content in healthy boys and girls aged 6–18 years: adjusted for size and puberty. *Acta Paediatr.* **87,** 244–249 (1998).
8. Seeman, E., Hopper, J. L., Young, N. R., Formica, C., Goss, P., and Tsalamandris, C. Do genetic factors contribute to associations between muscle strength, fat-free mass and bone density? *Am. J. Physiol.* **270,** E320–E327 (1996).
9. Seeman, E. Growth in bone mass and size—are racial and gender differences in bone mineral density more apparent than real? *J. Clin. Endocrinol. Metab.* **68,** 1414–1419 (1998).
10. Gilsanz, V., Skaggs, D. I., Kevanikaya, A., *et al.* Differential effects of race on the axial and appendicular skeleton of children. *J. Clin. Endocrinol. Metab.* 1420–1427 (1998).
11. Rosen, C. J., Dimai, H. P., Vereault, D., Donahue, L. R., Beamer, W. G., Farley, J., Linkhart, S., Linkhart, T., Mohan, S., and Baylink, D. J. Circulating and skeletal insulin-like growth factor-I (IGF-I) concentrations in two inbred strains of mice with different bone mineral densities. *Bone* **21,** 217–223 (1997).
12. Sainz, J., Van Tornout, J. M., Loro, M. L., Sayre, J., Roe, T. F., and Gilsanz, V. Vitamin D-receptor gene polymorphisms and bone density in prepubertal American girls of Mexican descent. *N. Engl. J. Med.* **337,** 77–82 (1997).
13. Gunnes, M., Berg, J. P., Halse, J., and Lehmann, E. H. Lack of relationship between vitamin D receptor genotype and forearm bone gain in healthy children, adolescents, and young adults. *J. Clin. Endocrinol. Metab.* **82,** 851–855 (1997).
14. Mizunuma, H., Hosoi, T., Okano, H., Soda, M., Tokizawa, T., Kagami, I., Miyamoto, S., Ibuki, Y., Inoue, S., Shiraki, M., and Ouchi, Y. Estrogen receptor gene polymorphism and bone mineral density at the lumbar spine of pre- and postmenopausal women. *Bone* **21,** 379–383 (1997).
15. Suarez, F., Zeghoud, F., Rossignol, C., Walrant, O., and Garabédian, M. Association between vitamin D receptor gene polymorphism and sex-dependent growth during the first two years of life. *J. Clin. Endocrinol. Metab.* **82,** 2966–2970 (1997).
16. Keen, R. W., Egger, P., Fall, C., Major, P. J., Lanchbury, J. S., Spector, T. D., and Cooper, C. Polymorphisms of the vitamin D receptor, infant growth, and adult bone mass. *Calcif. Tissue Int.* **60,** 233–235 (1997).
17. Han, K. O., Moon, I. G., Kang, Y. S., Chung, H. Y., Min, H. K., and Han, I. K. Nonassociation of estrogen receptor genotypes with bone mineral density and estrogen responsiveness to hormone replacement therapy in Korean postmenopausal women. *J. Clin. Endocrinol. Metab.* **82,** 991–995 (1997).
18. Han, Z.-H., Palnitka, S., Sudhaker, R. A. O., Nelson, D., and Parfitt, A. M. Effects of ethnicity and age or menopause on the remodeling and turnover of iliac bone: Implications for mechanisms of bone loss. *J. Bone Miner. Res.* **12,** 498–508 (1997).
19. Harris, S. S., Eccleshall, T. R., Gross, C., Dawson-Hughes, B., and Feldman, D. The vitamin D receptor start codon polymorphism (FokI) and bone mineral density in premenopausal American black and white women. *J. Bone Miner. Res.* **12,** 1043–1048 (1997).
20. Gross, C., Eccleshall, T. R., Malloy, P. J., Villa, M. L., Marcus, R., and Feldman, D. The presence of a polymorphism at the translation initiation site of the vitamin D receptor gene is associated with low bone mineral density in postmenopausal Mexican-American women. *J. Bone Miner. Res.* **11,** 1850–1855 (1996).
21. Arai, H., Miyamoto, K.-I., Taketani, Y., Yamamoto, H., Iemori, Y., Morita, K., Tonai, T., Nishisho, T., Mori, S., and Takeda, E. A vitamin D receptor gene polymorphism in the translation initiation codon: effect on protein activity and relation to bone mineral density in Japanese women. *J. Bone Miner. Res.* **12,** 915–921 (1997).
22. Eccleshall, T. R., Garnero, P., Gross, C., Delmas, P. D., and Feldman, D. Lack of correlation between start codon polymorphism of the vitamin D receptor gene and bone mineral density in premenopausal French women: the OFELY study. *J. Bone Miner. Res.* **13,** 31–35 (1998).
23. Flicker, L., Faulkner, K. G., Hopper, J. L., Green, R. M., Kaymakci, B., Nowson, C. A., Young, D., and Wark, J. D. Determinants of hip axis length in women aged 10–89 years: a twin study. *Bone* **18,** 41–45 (1996).
24. Slemenda, C. W., Turner, C. H., Peacock, M., Christian, J. C., Sorbel, J., Hui, S. L., and Johnston, C. C. The genetics of proximal femur geometry, distribution of bone mass and bone mineral density. *Osteopor. Int.* **6,** 178–182 (1996).
25. Arden, N. K., Baker, J., Hogg, C., Baan, K., and Spector, T. D. The heritability of bone mineral density, ultrasound of the calcaneus and hip axis length: a study of postmenopausal twins. *J. Bone Miner. Res.* **11,** 530–534 (1996).
26. Faulkner, K. G., Cummings, S. R., Black, D., Palermo, L., Gluer, C. C., and Genant, H. K. Simple measurement of femoral geometry predicts hip fracture in the study of osteoporotic fractures. *J. Bone Miner. Res.* **8,** 1211–1217 (1993).
27. Boonen, S., Koutri, R., Dequeker, J., Aerssens, J., Lowet, G., Nijs, J., Verbeke, G., Lesaffre, E., and Geusens, P. Measurement of femoral geometry in type I and type II osteoporosis: differences in hip axis length consistent with heterogeneity in the pathogenesis of osteoporotic fractures. *J. Bone Miner. Res.* **10,** 1908–1912 (1995).
28. Cummings, S. R., Cauley, J. A., Palermo, L., Ross, P. D., Wasnich, R. D., Black, D., and Faulkner, K. G. Racial differences in hip

axis lengths might explain racial differences in rates of hip fracture. *Osteoporosis Int.* **4,** 226–229 (1994).

29. Nelson, D. A., Jacobsen, G., Barondess, D. A., and Parfitt, A. M. Ethnic differences in regional bone density, hip axis length, and lifestyle variables among healthy black and white men. *J. Bone Miner. Res.* **10,** 782–787 (1995).
30. Mikhail, M. B., Vaswani, A. N., and Aloia, J. F. Racial differences in femoral dimensions and their relationship to hip fractures. *Osteopor. Int.* **6,** 22–24 (1996).
31. Nakamura, T., Turner, C. H., Yoshikawa, T., Slemenda, C. W., Peacock, M., Burr, D. B., Mizuno, Y., Orimo, H., Ouchi, Y., and Johnston, C. C., Jr. Do variations in hip geometry explain differences in hip fracture risk between Japanese and white Americans? *J. Bone Miner. Res.* **9,** 1071–1076 (1994).
32. Daniels, E. D., Pettifor, J. M., Schnitzler, C. M., Moodley, G. P., and Zachen, D. Differences in mineral homeostasis, volumetric bone mass and femoral neck axis length in black and white South African women. *Osteopor. Int.* **7,** 105–112 (1997).
33. Chin, K., Evans, M. C., Cornish, J., Cundy, T., and Reid, I. R. Differences in hip axis and femoral neck length in premenopausal women of Polynesian, Asian and European origin. *Osteopor. Int.* **7,** 344–347 (1997).
34. Reid, I. R., Chin, K., Evans, M. C., and Jones, J. G. Relation between increase in length of hip axis in older women between 1950s and 1990s and increase in age specific rates of hip fracture. *Br. Med. J.* **309,** 508–509 (1994).
35. Eisman, J. A. Vitamin D receptor gene alleles and osteoporosis: an affirmative view. *J. Bone Miner. Res.* **10,** 1289–1293 (1995).
36. Peacock, M. Vitamin D receptor gene alleles and osteoporosis: a contrasting view. *J. Bone Miner. Res.* **10,** 1294–1297 (1995).
37. Cooper, G. S. and Umbach, D. M. Are vitamin D receptor polymorphisms associated with bone mineral density? A metaanalysis. *J. Bone Min. Research* 1841–1849 (1996).
38. Ralston, S. H. The genetics of osteoporosis. *Q. J. Medicine* **90,** 247–251 (1997).
39. Morrison, N. A., Qi, J. C., Tokita, A., Kelly, P. J., Crofts, L., Nguyen, T. V., Sambrook, P. N., and Eisman, J. A. Prediction of bone density from vitamin D receptor alleles. *Nature* **367,** 284–287 (1994).
40. Morrison, N. A., Qi, J. C., Tokita, A., Kelly, P. J., Crofts, L., Nguyen, T. V., Sambrook, P. N., and Eisman, J. A. Prediction of bone density from vitamin D receptor alleles. *Nature* **387,** 106 (1997).
41. Hustmyer, F. G., Peacock, M., Hui, S., Johnston, C. C., Christian, J. Bone mineral density in relation to polymorphism at the vitamin D receptor gene locus. *J. Clin. Invest.* **94,** 2130–2134 (1994).
42. Spotila, L. D., Caminis, J., Johnston, R., Shimoya, K. S., O'Connor, M. P., Prockop, D. J., Tenenhouse, H. S. Vitamin D receptor genotype is not associated with bone mineral density in three ethnic/regional groups. *Calcif. Tissue Int.* **59,** 235–237 (1996).
43. Tsai, K. S., Hsu, S. H. J., Cheng, W. C., Chen, C. K., Chieng, P. U., Pan, W. H. Bone mineral density and bone markers in relation to vitamin D receptor gene polymorphisms in Chinese men and women. *Bone* **19,** 513–518 (1996).
44. McClure, L., Eccleshall, T. R., Gross, C., Luz Villa, M., Lin, N., Ramaswamy, V., Kohlmeier, L., Kels, J. L., Marcus, R., Feldman, D. Vitamin D receptor polymorphisms, bone mineral density, and body metabolism in postmenopausal Mexican–American women. *J. Bone Miner. Res.* **12,** 234–240 (1997).
45. Salamone, L. M., Ferrell, R., Black, D. M., Palermo, L., Epstein, R. S., Petro, N., Steadman, N., Kuller, L., Cauley, J. A. The association between vitamin D receptor gene polymorphisms and bone mineral density in the spine, hip and whole-body in premenopausal women. *Osteoporosis Int.* **6,** 63–68 (1996).
46. Houston, L. A., Grant, S. F. A., Reid, D. M., and Ralston, S. H. Vitamin D receptor polymorphism, bone mineral density, and osteoporotic vertebral fracture: studies in a UK population. *Bone* **18,** 249–252 (1996).
47. Uitterlinden, A. G., Burger, H., Huang, Q., Fang, Y., McGuigan, F. E. A., Grant, S. F. A., Hofman, A., van Leeuwen, J. P. T. M., Pols, H. A. P., and Ralston, S. H. Relation of alleles of the collagen type I alpha 1 gene to bone density and the risk of osteoporotic fractures in postmenopausal women. *N. Engl. J. Med.* **338,** 1016–1021 (1998).
48. Ferrari, S. L., Rizzoli, R., Slosman, D. O., and Bonjour, J.-P. Do dietary calcium and age explain the controversy surrounding the relationship between bone mineral density and vitamin D receptor gene polymorphisms? *J. Bone Miner. Res.* **13,** 363–370 (1998).
49. Krall, E. A., Parry, P., Lichter, J. B., and Dawson-Hughes, B. Vitamin D receptor alleles and rates of bone loss: influences of years since menopause and calcium intake. *J. Bone Miner. Res.* **10,** 978–984 (1995).
50. Yamagata, V., Miyamura, T., Iijima, S., Sasaki, M., Kato, J., and Koizumi, K. Vitamin D receptor gene polymorphism and bone mineral density in healthy Japanese women. *Lancet* **344,** 1027 (1994).
51. Ferrari, S., Rizzoli, R., Chevalley, T., Slosman, D., Eisman, J. A., and Bonjour, J.-P. Vitamin-D-receptor-gene polymorphisms and change in lumbar–spine bone mineral density. *Lancet* **345,** 423–424 (1995).
52. Kobayashi, S., Inoue, S., Hosoi, T., Ouchi, Y., Shiraki, M., and Orimo, H. Association of bone mineral density with polymorphism of the estrogen receptor gene. *J. Bone Miner. Res.* **11,** 306–311 (1996).
53. Willing, M., Sowers, M. F., Aron, D., Clark, M. K., Burns, T., Bunten, C., Crutchfield, M., D'Agostino, D., and Jannausch, M. Bone mineral density and its change in white women: Estrogen and vitamin D receptor genotypes and their interaction. *J. Bone Miner. Res.* **13,** 695–705 (1998).
54. Gennari, L., Becherini, L., Masi, L., Gonnelli, S., Cepollaro, C., Martini, S., Mansani, R., and Brandi, M. L. Vitamin D receptor genotypes and intestinal calcium absorption in postmenopausal women. *Calcif. Tissue Int.* **61,** 460–463 (1997).
55. Zmuda, J. M., Cauley, J. A., Danielson, M. E., Wolf, R. L., and Ferrell, R. E. Vitamin D receptor gene polymorphisms, bone turnover, and rates of bone loss in older African-American women. *J. Bone Miner. Res.* **12,** 1446–1452 (1997).
56. Dawson-Hughes, B., and Harris, S. S. Calcium absorption on high and low calcium intakes in relation to vitamin D receptor genotype. *J. Clin. Endocrinol. Metab.* **80,** 3657–3661 (1995).
57. Kinyamu, H. K., Gallagher, J. C., Knezetic, J. A., DeLuca, H. F., Prahl, J. M., and Lanspa, S. J. Effect of vitamin D receptor genotypes on calcium absorption, duodenal vitamin D receptor concentration, and serum 1,25 dihydroxyvitamin D levels in normal women. *Calcif. Tissue Int.* **60,** 491–495 (1997).
58. Francis, R. M., Harrington, F., Turner, E., Papiha, S. S., and Datta, H. K. Vitamin D receptor gene polymorphism in men and its effect on bone density and calcium absorption. *Clin. Endocrinol.* **46,** 83–86 (1997).
59. Barger-Lux, M. J., Heaney, R. P., Hayes, J., DeLuca, H. F., Johnson, M. L., and Gong, G. Vitamin D receptor gene polymorphism, bone mass, body size, and vitamin D receptor density. *Calcif. Tissue Int.* **57,** 161–162 (1995).
60. Garnero, P., Borel, O., Sornay-Rendu, E., and Delmas, P. D. Vitamin D receptor gene polymorphisms do not predict bone turnover and bone mass in healthy premenopausal women. *J. Bone Miner. Res.* **10,** 1283–1288 (1995).

61. Garnero, P., Borel, O., Sornay-Rendu, E., Arlot, M. E., and Delmas, P. D. Vitamin D receptor gene polymorphisms are not related to bone turnover, rate of bone loss, and bone mass in postmenopausal women: the OFELY study. *J. Bone Miner. Res.* **11,** 827–834 (1996).
62. Graafmans, W. C., Lips, P., Ooms, M. E., van Leeuwen, J. P. T. M., and Pols, H. A. P. The effect of vitamin D supplementation on the bone mineral density of the femoral neck is associated with vitamin D receptor genotype. *J. Bone Miner. Res.* **12,** 1241–1245 (1997).
63. Berg, J. P., Falch, J. A., and Haug, E. Fracture rate, pre- and postmenopausal bone mass and early and late postmenopausal bone loss are not associated with vitamin D receptor genotype in a high-endemic area of osteoporosis. *Eur. J. Endocrinol.* **135,** 96–100 (1996).
64. Riggs, B. L., Nguyen, T. V., Melton, L. J., III, Morrison, N. A., O'Fallon, W. M., Kelly, P. J., Egan, K. S., Sambrook, P. N., Muhs, J. M., and Eisman, J. A. The contribution of vitamin D receptor gene alleles to the determination of bone mineral density in normal and osteoporotic women. *J. Bone Miner. Res.* **10,** 991–996 (1995).
65. Kiel, D. P., Myers, R. H., Cupples, L. A., Kong, X. F., Zhu, X. H., Ordovas, J., Schaefer, E. J., Felson, D. T., Rush, D., Wilson, P. W. F., Eisman, J. A., and Holick, M. F. The BsmI vitamin D receptor restriction fragment length polymorphism (bb) influences the effect of calcium intake on bone mineral density. *J. Bone Miner. Res.* **12,** 1049–1057 (1997).
66. Vandevyver, C., Wylin, T., Cassiman, J.-J., Raus, J., Geusens, P., Dr. L. Willems-Inst, Diepenbeek, Belgium and two other centers. Influence of the vitamin D receptor gene alleles on bone mineral density in postmenopausal and osteoporotic women. *J. Bone Miner. Res.* **12,** 241–247 (1997).
67. Bakwin, H. Secular increase in height: Is the end in sight? *Lancet* **2,** 1195–1196 (1964).
68. Hopper, J. L. Variance components for statistical genetics: applications in medical research to characteristics related to human diseases and health. *Stat. Methods Med. Res.* **2,** 199–223 (1993).
69. Hopper, J. L. Heritability. *In* "Encyclopedia of Biostatistics" (P. Armitage and T. Colton, eds.). Wiley, New York, 1998.
70. Spector, T. D., Cicuttini, F., Baker, J., Loughlin, J., and Hart, D. Genetic influences on osteoarthritis in woman: a twin study. *Br. Med. J.* **312,** 940–943 (1996).
71. Smith, D. M., Nance, W. E., Kang, K. W., Christian, J. C., and Johnston, C. C., Jr. Genetic factors in determining bone mass. *J. Clin. Invest.* **52,** 2800–2808 (1973).
72. Hopper, J. L., Green, R. M., Nowson, C. A., Young, D., Sherwin, A. J., Kaymakci, B., Larkins, R. G., and Wark, J. D. Genetic, common environment, and individual specific components of variance for bone mineral density in 10- to 26-year-old females: a twin study. *Am. J. Epidemiol.* **147,** 17–29 (1998).
73. Flicker, L., Hopper, J. L., Rodgers, L., Kaymakci, B., Green, R. M., and Wark, J. D. Bone density determinants in elderly women: a twin study. *J. Bone Miner. Res.* **10,** 1607–1613 (1995).
74. Arden, N. K., and Spector, T. D. Genetic influences on muscle strength, lean body mass, and bone mineral density: a twin study. *J. Bone Miner. Res.* **12,** 2076–2081 (1997).
75. Nguyen, T. V., Howard, G. M., Kelly, P. J., and Eisman, J. A. Bone mass, lean mass, and fat mass: same genes or same environments? *Am. J. Epidemiol.* **147,** 3–16 (1998).
76. Geusens, P., Vandevyver, C., Vanhoof, J., Cassiman, J.-J., Boonen, S., and Raus, J. Quadriceps and grip strength are related to vitamin D receptor genotype in elderly nonobese women. *J. Bone Miner. Res.* **12,** 2082–2088 (1997).

Nutritional Determinants of Peak Bone Mass

TOM LLOYD AND DEBORAH CARDAMONE CUSATIS

The Department of Health Evaluation Sciences, Penn State College of Medicine and University Hospitals, M. S. Hershey Medical Center, Hershey, Pennsylvania 17033

Elucidation of the factors that lead to the development of peak bone mass is an essential step in the construction of strategies to prevent osteoporosis. However, our understanding of the nutritional determinants of peak bone mass is rudimentary at best. The average woman gains 40–50% of her skeletal mass, i.e., approximately 1000 g of bone mineral, during adolescence. In the past two decades the majority of our efforts to understand the relationships between bone gain and nutrient intake have focused on calcium intake during this period. From an evolutionary view, there is abundant evidence that the human species in the preagricultural era had larger and probably stronger bones than modern humans and had higher daily intakes of calcium (see Chapter 1). Our prehistoric ancestors also consumed many more calories as well as calcium to sustain their very much greater levels of daily physical activity [1–3].

In the past two decades, many cross-sectional observational epidemiologic studies have addressed the general question of calcium intake, bone health, and risk of osteoporotic fracture in women. To date, the findings have been inconsistent [4–9]. During the same time period, the possible roles of other minerals and macronutrients, particularly sodium, phosphate, and protein, on bone health have also been examined with cross-sectional retrospective studies [10–18]. In an attempt to resolve the many questions that have emerged on the relationships between nutrient intake and bone gain, a number of calcium supplementation trials with children and adolescents have been undertaken [19–29]. This chapter focuses on studies performed by others and by the authors on relationships between nutrient intake and bone gain among adolescent females during ages 12–18.

TIMING OF ADOLESCENT BONE GAIN

Normative data on bone gain in adolescent females are now available from a large number of cross-sectional studies and a much smaller number of longitudinal studies. These studies, which have been performed with several ethnic groups in the United States, as well as in Canada, Argentina, France, Denmark, Belgium, Finland, Sweden, and the Netherlands, all show that peak velocity for bone gain occurs between the ages of 12 and 14 [30–44], whereas peak height velocity occurs at age 11. Total body bone gain data from the longitudinal Penn State Young Women's Health Study show that 12-year-old females have, on average, a total body bone mineral content of 1317 g, which is approximately 57% of their expected adult skeletal mass. Between the ages of 12 and 14 they gain, on average, 489 g bone mineral, or 22% of their skeletal mass. For the interval ages 12–16, they gain, on average, 800 g of bone mineral, which is the equivalent to approximately 35% of their adult skeletal mass. Thus, by age 16, young women have achieved approximately 92% of their adult skeletal mass. Given the magnitude of bone gain during ages 12–16, and especially 12–14, modifiable determinants of peak bone mass may be most important during these years.

SECULAR TRENDS IN DIETS OF YOUNG WOMEN

The National Health and Nutrition Examination Surveys (NHANES I, II, and III) provide large, cross-sectional nutrient intake data bases [45]. In addition, dietary studies of children and adolescents have been performed with six cohorts of 10 year olds and two cohorts of 13 year olds as part of the Bogalusa Heart Study [46]. From these sources, we know that as children get older, mean intakes of vitamins and minerals per 1000 kcal decrease. Additionally, over the 14-year period between 1974 and 1988, 10 year olds in Bogalusa had unchanged total energy intakes, yet were 3 pounds heavier, indicating a decrease in physical activity. Furthermore, from a 24-hr recall dietary intake survey administered to 2772 college students at a large midwestern university, it was noted that 40% of the students had not eaten any fruit and 55% of the students had not eaten green salad or cooked vegetables in the previous 24 hr [47]. Thus, despite a probable increase in knowledge about nutrition among teenagers and well-founded national nutrition education efforts, U.S. teenagers do not appear to be improving their dietary behavior with time.

CANDIDATE NUTRIENT–BONE RELATIONSHIPS

Several calcium supplementation trials have been conducted with adolescent females in the United States, as well as in Switzerland, Hong Kong, Australia, and the United Kingdom [19–29]. In all cases, interventions were associated with increases in bone gain measurements during the time of the intervention period. However, there is no evidence to date that the interventions resulted in persistent or significant increases in peak bone mass.

It is well known that increases in dietary sodium chloride result in increased urinary calcium excretion in humans [10]. A number of investigations have been directed toward determining whether this salt-induced calciuria results in bone loss. A negative correlation between phosphorus intake and calcium absorption during calcium balance studies in teenage females has been reported. There has also been concern that elevated levels of dietary phosphorus, which could result from a diet high in protein or cola-type beverages, might lead to secondary hyperparathyroidism and subsequent bone loss or failure to attain peak bone mass [13,16].

NUTRIENT INTAKE ASSESSMENTS

Nearly all of the studies that have examined relationships among nutrient intakes and bone measurements in adolescent females have been cross-sectional in nature and have used food frequency, interview, and/or 24-hr recall diet assessment methods. A variety of potential data collection and statistical pitfalls may cloud the interpretation of results from these techniques. For example, Matkovic and co-workers studied 1061 women in two regions of Yugoslavia who did not differ in physical measurements and observed that hip fracture rates were higher in the region with low calcium intake. Diet data were obtained from only 100 of the 1061 women by only one observer using a variety of nonstandard nutrient intake techniques. In other words, a study that is often cited relied on a single, retrospective diet assessment of 10% of the study population, administered to all subjects by a nonblinded member of the research team [48]. It must be noted that cross-sectional studies such as the one described here [48] provide us with snapshot information regarding nutrient intake. In contrast, repeated assessments more closely reflect actual dietary practices.

RELATIONSHIPS AMONG ADOLESCENT BONE GAIN AND SPECIFIC NUTRIENTS

The lack of repeated measurements of nutrient intake has hindered past investigations of how and whether specific nutrients affect peak bone mass. Regularly scheduled repeated nutrient assessments are an integral part of the the Penn State Young Women's Health Study, which is an ongoing longitudinal study initiated in 1990 with a cohort of 112 twelve-year-old premenarchal female subjects. Details of recruitment, as well as baseline anthropometric, endocrine, and bone measurements of the subjects, the effects of a calcium supplementation trial on adolescent bone gain, and an investigation of fruit consumption levels in relation to fitness and cardiovascular health indices have been reported previously [19,24,49–51]. Comprehensive data were collected from the participants every 6 months for the first 4 years of the study and yearly thereafter. Data presented in this chapter were collected over the first 6 years of the study. Only data from the 81 subjects who remained in the cohort during this time are used. All subjects and their parents provided written, informed consent and all procedures were approved by the Institutional Review Board of the Pennsylvania State University College of Medicine.

The subjects completed 3-day food records, including 2 weekdays and 1 weekend day prior to each data collection visit. Subjects reported all food and drink they consumed over the 3 days, estimating serving sizes using everyday household measures and a metric scale. Detailed instructions concerning the completion of the records were provided to the subjects by a registered dietitian. The same dietitian reviewed the diet records, discussed any ambiguities in the records with the subjects, and entered the food items into a computer nutrient analysis program. Nutrient analysis was accomplished using Nutrition III and IV software [52].

Bone measurements were made initially with a Hologic QDR 1000W dual energy X-ray absorptiometer (DXA). This instrument was replaced with a QDR 2000W when the latter became available. A series of normal volunteers were scanned with both machines to validate the reproducibility of measurements. During the first 4 years of the study, participants were scanned at 6-month intervals, at which time total body and lumbar spine bone measurements were made. Thereafter (beginning at age 16) they were scanned yearly and dedicated hip measurements were added to the protocol. Data reported here are derived from a total of 968 whole body DXA scans and 162 dedicated hip scans of both hips made at age 18. Hip data are reported as the average of left and right hip measurements.

TOTAL BODY BONE GAIN AND CALCIUM INTAKE BY ADOLESCENT FEMALES DURING AGES 12–18

The longitudinal nutrient intake data set, which was derived from the 11 visits and therefore reflects 33 days of record keeping at regular intervals during ages 12–18, was used to determine each subject's average daily calcium intake during ages 12–18. These average daily calcium intakes are the sum of each individual's calcium intake and include dietary calcium sources and intake of the calcium supplement, if the subject received this intervention. Using these longitudinally derived individual calcium intakes, we established tertiles of average calcium intake over the 6-year period, as the cohort advanced from 12 to 18 years of age, as shown in Fig. 1. The bone gain and hip bone density of the individuals in the three tertiles were then compared and the results are presented in Fig. 2. The average calcium intake was 771 mg Ca^{2+}/day (n = 26) for the first tertile, 1100 mg Ca^{2+}/day (n = 29) for the second tertile, and 1398 mg Ca^{2+}/day (n = 26) for the third tertile. These three calcium intake tertiles had total body bone mineral gains between ages 12 and 18 of 902 ± 233, 914 ± 187, and 926 ± 183 g bone mineral, respectively, which were not statistically different from one another (p = 0.34). Hip bone density among the individuals in these three tertiles is shown in Fig. 2B. The lowest tertile of average calcium intake had a hip bone density of 0.96 ± 0.09 g/cm^2, 1.00 ± 0.10 g/cm^2 for the second tertile, and 0.99 ± 0.09 g/cm^2 for the third tertile. There were no statistical differences of hip bone density at age 18 (p = 0.35) relative to average calcium intake.

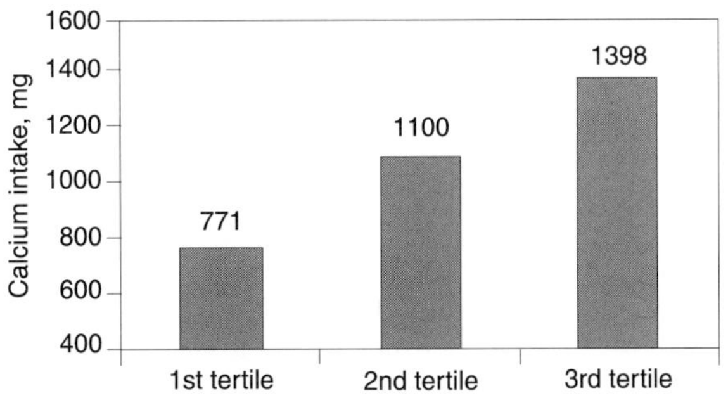

FIGURE 1 Mean daily calcium intake for first, second, and third tertiles at age 12.

TOTAL BODY BONE GAIN AND HIP DENSITY AS A FUNCTION OF SODIUM INTAKE

Using this cohort's longitudinal nutrient data base for sodium intake, we addressed the question of whether salt consumption during adolescence affects bone gain or hip density. The results presented in Fig. 3A show the relationship of each individual's averaged sodium intake per day over 6 years, ages 12–18, relative to her total body bone gain during ages 12–18 and expressed

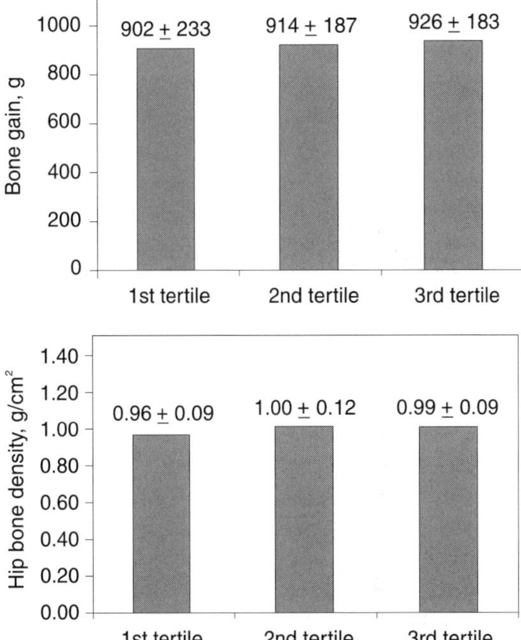

FIGURE 2 Total body bone gain and age 18 hip bone density by tertiles of calcium intake. Mean ± SD total body bone gain and age 18 hip bone density shown.

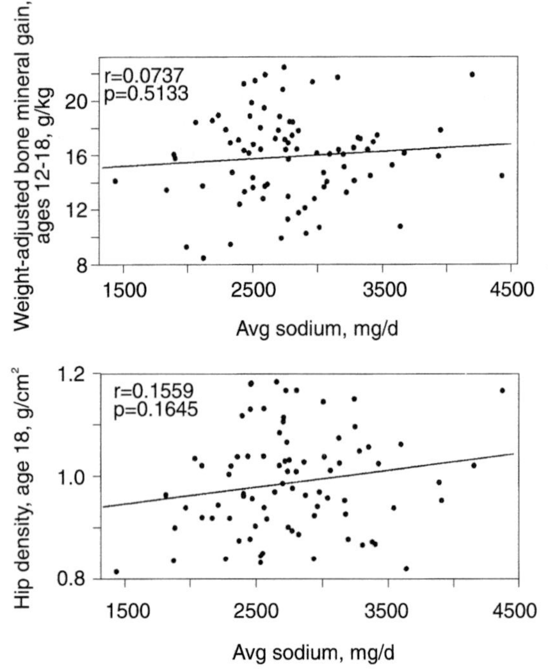

FIGURE 3 Total body bone gain and hip density as a function of sodium intake.

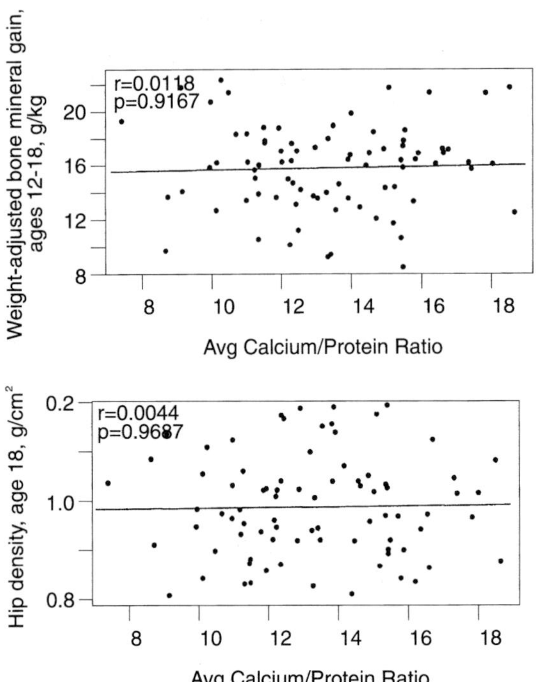

FIGURE 4 Total body bone gain and hip density as a function of the calcium/protein ratio.

as a function of her weight at age 18. The relationship is positive ($r = 0.07$) and is not significant ($p = 0.51$). Similarly, Fig. 3B shows each individual's average sodium intake as a function of her hip density at age 18. Again, there is a positive ($p = 0.16$) but insignificant relationship. Clearly these results do not support the notion that average daily sodium intakes ranging from 1500 to 4500 mg/day affect bone gain or hip bone density.

TOTAL BODY BONE GAIN AND HIP DENSITY AS A FUNCTION OF THE CALCIUM/PROTEIN RATIO

As before, we used the 6 years of nutrient intake data for each individual's total intake of calcium and total intake of protein to obtain time-averaged calcium/protein intake ratios for each of the 81 individuals. For example, a typical consumption of 900 mg/day of calcium and 65 g/day of protein would yield a ratio of 13.8:1. In contrast, consumption of only 600 mg/day calcium and 65 g/day protein would yield a ratio of 9.2:1. In our cohort the ratios ranged from just below 8:1 to just above 18:1. When these calcium/protein ratios were plotted as a function of total body bone gain adjusted for age 18 weight as shown in Fig. 4A, the relationship was slightly positive ($r = 0.01$) and insignificant ($p = 0.92$). When these calcium protein ratios were compared to hip density at age 18, as shown in Fig. 4B, again there was no relationship of consequence ($r = -0.004$ and $p = 0.97$).

TOTAL CALORIES PER KILOGRAM DURING AGES 12–18 AND BONE GAIN

To address the question of whether adolescent bone gain can be influenced by differences in total caloric intake, we first determined whether the cohort had consistent patterns of weight-adjusted caloric intake over time. Results of this analysis are presented in Fig. 5, where it can be seen that the three tertiles established at age 12 generally stay in rank for the following 6 years. As would be expected, linear growth slows as the individuals go from age 12–18, and the average weight-adjusted caloric intake of the three tertiles decreases over time. At only one time, at age 18, when the values of the three tertiles have become approximately equal, is there one tertile that is out of rank.

Given the fact that members of this cohort do track by weight-adjusted caloric intake and the fact that there have been suggestions that a reduction of caloric intake can restrict the achievement of maximum adult height and potentially restrict the achievement of peak bone

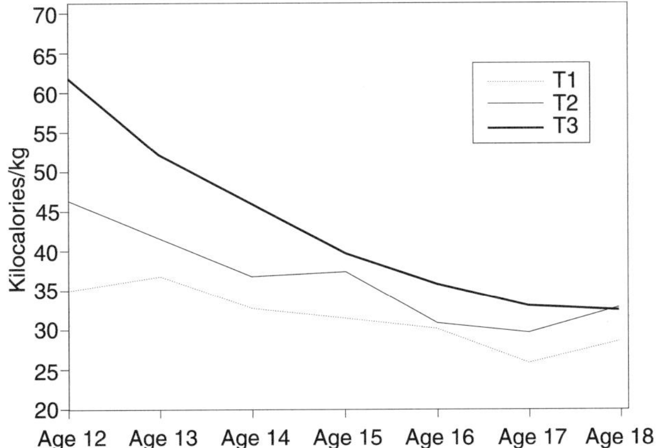

FIGURE 5 Mean kilocalorie intake per kilogram of body weight at ages 12–18 by subjects in tertiles 1–3 at age 12.

density, we analyzed adolescent bone gain and hip density at age 18 relative to the three tertiles of weight-adjusted caloric intake. Results of these analyses are presented in Figs. 6A and 6B. Figure 6A shows that total body bone gain over ages 12–18 for the first tertile of caloric intake was 891 ± 205 g bone mineral; total body bone mineral gain for the second caloric tertile was 943 ± 196 g total body gain; and total body bone mineral gain for the third caloric tertile was 908 ± 203 g. Thus, there is no difference in total body bone

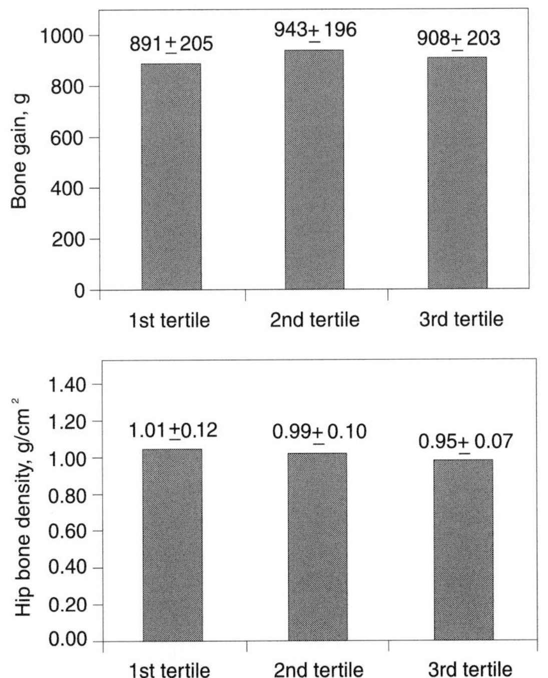

FIGURE 6 Total body bone gain and age 18 hip bone density by tertiles of kilocalories per kilogram of body weight. Mean ± SD shown. Mean kilocalories per kilogram body weight for the first, second, and third tertiles were 35.1, 46.4, and 62.1, respectively.

mineral gain made during adolescence as a function of weight-adjusted caloric intake during adolescence. The age 18 hip density values for the three caloric intake tertiles are presented in Fig. 6B where the value for the first tertile is 1.01 ± 0.12 g/cm^2, 0.99 g/cm^2 ± 0.10 for the second, and 0.95 ± 0.07 g/cm^2 for the third. A trend test shows that the level of significance for differences among these three groups is $p = 0.07$. It is noteworthy that the cohort with the highest age 18 hip density has the lowest weight-adjusted caloric intake.

DISCUSSION

The question of what is an adequate amount of calcium intake to support skeletal growth during adolescence and achievement of optimal peak bone mass remains largely unanswered [53]. Nutrient data from typical diets of healthy teenagers collected over the past 6 decades show several secular trends. First, as we have become an increasingly sedentary society, the total caloric intake for teenage women has decreased from about 2300 kcal/day in 1932 to 1700–1800 kcal/day in 1997 [54–63]. Second, with public recognition that high levels of saturated fat in the diet increase cardiovascular disease risk, there has been a reduction of total calories from fat from 42% in 1932 to 30–35% in the diets of teenage women today. During the same time frame there has been a decrease in dairy food consumption by teenagers, resulting in a decreased dietary calcium intake. According to NHANES II and NHANES III data, calcium intake by Caucasian teenage women has remained relatively constant, with mean values of 842 mg/day from NHANES II and 809 mg/day from NHANES III (64).

In recent years, several clinical trials of calcium supplementation with girls and adolescent women have been undertaken. Johnston and co-workers conducted a 3-year trial with 70 pairs of identical male and female twins ages 6–14 at entry. In their study, spontaneous calcium intake was 900 mg/day and the supplement added an additional 718 mg/day. The investigators observed significant increases in lumbar spine and radius bone density among those in the calcium-supplemented group who remained prepubertal during the trial [25]. This cohort has been followed for 4 years postintervention and the previously observed differences between supplemented and placebo groups disappeared by age 14 [26]. Lee and co-workers conducted an 18-month calcium supplementation trial with 84 seven-year-old male and female Chinese children who received an average of 567 mg/day dietary calcium and 240 mg/day in the calcium supplement. After the 18-month period, the supplemented group had a 22% increase in lumbar spine bone gain [21], yet when the cohort was restudied at 10 years of age (18 months postintervention), no differences in bone gain were observed [22,23].

Bonjour and coinvestigators studied 149 prepubertal girls who were 7.9 years at entry and were given additional calcium in the form of fortified food products. Significant increases were observed in femoral shaft width and content after 1 year only among the 49 subjects with spontaneous calcium intakes of less than 880 mg/day who consumed an additional 800 mg calcium/day from the fortified food. When this cohort was restudied 1 year after intervention at age 10, only the subgroup with a low spontaneous calcium intake continued to show an increase in femoral shaft width and shaft content compared to the placebo group. The extent of this gain decreased in the first postintervention year from 37 to 20% [20].

The Penn State Young Women's Health Study, which is the data source for the results presented in this chapter, included three arms of calcium supplementation and a placebo control group. One group received the calcium supplement for 2 years, ages 12–14, a second received the supplement for the 2 years between ages 14 and 16, and the third group received the supplementation for 4 years between ages 12 and 16. Although increases in bone gain were observed in each of the supplemented groups during their intervention periods, differences among the groups diminished quickly in the postintervention phase. When the cohort was 2 years beyond the intervention period at age 18, there were no significant differences in total body bone mineral content, total body bone mineral density, or hip bone density among the four study subgroups. However, final assessment of the effect of any nutrient or exercise modification program on peak bone mass cannot be made until the study cohort has reached skeletal maturity. Because approximately 95% of Caucasian women achieve greater than 95% of their peak bone mass by age 20, we and others studying the effects of calcium supplementation on peak bone mass must reevaluate our cohorts at or after this age.

OTHER NUTRIENTS AND ADOLESCENT BONE GAIN

Two dietary practices, namely high sodium consumption and a low calcium/protein intake ratio, have been proposed as having a negative impact on bone maintenance or achievement of peak bone density. Through examination of the nutrient and bone measurement data bases for the Penn State Young Women's Health Study, these practices were shown not to have any detrimental effect on bone acquisition in adolescence. In addition, the fact that adolescent bone gain was not affected by weight-adjusted caloric intake suggests that, at least during ages 12–18, physiologic adaptive mechanisms do not allow bone accretion to be perturbed by our current ranges of macronutrient and mineral intakes.

CALCIUM INTAKES, ABSORBABILITY, RETENTION, AND BONE ACCRETION

It seems logical to expect that optimizing calcium intake and absorbability would lead to optimal calcium retention and to maximum rates of bone accretion. It is, therefore, important to consider calcium kinetics that describe calcium absorbability and retention in adolescent women. Current technologies for these studies employ dual tracer isotope techniques [65–68]. Although these techniques do not involve ionizing radiation, they do require subjects to spend several days in metabolic research units. Accordingly, the studies are relatively expensive and only modest number of subjects can be studied at any one time. Results from these kinetic studies indicate that both calcium absorption and retention are highest in the early pubertal period [69]. During this time, mean dietary calcium absorption appears to be about 34% as compared to about 26% in late pubertal periods. In addition, calcium absorption varies according to health status and metabolic state. For example, whereas fractional calcium absorption among 9- to 17-year-old healthy females can be as high as 58% after short periods of reduced calcium intake [70], calcium absorption values for female adolescents with anorexia nervosa has been measured to be as low as 16% [71].

Inspection of individual fractional absorption rates and the resultant calculated calcium retention amounts may provide further insight into the factors affecting bone accretion. Two studies reported individual fractional absorption values from calcium carbonate for a total of 21 adolescents [72,73]. The mean fractional absorption rate for this group of 21 individuals was 26%. This mean value agrees with reports in the literature, but the individual fractional absorption values ranged widely from 12.8 to 39.6% [74]. Nine of the 21 subjects had values between 12.8 and 22.0% 6 subjects had fractional absorptions of 22.1–28.0%, and 6 subjects had fractional absorptions of 28.1–39.6%. Mean calcium fractional absorption rates for the low, moderate, and high groups just described are 19, 23, and 39%, respectively. Our data and those of Martin and co-workers [34] show that peak bone mineral accretion velocity occurs at the rate of about 240 g/year during ages 12–14 in females. At this rate, approximately 240 mg calcium is being added to the adolescent skeleton daily. Accordingly, in order to support bone mineral accretion at peak velocity of 240 mg calcium/day, the intakes of dietary calcium for individuals in these three groups would vary tremendously. Specifically, the low fractional absorption group would require 1300 mg calcium/day, the moderate fractional absorption group would require 1050 mg calcium/day, and the high fractional absorption group would require only 710 mg calcium/day. To what extent individual variation in fractional calcium absorption influences bone accretion rates remains to be determined.

The calcium supplementation trials conducted with young females that have been reviewed in this chapter indicate that increases in bone accretion seen during intervention periods do not appear to persist. Another caveat, however, is that different investigative teams have made bone measurements at different skeletal sites and with different instruments. Data presented here from the Penn State Young Women's Health Study refer only to total body and hip measurements. It is possible that positive persistent effects of calcium supplementation are evident at other sites. However, we have not observed any dose-dependent effect of average calcium intakes ranging from <500 to >1600 mg/day on total body adolescent bone gain or hip bone density at age 18. We do not believe that our results call into question the current United States recommended daily allowance for dietary calcium. Dairy products are the major source for dietary calcium in the United States, and these products, especially in their reduced fat forms, are excellent sources of important nutrients, including protein, vitamin D, magnesium, potassium, and zinc. In summary, results indicate that although calcium intake is a necessary ingredient in bone accrual, it is not rate limiting for female adolescent bone gain.

Acknowledgment

This study was supported by PHS RO-1-HD25973 and MO1-RR-10-732 (GCRC Grant).

References

1. Agarwal, S. C., and Grynpas, M. D. Bone quantity and quality in past populations. *Anat. Rec.* **246,** 423–432 (1996).
2. Nelson, D. A. An anthropological perspective on optimizing calcium consumption for the prevention of osteoporosis. *Osteopor. Intl.* **6,** 325–328 (1996).
3. Eaton, S. B., and Nelson, D. A. Calcium in the evolutionary perspective. *Am. J. Clin. Nutr.* **54,** 281S–287S (1991).
4. Cumming, R. G., Cummings, S. R., Nevitt, M. C., Scott, J., Ensrud, K. E., Vogt, T. M., and Fox, K. Calcium intake and fracture risk: results from the study of osteoporotic fractures. *Am. J. Epidemiol.* **145,** 926–934 (1997).
5. Cummings, S. R., Nevitt, M. C., Browner, W. S., Stone, K., Fox, K. M., Ensrud, K. E., Caulcy, J., Black, D., and Vogt, T. M. Risk factors for hip fractures in white women. Study of Osteoporotic Fractures Research Group. *N. Engl. J. Med.* **332,** 767–773 (1995).
6. Holbrook, T. L., Barrett-Connor, E., and Wingard, D. L. Dietary calcium and risk of hip fracture: 14 year prospective population study. *Lancet* **2,** 1046–1049 (1988).
7. Looker, A. C., Harris, T. B., Madans, J. H., and Sempos, C. T. Dietary calcium and hip fracture risk: The NHANES I Epidemiologic Follow-up Study. *Osteopor. Intl.* **3,** 177–184 (1993).
8. Johnell, O. T., Gullberg, B., Kanis, J. A., Allander, E., Elffors, L., Dequeker, J., Dilsen, G., Gennari, C., Vaz, A. L., Lyritis, G., Mazzuoli, G., Miravet, L., Passeri, M., Cano, R. P., Rapado, A., and Ribot, C. Risk factors for hip fracture in European women: the MEDOS Study. *J. Bone Miner. Res.* **10,** 1802–1815 (1995).
9. Chapuy, M. C., Arlot, M. E., Duboeuf, F., Brun, J., Crouzet, B., Arnaud, S., Delmas, P. D., and Meunier, P. J. Vitamin D3 and calcium to prevent hip fractures in elderly women. *N. Engl. J. Med.* **327,** 1637–1642 (1992).
10. Massey, L. K., and Whiting, S. J. Dietary salt, urinary calcium and bone loss. *J. Bone Miner. Res.* **11,** 731–736 (1996).
11. Goulding, A. Osteoporosis: why consuming less sodium chloride helps to conserve bone. *N. Z. Med. J.* **103,** 120–122 (1990).
12. Devine, A., Criddle, R. A., Dick, I. M., Kerr, D. A., and Prince, R. L. A longitudinal study of the effect of sodium and calcium intakes on regional bone density in post menopausal women. *Am. J. Clin. Nutr.* **62,** 740–745 (1995).
13. Matkovic, V., Ilich, J. Z., Andon, M. B., Hsieh, L. C., Tzagournis, M. A., Lagger, B. J., and Goel, P. K. Urinary calcium, sodium, and bone mass of young females. *Am. J. Clin. Nutr.* **62,** 417–425 (1995).
14. Greendale, G. A., Barrett-Connor, E., Edelstein, S., Ingles, S., and Haile, R. Dietary sodium and bone mineral density: Results of a 16 year follow-up study. *J. Am. Ger. Soc.* **42,** 1050–1055 (1994).
15. Barzel, U. S. The skeleton as an ion-exchange system: Implications for the role of acid-base imbalance in the genesis of osteoporosis. *J. Bone Miner. Res.* **10,** 1431–1436 (1995).
16. Calvo, M. S. Dietary phosphorus, calcium metabolism and bone. *J. Nutr.* **123,** 1627–1633 (1993).
17. Orwell, E. S. The effects of dietary protein insufficiency and excess on skeletal health. *Bone* **13,** 343–350 (1992).
18. Orwell, E., Ware, M., Stribrska, L., Bikle, D., Sanchez, T., Andon, M., and Li, H. Effects of dietary protein insufficiency on mineral metabolism and bone mineral density. *Am. J. Clin. Nutr.* **56,** 313–319 (1992).
19. Lloyd, T., Andon, M. A., Rollings, N., Martel, J. K., Landis, J. R., Demers, L. M., Eggli, D. F., Kieselhorst, K., and Kulin, H. E. Calcium supplementation and bone mineral density in adolescent girls. *JAMA* **270,** 841–844 (1993).
20. Bonjour, J-P., Carrie, A-L., Ferrari, S., Clavien, H., Slosman, D., and Theintz, G. Calcium enriched foods and bone mass growth in prepubertal girls: A randomized, double blind placebo-controlled trial. *J. Clin. Invest.* **99,** 1287–1294 (1997).
21. Lee, W. T. K., Leung, S. S. F., Leung, D. M. Y., Tsang, H. S. Y., Lau, J., and Cheung, J. C. Y. A randomized double-blind controlled calcium supplementation trial, and bone and height acquisition in children. *Br. J. Nutr.* **74,** 125–139 (1995).
22. Lee, W. T. K., Leung, S. S. F., Leung, D. M. Y., and Cheung, J. C. Y. A follow-up study on the effects of calcium-supplement withdrawal and puberty on bone acquisition of children. *Am. J. Clin. Nutr.* **64,** 71–77 (1996).
23. Lee, W. T., Leung, S. S., Leung, D. M., Wang, S. H., Xu, Y. C., Zeng, W. P., and Cheng, J. C. Bone mineral acquisition in low calcium intake children following the withdrawal of calcium supplement. *Acta Paediatr.* **86**(6), 570–576 (1997).

24. Lloyd, T., Martel, J. K., Rollings, N., Andon, M. B., Kulin, H., Demers, L. M., Eggli, D. F., Kieselhorst, K., and Chinchilli, V. M. The effect of calcium supplementation and Tanner stage on bone density content and area in teenage women. *Osteopor. Intl.* **6,** 276–283 (1996).
25. Johnston, C. C., Jr., Miller, J. Z., Slemenda, C., Reister, T. K., Hui, S., Christian, J. C., and Peacock, M. Calcium supplementation and increases in bone mineral density in children. *N. Engl. J. Med.* **327,** 82–87 (1992).
26. Slemenda, C., Reister, T. K., Peacock, M., and Johnston, C. C. Bone strength in children following the cessation of calcium supplementation. *J. Bone Miner. Res.* **8,** S154 (1993).
27. Cadogan, J., Eastell, R., Jones, N., and Barker, M. E. Milk intake and bone mineral acquisition in adolescent girls: randomized, controlled intervention trial. *Br. Med. J.* **315,** 1255–1260 (1997).
28. Nowson, C. A., Green, R. M., Hopper, J. L., Sherwin, A. J., Young, D., Kaymakei, B., Guest, C. S., Smid, M., Larkins, R. G., and Wark, J. D. A co-twin study of the effect of calcium supplementation on bone density during adolescence. *Osteopor. Intl.* **7,** 219–225.
29. Chan, G. M., Hoffman, K., and McMurray, M. Effects of dairy products on bone and body composition in prepubertal girls. *J. Pediatr.* **126,** 551–556 (1995).
30. DeSchepper, J., Derde, M. P., Van den Broeck, M., Piepsz, A., and Jonckheer, M. H. Normative data for lumbar spine bone mineral content in children: Influence of age, height, weight, and pubertal stage. *J. Nuclear Med.* **32**(2), 216–220 (1991).
31. Molgaard, C., Thomsen, B. L., Prentice, A., Cole, T. J., and Michaelsen, K. F. Whole body bone mineral content in healthy children and adolescents. *Arch. Dis. Child.* **76**(1), 9–15 (1997).
32. Sabatier, J. P., Guaydier-Souquieres, G., Laroche, D., Benmalek, A., Fournier, L., Guillon-Metz, F., Delavenne, J., and Denisay. Bone mineral acquisition during adolescence and early adulthood: A study of 574 healthy females 10–24 years of age. *Osteopor. Intl.* **6,** 141–148 (1996).
33. Gordon, C. L., and Webber, C. E. Body composition and bone mineral distribution during growth in females. *Can. Assoc. Radiol. J.* **44,** 112–116 (1993).
34. Martin, A. D., Bailey, D. A., McKay, H. A., and Whiting, S. Bone mineral and calcium accretion during puberty. *Am. J. Clin. Nutr.* **66,** 611–615 (1997).
35. Bonjour, J. P., Theintz, G., Buchs, G., Slosman, D., and Rizzoli, R. Critical years and stages of puberty for spinal and femoral bone mass accumulation during adolescence. *J. Clin. Endocrinol. Metab.* **73,** 555–563 (1991).
36. Glastre, C., Braillon, P., David, L., Cochat, P., Meunier, P. J., and Delmas, P. D. Measurement of bone mineral content of the lumbar spine by dual energy x-ray absorptiometry in normal children: Correlations with growth parameters. *J. Clin. Endocrinol. Metab.* **70,** 1330–1333 (1990).
37. Ellis, K. J., Abrams, S. A., and Wong, W. W. Body composition of a young multiethnic female population. *Am. J. Clin. Nutr.* **65,** 724–731 (1997).
38. Boot, A. M., de Ridder, M. A., Pols, H. A., Krenning, E. P., and de Muinck Keizer-Schrama, S. M. Bone mineral density in children and adolescents: relation to puberty, calcium intake, and physical activity. *J. Clin. Endocrinol. Metab.* **82,** 57–62 (1997).
39. Haapasalo, H., Kannus, P., Sievanen, H., Pasanen, M., Uusi-Rasi, K., Heinonen, A., Oja, P., and Vuori, I. Development of mass, density, and estimated mechanical characteristics of bones in Caucasian females. *J. Bone Miner. Res.* **11,** 1751–1760 (1996).
40. Zanchetta, J. R., Plotkin, H., and Alvarez Filgueira, M. L. Bone mass in children: Normative values for the 2–20 year old population. *Bone* **16,** 393S–399S (1995).
41. Nelson, D. A., Simpson, P. M., Johnson, C. C., Barondess, D. A., and Kleerekoper, M. The accumulation of whole body skeletal mass in third- and fourth-grade children: effects of age, gender, ethnicity, and body composition. *Bone* **20,** 73–78 (1997).
42. Faulkner, R. A., Bailey, D. A., Drinkwater, D. T., McKay, H. A., Arnold, C., and Wilkinson, A. A. Bone densitometry in Canadian children 8–17 years of age. *Calcif. Tissue Int.* **59,** 344–351 (1996).
43. Bhudhikanok, G. S., Wang, M.-C., Eckert, K., Matkin, C., Marcus, R., and Bachrach, L. K. Differences in bone mineral in young Asian and Caucasian Americans may reflect difference in bone size. *J. Bone Miner. Res.* **11,** 1545–1556 (1996).
44. Sundberg, M., Duppe, H., Gardsell, P., Johnell, O., Ornstein, E., and Sernbo, I. Bone mineral density in adolescents. *Acta Orthop. Scand.* **68,** 456–460 (1997).
45. McDowell, M. A., Briefel, R. R., Alaimo, K., Bischof, A. M., Caughman, C. R., Carroll, M. D., Loria, C. M., and Johnson, C. L. Energy and macronutrient intakes of persons ages 2 months and 45 over in the United States. *In* "The Third National Health and Nutrition Evaluation Survey, Phase 1, 1988–1991." National Center for Health Statistics, No. 255, 1994.
46. Nicklas, T. A. Dietary studies with children: The Bogalusa Heart Study experience. *J. Am. Diet. Assn.* **95,** 1127–1133 (1995).
47. Dinger, M. K., and Waigandt, A. Dietary intake and physical activity behaviors of male and female college students. *Am. J. Health Promot.* **11,** 360–362 (1997).
48. Matkovic, V., Kostial, K., Simonovic, J., Buzina, R., Brodarec, A., and Nordin, B. E. C. Bone status and fracture rates in two regions of Yugoslavia. *Am. J. Clin. Nutr.* **32,** 540–549 (1979).
49. Lloyd, T., Rollings, N., Andon, M. B., Demers, L. M., Eggli, D. F., Kieselhorst, K., Kulin, H. E., Landis, J. R., Martel, J. K., Orr, G., and Smith, P. Determinants of bone density in young women. I. Relationships among pubertal development, total body bone mass, and total body bone density in premenarchal females. *J. Clin. Endocrinol. Metab.* **75,** 383–387 (1992).
50. Lloyd, T., and Eggli, D. F. Measurement of bone mineral content and bone density in twelve year old Caucasian girls. *J. Nuclear Med.* **33,** 1143 (1992).
51. Lloyd, T., Chinchilli, V. M., Rollings, N., Kieselhorst, K., Tregea, D. F., Henderson, N. A., and Sinoway, L. I. Fruit consumption, fitness and cardiovascular risk factors in teenage women. *Am. J. Clin. Nutr.* in press.
52. Nutritionist III (Version 7.0), Nutritionist IV (Verson 3.0, 1994) n-Squared Computing, San Bruno, CA 94066.
53. Kanis, J. A. Calcium nutrition and its implications for osteoporosis. Part 1. Children and healthy adults. *Eur. J. Clin. Nutr.* **8,** 757–767 (1994).
54. Wait, B., and Roberts, L. J. Studies in the food requirement of adolescent girls. I. The energy intake of well nourished girls 10 to 16 years of age. *J. Am. Diet. Assoc.* **8,** 209–237 (1932).
55. McGregor-Hard, M., and Esselbaugh, N. C. Nutritional status of adolescent children. *Am. J. Clin. Nutr.* **8,** 346–352 (1960).
56. Wharton, M. A. Nutritive intake of adolescents. *J. Am. Diet. Assoc.* **42,** 306–310 (1963).
57. Hodges, R. E., and Krehl, W. A. Nutritional status of teenagers in Iowa. *Am. J. Clin. Nutr.* **17,** 200–210 (1965).
58. Hampton, M. C., Huenemann, R. L., Shapiro, L. R., and Mitchell, B. W. Caloric and nutrient intakes of teenagers. *J. Am. Diet. Assoc.* **50,** 385–396 (1967).
59. Durnin, J. V. G., Lonergan, M. S., Good, J., and Ewan, A. A cross-sectional nutritional and anthropometric study, with an interval of 7 years on 611 adolescent school children. *Br. J. Nutr.* **32,** 169–179 (1974).
60. Salz, K. M., Tamir, J., Ernst, N., Kwiterovich, P., Glueck, C., Christensen, B., Larsen, R., Pirhonen, D., Prewitt, T. E., and Scott,

L. W. Selected nutrient intakes of free-living white children ages 6–19 years. *Pediatr. Res.* **17,** 124–130 (1983).
61. Crawley, H. F. The energy, nutrient and food intakes of teenagers aged 16–17 years in Britain. *Br. J. Nutr.* **70,** 15–26 (1993).
62. Welten, D. C., Kemper, H. C. G., Post, G. B., Stavern, W. A. V., and Twisk, J. W. R. Longitudinal development and tracking of calcium and dairy intake from teenager to adult. *Eur. J. Clin. Nutr.* **51,** 612–618 (1997).
63. Hurson, M., and Corish, C. Evaluation of lifestyle, food consumption and nutrient intake patterns among Irish teenagers. *Irish J. Med. Sci.* **166,** 225–230 (1997).
64. Alaimo, K., McDowell, M. A., Briefel, R. R., *et al.* Dietary intakes of vitamins, minerals, and fiber of persons ages two months and over in the United States. *In* "Third National Health and Nutrition Examination Survey, Phase I, 1988–1991." National Center for Health Statistics, Hyattsville, MD, 1994.
65. Abrams, S. A., Esteban, N. V., Vieira, N. E., Sidbury, J. B., Specker, B. L., and Yergey, A. L. Developmental changes in calcium kinetics in children assessed using stable isotopes. *J. Bone Miner. Res.* **7,** 287–293 (1992).
66. Wastney, M. E., Ng, J., Smith, D., Martin, B. R., Peacock, M., and Weaver, C. M. Differences in calcium kinetics between adolescent girls and young women. *Am. J. Physiol.* **271,** R208–R216 (1996).
67. Jackman, L. A., Millane, S. S., Martin, B. R., Wood, O. B., McCabe, G. P., Peacock, M., and Weaver, C. M. Calcium retention in relation to calcium intake and postmenarchal age in adolescent females. *Am. J. Clin. Nutr.* **66,** 327–333 (1997).
68. Weaver, C. M. Age related calcium requirements due to changes in absorption and utilization. *J. Nutr.* **124,** 1418S–1425S (1994).
69. Abrams, S. A., and Stuff, J. E. Calcium metabolism in girls: current dietary intakes lead to low rates of calcium absorption and retention during puberty. *Am. J. Clin. Nutr.* **60,** 739–743 (1994).
70. O'Brien, K. O., Abrams, S. A., Liang, L. K., Ellis, K. J., and Gagel, R. F. Increased efficiency of calcium absorption during short periods of inadequate calcium intake in girls. *Am. J. Clin. Nutr.* **63,** 579–583 (1996).
71. Abrams, S. A., Silber, T. J., Esteban, N. V., Vieira, N. E., Stuff, J. E., Meyers, R., Majd, M., and Yergey, A. L. Mineral balance and bone turnover in adolescents with anorexia nervosa. *J. Pediatr.* **123,** 326–331 (1993).
72. Recker, R. R., Bammi, A., Barger-Lux, M. J., and Heaney, R. P. Calcium absorbability from milk products, an imitation milk, and calcium carbonate. *Am. J. Clin. Nutr.* **47,** 93–95 (1988).
73. Miller, J. Z., Smith, D. L., Flora, L., Slemenda, C., Jiang, X., and Johnston, C. C. Calcium absorption from calcium carbonate and a new form of calcium (CCM) in healthy male and female adolescents. *Am. J. Clin. Nutr.* **48,** 1291–1294 (1988).
74. Peacock, M. Calcium absorption efficiency and calcium requirements in children and adolescents. *Am. J. Clin. Nutr.* **54,** 2615–2655 (1991).

Mechanical Determinants of Peak Bone Mass

MARJOLEIN C. H. VAN DER MEULEN Sibley School of Mechanical and Aerospace Engineering, Cornell University, Ithaca, New York 14853

DENNIS R. CARTER Biomechanical Engineering Division, Stanford University, Stanford, California 94305; and Rehabilitation R&D Center, Department of Veterans Affairs, Palo Alto, California 94304

The skeleton provides structural support for the body and facilitates movement. The tissue stresses and strains created by these mechanical functions are extremely important in the growth, development, and mineral acquisition of the skeleton. Local tissue mechanical stimuli regulate the developing bone geometry, mineral content, and mineral distribution, which, in turn, determine the strength of the skeleton. Mechanical loading is critical to skeletal health throughout life, but particularly during the first 2 decades of life when the majority of an individual's lifetime bone mineral is acquired. During adolescence, growth in the length of bones causes an increase in body height. Increases in height result in even greater increases in body mass, which, under the influence of gravity, cause progressive increases in mechanical loading. The increase in body mass and the associated increase in mechanical loading are the primary determinants of adolescent bone mass acquisition. In cortical bone, mechanically regulated skeletogenesis is manifested by dramatic increases in diaphyseal size and changes in shape. In cancellous bone, mechanical stimuli associated with body mass and activity determine bone apparent density and trabecular architecture.

INTRODUCTION

In considering aging and the skeleton, no discussion is complete without considering the rapid increase in bone mass that is observed during adolescence. The dramatic growth of the skeleton during adolescence coincides with the period of peak bone mineral acquisition in both sexes. At least 50% of the peak adult bone mass is gained during these years [1]. The amount of bone gained during adolescence and the subsequent rate of bone loss are the primary factors that determine an individual's total bone mass in adulthood and during aging. Despite the importance of bone acquisition to achieving maximal peak bone mass, our knowledge of the factors that determine bone mass in healthy adolescents remains incomplete. The growth and structural development of the skeleton are the result of complex genetic and epigenetic processes. Some factors that are believed to influence bone accretion and resorption during development include age, pubertal stage, gender, genetics, nutrition, and ethnicity [2]. Among the most important factors in determining peak bone mass during development, however, are body mass and physical activity. These factors directly determine the mechanical loading that is imposed upon the developing bones.

This chapter focuses on the influences of mechanical loading on skeletal development and functional adaptation. When mechanics and the skeleton are considered, there are two related but different contexts to consider: (1) the role of mechanical loading on the development of bone geometry, total bone mass, and spatial distribution of bone tissue and (2) the resulting structural strength of the bones themselves.

Our understanding of the underlying mechanical mechanisms that control skeletal development has been enhanced by the use of analytical engineering approaches. These approaches, which are often implemented using computer models, allow for the simulation of the applied loading to the skeleton and predictions of the ensuing skeletal response. These results lead to meaningful explanations for the relationship between loading and bone mass acquisition during development, adolescence, maturity, and aging. These can be tested and evaluated using clinical and experimental data. The following sections will first explain these analytical approaches and then compare the results of computer emulations and predictions with clinical data on peak bone mass acquisition.

MECHANICAL MECHANISMS OF BONE MASS ACQUISITION

Skeletal structure in the adult reflects the diverse genetic and epigenetic contributions experienced throughout growth and development. To understand bone structure at a particular stage of development, such as adolescence, the preceding developmental history and critical influences leading up to the time of interest need to be considered. Mechanical influences first begin to guide skeletal development *in utero* and continue to influence the skeleton throughout life.

Skeletal formation is initiated in the embryo with the aggregation of mesenchymal tissue into a prepattern for skeletal development. While some of these aggregates differentiate directly to bone, many of the preskeletal mesenchymal aggregates chondrify, forming the cartilage anlagen of the skeletal elements. Early embryogenesis and pattern formation are clearly driven by intrinsic regulatory factors such as Hox genes and bone morphogenetic proteins.

Once the skeletal pattern is formed, ossification of the anlagen is initiated. This ossification begins at about the same time as the initiation of intermittent mechanical loading and movements that are caused by embryonic muscle contractions. At that point, skeletal development is no longer solely a biologically regulated growth process, but begins to be affected directly by mechanical events associated with muscular contractions. Mechanobiologically regulated growth processes play a major role in prenatal and postnatal skeletal development and continue throughout life. The mechanical forces imposed on the skeleton are dramatically increased after birth as a result of normal activity in Earth's gravitational field. The magnitude of the forces generated in bones and muscles is directly related to body mass and the associated gravitational forces created during these activities. During growth and maturation, additional factors such as diet and the extent of physical activity come into play [3,4]. In adolescence, changing hormone levels are another important consideration.

In 1892 in his "Law of Bone Remodeling," Julius Wolff stated: "Every change in the . . . function of bone . . . is followed by certain definite changes in . . . internal architecture and external conformation in accordance with mathematical laws" [5]. While Wolff never presented a quantitative relationship to predict bone development, the idea that bone adaptation to mechanical loading can be quantitatively described has come to be known as "Wolff's law." Based on this premise, numerous investigators have developed quantitative theories that relate *in vivo* mechanical loading to bone apposition or resorption [6–9]. A common feature of these theories is a feedback parameter associated with the local mechanical loading, a stress or strain stimulus, that drives the biological response of the system. For growth and adaptation, a response rule is implemented for which the mechanical stimulus parameter is compared to a desired reference value. The difference, or error, between the stimulus and the reference determines the system response (Fig. 1). At a given location, if the stimulus is greater than the reference level, bone apposition occurs; if the stimulus is less then the reference value, resorption will take place. Using this type of approach, mechanically regulated bone formation and adaptation can be simulated quantitatively.

In the long bones, growth and development occur by two different mechanisms, appositional growth and endochondral growth, which result in different developmental histories for bone in different regions (Fig. 2). The dense cortical bone of the diaphyses grows by direct apposition and resorption of existing cartilage and bone surfaces. The first embryonic bone, the bone collar, is deposited directly on the cartilage anlage at or near the center of the shaft. Subsequent growth of the shaft is

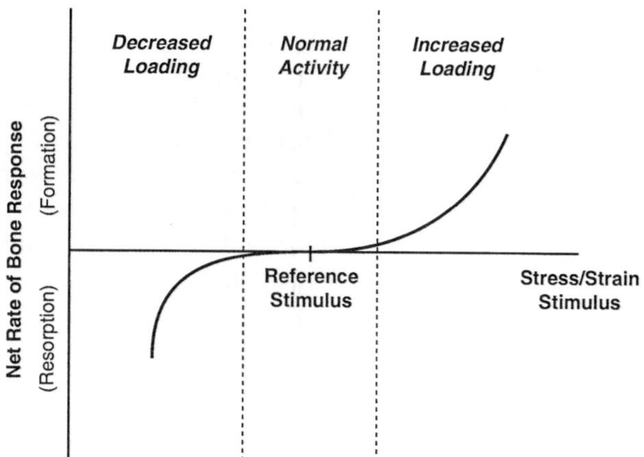

FIGURE 1 Hypothetical relationship between the applied stress or strain stimulus and the net rate of bone resorption or formation.

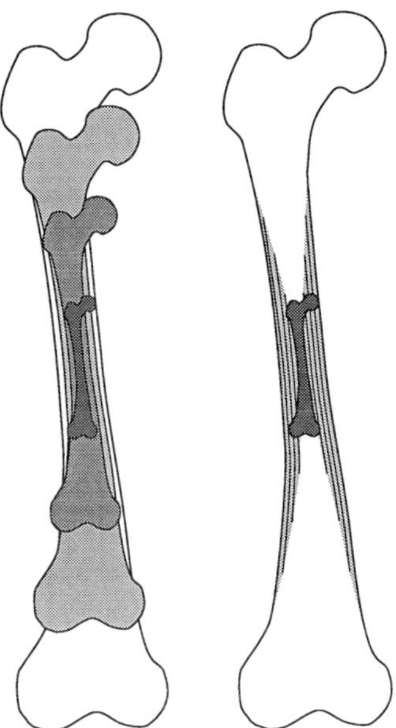

FIGURE 2 Illustration of two different mechanisms of long bone growth: endochondral growth (left) and appositional growth (right). Endochondral growth increases bone length. Appositional growth increases bone width.

achieved by the apposition of new bone directly on the perichondral and periosteal surfaces. The cancellous bone found in the epiphyses and metaphyses is formed during the final stage of endochondral growth and ossification. These two mechanisms of bone formation are the result of fundamentally different cellular processes and, while both are responsive to mechanical loading, the nature of the response to mechanical loading must be considered separately.

Appositional Growth

The first bone formed in the long bones is the primary bone collar, which appears concomitant with the first skeletal muscle contractions. The initial bone formation at this site will occur in the absence of any mechanical stimulus. Thereafter, however, further appositional growth is dependent on the mechanical forces generated by the embryonic muscles. Mechanical loading determines cortical periosteal and endosteal diameters, and the resulting bone cortical thickness [10–15].

Appositional growth can be modeled as a process controlled by a combination of (1) biological factors and (2) mechanobiological (mechanically mediated biological) factors. Based on this idea, an analytical model of long bone diaphyseal development was developed [16]. The femoral diaphysis is modeled as a circular cross section. In response to intrinsic growth and mechanically mediated stimuli, the periosteal and endosteal surfaces are "grown" over time. This model has been used to simulate normal development of the human femur as well as to predict development and adaptation under abnormal loading conditions.

In the computer implementation of the appositional bone development model, we view diaphyseal morphology as the result of biological and mechanobiological growth. Passive biological growth is present on the periosteum during early development and gradually reduces with time, disappearing by 6 years of age in our simulations of human femoral growth. Following the decay of the intrinsic growth rate, the mechanobiological stimulus dominates postnatal skeletal development and becomes the sole regulator of diaphyseal growth.

To predict cross-sectional morphology during growth and development, an age-dependent mechanical loading history must be assumed. As body size and mass increase, so do the loads borne by the skeleton. *In vivo* strain gage studies have demonstrated that the predominant strains on the surfaces of long bones are the result of bending and torsion [17,18]. These applied moments are produced by the actions of muscles, whose force is proportional to their cross-sectional area. The length of the moment arms increases in proportion to the length of the bones. These two factors suggest that mechanical moments applied to the long bones are, therefore, approximately proportional to the body height cubed. The body height cubed, however, is approximately proportional to the body mass. Human body mass data were used to construct an age-dependent loading history [19] by assuming simply that the magnitudes of the loading moments in the diaphyses are proportional to body mass.

The mechanical feedback parameter that stimulates bone formation or resorption is calculated from the loading history. We chose to implement the strain energy-based daily stress stimulus introduced by Carter and colleagues [6,20,21]. For a given load, this stimulus formulation takes into account both the cyclic load magnitude and the number of cycles during a day and weights the contribution of load magnitude relative to the number of load cycles. The difference between this stress stimulus and the reference stimulus determines the bone response.

The skeletal response to the mechanobiologic stimulus was derived from piecewise linear response rules for the periosteum and endosteum, similar to Fig. 1. A "lazy zone" was included in the region near the reference stimulus. Similar apposition rates and reference stimuli were modeled on both surfaces, but the periosteum was permitted to deposit bone only. For a stimulus greater than the reference stimulus on either surface, apposition would take place. When the stress stimulus was below the reference value, no response occurred on the periosteum and the endosteal surface resorbed. Values for the response rates, "lazy zone" width, reference stimulus, and maximum applied torsional moment were based on experimental data in the literature [16,20].

Based on the initial geometry for a primary bone collar and applying time-varying loads, simulations were performed to predict the cross-sectional morphological changes expected during normal human development (Fig. 3). As loading increases during growth, the simulated diaphysis displayed rapid periosteal expansion with slower endosteal expansion of the medullary canal. After maturity both surfaces showed reduced rates of expansion, but there was a continued expansion of the cross section and gradual thinning of the cortex with advancing age. These features of growth and aging parallel those measured experimentally [19,22,23]. In these simulations, adolescence is a critical period of bone development, and peak bone mass is achieved during this time. In our simulations, the greatest rates of loading occur during early infancy and adolescence, corresponding to high mineralization stages *in vivo* [24]. For the 70-kg adult male of our simulations, nearly 60% of the adult body mass is gained from age 10 to 20 years.

To validate our analytical approach, we compared our simulations of femoral development to dual energy X-ray absorptiometry (DXA) measurements of the human femur during adolescence and young adulthood [25]. We simulated the diaphyseal development of three different "phantom individuals" whose body masses were bounded by the subjects' masses and compared the predictions of femoral structure to this clinical cross-sectional data set [26]. These data documented femoral structure during growth in 101 healthy Caucasian subjects (48 males and 53 females) aged 9 to 26 years. Measurements included height, body mass, pubertal stage, and middiaphyseal linear bone mineral content (BMC in g/cm) and femoral width from DXA scans. Of age, pubertal stage, body mass, and height, body mass was shown to be the strongest predictor of femoral properties for these data, and the relationship was independent of gender.

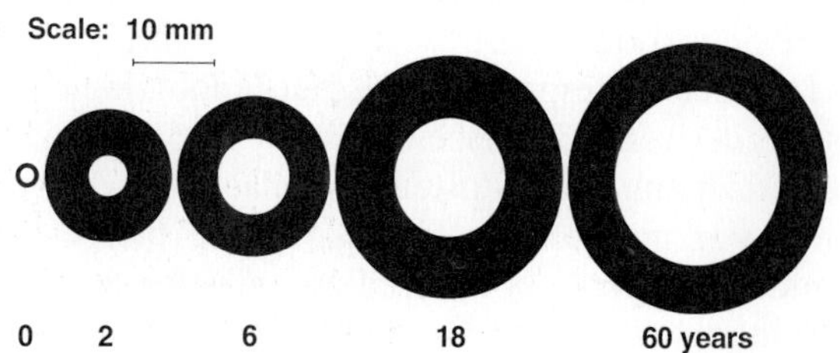

FIGURE 3 Simulation results for cross-sectional morphology of the human femoral diaphysis at 0, 2, 6, 18, and 60 years of age. Adapted from van der Meulen *et al.* [16].

Bone mineral content, the bone mineral mass per unit length, is commonly used to assess bone mass in the clinic and is determined directly from a DXA scan. To compare our simulations to these data, we needed to determine BMC for the simulations and cortical morphology for the DXA scans. Based on the approach of Martin and Burr [27], BMC can be estimated from the cortical bone area output from the simulation. Similarly, using the method of Martin and Burr [27], femoral cross-sectional and structural properties were calculated from the bone mineral properties, allowing us to compare the section modulus values. The section modulus reflects the ability of a cross section to withstand applied bending and torsional loads and indicates the strength of a circular section. For a circle, the section modulus is the ratio of the polar moment of inertia to the diameter.

Our model data for BMC showed no combined linear relationship with age and a single, strong linear relationship with body mass, similar to adolescent data (Fig. 4). Both the models and the clinical data each showed a strong linear relationship for section modulus with body mass. The relationship between age and section modulus was nonlinear in both cases. The strong correspondence of body mass with the model and DXA data, and the weak relationship with age, supports our hypothesis that the diaphyseal structure of long bones results from a biological response to *in vivo* mechanical loading, not simply a passive time-dependent growth process. In addition, this comparison demonstrates the utility of these simple models: the data show a strong relationship with body mass, and the simulations allow us to propose and evaluate a mechanism for this relation.

Endochondral Growth

The first endochondral bone forms within the long bone anlage in the cartilage surrounded by the primary bone collar. Primary ossification fronts form at this central location in the diaphysis, and ossification of the cartilage progresses slowly toward the bone ends. Endochondral ossification is accomplished by cell proliferation, extracellular matrix biosynthesis, and cell hypertrophy prior to cartilage calcification and replacement by cancellous bone. The process of endochondral ossification is, therefore, inextricably linked to the growth of bone in length.

Endochondral ossification proceeds in cartilage anlagen even when the normal mechanical loading is significantly diminished. However, the intermittent tissue stresses (or strains) caused by physical activities act to either accelerate or inhibit ossification in various locations within the anlage. The local mechanical modulation of endochondral growth and ossification is critical

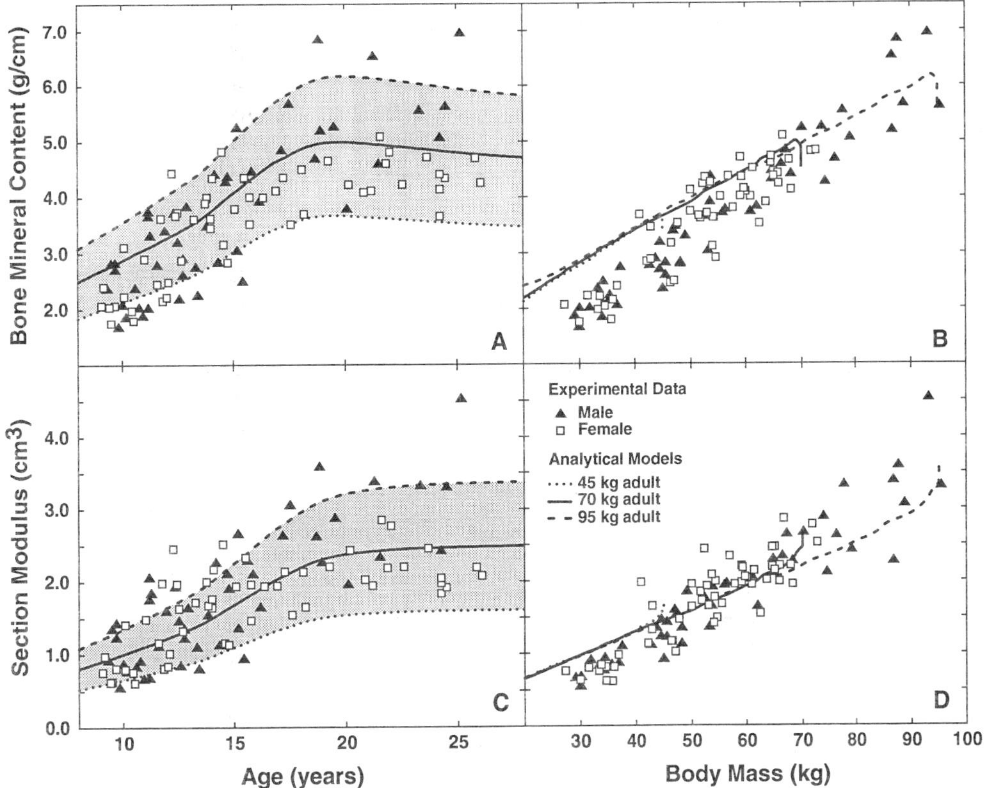

FIGURE 4 Correspondence between simulation results (lines) and clinical data (individual points) for bone mineral content (top row) and section modulus (bottom row) as a function of age (left column) and body mass (right column). The shaded region indicates the area bounded by the 45- and 95-kg simulations. From van der Meulen *et al.* [26].

in determining the geometry of the primary growth front and physis, the appearance and shape of secondary ossification centers, and the normal development of articular cartilage thickness and histomorphology [6,28,29].

In addition to regulating the pattern of endochondral growth and ossification, the local mechanical stress or strain stimulus influences the microstructural orientation and density of the cancellous bone that appears at the growth front. Furthermore, the local bone stress stimulus plays an important role in regulating the remodeling process and thus in determining the distribution of bone mass and the microstructural organization of the cancellous bone structure.

The local mechanical regulation of cancellous bone mass can be understood using the same basic analytical framework used for compact bone apposition and resorption [20,30–32]. With normal compact bone during development, the major changes in bone mass are due to bone apposition and resorption on the periosteal and endosteal surfaces. In cancellous bone, however, apposition and resorption take place on internal, trabecular surfaces. Variations in cancellous bone mass are therefore primarily a result of differences in bone porosity. Because the density of the mineralized tissue of cancellous bone is approximately the same as that of compact bone, the porosity of cancellous bone is inversely proportional to its apparent density [33].

The stresses in a region of cancellous bone are most commonly referred to in terms of an "apparent" or "continuum" stress that is averaged over a significant area of trabeculae and marrow spaces (e.g., 5×5 mm). Using this continuum stress definition, the failure stress of cancellous bone has been shown to be proportional to the square of its apparent density [33]. The strong dependence of failure stress on apparent density is a result of the fact that when forces are imposed on bone of low apparent density the trabecular struts are exposed to very high stresses on a microstructural level.

By regulating bone porosity during bone formation or remodeling, the mineralized tissue that comprises the trabecular struts may be exposed to increased stress (with increasing porosity) or decreased stress (with decreasing porosity) during normal physical activity. The stress stimulus at this microstructural, trabecular level is important in establishing the apparent density of cancellous bone during growth and development and in maintaining cancellous bone mass in adulthood and aging. At this microstructural level, the mechanical regulation of bone mass follows, in the first approximation, the same functional relationship as compact bone (Fig. 1). All mineralized bone tissue at the microstructural level tends to adapt so that it is exposed to some "normal" stress stimulus [21,31,34,35]. At the "apparent" or "continuum" stress level, however, this premise implies that cancellous bone will tend to adjust its apparent density so that the mechanical demands placed on the bone are similar at all cancellous and compact bone sites (Fig. 5).

The ability of the skeleton to develop and remodel in response to the local mechanical demands leads to a very efficient distribution of bone material in virtually all appendicular bones in all individuals. Computer-based demonstrations of the architectural construction of the proximal femur based on this fundamental concept were first implemented by Carter and colleagues [6,32,34,36,37] and were later refined and applied in many different remodeling applications [9,20,30,38–41].

The process of cancellous bone acquisition and adaptation in response to the mechanical loading caused by physical activity was illustrated using a time-dependent remodeling approach by Beaupre *et al.* [20,30] (Fig. 6). The proximal femur was represented as a two-dimensional finite element model, and it was initially assumed that the bone density was the same at every location throughout the model. The daily loading activity on the femur was simulated by applying three separate loading conditions on the model to represent the range of load magnitudes and orientations that would appear during normal physical activities. The stress stimulus was then calculated at every location in the model, and the bone remodeling rules (Figs. 2 and 5) were implemented in a stepwise fashion to simulate small time increments. After the first time increment, the density and material properties in the model were changed according to the new, remodeled bone density at each location. An additional time increment was then implemented and the stress stimulus at every location was calculated for the next remodeling step. Using this iterative approach, the entire proximal femur was remodeled and a rich, heterogeneous distribution of bone density was created (Fig. 6). Important bone features predicted by the model include dense cortical diaphyses, a dense compression column of cancellous bone through the femoral head, a trabecular band corresponding to the cancellous bone arcuate system of the lateral-superior neck, and the low bone density in the Ward's triangle region.

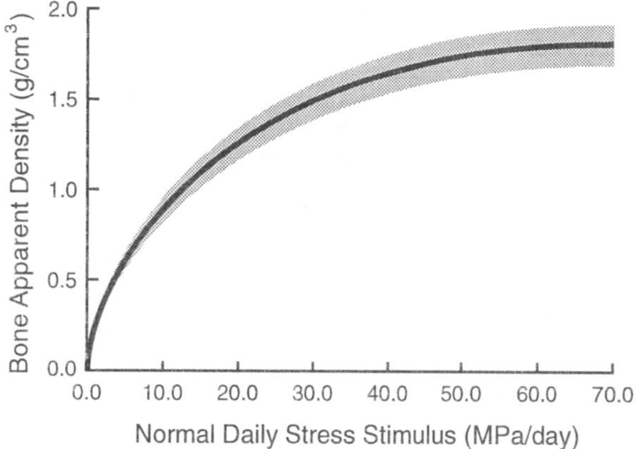

FIGURE 5 Theoretical relationship between the normal daily stress stimulus and the bone apparent density at any specific site in the postcranial skeleton. Adapted from Beaupré *et al.* [20].

Once the normal architecture of the proximal femur was created, the same incremental remodeling approach was used to predict the changes in bone density that could be expected if the magnitude of the forces imposed on the femur was increased or decreased by 20%. Reduced loading caused a general reduction in the apparent density of the cancellous bone throughout the proximal femur and a thinning of the cortices. Increased loading caused a systematic increase in cancellous bone density and a thickening of the cortices. In both cases, however, the general pattern of bone distribution remained relatively unchanged. These results are consistent with the changes in bone density predicted based on our approach of the influence of the stress stimulus on the steady state apparent density value of bone (Fig. 5).

CLINICAL STUDIES OF ACCRETION OF BONE MASS

Many clinical studies have measured bone mass in a variety of specific human populations. The lumbar spine and femoral neck are the most frequently studied sites because of their clinical relevance to age-related bone loss and fractures. The femoral shaft and distal radius have also been examined. In adolescents, understanding influences on bone mineral acquisition will give insights into the acquisition of peak bone mass. Most of the increase in bone mass during this time period is due to growth-related changes in skeletal size, not bone volumetric density (g/cm^3). Based on the mechanical mechanisms described previously, we would expect that an indicator of mechanical loading, such as body mass and/or physical activity, would strongly relate to clinical bone mass acquisition. As explained, the skeletal structure grows in response to increased mechanical loads due to increasing body size during growth.

Femoral structural behavior results from the interaction of material properties and geometry. During the

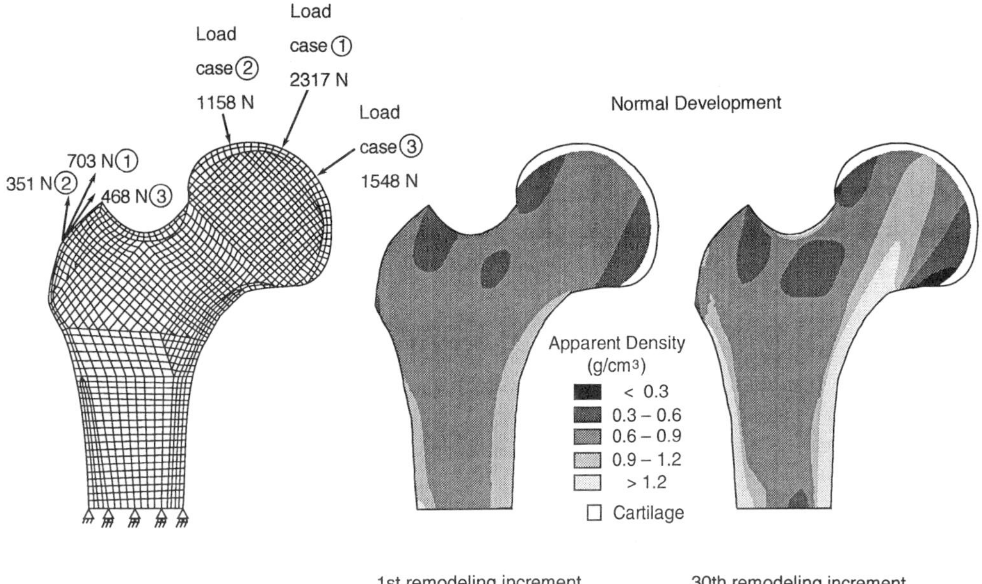

FIGURE 6 Finite element model demonstrating the computer predictions of bone apparent density distributions created by stress stimuli imposed during normal physical activity. Adapted from Beaupré *et al.* [30].

rapid growth period of adolescence, cortical bone tissue material properties change little [42,43] and are independent of gender [44]; however, significant changes in femoral length and cross-sectional dimensions occur [19,22]. Because of these rapid dimensional changes, investigations of children and adolescents generally focus on age or pubertal stage as primary correlates of bone mass [45–49]. These studies report significant relationships between age and bone mineral content or density of the spine and femoral neck, but they often do not consider body mass relationships.

Studies examining the relationship between bone mass and multiple developmental parameters, including age and body mass, have reported high positive correlations between body mass and bone mineral content (BMC, g) or bone mineral density (BMD, g/cm^2) in adolescent and young adult populations at both cortical and cancellous bone sites [25,50–52]. When both parameters are compared, the relationships with body mass are stronger than those with age.

In addition to changing hormone levels during adolescence, physical activity, diet, and genetic factors may also influence bone mass. Although many of these factors have not been well characterized, investigators examining the influence of physical activity and diet on bone mass have found mixed results, reporting a significant effect in some studies [53–56], but no detectable effect in others [1,52,57]. These different results may reflect differences in the method of physical activity assessment, but they may also reflect the primary role

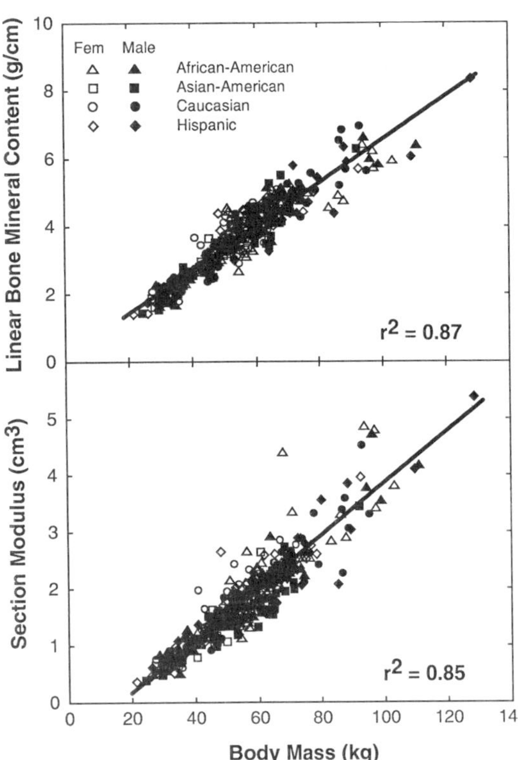

FIGURE 7 Linear regression between body mass and linear bone mineral content (top) or section modulus (bottom) for the middiaphysis of the femur in 375 adolescents. The relationships are independent of gender and ethnicity. From Moro *et al.* [57].

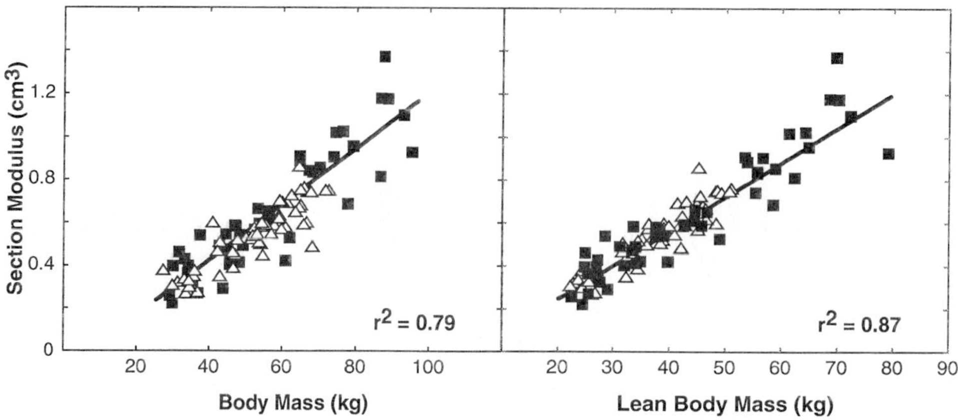

FIGURE 8 Linear regression between body mass (left) or lean body mass (right) and section modulus for the neck of the femur in 101 Caucasian adolescents. The relationships are independent of gender.

of body mass. Once body mass is accounted for, physical activity may add little additional explanatory power, whereas if only age is considered, physical activity may provide important additional information. The sensitivity of the skeleton to exercise may also be influenced by the stage of pubertal development [58].

In a cross-sectional cohort of 375 healthy, diverse adolescents, the midfemoral structural properties were characterized and the relative influences of age, body mass, pubertal status, ethnicity, gender, and physical activity on bone mass were examined [25,57]. Strong relationships of body mass with bone mineral content and section modulus were found (Fig. 7). For these relationships, body mass alone explained 85% of the variance in data, and it is not surprising, therefore, that accounting for additional factors, such as ethnicity, gender, age, pubertal stage, lean muscle mass, calcium, and weight-bearing, activity does not substantially improve the predictive power of the analysis. Also, the relationships with lean body mass may be a better indicator of physical activity than either questionnaires or body mass. At the midfemur, however, total body mass yielded stronger relationships than lean body mass, even when gender was accounted for. In the Caucasian subset of these subjects (53 females, 48 males), we also examined the structural behavior of the femoral neck. Lean body mass was found to be the strongest determinant of femoral neck section modulus (an indicator of bending strength) and the relationship was independent of gender (Fig. 8) [59]. The metabolic function of trabecular bone, as well as its development via endochondral ossification, not direct bone apposition, is different from the cortical midfemur and merits further consideration.

SUMMARY

The emphasis in this chapter is on the role that mechanics plays in the development and growth of the skeleton, leading to peak bone mass at maturity. Mechanical regulation of skeletal biology causes changes in skeletal mass, structure, and organization as a result of age-related changes in skeletal loading. The magnitude of this loading can be directly related to body mass and physical activity. While we have focused on mechanical regulation, genetic, dietary, and hormonal influences are also important and are addressed in the further chapters in this section. Much remains to be learned about those factors, particularly their interactions with the mechanical regulation of bone mineral acquisition during development. Within Earth's gravitational environment, however, the mechanical function of the skeleton in supporting the body weight and facilitating movement appears to be the primary, limiting regulator in determining peak bone mass.

Acknowledgments

We acknowledge the significant contributions of Gary Beaupré to both the ideas and work presented here. This work has been supported in part by the Department of Veterans Affairs, the National Institutes of Health, and the National Aeronautics and Space Administration.

References

1. Katzman, D. K., Bachrach, L. K., Carter, D. R., and Marcus, R. Clinical and anthropometric correlates of bone mineral acquisition in healthy adolescent girls. *J. Clin. Endocrinol. Metab.* **73,** 1332–1339 (1991).
2. Ott, S. Bone density in adolescents. *N. Engl J. Med.* **325,** 1646–1647 (1991).
3. Heaney, R. P. Nutrition and risk for osteoporosis. *In* "Osteoporosis" (R. Marcus, D. Feldman and J. Kelsey, eds.), pp. 483–509. Academic Press, San Diego, 1996.
4. Marcus, R., and Carter, D. R. The role of physical activity in bone mass regulation. *Adv. Sports Med. Fitness* **1,** 63–82 (1988).
5. Wolff, J., "The Law of Bone Remodeling." Springer-Verlag, Berlin, 1892.

6. Carter, D. R. Mechanical loading history and skeletal biology. *J. Biomech.* **20,** 1095–1109 (1987).
7. Cowin, S. C., Hart, R. T., Balser, J. R., and Kohn, D. H. Functional adaptation in long bones: establishing in vivo values for surface remodeling rate coefficients. *J. Biomech.* **18,** 665–684 (1985).
8. Hart, R. T., Davy, D. T., and Heiple, K. G. Mathematical modeling and numerical solutions for functionally dependent bone remodeling. *Calcif. Tissue Int.* **36,** S104–S109 (1984).
9. Huiskes, R., Weinans, H., Grootenboer, H. J., Dalstra, M., Fudala, B. and Sloof, T. J. Adaptive bone-remodeling theory applied to prosthetic-design analysis. *J. Biomech.* **20,** 1135–1150 (1987).
10. Biewener, A. A., and Bertram, J. E. A. Structural response of growing bone to exercise and disuse. *J. Appl. Physiol.* **76,** 946–955 (1994).
11. Dietz, F. R. Effect of denervation on limb growth. *J. Orthop. Res.* **7,** 292–303 (1989).
12. Hall, B. K., and Herring, S. W. Paralysis and growth of the musculoskeletal system in the embryonic chick. *J. Morphol.* **206,** 45–56 (1990).
13. Rodríguez, J. I., Garcia-Alix, A., Palacios, J., and Paniagua, R. Changes in long bones due to fetal immobility caused by neuromuscular disease. *J. Bone Joint Surg.* **70A,** 1052–1060 (1988).
14. van der Meulen, M. C. H., Morey-Holton, E. R., and Carter, D. R. Hindlimb suspension diminishes femoral cross-sectional growth in the rat. *J. Orthop. Res.* **13,** 700–707 (1995).
15. Wong, M., Germiller, J., Bonadio, J., and Goldstein, S. A. Neuromuscular atrophy alters collagen gene expression, pattern formation, and mechanical integrity of the chick embryo long bone. *Prog. Clin. Biol. Res.* **383B,** 587–597 (1993).
16. van der Meulen, M. C. H., Beaupré, G. S., and Carter, D. R. Mechanobiologic influences in long bone cross-sectional growth. *Bone* **14,** 635–642 (1993).
17. Gross, T. S., McLeod, K. J., and Rubin, C. T. Characterizing bone strain distributions *in vivo* using three triple rosette strain gages. *J. Biomech.* **25,** 1081–1087 (1992).
18. Keller, T. S., and Spengler, D. M. Regulation of bone stress and strain in the immature and mature rat femur. *J. Biomech.* **22,** 1115–1127 (1989).
19. McCammon, R. W., "Human Growth and Development." Thomas, Springfield, IL, 1970.
20. Beaupré, G. S., Orr, T. E., and Carter, D. R. An approach for time-dependent bone modeling and remodeling—theoretical development. *J. Orthop. Res.* **8,** 651–661 (1990).
21. Fyhrie, D. P., and Carter, D. R. A unifying principle relating stress to trabecular bone morphology. *J. Orthop. Res.* **4,** 304–317 (1986).
22. Martin, R. B., and Atkinson, P. J. Age and sex-related changes in the structure and strength of the human femoral shaft. *J. Biomech.* **10,** 223–231 (1977).
23. Smith, R. W., and Walker, R. R. Femoral expansion in aging women: implications for osteoporosis and fractures. *Science* **145,** 156–157 (1964).
24. Hillman, L. Nutrition and risk for osteoporosis. *In* "Osteoporosis" (R., Marcus, D. Feldman and J. Kelsey, eds.), pp. 449–464. Academic Press, San Diego, 1996.
25. van der Meulen, M. C. H., Ashford, M. W., Jr., Kiratli, B. J., Bachrach, L. K., and Carter, D. R. Determinants of femoral geometry and structure during adolescent growth. *J. Orthop. Res.* **14,** 22–29 (1996).
26. van der Meulen, M. C. H., Marcus, R., Bachrach, L. K., and Carter, D. R. Correspondence between theoretical models and DXA measurements of femoral cross-sectional growth during adolescence. *J. Orthop. Res.* **15,** 473–476 (1997).
27. Martin, R. B., and Burr, D. B. Non-invasive measurement of long bone cross-sectional moment of inertia by photon absorptiometry. *J. Biomech.* **17,** 195–201 (1984).
28. Carter, D. R., Orr, T. E., Fyhrie, D. P., and Schurman, D. J. Influences of mechanical stress on prenatal and postnatal skeletal development. *Clin. Orthop.* **219,** 237–250 (1987).
29. Carter, D. R. The role of mechanical loading histories in the development of diarthrodial joints. *J. Orthop. Res.* **6,** 804–816 (1988).
30. Beaupré, G. S., Orr, T. E., and Carter, D. R. An approach for time-dependent bone modeling and remodeling—application: a preliminary remodeling situation. *J. Orthop. Res.* **8,** 662–670 (1990).
31. Carter, D. R., Fyhrie, D. P., and Whalen, R. T. Trabecular bone density and loading history: regulation of connective tissue biology by mechanical energy. *J. Biomech.* **20,** 785–794 (1987).
32. Carter, D. R., Orr, T. E., and Fyhrie, D. P. Relationships between loading history and femoral cancellous bone architecture. *J. Biomech.* **22,** 231–244 (1989).
33. Carter, D. R., and Hayes, W. C. The compressive behavior of bone as a two-phase porous structure. *J. Bone Joint Surg.* **59A,** 954–962 (1977).
34. Fyhrie, D. P., and Carter, D. R. Femoral head apparent density distribution predicted from bone stresses. *J. Biomech.* **23,** 1–10 (1990).
35. Whalen, R. T., Carter, D. R., and Steele, C. R. Influence of physical activity on the regulation of bone density. *J. Biomech.* **21,** 825–837 (1988).
36. Orr, T. E., "The Role of Mechanical Stresses in Bone Remodeling." Ph.D. thesis, Department of Mechanical Engineering, Stanford University, Stanford, CA, 1990.
37. Orr, T. E., Beaupré, G. S., Carter, D. R., and Schurman, D. J. Computer predictions of bone remodeling around porous-coated implants. *J. Arthrop.* **5,** 191–200 (1990).
38. Jacobs, C. R., Simo, J. C., Beaupré, G. S., and Carter, D. R. A principal stress-based approach to the simulation of anisotropic bone adaptation to mechanical loading. *In* "Bone Structure and Remodeling" (H. Wienans and A. Odgaard, eds.), pp. 225–239. World Scientific Publishing Co., Singapore, 1995.
39. Levenston, M. E., Beaupre, G. S., Jacobs, C. R., and Carter, D. R. The role of loading memory in bone adaptation simulations. *Bone* **15,** 177–186 (1994).
40. Prendergast, P. J., and Taylor, D. Prediction of bone adaptation using damage accumulation. *J. Biomech.* **27,** 1067–1076 (1994).
41. Weinans, H., Huiskes, R., van Rietbergen, B., Sumner, D. R., Turner, T. M., and Galante, J. O. Adaptive bone remodeling around bonded noncemented total hip arthroplasty: a comparison between animal experiments and computer simulation. *J. Orthop. Res.* **11,** 500–513 (1993).
42. Atkinson, P., and Weatherell, J. A. Variation in the density of the femoral diaphysis with age. *J. Bone Joint Surg.* **49B,** 781–788 (1967).
43. Currey, J. D., and Butler, G. The mechanical properties of bone tissue in children. *J. Bone Joint Surg.* **57A,** 810–814 (1975).
44. Burstein, A. H., Reilly, D. T., and Martens, M. Aging of bone tissue: mechanical properties. *J. Bone Joint Surg.* **58A,** 82–86 (1976).
45. Bonjour, J.-P., Theintz, G., Buchs, B., Slosman, D., and Rizzoli, R. Critical years and stages of puberty for spinal and femoral bone mass accumulation during adolescence. *J. Clin. Endocrin. Metab.* **73,** 555–563 (1991).
46. Glastre, C., Braillon, P., David, L., Cochat, P., Meanier, P. J., and Delmas, P. D. Measurement of bone mineral content of the lumbar spine by dual energy x-ray absorptiometry in normal children: correlations with growth parameters. *J. Clin. Endocrin. Metab.* **70,** 1330–1333 (1990).
47. Henderson, R. C. Assessment of bone mineral content in children. *J. Pediatr. Orthop.* **11,** 314–317 (1991).

48. Kröger, H., Lotaniemi, A., Vainio, P., and Alhava, E. Bone densitometry of the spine and femur in children by dual-energy x-ray absorptiometry. *Bone Miner.* **17,** 75–85 (1992).
49. Rico, H., Revilla, M., Hernandez, E. R., Villa, L. F., and Alvarez der Buergo. Sex differences in the acquisition of total bone mineral mass peak assessed through dual-energy x-ray absorptiometry. *Calcif. Tissue Int.* **51,** 251–254 (1992).
50. Gilsanz, V., Kovanlikaya, A., Costin, G., Roe, T. F., Sayre, J., and Kaufman, F. Differential effect of gender on the sizes of the bones in the axial and appendicular skeletons. *J. Clin. Endocrin. Metab.* **82,** 1603–1607 (1997).
51. Ponder, S. W., McCormick, D. P., Fawcett, H. D., Palmer, J. L., McKernan, G., and Brouhard, B. H. Spinal bone mineral density in children age 5.00 through 11.99 years. *Am. J. Dis. Child.* **144,** 1346–1348 (1990).
52. Southard, R. N., Morris, J. D., Mahan, N. D., Hayes, J. R., Torch, M. A., Sommer, A., and Zipf, W. B. Bone mass in healthy children: measurement with quantitative DXA. *Radiology* **179,** 735–738 (1991).
53. Henderson, N. K., Price, R. I., Cole, J. H., Gutteridge, D. H., and Bhagat, C. I. Bone density in young women is associated with body weight and muscle strength but not dietary intakes. *J. Bone Miner. Res.* **10,** 384–393 (1995).
54. Pocock, N., Eisman, J., Gwinn, T., Sambrook, P., Kelly, P., Freund, J., and Yeates, M. Muscle strength, physical fitness, and weight but not age predict femoral neck bone mass. *J. Bone Miner. Res.* **4,** 441–448 (1989).
55. Slemenda, C. W., Miller, J. Z., Hui, S. L., Reister, T. K., and Johnston, C. C. J. Role of physical activity in the development of skeletal mass in children. *Bone Miner. Res.* **6,** 1227–1233 (1991).
56. Welten, D. C., G, K. H. C., Post, G. B., van Michelen, W., Twisk, J., Lips, P., and Teule, G. J. Weight-bearing activity during youth is a more important factor for peak bone mass than calcium intake. *J. Bone Miner. Res.* **9,** 1089–1096.
57. Moro, M., van der Meulen, M. C. H., Kiratli, B. J., Marcus, R., Bachrach, L. K., and Carter, D. R. Body mass is the primary determinant of midfemoral bone acquisition during adolescent growth. *Bone* **19,** 519–526.
58. Haapasalo, H., Kannus, P., Sievänen, H., Pasanen, M., Uusi-Rasi, K., Heinonen, A., Oja, P., and Vuori, I. Effect of long-term unilateral activity on bone mineral density of female junior tennis players. *J. Bone Miner. Res.* **13,** 310–319 (1998).
59. van der Meulen, M., Moro, M., Kiratli, B. J., Marcus, R., Bachrach, L. K., and Carter, D. R. Determinants of femoral neck structure during adolescence. *J. Bone Miner. Res.* **12** (Suppl. 1), S252 (1997).

CHAPTER 11

Hormonal Influences on the Establishment of Peak Bone Mass

MICHELLE P. WARREN Department of Medicine and Obstetrics and Gynecology, Columbia University College of Physicians and Surgeons, New York, New York 10032

INTRODUCTION

The attainment of peak bone mass sets the stage for the prevention of osteoporosis in later life. Understanding the factors that lead to maximal bone accretion is critical as it presents an important opportunity for intervention. Bone accretion has a unique sensitivity to metabolic, hormonal, environmental, and genetic factors. Adolescence and young adulthood represent an important window of time when bone mass reaches its peak because up to 80% of total mass is accrued by this time. Thus understanding the mechanisms leading to peak bone mass may lead to strategies to improve the quality and quantity of bone accrued during this critically important period. This chapter focuses on the hormonal factors that are importance in the establishment of peak bone mass. Since a consideration of hormonal influences must necessarily take into account other factors, such as exercise and nutrition, they will be correct but only in the context of interrelationships.

FORMATION OF BONE MASS

General Influences on Peak Bone Mineral Density

Bone mass formation increases dramatically at puberty (up to 40%) [1–10] (Fig. 1) and continues into the 30s [11], although recent studies have shortened this incremental period to the early 20's [9,12–16]. Lloyd *et al.* [9] have shown that premenarcheal girls attained 83% of adult bone mineral density (BMD) by early puberty, whereas other studies suggest that women have the potential of increasing bone mass up to age 30 [17]. As noted, the exact age at which peak bone mass is achieved, is maintained, and begins to decline is uncertain and is likely to encompass a range of ages. After age 40, nevertheless, if there is no intervention, bone mass begins to decline [18]. Factors affecting peak bone mass include age [19], weight [2,9,20–22], body surface area [23], body mass [24], physical activity [25–28] (Fig. 2), calcium intake [28,29], genetics [30], sex hormone exposure [9,31], and pubertal development [3,21,31,32]. The influence of pubertal development on peak bone mass is critically important. The relationship between bone density and pubertal development has been emphasized in several studies because of the acceleration of BMD increases at this time. Not all studies, however, suggest that pubertal development is the major determinant in both sexes. The major determinant in one study was pubertal development in girls but weight for boys [21].

Biochemical markers of bone formation [33,34] and bone resorption [35] increase with the growth spurt. When biochemical markers of bone formation were examined and correlated with the pubertal stage, all formation markers were maximal in Tanner stages II and III and decreased in stages IV and V. All markers were lower after menarche [36] (Fig. 3). Thus, markers of bone resorption varied significantly with pubertal stage.

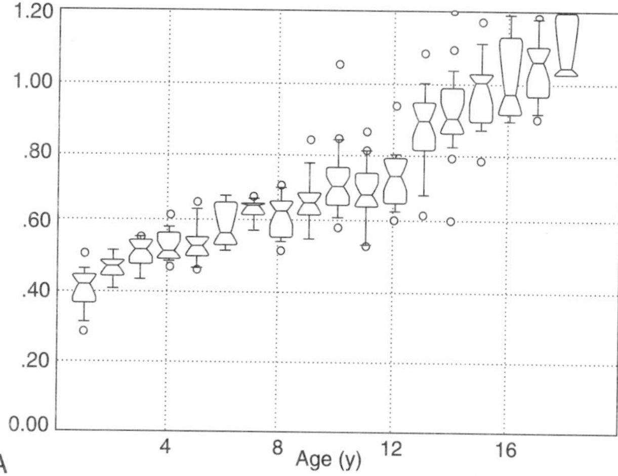

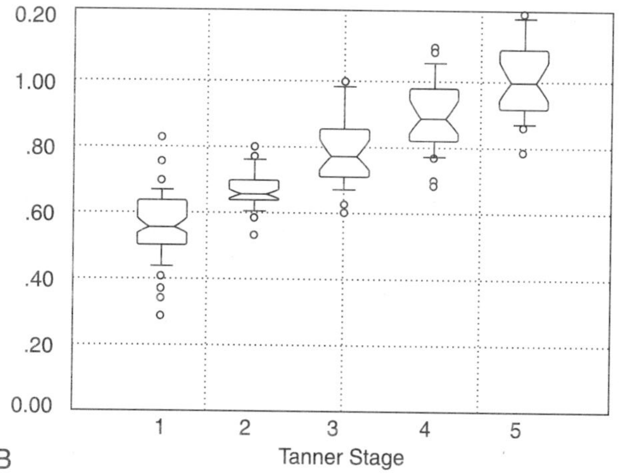

FIGURE 1 (A) Box plot of total bone density (grams per square centimeter) versus age for 218 children. (B) Box plot of total bone density versus Tanner stage for 218 children. The bottom, middle, and top of each box represent the 25th, 50th, and 75th percentiles; the extension lines represent the 10th and 90th percentiles. Notches represent a median test at the $P < 0.05$ level so that nonoverlapping notches are significantly different. Individual subjects' data points outside the 10th and 90th percentiles are represented as circles (o). From Southard *et al.* [10].

This study also demonstrated a negative correlation between estradiol levels and markers of bone turnover in pubertal subjects. There was no evidence for a positive relationship between bone turnover and plasma levels of insulin-like growth factor-1 (IGF-1) and insulin-like growth factor-binding protein-3 (IGFBP-3). This is of interest as the early phase of the pubertal growth spurt is related, at least in part, to sex steroid augmentation of growth hormone secretion [37,38]. A positive correlation between IGF-1 and osteocalcin has been noted with age [39].

Exercise

Exercise is also an important consideration in the establishment of peak bone mass. One study (see Chapter 39) [26] showed a relationship between exercise and radius and hip BMD in both sexes aged 5–14 years. Others have shown a relationship to lumbar spine [27] and femoral neck [40] in children. In ballet dancers, a relationship between spine and foot BMD and exercise has been demonstrated [41]. One prospective study has shown that those who perform the most exercise at age 9–18 had higher femoral BMD at the ages of 20–29 in both sexes. Higher exercise levels affected BMD in the spine only in boys, however [28]. The absence of a similar correlation may be due to the low variance of exercise in girls. Because weight and physical activity both have positive effects on bone, children who are underweight and inactive may be at risk for low BMD.

Nutrition

GENERAL INFLUENCES

Peak bone mass is influenced by nutrition, particularly protein for matrix formation and calcium and phosphorus for mineralization [42]. Weaver [42a] showed that serum osteocalcin as well as postmenarcheal age accounted for 75% of the variability in calcium retention. Another study examining osteocalcin in adolescence showed a rise with age in both sexes and a decline 2 years earlier for girls, with a peak at 15–16 years [43].

MODELS WHERE PEAK BONE MASS IS ALTERED

Processes that disturb hormonal or metabolic regulation prior to the attainment of peak bone mass also lend insight into the normal mineralization process.

Delayed Puberty

Because bone mass increases throughout childhood and accretion accelerates during puberty, a delay in puberty significantly delays this process. However, "catch up" may be seriously compromised as recovery from processes that delay puberty does not lead to normalization of bone density. A delay in puberty significantly affects peak bone mass [1,3,31], indicating a critical role for the timing of hormonal sufficiency during

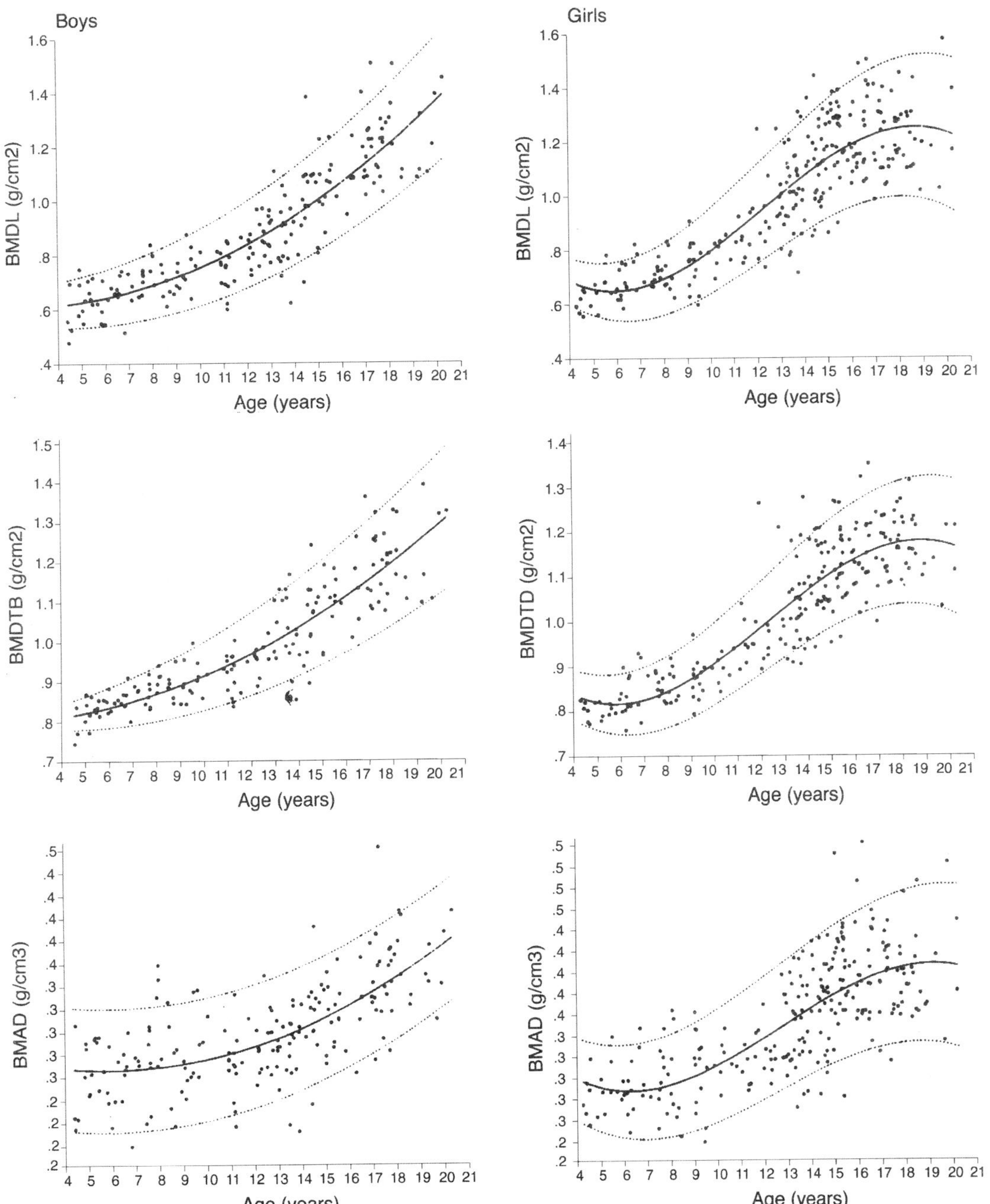

FIGURE 2 Relationship between age and BMD of the lumbar spine (BMDL; grams per cm^2), total body BMD (BMDTB; grams per cm^2), and BMAD of the lumbar spine (grams per cm^3) in boys and girls. The line shows the best-fitted function with the factors age, age^2, age^3 for girls, and age and age^2 for boys. Dotted lines represent the 5 and 95% prediction limits. From Boot *et al.* [21].

puberty [5]. Adult men who have a history of constitutional delay have decreased BMD compared to men with normal sexual development [44]. Treatment for delayed puberty in boys with idiopathic hypogonadotrophic hypogonadism at an older age does not lead to normalization of bone mass [45].

Exercise at Times of Bone Accretion

It has been hypothesized that mechanical loading may enhance bone formation in a synergistic fashion in the presence of developing estrogen "competence" (i.e., puberty). The difference in bone mass of tennis and

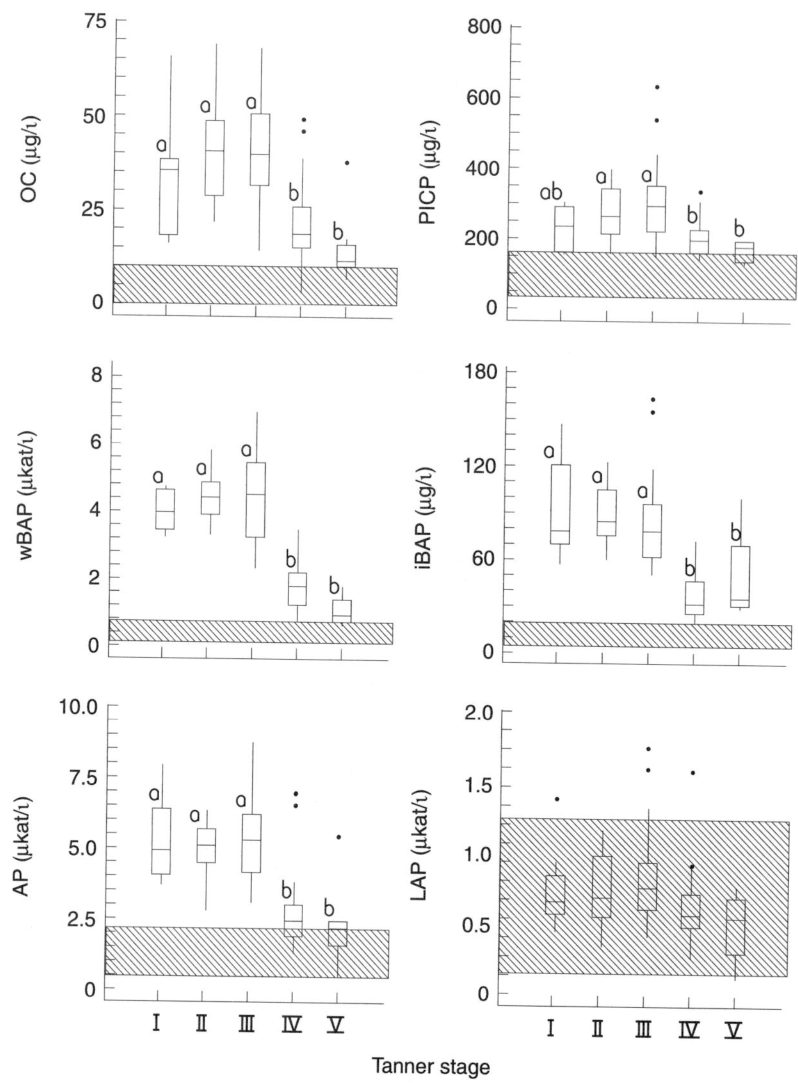

FIGURE 3 Levels of biochemical markers of bone formation according to Tanner stage in girls. In this and other figures, the enclosed boxes indicate the interquartile range of data, and the horizontal lines indicate the median. The whiskers indicate the range between highest and lowest values, excluding the outliers, the positions of which are shown (•). The shaded area indicates the 95% reference range for healthy adult women. Overall significance of the differences between groups by analysis of variance are as follows: OC (serum osteocalcin), $P < 0.0001$; PICP (serum type I procollagen carboxyterminal propeptide), $P < 0.0001$; wBAP (wheat-germ lectin precipitated AP), $P < 0.0001$; iBAP (immunoreactive bone isoenzyme of AP), $P < 0.0001$; AP (serum total alkaline phosphatase), $P < 0.0001$; LAP (liver AP), $P =$ NS. Bars without a common letter are significantly different ($P < 0.05$, Scheffe test). From Blumsohn *et al.* [36].

squash players was two to four times higher in those players who had started training before or at menarche compared to those who started 15 years after menarche [46]. This group has also reported that the osteotrophic effect may be the greatest during a relatively short pubertal period [47]. Analysis of pre-, peri-, and postpubertal female tennis players (aged 7 to 17 years) showed that bilateral differences in bone density of the arms of the players began to differ from controls at Tanner stage III.

Even before estrogen levels rise, the prepubertal years may be a uniquely opportune time when the skeleton is responsive to exercise. This effect may be growth hormone dependent as exercise is a potent stimulus for growth hormone secretion [48,49]. The relative advantage of the sex hormone-independent prepubertal years may pertain to the intensity of exercise needed to exert an anabolic effect on bone mass. It may reach the intensity associated with the interference with sex hormone cyclicity and a delay in pubertal maturation. Large increases in bone density have been reported in elite prepubertal gymnasts [50,51], and positive associations with moderate exercise and bone density have been reported in prepubertal girls. This is not the case for pubertal girls as noted below [52,53,54].

The relative advantage of the pre- and peripubertal years over the postpubertal period may also relate to the fact that the rapidly remodeling skeleton is affected per se by sex hormones. In the postpubertal years of adolescence and young adulthood, the osteotrophic response is tempered by sex hormones [55–57].

Amenorrhea: Influences of Poor Nutrition and Exercise

Bachrach, *et al.* [58] found that one-third of females who recovered from anorexia nervosa during adolescence had persistent osteopenia. Women where anorexia nervosa began in adolescence had lower spinal BMD compared to those where the disease began in adulthood [59]. A number of studies have documented osteopenia associated with amenorrhea in premenopausal women, including athletes, ballet dancers, and women with anorexia nervosa [60].

A major complication of amenorrhea is the loss of bone mineral content (density) and bone strength [31,41,61,62,63–67]. Compromised bone accretion in adolescence and young adulthood results in women entering menopause with a greatly reduced bone mass. Amenorrheic young women have persistently lower BMD [31,41,17,68] when compared to normal controls. This effect is particularly significant when delayed menarche is associated with amenorrhea [31,41,69]. Considered by itself, delayed menarche is a strong predictor of reduced bone density. The effect persists when controlling for age and weight [41]. Interestingly, amenorrheic dancers showed the greatest increase (12% spine, 11% wrist, 5% foot) in BMD over 2 years. Their BMD values, however, still remained significantly below normal controls for the duration of the study [17] (Fig. 4).

In these subjects, estrogen deficiency has been treated with hormonal therapy. Estrogen replacement therapy shows a small and insignificant effect on bone mineral density, with treated amenorrheic subjects remaining below normals. Thus, prolonged hypoestro-

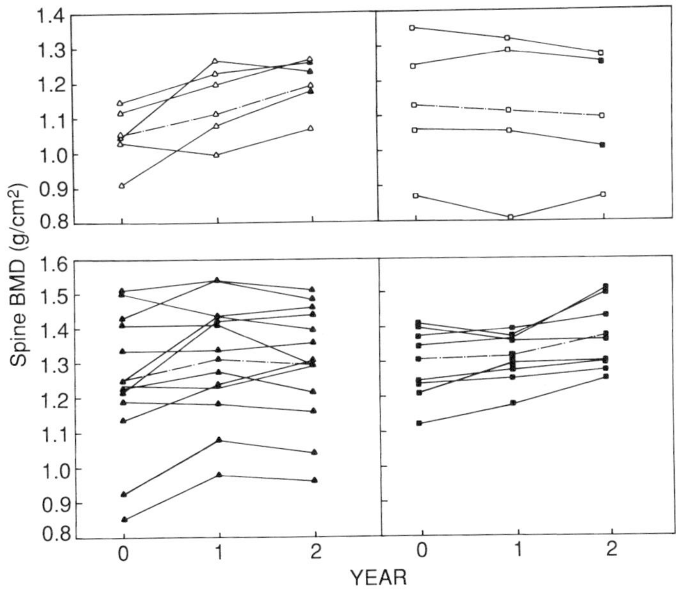

FIGURE 4 Spine bone mineral density (BMD) in normal and amenorrheic subjects over 2 years. Groups are divided into dancers and nondancer controls. Changes from an open symbol to a solid one denote changes from amenorrheic to eumenorrheic status. Dotted lines represent the mean of all values. △, amenorrheic dancers; □, amenorrheic controls; ▲, cycling dancers; ■, cycling controls. From Jonnavithula *et al.* [17].

genism in adolescence appears to be associated with a persistent lowering of BMD that does not appear to be easily reversible with estrogen therapy at the doses employed [70]. Severe nutritional aberrations and subtle eating disorders in both exercising and nonexercising amenorrheics [71,72] may contribute to the persistently low BMD.

Exercise

The loss of bone mass and lack of bone accretion seen in young amenorrheic athletes [31,41,61–65,69], in other amenorrheic groups [31,41,73], and in groups with delayed menarche and delayed development [12,41,70,74] (Fig. 5) may be important determinants of osteoporosis. The incidence of stress fractures, scoliosis [75], vertebral compression fractures [76] and femoral head collapse [77] in young women may all be related to hypoestrogenesis in adolescence or later. Stress fractures are a particular problem for the amenorrheic athlete. The ballet dancer with amenorrheic exemplifies the osteopenic state, despite risorous exercise (Fig. 6). This reduction in bone mass may also be irreversible [78] and is associated with significant clinical problems. (Table I). Data indicate that exercise improves a bone mass in normal adolescents, but in the hypoestrogenic state, exercise cannot serve as a substitute for the protective effect of a euestrogenic state, nor can it reverse the osteopenia.

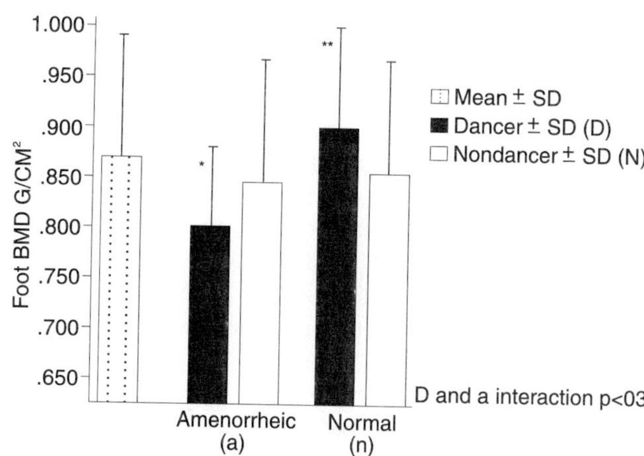

FIGURE 6 Foot bone mineral densities in normal and amenorrheic subjects. Groups are divided into dancers and nondancers. Significance determined by ANOVA. $P < 0.05$. Stippled bar, mean of all values. Two-way ANOVA shows a significant effect of amenorrhea on BMD when controlling for age but was eliminated by controlling for weight. *, Multiple comparisons show that amenorrheic dancers differ from normal dancers even when controlling for age and weight. **, Normal dancers were higher than both amenorrheic groups when controlling for age. Interaction was eliminated when controlling for age but not weight. From Warren *et al.* [41].

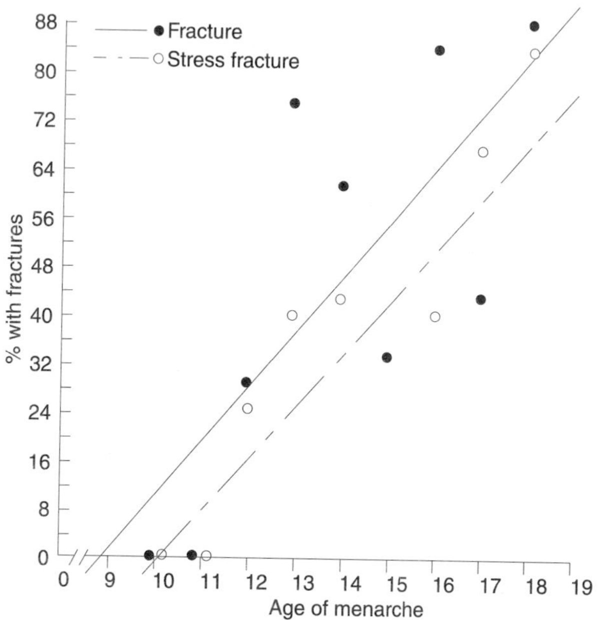

FIGURE 5 Relation between age at menarche and the percentage of subjects with fractures and stress fractures ($N = 75$). When the type of fracture was specified, the correlations for frequency distribution versus age at menarche were found to be greatest among those reporting stress fractures ($n = 40$), despite the smaller number of dancers in that group. From Warren *et al.* [75].

Hormone Replacement in Amenorrhea

Studies in young dancers suggest that increases in bone mass do occur in young individuals even prior to the return of normal menses, but bone density remains below normal [17,31,70]. Clinical trials to demonstrate the benefit of exogenous estrogen in this age group have not been done [1,79]. An overall paucity of research regarding sex steroid replacement has plagued this field

TABLE I Incidence of Stress Fractures in Amenorrheic and Eumenorrheic Athletes[a]

Study	Sport	Amenorrheic $(N)^b$	Eumenorrheic (N)
Lindberg 1984	Runner	49% (11)	0% (15)
Warren 1986	Dancers	20% (25)	13% (31)
Lloyd 1986	Mixed	15% (41)	4% (158)
Barrow 1988	Runners	49% (69)	29% (120)
Marcus 1985	Runners	55% (11)	17% (6)
Clark 1988	Runners	72% (18)	36% (75)

[a] Adapted, with permission, from Constantini [123].
[b] Total number of subjects.

[80]. Estrogen therapy and oral contraceptives continue to be used in young women with amenorrhea. Several authors have suggested that estrogen may have an independent effect on bone mass, with weight gain affecting bone mass separately [73,81].

No long-term study on estrogen replacement has been reported, although a number of cross-sectional studies suggest that estrogen therapy may be effective in the pure hypogonadal state. Improvement has been seen in premature ovarian failure [82], after oophorectomy [83], in women treated with gonadotropin-releasing hormone (GnRH) analogs [84–86], and in Turner's syndrome [87], although data are admittedly conflicting [81,88]. One study reports that women undergoing medical castration with GnRH and replaced via oral contraceptive therapy show no effect on bone [88]. However, another study shows that although the standard dose of conjugated estrogen (0.625 Premarin) in GnRH-treated women is not sufficient to protect against bone loss, a doubling of that dose to 1.25 mg does afford protection [89].

Reversal of amenorrhea might be expected to improve bone density [1,90–92]. Such expectations are bolstered by observations that normal women who use oral contraceptives may have higher bone mass [84–86,88]. Some studies have shown little [93–95] or no [96] reversal whereas others have suggested that increases occur even prior to reversal of the hypogonadal state. Preliminary studies on small numbers of subjects ($N = 4$) suggest that oral contraceptives may be effective in athletic amenorrhea [97], although a report that included subjects on estrogens and oral contraceptives indicated no effect resulting from the contraceptives [73]. One report showed significantly greater improvements in amenorrheic females randomly assigned to oral contraceptives (0.5 to 1.0 mg of norethindrone/0.035 mg ethinyl estradiol) vs 10 mg medroxyprogesterone or placebo for 12 months [73a]. Others have suggested that the hypercortisolemia seen in anorexia nervosa [98,99] and athletically induced amenorrhea [100–102] is related to osteopenia. Alternatively, the estrogen doses used to replace adolescent hypoestrogenism in our study and that by Biller *et al.* [98] may be less than optimal to compensate for the rapid increase in bone density that occurs during puberty. One study that specifically examined estrogen-replaced adolescents and young adults noted lowered BMD in this group, despite estrogen. This study suggested that daily and/or higher levels of estrogen replacement may be needed for adolescents and that unidentified factors may be responsible for the poor outcome in estrogen-deficient patients [81]. Thus, pharmacologic amount of estrogen may be needed to achieve an effect in these individuals. Oral contraceptives are commonly used in this age group for estrogen replacement. Oral contraceptives have considerably more estrogen than Premarin in doses generally used for replacement. Estrogenicity, measured in terms of vaginal cornification, antigonadotropin effect, anti-implantation, and antiovulation effects, reflects a greater value for doses of estrogens in oral contraceptive medication on a per weight basis than Premarin [103]. Doses of estrogen required to achieve similar biologic effects are 3.75 mg conjugated estrogen, 0.08 mg mestranol, and 0.05 mg ethinyl estradiol [103]. The progestin in oral contraceptives may also have an effect on bone density. One study has shown that low bone density was related to a lack of progesterone secretion and inadequate luteal phases [104]. Thus, the daily dose of a progestin in an oral contraceptive may also have important effects on bone, which may be independent of estrogen-induced effects. This has been suggested in patients treated with GnRH and a progestin to preserve bone loss [105,106]. However, a study with Depo-Provera, when used alone, suggests that a bone loss up to 1.5% may occur. This may be due to the concomitant hypoestrogenism [107] induced by a progestational agent. Interestingly, Norplant, a 19-norprogestin, was associated with a BMD gain of 2.5%. Thus different progestins may have varying effects. This may relate, in part, to their androgenicity. The 19-nor compounds are derivatives of testosterone and thus might be expected to exert a greater anabolic effect on bone mass.

Lack of a skeletal response to exogenous estrogen in subjects with hypothalamic amenorrhea suggests that bone metabolism, both exercising and nonexercising, is unresponsive to the antiresorptive effect of estrogen. Indices of bone turnover have not been examined systematically in this group, but indicators of bone formation and resorption have generally been low in dieting groups with hypothalemic amenorrhea [96,108]. Recent work on exercise and hypothalemic amenorrhea, as well as physiologic studies on normal women [72,109], suggests that reproductive dysfunction occurs when the caloric intake is insufficient for the level of activity [72,109–111]. A high incidence of abnormal eating patterns appears among women with exercise and weight loss-induced or idiopathic amenorrhea [40,72,112,113]. Abnormal eating and high energy output may be associated with an altered metabolic state, inducing changes in the microenvironment of bone. The presence of disordered eating, amenorrhea, and osteoporosis is now an established association, known as "The female athletic triad" [71,113,114].

Nutritional Influences

The triad of disordered eating, amenorrhea, and osteopenia has been the source of much concern in the athlete [71,113,114]. The mechanism by which caloric restriction and abnormal eating may compromise bone mass is unclear. Multiple factors are affected by dietary restriction [110,111,115] and hypothalamic amenorrhea, including the suppression of thyroid [109,116–119] and growth hormones [119]. Triiodothyronine is a potent stimulator of bone turnover [80]. Growth hormone has stimulatory effects on bone formation *in vivo* and is necessary for the maintenance of normal bone mass [120,121]. Growth hormone is thought to stimulate IGF-1 by skeletal cells and, through this local factor, growth hormone may regulate bone formation. IGF-1 is reduced in starvation and in turn is associated with decreases in bone collagen formation. This may be responsible for the lower peak bone mass seen in malnourished patients with anorexia nervosa. These multiple processes of bone metabolism may be affected in the nutritionally restricted model [122].

SUMMARY

Peak bone mass is affected by multiple processes, both metabolic and genetic. Environmental influences also appear to affect bone mass and may suppress bone accretion greatly, particularly in adolescents. Further research is needed to understand the physicochemical as well as the molecular influences on bone remodeling so that interventions may lead to the establishment of optimum bone mass.

References

1. Ott, S. M. Editorial: Attainment of peak bone mass. *J. Clin. Endocrinol. Metab.* **71,** 1082A–1082C.
2. Ponder, S. W., McCormick, D. P., Fawcett, H. D., Palmer, J. L., McKerna, M. G., and Brouhard, B. H. Spinal bone mineral density in children aged 5.00 through 11.99 years. *Am. J. Dis. Child.* **144,** 1346–1348 (1990).
3. Glastre, C., Braillon, P., David, L., Cochat, P., Meunier, P. J., and Delmas, P. D. Measurement of bone mineral content of the lumbar spine by dual energy x-ray absorptiometry in normal children: Correlations with growth parameters. *J. Clin. Endocrinol. Metab.* **70,** 1330–1333.
4. Gilsanz, V., Gibbens, D. T., Carlson, M., Boechat, M. I., Cann, C. E., and Schulz, E. E. Peak trabecular vertebral density: A comparison of adolescent and adult females. *Calcif. Tissue Int.* **43,** 260–262 (1988).
5. Gilsanz, V., Gibbens, D. T., Roe, T. F., Carlson, M., Senac, M. O., Boechat, M. I., Huang, H. K., Schulz, E. E., Libanati, C. R., and Cann, C. C. Vertebral bone density in children: Effect of puberty. *Radiology* **166,** 847–50 (1988).
6. McCormick, D. P., Ponder, S. W., Fawcett, H. D., and Palmer, J. L. Spinal bone mineral density in 335 normal and obese children and adolescents: Evidence for ethnic and sex differences. *J. Bone Miner. Res.* **6,** 507–513 (1991).
7. Bonjour, J. P., Theintz, G., Buchs, B., Slosman, D., and Rizzoli, R. Critical years and stages of puberty for spinal and femoral bone mass accumulation during adolescence. *J. Clin. Endocrinol Metab.* **73,** 555–563.
8. Gilsanz, V., Roe, T. F., Mora, S., Costin, G., and Goodman, W. G. Changes in vertebral bone density in black girls and white girls during childhood and puberty. *N. Engl. J. Med.* **325,** 1597–1600 (1991).
9. Lloyd, T., Rollings, N., Andon, M. B., Demers, L. M., Eggli, D. F., Keiselhorst, K., Kulin, H., Landis, J. R., Martel, J. K., Orr, G. *et al.* Determinants of bone density in young women. I. Relationships among pubertal development, total body bone mass, and total body bone density in premenarchal females. *J. Clin. Endocrinol. Metab.* **75,** 383–387 (1992).
10. Southard, R. N., Morris, J. D., Mahan, J. D., *et al.* Bone mass in healthy children: Measurement with quantitative DXA. *Radiology* **179,** 735–738 (1991).
11. Krolner, B., and Pors Nielsen, S. Bone mineral content of the lumbar spine in normal and osteoporotic women: Cross-sectional and longitudinal studies. *Clin. Sci.* **62**(3), 329–336 (1982).
12. Rosenthal, D. I., Mayo-Smith, W., Hayes, C. W., Khurana, J. S., Biller, B. M. K., Neer, R. M., and Klibanski, A. Age and bone mass in premenopausal women. *J. Bone Miner. Res.* **4**(4), 533–538 (1989).
13. Sowers, M. F., Kshirsagar, A., Crutchfield, M., and Updike, S. Body composition, age, and femoral bone mass of young adult women. *Ann. Epidemiol.* **1,** 245–254 (1991).
14. Mazess, R. B., and Barden, H. S. Bone density in premenopausal women: Effects of age, dietary intake, physical activity, smoking, and birth-control pills. *Am. J. Clin. Nutr.* **53,** 132–142 (1991).
15. Buchanan, J. R., Myers, C., Lloyd, T., and Greer, R. B. Early vertebral trabecular bone loss in normal premenopausal women. *J. Bone Miner. Res.* **3,** 583–587 (1988).
16. Theintz, G., Buchs, B., Rizzoli, R., Slosman, D., Clavien, H., Sizonenko, P. C., and Bonjour, J. P. Longitudinal monitoring of bone mass accumulation in healthy adolescents: Evidence for a marked reduction after 16 years of age at the levels of lumbar spine and femoral neck in female subjects. *J. Clin. Endocrinol. Metab.* **75,** 1060–1065 (1992).
17. Jonnavithula, S., Warren, M. P., Fox, R. P., and Lazaro, M. I. Bone density is compromised in amenorrheic women despite return of menses: A 2-year study. *Obstet. Gynecol.* **81,** 669–674 (1993).
18. Arnaud, C. D. Osteoporosis. Using "bone markers" for diagnosis and monitoring. *Geriatics* **51,** 24–30 (1996).
19. Mazess, R. B., and Cameron, J. R. Growth of bone in school children: comparison of radiographic morphometry and photon absorptiometry. *Growth* 3677–3692 (1972).
20. Picard, D., Ste-Marie, L. G., Coutu, D., Carrier, L., Chartrand, R., Lepage, R., Fugere, P., and D'Amour, P. Premenopausal bone mineral content relates to height, weight and calcium intake during early adulthood. *Bone Miner.* **4**(3), 299–309 (1988).
21. Boot, A. M., DeRidder, M. A. J., Pols, H. A. P., Krenning, E. P., and DeMuinck Keizer-Schrama, S. M. P. F. Bone mineral density in children and adolescents: Relation to puberty, calcium intake, and physical activity. *J. Clin. Endocrinol. Metab.* **82,** 57–62 (1997).
22. Lowrey, G. H., ed., *in* "Growth and development of Children," 7th Ed., pp. 279–295. Year Book, Chicago, 1978.
23. Riggs, B. L., Wahner, H. W., Dunn, W. L., Mazess, R. B., Offord, K. P., and Melton, L. J. Differential changes in bone density of the appendicular and axial skeleton with aging. *J. Clin. Invest.* **67,** 328–335 (1981).

24. Dequeker, J., Goris, P., and Uyherhoeven, R. Osteoporosis and osteoarthritis: Anthropometric distinctions. *JAMA* **249,** 1448–1451 (1983).
25. Aloia, J. F., Vaswani, A. N., Yeh, J. K., and Cohn, S. H. Premenopausal bone mass is related to physical activity. *Arch. Intern. Med.* **148,** 121–123 (1988).
26. Slemenda, C. W., Miller, J. Z., Hui, S. L., Reister, T. K., and Johnston, C. C. Role of physical activity in the development of skeletal mass in children. *J. Bone Miner. Res.* **6,** 1227–1233 (1991).
27. Rubin, K., Schirduan, V., Gendreau, P., Sarfarazi, M., Mendola, R., and Dalsky, G. Predictors of axial and peripheral bone mineral density in healthy children and adolescents, with special attention to the role of puberty. *J. Pediatr.* **123,** 863–870 (1993).
28. Valimaki, M. J., Karkkainen, M., Lamberg-Allardt, C., *et al.* Exercise, smoking and calcium intake during adolescence and early adulthood as determinants of peak bone mass. *Br. Med. J.* **309,** 230–235 (1994).
29. Kanders, B., Dempster, D. W., and Lindsay, R. Interaction of calcium nutrition and physical activity on bone mass in young women. *J. Bone Miner. Res.* **3**(2), 145–149 (1988).
30. Matkovic, V., Fontana, D., Tominac, C., Goel, P., and Chesnut, C. H., III. Factors that influence peak bone mass formation. A study of calcium balance and the inheritance of bone mass in adolescent females. *Am. J. Clin. Nutr.* **52,** 878–888 (1990).
31. Dhuper, S., Warren, M. P., Brooks-Gunn, J., and Fox, R. P. Effects of hormonal status on bone density in adolescent girls. *J. Clin. Endocrinol. Metab.* **71,** 1083–1088 (1990).
32. Kleerkoper, M., Tolia, K., and Parfitt, A. M. Nutritional, endocrine and demographic aspects of osteoporosis. *Orthop. Clin. North Am.* **12,** 547–558 (1981).
33. Bennett, D. L., Ward, M. S., and Daniel, W. A. The relationship of serum alkaline phosphatase concentrations to sex maturity ratings in adolescents. *J. Pediatr.* **88,** 633–636 (1976).
34. Cole, D. E. C., Carpenter, T. O., and Gundberg, C. M. Serum osteocalcin concentrations in children with metabolic bone disease. *J. Pediatr.* **106,** 770–776 (1985).
35. Jasin, H. E., Fink, C. W., Wise, W., and Ziff, M. Relationship between urinary hydroxyproline and growth. *J. Clin. Invest.* **41,** 1928–1935 (1962).
36. Blumsohn, A., Hannon, R. A., Wrate, R., Barton, J., Al-Dehaimi, A. W., Colwell, A., and Eastell, R. Biochemical markers of bone turnover in girls during puberty. *Clin. Endocrinol. (Oxford)* **40,** 663–670 (1994).
37. Moll, G. W., Jr., Rosenfield, R. L., and Fang, V. S. Administration of low dose estrogen rapidly and directly stimulates growth hormone production. *Am. J. Dis. Child.* **140,** 124–127 (1986).
38. Stanhope, R., Preece, M. A., Grant, D. B., and Brook, C. G. D. New concepts of the growth spurt of puberty. *Acta Paediatr. Scand.* **347**(Suppl.), 30–37 (1988).
39. Johansen, J. S., Giwercman, A., Hartwell, D., Nielsen, C. T., Price, P. A., Christiansen, C., and Skakkebaek, N. E. Serum bone glaprotein as a marker of bone growth in children and adolescents: correlation with age, height, serum insulin-like growth factor I and serum testosterone. *J. Clin. Endocrinol. Metab.* **67,** 273–278 (1988).
40. Kroger, H., Kotameini, A., Vainio, P., and Alhava, E. Bone densitometry of the spine and femur in children by dual energy x-ray absorptiometry. *Bone Miner.* **17,** 75–85 (1992).
41. Warren, M. P., Brooks-Gunn, J., Fox, R. P., Lancelot, C., Newman, D., and Hamilton, W. G. Lack of bone accretion and amenorrhea: Evidence for a relative osteopenia in weight bearing bones. *J. Clin. Endocrinol. Metab.* **72,** 847–853 (1991).
42. Forbes, G. B. Some remarks on bone mineralization. *J. Pediatr.* **113,** 167–171 (1988).
42a. Weaver, C. M., Peacock, M., Martin, B. R., Plawecki, K. L., and McCabe, G. P. Calcium retention estimated from indicators of skeletal status in adolescent girls and young women. *Am. J. Clin. Nutr.* **64,** 67–70 (1996).
43. Magnusson, P., Hager, A., and Larsson, L. Serum osteocalcin and bone and liver alkaline phosphatase isoforms in healthy children and adolescents. *Pediatr. Res.* **38,** 955–961 (1995).
44. Finkelstein, J. S., Neer, R. M., Biller, B. M. K., Crawford, J. D., and Klibanski, A. Osteopenia in men with a history of delayed puberty. *N. Engl. J. Med.* **326,** 600–604 (1992).
45. Finkelstein, J. S., Klibanski, A., Neer, R. M., Doppelt, S. H., Rosenthal, D. I., Segre, G. V., and Crowley, W. F., Jr. Increases in bone density during treatment of men with idiopathic hypogonadotropic hypogonadism. *J. Clin. Endocrinol. Metab.* **69,** 776–783 (1989).
46. Kannus, P., Haapasalo, H., Sankelo, M., Sievanen, H., Pasanen, M., Heinonen, A., Oja, P., and Vuori, I. Effect of starting age of physical activity on bone mass in the dominant arm of tennis and squash players. *Ann. Intern. Med.* **123,** 27–31 (1995).
47. Haapasalo, H., Kannus, P., Sievanen, H., Pasanen, M., Uusi-Rasi, K., Heinonen, A., Oja, and P., Vuori. Effect of long-term unilateral activity on bone mineral density of female junior tennis players. *J. Bone. Miner. Res.* **13**(2), 310–319 (1998).
48. Borer, K. T., "Exercise-Induced Facilitation of Pulsatile Growth Hormone (GH) Secretion and Somatic Growth." Serono Symposium from Raven Press, New York, 1989.
49. Eliakim, A., Brasel, J. A., Mohan, S., Barstow, T. J., Berman, N., and Cooper, D. M. Physical fitness, endurance training, and the growth hormone insulin-like growth factor I system in adolescent females. *J. Clin. Endocrinol. Metab.* **81**(11), 3986–3992 (1996).
50. Bass, S., Pearce, G., Bradney, M., Hendrick, E., Delmas, P., Harding, A., and Seeman, E. Exercise before puberty may confer residual benefits in bone density in adulthood: studies in active prepubertal and retired female gymnasts. *J. Bone. Miner. Res.* **13**(2), 500–507 (1998).
51. Dyson, K., Blimkie, C. J. R., Davison, S., Webber, C. E., and Adachi, J. D. Gymnastic training and bone density in preadolescent females. *Med. Sci. Sports. Exerc.* **29**(4), 443–450 (1997).
52. Gunnes, M., and Lehman, E. H. Physical activity and dietary constituents as predictors of forearm cortical and trabecular bone gain in healthy children and adolescents: a prospective study. *Acta Paediatr.* **85,** 19–25 (1996).
53. Slemenda, C. W., Reister, T. K., Hui, S. L., Miller, J. Z., Christian, J. C., and Johnston, C. C. Influences of skeletal mineralization in children and adolescents: Evidence for varying effects of sexual maturation and physical activity. *J. Pediatr.* **125**(2), 201–207 (1994).
54. Morris, F. L., Naughton, G. A., Gibbs, J. L., Carlson, J. S., and Wark, J. D. Prospective ten-month exercise intervention in premenarchel girls: positive effects on bone and lean mass. *J. Bone Miner. Res.* **12**(9), 1453–1462 (1997).
55. Robinson, T. L., Snow-Harter, C., Taaffee, D. R., Gills, D., Shaw, J., and Marcus, R. Gymnasts exhibit higher bone mass than runners despite similar prevalence of amenorrhea and oligomenorrhea. *J. Bone Miner. Res.* **10**(1), 26–35 (1995).
56. Taaffee, D. R., Robinson, T. L., Snow, C. M., and Marcus, R. High-Impact exercise promotes bone gain in well-trained female athletes. *J. Bone. Miner. Res.* **12**(2), 255–260 (1997).
57. Blimkie, C. J. R., Rice, S., Webber, C. E., Martin, J., Levy, D., and Gordon, C. L. Effects of resistance training on bone mineral content and density in adolescent females. *Can. J. Physiol. Pharmacol.* **74,** 1025–1033 (1996).

58. Bachrach, L. K., Katzman, D. K., Litt, I. F., *et al.* Recovery from osteopenia in adolescent girls with anorexia nervosa. *J. Clin. Endocrinol. Metab.* **72,** 602–606 (1991).
59. Biller, B. M. K., Saxe, V., Herzog, D. B., Rosenthal, D. I., *et al.* Mechanisms of osteoporosis in adult and adolescent women with anorexia nervosa. *J. Clin. Endocrinol. Metab.* **68,** 548–554 (1989).
60. Constantini, N. W., and Warren, M. P. Menstrual dysfunction in swimmers: A distinct entity. *J. Clin. Endocrinol. Metab.* **80,** 2740–2744 (1995).
61. Drinkwater, B. L., Nilson, K., Chesnut, C. H., III, Bremner, W. J., Shainholtz, S., and Southworth, M. B. Bone mineral content of amenorrheic and eumenorrheic athletes. *N. Engl. J. Med.* **311**(5), 277–281 (1984).
62. Lindberg, J. S., Fears, W. B., Hunt, M. M., Powell, M. R., Boll, D., and Wade, C. E. Exercise-induced amenorrhea and bone density. *Ann. Intern. Med.* **101,** 647–648 (1984).
63. Marcus, R., Cann, C. E., Madvig, P., Minkoff, J., Goddard, M., Bayer, M., Martin, M. C., Gaudiani, L., Haskell, W., and Genant, H. K. Menstrual function and bone mass in elite women distance runners. *Ann. Intern. Med.* **102,** 158–163 (1985).
64. Lloyd, T., Buchanan, J. R., Bitzer, S., Waldman, C. J., Myers, C., and Ford, B. G. The relationship of diet, athletic activity, menstrual status and bone density among collegiate women. *Am. J. Clin. Nutr.* **46,** 681–684 (1987).
65. Cann, C. E., Martin, M. C., Genant, H. K., and Jaffe, R. B. Decreased spinal mineral content in amenorrheic women. *JAMA* **251,** 626–629 (1984).
66. Schlechte, J. A., Sherman, B., and Martin, R. Bone density in amenorrheic women with and without hyperprolactinoma. *J. Clin. Endocrinol. Metab.* **56,** 1120–1123 (1983).
67. Rigotti, N. A., Nussbaum, S. R., Herzog, D. B., and Neer, R. M. Osteoporosis in women with anorexia nervosa. *N. Engl. J. Med.* **311,** 1601–1606 (1984).
68. Myerson, M., Gutin, B., Warren, M. P., Wang, J., Lichtman, S., and Pierson, R. N. Total body bone density in amenorrheic runners. *Obstet. Gynecol.* **79**(6), 973–978 (1992).
69. Drinkwater, B. L., Bruemner, B., and Chesnut, C. H., III. Menstrual history as a determinant of current bone density in young athletes. *JAMA* **263,** 545–548 (1990).
70. Warren, M. P., and Holderness, C. C. Estrogen replacement does not affect bone density with one year of replacement. *Endocr. Soc. Annu. Meet.* (1992). [Abstract]
71. Frusztajer, N. T., Dhuper, S., Warren, M. P., Brooks-Gunn, J., and Fox, R. P. Nutrition and the incidence of stress fractures in ballet dancers. *Am. J. Clin. Nutr.* **51,** 779–783 (1990).
72. Warren, M. P., Holderness, C. C., Lesobre, V., Tzen, R., Vossoughian, F., and Brooks-Gunn, J. Hypothalamic amenorrhea and hidden nutritional insults. *J. Soc. Gynecol. Invest.* **1,** 84–88 (1994).
73. Biller, B. M. K., Schoenfeld, D., and Klibanski, A. Premenopausal osteopenia: Effects of estrogen administration. *Endocr. Soc. Annu. Meet.* **75,** 454 (1993). [Abstract]
74. Finkelstein, J. S., Neer, R. M., Biller, B. M. K., Crawford, J. D., and Klibanski, A. Osteopenia in men with a history of delayed puberty. *N. Engl. J. Med.* **326,** 600–604 (1992).
75. Warren, M. P., Brooks-Gunn, J., Hamilton, L. H., Warren, L. F., and Hamilton, W. G. Scoliosis and fractures in young ballet dancers: Relation to delayed menarche and secondary amenorrhea. *N. Engl. J. Med.* **314,** 1348–1353 (1986).
76. Ayers, J., Gidwani, G. P., Schmidt, I. M., and Gross, M. Osteopenia in hypoestrogenic women with anorexia nervosa. *Fertil. Steril.* **41,** 224–228 (1984).
77. Warren, M. P., Shane, E., Lee, M. J., Lindsay, R., Dempster, D. W., Warren, L. F., and Hamilton, W. G. Femoral head collapse associated with anorexia nervosa in a twenty-year-old ballet dancer. *Clin. Orthop.* **251,** 171–176 (1990).
78. Cann, C. E., Martin, M. C., and Jaffe, R. B. Duration of amenorrhea affects rate of bone loss in women runners: Implications for therapy. *Med. Sci. Sports. Exerc.* **17,** 214 (1985).
79. Lindsay, R., Nieves, J., Golden, A., and Kelsey, J. Bone mass among premenopausal women. *Int. J. Fertil. Menopausal Studies* **38,** 83–87 (1993).
80. Riggs, B. L., and Eastell, R. Exercise, hypogonadism and osteopenia. *JAMA* **256,** 392–393 (1986).
81. Emans, S. J., Grace, E., Hoffer, F. A., Gundberg, C., Ravnikar, V., and Woods, E. R. Estrogen deficiency in adolescents and young adults: Impact on bone mineral content and effects of estrogen replacement therapy. *Obstet. Gynecol.* **76,** 585–592 (1990).
82. Metka, M., Holzer, G., Heytmanek, G., and Huber, J. Hypergonadotropic hypogonadic amenorrhea (World Health Organization III) and osteoporosis. *Fertil. Steril.* **57,** 37–41 (1992).
83. Genant, H. K., Cann, C. E., Ettinger, B., and Gordan, G. S. Quantitative computed tomography of vertebral spongiosa: A sensitive method for detecting early bone loss after oophorectomy. *Ann. Intern. Med.* **97,** 699–705 (1982).
84. de Aloysio, D., Mauloni, M., Roncuzzi, A., Altieri, P., Bottiglioni, F., Trossarelli, G. F., Fanizza, G., and Covelli, A. Effects of an oral contraceptive combination containing 0.150 mg desogestrel plus 0.020 mg ethinyl estradiol on healthy premenopausal women. *Arch. Gynecol. Obstet.* **253,** 15–19 (1993).
85. Laitinen, K., Valimaki, M., and Keto, P. Bone mineral density measured by dual-energy x-ray absorptiometry in healthy Finnish women. *Calcif. Tissue Int.* **48,** 224–231 (1991).
86. Recker, R. R., Davies, K. M., Hinders, S. M., Heaney, R. P., Stegman, M. R., and Kimmel, D. B. Bone gain in young adult women. *JAMA* **268,** 2403–2408.
87. Neely, E. K., Marcus, R., Rosenfeld, R. G., and Bachrach, L. K. Turner syndrome adolescents receiving growth hormone are not osteopenic. *J. Clin. Endocrinol. Metab.* **76,** 861–866 (1993).
88. Gambacciani, M., Spinetti, A., Taponeco, F., Cappagli, B., Piaggesi, L., and Fioretti, P. Longitudinal evaluation of perimenopausal vertebral bone loss: effects of a low-dose oral contraceptive preparation on bone mineral density and metabolism. *Obstet. Gynecol.* **83,** 392 (1994).
89. Sugimoto, A. K., Hodsman, A. B., and Nisker, J. A. Long term gonadotropin releasing hormone agonist with standard postmenopausal estrogen replacement failed to prevent vertebral bone loss in premenopausal women. *Fertil. Steril.* **60,** 672–674 (1993).
90. Johnston, C. C., Jr., and Longcope, C. Premenopausal bone loss: A risk factor for osteoporosis. *JAMA* **323**(18), 1271–1272 (1990).
91. Salisbury, J. J., and Mitchell, J. E. Bone mineral density and anorexia nervosa in women. *Am. J. Psychiatr.* **148,** 768–774 (1991).
92. Davies, M. C., Hall, M. L., and Jacobs, H. S. Bone mineral loss in young women with amenorrhea. *Br. Med. J.* **301,** 790–793 (1990).
93. Drinkwater, B. L., Nilson, K., Ott, S., and Chesnut, C. H., III. Bone mineral density after resumption of menses in amenorrheic athletes. *JAMA* **256,** 380–382 (1986).
94. van Binsbergen, C. J. M., Coelingh-Bennink H. J. T., Odink, J., Haspels, A. A., and Koppeschaar, H. P. F. A comparative and longitudinal study on endocrine changes related to ovarian function in patients with anorexia nervosa. *J. Clin. Endocrinol. Metab.* **71,** 705–711 (1990).

95. Bachrach, L. K., Katzman, D. K., Litt, I. F., Guido, D., and Marcus, R. Recovery from osteopenia in adolescent girls with anorexia nervosa. *J. Clin. Endocrinol. Metab.* **72,** 602–606 (1991).
96. Rigotti, N. A., Neer, R. M., Skates, S. J., Herzog, D. B., and Nussbaum, S. R. The clinical course of osteoporosis in anorexia nervosa: A longitudinal study of cortical bone mass. *JAMA* **265,** 1133–1138 (1991).
97. DeCree, C., Lewin, R., and Ostyn, M. Suitability of cyproterone acetate in the treatment of osteoporosis associated with athletic amenorrhea. *Int. J. Sports Med.* **9,** 187–192 (1988).
97a. Hergenroeder, A. C., O'Brian Smith, E., Shypailo, R., *et al.* Bone mineral changes in young women with hypothalamic amenorrhea treated with oral contraceptives, medroxyprogesterone, or placebo over 12 months. *Am. J. Obstet. Gynecol.* **176,** 1017–1025 (1997).
98. Biller, B. M. K., Saxe, V., Herzog, D. B., Rosenthal, D. I., Holzman, S., and Klibanski, A. Mechanisms of osteoporosis in adult and adolescent women with anorexia nervosa. *J. Clin. Endocrinol. Metab.* **68,** 548–554 (1989).
99. Newman, M. M., and Halmi, K. A. Relationship of bone density to estradiol and cortisol in anorexia nervosa and bulimia. *Psychiatr. Res.* **29,** 105–112 (1989).
100. Loucks, A. B., Mortola, J. F., Girton, L., and Yen, S. S. C. Alterations in the hypothalamic–pituitary–ovarian and the hypothalamic–pituitary–adrenal axes in athletic women. *J. Clin. Endocrinol. Metab.* **68,** 402–411 (1989).
101. Villaneuva, A. L., Schlosser, C., Hopper, B., Liu, J. H., Hoffman, D. I., and Rebar, R. W. Increased cortisol production in women runners. *J. Clin. Endocrinol. Metab.* **63,** 133–136 (1986).
102. Hohtari, H., Salminen-Lappalainen, K., and Laatikainen, T. Response of plasma endorphins, corticotropin, cortisol, and luteinizing hormone in the corticotropin-releasing hormone stimulation test in eumenorrheic and amenorrheic athletes. *Fertil. Steril.* **55,** 276–280 (1991).
103. Hammond, C. B., and Maxson, W. S. Current status of estrogen therapy for menopause. *Fertil. Steril.* **37,** 5–25 (1982).
104. Prior, J. C., Vigna, Y. M., Schechter, M. T., and Burgess, A. E. Spinal bone loss and ovulatory disturbances. *N. Engl. J. Med.* **323,** 1221–1227 (1990).
105. Cedar, M. I., Lu, J. K. H., Meldrum, D. R., and Judd, H. L. Treatment of endometriosis with a long-acting gonadotropin-releasing hormone agonist plus medroxyprogesterone acetate. *Obstet. Gynecol.* **75,** 641–645 (1990).
106. Surrey, E. S., Gambone, J. C., Lu, J. K. H, and Judd, H. L. The effects of combining norethindrone with a gonadotropin-releasing hormone agonist in the treatment of symptomatic endometriosis. *Fertil. Steril.* **53,** 620–626 (1990).
107. Cromer, B. A., Blair, J. M., Mahan, J. D., Zibners, L., and Naumovski, Z. A prospective comparison of bone density in adolescent girls receiving depot medroxyprogesterone acetate (Depo-Provera), levonorgestrel (Norplant), or oral contraceptives. *J. Pediatr.* **129,** 671–676 (1996).
108. Davies, K. M., Pearson, P. H., Huseman, C. A., Greger, N. G., Kimmel, D. K., and Recker, R. R. Reduced bone mineral in patients with eating disorders. *Bone* **11,** 143–147 (1990).
109. Myerson, M., Gutin, B., Warren, M. P., May, M., Contento, I., Lee, M., Pi-Sunyer, F. X., Pierson, R. N., and Brooks-Gunn, J. Resting metabolic rate and energy balance in amenorrheic and eumenorrheic runners. *Med. Sci. Sports Exerc.* **23**(1), 15–22 (1991).
110. Loucks, A. B., and Heath, E. M. Induction of low-T3 syndrome in exercising women occurs at a threshold of energy availability. *Am. J. Physiol.* **266,** R817–R823 (1994).
111. Loucks, A. B., Brown, R., King, K., Thuma, J. R., and Verdun, M. A combined regimen of moderate dietary restriction and exercise training alters luteinizing hormone pulsatility in regularly menstruating young women. *Endocr. Soc. Annu. Meet.* **558** (1995).
112. Brooks-Gunn, J., Warren, M. P., and Hamilton, L. H. The relation of eating problems and amenorrhea in ballet dancers. *Med. Sci. Sports Exerc.* **19**(1), 41–44 (1987).
113. Myerson, M., Gutin, B., Warren, M. P., *et al.* Energy balance of amenorrhea and eumenorrheic runners. *Med. Sci. Sports Exerc.* **19**(Suppl), S37 (1987). [Abstract]
114. Snead, D. B., Stubbs, C. C., Weltman, J. Y., Evans, W. S., Veldhuis, J. D., Rogol, A. D., Teates, C. D., and Weltman, A. Dietary patterns, eating behaviors, and bone mineral density in women runners. *Am. J. Clin. Nutr.* **56,** 705–711 (1992).
115. Bosello, O., Fervari, F., Tonon, M., Cigolini, M., Micciolo, R., and Renoffio, W. Serum thyroid hormone concentration during semi-starvation and physical exercise. *Horm. Metab. Res.* **13,** 651–652 (1981).
116. Loucks, A. B., Laughlin, G. A., Mortola, J. F., Girton, L., Nelson, J. C., and Yen, S. S. C. Hypothalamic pituitary thyroidal function in eumenorrheic and amenorrheic athletes. *J. Clin. Endocrinol. Metab.* **75,** 514–518 (1992).
117. Berga, S. L., Mortola, J. F., Girton, L., Suh, B. Y., Laughlin, G. A., Pham, P., and Yen, S. S. C. Neuroendocrine aberrations in women with functional hypothalamic amenorrhea. *J. Clin. Endocrinol. Metab.* **68,** 301–308 (1989).
118. Warren, M. P., Vossoughian, F., Geer, E. B., Adberg, C. L., and Ramos, R. H. Thyroidal changes in functional hypothalamic amenorrhea. *J. Clin. Endocrinol. Metab.,* in press.
119. Yen, S. S. C. Female hypogonadotropic hypogonadism. *Neuroendocrinology* 2229–2258 (1993).
120. Saggese, G., Baroncelli, G. I., Bertelloni, S., Cinquanta, L., and Di Nero, G. Effects of long-term treatment with growth hormone on bone and mineral metabolism in children with growth hormone deficiency. *J. Pediatr.* **122,** 37–45 (1993).
121. Kaufman, J. M., Taelman, P., Vermeulen, A., and Vandeweghe, M. Bone mineral status in growth hormone-deficient males with isolated and multiple pituitary deficiencies of childhood onset. *J. Clin. Endocrinol. Metab.* **74,** 118–123 (1992).
122. Canalis, E., and Favus, M. J., eds. Primer on the Metabolic Bone Diseases and Disorders of Mineral Metabolism. *In* "Regulation of Bone Remodeling" 2nd Ed., pp. 33-37. Raven Press, New York, 1993.
123. Constantini, N. W. *Sports Med.* **17,** 213–223 (1994).

CHAPTER 12

Racial Determinants of Peak Bone Mass

L. LYNDON KEY AND NORMAN H. BELL
Department of Pediatrics, Medicine and Pharmacology, Medical University of South Carolina and Department of Veterans Affairs Medical Center, Charleston, SC 29401

INTRODUCTION

Race is a major determinant of peak bone mass, bone density, and fracture. Available evidence indicates that Caucasian women and men have a lower bone mineral density and a higher risk of hip fracture than African American women and men. Whereas Asian women have a bone mineral density similar to that of Caucasian women, their risk of fracture is less. African American, Hispanic, and Asian women have at least a 40% lower incidence of hip fracture and 50% lower incidence of fractures at other sites than Caucasian women. The difference in fracture rates appears to be related to a variety of hormonal, biochemical, and life-style differences between Caucasian and other racial groups. The fact that differences in bone mineral density, especially between African Americans and Caucasians, can be traced to early childhood provides evidence that bone mass may be determined by genetic as well as by environmental factors. Bone mass appears to be a major, although not the sole, determinant of fracture risk. A comprehensive review of the relationship between race and age-related bone loss is covered in Chapter 22.

AFRICAN AMERICANS

Peak Bone Mass

Based on radiographic measurements of metacarpal cortical area, African Americans were found to have a greater skeletal mass than Caucasians throughout life [1,2], a finding that can be traced to childhood [3,4]. Bone mineral density of the midradius, lumbar spine, trochanter, and femoral neck is higher in African American than in Caucasian boys and girls [4,5]. Bone mineral density of the lumbar spine, trochanter and femoral neck are higher in African American than in Caucasian premenopausal and postmenopausal women [6–13] and young adult men [14–16]. Thus, peak bone mass is higher in African American than in Caucasian women and men. The magnitude of the differences in the prevalence of osteoporosis between African Americans and Caucasians and bone density between these races has led to a search for differences that explain these observations. However, the mechanisms for increased bone mineral density in African Americans are not yet established. As summarized in Table I, a number of factors, some of which are controversial, have been proposed that would contribute to or be responsible for the racial difference in bone density. These include (a) differences in metabolism of vitamin D and calcium, (b) skeletal resistance to parathyroid hormone, (c) lower rate of skeletal remodeling, (d) higher serum leptin and earlier puberty in girls and higher serum testosterone, 17β-estradiol, and rate of secretion of growth hormone in men, and (e) differences in distribution of alleles of the vitamin D receptor. Each of these proposed factors will be discussed separately.

Vitamin D and Calcium Metabolism

A number of studies have shown that urinary calcium is lower in African Americans than in Caucasians [11,12,17,18]. This may explain, in part, a reduced incidence of calcium-containing renal stones [19]. Reduction in urinary calcium is attributed to a certain extent to diminished dermal synthesis of vitamin D_3, a conse-

TABLE I Factors That May Account for Greater Bone Density in African Americans

Differences in vitamin D and calcium metabolism
Low urinary calcium
Increased intestinal absorption of calcium
Skeletal resistance to parathyroid hormone
Diminished rate of skeletal remodeling
Earlier puberty and increased secretion of hormones
Leptin
Sex hormones
Growth hormone
Difference in distribution of alleles of the vitamin D receptor

quence of increased skin pigment. Reduced amounts of substrate vitamin D_3 could account for diminished synthesis of 25-hydroxyvitamin D [17,20]. Melanin absorbs ultraviolet light and prevents the formation of previtamin D_3 from 7-dehydrocholesterol. Near the equator, darkly pigmented skin protects against increased dermal production of vitamin D_3, subsequent hepatic production of 25-hydroxyvitamin D, and possible vitamin D intoxication. Because of exposure to less intense sunlight, decreases in dermal production of vitamin D_3 occur when blacks move away from the equator. This results in reductions in serum 25-hydroxyvitamin D and compensatory increases in the secretion of parathyroid hormone [21]. In African Americans, alteration of the vitamin D–endocrine system is characterized by low serum vitamin D_3, 25-hydroxyvitamin D, and urinary calcium. An increased circulating parathyroid hormone is associated with an increased renal production of 1,25-dihydroxyvitamin D and cyclic adenosine 3′,5′-monophosphate, an index of parathyroid hormone secretion [9,11,12,17]. Further evidence for a compensatory increase in parathyroid hormone is the finding of an altered dynamic secretory pattern of parathyroid hormone in response to changes in serum calcium produced by the infusion of calcium and EDTA [22], as well as the greater weight of parathyroid glands at postmortem examination in African Americans [23]. Changes resulting from alteration of the vitamin D–endocrine system are reversed by 25-hydroxyvitamin D_3 [24]. Thus, short-term administration of 25-hydroxyvitamin D_3 increases serum 25-hydroxyvitamin D and urinary calcium and decreases serum 1,25-dihydroxyvitamin D and urinary cyclic adenosine 3′,5′-monophosphate [24].

A number of studies indicate that serum 25-hydroxyvitamin D is reduced by about 50% in African Americans [24]. As anticipated because of vitamin D deficiency, turnover studies of [^{3}H]-25-hydroxyvitamin D_3 indicate that low serum 25-hydroxyvitamin D in African Americans compared to Caucasians probably results from decreased production rate and not to an increased metabolic clearance rate [25]. This likelihood is strengthened by the fact that the precursor vitamin D circulates at concentrations that are almost 90% lower in African Americans compared to Caucasians [25]. In these studies it was found that activity of 25-hydroxyvitamin D-24-hydroxylase, the rate-limiting enzyme for further metabolism of 25-hydroxyvitamin D, in skin fibroblasts is 40% higher in African Americans than Caucasians. Even so, there was no racial difference in the rate of metabolic clearance of the metabolite. Interpretation of results was complicated by the wide range of values for metabolic clearance rate, eightfold in Caucasians and fourfold in African Americans.

In one study, the greater accumulation of bone mass during childhood and adolescence in African American compared to Caucasian girls was attributed to a higher intestinal absorption of calcium in African American females [26]. In another study, however, no racial difference in the intestinal absorption of calcium was found, and the greater bone mineral density in African American compared to Caucasian children was attributed to a lower urinary calcium, which would result in a more positive calcium balance and contribute to a greater bone mass [18]. No racial difference in the intestinal absorption of calcium was found in two studies in premenopausal African American and Caucasian women [27,28]. Low urinary calcium is a consistent finding in African Americans. Whether it contributes to or is responsible for skeletal conservation of calcium and greater bone mineral density in African Americans remains to be determined.

Because of maternal vitamin D depletion, African American infants, especially when they are breast fed, are at risk for developing nutritional rickets [29–33]. Since 25-hydroxyvitamin D is stored in milk and provides a major source for 25-hydroxyvitamin D in infants, low concentrations of maternal serum 25-hydroxyvitamin D result in low concentrations of 25-hydroxyvitamin D in mother's milk. Neonatal rickets can be prevented by supplemental vitamin D to mothers. Despite the propensity toward a reduced amount of vitamin D and rachitic changes in the skeleton, bone mass increases in African American children more rapidly than in Caucasian children from infancy to adulthood. This indicates that factors other than availability of vitamin D must be important.

Skeletal Resistance to Parathyroid Hormone

In the first study demonstrating alteration of the vitamin D–endocrine system in African Americans, it was found that compared to Caucasian women and men, serum parathyroid hormone and urinary cyclic 3′,5′-monophosphate, an index of secretion of parathyroid hormone, were increased and serum osteocalcin, a marker for bone formation, was decreased [17]. Based on these findings, it was proposed that the greater bone mass in African Americans could result from skeletal resistance to parathyroid hormone. This possibility is supported by a subsequent study which showed that increments in bone markers, including urinary cross-linked N-telopeptide of type I collagen, C-telopeptide of type I collagen and free deoxypyridinoline in response to human [1–34]parathyroid hormone, were reduced in African American compared to Caucasian premenopausal women [34]. It should be emphasized that a reduced rate of skeletal remodeling (see later) may be associated with skeletal resistance to parathyroid hormone and be a key factor in the racial difference in bone density.

A question that arises from this investigation is whether the skeletal resistance to parathyroid hormone is a primary event or whether it results from depletion of 25-hydroxyvitamin D. Because administration of 25-hydroxyvitamin D_3 in African Americans increases serum 25-hydroxyvitamin D and reduces urinary cyclic adenosine 3′,5′-monophosphate, it is possible that correction of the changes in the vitamin D–endocrine system could correct the diminished skeletal response to [1-34]parathyroid hormone in African Americans. An argument against this hypothesis is that the vitamin D–endocrine system is similarly altered in obese Caucasian subjects in whom serum osteocalcin and skeletal remodeling are not reduced compared to nonobese Caucasian men and women [35]. In these individuals, serum vitamin D is strikingly low [36]. The cause for this is not known. Because vitamin D, a fat-soluble vitamin, is stored in fat [37,38], it may preferentially be diverted to fat or distributed in a larger amount of fat in obese individuals. As a consequence of low serum vitamin D, serum 25-hydroxyvitamin D and urinary calcium are significantly reduced, whereas serum immunoreactive parathyroid hormone, serum 1,25-dihydroxyvitamin D, and urinary cyclic adenosine 3′,5′-monophosphate are increased. In any event, low serum 25-hydroxyvitamin D and increased circulating parathyroid hormone return to normal after weight loss. In obese subjects, administration of 25-hydroxyvitamin D_3 increases serum 25-hydroxyvitamin D and urinary calcium and lowers serum 1,25-dihydroxyvitamin D and urinary cyclic adenosine 3′,5′-monophosphate, as occurs in nonobese African Americans [39].

Skeletal Remodeling

Histomorphometric analysis of biopsies of the iliac crest after double-tetracycline labeling indicated a marked reduction in the bone formation rate in African American compared to Caucasian subjects [40]. There was no difference in static measurements. Based on these findings and the lower serum osteocalcin in African Americans, it was proposed that the greater bone mass in African Americans results from diminished bone turnover [40]. A subsequent histomorphometric study confirmed that the bone formation rate is lower in African American than in Caucasian pre- and postmenopausal women [41]. It should be noted, however, that in another histomorphometric study in premenopausal women, no racial difference was found in the bone formation rate [42]. However, it was found that African American women had a lower rate of mineralized matrix apposition within each modeling unit and a longer total formation period than white women. It was concluded that these differences may allow a greater overall deposition of bone mineral and provide a greater bone mass and bone quality in African American women.

Studies demonstrating that serum osteocalcin and urinary hydroxyproline, an index of bone resorption, are lower in African American than in Caucasian women provide additional evidence that bone formation and resorption are lower in African Americans [11,12,17]. A more recent study in twins found that bone mineral density was significantly higher and that markers of bone turnover were significantly lower in African American than in Caucasian adolescent boys and girls [5]. In this study, it was concluded that the greater peak bone mass in African Americans likely results from a lower rate of skeletal remodeling.

In Caucasian women, increased bone resorption itself was found to be an independent risk factor for osteoporosis and fractures [43]. It remains to be determined whether a lower rate of skeletal remodeling is an independent negative risk factor to the lower incidence of osteoporosis and fractures in African Americans.

Hormones

There is evidence that sexual development and menses begin 1 to 2 years earlier in African American than in Caucasian girls [44]. A rise in serum leptin was found to precede the rise in sex hormones in normal children [45]. More recently, it was found that serum leptin and body fat are higher in African American than in Caucasian girls [46]. Thus, serum leptin correlates with sexual development and racial differences in sexual development in girls.

Endogenous 17β-estradiol is a major determinant of growth hormone secretion in both men and women, and serum 17β-estradiol was found to be higher in African American than in Caucasian boys during the latter stages of puberty [47]. It was found that serum 17β-estradiol and production of growth hormone were higher in African American than in Caucasian men [15]. Serum testosterone was not different in the two groups. Because serum 17β-estradiol inhibits bone resorption in postmenopausal women [48] and is a major determinant of bone mineral density in older men [49], the higher serum 17β-estradiol in African American men could contribute to the higher bone mass in them by reducing bone turnover. The greater secretion of growth hormone also could contribute to the greater bone mass in African American men. In premenopausal women, however, no racial difference was found in either serum 17β-estradiol or secretion of growth hormone even though bone mineral density of the total body, hip, and forearm was higher in African American than Caucasian women [13]. Further, there was no racial difference in serum testosterone, serum 17β-estradiol and growth hormone secretion in prepubertal boys, despite the fact that bone mineral density of the forearm, hip, trochanter, and femoral neck was higher in African American than in Caucasian males [50]. Thus, the racial difference in bone density is present before puberty so that it is unlikely that sex hormones or growth hormone contribute to the racial difference in bone mass at this age. It should be noted that another study found that serum testosterone was significantly higher in African American than in Caucasian young men [51]. The significance, if any, of the racial difference in serum testosterone in terms of bone mass remains to be determined.

Polymorphisms of the Vitamin D Receptor

Although controversial, a number of studies have shown that alleles of the vitamin D receptor determined by restriction fragment length polymorphism analysis predict bone mineral density. Studies in premenopausal African American and Caucasian women showed that alleles of the vitamin D receptor, determined with endonuclease *Bsm*I, were associated with significant differences in bone mineral density of the femoral neck and no racial difference in distribution of the alleles [52]. Subsequent studies in the same women showed a significant and major racial difference in the distribution of alleles of the vitamin D receptor determined with endonuclease *Fok*I, which identifies a start codon polymorphism at the translation initiation site of the receptor [53]. There was a significant correlation between alleles of the receptor and bone mineral density of the femoral neck in African American and Caucasian women together, in Caucasian women alone, but not in the African American women alone [54]. However, there was no significant interaction between race and bone mineral density. It was concluded that racial differences in the *distribution* of the *Fok*I alleles may account for some of the racial differences in bone mineral density of the femoral neck.

In young men, alleles of the vitamin D receptor, determined with endonuclease *Apa*I, were significantly associated with bone mineral density of the lumbar spine (N. H. Bell and J. Eisman, unpublished observations). In this study, bone mineral density of the total body, lumbar spine and femoral neck was higher in African American than in Caucasian men. However, there was no racial difference in distribution of the alleles, and alleles of the receptor did not account for the racial difference in bone mineral density.

Osteoporosis and Fractures

The incidence of osteoporosis and atraumatic fractures is lower in African American than in white subjects. In the United States, hip fracture rates for African American women are 40 to 60% lower than those for Caucasian women and the incidence of fractures also is lower in African American than in Caucasian men [54–62]. As noted already, the lower incidence of fractures in African Americans compared to Caucasians is attributed, at least in part, to higher bone mass (see earlier discussion). As also indicated, lower rate of bone resorption could be a contributing factor. Despite the higher bone mass, bone loss occurs in African Americans. Low values for vertebral bone mineral density, in African American women, even below mean values for age-matched Caucasian women, were reported [10]. Additionally, a small but significant number of healthy African American women were found to have bone density below the theoretical fracture threshold [10], suggesting that there may be a subgroup of African American women at a higher risk for osteoporotic fractures. Risk factors for fractures in women, both African American and Caucasian, include low body weight [60], previous stroke, use of aids in walking, and consumption of alcohol [61]. A shorter hip axis length may contribute to the lower incidence of fractures in African American women [62]. The incidence of obesity is twice as high in African American than in Caucasian women. Obesity is a negative risk factor for fractures because body weight is a major determinant of bone mass and, by cushioning falls, increased body fat helps to prevent fractures.

ASIAN INDIANS AND PAKISTANIS

Peak Bone Mass

Asian Indians are smaller in body size than Caucasians [63,64]. Available evidence indicates that when the body mass index and the area over which the X-ray beam is projected are taken into account, there is no difference in bone mass between Asian Indians and Caucasians [64].

Calcium and Vitamin D Metabolism

Asian Indians and Pakistanis who migrate to Europe develop vitamin D deficiency, rickets, and osteomalacia [65–75]. Vitamin D deficiency is attributed to reduced intake of vitamin D [67,71,72], increased skin pigmentation [20], consumption of a vegetarian diet [66,70,74], and diminished exposure to sunlight [76]. Vitamin D deficiency also occurs in Asian Indians in the United States [63]. Decreases in serum vitamin D, serum 25-hydroxyvitamin D, and urinary calcium and increases in serum-intact immunoreactive parathyroid hormone and 1,25-dihydroxyvitamin D occur, changes in vitamin D and calcium metabolism that are similar to those that occur in African Americans. Unlike African Americans, however, administration of 25-hydroxyvitamin D_3 increases serum 25-hydroxyvitamin D and urinary calcium but does not lower serum parathyroid hormone or serum 1,25-dihydroxyvitamin D [63]. Activity of 25-hydroxyvitamin D-24-hydroxylase, the rate-limiting enzyme for degradation of 25-hydroxyvitamin D, in cultured skin fibroblasts of Asian Indians is markedly increased compared to activity from skin fibroblasts of Caucasians [63]. Whether increased activity of the enzyme plays a role or the extent to which it may play a role in vitamin D deficiency in Asian Indians is not known.

Osteoporosis and Fractures

The predilection in Asian Indians for development of vitamin D deficiency, rickets, and osteomalacia during infancy and childhood, especially when a vegetarian diet is consumed, has not translated into a decreased bone mineral density and increased incidence of osteoporosis and fractures in adulthood. In England, no difference in the incidence of hip fractures was found in Asian Indians compared to the incidence in Caucasians [77].

OTHER RACES

Asians

During adolescence, Asian males have a greater spine bone mineral content at midpuberty and a lower total body bone mineral content than Caucasian males at maturity [78]. Asian refers to persons of Chinese, Japanese, and Vietnamese ancestry. Asian girls have lower femoral neck bone mineral content through midpuberty and lower whole body bone mineral content in prepuberty and early puberty [78]. Multivariate regression analysis indicates that racial differences in bone mass between Asian and Caucasian individuals are attributable to differences in weight and pubertal stage and, at the femoral neck, to differences in weight-bearing activity [78]. Bone mineral density of the total body, arm, lumbar spine, hip, pelvis, and leg are 4 to 6 percent lower in Asian than in Caucasian women [79]. However, the difference can be accounted for by differences in body size. In this study, Asian refers to women of Chinese, Japanese, or Korean ancestry.

Bone mineral density of the lumbar spine is lower in Japanese than in Caucasian women and declines more rapidly after menopause [80]. The fracture threshold is lower in Japanese than in Caucasian women. The incidence of hip fracture is lower and of spine fracture is higher in native Japanese women than in Japanese women who are immigrants to Hawaii and Caucasian women [81]. In the United States, the incidence of hip fracture is lower in Japanese and Chinese than in Caucasians [82]. Because the incidence of hip fracture is lower in Asians than in Caucasians, despite a lower bone mineral density related to body size, factors other than bone mass must account for the difference in incidence. In this regard, it was found that the incidence of falls is lower in Japanese than in Caucasian men and women in Hawaii [83].

Bone mineral density of the lumbar spine is lower in Chinese women in Hong Kong than in Caucasian women [84]. However, the incidence of vertebral fracture is not different in the two groups.

Mexican Americans

Because bone mineral density is not different in Mexican American compared to Caucasian postmenopausal women [85], peak bone mass must not be racially different. However, the incidence of hip fracture is only half as high in Mexican American compared to Caucasian women [56,86]. Hip axis length is significantly shorter in Mexican American compared to Caucasian women and could account for the lower incidence of hip fractures [86]. Differences in body fat and distribution of body fat also may be contributing factors to the racial difference in fracture incidence. In postmenopausal Mexican American women, no correlation was found between vitamin D genotype and bone mineral density [87]. However, in this study the sample size was not sufficient to demonstrate a significant relationship.

Because of increased skin pigment, serum vitamin D and 25-hydroxyvitamin D are lower and the serum immunoreactive parathyroid hormone is higher in Mexican American than in Caucasian men and women [88]. In contrast to African Americans, no differences were found in serum osteocalcin, urinary calcium, or urinary cyclic adenosine 3′,5′-monophosphate [88].

It is interesting to note that in prepubertal Mexican American girls, *Apa*I and *Bsm*I alleles of the vitamin D receptor predict bone mineral density of the lumbar spine and femoral shaft [89]. This is the first study in children to show a significant relationship between genetic markers and bone mineral density, and the results support the controversial hypothesis that the vitamin D receptor in this population may be a determinant of peak bone mass.

Polynesians

Bone mineral content of the forearm is significantly higher in Polynesians than in Caucasians [90,91]. Serum 25-hydroxyvitamin D is lower in Polynesians than in Caucasians as a consequence of increased skin pigment. However, there is no racial difference in serum parathyroid hormone, 1,25-dihydroxyvitamin D, osteocalcin, and alkaline phosphatase or urinary calcium and hydroxyproline [91]. The incidence of hip fracture is lower in Polynesian than in Caucasian women [92]. This difference could be related to the difference in bone mass.

SUMMARY

The effects of race on bone mass and fracture incidence are summarized in Table II. Only African Americans and Polynesians have a greater bone mass than Caucasians, which may account for the lower incidence of osteoporosis and fractures in them. A number of factors have been proposed that may account for the difference in bone mass between African Americans and Caucasians. These are summarized in Table I and are discussed at length in the text. Bone mass is the same in Mexican Americans compared to Caucasians, but the incidence of hip fractures is lower in Mexican Americans. The lower bone mass in Asians is accounted for by smaller body size. However, the incidence of hip fracture is lower in Asians. The incidence in vertebral fractures is higher and the incidence in hip fractures is lower in Japanese compared to Caucasian women. Despite considerable information about bone mass and the incidence of fractures, very little is known about why racial differences in bone density and fracture incidence occur.

TABLE II Bone Mass and Incidence of Fracture in Different Races Compared to Caucasians

Race	Bone mass	Fracture incidence
Asian Indians	Same	Same
African Americans	Increased	Decreased
Chinese	Decreased	Decreased
Japanese	Decreased; decreases with aging	Increased at spine Decreased at hip
Mexican Americans	Same	Decreased
Polynesians	Increased	Decreased

References

1. Garn, S. M., and Clark, D. C. Nutrition, growth, development and maturation: findings from the ten-state survey 1968–70. *Pediatrics* **56,** 306–319 (1975).
2. Garn, S. M. Bone loss and aging. *In* "Physiology and Pathology of Human Aging." (R. Goldman, ed.), pp. 39–57. Academic Press, New York, 1975.
3. Li, J.-Y., Specker, B. L., Ho, M. L., and Tsang, R. C. Bone mineral content in black and white children 1 to 6 years of age. Early appearance of race and sex differences. *Am. J. Dis. Child.* **143,** 1346–1349 (1989).
4. Bell, N. H., Shary, J., Stevens, J., Garza, M., Gordon, L., and Edwards, J. Demonstration that bone mass is greater in black than in white children. *J. Bone Miner. Res.* **6,** 719–723 (1991).
5. Slemenda, C. W., Peacock, M., Zhou, L., and Johnston, C. C. Reduced rates of skeletal remodeling are associated with increased bone mineral density during the development of peak skeletal mass. *J. Bone Miner. Res.* **12,** 676–682 (1997).
6. Cohn, S. H., Abesamis, C., Yasumara, S., Aloia, J. F., Zanai, I., and Ellis, K. J. Comparative skeletal mass and radial bone mineral content in black and white women. *Metabolism* **26,** 171–178 (1977).
7. Liel, Y., Edwards, J., Shary, J., Spicer, K. M., Gordon, L., and Bell, N. H. The effects of race and body habitus on bone mineral density of the radius, hip and spine in premenopausal women. *J. Clin. Endocrinol. Metab.* **66,** 1247–1250 (1988).

8. DeSimone, D. P., Stevens, J., Edwards, J., Shary, J., Gordon, L., and Bell, N. H. Influence of body habitus and race on bone mineral density of the midradius, hip and spine in aging women. *J. Bone Miner. Res.* **4,** 827–830 (1989).
9. Meier, D. E., Luckey, M. M., Wallenstein, S., Clemens, T. L., Orwoll, E. S., and Waslien, C. I. Calcium, vitamin D and parathyroid hormone status in young white and black women: association with racial differences in bone mass. *J. Clin. Endocrinol. Metab.* **72,** 703–710 (1991).
10. Luckey, M. M., Meier, D. E., Mandeli, J. P., DaCosta, M. C., Hubbard, M. L., and Goldsmith, S. J. Radial and vertebral bone density in white and black women: evidence for racial differences in premenopausal bone homeostasis. *J. Clin. Endocrinol. Metab.* **69,** 762–770 (1989).
11. Meier, D. E., Luckey, M. M., Wallenstein, S., Lapinski, R. H., and Catherwood, B. Racial differences in pre- and postmenopausal bone homeostasis: association with bone density. *J. Bone Miner. Res.* **7,** 1181–1189 (1992).
12. Kleerekoper, M., Nelson, D. A., Peterson, E. L., Flynn, M. J., Pawluszka, A. S., Jacobsen, G., and Wilson, P. Reference data for bone mass, calciotropic hormones, and biochemical markers of bone remodeling in older (55–75) postmenopausal white and black women. *J. Bone Miner. Res.* **8,** 1267–1276 (1994).
13. Wright, N. M., Papadea, N., Willi, S., Veldhuis, J. D., Pandey, J. P., Key, L. L., and Bell, N. H. Demonstration of a lack of racial difference in secretion of growth hormone despite a racial difference in bone mineral density in premenopausal women—a clinical research center study. *J. Clin. Endocrinol. Metab.* **81,** 1023–1026 (1996).
14. Bell, N. H., Gordon, L., Stevens, J., and Shary, J. Demonstration that bone mineral density of the lumbar spine, trochanter and femoral neck is higher in black than in white young men. *Calcif. Tissue Int.* **56,** 11–13 (1995).
15. Wright, N. M., Renault J., Willi S., Veldhuis, J. D., Pandey, J. P., Gordon, L., Key, L. L., and Bell, N. H. Greater secretion of growth hormone in black than in white men: possible factor in greater bone mineral density—a clinical research center study. *J. Clin. Endocrinol. Metab.* **80,** 2291–2297 (1995).
16. Nelson, D. A., Jacobsen, G., Barondess, D. A., and Parfitt, A. M. Ethnic differences in regional bone density, hip axis length, and lifestyle variables among healthy black and white men. *J. Bone Miner. Res.* **10,** 782–787 (1995).
17. Bell, N. H., Greene, A., Epstein, S., Oexmann, M. J., Shaw, S., and Shary, J. Evidence for alteration of the vitamin D endocrine system in blacks. *J. Clin. Invest.* **76,** 470–473 (1985).
18. Bell, N. H., Yergey, A. L., Vieira, N. E., Oexmann, M. J., and Shary, J. R. Demonstration of a difference in urinary calcium, not calcium absorption, in black and white adolescents. *J. Bone Miner. Res.* **8,** 1111–1115 (1993).
19. Sarmina, I., Spirnak, J. P., and Resnick, M. Urinary lithiasis in the black population: an epidemiological study and review of the literature. *J. Urol.* **138,** 14–17 (1987).
20. Clemens, T. L., Henderson, S. L., Adams, J. S., and Holick, M. F. Increased skin pigment reduces the capacity of skin to synthesize vitamin D_3. *Lancet* **1,** 74–76 (1982).
21. M'Buyamba-Kabangu, J. R., Fagard, R., Lijnen, P., Bouillon, R., Lissens, W., and Amery, A. Calcium, vitamin D-endocrine system and parathyroid hormone in black and white males. *Calcif. Tissue Int.* **1,** 70–74 (1987).
22. Fuleihan, G. E. H., Gundberg, C. M., Gleason, R., Brown, E. M., Stromski, M. E., Grant, F. D., and Conlin, P. R. Racial differences in parathyroid hormone dynamics. *J. Clin. Endocrinol. Metab.* **79,** 1642–1647 (1994).
23. Ghandur-Mnaymneh, L., Cassady, J., Hajanpour, M. A., and Reiss, E. The parathyroid gland in health and disease. *Am. J. Pathol.* **125,** 292–299 (1986).
24. Bell, N. H. 25-Hydroxyvitamin D_3 reverses alteration of the vitamin D-endocrine system in blacks. *Am. J. Med.* **99,** 597–599 (1995).
25. Awumey, E., Hollis, B. W., Bell, N. H. Evidence that decreased production rate and not increased metabolic clearance rate is probably responsible for low serum 25-hydroxyvitamin D in African Americans. *In* "Vitamin D: Chemistry, Biology and Clinical Applications of the Steroid Hormone." A. W. Norman, R. Bouillon, and M. Thomasset (eds.), pp. 701–708. University of Riverside, Riverside, 1997.
26. Abrams, S. A., O'Brien, K. O., Liang, L. K., and Stuff, J. E. Differences in calcium absorption and kinetics between black and white girls aged 5–16 years. *J. Bone Miner. Res.* **10,** 829–833 (1995).
27. Dawson Hughes, B., Harris, S., Kramich, C., Dallal, G., and Rasmussen, H. M. Calcium retention and hormone levels in black and white women on high and low calcium diets. *J. Bone Miner. Res.* **8,** 779–787 (1993).
28. Dawson Hughes, B., Harris, S., Fineran, S., and Rasmussen, H. M. Calcium absorption responses to calcitriol in black and white premenopausal women. *J. Clin. Endocrinol. Metab.* **80,** 3068–3072 (1993).
29. Bachrach, S., Fisher, J., and Parks, J. S. An outbreak of vitamin D deficiency rickets in a susceptible population. *Pediatrics* **64,** 277–283 (1980).
30. Edidin, D. V., Levitsky, L. L., Schey, W., *et al.* Resurgence of nutritional rickets associated with breast-feeding and special dietary practices. *Pediatrics* **65,** 232–235 (1980).
31. Kruger, D. M., Lyne, E. D., and Kleerekoper, M. Vitamin D deficiency rickets. A report of three cases. *Clin. Orthop.* **224,** 277–283 (1987).
32. Key, L. L. Vitamin D deficiency rickets. *Trends Endocrinol. Metab.* **2,** 81–85 (1992).
33. Chang, Y. T., Germain-Lee, E. L., Doran, T. F., Migeon, C. J., Levine, M. A., and Berkovitz, G. D. Hypocalcemia in nonwhite breast-fed infants. *Clin. Pediatr.* **31,** 695–698 (1992).
34. Cosman, F., Morgan, D. C., Nieves, J. W., Shen, V., Luckey, M. M., Dempster, D. W., Lindsay, R., and Parisien, M. Resistance to bone resorbing effects of PTH in black women. *J. Bone Miner. Res.* **12,** 958–966 (1997).
35. Bell, N. H., Epstein, S., Greene, A., Shary, J., Oexmann, M. J., and Shaw, S. Evidence for alteration of the vitamin D-endocrine system in obese subjects. *J. Clin. Invest.* **76,** 370–373 (1985).
36. Liel, Y., Ulmer, E., Shary, J., Hollis, B. W., and Bell, N. H. Low circulating vitamin D in obesity. *Calcif. Tissue Intl.* **43,** 199–201 (1988).
37. Rosenstreich, S. J., Rich, C., and Volwiler, W. Deposition in and release of vitamin D_3 from body fat: evidence for a storage site in the rat. *Clin. Invest.* **50,** 679–687 (1971).
38. Mawer, E. B., Backhouse, J., Holman, C. A., Lumb, G. A., Stanbury, S. W. The distribution and storage of vitamin D and its metabolites in human tissues. *Clin. Sci.* **43,** 414–431 (1972).
39. Bell, N. H., Epstein, S., Shary, J., Greene, V., Oexmann, M. J., and Shaw, S. Evidence of a probable role for 25-hydroxyvitamin D in the regulation of calcium metabolism in man. *J. Bone Miner. Res.* **3,** 489–495 (1988).
40. Weinstein, R. S., and Bell, N. H. Diminished rates of bone formation in normal black adults. *N. Engl. J. Med.* **319,** 1698–1701 (1988).
41. Han, Z.-H., Palmitkar, S., Rao, D. S., Nelson, D., and Parfitt, A. M. Effects of ethnicity and age or menopause on the remodeling and turnover of iliac bone: implications for mechanisms of bone loss. *J. Bone Miner. Res.* **12,** 498–508 (1997).

42. Parisien, M., Cosman, F., Morgan, D., Schnitzer, M., Liang, X., Nieves, J., Forese, L., Luckey, M., Meier, D., Shen, V., Lindsay, R., Dempster, D. Histomorphometric assessment of bone mass, structure and remodeling: a comparison between healthy black and white premenopausal women. *J. Bone Miner. Res.* **12,** 948–957 (1997).
43. Melton, L. J., Khosla, S., Atkinson, E. J., O'Fallon, W. M., and Riggs, B. L. Relationship of bone turnover to bone density and fractures. *J. Bone Miner. Res.* **12,** 1283–1091 (1997).
44. Herman Giddens, M. E., Stora, E. J., Wasserman, R. C., Bourdony, C. J., Bhapkar, M. V., Koch, G. G., and Hasemeier, C. M. Secondary sexual characteristics and menses in young girls seen in office practice: a study from the Pediatric Research in Office Settings Network. *Pediatrics* **99,** 505–512 (1997).
45. Garcia-Mayor, R. V., Andrade, M. A., Rios, M., Lage, M., Dieguez, C., and Casanueva, F. F. Serum leptin levels in normal children: relationship to age, gender, body mass index, pituitary-gonadal hormones, and pubertal stage. *J. Clin. Endocrinol. Metab.* **82,** 2849–2855 (1997).
46. Wong, W. W., Nicolson, M., Stuff, J. E., Butte, N. F., Ellis, K. J., Hergenroeder, A. C., Hill, R. B., and Smith, E. O. Serum leptin concentrations in Caucasian and African American girls. *J. Clin. Endocrinol. Metab.* **83,** 3574–3577 (1998).
47. Richards, R. J., Svec, F., Bai, W., Srinivasan, S. R., and Berenson, G. S. Steroid hormones during puberty:racial (black–white) differences in androstenedione and estradiol the Bogalusa Heart Study. *J. Clin. Endocrinol. Metab.* **75,** 624–631 (1992).
48. Bell, N. H., Hollis, B. W., Shary, J. R., Eyre, D. R., Eastell, R., Colwell, A., and Russell, R. G. G. Diclofenac sodium inhibits bone resorption in postmenopausal women. *Am. J. Med.* **96,** 349–353 (1995).
49. Slemenda, C. W., Longcope, C., Zhou, L., Hui, S. L., Peacock, M., and Johnston, C. C. Sex steroids and bone mass in older men: positive associations with serum estrogens and negative associations with androgens. *J. Clin. Invest.* **100,** 1755–1759 (1997).
50. Wright, N. M., Papadea, N., Veldhuis, J. D., Pandey, J. P., and Bell, N. H. Evidence that racial differences in bone mineral density do not result from differences in growth hormone secretion in prepubertal boys. Submitted.
51. Ross, R., Bernstein, L., Judd, H., Hanisch, R., Pike, M., and Henderson, B. Serum testosterone levels in healthy young black and white men. *J. Natl. Cancer Inst.* **76,** 45–48 (1986).
52. Fleet, J. C., Harris, S. S., Wood, R. J., and Dawson-Hughes, B. The *Bsm*I vitamin D receptor restriction fragment length polymorphism (BB) predicts low bone density in premenopausal black and white women. *J. Bone Miner. Res.* **10,** 985–990 (1995).
53. Harris, S. S., Eccleshall, T. R., Gross, C., Dawson-Hughes, B., and Feldman, D. The vitamin D receptor start codon polymorphism (*Fok*1) and bone mineral density in premenopausal American black and white women. *J. Bone Miner. Res.* **12,** 1043–1048 (1997).
54. Gyepes, M., Melliaz, H. Z., and Katz, I. The low incidence of fracture of the hip in the Negro. *JAMA* **181,** 1073–1074 (1962).
55. Bollet, A. J., Engh, G., and Parson, W. Epidemiology of osteoporosis. *Arch. Intern. Med.* **116,** 191–194 (1965).
56. Farmer, M. E., White, L. R., Brody, J. A., and Bailey, K. R. Race and sex differences in hip fracture incidence. *Am. J. Public Health* **74,** 1374–1380 (1984).
57. Silverman, S. L., and Madison, R. E. Decreased incidence of hip fracture in Hispanics, Asians and Blacks: California hospital discharge data. *Am. J. Public Health* **78,** 1482–1483 (1988).
58. Kellie, S. E., and Brody, J. A. Sex-specific and race-specific hip fracture rates. *Am. J. Public Health* **80,** 326–328 (1990).
59. Griffin, M. R., Ray, W. A., Fought, R. L., and Melton, L. J., III Black-white differences in fracture rates. *Am. J. Epidemiol.* **136,** 1378–1385 (1992).
60. Pruzansky, M. E., Turano, M., Luckey, M., and Senie, R. Low body weight is a risk factor for hip fracture in both black and white women. *J. Orthop. Res.* **7,** 192–197 (1989).
61. Grisso, A. J., Kelsey, J. L., Strom, B. L., O'Brien, L. A., Maislin, G., La Pann, K., Samelson, L., and Hoffman, S. Risk factors for hip fracture in black women. The Northeast Hip Fracture Study Group. *N. Engl. J. Med.* **330,** 1555–1559 (1994).
62. Cummings, S. R., Cauley, J. A., Paleremo, L., Ross, P. D., Wasnich, R. D., Black, D., and Faulkner, K. G. Racial differences in hip axis lengths might explain racial differences in rates of hip fracture. *Osteopor. Int.* **4,** 226–229 (1994).
63. Mitra, D. A., Hollis, B. W., Kumar, R., and Bell, N. H. Vitamin D metabolism is altered in Asian Indians in the Southern United States: a clinical research center study. *J. Endocrinol. Metab.* **83,** 169–173 (1998).
64. Cundy, C., Cornish, J., Evans, M. C., Gamble, G., Stapleton, J., and Reid, I. R. Sources of interracial variation of bone mineral density. *J. Bone Miner. Res.* **10,** 368–373 (1995).
65. Holmes, A. M., Enoch, B. A., Taylor, J. L., and Jones, M. E. Occult rickets and osteomalacia amongst the Asian immigrant population. *Q. J. Med.* **42,** 125–149 (1973).
66. Preece, M. A., Ford, J. A., McIntosh, W. B., Dunnigan, M. G., Tomlinson, S., and O'Riordan, J. L. H. Vitamin D deficiency among Asian immigrants to Britain. *Lancet* **1,** 907–910 (1973).
67. Dent, C. E., and Gupta, M. M. Plasma 25-hydroxyvitamin-D levels during pregnancy in Caucasians and in vegetarian and non-vegetarian Asians. *Lancet* **2,** 1057–1060 (1975).
68. Hunt, S. P., O'Riordan, J. L. H., Windo, J., and Truswell, A. S. Vitamin D status in different sub-groups of British Asians. *Br. Med. J.* **2,** 1351–1354 (1976).
69. Heckmatt, J. Z., Peacock, M., Davies, A. E. J., McMurray, J., and Isherwood, D. M. Plasma 25-hydroxyvitamin D in pregnant Asian women and their babies. *Lancet* **2,** 546–548 (1979).
70. Brooke, O. G., Brown, I. R. F., Cleeve, H. J. W., and Sood, A. Observations on the vitamin D state of pregnant Asian women in London. *Br. J. Obstet. Gynaecol.* **88,** 18–26 (1981).
71. Ford, J. A., Davidson, D. C., McIntosh, W. B., Fyfe, W. M., and Dunnigan, M. G. Neonatal rickets in Asian immigrant population. *Br. Med. J.* **3,** 211–212 (1973).
72. Goel, K. M., Sweet, E. M., Logan, R. W., Warren, J. M., Arneil, G. C., and Shanks, R. A. Florid and subclinical rickets among immigrant children in Glasgow. *Lancet* **1,** 1141–1145 (1976).
73. Dent, C. E., Rowe, D. J. F., Round, J. M., and Stamp, T. C. B. Effect of chapattis and ultraviolet irradiation on nutritional rickets in an Indian immigrant. *Lancet* **1,** 1282–1284 (1973).
74. Preece, M. A., Tomlinson, S., Ribot, C. A., Pietrek, J., Korn, H. T., Davies, D. M., Ford, J. A., Dunnigan, M. G., and O'Riordan, J. L. H. Studies of vitamin D deficiency in man. *Q. J. Med.* **44,** 575–589 (1975).
75. Ashby, J. P., Newman, D. J., and Rinsler, M. G. Is intact PTH a sensitive biochemical marker of deranged calcium homeostasis in vitamin D deficiency? *Ann. Clin. Biochem.* **26,** 24–327 (1989).
76. Henderson, J. B., Dunnigan, M. G., McIntosh, W. B., Motaal, A. A., and Hole, D. Asian osteomalacia is determined by dietary factors when exposure to ultraviolet radiation is restricted: a risk factor model. *Q. J. Med.* **76,** 923–933 (1990).
77. Parker, M., Anand, J. K., Myles, J. W., and Lodwick, R. Proximal femoral fractures: prevalence in different racial groups. *Eur. J. Epidemiol.* **8,** 730–732 (1992).
78. Bhudhikanok, G. S., Wang, M. C., Eckert, K., Matkin, C., Marcus, R., and Bachrach, L. K. Differences in bone mineral in young Asian and Caucasian Americans may reflect differences in bone size. *J. Bone Miner. Res.* **11,** 1545–1556 (1996).

79. Ross, P. D., He, Y.-F., Yates, A. J., Coupland, C., Ravn, P., McClung, M., Thompson, D., and Wasnich, R. D. Body size accounts for most differences in bone density between Asian and Caucasian women. *Calcif. Tissue Int.* **59,** 339–343 (1996).
80. Ito, M., Lang, T. F., Jergas, M., Ohki, M., Takada, M., Nakamura, T., Hayashi, T., and Genant, H. K. Spinal trabecular bone loss and fracture in American and Japanese women. *Calcif. Tissue Int.* **61,** 123–128 (1997).
81. Ross, P. D., Fujiwara, S., Huang, C., Davis, J. W., Epstein, R. S., Wasnich, R. D., Kodama, K., and Melton, L. J., III. Vertebral fracture prevalence in women in Hiroshima compared to Caucasians or Japanese in the U.S. *Int. J. Epidemiol.* **24,** 1171–1177 (1995).
82. Lauderdale, D. S., Jacobsen, S. J., Furner, S. E., Levy, P. S., Brody, J. A., and Goldberg, J. Hip fracture incidence among elderly Asian-American populations. *Am. J. Epidemiol.* **146,** 502–509 (1997).
83. Davis, J. W., Ross, P. D., Nevitt, M. C., and Wasnich, R. D. Incidence rates of falls among Japanese men and women living in Hawaii. *J. Clin. Epidemiol.* **50,** 589–594 (1997).
84. Lau, E. M. C., Chan, H. H. L., Woo, J., Sham, A., and Leung, P. C. Body composition and bone mineral density of Chinese women with vertebral fracture. *Bone* **19,** 657–662 (1996).
85. Villa, M. L., Marcus, R., Delay, R. R., and Kelsey, J. L. Factors contributing to skeletal health of postmenopausal Mexican-American women. *J. Bone Miner. Res.* **10,** 1233–1242 (1995).
86. Bauer, R. L. Ethnic differences in hip fracture: a reduced incidence in Mexican Americans. *Am. J. Epidemiol.* **127,** 145–149 (1988).
87. McClure, L., Eccleshall, T. R., Gross, C., Villa, M. L., Lin, N., Ramaswamy, V., Kohlmeier, L., Kelsey, J., Marcus, R., and Feldman, D. Vitamin D receptor polymorphisms, bone mineral density, and bone metabolism in postmenopausal Mexican American women. *J. Bone Miner. Res.* **12,** 134–240 (1997).
88. Reasoner, C. A., III, Dunn, J. F., Fetchik, D. A., Leil, Y., Hollis, B. W., Epstein, S., Shary, J., Mundy, G. R., and Bell, N. H. Alteration of vitamin D metabolism in Mexican Americans. *J. Bone Miner. Res.* **5,** 13–17 (1990).
89. Sainz, J., Van Tornout, J. M., Loro, L. M., Sayre, J., Roe, T. F., and Gilsanz, V. Vitamin D receptor gene polymorphisms and bone density in prepubertal American girls of Mexican descent. *N. Engl. J. Med.* **337,** 77–82 (1997).
90. Reid, I. R., Mackey, M., Ibbertson, H. K. Bone mineral content in Polynesian and white New Zealand women. *Br. Med. J.* **2,** 1457–1458 (1986).
91. Reid, I. R., Cullen, S., Schooler, B. A., Livingstone, N. E., and Evans, M. C. Calciotropic hormone levels in Polynesians, evidence against their role in inter-racial differences in bone mass. *J. Clin. Endocrinol. Metab.* **70,** 1452–1456 (1990).
92. Stott, S., and Gray, D. H. The incidence of femoral neck fractures in New Zealand. *N. Z. Med. J.* **91,** 6–9 (1980).

CHAPTER 13

Determinants of Maintenance of Bone Mass

DANIEL T. BARAN Department of Orthopedics and Physical Rehabilitation, University of Massachusetts Medical School, Worcester, Massachusetts 01655

INTRODUCTION

Osteoporosis, which has been linked to inadequate calcium intake as well as other factors [1], is an important health problem in the United States. It is estimated that 23 million women over the age of 45 have low bone mass or osteoporosis [2]. The condition is manifested by a decrease in bone substance and strength. The resulting diminution of bone tissue is expressed as a reduction in bone mineral density. The incidence of osteoporosis could be reduced by maximizing peak bone mass and/or minimizing subsequent bone loss. Most studies suggest that peak bone mass at the various skeletal sites in women is attained by the age of 35. Likewise, investigators concur that bone loss occurs after menopause. Although there is disagreement in the literature regarding bone loss in women after attainment of peak bone mass but before menopause, most studies indicate that both axial and appendicular bone mineral density decline in premenopausal women and that the bone mineral density of women entering menopause is significantly lower than their peak bone mineral density. Prevention or amelioration of bone loss during this period of time would allow women to enter menopause with greater bone mass, thereby reducing future risk of fracture.

PREMENOPAUSAL BONE LOSS

Numerous cross-sectional studies have demonstrated that bone mass decreases in premenopausal women between the time that peak bone mass is attained and menopause [3–19]. Reductions in bone mineral density have been observed at the spine [4,7,11,13,19], femoral neck [3,5–9,11–19], Ward's area [3,5,6,8,9,13–16,19], trochanter [3,8,14], and forearm [10]. In general, these cross-sectional studies have noted greater bone loss at sites rich in trabecular bone. Ward's area bone mineral density declined at a rate of 0.6–1.0%/year, whereas reductions at the femoral neck ranged between 0.3 and 0.9%/year and at the trochanter between 0.3 and 0.6%/year. Vertebral (anterior–posterior) bone mineral density has been reported to decrease at rates of 1.0%/year, although many of the cross-sectional studies showing loss at femoral sites have been unable to document vertebral bone loss as well [3,6,9,14]. The trabecular component of vertebral bone has been reported to decline at a rate of 0.7%/year [4]. Forearm bone mineral density was reduced more rapidly in the ultradistal trabecular region (0.6%/year) than in the proximal cortical region (0.4%/year).

More recent cross-sectional surveys have supported the concept that bone mineral density is not maintained during premenopausal years. In a survey of 1708 women between the 3rd and 5th decades in the United States, Ward's area bone mineral density declined by 0.7%/year in non-Hispanic white women, by 0.5%/year in non-Hispanic black women, and by 0.45%/year in Mexican-American women. Femoral neck bone mineral density declined by 0.3%/year in non-Hispanic white women during the same period. Losses in bone mineral density at the femoral neck were not observed in non-Hispanic black or Mexican-American women [16]. A cross-sectional survey of 330 healthy Finnish girls and premenopausal women, aged 7–47 years, noted no change in bone mineral density at the spine or radius after age 20. However, femoral neck bone mineral density declined at a rate between 0.3 and 0.5%/year. The investigators observed that, although this loss might not seem high, it could cumulatively represent a significant loss over the 30 years between the attainment of peak bone mass and menopause [18]. Similarly, a survey of 246 premenopausal women (range 31–55 years) in France showed a 0.6%/year loss in bone mineral density at Ward's area and a 0.4%/year loss in bone mineral density at the lateral spine. Femoral neck bone mineral density declined by only 0.2%/year, whereas there was no change in vertebral (anterior–posterior) density [19].

Longitudinal studies [20–23] have also confirmed that premenopausal bone loss occurs. In 3-year prospective study, vertebral (anterior–posterior) bone mineral density decreased at a rate of 1%/year in premenopausal women between the ages of 30 and 42 years [20]. A more recent 4-year prospective study by Citrimi *et al.* [21] has observed that vertebral trabecular bone mineral density declined at a rate of 0.86%/year in premenopausal women who were 38–42 years old at the onset of the study. These investigators noted no change in radial bone mineral density. In contrast, Sowers *et al.* [22] showed in a 5-year prospective study of 108 premenopausal women that radial bone mineral density declined at a rate of 0.9%/year. Likewise, a 4-year prospective study of 19 premenopausal women reported that radial bone mineral density decreased at a rate of 1%/year [23]. Thus, both cross-sectional and prospective studies indicate that premenopausal bone loss occurs in the axial and appendicular skeleton. Prospective studies have reported rates of loss that are consistently slightly greater than those observed in cross-sectional surveys.

Not all studies have been able to document changes in bone mass in premenopausal women [24–28]. A cross-sectional survey of 69 premenopausal women between the ages of 29 and 55 years showed no changes in bone mineral density of the proximal or distal radius, vertebrae, or total body bone mineral [24]. A cross-sectional study of 186 premenopausal Finnish women by Laitinen *et al.* [25] showed no changes in bone mineral density at the lumbar vertebrae, femoral neck, Ward's area, or trochanter. Likewise, a cross-sectional study of 200–300 premenopausal women between the ages of 20 and 39 years in the United States showed no significant decline in bone mineral density at the spine, femoral neck, Ward's area, trochanter, or radius [26]. Similarly, two longitudinal studies in the United States and Europe have been unable to demonstrate premenopausal bone loss [27,28]. A 2-year study of 75 women nearing menopause (average age 49 years) observed no changes in bone mineral density of the spine or total body [27]. A 1-year prospective study of 30 premenopausal women between the ages of 20 and 35 years noted no changes in bone mass of the spine, femoral neck, Ward's area, trochanter, or total body [28].

Potential explanations for the differences in the studies demonstrating premenopausal bone loss and those unable to show differences may relate to dietary calcium intake and/or exercise levels of the women. Longitudinal studies that showed premenopausal bone loss [20–23] were longer in duration than those that did not [27,28]. Similarly, cross-sectional studies observing premenopausal bone loss [3–19] have tended to be larger and to involve women with greater ranges in age than those studies that observed no change [24–26].

DIETARY CALCIUM AND PREMENOPAUSAL BONE LOSS

The impact of dietary calcium on bone mineral density after peak bone mass is reached but before menopause is unclear. Increased dietary calcium intake has been reported to positively affect vertebral bone mass in women between the ages of 25 and 35 years [29]. In the 31 women in this study consuming more than 800 mg calcium/day (average intake 1071 mg/day), vertebral bone mineral density was 6.7% higher ($p < 0.05$) than in the 29 women consuming less than 800 mg/day (average intake 638 mg/day). Likewise, milk consumption has been shown to be positively correlated with proximal radius bone mineral density in women aged 25–34 years [30]. In a cross-sectional study of 139 women aged 30–39 years, the current calcium intake was modestly correlated with femoral neck bone mineral density. However, the intake of calcium as a teenager was more highly correlated with bone mass [31]. Given the age of the women in these three studies, it is reasonable to postulate that calcium has an effect on the acquisition of peak bone mass rather than on its maintenance. Conversely, other studies of women in this same age group (less than age 40 years) have shown no correlation between current dietary calcium intake and bone mineral density. In women between the ages of 20 and 29 years, dietary calcium intake was reported to have no correlation with bone mineral density of the spine or femur [26]. Similarly, neither current dietary calcium intake nor caloric intake was associated with the bone mineral density of women between the ages of 30 and 40 years [32].

Studies examining the impact of dietary calcium intake in older premenopausal women have also been inconclusive. In a study of 72 premenopausal women over the age of 30 years (mean age 39 years), calcium intake was positively associated with distal radius bone mineral density, but not with density of the lumbar spine, femoral neck, trochanter, or midradius [33]. Conversely, in a study of 88 premenopausal women over the age of 23 years (mean age 38 years), calcium was not correlated with spine, femoral neck, or forearm bone mineral density [34].

Retrospective studies have suggested that increased dietary calcium in the premenopausal years is associated with greater bone mass. In an analysis of premenopausal bone mineral content [35], subjects were divided into three groups according to their calcium intake (less than 500 mg/day, between 500 and 1000 mg/day, and more than 1000 mg/day). The mean vertebral bone mineral density adjusted for the covariates of height and weight was significantly greater in the high compared to the low calcium intake group. Other studies have indicated that a lifetime of adequate calcium intake coupled with adequate levels of serum estrogens could maximize bone density after menopause [36]. Women who reported having had higher calcium intakes during early adulthood had greater forearm bone mineral content after menopause than did those reporting lower intakes early in life [37,38]. Given the difficulties with retrospective analyses, these studies do little to resolve the controversy.

Two prospective studies have addressed the effect of dietary calcium on the maintenance of bone mineral density in premenopausal women: one demonstrated a beneficial effect [20] whereas the other reported no effect [39]. In a randomized study, the effect of calcium supplementation on vertebral bone mineral density in 30- to 42-year-old premenopausal women over a 3-year period was investigated [20]. Dietary calcium was supplemented in the form of dairy products, and as a result the study was not blinded. Twenty women increased their dietary calcium intake by an average of 610 mg/day ($p < 0.03$) (from 962 to 1572 mg/day), whereas 17 age- and weight-matched women served as controls (dietary calcium 892 mg/day initially and 810 mg/day after 3 years). Urinary calcium excretion increased by 28% ($p < 0.03$) in the supplemented women, confirming increased dietary calcium intake. The vertebral bone mineral density in the women consuming increased calcium did not change over the 3-year period. In contrast, the vertebral bone mineral density in the control group declined by 2.9% ($p < 0.001$), and was significantly lower than the supplemented group at 30 and 36 months. In contrast, in an observational study with a duration on average of 4.1 years, dietary calcium had no effect on the rate of change of vertebral bone mineral density [39]. Women in the lower (mean, 501 mg/day) and in the upper (mean, 1397 mg/day) quartiles of dietary calcium intake had similar rates of change in bone mass. Women in the lowest quartile of intake lost vertebral bone mineral density at the rate of 1.06%/year, whereas those in the highest quartile lost bone mineral density at the rate of 0.98%/year. Thus, both studies document decreases in vertebral bone mineral density during the premenopausal years, but differ with regard to the effect of dietary calcium on these losses. These differences may relate to study design. The latter study was not a randomized or an interventional study and did not document the stability of calcium intake over the study period. A randomized, blinded, prospective, controlled trial is needed to address these issues.

Differences in vitamin D intake and levels may also affect changes in bone mineral density in premenopausal women. Vitamin D intake has been shown to modify bone loss in perimenopausal women [40]. Thus, vitamin D levels may be important in assessing the skeletal response of premenopausal women to calcium supplementation.

EXERCISE, MENSTRUAL STATUS, AND PREMENOPAUSAL BONE MASS

Other potential influences on bone loss in premenopausal women include life-style and physiological factors such as exercise and menstrual status. In some cross-sectional studies, exercise has been associated with greater bone mass in premenopausal women compared to sedentary controls [29,41,42]. Other studies have found no correlation between the intensity of physical activity and bone mineral density [22,26,30].

A 4-year exercise program consisting of aerobic activities (three sessions/week, 45 min/session) reduced bone loss in the arms of premenopausal women, but did not increase bone mass [43]. A 1-year prospective intervention trial examined the effect of weight lifting on vertebral and calcaneus bone mineral density in premenopausal women between the ages of 23 and 46 years [44]. To enhance compliance the groups were formed based on choice rather than random assignment. Sixty-seven women chose to be weight lifters, and 44 women served as controls. Subjects were given a daily 500-mg calcium supplement. Strength in the weight-lifting group increased by 83% during the year. The weight-lifting group had a nonsignificant increase in vertebral bone mineral density of 0.81%, and the control group exhibited a nonsignificant decrease of 0.5%. There was a significant difference in the percentage change in bone mineral density between the two groups. There were no significant differences in calcaneus bone mineral density between the groups. The investigators concluded that the relatively small changes seen as a result of this exercise program might prevent weight lifting from being a practical solution to the problem of osteoporosis [44]. Although increases in bone mass were not significant, it should be noted that bone loss was prevented by this exercise program.

In contrast, a 9-month intervention trial examining the effect of weight lifting in a smaller group of premenopausal women (mean age 38 years) reported a 3.96% decrease in the vertebral bone mineral density of the exercising group [45]. Groups were formed based on choice to enhance compliance. Ten women chose to exercise, whereas seven remained relatively sedentary. Despite a 57% increase in strength, the exercising group had a decrease in vertebral bone mineral density and no change at the femoral neck. Confounders in this study include its small size and the lack of randomization: women choosing exercise had greater vertebral and femoral neck bone mineral density at the start of the study than did controls.

A more recent study has more rigorously evaluated the effect of exercise intervention on bone mass [46]. A 2-year randomized, intervention trial investigated the efficacy of exercise and calcium supplementation on increasing bone mineral density in 127 premenopausal women between the ages of 20 and 35 years. During the course of the study, there was a 50% attrition rate. Thirty-two women completed the exercise program that consisted of both aerobic and strength training, whereas 31 women completed the control program of stretching exercises. The exercise program produced significant gains in all fitness parameters and resulted in significant increases in vertebral (anterior–posterior) (1.3%), trochanter (2.6%), and calcaneus (5.6%) bone mineral density. There were significant positive differences in bone mineral density between the exercise and the stretching groups for vertebral trabecular (2.5%), femoral neck (2.4%), trochanter (2.3%), and calcaneus (6.4%). Calcium supplementation (up to 1500 mg/day) had no effect on bone mineral density in either group, although these subgroup analyses were small with 14 to 17 women/group.

Intense physical training in female athletes can lead to a decrease in circulating estradiol levels and altered menstrual patterns. Despite the physical activity, the altered menstrual patterns are accompanied by a decrease in vertebral bone mineral density [47]. Vertebral bone mineral density increases after the resumption of menses in amenorrheic athletes [48]. Regardless of the resumption of normal menstruation, retrospective analysis suggests that extended periods of oligomenorrhea/amenorrhea may have a residual negative effect on bone mineral density [49]. Exercises that load a particular skeletal area can partially compensate for the adverse effect of low estradiol levels on bone mass, attesting to the positive role of mechanical forces on skeletal health [50].

SUMMARY

The majority of studies suggest that bone mass is lost during the period after the attainment of peak bone mineral density and prior to menopause. Vertebral bone mineral density decreases at rates between 0.4 and 1%/year. Femoral neck bone mineral density decreases at rates between 0.2 and 0.9%/year. Dietary calcium, exercise, and menstrual status can affect premenopausal bone loss, but the impact of these factors is unclear. Preventing this bone loss in premenopausal women would allow them to enter menopause with greater vertebral and femoral bone mass. Given the inverse relationship between bone mineral density and fracture risk, these women would be at a lower fracture risk in later life.

References

1. Heaney, R. P. Nutritional factors in osteoporosis. *Annu. Rev. Nutr.* **13,** 287–316 (1993).
2. National Osteoporosis Foundation. "Osteoporosis Prevalence Figures State-by State Report." Washington, DC (1997).
3. Mazess, R. B., Barden, H. S., Ettinger, M., Johnston, C., Dawson-Hughes, B., Baran, D., Powell, M., and Notelovitz, M. Spine and femur density using dual-photon absorptiometry in US white women. *Bone Miner.* **2,** 211–219 (1987).
4. Buchanan, J. R., Myers, C., Lloyd, T., and Greer, R. B., III, Early vertebral trabecular bone loss in normal premenopausal women. *J. Bone Miner. Res.* **3,** 583–587 (1988).
5. Hedlund, L. R., and Gallagher, J. C. The effect of age and menopause on bone mineral density of the proximal femur. *J. Bone Miner. Res.* **4,** 639–642 (1989).
6. Elliot, J. R., Gilchrist, N. L., Wells, J. E., *et al.* Effects of age and sex on bone density at the hip and spine in a normal caucasian New Zealand population. *New Zeal. Med. J.* **103,** 35–38 (1990).
7. Rodin, A., Murby, B., Smith, M. A., Caleffi, M., Fentiman, I., Chapman, M. G., and Fogelman, I. Premenopausal bone loss in the lumbar spine and neck of femur: a study of 225 Caucasian women. *Bone* **11,** 1–5 (1990).
8. Sowers, M.-F., Kshirsagar, A., Crutchfield, M., and Updike S. Body composition by age and femoral bone mass of young adult women. *Ann. Epidemiol.* **1,** 245–254 (1991).
9. Lindsay, R., Cosman, F., Herrington, B. S., and Himmelstein, S. Bone mass and body composition in normal women. *J. Bone Miner. Res.* **7,** 55–63 (1992).
10. Duppe, H., Bardsell, P., Johnell, O., *et al.* Bone mineral content in women: trends of change. *Osteopor. Int.* **2,** 262–265 (1992).
11. Kruger, H., Heikkinene, J., Laitinen, K., *et al.* Dual energy x-ray absorptiometry in normal women: A cross-sectional study of 717 Finnish volunteers. *Osteopor. Int.* **2,** 135–140 (1992).
12. Beck, T. J., Ruff, C. B., Scott, W. W., Jr., Plato, C. C., Tobin, J. D., and Quan, C. A. Sex differences in geometry of the femoral neck with aging: A structural analysis of bone mineral data. *Calcif. Tissue Int.* **50,** 24–29 (1992).

13. Ho, S. C., Hsu, S. Y. C., Leung, P. C., Chan, C., Swaminathan, R., Fan, Y. K., and Chan, S. S. G. A longitudinal study of the determinants of bone mass in Chinese women aged 21 to 40. *Ann. Epidemiol.* **3,** 256–263 (1993).
14. Matkovic, V., Jelic, T., Wardlaw, G. M., *et al.* Timing of peak bone mass in Caucasian females and its implications for the prevention of osteoporosis. *J. Clin. Invest.* **93,** 799–808 (1994).
15. Ravn, P., Hetland, M. L., Overgaard, K., and Christiansen, C. Premenopausal and postmenopausal changes in bone mineral density of the proximal femur measured by dual energy x-ray absorptiometry. *J. Bone Miner. Res.* **9,** 1975–1980 (1994).
16. Looker, A. C., Wahner, H. W., Dunn, W. L., *et al.* Proximal femur bone mineral levels of US adults. *Osteopor. Int.* **5,** 389–409 (1995).
17. Johnston, C. C., Jr., and Slemenda, C. W. Pathogenesis of osteoporosis. *Bone* **17,** 19S–22S (1995).
18. Haapasalo, H., Kannus, P., Sievanen, H., Pasanen, M., Uusi-Rasi, K., Heinonen, A., Oja, P., and Vuori, I. Development of mass, density, and estimated mechanical characteristics of bones in Caucasian females. *J. Bone Miner. Res.* **11,** 1751–1760 (1996).
19. Arlot, M. E., Sornay-Rendu, E., Garnero, P., Vey-Marty, B., and Delmas, P. D. Apparent pre- and postmenopausal loss evaluated by DXA at different skeletal sites in women: the OFELY Cohort. *J. Bone Miner. Res.* **12,** 683–690 (1997).
20. Baran, D., Sorensen, A., Grimes, J., Lew, R., Karellas, A., Johnson, B., and Roche, J. Dietary modification with dairy products for preventing vertebral bone loss in premenopausal women: A three-year prospective study. *J. Clin. Endocrinol. Metab.* **70,** 264–270 (1989).
21. Citron, J. T., Ettinger, B., and Genant, H. K. Spinal bone mineral loss in estrogen-replete, calcium-replete premenopausal women. *Osteopor. Int.* **5,** 228–233 (1995).
22. Sowers, M. R., Clark, K., Hollis, B., Wallace, R. B., and Jannausch, M. Radial bone mineral density in pre- and perimenopausal women: a prospective study of rates and risk factors for loss. *J. Bone Miner. Res.* **7,** 647–657 (1992).
23. Smith, E. L., Gilligan, C., Smith, P. E., *et al.* Calcium supplementation and bone loss. *Am. J. Clin. Nutr.* **50,** 833–842 (1989).
24. Nilas, L., and Christiansen, C. Bone mass and its relationship to age and the menopause. *J. Clin. Endocrinol. Metab.* **65,** 697–702 (1987).
25. Laitinen, K., Valimaki, M., and Keto, P. Bone mineral density measured by dual-energy x-ray absorptiometry in healthy Finnish women. *Calcif. Tissue Int.* **48,** 224–231 (1991).
26. Mazess, R. B., and Barden, H. S. Bone density in premenopausal women: effects of age, dietary intake, physical activity, smoking, and birth-control pills. *Am. J. Clin. Nutr.* **53,** 132–142 (1991).
27. Recker, R. R., Lappe, J. M. Davies, K. M., and Kimmel, D. B. Change in bone mass immediately before menopause. *J. Bone Miner. Res.* **7,** 857–862 (1992).
28. Slosman, D. O., Rizzoli, R., Pichard, C., Donath, A., and Bonjour, J.-P. Longitudinal measurement of regional and whole body bone mass in young healthy adults. *Osteopor. Int.* **4,** 185–190 (1994).
29. Kanders, B., Dempster, D. W., Lindsay, R., *et al.* Interaction of calcium nutrition and physical activity on bone mass in young women. *J. Bone Miner. Res.* **3,** 145–149 (1988).
30. Davis, J. W., Novotny, R., Ross, P. D., and Wasnich, R. D., Anthropometric, lifestyle and menstrual factors influencing size-adjusted bone mineral content in a multiethnic population of premenopausal women. *J. Nutr.* **126,** 2968–2976 (1996).
31. Nieves, J. W., Golden, A. L., Siris, E., Kelsey, J. L., and Lindsay, R. Teenage and current calcium intake are related to bone mineral density of the hip and forearm in women aged 30–39 years. *Am. J. Epidemiol.* **141,** 342–351 (1995).
32. Desai, S. S., Baran, D. T., Grimes, J., Gionet, M., and Milne, M. Relationship of diet, axial, and appendicular bone mass in normal premenopausal women. *Am. J. Med. Sci.* **293,** 218–220 (1987).
33. Cooper, C., Atkinson, E. J., Hensrud, D. D., Wahner, H. W., O'Fallon, W. M. Riggs, B. L., Melton, L. J., III, Dietary protein intake and bone mass in women. *Calcif. Tissue Int.* **58,** 320–325 (1996).
34. Angus, R. M., Sambrook, P. N., Pocock, N. A., and Eisman, J. A. Dietary intake and bone mineral density. *Bone Miner.* **4,** 165–277 (1988).
35. Picard, D., Ste-Marie, L. G., Coutu, D., *et al.* Premenopausal bone mineral content relates to height, weight, and calcium intake during early adulthood. *Bone Miner.* **4,** 299–309 (1988).
36. Cauley, J. A., Gutai, J. P., Kuller, L. H., *et al.* Endogenous estrogen levels and calcium intakes in premenopausal women: relationships with cortical bone measures. *JAMA* **260,** 3150–3155 (1988).
37. Sandler, R. B., Slemenda, C. W., LaPorte, R. E., *et al.* Postmenopausal bone density and milk consumption in childhood and adolescence. *Am. J. Clin. Nutr.* **42,** 270–274 (1985).
38. Bauer, D. C., Browner, W. S., Cauley, J. A., *et al.* Factors associated with appendicular bone mass in older women. *Ann. Intern. Med.* **118,** 657–665 (1993).
39. Riggs, B. L., Wahner, H. W., Melton, L. J., III, Richelson, L. S., Judd, H. L., and O'Fallon, W. M. Dietary calcium intake and rates of bone loss in women. *J. Clin. Invest.* **80,** 979–982 (1987).
40. Lukert, B., Higgins, J., and Stoskop, J. M. Menopausal bone loss is partially regulated by dietary intake of vitamin D. *Calcif. Tissue Int.* **51,** 173–179 (1992).
41. Drinkwater, B. L. Exercise in the prevention of osteoporosis. *Osteopor. Int.* **1,** S169–S171 (1993).
42. Gutin, B., and Kasper, M. J. Can vigorous exercise play a role in osteoporosis prevention? *Osteopor. Int.* **2,** 55–69 (1992).
43. Smith, E. L., Gilligan, C., McAdam, M., Ensign, C. P., and Smith, P. E. Deterring bone loss by exercise intervention in premenopausal and postmenopausal women. *Calcif. Tissue Int.* **44,** 312–321 (1989).
44. Gleeson, P. B., Protas, E. J., LeBlanc, A. D., Schneider, V. S., and Evans, H. J. Effects of weight lifting on bone mineral density in premenopausal women. *J. Bone Miner. Res.* **5,** 153–158 (1990).
45. Rockwell, J. C., Sorensen, A. M., Baker, S., Leahey, D., Stock, J. L., Michaels, J., and Baran, D. T. Weight training decreases vertebral bone density in premenopausal women: A prospective study. *J. Clin. Endocrinol. Metab.* **71,** 988–993 (1990).
46. Friedlander, A. L., Genant, H. K., Sadowsky, S., Byl, N. N., and Gluer, C.-C. A two-year program of aerobics and weight training enhances bone mineral density of young women. *J. Bone Miner. Res.* **10,** 574–585 (1995).
47. Drinkwater, B. L., Nilson, K., Chestnut, C. H., III, Bremner, W. J., Shainholtz, S., and Southworth, M. B. Bone mineral content of amenorrheic and eumenorrheic athletes. *N. Engl. J. Med.* **311,** 277–281 (1984).
48. Drinkwater, B. L., Nilson, K., Ott, S., and Chestnut, C. H., III, Bone mineral density after resumption of menses in amenorrheic athletes. *JAMA* **256,** 380–382 (1986).
49. Drinkwater, B. L., Bruemner, B., and Chestnut, C. H., III, Menstrual history as a determinant of current bone density in young athletes. *JAMA* **263,** 545–548 (1990).
50. Wolman, R. L., Clark, P., McNally, E., Harries, M., and Reeve, J. Menstrual state and exercise as determinants of spinal trabecular bone density in female athletes. *Br. Med. J.* **301,** 516–518 (1990).

PART III

Mechanisms of Age-Related Bone Loss

CHAPTER 14

Cellular Mechanisms of Age-Related Bone Loss

PAMELA GEHRON ROBEY Craniofacial and Skeletal Diseases Branch, National Institute of Dental Research, National Institutes of Health, Bethesda, Maryland 20892

PAOLO BIANCO Dipartimento di Medicina Sperimentale, Universita dell'Aquila, L'Aquila, Italy

INTRODUCTION

Peak bone mass is attained during the third decade of life. Subsequently, bone mass declines slowly with advancing age. Although there is currently intense activity to determine the cause of acute bone loss associated with sex steroid deficiency and development of osteoporosis, there is little understanding of the mechanism by which bone is lost solely as attributed to the aging process. This chapter will not address the issue of "acute" bone loss, generated by the suppression of gonadal function and typically associated with, and determined by, a significant increase in bone remodeling. Rather, it will focus on what is currently known about the aging of bone that is independent of acute loss of sex hormones, leading to the so-called "senile osteoporosis." Emphasis will be on reviewing current knowledge about the changes in the biology of bone cells that can be traced to the effects of aging. "Bone cells" with which this discussion will deal include cells that are found in the marrow, that is, cells of bone as an organ, rather than cells in bone tissue only. This is justified not only by the current dominant view of the marrow stromal system as a reservoir of bone cells, but also by the circumstance that aging affects bone as an organ. Structural changes in bone are accompanied by structural changes in the marrow and both reflect changes in a continuous cellular system encompassing cell types found in the two tissues.

BONE TURNOVER AND AGING

Bone turnover is a necessary event in order to maintain calcium homeostasis to replace hypermineralized foci with "younger," tougher tissue and to restore bone that has become defective through development and propagation of microfractures (see Chapter 25). Bone turnover is initiated by the formation of an osteoclast on the surface of bone that has been targeted for resorption by factors that have yet to be fully characterized. Endosteal surface cells retract, thereby exposing the underlying matrix. This surface must be modified either by the osteoclast itself or by nearby cells such that the thin layer of unmineralized osteoid is removed prior to the attachment and fusion of osteoclastic precursor cells to form a fully mature osteoclast, which excavates a packet of bone that must then be refilled. After a phase in which monocytic cells of unknown origin follow in the trail of the osteoclast, osteogenic precursor cells repopulate the gap and, when turnover is in balance, the amount of bone that is deposited is equivalent to the amount that was removed. Age-related bone loss, like other circumstances characterized by a change in skeletal mass, can be seen as the result of an alteration in bone turnover. With aging, the process of bone turnover becomes attenuated [1]. Consequently, the half-life of the bone matrix is extended, as is its exposure to fatigue damage and microfracture, resulting in inferior material properties [2]. In addition, turnover becomes unbalanced such that the amount of bone that is deposited is less than what was removed (Fig. 1). There are several possible scenarios by which both the attenuation of bone turnover and the lack of complete filling can occur, mediated by osteoclastic cells, osteogenic cells, or both.

OSTEOBLASTIC CELLS

Bone Formation, Osteogenic Cells, and the Marrow Stromal System

Commonly, bone formation is alluded to as a single uniform process initiated by a specialized cell type—the osteoblast—which differentiates from committed precursors within the osteogenic lineage. Indeed, there are several variants (patterns) of the process that take place in, and characterize, specific events in the physiology of the organism; all are marked by the common denominator of *bone formation.* Some of these patterns (membranous bone formation, subperiosteal bone formation, and endochondral bone formation) are specifically related to bone growth, either during development or postnatally. They provide the means whereby bone is formed *de novo* in order to secure the basis for bone shaping (modeling) and growth. They involve the differentiation of osteoblasts from committed precursor cells associated with specific tissues (the periosteum or the osteogenic mesenchyme) and result in the deposition of a mineralized bone matrix that is chemically, structurally, and kinetically peculiar (collagen poor, fast mineralizing, woven, or primary bone). Bone formation that occurs during postnatal remodeling, in contrast, does not generate bone *de novo,* is characterized by a different matrix stoichiometry and structure (lamellar bone) [3,4], and takes place, as far as trabecular bone is concerned, in a special environment provided by the bone marrow, with which the bone trabeculae are interfaced [5] (Fig. 2).

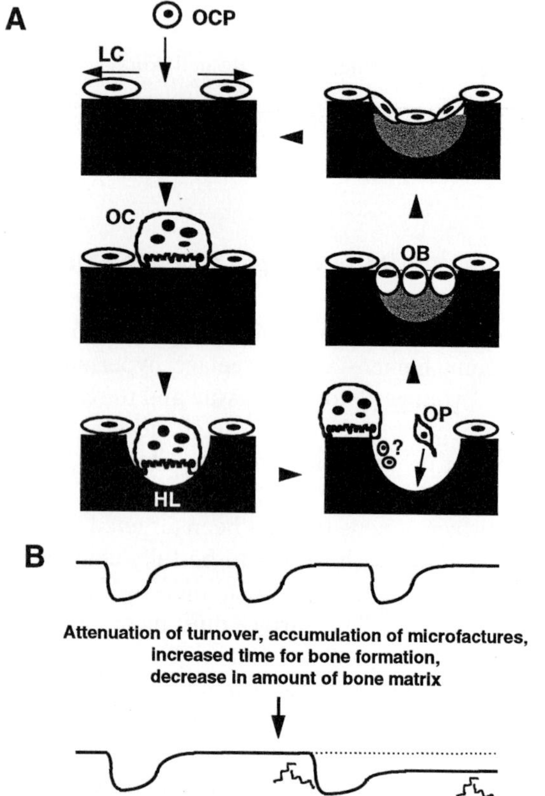

FIGURE 1 Changes in bone turnover with aging. (A) Bone turnover is a cycling process that is initiated when lining cells (LC) retract, exposing the surface of bone to osteoclast precursor cells (OCP), which fuse on the surface of bone to form a mature osteoclast (OC). The osteoclast resorbs a packet of bone forming a Howship's lacuna (HL). As the OC migrates away, the resorption bay is temporarily populated by monocytic cells of unknown origin (?), followed by osteoprogenitors (OP) from the bone marrow stroma. The progenitors form fully functioning osteoblastic cells (OB) that synthesize new bone matrix (shaded area). However, in aging, the amount of bone synthesized is not equivalent to the amount removed, and a net bone loss occurs. (B) In addition to the deficiency in bone formation, there is also a slowing of the rate of bone turnover such that the matrix is exposed for longer periods of time to damage before it is replaced, thereby leading to bone of inferior quality.

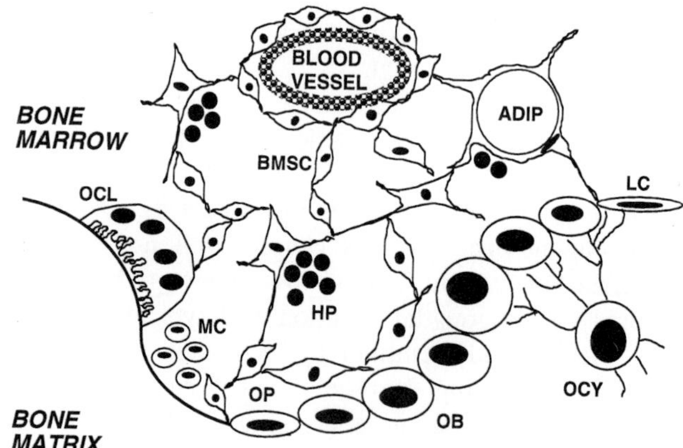

FIGURE 2 Pattern of bone formation during remodeling. Although patterns of bone formation during development and postnatal remodeling are similar, they are not identical in that they occur in different microenvironments. Bone formation during bone turnover occurs in the presence and is dependent on bone marrow, which, in addition to hematopoietic components, contains a continuous stroma that originates from marrow blood vessels. During development, cells from the presumptive periosteum/perichondrium associate with blood vessels that grow into the bond rudiment. These cells further elaborate the bone marrow stroma. This stroma is composed of uncommitted bone marrow stromal cells (BMSCs) that support hematopoiesis (HP) and adipocytes (ADIP). Following a resorptive event by an osteoclast (OCL), the resorbed area is populated by osteoprogenitors (OP) and new bone is formed by cells that subsequently go through various stages of osteoblastic maturation: preosteoblasts (POB), mature osteoblasts (OB), osteocytes (OCY), and finally quiescent osteoblasts, or lining cells (LC).

It has been recognized from the pioneering work of Friedenstein in the 1960s and Owen that bone marrow contains a population of cells that serve as a pool of progenitors that have the ability to form bone, cartilage, hematopoiesis-supportive stroma, and adipocytes [6,7]. From this basis, the view that these cells represent the local reservoir of osteoblasts to be enrolled in the process of trabecular bone remodeling has gained wide acceptance.

It is also now well accepted that this population of progenitors originates from the bone marrow stroma. This *in vivo* stroma provides not only mechanical support for the formation of blood components, but also functional support through the expression of various cytokines and growth factors [8]. Furthermore, after activation, they secrete autocrine and paracrine factors that regulate how they participate in endochondral bone formation following fracture and bone formation following a resorptive event. The physical stroma is a continuous network composed of apparently distinct cell phenotypes, including adipocytes, cells lining the bone surface (lining cells, or inactive osteoblasts), and what has been described as "reticular cells." One of the most notable features of this stroma is that although it is a connective tissue, unlike other connective tissues, it is relatively devoid of extracellular matrix, and its architecture is primarily one of cell surface interfaces. It is a highly sophisticated structure designed for the optimization of direct cell–cell interactions and cell signaling by soluble factors [9].

Identification of cell types within the physical stroma *in vivo* has remained elusive, clouded by the presence of hematopoiesis and by the highly complicated morphology of its constituent cell types. Furthermore, there is a paucity of techniques to adequately image them. Perhaps the most useful marker to date was first described by Westen and Bainton, who used alkaline phosphatase activity to highlight bone marrow reticular cells upon which hematopoiesis occurs [10]. These "Westen–Bainton" cells are clearly a key cellular element in the bone marrow stroma. However, as we still do not know what regulates alkaline phosphatase activity in stromal cells, the sensitivity of alkaline phosphatase activity for identifying all stromal cells may be lower than desirable. There is one marker, STRO-1, that has been used for sorting of stromal cells from the bone marrow population [11]; however, its utility in marking stromal cells *in situ* has not been determined to date. Complete identification of the stromal population may require the development of more specific markers and techniques that will allow for their imaging *in vivo* [9].

The situation becomes even more unclear when stroma is studied *in vitro*. When single cell suspensions of bone marrow are explanted, the adherent population contains macrophages, endothelial cells, and mature adipocytes (of which the latter two generally do not survive for prolonged periods of time) and a cell that has been termed a colony forming unit-fibroblast (CFU-F) based on its ability to form colonies of cells that have some, but not all, fibroblastic characteristics. It is these cells, the CFU-F, that have been found to proliferate and produce bone, cartilage, hematopoiesis-supportive stroma, and adipocytes based on a large number of *in vivo* and *in vitro* studies [12]. It is not clear, however, whether CFU-Fs represent the entire population of stromal cells present *in vivo*. Likewise, the diversity in terms of the differentiation potential of CFU-Fs is beginning to emerge from studies using clonal strains in *in vivo* or *in vitro* differentiation assays. Their diversity in proliferation potential is still largely unexplored, despite the major relevance that this property has with respect to their putative "stem" cell character. Furthermore, as the very concept of CFU-F relates to *in vitro* studies, and a reasonable panel of *in vivo* markers is missing to date, it has not been possible to unequivocally match the *in vitro* clonogenic ability to any defined *in vivo* counterpart. Consequently, there is a gap in our knowledge of the cells in the stroma, both *in vivo* and *in vitro*. Based on prevailing evidence to date, the multipotential stromal cell is best defined as a cell present in the extravascular marrow spaces that is part of the physical stroma. It is not of hematopoietic origin, although it supports hematopoiesis (both physically and functionally) and can give rise (in appropriate assays) to one or more of a variety of connective tissues. Although these cells have been termed "mesenchymal stem cells" by some [13], their true *stem* cell character (i.e., the ability to self-replicate and remain multipotential for the life span of the organism) has never been formally determined. Consequently, for lack of a better term, these cells are perhaps best referred to using the operational label of bone marrow stromal cells (BMSCs). Further discussion of marrow cultures as a model for skeletal aging can be found in Chapter 7.

The Balance of Phenotypes within the Stromal System

Phenotypes observed in the bone marrow stroma *in vivo* or generated from CFU-F in appropriate assays (fibroblastic/reticular cells, adipocytes, osteogenic cells) comprise the so-called stromal system [14]. Plasticity, meaning the reversible nature of individual phenotypes and their ability to convert to other phenotypes comprised in the system, is a unique feature of the stromal system. Evidence for this has been obtained both *in vivo* and *in vitro*. *In vivo,* alkaline phosphatase-positive reticular cells can become adipocytes upon reduction of the marrow hematopoietic activity, as has been observed in leukemia patients treated with chemotherapeutic agents [15]. *In vitro,* clonally derived cells that display an adipocytic phenotype have been shown to form bone when transplanted in diffusion chambers *in vivo* [16]. Furthermore, these clonally derived adipocytes can resume proliferation and switch directly to an osteogenic phenotype *in vitro* and vice versa [17]. Several additional pieces of evidence for important lineage links between osteogenic and adipocytic cells can also be found in more recent *in vitro* studies (reviewed in Ref. 18).

In vivo, adipocytes appear in the bone marrow stroma postnatally and progressively increase in number as a function of bone growth and age [9]. Increased numbers of adipocytes in the marrow thus represent the most obvious change in the stromal cell composition *in vivo* that occurs with aging. Histomorphometric analysis indicates that there is a decrease in the number of mature osteoblasts with decreased activity [2,19,20]. The increased numbers of adipocytes observed in osteoporosis [21] and age-related bone loss [22] reflect the increased space made available by the relative reduction in hematopoietic cell mass, and even bone mass per se (Fig. 3). Adipocytes represent a direct conversion of alkaline phosphatase-positive reticular (Westen–Bainton) cells, which are able to accumulate fat while losing alkaline phosphatase activity and appear to be in a quantitative inverse relationship with them [23]. A number of animal studies, and observations from human specimens, point to the possibility that the osteogenic potential of the bone marrow stroma diminishes with age. This may be linked to the observed reduction in CFU-F that also occurs with age (reviewed later). The prospect that increased adipogenesis and reduced osteogenic potential of the aging marrow are linked to one another would fit with *in vivo* and *in vitro* observations and with the notion of stromal cell plasticity and balance between different phenotypes. The extent to which these altered balances could be reversed *in vivo* obviously represents an important unanswered question. The recognition of factors regulating the balance between stromal phenotypes (and as a result also of the relative cellular composition of the stromal system and its osteogenic efficacy) is of critical importance in addressing this question. Such information would also clarify how much of the changes in the biology of the stroma occurring with age reflect an altered systemic milieu versus inherent changes of the aging cells themselves.

Extrinsic Regulation of Differentiation within the Stromal System

In the postnatal organism, changes in the balance of systemic factors (such as parathyroid hormone (PTH), vitamin D metabolites, sex steroids, growth factors, and cytokines, which are likely to change in aging) alter

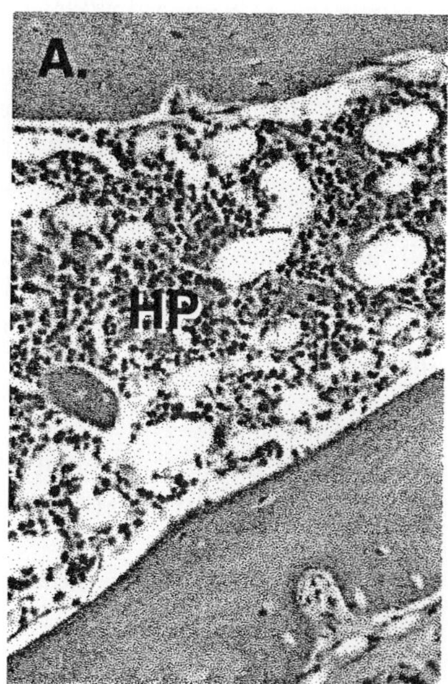

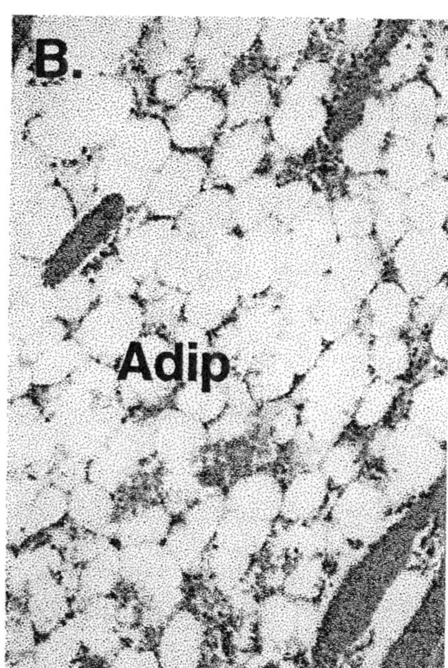

FIGURE 3 Conversion of red marrow to yellow marrow during aging. (A) During postnatal growth, the bone marrow stroma supports hematopoiesis (HP). In addition, stroma supports osteoblastogenesis and osteoclastogenesis during bone turnover, which is essential for maintaining normal skeletal functions. (B) With aging, the stroma shifts its phenotype to one primarily of adipocytes, thereby causing a defect in osteoblastogenesis and possibly osteoclastogenesis.

bone metabolism through direct effects on BMSCs [24]. *In vitro* studies, using primarily mouse and rat cells, have more clearly delineated the factors mediating changes in the phenotypic balance of BMSCs. These studies have focused on the expression of osteoblastic and adipogenic markers [alkaline phosphatase activity, expression of bone matrix proteins, generation of "bone nodules" versus aP2, lipoprotein lipase (LPL), peroxisome proliferator-activated receptors (PPAR-γ), and accumulation of fat], as well as the ability to support the formation of hematopoietic lineages (Fig. 4). Based on studies from numerous cell lines (transformed or spontaneously immortalized) and normal cells [25], the regulation of conversion from an osteogenic to an adipogenic phenotype and vice versa and support of hematopoiesis appear to be mediated by steroids and peptide hormones, members of the transforming growth factor β (TGF-β) superfamily, and proinflammatory cytokines. However, there is a great deal of variability in requirements for the expression of one phenotype versus another. This may be due to differences between animal species or to the timing at which point factors are added to the *in vitro* stromal culture systems. This latter point reemphasizes

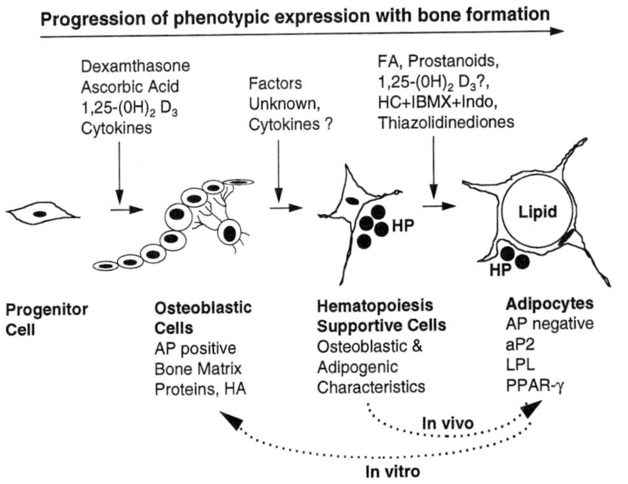

FIGURE 4 Constituent cells of the bone marrow stromal system: a potential model. The bone marrow stroma contains a family of progenitor cells that give rise to a number of phenotypes, including osteogenic cells [characterized by alkaline phosphatase activity and the production of bone matrix proteins and deposition of hydroxyapatite (HA)], hematopoiesis supportive stroma (which exhibits osteoblastic and adipogenic character), and adipocytes (which express aP2, LPL and PPAR-γ, with lipid accumulation). *In vitro* studies have characterized some of the factors that may regulate the sequential expression of these different phenotypes as a bone/bone marrow organ is formed. In addition, *in vivo* and *in vitro* evidence suggests that this lineage is very "plastic" and is able to convert from one phenotype to another directly. This plasticity of bone marrow stromal cells allows for changes in bone marrow to accomodate the metabolic needs of the organism and can be the cause or the result of a disease state.

that BMSCs at different stages of maturation or commitment may have different responses to these factors.

When single cell suspensions of human bone marrow are plated at high density, a monolayer of adherent cells develops rapidly and both osteogenic and adipogenic markers are expressed concomitantly [26]. If the nonadherent cell population is not removed, and the culture medium is appropriate, hematopoiesis is supported, although it is not exuberant in human bone marrow cultures. If rodent or human bone marrow suspensions are plated at lower densities such that single colonies are formed, colonies with osteoblastic features, enumerated by alkaline phosphatase and accumulation of calcium phosphate (Alizarin Red or von Kossa staining), can be readily distinguished from adipocytic colonies that are identified by Oil Red O staining for lipid. Colonies negative for either set of markers are also regularly formed [17,27] (Kuznetsov and Gehron Robey, unpublished results). By including dexamethasone and ascorbic acid-2-phosphate in the culture medium at the time of initial plating, there is an increase in osteoblastic character [17] (Kuznetsov and Gehron Robey, unpublished results), which, in rat cultures, is further enhanced by the later addition of 1,25-dihydroxyvitamin D_3 [28]. The stimulation of osteogenesis by dexamethasone *in vitro* is somewhat enigmatic since long-term glucocorticoid therapy is associated with a decrease in bone mass in humans. Consequently, the interaction of other factors in the *in vivo* environment most likely mitigates the positive effect of glucocorticoids found *in vitro.* Estrogen [29–31], TGF-β super family members [32–36], Interleukin-1 (IL-1), Tumor Necrosis Factor-α (TNF), and members of the IL-6 cytokine family [37] also exert positive effects on osteoblastogenesis at the expense of adipogenesis in BMSCs *in vitro,* as demonstrated primarily in rodent cell cultures (reviewed in Ref. 37).

Conversion of progenitor cells to the adipogenic phenotype has been noted by changing the type of serum that is used in the culture medium [17,38]; it has been found that fatty acids in rabbit serum increase adipogenesis [39]. In general, factors that activate PPAR-γ or induce CAAT/enhancer-binding protein (C/EBP) (a transcription factor essential for adipogenesis), such as fatty acids and prostaglandins, induce adipogenesis (reviewed in Ref. 18). Routinely, the addition of hydrocortisone, isobutyl methylxanthine (IBMX), and indomethasone to BMSC cultures induces the adipogenic phenotype [37], as does a class of antidiabetic compounds, the thiazolidinediones [18,37]. Pharmacological doses of dexamethasone may also induce adipocyte formation [40]. The role of 1,25-dihydroxyvitamin D_3 in adipogenesis is unclear in that it has been reported to induce adipocyte formation when added alone or simultaneously with dexamethasone [41] or to block adipogenesis induced by the cocktail of hydrocortisone, IBMX, and indomethacin [42]. Members of the TGF-β superfamily also have pleiomorphic effects, with low concentrations being inductive and higher concentrations being inhibitory [43].

In long-term Dexter-type cultures that support hematopoiesis, the underlying adherent cell layer has been found to have osteoblastic and adipocytic character [44,45]. It is not known whether different members of the BMSC family support the differentiation of different types of hemopoietic cells. Few studies have addressed the issue of what factors modulate the ability of BMSCs to support specific hematopoietic lineages, but the addition of IL-11 to long-term Dexter-type cultures has been reported to increase the expansion of myeloid and mixed progenitors, but not of erythroid progenitors. This change in hematopoietic potential was concomitant with changes in the nature of the stromal cell layer, including a decrease in adipogenesis [46]. The donor age of stromal cells seems to influence the type of hematopoietic lineage that is preferentially supported [47]. In *in vitro* studies of long-term Dexter-type cultures from a mouse model of osteopenia, the supportive stromal layer was primarily adipogenic and supported myelopoiesis [48]. Aging stroma seems less capable of supporting B cell lymphopoiesis *in vitro* [49].

Intrinsic Properties of the Aging Stromal System

There is no doubt that extrinsic factors have a profound effect on cells in the BMSC lineage and alter their metabolism in a way that leads to decreased bone mass. It is also clear that the behavior of the cells themselves changes as a function of age as well. *In vitro* studies directly comparing metabolic activities of cells derived from donors of different ages eliminate the varying systemic milieu that cells are exposed to *in vivo* (see Chapter 6). These types of studies indicate that bone-forming cells do indeed have a "memory" of what their functional status was *in situ* and that the aging cell has altered responsiveness to external signals, perhaps through changes in receptor content, receptor activity, intracellular signaling pathways, and regulation of gene expression. It is not known how such changes are stabilized within the genome of the cell, but this is clearly an area that requires far more research in order to derive new methodologies for cell "rejuvenation." For the time being, however, avenues of investigation include (1) quantitative changes in precursor cells in the marrow stroma, (2) altered rates of cell proliferation, (3) an intrinsically altered balance of differentiation within the stromal system, and (4) changes in the matrix secreted by osteogenic cells.

Decreased Number of Precursor Cells The possibility of an intrinsic cell defect is supported by the observation that there are fewer progenitors present in aged bone marrow [27,50–53]. These observations are based on colony-forming efficiency assays, whereby single cell suspensions of marrow are plated at a low density in the presence of an appropriate feeder cell layer and allowed to generate as separate colonies that are the progeny of CFU-F. These data imply that the "stem" cell compartment has lost its ability to replenish itself with age (which, in fact, would warrant a reexamination of the term mesenchymal "stem" cell).

However, there are a number of caveats in this type of analysis. First, it is not clear what the CFU-F that proliferates *in vitro* represents *in vivo*. Some studies have used AP as the marker by which colonies are identified, but this may lead to an underestimation of the colony-forming efficiency and the number of progenitor cells present *in situ*. Another potential caveat is the manner by which the marrow is obtained. If a bone marrow aspirate is used, it is very difficult to determine the amount of peripheral blood that contaminates the true marrow, even when using various correction factors. Furthermore, it has been found that peripheral blood may exert a negative effect on colony formation [54]. In addition, the way in which the colony-forming efficiency assay is established *in vitro* has a profound effect on the enumeration of CFU-F. Methods that utilize the separation of different cell populations prior to plating by centrifugation through various forms of media, or any other type of manipulation, may result in an underestimate of CFU-F due to their highly adhesive nature. It is also known that the factors that stimulate the proliferation of CFU-F to form colonies are produced by the nonadherent, hematopoietic population of bone marrow. Consequently, complete colony-forming efficiency in many animal species (with the exception of human) requires appropriate nonadherent feeder cells [55], and there are different requirements for the number of feeder cells depending on the animal species [56]. If autologous feeder cells are used, it must be recognized that aging also has an impact on them and could influence their ability to support complete colony formation. Despite these potential caveats, it would appear that the number of BMSCs is decreased as a function of age and is a contributing factor to age-related bone loss (Fig. 5). The decreased number of CFU-F has been linked to a decrease in osteoblastogenesis and to a decrease in bone mass as a function of age [27]. In addition, because osteoclastogenesis is also dependent on this population of cells, it is also likely that decreased numbers of CFU-F are also linked to the attenuation of bone turnover noted with age [27].

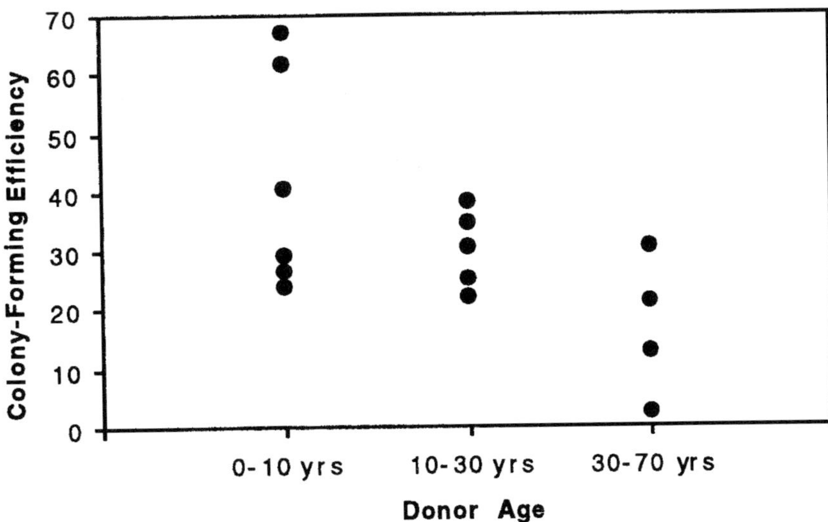

FIGURE 5 Colony-forming efficiency of human CFU-F as a function of age. Although there are a number of caveats in determining colony-forming efficiency, colony-forming efficiency generally decreases as a function of aging (S. A. Kuznetsov and P. Gehron Robey, unpublished results).

Proliferation Rate After activation of BMSCs, the rate at which they proliferate may also contribute to reduced bone formation in aging. The limited studies that have evaluated the doubling time of cells in the BMSC lineage *ex vivo* as a function of donor age do not provide a clear indication of the role that the proliferation rate plays in age-related bone loss. In rodent BMSC cultures, doubling time has been reported to be unchanged under normal culture conditions [57], but is decreased with serum starvation [53] or slower with age [47]. In cultures derived from more mature human cells from trabecular bone, there is a trend toward an increase in doubling time with increasing age of the donor [58–60]. Aged rodent cells have been found to be less responsive to mitogenic stimuli such as basic Fibroblast Growth Factor (bFGF) [61]. The reason for this decrease in the proliferation rate may be related to reduced synthesis and secretion of autocrine and paracrine factors, number or activity of cognate receptors, or to changes in the intracellular signaling pathways that lead to cell division in the aging cell.

Intrinsic Changes in the Balance between Different Phenotypes within the BMSC Lineage Although the shift in phenotypes of the BMSC lineage is highly dependent on the systemic factors to which they are exposed, it is also possible that there is a level of commitment that limits their ability to shift from one phenotype to another. Studies using single colony derived strains of human BMSCs have showed that upon *in vivo* transplantation in an open system, the colonies vary remarkably in their ability to give rise to different/multiple phenotypes. Approximately 56% of the clones were able to generate bone, while others formed only fibrous tissue. Of the bone-forming clones, only 24% formed a complete "ossicle" (i.e., a miniature organ including hematopoiesis-supportive stroma and associated adipocytes) [62]. Because these experiments were performed *in vivo,* where presumably all of the necessary extrinsic factors would be available to the cells, these data imply that there are intrinsic differences in the differentiation potential of members of the BMSC population. How these differences are affected by age and to what extent they might be reversed remain to be determined.

Reduced Cellular Activity Although few published studies compare cellular activities of bone-forming cells as a function of age, available evidence indicates that a number of metabolic parameters are altered in aging bone cells. Aged rodent cells with osteoblastic phenotype are less responsive to PTH's stimulation of cAMP production (despite equivalent binding of PTH compared to young cells), presumably due to the downregulation of the G protein that regulates adenylyl cyclase activity, Gs-α [63]. A decrease in the secretion of several autocrine and paracrine factors has also been reported in rodent cells [64]. With increasing donor age, a decrease in alkaline phosphatase has been noted *in vitro* in rodents [52,57].

Inasmuch as a primary function of osteoblastic cells is to make mineralized matrix, a decrease in their ability to do so would clearly influence bone mass and contribute to age-related bone loss. At the cellular level *in vivo* in rodents, mRNA for various bone matrix proteins as measured by *in situ* hybridization in morphologically identifyable osteoblasts was decreased with age [19]. This leads to a decreased percentage of mineralizable osteoid [65]. Further analysis in rodents indicates that there is initially a decrease in osteoblastic activity during aging, which is then followed by a decrease in osteoblast number [66].

In vitro, the rate at which rodent and human osteoblastic cells synthesize bone matrix proteins (collagen, versican, decorin, biglycan, osteonectin [58,59], and osteocalcin [57,67]) decreases with age on a per cell basis. Postnatally in humans, the maximum rates of synthesis on a per cell basis were noted during puberty, at which point they gradually decreased to a baseline level by the third decade [58,59]. Consequently, the time that it would take to completely fill in a resorbed area would be longer, and with advancing age, the cells may never complete their task. This decreased capacity for bone matrix synthesis has been verified whereby demineralized bone matrix induced less bone in old rodents than in young ones [68], and BMSCs from aged donors produced less bone when transplanted *in vivo* in rodents [52].

Changes in Matrix Composition It has long been recognized that as bone ages, the protein content decreases. Bone matrix constituents (with the exception of highly cross-linked collagen) are slowly degraded by enzymes that are present in the matrix, secreted either locally or adsorbed from the circulation by virtue of their affinity to hydroxyapatite [69]. The removal of these noncollagenous proteins is thought to influence the size and shape of the mineral. It has been found that in humans that the mineral crystals become larger, fuse, and form plates with age [70]. From a biomechanical point of view, this causes a change in the material properties of bone such that it becomes more brittle. In addition, the relative percentages of bone matrix proteins synthesized during bone turnover also change with age. During puberty, when matrix synthesis reaches its maximum rate, the secreted proteins are primarily collagenous in nature, and there is relatively more biglycan than decorin and osteonectin. After approximately the third decade, the synthesis of many of the matrix proteins reaches a baseline rate. Their relative ratio is quite different, with collagen representing a lower percentage, and biglycan, decorin, and osteonectin being nearly equivalent [58,59]. It has also been found that extracts of bone isolated from aged donors have a reduced calcium-binding capacity [71]. This change in matrix composition as a function of age has an impact on the biomechanical properties of bone, as reflected by changes in strength, resilience, and distribution of stress and strain (see Chapter 25). It must also be recognized that while bone matrix proteins play a major structural role in bone formation, they also play major roles in mediating cell metabolism [72] (reviewed in Ref. 73). Decreased levels and changes in relative ratios very likely influence the activity of cells in the bone microenvironment. For example, advanced glycation end products (AGE) accumulate on long-lived proteins, such as collagen, as a function of age. Bone cell differentiation *in vitro* is inhibited by AGEs [74], and these metabolites stimulate osteogenic cells to secrete higher levels of IL-6 [75].

OSTEOCLASTS

Maturation of Osteoclasts from Hematopoietic Progenitors

Osteoclasts are generated from hematopoietic precursor cells that are present in the bone marrow [76], under the control of systemic osteotropic hormones and of local factors that are produced by cells of the BMSC lineage and by other cell types in the marrow microenvironment (Fig. 6). Prevailing evidence indicates that the CFU-GM (granulocyte–macrophage) lineage not only gives rise to monocytes and macrophages, but also to osteoclastic precursor cells (reviewed in Refs. 77 and 78).

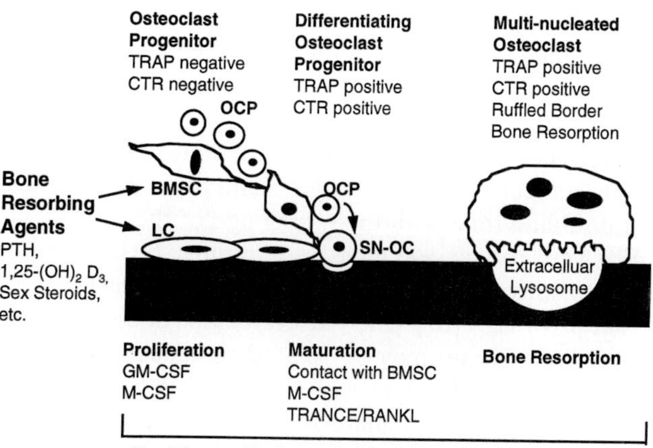

FIGURE 6 Osteoclastogenesis. Induction of osteoclastogenesis is mediated by members of the bone marrow stromal cell (BMSC) population, which may also include lining cells (LC). Osteoclast precursors (OCP) are stimulated to proliferate by factors that are synthesized by BMSCs, including M-CSF. Further maturation requires cell–cell contact and appears to be dependent on the production of TRANCE/RANKL (osteoclast differentiation factor). A mononuclear osteoclast (SN-OC) (more or less apparent, depending on the animal species) fuses with other mature progenitors, forms a ruffled border, and establishes an extracellular lysosomal compartment into which acid and lysosomal enzymes are secreted to degrade bone. Many other factors influence this process, but may have varying effects depending on what stage of the process they become available to the osteoclastic cells.

INFLUENCE OF STROMAL CELLS AND THEIR PROGENY

The regulation of osteoclasts in bone resorption is indirect. Osteoclastic precursor cells and mature osteoclasts do not bear receptors for many of the factors that stimulate bone resorption. This fact led to the commonly held belief that "osteoblasts" are the mediators of bone resorption [79]. However, based on current understanding of the bone marrow stroma and recent studies elucidating the role of stromal cells in osteoclastogenesis (reviewed extensively in Ref. 78), it is likely that members of the BMSC lineage are major regulators of osteoclast formation and activity [77]. Supportive cells include hematopoiesis-supportive BMSCs and those committed to the osteogenic phenotype, including osteocytes, and perhaps even those with an adipocytic phenotype [18].

In the first stages of osteoclastogenesis, proliferation of the CFU-GM lineage and initial commitment requires CSF-1 (M-CSF) [80] synthesized by BMSCs. Subsequent osteoclast formation requires direct cell to cell contact of the precursor cells with BMSCs [81,82]. The nature of this association is not yet known but is mediated by various forms of cell surface molecules on both stromal cells and osteoclast precursor cells such as integrins (α_v β_3) [83], cadherins (E-cadherin) [84], and cell adhesion molecules (CAMs) [85].

Other data imply the existence of a stromal cell surface protein that would be required for osteoclastogenesis ("osteoclast differentiation factor"). This potentially critical factor has been isolated via its association with the osteoprotergin/osteoclast inhibitory factor and was identified as TRANCE/RANKL, a member of the membrane-associated TNF ligand family. It is speculated that osteoprotegerin/osteoclast inhibitory factor acts as a soluble inhibitor of TRANCE/RANKL. In the absence of osteoprotegerin, this molecule binds to a putative receptor on the membrane of the osteoclast precursor [86].

BONE RESORPTION

Prior to osteoclastic resorption, endosteal lining cells retract by mechanisms that are not well understood, but may be related to exposure of these cells to PTH in some cases. Furthermore, these lining cells may provide signals (some of which have been described earlier) that cause osteoclastic cells to adhere and fuse with one another on the bone surface to form a resorption pit (Howship's lacuna). Howship's lacuna results from the formation of what is functionally speaking an extracellular lysosomal compartment, the integrity of which is maintained by the establishment of a sealing zone. The apical surface of the osteoclast in apposition to the bone is highly invaginated to form a ruffled border. After acidification of this extracellular compartment by the action of carbonic anhydrase II to partially demineralize the bone surface, large quantities of lysosomal enzymes, including cathepsins, are secreted to degrade bone matrix [87].

After removal of a quantity of bone, the osteoclast moves to an adjacent area of bone and extends the resorptive area or disappears from the resorption pit that it has created, possibly undergoing apoptosis. Factors that regulate the cessation of a cycle of resorption in a particular site are not clearly delineated, but may be related to an increase in the local concentration of calcium and phosphate, binding of calcitonin, glucocorticoid status, interferon-γ levels, and release of factors, such as TGF-β, from the degraded mineralized matrix. Regulation of the demise of osteoclasts is not well understood to date, but may be modulated by sex hormones. It is also not known whether aging influences the length of the life span of an osteoclast.

Factors That Regulate Osteoclastic Activity

Maturation of precursors and activity of fused cells are further stimulated by systemic factors such as PTH, vitamin D analogs, sex hormones, and local factors (IL-1, IL-3, IL-4, IL-6, IL-11, LIF, OSM, TNF-α, TGF-α, and prostaglandins, to name but a few). IL-1, IL-6, and TNF-α are produced by monocytes and macrophages in the bone microenvironment. BMSCs also produce these cytokines along with M-CSF, GM-CSF, LIF, OSM, IL-3, IL-11, and the third component of complement, C3. The long list of factors that have been shown to modulation the process of osteoclast formation and activity *in vitro* is indicative of a complicated regulatory pathway. Furthermore, these factors have different effects of osteoclast generation, depending on when they are available to the system (reviewed in Refs. 77, 78). They may ultimately lead into a common pathway that results in the activity of the putative osteoclast differentiation factor, TRANCE/RANKL.

Changes in Bone Resorption with Aging

INFLUENCE OF HEMATOPOIETIC STATUS

Keeping in mind the hematopoietic origin of osteoclastic precursor cells and the fact that cells in the hematopoietic lineages produce factors that influence members of the BMSC lineage, it is apparent that the hematopoietic status of the organism may also be reflected in changes in the rate of bone turnover. With aging, many factors have an impact on hematopoietic status due to hormonal abnormalities, disease(s), and treatment for a variety of disorders [88]. However, there may be decreases in the level of peripheral blood stem cells [89] and in the hematopoietic reserve capacity [90] as a function of age. The activity of hematopoietic cells, such as macrophages, also varies with aging [91]. An impaired ability of stromal cells to support the differentiation of certain types of blood cells has been noted [49] due to the decreases in factors produced by stromal cells that are responsible for stimulating the generation of hematopoietic components [92]. It has been reported that there is an increase in myelopoiesis in an animal model of age-related osteopenia [48].

Regulation by Stromal Cells

Because members of the BMSC lineage are responsible for the generation of osteoclasts, the combined effects of extrinsic and intrinsic factors that impinge on stromal cell activity as a function of aging also impinge on their ability to stimulate osteoclast formation. As discussed earlier, the probability that there are fewer stromal cells in aging marrow may also dictate the reduced ability of aging marrow to generate osteoclasts. This has been reported in a murine model of accelerated age-related bone loss [27]. However, attenuated osteoclastogenesis may also be due to quantitative and qualitative changes in the bioactive factors that aged BMSCs secrete. It has been reported that aged BMSCs secrete decreased levels of GM-CSF, a factor necessary for the proliferation of osteoclastic precursor cells [93]. In addition, there is an age-dependent increase in IL-6 and IL-11 by human marrow stromal cell *in vitro* [94]. It is of interest that in a transgenic mouse model that overproduces human IL-6, osteoblastogenesis and osteoclastogenesis were decreased [95]. Although increased levels of IL-6 are thought to lead to an increase in bone turnover noted with a loss of gonadal function [24], in certain situations (the circumstances of which are not yet clear) IL-6 may also contribute to the attenuation of bone turnover. More data are needed to resolve whether these processes play a role in human skeletal aging.

Changes in Osteoclast Activity

In general, studies on the regulation of osteoclastic activity are based on the histomorphometric analysis of osteoclastic number and surface and on the release of biochemical markers indicative of bone resorption (collagen cross-links, for example). These studies are indicative of osteoclastic activity as a whole and do not comment directly on the activity of an osteoclast on a per cell basis. It has been postulated that in age-related bone loss, osteoclasts are more active on a per cell basis and remove more bone during a cycle of resorption [1]. Prevailing evidence strongly suggests that it is primarily reduced osteoblastic activity and number that lead to decreased bone mass in the aging skeleton.

SUMMARY

The mechanisms that cause the attenuation of bone turnover and ultimately the loss of bone and bone fragility with age have not been fully elucidated to date. However, it is clear that aging has a major impact on the structure and function of bone marrow that contains the progenitors for both osteogenic and osteoclastic cells. Bone marrow stroma contains progenitors that give rise to several different phenotypes, including osteogenic cells, hematopoiesis-supportive cells, and adipocytes. With aging there is a shift in balance from a stroma that actively supports osteogenesis and exuberant hematopoiesis to one that is primarily adipogenic and supports an altered form of hematopoiesis. The cause for this shift in phenotypic expression may be due, in part, to changes in the systemic and local factors (extrinsic factors) to which the cells are exposed as aging progresses. However, there are also factors intrinsic to stromal cells that change with age. These intrinsic factors include their lack of self-renewal (decrease in number of progenitors), decreased cellular activity (reduced responsiveness, reduced production of bone matrix proteins, and other cell products), and the apparent loss of plasticity (inability to convert from one phenotype to another). Furthermore, the combined effect of these extrinsic and intrinsic factors on bone marrow stromal cells decreases their ability to support osteoclast formation. Based on current evidence, it would appear that the primary cause of age-related bone loss is based on the inability of bone marrow stromal cells to deposit adequate amounts of bone to compensate for the amount removed by osteoclasts. Furthermore, it is possible that decreases in osteoclastic resorption lead to the accumulation of bone of inferior quality due to changes in the material properties and microfractures. Clearly, bone marrow stroma is a primary target for the development of new therapeutic modalities that could maintain an adequate number of progenitor cells, optimize their metabolic activities, and thereby establish a normal, balanced rate of bone turnover.

References

1. Eriksen, E. F. Normal and pathological remodeling of human trabecular bone: three dimensional reconstruction of the remodeling sequence in normals and in metabolic bone disease. *Endocr. Rev.* **7,** 379–408 (1986).
2. Parfitt, A. M. Bone age, mineral density, and fatigue damage. *Calcif. Tissue Int.* **53**(Suppl. 1), S82–S85 (1993).

3. Gehron Robey, P. *In* "Bone Formation and Repair" (C. T. Brighton, G. Friedlaender, and J. M. Lane, eds.), pp. 253–260. AAOS, Rosement, IL, 1994.
4. Gehron Robey, P. *In* "Bone Formation and Repair" (C. T. Brighton, G. Friedlaender, and J. M. Lane, eds.). AAOS, Rosemont, IL, 1994.
5. Gehron Robey, P., Bianco, P., and Termine, J. D. *In* "Disorders of Mineral Metabolism" (M. J. Favus, and F. L. Coe, eds.), pp. 241–263. Raven Press, New York, 1992.
6. Friedenstein, A. J., Piatetzky, S., II, and Petrakova, K. V. Osteogenesis in transplants of bone marrow cells. *J. Embryol. Exp. Morphol.* **16,** 381–90 (1966).
7. Owen, M. The origin of bone cells. *Int. Rev. Cytol.* **28,** 213–238 (1970).
8. Chailakhyan, R. K., Gerasimov, Y. V., and Friedenstein, A. J. Transfer of bone marrow microenvironment by clones of stromal mechanocytes. *Bull. Exp. Biol. Med.* **86,** 1633–1635 (1978).
9. Bianco, P., and Riminucci, M. *In* "Marrow Stromal Cell Cultures" (J. N. Beresford and M. Owen, eds.), pp. 10–25. Cambridge Univ. Press, Cambridge, UK, 1998.
10. Westen, H., and Bainton, D. F. Association of alkaline phosphatase positive reticulum cells in the bone marrow with granulocytic precursors. *J. Exp. Med.* **150,** 919–937 (1979).
11. Simmons, P. J., and Torok-Storb, B. Identification of stromal cell precursors in human bone marrow by a novel monoclonal antibody, STRO-1. *Blood* **78,** 55–62 (1991).
12. Friedenstein, A. J., Gorskaja, J. F., and Kulagina, N. N. Fibroblast precursors in normal and irradiated mouse hematopoietic organs. *Exp. Hematol.* **4,** 267–274 (1976).
13. Caplan, A. I. Mesenchymal stem cells. *J. Orthop. Res.* **9,** 641–650 (1991).
14. Owen, M., and Friedenstein, A. J. Stromal stem cells: marrow-derived osteogenic precursors. *Ciba Found. Symp.* **136,** 42–60 (1988).
15. Bianco, P., Costantini, M., Dearden, L. C., and Bonucci, E. Alkaline phosphatase positive precursors of adipocytes in the human bone marrow. *Br. J. Haematol.* **68,** 401–403 (1988).
16. Bennett, J. H., Joyner, C. J., Triffitt, J. T., and Owen, M. E. Adipocytic cells cultured from marrow have osteogenic potential. *J. Cell Sci.* **99,** 131–139 (1991).
17. Beresford, J. N., Bennett, J. H., Devlin, C., Leboy, P. S., and Owen, M. E. Evidence for an inverse relationship between the differentiation of adipocytic and osteogenic cells in rat marrow stromal cell cultures. *J. Cell Sci.* **102,** 341–351 (1992).
18. Gimble, J. M., Robinson, C. E., Wu, X., and Kelly, K. A. The function of adipocytes in the bone marrow stroma: an update. *Bone* **19,** 421–428 (1996).
19. Ikeda, T., Nagai, Y., Yamaguchi, A., Yokose, S., and Yoshiki, S. Age-related reduction in bone matrix protein mRNA expression in rat bone tissues: application of histomorphometry to *in situ* hybridization. *Bone* **16,** 17–23 (1995).
20. Roholl, P. J., Blauw, E., Zurcher, C., Dormans, J. A., and Theuns, H. M. Evidence for a diminished maturation of preosteoblasts into osteoblasts during aging in rats: an ultrastructural analysis. *J. Bone Miner. Res.* **9,** 355–366 (1994).
21. Meunier, P., Aron, J., Eduoard, C., and Vignon, G. Osteoporosis and the replacement of cell populations of the marrow by adipose tissue: a quantitative study of 84 iliac bone biopsies. *Clin. Orthop.* **80,** 147–154 (1971).
22. Rozman, C., Feliu, E., Berga, L., Reverter, J. C., Climent, C., and Ferran, M. J. Age-related variations of fat tissue fraction in normal human bone marrow depend both on size and number of adipocytes: a stereological study. *Exp. Hematol.* **17,** 34–37 (1989).
23. Bianco, P., Bradbeer, J. N., Riminucci, M., and Boyde, A. Marrow stromal (Western-Bainton) cells: identification, morphometry, confocal imaging and changes in disease. *Bone* **14,** 315–320 (1993).
24. Manolagas, S. C., and Jilka, R. L. Bone marrow, cytokines, and bone remodeling. Emerging insights into the pathophysiology of osteoporosis. *N. Engl. J. Med.* **332,** 305–311 (1995).
25. Deryugina, E. I., and Muller-Sieburg, C. E. Stromal cells in long-term cultures: keys to the elucidation of hematopoietic development? *Crit. Rev. Immunol.* **13,** 115–150 (1993).
26. Rickard, D. J., Kassem, M., Hefferan, T. E., Sarkar, G., Spelsberg, T. C., and Riggs, B. L. Isolation and characterization of osteoblast precursor cells from human bone marrow. *J. Bone Miner. Res.* **11,** 312–324 (1996).
27. Jilka, R. L., Weinstein, R. S., Takahashi, K., Parfitt, A. M., and Manolagas, S. C. Linkage of decreased bone mass with impaired osteoblastogenesis in a murine model of accelerated senescence. *J. Clin. Invest.* **97,** 1732–1740 (1996).
28. Rickard, D. J., Kazhdan, I., and Leboy, P. S. Importance of 1,25-dihydroxyvitamin D3 and the nonadherent cells of marrow for osteoblast differentiation from rat marrow stromal cells. *Bone* **16,** 671–678 (1995).
29. Benayahu, D. Estrogen effects on protein expressed by marrow stromal osteoblasts. *Biochem. Biophys. Res. Commun.* **233,** 30–35 (1997).
30. Shamay, A., Knopov, V., and Benayahu, D. The expression of estrogen receptor and estrogen effect in MBA-15 marrow stromal osteoblasts. *Cell Biol. Int.* **20,** 401–405 (1996).
31. Zhang, R. W., Supowit, S. C., Xu, X., Li, H., Christensen, M. D., Lozano, R., and Simmons, D. J. Expression of selected osteogenic markers in the fibroblast-like cells of rat marrow stroma. *Calcif. Tissue Int.* **56,** 283–291 (1995).
32. Benayahu, D., Zipori, D., and Wientroub, S. Marrow adipocytes regulate growth and differentiation of osteoblasts. *Biochem. Biophys. Res. Commun.* **197,** 1245–1252 (1993).
33. Gazit, D., Ebner, R., Kahn, A. J., and Derynck, R. Modulation of expression and cell surface binding of members of the transforming growth factor-beta superfamily during retinoic acid-induced osteoblastic differentiation of multipotential mesenchymal cells. *Mol. Endocrinol.* **7,** 189–198 (1993).
34. Gordon, E. M., Skotzko, M., Kundu, R. K., Han, B., Andrades, J., Nimni, M., Anderson, W. F., and Hall, F. L. Capture and expansion of bone marrow-derived mesenchymal progenitor cells with a transforming growth factor-beta1-von Willebrand's factor fusion protein for retrovirus-mediated delivery of coagulation factor IX. *Hum. Gene Ther.* **8,** 1385–1394 (1997).
35. Yamaguchi, A., Katagiri, T., Ikeda, T., Wozney, J. M., Rosen, V., Wang, E. A., Kahn, A. J., Suda, T., and Yoshiki, S. Recombinant human bone morphogenetic protein-2 stimulates osteoblastic maturation and inhibits myogenic differentiation in vitro. *J. Cell Biol.* **113,** 681–687 (1991).
36. Yamaguchi, A. Regulation of differentiation pathway of skeletal mesenchymal cells in cell lines by transforming growth factor-beta superfamily. *Semin. Cell Biol.* **6,** 165–173 (1995).
37. Gimble, J. M., Wanker, F., Wang, C. S., Bass, H., Wu, X., Kelly, K., Yancopoulos, G. D., and Hill, M. R. Regulation of bone marrow stromal cell differentiation by cytokines whose receptors share the gp130 protein. *J. Cell Biochem.* **54,** 122–133 (1994).
38. Lanotte, M., Scott, D., and Dexter, T. M. Clonal preadipocyte cell lines of different phenotypes derived from murine marrow stroma: factors influencing growth and adipogenesis *in vitro*. *J. Cell Physiol.* **111,** 177–186 (1982).
39. Diascro, D. D., Jr., Vogel, R. L., Johnson, T. E., Witherup, K. M., Pitzenberger, S. M., Rutledge, S. J., Prescott, D. J., Rodan, G. A., and Schmidt, A. High fatty acid content in rabbit serum

is responsible for the differentiation of osteoblasts into adipocyte-like cells. *J. Bone Miner. Res.* **13,** 96–106 (1998).

40. Cui, Q., Wang, G. J., and Balian, G. Steroid-induced adipogenesis in a pluripotential cell line from bone marrow. *J. Bone Joint Surg. Am.* **79,** 1054–1063 (1997).
41. Grigoriadis, A. E., Heersche, J. N., and Aubin, J. E. Differentiation of muscle, fat, cartilage, and bone from progenitor cells present in a bone-derived clonal cell population: effect of dexamethasone. *J. Cell Biol.* **106,** 2139–2151 (1988).
42. Kelly, K. A., and Gimble, J. M. 1,25-Dihydroxy vitamin D3 inhibits adipocyte differentiation and gene expression in murine bone marrow stromal cell clones and primary cultures. *Endocrinology* **139,** 2622–2628 (1998).
43. Asahina, I., Sampath, T. K., and Hauschka, P. V. Human osteogenic protein-1 induces chondroblastic, osteoblastic, and/or adipocytic differentiation of clonal murine target cells. *Exp. Cell Res.* **222,** 38–47 (1996).
44. Dorheim, M. A., Sullivan, M., Dandapani, V., Wu, X., Hudson, J., Segarini, P. R., Rosen, D. M., Aulthouse, A. L., and Gimble, J. M. Osteoblastic gene expression during adipogenesis in hematopoietic supporting murine bone marrow stromal cells. *J. Cell Physiol.* **154,** 317–328 (1993).
45. Hangoc, G., Daub, R., Maze, R. G., Falkenburg, J. H., Broxmeyer, H. E., and Harrington, M. A. Regulation of myelopoiesis by murine fibroblastic and adipogenic cell lines. *Exp. Hematol.* **21,** 502–507 (1993).
46. Keller, D. C., Du, X. X., Srour, E. F., Hoffman, R., and Williams, D. A. Interleukin-11 inhibits adipogenesis and stimulates myelopoiesis in human long-term marrow cultures. *Blood* **82,** 1428–1435 (1993).
47. Jiang, D., Fei, R. G., Pendergrass, W. R., and Wolf, N. S. An age-related reduction in the replicative capacity of two murine hematopoietic stroma cell types. *Exp. Hematol.* **20,** 1216–1222 (1992).
48. Kajkenova, O., Lecka-Czernik, B., Gubrij, I., Hauser, S. P., Takahashi, K., Parfitt, A. M., Jilka, R. L., Manolagas, S. C., and Lipschitz, D. A. Increased adipogenesis and myelopoiesis in the bone marrow of SAMP6, a murine model of defective osteoblastogenesis and low turnover osteopenia. *J. Bone Miner. Res.* **12,** 1772–1779 (1997).
49. Stephan, R. P., Reilly, C. R., and Witte, P. L. Impaired ability of bone marrow stromal cells to support B-lymphopoiesis with age. *Blood* **91,** 75–88 (1998).
50. Egrise, D., Vienne, A., Martin, D., and Schoutens, A. Trabecular bone cell proliferation *ex vivo* increases with donor age in the rat: it is correlated with the extent of bone loss and not with histomorphometric indices of bone formation. *Calcif. Tissue Int.* **59,** 45–50 (1996).
51. Kahn, A., Gibbons, R., Perkins, S., and Gazit, D. Age-related bone loss. A hypothesis and initial assessment in mice. *Clin. Orthop.* 69–75 (1995).
52. Quarto, R., Thomas, D., and Liang, C. T. Bone progenitor cell deficits and the age-associated decline in bone repair capacity. *Calcif. Tissue Int.* **56,** 123–129 (1995).
53. Bergman, R. J., Gazit, D., Kahn, A. J., Gruber, H., McDougall, S., and Hahn, T. J. Age-related changes in osteogenic stem cells in mice. *J. Bone Miner. Res.* **11,** 568–577 (1996).
54. Kharlamova, L. A. Inhibition of formation of stromal cell colonies of human bone marrow by a factor formed *in vitro* by peripheral blood leukocytes. *Bull. Exp. Biol. Med.* **80,** 811–812 (1975).
55. Friedenstein, A. J., Latzinik, N. V., Gorskaya Yu, F., Luria, E. A., and Moskvina, I. L. Bone marrow stromal colony formation requires stimulation by haemopoietic cells. *Bone Miner.* **18,** 199–213 (1992).
56. Kuznetsov, S., and Gehron Robey, P. Species differences in growth requirements for bone marrow stromal fibroblast colony formation in vitro. *Calcif. Tissue Int.* **59,** 265–270 (1996).
57. Tsuji, T., Hughes, F. J., McCulloch, C. A., and Melcher, A. H. Effects of donor age on osteogenic cells of rat bone marrow in vitro. *Mech. Ageing Dev.* **51,** 121–132 (1990).
58. Fedarko, N. S., Vetter, U. K., Weinstein, S., and Gehron Robey, P. Age-related changes in hyaluronan, proteoglycan, collagen, and osteonectin synthesis by human bone cells. *J. Cell Physiol.* **151,** 215–227 (1992).
59. Fedarko, N. S., Robey, P. G., and Vetter, U. K. Extracellular matrix stoichiometry in osteoblasts from patients with osteogenesis imperfecta. *J. Bone Miner. Res.* **10,** 1122–1129 (1995).
60. Battmann, A., Battmann, A., Jundt, G., and Schulz, A. Endosteal human bone cells (EBC) show age-related activity *in vitro. Exp. Clin. Endocrinol. Diab.* **105,** 98–102 (1997).
61. Kato, H., Matsuo, R., Komiyama, O., Tanaka, T., Inazu, M., Kitagawa, H., and Yoneda, T. Decreased mitogenic and osteogenic responsiveness of calvarial osteoblasts isolated from aged rats to basic fibroblast growth factor. *Gerontology* **41** (Suppl. 1), 20–27 (1995).
62. Kuznetsov, S. A., Krebsbach, P. H., Satomura, K., Kerr, J., Riminucci, M., Benayahu, D., and Robey, P. G. Single-colony derived strains of human marrow stromal fibroblasts form bone after transplantation *in vivo. J. Bone Miner. Res.* **12,** 1335–1347 (1997).
63. Donahue, H. J., Zhou, Z., Li, Z., and McCauley, L. K. Age-related decreases in stimulatory G protein-coupled adenylate cyclase activity in osteoblastic cells. *Am. J. Physiol.* **273,** E776–E781 (1997).
64. Wong, G. L., and Ng, M. C. Maturation-associated changes in the cellular composition of mouse calvariae and in the biochemical characteristics of calvarial cells separated into subclasses on Percoll density gradients. *J. Bone Miner. Res.* **7,** 701–708 (1992).
65. Nimni, B. S., Bernick, S., Paule, W., and Nimni, M. E. Changes in the ratio of non-calcified collagen to calcified collagen in human vertebrae with advancing age. *Connect. Tissue Res.* **29,** 133–140 (1993).
66. Turner, R. T., and Spelsberg, T. C. Correlation between mRNA levels for bone cell proteins and bone formation in long bones of maturing rats. *Am. J. Physiol.* **261,** E348–E353 (1991).
67. Chavassieux, P. M., Chenu, C., Valentin-Opran, A., Merle, B., Delmas, P. D., Hartmann, D. J., Saez, S., and Meunier, P. J. Influence of experimental conditions on osteoblast activity in human primary bone cell cultures. *J. Bone Miner. Res.* **5,** 337–343 (1990).
68. Nimni, M. E., Bernick, S., Ertl, D., Nishimoto, S. K., Paule, W., Strates, B. S., and Villaneuva, J. Ectopic bone formation is enhanced in senescent animals implanted with embryonic cells. *Clin. Orthop.* **2434,** 255–266 (1988).
69. Fisher, L. W., and Termine, J. D. *In* "Current Advances in Skeleteogenesis" (A., Ornoy, A., Harell, and J. Sela, eds.), pp. 188–196. Elsevier, Amsterdam, 1985.
70. Traub, W., Arad, T., Vetter, U., and Weiner, S. Ultrastructural studies of bones from patients with osteogenesis imperfecta. *Matrix Biol.* **14,** 337–345 (1994).
71. Pinto, M. R., Gorski, J. P., Penniston, J. T., and Kelly, P. J. Age-related changes in composition and $Ca2^+$-binding capacity of canine cortical bone extracts. *Am. J. Physiol.* **255,** H101–H110 (1988).
72. Termine, J. D. Cellular activity, matrix proteins, and aging bone. *Exp. Gerontol.* **25,** 217–221 (1990).
73. Gehron Robey, P., and Boskey, A. L. *In* "Osteoporosis" (R. Marcus and D. Feldman, eds.), pp. 95–184. Raven Press, New York, 1996.

74. Fong, Y., Edelstein, D., Wang, E. A., and Brownlee, M. Inhibition of matrix-induced bone differentiation by advanced glycation end-products in rats. *Diabetologia* **36,** 802–807 (1993).
75. Takagi, M., Kasayama, S., Takehisa, Y., Motomura, T., Hashimoto, K., Yamamoto, T., Sato, B., Okada, S., and Tadamitsu, K. Advanced glycation end-products stimulate interleukin-6 production by human bone-derived cells. *J. Bone Miner. Res.* **12,** 439–446 (1997).
76. Kahn, J. J., and Simmons, D. J. Investigation of the cell lineage in bone using a chimera of chick and quail embryonic tissue. *Nature* **258,** 325–327 (1975).
77. Martin, T. J., and Ng, K. W. Mechanisms by which cells of the osteoblast lineage control osteoclast formation and activity. *J. Cell Biochem.* **56,** 357–366 (1994).
78. Suda, T., Udagawa, N., and Takahashi, N. *In* "The Principles of Bone Biology" (J. P. Bilezikian, L. G. Raisz, and G. A. Rodan, eds.), pp. 87–102. Academic Press, New York, (1996).
79. Rodan, G. A., and Martin, T. J. Role of osteoblasts in hormonal control of bone resportion—a hypothesis. *Calcif. Tissue Int.* **33,** 349–351 (1981).
80. Felix, R., Cecchini, M. G., and Fleisch, H. Macrophage colony stimulating factor restores *in vivo* bone resorption in the op/op osteopetrotic mouse. *Endocrinology* **127,** 2592–2594 (1990).
81. Takahashi, N., Akatsu, T., Udagawa, N., Sasaki, T., Yamaguchi, A., Moseley, J. M., Martin, T. J., and Suda, T. Osteoblastic cells are involved in osteoclast formation. *Endocrinology* **123,** 2600–2602 (1988).
82. Udagawa, N., Takahashi, N., Akatsu, T., Sasaki, T., Yamaguchi, A., Kodama, H., Martin, T. J., and Suda, T. The bone marrow-derived stromal cell lines MC3T3-G2/PA6 and ST2 support osteoclast-like cell differentiation in cocultures with mouse spleen cells. *Endocrinology* **125,** 1805–1813 (1989).
83. Mimura, H., Cao, X., Ross, F. P., Chiba, M., and Teitelbaum, S. L. 1,25-Dihydroxyvitamin D3 transcriptionally activates the beta 3-integrin subunit gene in avian osteoclast precursors. *Endocrinology* **134,** 1061–1066 (1994).
84. Mbalaviele, G., Chen, H., Boyce, B. F., Mundy, G. R., and Yoneda, T. The role of cadherin in the generation of multinucleated osteoclasts from mononuclear precursors in murine marrow. *J. Clin. Invest.* **95,** 2757–2765 (1995).
85. Feuerbach, D., and Feyen, J. H. Expression of the cell-adhesion molecule VCAM-1 by stromal cells is necessary for osteoclastogenesis. *FEBS Lett.* **402,** 21–24 (1997).
86. Yasuda, H., Shima, N., Nakagawa, N., Yamaguchi, K., Kinosaki, M., Mochizuki, S., Tomoyasu, A., Yano, K., Goto, M., Murakami, A., Tsuda, E., Morinaga, T., Higashio, K., Udagawa, N., Takahashi, N., and Suda, T. Osteoclast differentiation factor is a ligand for osteoprotegerin/osteoclastogenesis-inhibitory factor and is identical to TRANCE/RANKL. *Proc. Natl. Acad. Sci. USA* **95,** 3597–3602 (1998).
87. Baron, R., Chakhraborty, M., Chatterjee, D., Horne, W., Lomri, D., and Ravesboot, J.-H. *In* "Handbook of Experimenta Pharmacology" (G. R. Mundy, ed.), pp. 362–370. Elsevier, Amsterdam, (1993).
88. Quaglino, D., Ginaldi, L., Furia, N., and De Martinis, M. The effect of age on hemopoiesis. *Aging (Milano)* **8,** 1–12 (1996).
89. Egusa, Y., Fujiwara, Y., Syahruddin, E., Isobe, T., and Yamakido, M. Effect of age on human peripheral blood stem cells. *Oncol. Rep.* **5,** 397–400 (1998).
90. Lipschitz, D. A. Age-related declines in hematopoietic reserve capacity. *Semin. Oncol.* **22,** 3–5 (1995).
91. Faust, N., Huber, M. C., Sippel, A. E., and Bonifer, C. Different macrophage populations develop from embryonic/fetal and adult hematopoietic tissues. *Exp. Hematol.* **25,** 432–444 (1997).
92. Buchanan, J. P., Peters, C. A., Rasmussen, C. J., and Rothstein, G. Impaired expression of hematopoietic growth factors: a candidate mechanism for the hematopoietic defect of aging. *Exp. Gerontol.* **31,** 135–144 (1996).
93. Van den Heuvel, R., Mathieu, E., Schoeters, G., Leppens, H., and Vanderborght, O. Stromal cells from murine developing hemopoietic organs: comparison of colony-forming unit of fibroblasts and long-term cultures. *Int. J. Dev. Biol.* **35,** 33–41 (1991).
94. Cheleuitte, D., Mizuno, S., and Glowacki, J. *In vitro* secretion of cytokines by human bone marrow: effects of age and estrogen status. *J. Clin. Endocrinol. Metab.* **83,** 2043–2051 (1998).
95. Kitamura, H., Kawata, H., Takahashi, F., Higuchi, Y., Furuichi, T., and Ohkawa, H. Bone marrow neutrophilia and suppressed bone turnover in human interleukin-6 transgenic mice. A cellular relationship among hematopoietic cells, osteoblasts, and osteoclasts mediated by stromal cells in bone marrow. *Am. J. Pathol.* **147,** 1682–1692 (1995).

Sex Steroids, Bone, and Aging

MERYL S. LEBOFF* AND JULIE GLOWACKI*,†
*Brigham and Women's Hospital, Harvard Medical School; and †Massachusetts General Hospital, Harvard School of Dental Medicine, Boston Massachusetts 02115

INTRODUCTION

Aging is associated with declines in the sex steroids estrogen, testosterone, and the adrenal androgen dehydroepiandrosterone (DHEA). Individual variations in circulating levels of sex steroids with aging may have important effects on the bone. This chapter reviews the role of changes in levels of estrogen (menopause), testosterone (andropause), and the adrenal androgen DHEA and its sulfated derivative DHEA(S) (adrenopause) on skeletal aging in women and men.

MENOPAUSE

Effect of Aging on Serum Estrogens

ESTROGENS IN WOMEN

Aging of the ovary starts before birth when oogenesis ceases [1]. Follicular development, ovulation, and reproduction in women involve the complex interaction between the ovary and the hypothalmic–pituitary axis. With advancing age and progressive loss of follicular function and follicular atresia, there is a reduction in the generation of inhibin from the granulosa cells and a rise in follicle-stimulating hormone (FSH) levels. The more abrupt transition into menopause is a process that occurs over nearly 4 years with declining ovarian function [2]. Amenorrhea for 1 year and an elevated FSH level indicate menopause. The average age of menopause is 51 years. Currently, women spend one-third of their lives after menopause.

Before menopause, estradiol is the major estrogen produced by granulosa cells of the ovary. In the postmenopausal woman, there is a generalized decrease in estradiol produced by the ovary and adrenal androgens become the predominant precursor of estrogen. At menopause, however, the ovarian interstitial production of androstenedione decreases by approximately 50%, but ovarian testosterone production continues at a higher rate than in premenopausal women [1,3]. The net result is a gradual decline in circulating levels of estradiol (Fig. 1A). Compared with premenopausal values, circulating estradiol levels decrease from 40–350 to 13 pg/ml and estrone levels decrease from 40–200 to 35 pg/ml after menopause [4]. The availability of free estrogen and testosterone concentrations is affected by levels of sex hormone-binding globulin (SHBG) that binds these sex steroids. High levels of estrogen increase SHBG and androgens decrease circulating concentrations of SHBG. The adrenal gland accounts for 70% of circulating androstenedione after menopause [5]. The adrenal androgens androstenedione and DHEA(S) and, to a lesser extent, the ovarian androgens are converted to estrogen through aromatases in fat, liver, kidney, and bone marrow [6,7]. The weaker estrogen estrone is generated from androstenedione and testosterone; estradiol, in turn, is produced in low concentrations from testosterone and estrone. It is now recognized that adipose tissue is the primary source of estrogen both in postmenopausal women and in men. The precursor is circulating androstenedione derived from the adrenal; the enzyme that catalyzes estrogen synthesis in fat is aromatase cytochrome P450. This enzyme is found in other tissues, such as the placenta and brain. In the placenta, the precursor is 16α-hydroxydehydroepiandrosterone sulfate derived from fetal adrenals and liver. Different estrogens are produced in the different sites:

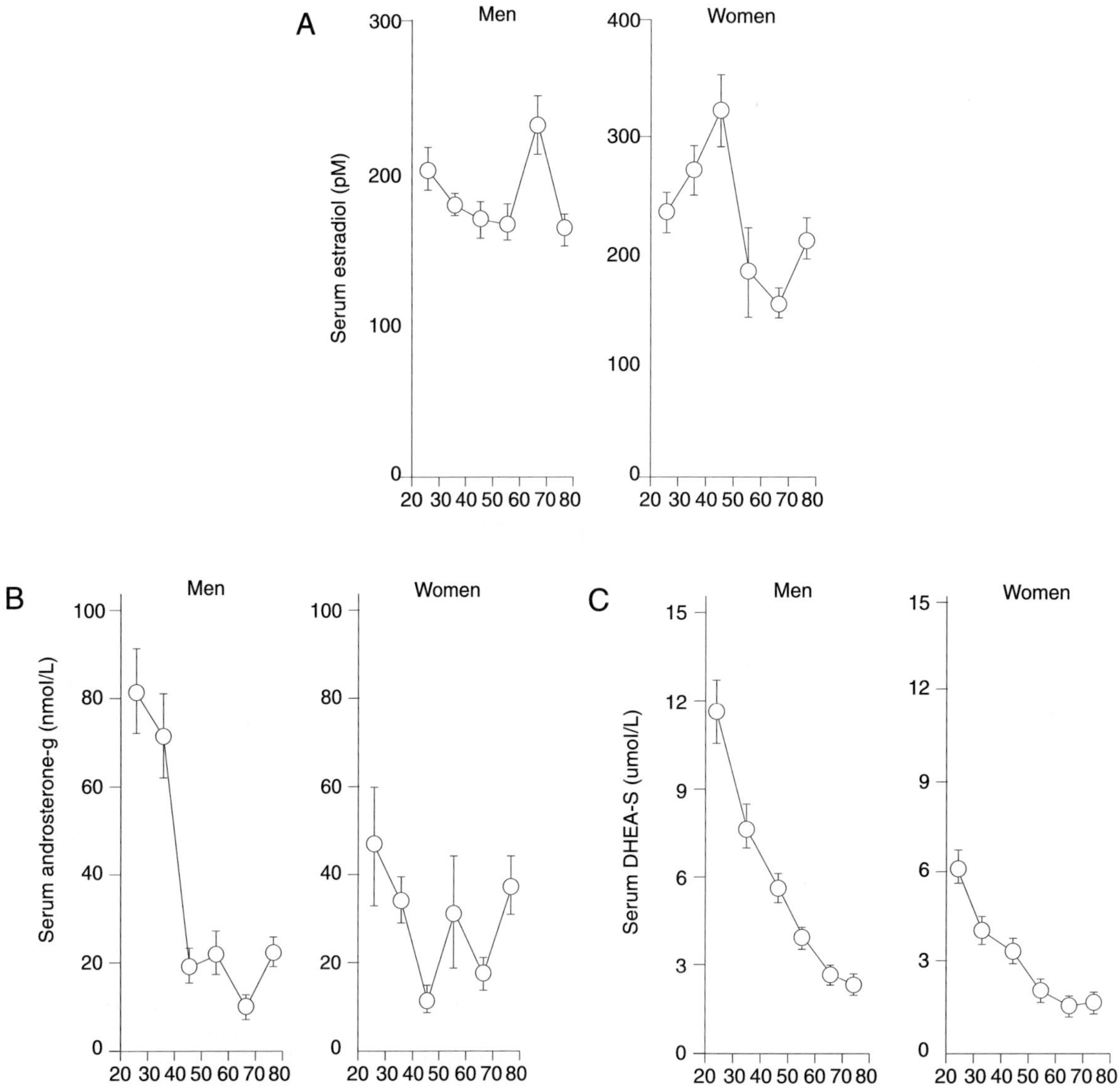

FIGURE 1 Effect of decade of age for men and women on serum concentration of estradiol (A), androsterone-glucoronidated derivative (B), and DHEA(S) (C). Modified from Labrie *et al.* [76].

estrone in fat, estriol in the placenta, and estradiol in the ovary. In fat, aromatase is expressed in both adipocytes and stromocytes [8]. Aromatase-specific activity increases as a function of age, with women older than 50 years having activity on a per cell basis nearly twice that of younger women [9]. That increase appears to be independent of menopausal status because the level of aromatase activity in fat from young women who had oophorectomy was comparable to nonoophorectomized women of the same age. Thus, with obesity, there is increased aromatase activity because of an increase in the number of fat cells, but the increase with aging is attributable to an increase in specific activity per cell. Whether the age-related increase in aromatase activity is due to a decline in an inhibitory factor or in receptor responsiveness to an inhibitor is not clear.

Serum estrone levels are 40% higher in obese women compared with nonobese women. Obesity is a determinant of estradiol concentrations [10] because body fat is a significant extraovarian source of estrogen. Increased body fat is further associated with lower levels of sex hormone-binding globulin and thus higher percentages of free serum estrogen [11,12].

Sex steroids may be involved in the regulation of insulin-like growth factors (IGFs) [13]. During puberty, there is a relationship between concentrations of sex steroids and IGF-I [14]. Sex steroids may interact with the IGF axis after menopause. According to cross-sectional and longitudinal studies, serum IGF levels decrease in postmenopausal women and are correlated with bone mineral density (BMD) [15,16]. It is uncertain, however, whether the decrement in IGF-I levels is directly related to a drop in serum estrogens or other steroids. For example, several studies show a strong correlation between serum DHEA(S) and IGF-I in postmenopausal women [17–19]. In postmenopausal women, estrogen therapy is associated with a rise in serum IGF-I [18,20]. New data, however, suggest that IGF-I levels decline with oral estrogen therapy. These differences may be explained by differences in basal IGF-I values [Ref 20a]. A study of IGF-I serum levels during transdermal estradiol treatment in postmenopausal women showed that estrogen increased IGF-I levels in a subset of women with low basal levels, but that estrogen decreased IGF-I and SHBG in women with highest basal IGF-I values and had no effect in the intermediate group. These findings suggest that there may be bimodal effects depending upon individual responses to estrogen or to contributions by other steroids (Fig. 2). Thus, sex steroids may play an important role in the regulation of IGF-I availability, although the relationship between estrogen and IGF-I may be complicated. Estrogen receptors have been identified in bone cells [21,22], and investigations of mechanisms suggest that estrogen treatment may directly suppress cytokine-mediated osteoclastic differentiation and bone resorption [23]. Estrogens generated locally in marrow through aromatases may prevent bone loss through paracrine interactions in bone and/or through growth factors or cytokines that affect skeletal remodeling [7,23].

ESTROGENS IN MEN

Emerging data indicate that estrogen is critically important for the male skeleton. It has been shown that

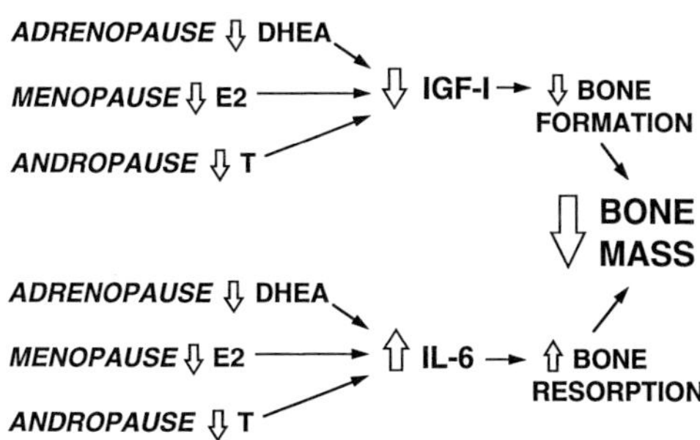

FIGURE 2 An hypothesis on the mechanisms of bone loss associated with age-related declines in sex steroids. With aging and decline of ovarian, testicular, and adrenal production of estradiol (E2), testosterone (T), and dehydroepiandrosterone (DHEA), subsequent changes in anabolic and osteolytic factors may contribute to changes in bone metabolism. Decreased IGF-I may be responsible for decreased osteoblastic bone formation. Increased IL-6 may contribute to increased osteoclast formation and bone resorption.

human adipose tissue [24], marrow [7], and hair follicles [25], as well as brain and other tissues in experimental animals, express aromatase in males. There are different levels of 5α-reductase type I and II, aromatase, and androgen receptor in hair follicles.

Smith *et al.* [26] reported on a male with a mutation in the estrogen receptor gene who was unresponsive to circulating estrogen. The subject presented with increased linear growth, unfused epiphyses, accelerated bone turnover, and osteoporosis [26]. In addition, individuals with aromatase deficiency and a mutation of the cyp 19 gene also have low estrogen levels and increased concentrations of androgens [27,28]. A male with aromatase deficiency was reported to have delayed skeletal maturation, low bone mass, and high bone turnover [28]. These data underscore the important role that estrogen plays in males for both bone accretion and fusion of the epiphyses. Serum estradiol stays relatively constant in men from young adulthood to old age (Fig. 1A). Estrogen deficiency, however, may contribute to age-related bone loss in men [29,30].

Age-Related Bone Loss in Women

Osteoporosis rises exponentially with age, and osteoporotic-related hip fractures are increasing worldwide as men and women live longer. Bone mass is normally maintained by the tight coupling of bone remodeling, with areas of bone resorption by osteoclasts being replaced by new bone laid down by osteoblasts. Bone mass increases about 50% during puberty, with peak bone mass normally achieved by the third decade. Men and women have an age-related bone loss of approximately 0.7 to 1% per year [31–33]. Some women show an early menopausal acceleration of bone loss of ~1 to 3% per year [34–36]. Data show that rates of bone loss increase in the eighth and ninth decades in women and men [37,38]. From young adulthood to extreme old age, women lose 42% of their spinal and 58% of femoral neck bone mass; in the spine and hip, men lose one-fourth and two-thirds that of women, respectively [39].

Relationship between BMD and Circulating Levels of Estrogen

BMD AND ESTROGEN DEFICIENCY IN WOMEN

Estrogen deficiency is an important determinant of postmenopausal bone loss. After menopause there is accelerated bone loss over 8 to 10 years [35]. On average, women may lose between one-third to one-half of their bone density during menopause. Some studies indicate that vertebral bone loss starts before menstrual function stops [40], although other investigators have not found a decrease in bone density before menopause [35,38,41,42]. In a longitudinal study of premenopausal women, there was a loss of hip bone density of 0.3% per year and a gain in the spine and radius [43]. Bone loss in the hip in premenopausal woman was weakly associated with androgens [44]. This decrease in hip bone density premenopausally is consistent with the results of the National Health and Nutrition Examination Survey III data analysis of American women [45]. Bone loss in postmenopausal women was related to serum levels of both androgens and estrogens [44].

Another model for illustrating the effects of estrogen deficiency on bone is the use of gonadotropin releasing hormone (GnRH) agonists in premenopausal women. Use of GnRH agonists for the treatment of endometriosis or fibroids leads to acute estrogen deficiency and a rapid and substantial loss of bone density of as much as 3% in 3 months and to between 5.9 and 8.2% after 6 months of treatment [46–49]. It has been shown that low-dose estrogen and progesterone add-back regimens prevent this GnRH-induced bone loss. Thus a rapid decline in ovarian function leads to accelerated bone loss that can be prevented with estrogen replacement. This model for the effects of estrogen deficiency on bone differs from normal menopause in which estrogen deficiency may develop more gradually. Among perimenopausal women, however, those with the highest rates of bone loss have the lowest estrogen concentrations [42,50].

Although the greatest decrements in estrogen occur in the perimenopausal period, low estrogen levels contribute to bone loss and fracture risk later in life [29,50,51]. In a cross-sectional study of 617 postmenopausal women, Rozenberg *et al.* [52] found that estradiol levels were correlated with trabecular bone mass in the spine. Concentrations of DHEA(S) that also reach low levels by the age of 50 to 60 years were related to changes in cortical bone mass in the forearm [52]. In a longitudinal study of 84 women between the ages of 42 and 58, over 3 years, Slemenda *et al.* [42] showed that estrogen levels in perimenopausal and postmenopausal women predicted the rate of menopausal bone loss in the forearm, in association with changes in skeletal turnover. In the same group, testosterone levels were related to changes in bone density in the distal forearm. In a larger prospective study of 231 women between the ages of 32 and 77 years, Slemenda *et al.* [43] examined the role of sex steroids on bone mass of the spine, hip, and forearm in peri- and postmenopausal women up to 25 years after menopause. In postmenopausal women, estrogen and androgens were independent factors, both affecting bone loss. In women over 60 years, estrogen levels were lower in those losing more bone in the spine and forearm, although testosterone levels were related to hip bone loss [43]. Years since menopause is a major determinant of postmenopausal bone loss [41] and, in conjunction with body weight, may account for as much as 60% of the variance in bone density [53]. Further, the rate and magnitude of estrogen deficiency in postmenopausal women may determine the rate and extent of bone loss.

Relationship between Circulating Concentrations of Estrogen and Bone Density in Women

In cross-sectional and case-controlled studies, measurement of estrogen levels in osteoporotic and nonosteoporotic women and studies of the relationship of estrogen levels to bone density show contradictory results. Newer data from large population-based studies have shown that very low concentrations of endogenous estrogen levels in older women are associated with low bone density or increased fracture risk. According to earlier studies, total estrogen levels did not distinguish osteoporotic from postmenopausal control women [54–56]. In some studies, it was the level of circulating estrone that was correlated with bone density [42,57]. The high concentrations of sex steroids in fat ranging from 20 to 400 times the circulating levels for estrogens and androgens may account for the observations that estrone levels, for example, are poor predictors of bone density [58].

The availability of large population-based studies has made it possible to clarify some of the discrepant results about the relationships between circulating estrogen levels and osteoporosis in women. In the Rancho Bernardo study, an observational study of 457 older women with a mean age of 72.1 years, multivariate analyses adjusting for body mass index and other confounding variables showed a strong and significant relationship between bioavailable estradiol and bone density at the spine, hip, and forearm (Table I) [59]. Total estrogen levels were also related to bone density at each of these sites, although the effect was not as great as that of bioavailable estradiol [59] (Table I). Estrone levels were also correlated with bone mass in the women, but the effect was less than that of free estradiol. Concentrations of DHEA(S), weak precursors to estrogens and androgens in peripheral tissues, were associated with bone density at the spine, hip, and midradius in women; DHEA(S) levels were not associated with bone density in men.

Data indicate an important role for very low endogenous estradiol levels in the reduction in bone density later in life and the increased risk of hip fractures [29,51,59]. On the basis of the detection limits of estradiol assays, women in the lowest postmenopausal ranges for estradiol may have undetectable estradiol levels. Cauley *et al.* [60], for example, found undetectable estradiol levels in as many as 50% of postmenopausal women.

TABLE I Presence (+) or Absence (−) of a Significant Relationship between Circulating Levels of Estrogen and Androgens and Bone Mineral Density (Spine, Hip, and Forearm)[a]

	Women	Men
Total estrogen	+	+[b]
Bioavailable estrogen	+	+
DHEA	−[b]	+

[a] Modified from Greendale *et al.* [S9].
[b] Except UD radius. Ranges of the R^2 for the relationship between bioavailable estrogen and bone density at the spine, hip, and forearm were 0.193–0.358 in women and 0.111–0.294 in men (R^2 for total estrogen was not presented in reference and was less significant than bioavailable estrogen). Ranges of the R^2 for the relationship between DHEAS in women or bioavailable testosterone in men and bone density sites were 0.170–0.344 and 0.092–0.248, respectively.

In other studies, 13% [59] or 33% [51] of the estradiol levels in postmenopausal women were below the detection limit. New data from the Study of Osteoporotic Fractures (SOF), a longitudinal cohort study of women 65 years or older, underscore the importance of low sex steroid levels in older postmenopausal women. Undetectable estradiol levels below the limit of detection (<5 pg/ml estradiol) were associated with a 2.5-fold increased risk for hip and spine fracture, and high concentrations of SHBG was associated with a 1.4-fold increased fracture risk. Postmenopausal women with both undetectable estradiol levels and high SHBG levels ≥1 μg/dl had a 6.9-fold increased risk of a hip fracture and a 7.9-fold greater risk of a spine fracture. These data from the SOF show that very low free estradiol levels and high concentrations of SHBG that decrease bioavailable estradiol were associated with a markedly increased risk of fractures [51].

RELATIONSHIP BETWEEN CIRCULATING CONCENTRATIONS OF ESTROGEN AND BONE DENSITY IN MEN

It has been shown in numerous studies that free serum E rather than free serum T was strongly correlated with bone mass in men [44,59,61]. Greendale and coworkers [59] examined sex steroids in a large defined population-based cohort and showed that in 534 older men (mean age 68.6 years), bioavailable estrogen was the sex steroid most strongly associated with bone density at the spine, hip, and forearm. In these older men, total estrogen levels were correlated with bone density in the spine and hip but not in the ultradistal radial site; bioavailable testosterone, but not total testosterone, was positively correlated with hip, spine, and ultradistal radial bone density (Table I). In another study that was performed in eugonadal men with vertebral fractures, testosterone therapy led to a rise in both testosterone and estradiol levels, a reduction in SHBG, and a concomitant rise in free sex steroids [62]. The increase in bone density in these osteoporotic men was significantly related to estradiol, but not testosterone, levels. Thus for the male skeleton, estrogen appears to have important skeletal effects on bone maturation, accretion, and aging.

ESTROGEN THERAPY FOR OSTEOPOROSIS IN WOMEN

In postmenopausal women, it is well established that estrogen replacement therapy prevents bone loss and is very effective in older women many years after the onset of menopause. In older women, estrogen therapy increases bone mass [33,63,64], and current users have a 33% more age-adjusted bone mass than nonusers [37]. In addition, Schneider *et al.* [65] showed that long-term and continuous therapy resulted in a high bone mass later in life than earlier or short-term estrogen replacement therapy. Further, Cauley *et al.* [66] showed in older women that estrogen therapy for more than 10 years was associated with a reduction in fractures by about 75% [66]. The effects of estrogen therapy on bone density in women are reviewed in detail in Chapter 41.

ANDROPAUSE

Effect of Aging on Serum Androgens

ANDROGENS IN MEN

Controversy remains about the existence of a male menopause, the andropause. Nevertheless, it is generally accepted that androgen levels decline with aging [67]. Aging in men is accompanied by decreased function of the Leydig and Sertoli cells. Plasma testosterone reflects the testicular level and is influenced by the hypothalamic–pituitary axis. Although sperm production, sperm quality, and testicular production of testosterone decrease with age, fertility may be preserved until senescence [68]. Most men and many physicians are not familiar with the changes that occur as men age unless symptoms of hypogonadism are manifest [69]. Studies show that aging in men is associated with reductions in circulating levels of testosterone [67,70]. In a longitudinal study of 66 men ages 41 to 61 years, total serum testosterone levels decreased by 41 ng/dl over a 13-year period. That decrease was correlated with an increase in triglycerides and a decrease in high-density lipoprotein cholesterol but not with age, body weight, or alcohol intake [71]. In a cross-sectional study of 62 healthy men 30 to 92 years old, there was a significant decrease in free testosterone levels with age [72]. The Massachusetts Male Aging Study reported that in men between 39 and 70 years, free testosterone declined by 1.2% per year and albumin-bound testosterone by 1.0% per year. SHBG, the major carrier of testosterone, increased by 1.2% per year, with the net effect that total serum testosterone declined more slowly than the other pools, by 0.4% per year [70]. Many other reports concur that with aging, there is an increase in SHBG and a decrease in total and in free or bioavailable testosterone [73,74]. By other estimates, free testosterone decreases by 1% per year between the ages of 40 and 70 years, but that rate is greater in men at a high risk of cardiovascular disease. Studies showing slight [75] or inconsistent [76] decreases in circulating testosterone/dihydrotestosterone (DHT) point out that levels of those androgens reflect primarily the synthetic and secretory activity of the testes.

Serum testosterone and DHT are useful markers of testicular secretion in men and interstitial ovarian secretion in women. However, because of other sources of androgens and wide ranges of normal values, it has been proposed that glucuronidated derivatives of androsterone may be more meaningful measures of androgen status [76]. In men, other androgens are formed in peripheral tissues from the adrenal precursors: DHEA and DHEA(S). During the first 6 months of life, the adrenals are the main source of testosterone, and during the first 2 years of life, they are also the main source of androstenedione [77] (Fig. 1). It has been estimated that the adrenals contribute 40–50% of total androgens in 60- to 70-year-old men [78]. The most reliable estimate of the total androgen pool is the measurement of serum glucuronidated derivatives of androsterone (ADT-G), androstane-3α, 17β-diol (3α-diol-G), and androstane-3β, 17β-diol(3β-diol-G) [76]. Those androgens showed striking associations with age; compared to men in the third decade of life, serum ADT-G, 3α-diol-G, and 3β-diol-G were lower in men in the eighth decade, to 27, 60, and 53%, respectively (Fig. 1B). Most of the decline occurs between the third and sixth decade, with smaller changes thereafter. Similar age-associated decreases were seen in unconjugated metabolites.

Some information is available concerning age-related changes in secretory reserve and in the gonadostat. One study showed preserved hypothalamic–pituitary responsiveness in elderly men, but diminished androgen secretion following the administration of clomiphene citrate, compared to younger men [79]. Compared to young men, elderly men show a significantly lower frequency of high-amplitude pulses for both leutinizing hormone and testosterone [67]. In addition, the sensitivity of the gonadostat to feedback by androgens is significantly greater in elderly men [67]. Both food restriction and obesity, as well as smoking and alcohol, have negative effects on the GnRH pulse generator [68].

Investigations on the physiology of the somatopause frequently examine interactions of the hypothalamic/pituitary axis with sex hormones. A small study of men between 18 and 63 years of age concluded that testosterone was a robust determinant of pulsatile and mean serum GH [80]. That series also showed the expected positive relationship between total pulsatile GH secretion and serum IGF-I. Another study of men between 50 and 80 years of age examined interactions between androgens and the somatotrophic axis [81]. The most striking association in that report was between components of the skeletal IGF system (IGF-I, IGF-II, and IGFBP-3) and SHBG. Consistent with this, free testosterone, but not total testosterone, was positively associated with components of the IGF system (Fig. 2).

Nutritional and life-style factors influence circulating levels of androgens. In a detailed study of middle-aged men, it was found that serum sex and adrenal steroid hormone concentrations were increased in cigarette smokers and that androgens and SHBG were negatively correlated with age and weight [82]. Men on chronic glucocorticoid therapy were found to have a significantly reduced ratio of testosterone to SHBG compared to age-matched controls [83]. Reduction of free testosterone may contribute to the pathophysiology of glucocorticoid-induced osteoporosis.

In men, a decrease in testosterone has unfavorable consequences on muscle, fat, hematopoiesis, fibrinolysis, insulin sensitivity, the central nervous system, mood, sexual function, and on bone. In a study of 145 healthy men aged 60 to 91, 46% had normal levels of androgens and gonadotropins [84]. However, 22% were found with hypergonadotropic hypogonadism (elevated LH and low T) and 17% had hypogonadotrophic hypogonadism (low LH and low T). Another study reported that 39% of older impotent men were hypogonadal compared with 48% of a group of older potent men [85]. A set of the older men and younger controls underwent GnRH testing. Older subjects showed impaired responsiveness to GnRH, with a high correlation with basal levels of LH. These data show that hypogonadism and impotence are common, yet independent conditions of older men. Thus, andropause is not an obligatory event in men and varies when it does occur.

ANDROGENS IN WOMEN

A number of studies have examined circulating androgens in women, with apparently conflicting results. In a small study of 33 healthy premenopausal women, both total and free plasma testosterone showed steep declines with age [86]. According to that study, a women of 40 would have half the total testosterone concentration of a woman of 21. In those premenopausal women, plasma DHEA and DHEA(S) also declined steeply with age.

In a cross-sectional analysis of 60 women, 10 in each decade from the third to eighth decades, there were no age-related changes in serum testosterone [76]. A gradual 44% decline in serum DHT was seen in those women. As with men, androgen status in women may not be fully reflected by free plasma testosterone or DHT. As with men, however, the women showed age-related decreases in serum glucuronidated derivatives of androgens (Fig. 1B). Clearly, women also pass through an andropause with aging. It was reported that women produce approximately 66% of the total androgens found in men. In women, 67% of serum testosterone is secreted from the ovaries. The postmenopausal ovary continues to produce testosterone from stromal and hilar cells. After menopause, the ovarian production of androstenedione markedly declines and the adrenal glands are the predominant source of androstenedione. Androgens are also derived from the conversion of androstenedione or DHEA and DHEA(S) into testosterone and DHT.

Age-Related Bone Loss in Men

There are well-documented differences in age-related fractures in men and women [87]. Men do not show age-related increases in Colles' fractures as do women. Although both men and women show striking age-related increases in femoral fractures, the incidence is greater for women than men at all ages after 50 years. In addition, among men, the incidence of fractures of the pelvis and proximal humerus does not rise as rapidly with age as is the case for fracture, of the proximal femur. From many large studies with different measures, it is clear that there is a decline in bone mineral density that begins before middle age in both genders. Subsequently, women show an increased rate of loss in the postmenopausal period, with both men [39] and women [37] showing increased rates of loss after 70 years of age.

Boonen *et al.* [88] studied levels of testosterone, estradiol, and calciotropic hormones in 40 men who developed a hip fracture (mean age 73 years) and in 40 age-matched controls. Compared with the control subjects, men with fractures had significantly lower serum concentrations of total and free testosterone and DHEA(S). Although the concentrations of estradiol were not lower in men with hip fractures, the free estradiol index (unbound free estradiol calculated from the total serum level of estradiol and SHBG) was also significantly lower in men with hip fractures.

Relationship between BMD and Circulating Levels of Testosterone

BMD and Hypogonadism in Men

Bone is an androgen-dependent tissue. Hypogonadism is associated with reduced bone mass in men. Hypogonadal adolescent males with Tanner stages I to II showed striking increases in bone density with testosterone treatment [89]. Hypogonadism is associated with impaired skeletal growth and maintenance with most, but not all, patients with idiopathic hypogonadotropic hypogonadism having low turnover osteoporosis [90]. Testosterone replacement ranging from 12 to 31 months was shown to increase BMD, but not to normal levels. Some information is available about long-term testosterone therapy [91]. It was concluded that long-term testosterone treatment can increase and maintain BMD, with the greatest increase during the first year of therapy for either primary or secondary hypogonadism.

Men with hyperprolactinemic hypogonadism underwent various regimens of surgical, radiation, or bromocriptine therapy for hyperprolactinemia [92]. Those in whom gonadal function was restored showed significant increases in radial and vertebral bone density in comparison with those who remained hypogonadal. The increases in radial and vertebral bone density were positively correlated with the change in the testosterone level. Testosterone therapy improved body composition and bone density in a group of 36 adult men with acquired hypogonadism [93]. They were compared to 29 men with central hypogonadism and to 44 age-matched control men. Both groups of hypogonadal men showed elevated body fat and low spinal BMD compared to controls.

A small metabolic study showed a relationship between hypogonadism and vitamin D homeostasis. Seven men with vertebral crush fractures had lower 1,25-dihydroxyvitamin D levels and malabsorption of calcium compared to 6 controls [94]. Treatment with testosterone led to an increase in total and free plasma 1,25-dihydroxyvitamin D and improved calcium absorption. It was concluded that hypogonadism can contribute to the risk of osteoporotic fractures by effects on calcium homeostasis.

Relationship between Circulating Concentrations of Androgens and Bone Density in Eugonadal Men

It is not clear whether the age-related decline in bone mineral density in men is in large measure a result of declining concentrations of circulating androgens. In a cross-sectional study of 62 healthy men, 30 to 92 years old, an age-related decline in radial bone mineral content was calculated at a loss of 2–3.4% per decade [72]. An even more rapid loss was calculated for vertebral trabecular bone mineral content at 12% per decade. Free serum testosterone concentrations fell with age and were significantly correlated with vertebral bone mineral density, but not with radial sites. Multiple regression analysis revealed that age was the major variable associated with bone mineral content and that testosterone levels added no further association. It was therefore concluded that age-related declines in male gonadal function were not of primary importance in male age-related bone loss. From a study of 112 elderly men (average age of 71.7 years), it was also concluded that there was no relationship between free testosterone and bone density [95]. That report duly noted that free testosterone levels may not fully define the androgen status of an individual.

There are data supporting the view that androgen status is related to bone density. A study of 134 men of average age 69.5 years showed an association between free androgen index and hip bone mineral density after adjustment for age and body mass index [96]. Another analysis with normal men concluded that the age-related decrease in serum-free testosterone was an additional factor contributing to the effect of age on bone mineral density at the femoral neck and Ward's triangle [97]. Another study of 48 men between 21 and 79 years of age demonstrated that radial but not lumbar spine or femoral neck bone density was predicted by an index of free testosterone and weight and not by dietary calcium [98].

Despite the limited value of measurements of only serum testosterone, there is additional evidence of a relationship between free testosterone and bone density in normal men. A study of 90 healthy, nonsmoking Thai men showed a correlation between testosterone levels and bone mineral density, even after correcting for age [97]. Other data indicate a correlation between bone density and serum estradiol concentrations in men [44]. Men in that study were older than 65 years and all had testosterone levels within the normal range. These and other data indicate that a deficiency of estrogen may be as important a determinant of bone loss in men as testosterone deficiency [29]. In a large study, analysis of 534 men in the Rancho Bernardo Study demonstrated a positive correlation between bioavailable estradiol and BMD at all sites, with smaller, significant relationships between bioavailable testosterone (but not total testosterone) and BMD of the spine and hip and distal radius (Table I) [59]. Clearly individual variations in bone mass can be accounted for by differences in sex hormone levels.

Hip fractures increase exponentially with age in men. Several studies indicate the role of occult hypogonadism in osteoporotic fractures in men. It was reported that 59% of elderly men with "minimal trauma hip fractures" were hypogonadal compared to 18% in matched controls [99]. However, a large prospective study of 242 Scandinavian men followed for 7 years showed that BMD, skinfold thickness, and alcohol abuse, but not testosterone or SHBG, were risk factors for subsequent hip fractures [100].

BMD and Androgens in Women

It is now clear that both endogenous estrogens and androgen levels influence bone and mineral metabolism in women [101]. Data in premenopausal and postmenopausal women indicate that androgens may exert positive effects on bone [59,102–104]. Analysis of 457 postmenopausal women in the Rancho Bernardo Heart and Chronic Disease Study indicated a positive correlation between endogenous bioavailable estradiol and BMD at all sites and positive correlations between DHEA(S) or bioavailable testosterone and BMD at some sites (Table I) [59]. In some cross-sectional studies, androgen levels are low in women with hip or vertebral fractures [56,105], although results are conflicting [54].

Some information is available from women with excess androgens. Supraphysiological levels of endogenous androgens were found to be associated with increased trabecular bone density [102]. Nineteen women with androgen excess were compared with 27 normal women, aged 21 to 48 years. In that group of normal women, cortical bone density was correlated with serum testosterone, both total and free levels. In the other group, serum androstendione was the most strongly correlated with trabecular BMD. In another report, it was demonstrated that 20 hirsute women had high BMD, although they lost bone during 9 months of treatment with the GnRH agonist [106]. Addition of estrogen/progestin replacement therapy protected the spine and trochanter against bone loss.

In an evaluation of the effects of smoking on bone density and sex steroids in women, it was shown that SHBG was higher and free testosterone and bone density were lower in the group of smokers [107]. Further, concentrations of DHEA(S) and free testosterone were correlated with BMD at the femoral neck. Smokers also have increased metabolism of estrogen, earlier menopause, and increased osteoporotic fractures [108].

Androgen Therapy for Men and Women

Successes in preventing bone loss in hypogonadal men and men treated with glucocorticoids have led to the possibility of preventing age-related bone loss in men [109]. A number of studies evaluating testosterone replacement/supplementation therapy support the potential for improvements in bone mass, muscle mass, and muscle strength, but other benefits are not clear and long-term risks of prostate cancer are of concern [110]. Short-term treatment of 13 men, 57 to 76 years old, who had low or borderline-low serum testosterone levels were evaluated before and after 3 months of treatment with weekly intramuscular injections of testosterone enanthate or placebo [111]. With treatment, there was an increase in lean body mass and a decrease in urinary hydroxyproline excretion. However, there was an increase in serum prostate-specific antigen (PSA) levels and in hematocrit, as well as a decline in total cholesterol and low-density lipoprotein cholesterol.

Very few studies have sought to "treat" andropause with replacement testosterone. Nevertheless, several studies provide some information about the effects of testosterone treatment on BMD in men. A 6-month trial of testosterone enanthate showed a modest reduction in fat mass and small increases in fat-free mass, muscle strength, and bone density compared to controls [112]. Changes in bone density varied with sites, with significant increases at four of the nine sites measured.

Short-term testosterone therapy has been shown to increase BMD in men with idiopathic osteoporosis [62,113]. Yet increases in hematocrit and plasma viscosity suggest that care should be taken in patient selection and monitoring [113].

Bone density and sex hormones have been evaluated in men with rheumatoid arthritis (RA) [114]. Compared to a group of 68 age-matched men, 99 men with RA showed reduced lumbar and femoral BMD, with significant correlations with salivary, not serum, testosterone. A cumulative dose of corticosteroids was a strong predictor for BMD as were reductions in serum androstenedione and DHEA(S). Other data show that men who take glucocorticoids may show reduced circulating concentrations. In a prospective, crossover study, the effects of testosterone therapy on bone density and body composition in asthmatic men receiving long-term glucocorticoid treatment were evaluated [115]. That study showed that testosterone reversed the deleterious effects of glucocorticoid drugs on skeletal and soft tissues in men. Bone density and body composition were measured by dual-energy X-ray absorptiometry. However, no beneficial effects were found in a small trial of testosterone versus placebo in 35 men with RA [116]. In that study, 30% of the subject had at least one vertebral fracture and all subjects in the treatment group showed significant increases in serum androgens and estradiol.

Anabolic androgens have been shown to increase bone mass in postmenopausal women [117]. Testosterone implants and percutaneous estrogen therapy raised bone mass in women previously treated with estrogen [118], although another report showed no additional bone-sparing benefit of testosterone for postmenopausal women treated with estrogen [119]. A short-term study in postmenopausal women treated with conjugated estrogen or conjugated estrogen and 2.5 mg methyltestosterone showed that estrogen led to a reduction of markers of bone resorption and formation and that the addition of testosterone increased indices of bone formation [120]. Further, in women who had a surgical oophorectomy, estrogen plus androgen produced a greater increase in bone mass than estrogens alone. Finally, testosterone has been shown to preserve bone density and architecture in women who have undergone bilateral ovariectomy for female-to-male transsexual reconstruction [118]. Use of androgens in postmenopausal women is limited by the potential reduction in high density lipoprotein (HDL) levels and possible adverse effects on cardiovascular risk. Large prospective studies are needed to resolve whether androgens have beneficial effects on bone density and fractures in women.

ADRENOPAUSE

Aging of the Adrenal Gland

Compared to the adrenal gland of other species, the human adrenal is unusual in its high synthesis and secretion of the androgens: DHEA, DHEA(S), and androstenedione. The human adrenal glands show remarkable functional and morphological changes during growth and aging. The fetal adrenal cortex produces large quantities of androgens and estrogen precursors; the transient fetal tissue involutes after birth as a result of the combined effects of ACTH, prolactin, and growth hormone. At birth, the DHEA(S) concentration is four times higher than cortisol. Serum levels of DHEA(S) plummet after birth and remain low until adrenarche. Between 6 and 8 years of age, serum levels of adrenal androgens begin to increase in both boys and girls [121]. The ratio of DHEA(S) to cortisol increases during this period and through puberty. Pubertal secretion of the gonadotropin-releasing hormone causes large increases in testosterone and estrogen levels in boys and girls. DHEA, DHEA(S), and androstenedione continue to increase whereas ACTH and cortisol remain constant.

The effects of aging on adrenal function need to be dissociated from other factors. Acute stress situations due to illnesses cause increases in cortisol, DHEA, and

DHEA(S) concentrations. In healthy populations, serum levels of adrenal adrenogens decline with aging, a phenomenon named by Albright as "adrenopause" [122]. Aging of the adrenal gland appears to be restricted to synthesis and secretion of the androgens. During aging, serum levels of aldosterone, cortisol, and corticosterone show little change, whereas serum DHEA and DHEA(S) decline from a peak at age 25 to less than 20% of that by the age of 70 [123]. Moreover, the response of DHEA to acute ACTH stimulation also decreases with age, whereas the responses of cortisol and aldosterone are preserved with age [124].

The adult adrenal is composed of functionally distinct zones: the zona glomerulosa is the site of aldosterone production, the zona fasciculata is the site of cortisol synthesis, and the zona reticularis is the site of DHEA and DHEA(S) synthesis. The fasciculata has high levels of 3β-hydroxysteroid dehydrogenase-isomerase (3β-HSD), which advances substrates along the major pathway of cortisol or androstenedione biosynthesis, away from the DHEA(S) pathway; the reticularis has low levels of 3β-HSD and high DHEA sulfotransferase activity, the appropriate enzyme machinery for DHEA(S) synthesis. The centripetal flow of blood from the zona fasciculata toward the reticularis is the basis for the theory that high levels of cortisol or other products from the fasciculata may alter the regulation of steroid synthesis in the reticularis, thereby explaining the dissociation of the effects of aging or responses to ACTH, for example. Adrenal microanatomy and histogenesis can account for the changes in androgen synthesis throughout life [125]. In the fetus, the adrenal cortex is composed of transient tissue that produces androgens and estrogens and that involutes after birth. The development of a morphologically distinct zona reticularis coincides with adrenarche; suppression of 3β-HSD in this zone changes production toward DHEA and DHEA(S). The simplest theory to explain adrenopause is that there is a progressive decrease in the number of functional reticularis cells, although this is not supported by direct morphological evidence. Thus, the term andropause is not accurate because aging does not affect all products of the gland.

Age-Related Changes in DHEA(S)

Levels of DHEA and its sulfated ester DHEA(S) rise sharply during puberty, achieve a maximal level in the early twenties, and markedly decrease to about 30% of the young adult values by age 50 to 60 years and to 10 to 20% of young adult levels by age 70 [76,123,126,127]. DHEA is the most abundant steroid produced by the adrenals and the age-related changes in DHEA contrast that of cortisol, which does not decrease with age. In primates, DHEA circulates at a 10-fold higher concentration than cortisol and is converted to androgens and estrogens in peripheral tissues [12,127–129]. The fall in DHEA(S) levels with age is associated with a reduction in the synthesis of the 17,20-desmolase enzyme. Its major form in the circulation is sulfated [DHEA(S)]. It is activated in peripheral tissues that have sulfatase. Bone density also rises during adolescence in association with the rise in adrenal androgens and gonadal steroids and declines with menopause in women and with age in men and women. Mean values of DHEA and DHEAS are higher for men than women at all ages. Data show that DHEA treatment given to young women with low DHEA levels and anorexia [130] may reduce markers of bone resorption and stimulate indices of bone formation [131].

Androgens and sex steroids exert independent and positive effects on peak bone mass [132]. In addition, androgens are the predominant source of estrogen in postmenopausal women and account for one-third of the estrogen generated before menopause [12]. Low adrenal androgen levels are of potential risk for the skeleton for three reasons. First, androgens have a direct, anabolic effect on bone mass. According to some studies, circulating DHEA levels are positively correlated with bone mass measurements [133,134] and are lower in patients with osteoporosis [88,133]. Second, these androgens (DHEA and androstenedione) are steroid precursors to estrogens through aromatization in adipose and other tissues [12,129,135,136]. DHEA lowers SHBG that results in a net increase in bioactive estrogen levels. Third, the adrenal androgen DHEA stimulates human osteoblastic cell proliferation through androgen receptor-mediated mechanisms and alkaline phosphatase production through transforming growth factor (TGFβ) [137].

In a recent cross-sectional study of 102 healthy women, serum DHEAS levels showed a striking decrease with age ($r = -0.52$, $p = 0.0001$) [137a]. There was a strong positive correlation between circulating DHEAS and IGF-I levels ($r = 0.43$, $p = 0.0001$) and a negative correlation between DHEAS and IL-6 ($r = -0.32$, $p = 0.02$). These data are consistent with the hypothesis that with age, declining adrenal function and DHEAS production contribute to lower IGF-I and higher IL-6 production (Fig. 2).

DHEA Replacement

Epidemiological data show an inverse relationship between DHEA(S) levels and cardiovascular mortality in men [138] and breast cancer in women. Previous research, including studies in animals, shows that DHEA has protective effects on bodily functions and diseases such as bone loss, atherogenesis, immune senescence, systemic lupus, cancer, and diabetes [126,139–142]. Because DHEA circulates in low concentrations in rodents, the effects of DHEA in rodent models may not be applicable to humans. In humans, some studies show a significant correlation between DHEA levels and bone density [103,133,134,143], although results are contradictory. One population-based study in an older community showed no relationship between DHEA and bone density in elderly residents of the Rancho Bernardo retirement community [144]. However, newer data from the same group that included a larger number of women and men between the ages of 50 and 89 found that circulating DHEA(S) in women was associated with BMD in the forearm, spine, and hip but that DHEA(S) was not associated with bone density in men [59] (Table I). These data indicate gender differences in the relationship between DHEA(S) and bone in women and men.

To date, research examining the effects of DHEA on clinical parameters has been carried out in short-term studies in older patients. Replacement studies in humans include a study of pharmacological doses of DHEA (1600 mg/day) for 28 days on the production of endogenous androgens and estrogens in six postmenopausal women. Mortola and Yen [135] showed that this high-dose DHEA therapy produced a marked rise in testosterone and androstenedione, a rise in basal estradiol levels to 30–40 pg/ml (slightly above postmenopausal values), and a reduction in sex hormone-binding globulin (which leads to higher free androgen and estrogen levels). Studies have examined the effects of short-term DHEA replacement or "add-back" therapy with 50 mg of crystalline DHEA to achieve young adult DHEA(S) levels. Morales and co-workers [145] showed that restoration of DHEA to young adult levels with 50 mg DHEA produced a two-fold rise in serum androgens (androstenedione, testosterone) and no change in sex hormone-binding globulin, estrogen, or cholesterol, although HDL was decreased slightly. Of particular relevance to potential anabolic effects on bone, DHEA produced a rise in IGF-I and free IGF levels because of a decline in IGF-BP1 levels. DHEA therapy was without adverse effects [145–147] and in 70–80% of the patients produced an increase in the sense of "well-being" according to tests of quality of life variables. DHEA also may decrease dysregulated serum interleukin (IL)-6 levels [140,148,149]. The finding in older 60- to 70-year-old women that 10% DHEA cream increased bone density of the hip by ~2.0% in 1 year, in association with a suppression of bone resorption markers and stimulation of bone formation, suggests that DHEA may have beneficial effects on the aging skeleton through conversion to estrogen and/or androgens or through androgenic effects on bone [147]. Treatment of postmenopausal women with oral androgen (testosterone) and estrogen for 6 weeks not only had antiresorptive effects on markers of bone breakdown similar to those of estrogen, but also stimulated bone formation [120]. Furthermore, preliminary data indicate that a combination of topical DHEA (10 mg/day) and an estrogen receptor modulator (antiestrogen) for 282 days produced large increments in spine and hip bone density of 10.6 and 8.2%, respectively [150]. Use of androgens in combination with other agents may produce a heightened effect on bone density, although large prospective studies would be necessary to demonstrate an effect on fractures.

SUMMARY

After the age of 50, there is an exponential rise in osteoporotic fractures as bone density decreases with age in women and men and with menopause in women. With the onset of menopause, estrogen deficiency is associated with a rapid bone loss, which estrogen therapy prevents by inhibiting bone resorption. Recent data indicate that low estradiol levels and high levels of SHBG in older women are associated with reduced bone density and increased fracture risk. Estrogen is important for bone maturation and accretion in men, and bioavailable estradiol levels are significantly correlated with bone density in older men. In men, some reports indicate that with aging there is an increase in SHBG and a decrease in total and in free, or bioavailable testosterone. Levels of free testosterone have been associated with bone density in men. In addition, several studies indicate a role of occult hypogonadism in osteoporotic fractures in men. DHEA(S) is the most abundant steroid in the circulation. Mean values are higher for men than women at all ages. For both genders, values decline from a peak in young adulthood with low levels to 10–20% of peak levels by age 70. Low DHEA adrenal androgen levels are of potential risk for the skeleton for two reasons. First, androgens provide an anabolic effect on bone mass. Second, these androgens [DHEA(S) and androstenedione] are precursors of estrogens by aromatization in peripheral tissues. Some studies show that DHEA(S) levels are correlated with bone density in women and are lower in patients with osteoporosis, although results are conflicting. In summary, low levels of sex steroids, particularly levels of bioavailable hormones, can contribute to age-related bone loss and increased osteoporotic fractures. Estrogen is an important determinant of bone mass in both women and men.

A unified hypothesis has been formulated to suggest possible mechanisms by which the menopause, andropause, and adrenopause contribute to age-related bone loss (Fig. 2). Changes in these circulating sex steroids may effect dramatic changes in local mediators that control rates of bone formation and bone resorption. It is not known whether replacement therapy can reverse all of these processes for significant periods of time or how the contribution of other age-related physiological changes and diseases would alter tissue responses to sex steroids and pose additional risks for hormone-dependent cancers, for example. Nevertheless, the striking relationships between sex steroids and aspects of bone metabolism and the demonstrated beneficial effects of estrogen to protect skeletal mass indicate that sex steroids play a significant role in age-related bone loss. Chapters 7, 14, 18, 19, and 47 include detailed information on other aspects of these processes.

Acknowledgments

We greatly appreciate the expert secretarial assistance of Irma Sabbag and Karen Aneshansley for assistance with the figures. Support was provided in part by NIH Grants ROI AG12271 and RO1 AG 13519.

References

1. Schiff, I., and Walsh, B. Menopause. *In* "Principles and Practice of Endocrinology and Metabolism." (K. Beck, ed.), 2nd Ed., pp. 915–916. Lippincott, Philadelphia, 1995.
2. McKinlay, S. M., Brambilla, D. J., and Posner, J. G. The normal menopause transition. *Maturitas* **14,** 103–115 (1992).
3. Bellantoni, M. F., and Blackman, M. R. Menopause and its consequences. *In* "Handbook of the Biology of Aging" (E. L. Schneider and J. W. Rowe, eds.), 4th Ed., pp. 415–444. Academic Press, San Diego, 1996.
4. Korenman, S. G. Menopausal endocrinology and management. *Arch. Intern. Med.* **142,** 1131–1136 (1982).
5. Lipsett, M. B. Steroid hormones. *In* "Reproductive Endocrinology: Physiology, Pathophysiology and Clinical Management" (S. S. C. Yen and R. B. Jaffe, pp. 140–153. Saunders Company, Philadelphia, 1986.
6. Grodin, J. N., Siiteri, P. K., and MacDonald, P. C. Sources of estrogen production in post-menopausal women. *J. Clin. Endocrinol. Metab.* **36,** 207 (1973).
7. Frisch, R. E., Canick, J. A., and Tulchinsky, D. Human fatty marrow aromatizes androgens to estrogens. *J. Clin. Endocrinol. Metab.* **51,** 394–396 (1980).
8. Ackerman, G. E., Smith, M. E., Mendelson, C. R., *et al.* Aromatization of androstenedione by human adipose tissue stromal cells and adipocytes in monolayer culture. *J. Clin. Endocrinol. Metab.* **53,** 412–417 (1981).
9. Cleland, W. H., Mendelson, C. R., and Simpson, E. R. Effects of aging and obesity on aromatase activity of human adipose cells. *J. Clin. Endocrinol. Metab.* **60,** 174–177 (1985).
10. Cauley, J. A., Gutai, J. P., Kuller, L. H., LeDonne, D., and Powell, J. G. The epidemiology of serum sex hormones in postmenopausal women. *Am. J. Epidemiol.* **129,** 1120–1131 (1989).
11. Siiteri, P. K. Extragonadal oestrogen formation and serum binding of oestradiol: relationship to cancer. *J. Endocrinol.* **89,** 119–129 (1981).
12. Frisch, R. E. Body fat, menarche, fitness and fertility. *Prog. Reprod. Biol. Med.* **14,** 1–26 (1990).
13. Rosen, C. J., Glowacki, J., and Craig, W. Sex steroids, the insulin-like growth factor regulatory system, and aging: implications for the management of older postmenopausal women. *J. Nutr. Health Aging,* **2,** 1–6 (1998).
14. Clark, P. A., and Rogol, A. D. Growth hormone and sex steroid interactions at puberty. *Endocrinol. Metab. Clin.* **25,** 665–670 (1996).
15. Itastu, S., Kudo, Y., Iguchi, T., and Takeda, Y. Studies on the bone metabolism in either natural menopause or surgical menopause: implications of the IGF-IGFBP system for postmenopausal osteoporosis. *Acta Obstetr. Gynaecol. Japon.* **47,** 1329–1336 (1995).
16. Poehlman, E. T., Toth, M. J., Ades, P. A., and Rosen, C. J. Menopause-associated changes in plasma lipids, insulin-like growth factor-1 and blood pressure: a longitudinal study. *Eur. J. Clin. Invest.* **27,** 322–326 (1997).
17. LeBoff, M. S., Rosen, C. J., Rightmire, E., and Glowacki, J. Changes in growth factors and cytokines in postmenopausal women. *J. Bone Miner. Res.* **10,** 241 (1995).
18. Hartmann, B., Hirchengast, T., Albrecht, A., Laml, T., Bikas, D., and Huber, J. Effects of hormone replacement therapy on GH secretion patterns in correlation to somatometric parameters in healthy postmenopausal women. *Maturitas* **22,** 239–246 (1995).
19. Ravn, P., Overgaard, K., Spencer, E. M., and Christiansen, C. IGF-I and IGF-II in healthy women with and without established osteoporosis. *Eur. J. Endocrinol.* **132,** 313–319 (1995).
20. Slowinska-Srzednicka, J., Zgliczynski, S., Jeske, W., Stopinska-Gluszak, U., Srednick, M., Brzezinska, A., Zgliczynski, W., and Sadowski, Z. Transdermal 17 beta estradiol combined with oral progestogen increases plasma levels of IGF-I in postmenopausal women. *J. Endocrinol. Invest.* **15,** 533–538 (1992).
20a. Campagnoli, C., Biglia, N., Cantamessa, C., Lesca, L., Lotano, M. R., and Sismondi, P. Insulin-like growth factor I (IGF-I) serum level modifications during transdermal estradiol treatment in postmenopausal women: A possible bimodal effect depending on basal IGF-I values. *Gynecol. Endocrinol.* **12,** 259–266 (1998).
21. Eriksen, E. F., Colvard, D. S., Berg, N. G., Graham, M. L., Mann, K. G., Spelsberg, T. C., and Riggs, B. L. Evidence of estrogen receptors in normal human osteoblast-like osteosarcoma cells. *Science* **241,** 84–86 (1988).
22. Komm, B. S., Terpening, C. M., Benz, D. J., Graeme, K. A., Gallagos, A., Korc, M., Greene, G. L., O'Malley, B. W., Hausler, M. R. Estrogen binding receptors in normal human osteoblast-like osteosarcoma cells. *Science* **241,** 81–84 (1988).
23. Horowitz, M. C. Cytokines and estrogen in bone: Anti-osteoporotic effects. *Science* **260,** 626–627 (1993).
24. Lueprasitsakul, P., Latour, D., and Longcope, C. Aromatase activity in human adipose tissue stromal cells: effect of growth factors. *Steroids* **55,** 540–544 (1990).
25. Sawaya, M. E., and Price, V. Different levels of 5a-reductase type I and II, aromatase, and androgen receptor in hair follicles in women and men with androgenetic alopecia. *J. Invest. Derm.* **109,** 296–300 (1997).

26. Smith, E. P., Boyd, J., Frank, G. R., Takahashi, H., Cohen, R. M., Specker, B., Williams, T. C., Lubahn, D. B., and Korach, K. S. Estrogen resistance caused by a mutation in the estrogen-receptor gene in man. *N. Engl. J. Med.* **331,** 1056–1061 (1994).
27. Morishima, A., Grumbach, M. M., Simpson, E. R., Fisher, C., and Qin, K. Aromatase deficiency in male and female siblings caused by a novel mutation and the physiological role of estrogens. *J. Clin. Endocrinol. Metab.* **80,** 3689–3698 (1995).
28. Conte, F. A., Grumbach, M. M., Ito, Y., Fisher, C. R., and Simpson, E. R. A syndrome of female pseudohermaphroditism, hypergonadotropic hypogonadism, and multicystic ovaries associated with missense mutations in the gene encoding aromatase (P450arom). *J. Clin. Endocrinol. Metab.* **78,** 1287–1292 (1994).
29. Riggs, B. L., Khosla, S., and Melton, L. J., III, A unitary model for involutional osteoporosis: Estrogen deficiency causes both Type I and Type II osteoporosis in postmenopausal women and contributes to bone loss in aging man. *J. Bone Miner. Res.* **13,** 763–773 (1998).
30. Bilezikian, J. P. Estrogens and postmenopausal osteoporosis. Was Albright right after all? *J. Bone Miner. Res.* **13,** 774–776 (1998).
31. Dawson-Hughes, B., Dallal, G. E., Krall, E. A., Sadowski, L., Sahyoun, N., and Tannenbaum, S. A controlled trial of the effect of calcium supplementation on bone density in postmenopausal women. *N. Engl. J. Med.* **323,** 878–883 (1990).
32. Greenspan, S. L., Maitland, L. A., Myers, E. R., Krasnow, M. B., and Kido, T. H. Femoral bone loss progresses with age: A longitudinal study in women over age 65. *J. Bone Miner. Res.* **9,** 1959–1965 (1994).
33. The Writing Group for the PEPI Trial. Effects of estrogen or estrogen/progestin regimens on heart disease risk factors in postmenopausal women. The postmenopausal estrogen/progestin interventions (PEPI) Trial. *JAMA* **273,** 199–208 (1995).
34. Mazess, R. B., Barden, H. S., Ettinger, M., Johnston, C., Dawson-Hughes, B., Baran D., Powell, M., and Notelovitz, M. Spine and femur density using dual-photon absorptiometry in U.S. white women. *Bone Miner.* **2,** 211–219 (1987).
35. Mazess, R. B. On aging bone loss. *Clin. Orthop. Related Res.* **165,** 239–252 (1982).
36. Ravn, P., Hetland, M. L., Overgaard, K., and Christiansen, C. Premenopausal and postmenopausal changes in bone mineral density of the proximal femur measured by dual-energy x-ray absorptiometry. *J. Bone Miner. Res.* **9,** 1975 (1994).
37. Ensrud, K. E., Palermo, L., Black, D. M., Cauley, J., Jergas, M., Orwoll, E. S., Nevitt, M. C., Fox, K. M., and Cummings, S. R. Hip and calcaneal bone loss increase with advancing age: Longitudinal results from the study of osteoporotic fractures. *J. Bone Miner. Res.* **10,** 1778–1787 (1995).
38. Riggs, B. L., Wahner, H. W., Dunn, W. L., Mazess, R. B., Offord, K. P., and Melton, L. J., III. Differential changes in bone mineral density of the appendicular and axial skeleton with aging. *J. Clin. Invest.* **67,** 328–335 (1981).
39. Riggs, B. L., Wahner, W., Seeman, E., Offord, K. P., Dunn, W. L., Mazezz, R. B., Johnson, K. A., and Melton, L. J., III, Changes in bone mineral density of the proximal femur and spine with aging: differences between the postmenopausal and senile osteoporosis syndromes. *J. Clin. Invest.* **70,** 716–723 (1982).
40. Johnston, C. C., Jr., Hui, S. L., Witt, R. M., Appledorn, R., Baker, R. S., and Longcope, C. Early menopausal changes in bone mass and sex steroids. *J. Clin. Endocrinol. Metab.* **61,** 905–911 (1985).
41. Nilas, L., and Christiansen, C. Bone mass and its relationship to age and the menopause. *J. Clin. Endocrinol. Metab.* **65,** 697 (1987).
42. Slemenda, C., Hui, S. L., Longcope, C., and Johnston, C. C. Sex steroids and bone mass: A study of changes about the time of menopause. *J. Clin. Invest.* **80,** 1261–1269 (1987).
43. Slemenda, C., Longcope, C., Peacock, M., Hui, S., and Johnston, C. C. Sex steroids, bone mass, and bone loss: A prospective study of pre-, peri-, and postmenopausal women. *J. Clin. Invest.* **97,** 14–21 (1996).
44. Slemenda, C. W., Longcope, C., Zhou, L., Hui, S., Peacock, M., and Johnston, C. C. Sex steroids and bone mass in older men. Positive associations with serum estrogens and negative associations with androgens. *J. Clin. Invest.* **100,** 1755–1759 (1997).
45. Looker, A. C., Johnston, C. C. J., Wahner, H. W., Dunn, W. L., Calvo, M. S., Harris, T. B., Heyse, S. P., and Lindsay, R. L. Prevalence of low femoral bone density in older U.S. women from NHANES III. *J. Bone Miner. Res.* **10,** 796–802 (1995).
46. Riis, B. J., Christiansen, C., Johansen, J. S., and Jacobson, J. Is it possible to prevent bone loss in young women treated with luteinizing hormone-releasing hormone agonists? *J. Clin. Endocrinol. Metab.* **70,** 920–924 (1990).
47. Matta, W. H., Shaw, R. W., Hesp, R., and Evans, R. Reversible trabecular bone density loss following induced hypo-oestrogenism with the GnRH analogue buserelin in premenopausal women. *Clin. Endocrinol.* **29,** 45–51 (1988).
48. Friedman, A. J., Daly, M., Juneau-Norcross, M., Gleason, R., Rein, M. S., and LeBoff, M. S. Long-term medical therapy for leiomyomata uteri: a prospective randomized study of leuprolide acetate depot plus either oestrogen-progestin or progestin add-back for 2 years. *Hum. Reprod.* **9,** 1618–1625 (1994).
49. Friedman, A. J., Daly, M., Juneau-Norcross, M., Rein, M. S., Fine, C., Gleason, R., and LeBoff, M. A prospective, randomized trial of gonadotropin-releasing hormone agonist plus estrogen-progestin or progestin "add-back" regimens for women with leiomyomata uteri. *J. Clin. Endocrinol. Metab.* **76,** 1439–1445 (1993).
50. Riis, B. J., Christiansen, C., Deftos, L. J., and Catherwood, B. D. The role of serum concentrations of estrogens on postmenopausal osteoporosis and bone turnover. *In* "Osteoporosis" (C. Christiansen, C. D. Arnaud, B. E. C. Nordin, A. M. Parfitt, W. A. Peck, and B. L. Riggs, eds.), p. 333, Glostrup, 1984.
51. Cummings, S. R., Browner, W. S., Bauer, D. B., Stone, K., Ensrud, K., and Jamal, S., Ettinger, B. Endogenous sex and calciotropic hormones and the risk of hip and vertebral fractures in older women: The study of osteoporotic fractures. *N. Engl. J. Med.* **339,** 733–738 (1998).
52. Rozenberg, S., Ham, H., Bosson, D., Peretz, A., and Robyn, C. Age, steroids and bone mineral content. *Maturitas* **12,** 137–143 (1990).
53. Carroll, J., Testa, M. A., Erat, K., LeBoff, M. S., El-Hajj, and Fuleihan, G. Modeling fracture risk using bone density, age, and years since menopause. *Am. J. Prev. Med.* **13,** 447–452 (1997).
54. Davidson, B. J., Riggs, B. L., Wahner, H. W., and Judd, H. L. Endogenous cortisol and sex steroids in patients with osteoporotic spinal fractures. *Obstet, Gynecol.* **61,** 275–278 (1983).
55. Riggs, B. L., Ryan, R. J., Wahner, H. W., Jiang, N. S., and Mattox, V. R. Serum concentrations of estrogen, testosterone, and gonadotropins in osteoporotic and nonosteoporotic postmenopausal women. *J. Clin. Endocrinol. Metab.* **36,** 1097–1099 (1982).
56. Longcope, C., Baker, R. S., Hui, S. L., and Johnston, C. C. J. Androgen and estrogen dynamics in women with vertebral crush fractures. *Maturitas* **6,** 309–318 (1984).
57. Harris, S., Dallal, G. E., and Dawson-Hughes, B. Influence of body weight on rates of change in bone density of the spine, hip, and radius in postmenopausal women. *Calcif. Tissue Int.* **50,** 19–23 (1992).

58. Desplypere, J. P., Verdonck, L., and Vermeulen, A. Fat tissue: A steroid reservoir and site of steroid metabolism. *J. Clin. Endocrinol. Metab.* **61,** 564–570 (1985).
59. Greendale, G. A., Edelstein, S., and Barrett-Connor, E. Endogenous sex steroids and bone mineral density in older women and men: The Rancho Bernardo Study. *J. Bone Miner. Res.* **12,** 1833–1843 (1997).
60. Cauley, J. A., Gutai, J. P., Kuller, L. H., and Powell, J. G. Reliability and interrelations among serum sex hormones in postmenopausal women. *Am. J. Epidemiol.* **133,** 50–57 (1991).
61. Khosla, S., Melton, L. J. I., Atkinson, E. J., Klee, G. G., O'Fallon, W. M., and Riggs, B. L. Relationship of serum sex steroid levels with bone mineral density in aging women and men: A key role for bioavailable estrogen. *J. Clin. Endocrinol. Metab.* **83,** 2266–2274 (1998).
62. Anderson, F. H., Francis, R. M., Peaston, R. T., and Wastell, H. J. Androgen supplementation in eugonadal men with osteoporosis: Effects on six months' treatment on markers of bone formation and resportion. *J. Bone Miner. Res.* **12,** 472–478 (1997).
63. Lindsay, R., and Tohme, J. F. Estrogen treatment of patients with established postmenopausal osteoporosis. *Obstet. Gynecol.* **76,** 290–295 (1990).
64. Lindsay, R., Bush, T. L., Grady, D. G., Speroff, L., and Lobo, R. A. Therapeutic controversy: Estrogen replacement in menopause. *J. Clin. Endocrinol. Metab.* **81,** 3829–3838 (1996).
65. Schneider, D. L., Barrett-Connor, E., and Morton, D. J. Timing of postmenopausal estrogen for optimal bone density: The Rancho Bernardo Study. *JAMA* **277,** 543–547 (1997).
66. Cauley, J. A., Seeley, D. G., Ensrud, K., Ettinger, B., Black, D., and Cummings, S. R. Estrogen replacement therapy and fractures in older women. *Ann. Intern. Med.* **122,** 9–16 (1995).
67. Vermeulen, A., Deslypere, J. P., and DeMeirleir, K. A new look to the andropause: altered function of the gonadotrophs. *J. Steroid Biochem.* **32,** 163–165 (1989).
68. Vermeulen, A. Environment, human reproduction, menopause, and andropause. *Environ. Health Perspect.* **101,** 91–100 (1993).
69. Schow, D. A., Redmon, B., and Pryor, J. L. Male menopause. How to define it, how to treat it. *Postgrad. Med.* **101,** 62–64 (1997).
70. Gray, A., Feldman, H. A., McKinlay, J. B., and Longcope, C. Age, disease, and changing sex hormone levels in middle-aged men: results of the Massachusetts Male Aging Study. *J. Clin. Endocrinol. Metab.* **73,** 1016–1025 (1991).
71. Zmuda, J. M., Cauley, J. A., Kriska, A., Glynn, N. W., Gutai, J. P., and Kuller, L. H. Longitudinal relation between endogenous testosterone and cardiovascular disease risk factors in middle-aged men. A 13-year follow-up of former Multiple Risk Factor Intervention Trial participants. *Am. J. Epidemiol* **146,** 609–617 (1997).
72. Meier, D. E., Orwoll, E. S., Keenan, E. J., and Fagerstrom, R. M. Marked decline in trabecular bone mineral content in healthy men with age: lack of association with sex steroid levels. *J. Am. Geriatr. Soc.* **35,** 189–197 (1987).
73. deLignieres, B. Transdermal dihydrotestosterone treatment of "andropause." *Ann. Med.* **25,** 235–241 (1993).
74. Nankin, H. R., and Calkins, J. H. Decreased bioavailable testosterone in aging normal and impotent men. *J. Clin. Endocrinol. Metab.* **63,** 1418–1420 (1986).
75. Vermeulen, A. Clinical review 24: Androgens in the aging male. *J. Clin. Endocrinol. Metab.* **73,** 221–224 (1991).
76. Labrie, F., Belanger, A., Cusan, L., Gomez, J.-L., and Candas, B. Marked decline in serum concentrations of adrenal C19 sex steroid precursors and conjugated androgen metabolites during aging. *J. Clin. Endocrinol. Metab.* **82,** 2396–2402 (1997).
77. Bidlingmaier, R., Dorr, H. G., Eisenmenger, W., Kuhnle, U., and Knorr, D. Contribution of the adrenal gland to the production of androstenedione and testosterone during the first two years of life. *J. Clin. Endocrinol. Metab.* **62,** 331–335 (1986).
78. Labrie, F., Belanger, A., Dupont, A., *et. al.* Science behind total androgen blockade: from gene to combination therapy. *Clin. Invest. Med.* **16,** 475–492 (1993).
79. Tenover, J. S., Metsumoto, A. M., Plymate, S. R., and Bremner, W. J. The effects of aging in normal men on bioavailable testosterone and luteinizing hormone secretion: response to clomiphene citrate. *J. Clin. Endocrinol. Metab.* **65,** 1118–1126 (1987).
80. Veldhuis, J. D., Liem, A. Y., South, S., Weltman, A., Weltman, J., Clemmons, D. A., Abbott, R., Mulligan, T., Johnson, M. L., Pincus, S., *et al.* Differential impact of age, sex steroid hormones, and obesity on basal versus pulsatile growth hormone secretion in men as assessed in an ultrasensitive chemiluminescence assay. *J. Clin. Endocrinol. Metab.* **80,** 3209–3222 (1995).
81. Pfeilschifter, J., Scheidt-Nave, C., Leidig-Bruckner, G., Woitge, H. W., Blum, W. F., Wuster, C., Haack, D., and Ziegler, R. Relationship between circulating insulin-like growth factor components and sex hormones in a population-based sample of 50- to 80-year-old men and women. *J. Clin. Endocrinol. Metab.* **81,** 2534–2540 (1996).
82. Field, A. E., Colditz, G. A., Willett, W. C., Longcope, C., and McKinlay, J. B. The relation of smoking, age, relative weight, and dietary intake to serum adrenal steroids, sex hormones, and sex hormone-binding globulin in middle-aged men. *J. Clin. Endocrinol. Metab.* **79,** 1310–1316 (1994).
83. Fitzgerald, R. C., Skingle, S. J., and Crisp, A. J. Testosterone concentrations in men on chronic glucocorticosteroid therapy. *J. R. Coll. Phys. Lond.* **31,** 168–170 (1997).
84. Mastrogiacomo, I. Andropause: incidence and pathogenesis. *Arch. Androl.* **69,** 293–296 (1982).
85. Korenman, S. G., Morley, J. E., Mooradian, A. D., Davis, S. S., Kalser, F. E., Silver, A. J., Viosca, S. P., and Garza, D. Secondary hypogonadism in older men: its relation to impotence. *J. Clin. Endocrinol. Metab.* **71,** 963–969 (1990).
86. Zumoff, B., Strain, G. W., Miller, L. K., and Rosner, W. Twenty-four hour mean plasma testosterone concentration declines with age in normal premenopausal women. *J. Clin. Endocrinol. Metab.* **80,** 1429–1430 (1995).
87. Melton, L. J., III, and Riggs, B. L. The epidemiology of age-related fractures. *In* "The Osteoporotic Syndrome" (L. V. Avioli, ed.), pp. 45–72 Grune and Stratton, Orlando, 1993.
88. Boonen, S., Vanderschueren, D., Cheng, X. G., Verbeke, G., Dequeker, J., Geusens, P., Broos, P., and Bouillon, R. Age-related (Type II) femoral neck osteoporosis in men: biochemical evidence for both hypovitaminosis D and androgen deficiency-induced bone resorption. *J. Bone Miner. Res.* **12,** 2119–2126 (1997).
89. Arisaka, O., Arisaka, M., Nakayama, Y., Fujiwara, S., and Yabuta, K. Effect of testosterone on bone density and bone metabolism in adolescent male hypogonadism. *Metabolism* **44,** 418–423 (1995).
90. Finklestein, J. S., Klibanski, A., Neer, R. M., Doppelt, S. H., Rosenthal, D. I., Segre, G. V., and Crowley, Jr. W. F. Increases in bone density during treatment of men with idiopathic hypogonadotropic hypogonadism. *J. Clin. Endocrinol. Metab.* **69,** 776–783 (1989).
91. Behre, H. M., Klesch, S., Leifke, E., Link, T. M., and Nieschlag, E. Long-term effect of testosterone therapy on bone mineral density in hypogonadal men. *J. Clin. Endcrinol. Metab.* **82,** 2386–2390 (1997).

92. Greenspan, S. L., Oppenheim, D. S., and Klibanski, A. Importance of gonadal steroids to bone mass in men with hyperprolactinemic hypogonadism. *Ann. Intern. Med.* **110,** 526–531 (1989).
93. Katznelson, L., Finklestein, J. S., Schoenfeld, D. A., Rosenthal, D. I., Anderson, E. J., and Klibanski, A. Increase in bone density and lean body mass during testosterone administration in men with acquired hypogonadism. *J. Clin. Endocrinol. Metab.* **81,** 4358–4365 (1993).
94. Francis, R. M., Peacock, M., Aaron, J. E., Selby, P. L., Taylor, G. A., Thompson, J., Marshall, D. H., and Horsman, A. Osteoporosis in hypogonadal men: Role of decreased plasma 1,25-dihydroxyvitamin D, calcium malabsorption, and low bone formation. *Bone* **7,** 261–268 (1986).
95. Drinka, P. J., Olson, J., Bauwens, S., Voeks, S. K., Carlson, I., and Wilson, M. Lack of association between free testosterone and bone density separate from age in elderly males. *Calcif. Tissue Int.* **52,** 67–69 (1993).
96. Murphy, S., Khaw, K. T., Cassidy, A., and Compston, J. E. Sex hormones and bone mineral density in elderly men. *Bone Miner.* **20,** 133–140 (1993).
97. Ongphiphadhanakul, B., Rajatanavin, R., Chailurkit, L., Piaseu, N., Teerarungsikul, K., Sirisriro, R., Komindr, S., and Puavilai, G. Serum testosterone and its relation to bone mineral density and body composition in normal males. *Clin. Endocrinol.* **43,** 727–733 (1995).
98. Kelly, P. J., Pocock, N. A., Sambrook, P. N., and Eisman, J. A. Dietary calcium, sex hormones, and bone mineral density in men. *Br. Med. J.* **300,** 1361–1364 (1990).
99. Stanley, H. L., Schmitt, B. P., Poses, R. M., and Deiss, W. P. Does hypogonadism contribute to the occurrence of a minimal trauma hip fracture in elderly men? *J. Am. Geriatr. Soc.* **39,** 766–771 (1991).
100. Nyquist, F., Gardsell, P., Sernbo, I., Jeppson, J. O., and Johnell, O. Assessment of sex hormones and bone mineral density in relation to occurrence of fracture in men: A prospective population-based study. *Bone* **22,** 147–151 (1998).
101. Gasperino, J. Androgenic regulation of bone mass in women. *Clin. Orthop.* **311,** 278–286 (1995).
102. Buchanan, J. R., Hospodar, P., Myers, C., Leuenberger, P., and Demers, L. M. Effect of excess endogenous androgens on bone density in young women. *J. Clin. Endocrinol. Metab.* **67,** 937–943 (1988).
103. Wild, R. A., Buchanan, J. R., Myers, C., and Demers, L. M. Declining adrenal androgens: An association with bone loss in aging women (42625). *Proc. Soc. Exp. Biol. Med.* **186,** 355–360 (1987).
104. Nordin, B. E. C., Cleghorn, D. B., Chatterton, B. E., Morris, H. A., and Need, A. G. A 5-year longitudinal study of forearm bone mass in 307 postmenopausal women. *J. Bone Miner. Res.* **8,** 1427–1432 (1993).
105. Davidson, B. J., Ross, R. K., Paganini-Hill, A., Hammond, G. D., Siiteri, P. K., and Judd, H. L. Total and free estrogens and androgens in postmenopausal women with hip fractures. *J. Clin. Endocrinol. Metab.* **54,** 115–120 (1982).
106. Simberg, N., Tiitinen, A., Silfvast, A., Viinikka, L., and Ylikorkala, O. High bone density in hyperandrogenic women: effect of gonadotropin-releasing hormone agonist alone or in conjunction with estrogen-progestin replacement. *J. Clin. Endocrinol. Metab.* **81,** 646–651 (1996).
107. Ortego-Centeno, N., Munoz-Torres, M., Hernandez-Quero, J., Jurado-Duce, A., and Torres-Puchol, J. Bone mineral density, sex steroids, and mineral metabolism in premenopausal smokers. *Calcif. Tissue Int.* **55,** 403–407 (1994).
108. Michnovicz, J. J., Hershcopf, R. J., Naganuma, H., Bradlow, H. L., and Fishman, J. Increased 2-hydroxylation of estradiol as a possible mechanism for the anti-estrogenic effect of cigarette smoking. *N. Engl. J. Med.* **315,** 1305–1309 (1986).
109. Niewoehner, C. B. Osteoporosis in men. Is it more common than we think? *Postgrad. Med.* **93,** 59–60, 63–70 (1993).
110. Tenover, J. L. Testosterone and the aging male. *J. Androl.* **18,** 103–106 (1997).
111. Tenover, J. S. Effects of testosterone supplementation in the aging male. *Clin. Endocrinol. Metab.* **75,** 1092–1098 (1992).
112. Young, N. R., Baker, H. W., Liu, G., and Seeman, E. Body composition and muscle strength in healthy men receiving testosterone enanthate. *J. Clin. Endocrinol. Metab.* **77,** 1028–1032 (1993).
113. Anderson, F. H., Francis, R. M., and Faulkner, K. Androgen supplementation in eugonadal men with osteoporosis—effects of 6 months of treatment on bone mineral density and cardiovascular risk factors. *Bone* **18,** 171–177 (1996).
114. Mateo, L., Nolla, J. M., Bonnin, M. R., Navarro, M. A., and Roig-Escofet, D. Sex hormone status and bone mineral density in men with rheumatoid arthritis. *J. Rheumatol.* **22,** 1455–1460 (1955).
115. Reid, I. R., Wattie, D. J., Evans, M. C., and Stapleton, J. P. Testosterone therapy in glucocorticoid-treated men. *Arch. Intern. Med.* **156,** 1173–1177 (1996).
116. Hall, G. M., Larbre, J. P., Spector, T. D., Perry, L. A., and DaSilva, J. A. A randomized trial of testosterone therapy in males with rheumatoid arthritis. *Br. J. Rheumatol.* **35,** 568–573 (1996).
117. Chesnut, C. H., Ivey, J. L., Gruber, H. E., Matthews, M., Nelp, W. B., Sisom, K., and Baylink, D. J. Stanozolol in postmenopausal osteoporosis: therapeutic efficacy and possible mechanisms of action. *Metabolism* **32,** 571–580 (1983).
118. Savvas, M., Studd, J. W. W., Norman, S., Leather, A. T., Garnett, T. J., and Fogelman, I. Increase in bone mass after one year of percutaneous oestradiol and testosterone implants in postmenopausal women who have previously received long-term oral estrogens. *Br. J. Obstet. Gynaecol.* **99,** 757–760 (1992).
119. Garnett, T., Studd, J., Watson, N., Savvas, M., and Leather, A. The effects of plasma estradiol levels on increases in vertebral and femoral bone density following therapy with estradiol and estradiol with testosterone implants. *Obstet. Gynecol.* **79,** 968–972 (1992).
120. Raisz, L. G., Wita, B., Artis, A., Bowen, A., Schwartz, S., Trahiotis, M., Shoukri, K., and Smith, J. Comparison of the effects of estrogen alone and estrogen plus androgen on biochemical markers of bone formation and resorption in postmenopausal women. *J. Clin. Endocrinol. Metab.* **81,** 37–43 (1996).
121. Babalola, A., and Ellis, G. Serum DHEAS in a normal pediatric population. *Clin. Biochem.* **18,** 184–189 (1985).
122. Allbright, F. Osteoporosis. *Ann. Intern. Med.* **27,** 861 (1947).
123. Orentreich, N., Brind, J. L., Rizer, R. L., and Vogelman, J. H. Age changes and sex differences in serum dehydroepiandrosterone sulfate concentrations throughout adulthood. *J. Clin. Endocrinol. Metab.* **59,** 551–555 (1984).
124. Parker, L., Gral, T., Perrigo, V., and Skowsy, R. Decreased adrenal androgen sensitivity to ACTH during aging. *Metab. Clin. Exp.* **30,** 601–604 (1981).
125. Hornsby, P. J. Biosynthesis of DHEAS by the human adrenal cortex and its age-related decline. *Ann. N.Y. Acad. Sci.* **774,** 29–46 (1995).
126. Herbert, J. The age of dehydroepiandrosterone. *Lancet* **345,** 1193–1194 (1995).

127. Meikle, A. W., Daynes, R. A., and Araneo, B. A. Adrenal androgen secretion and biological effects. *Endocr. Metab. Clin. N. Am.* **20,** 381 (1991).

128. Labrie, F., Belanger, A., Cusan, L., and Candas, B. Physiological changes in dehydroepiandrosterone are not reflected by serum levels of active androgens and estrogens but of their metabolites: intracrinology. *J. Clin. Endocrinol. Metab.* **82,** 2403–2409 (1997).

129. Nimrod, A., and Ryan, K. J. Aromatization of androgens by human abdominal and breast fat tissue. *J. Clin. Endocrinol. Metab.* **40,** 367–372 (1975).

130. Zumoff, B., Walsh, B. T., Katz, J. L., Levin, Rosenfeld, R. S., Kream, J., and Weiner, H. Subnormal plasma dehydroepiandrosterone to cortisol ratio in anorexia nervosa: a second hormonal parameter of ontogenic regression. *J. Clin. Endocrinol. Metab.* **56,** 668–671 (1983).

131. Gordon, C. M., Grace, E., Emans, J., Goodman, E., Crawford, M. H., and LeBoff, M. S. Use of DHEA to prevent osteoporosis in patients with anorexia nervosa. *Soc. Adolesc. Med.* (1998). [Abstract]

132. Buchanan, J. R., Myers, C., Lloyd, T., Leuenberger, P., and Demers, L. M. Determinants of peak trabecular bone density in women: The role of androgens, estrogen and exercise. *J. Bone Miner. Res.* **3,** 673–680 (1988).

133. Nordin, B. E. C., Robertson, A., Sezmark, R. F., Bridges, A., Philcox, J. C., Need, A. G., Horowitz, M., Morris, H. A., and Deam, S. The relation between calcium absorption, serum dehydroepiandrosterone and vertebral mineral density in postmenopausal women. *J. Clin. Endocrinol. Metab.* **60,** 651–657 (1985).

134. Taelman, P., Kaufman, J. M., Janssens, X., and Vermeulen, A. Persistence of increased bone resorption and possible role of dehydroepiandrosterone as a bone metabolism determinant in osteoporotic women in late post-menopause. *Maturitas* **11,** 65–73 (1989).

135. Mortola, J. F., and Yen, S. S. C. The effects of oral dehydroepiandrosterone (DHEA) on endocrine-metabolic parameters in postmenopausal women. *J. Clin. Endocrinol. Metab.* **71,** 696–704 (1990).

136. Labrie, F., Belanger, A., Simard, J., Van, L.-T., and Labrie, C. DHEA and peripheral androgen and estrogen formation: intracrinology. *Ann. N. Y. Acad. Sci.* **774,** 16–28 (1995).

137. Kasperk, C. H., Wakley, G. K., Hierl, T., and Ziegler, R. Gonadal and adrenal androgens are potent regulators of human bone cell metabolism *in vitro*. *J. Bone Miner. Res.* **12,** 464–471 (1997).

137a. Haden, S. T., Hurwitz, S. Glowacki, J., Rosen, C. J., and LeBoff, M. S. Effects of age on serum dehydroepiandrosterone, IGF-I and IL-6 levels. *Bone* **23,** S620 (1998).

138. Barrett-Connor, E., Khaw, K., and Yen, S. S. C. A prospective study of dehydroepiandrosterone sulphate, mortality and cardiovascular disease. *N. Engl. J. Med.* **315,** 1519–1524 (1986).

139. Nestler, J. E. Regulation of human dehydroepiandrosterone metabolism by insulin. *Ann. N. Y. Acad. Sci.* **774,** 73–81 (1995).

140. Daynes, R. A., and Araneo, B. A. Prevention and reversal of some age-associated changes in immunologic responses by supplemental dehydroepiandrosterone sulfate therapy. *Immun. Infect. Dis.* **3,** 135–154 (1992).

141. Daynes, R. A., Araneo, B. A., Ershler, W. B., *et al.* Altered regulation of IL-6 production with normal aging. Possible linkage to the age-associated decline in DHEA and its sulphated derivative. *J. Immunol.* **150,** 5219–5230 (1993).

142. Turner, R. T., Wakley, G. K., and Hannon, K. S. Differential effect of androgens on cortical bone histomorphometry in gonadectomized male and female rats. *J. Orthop. Res.* **8,** 612–617 (1990).

143. Steinberg, K. K., Freni-Titulaer, L. W., DePuey, E. G., Miller, D. T., Sgoutas, D. S., Coralli, C. H., Phillips, D. L., Rogers, T. N., and Clark, R. V. Sex steroids and bone density in premenopausal and perimenopausal women. *J. Clin. Endocrinol. Metab.* **69,** 533–539 (1989).

144. Barrett-Connor, E., Kritz-Silvertein, D., and Edelstein, S. L. A prospective study of dehydroepiandrosterone sulphate (DHEAS) and bone mineral density in older men and women. *Am. J. Epidemiol.* **137,** 201–206 (1993).

145. Morales, A. J., Nolan, J. J., Nelson, J. C., and Yen, S. S. C. Effects of replacement dose of dehydroepiandrosterone in men and women of advancing age. *J. Clin. Endocrinol. Metab.* **78,** 1360–1367 (1994).

146. Deleted in proof.

147. Labrie, F., Diamond, P., Cusan, L., Gomez, J-L., Belanger, A., and Candas, B. Effect of 12-month dehydroepiandrosterone replacement therapy on bone, vagina, and endometrium in postmenopausal women. *J. Clin. Endocrinol. Metab.* **82,** 3498–3505 (1997).

148. Araneo, B. A., Woods, M. L., II, and Daynes, R. A. Reversal of the immunosenescent phenotype by dehydroepiandrosterone: hormonal treatment provides an adjuvant effect on the immunization of aged mice with recombinant hepatitis B surface antigen. *J. Infect. Dis.* **167,** 830–840 (1993).

149. Casson, P. R., Faquin, L. C., Stentz, F. B., Straughn, A. B., Andersen, R. N., and Buster, J. E. Replacement of dehydroepiandrosterone enhances T-lymphocyte insulin binding in postmenopausal women. *Fertil. Steril.* **63,** 1027–1031 (1995).

150. Luo, S., Labrie, C., Belanger, A., and Labrie, F. Effect of DHEA and the pure antiestrogen EM-800 on bone mass serum lipids, and the development of dimethylbenz(A)-anthracene (DMBA)-induced mammary carcinoma in the rat. *Endoc. Soc.* 1997. [Abstract 1527]

CHAPTER 16

Parathyroid Hormone

SHONNI J. SILVERBERG* AND JOHN P. BILEZIKIAN*,†
Departments of *Medicine and †Pharmacology, College of Physicians & Surgeons, Columbia University, New York, New York 10032

INTRODUCTION

The aging process is associated with many changes in important elements of mineral metabolism. They lead, in the aggregate, to age-related reductions in bone mass. Processes associated with age-related bone loss are accelerated by menopause and the attendant estrogen deficiency state. This book covers a number of critically important features of the aging process that lead to a state of negative calcium balance. The efficiency and the quantity of calcium absorbed from the gastrointestinal tract wane with age (see Chapter 3). Major alterations in vitamin D formation, metabolism, and action have profound effects on the maintenance of calcium homeostasis in the later years (see Chapter 17). Not so clearly implicated in the events associated with age-related bone loss is parathyroid hormone. It is important to consider parathyroid hormone because it is such a pivotal regulator of calcium metabolism. Its actions influence bone remodeling, vitamin D metabolism, renal handling of calcium, and gastrointestinal absorption of calcium. Changes in parathyroid hormone concentrations, action, or glandular function could have key implications for the pathophysiological events associated with bone loss and aging. This chapter reviews what is known about how aging effects parathyroid hormone and how, in turn, parathyroid hormone may be associated with events related to age-related bone loss as well as to those associated with menopause.

PARATHYROID HORMONE AND NORMAL AGING

Since the early 1980s, a plethora of studies have documented that circulating concentrations of parathyroid hormone increase with advancing age [1–6]. Interpretations of earlier reports were complicated by the use of assays that detected fragments of parathyroid hormone, not the intact 1-84 peptide. These midmolecule and carboxy-terminal radioimmunoassays can show increases with the aging process simply because the aging kidney is less able to clear these fragments [1–4]. Nevertheless, other data were consistent with greater biological effects of parathyroid hormone in the elderly, suggesting an increase in intact hormone with age. Urinary cyclic AMP excretion increases with age, and urinary phosphorus excretion decreases, which are both features of increased bioactive parathyroid hormone [2,3,6]. These measures of parathyroid hormone bioactivity indicate that the mere retention of inactive hormone fragments is an inadequate explanation for the increase in parathyroid hormone levels. More recently, assays that measure the intact molecule [immunoradiometric assay (IRMA)] have confirmed that parathyroid hormone levels in fact rise with age [7–11]. The association between the increase in parathyroid hormone levels and the rates of bone loss with aging, along with the known physiological actions of parathyroid hormone to cause increased bone turnover, has led to efforts to elucidate the etiology of this age-related rise in parathyroid hormone concentration. Several possibilities are listed.

Altered Calcium Absorption and Vitamin D Metabolism

The increase in parathyroid hormone levels in normal aging individuals is attributable, at least in part, to alterations in gastrointestinal absorption of calcium. Decreased intestinal calcium in the elderly has been reported in studies of fractional calcium absorption and metabolic balance [12–16]. The decrease in intestinal calcium absorption leads to a subtle reduction in serum calcium concentration, which induces a secondary increase in parathyroid hormone.

Putative mechanisms for reduced calcium absorption in the elderly have focused on changes in the vitamin D axis leading to decreased vitamin D levels. With aging, the sun becomes less of a source of vitamin D because of reduced sun exposure among the elderly per se and also because of a reduction in the skin levels of the vitamin D precursor, 7-dehydrocholesterol. In addition, subsequent mechanisms of vitamin D activation, particularly the conversion of 25-hydroxyvitamin D to 1,25-dihydroxyvitamin D in the kidney, are relatively impaired with aging.

Alterations in intestinal calcium absorption could also be due to vitamin D action in the gastrointestinal tract. An element of intestinal resistance to 1,25-dihydroxyvitamin D is known to emerge with age [17,18]. This could be due to a reduction in 1,25-dihydroxyvitamin D receptors in the small intestine [18,19]. In 44 healthy women, aged 20–87, a decrease in the concentration of duodenal 1,25-dihydroxyvitamin D receptors was shown to occur as a function of age. Altered vitamin D metabolism with aging may involve impaired binding of 1,25-dihydroxyvitamin D to its intestinal receptors [20] rather than a decrease in receptor number. A postreceptor defect in 1,25-dihydroxyvitamin D action is possible as well. Any of these mechanisms could lead to a reduction in gastrointestinal tract calcium absorption and to a subsequent increase in parathyroid hormone concentration.

Renal Resistance to Parathyroid Hormone

Another explanation for the increase in parathyroid hormone levels with advancing age is based on the progressive decline in renal function associated with aging. However, even in elderly individuals with intact renal function (glomerular filtration rate > 70 cc/min), parathyroid hormone levels are increased [21]. While parathyroid hormone levels increase with age, no similar increment is seen in levels of 1,25-dihydroxyvitamin D_3 concentrations. This observation suggests a possible explanation. If aging per se (in the absence of renal insufficiency or osteoporosis) impairs the ability of the kidney to respond to parathyroid hormone, higher levels of the latter would be required to maintain vitamin D homeo stasis. Halloran *et al.* [9] compared the ability of the kidney to respond to infusions of human parathyroid hormone among healthy young and healthy elderly men. These authors elegantly confirmed that maximal renal responsiveness to parathyroid hormone is not impaired in elderly men. This observation, however, does not simulate physiological conditions in which the kidney may in fact be less functional and is normally not exposed to such high concentrations of parathyroid hormone.

One formulation that could account for the inability of the kidney to maintain 1,25-dihydroxyvitamin D_3, despite the age-related compensatory increase in parathyroid hormone (PTH), implicates growth hormone (GH) and insulin-like growth factor-1 (IGF-1). These agents, which stimulate the renal 1-α hydroxylase enzyme, decline with advancing age [22–24]. Halloran and Portale [25] have theorized that the decrease in GH and IGF-I tends to impair the renal production of 1,25-dihydroxyvitamin D_3, an effect that counterbalances the effect of increased parathyroid hormone to raise levels of 1,25-dihydroxyvitamin D_3.

Depending on whether the compensatory increase in PTH is dominant or not with respect to the counterforce generated by GH and IGF-I, 1,25-dihydroxyvitamin D levels could be normal or reduced in the elderly. This hypothesis is predicated on the documentation of direct effects of IGF-I and/or GH on the renal 1-α hydroxylase enzyme, evidence that has not been definitely established. Data from Favus *et al.* support an effect of age-related loss of IGF-I action on rat 1-α hydroxylase activity. IGF-I administration to older rats reverses the age-acquired defect in 1,25-dihydroxyvitamin D production [25a]. Even if GH and IGF-I are not shown to be pivotal regulators of this enzyme, renal function per se does decline as part of the aging process and thus the 1-α hydroxylase enzyme is going to become less active with aging, even if it is not further compromised by GH and IGF-I. Whatever the mechanisms for a tendency for 1,25-dihydroxyvitamin D levels to decline in the elderly, this reduction produces another stimulus for increased parathyroid hormone levels. 1,25-Dihydroxyvitamin D is a key regulator of parathyroid hormone gene function. When levels decline, the parathyroid hormone gene is stimulated by virtue of the loss of 1,25-dihydroxyvitamin's tonic inhibition of gene transcription. When the inhibitory effect is lessened, parathyroid hormone synthesis is stimulated and parathyroid hormone levels rise.

Parathyroid Resistance/Altered Set Point

Another mechanism implicated in the age-related increase in parathyroid hormone is a change in the parathyroid cell itself. Aging could be associated with an emerging resistance of parathyroid tissue to tonic inhibition by 1,25-dihydroxyvitamin D_3 at the level of the parathyroid hormone gene. Ledger *et al.* [10] found that elderly women have greater basal, maximal, and nonsuppressible levels of parathyroid hormone secretion than young women. However, no alteration in set point for parathyroid hormone secretion could be documented. It was their conclusion that the change in parathyroid secretory dynamics to calcium could be explained by a chronic parathyroid hyperfunctioning state (secondary hyperparathyroidism) in response to the primary abnormality, namely a reduction in intestinal calcium absorption.

The question of parathyroid gland resistance with aging has not been definitively resolved, as results of studies from other groups have met with divergent results [21,26]. In elderly men, Portale *et al.* [21] suggested that there is an increase in the calcium set-point for parathyroid hormone release [21]. Although the molecular mechanism for this alteration is unknown, the calcium-sensing receptor of the parathyroid cell might be a factor. In aging rats, calcium receptor mRNA and receptor protein concentration both increase.

If the increase in calcium receptors in the parathyroid cell is to be etiologically linked to the processes associated with increased parathyroid hormone secretion, one has to postulate that the affinity of these receptors is reduced. Otherwise, increases in calcium receptors without any change in affinity might be expected to reduce parathyroid hormone levels by virtue of greater binding by calcium ion to this receptor.

PARATHYROID HORMONE AND OSTEOPOROSIS

We have reviewed the processes that have been implicated in the generally understood and pervasive observation that parathyroid hormone levels increase with age. While the exact mechanisms by which this increase occurs is unclear, the fact that it does occur, under normal circumstances, is incontrovertible. Because the increase in parathyroid hormone with age is a universal finding, it has been tempting to link that finding with age-associated osteoporosis. The assumption here is that in osteoporosis too, parathyroid hormone levels rise. Further, the implication is that elevated levels of parathyroid hormone as a function of aging or in association with osteoporosis are necessarily a negative influence on bone balance. Such assumptions and implications will be explored in this section.

First, it should be pointed out that in osteoporosis, increases in the parathyroid hormone have not been demonstrated consistently. Basal levels of parathyroid hormone have been reported to be increased [28–30], normal [31,32], or decreased [13,33] relative to age-matched control subjects. Using the immunoradiometric assay for intact parathyroid hormone, no difference was documented between osteoporotic and normal women [34,30], while the even more sensitive immunochemiluminometric assay has shown reduced basal parathyroid hormone levels in some series of osteoporotic patients [34,36]. Several studies, beginning with those of Jowsey and Riggs in 1973, have described a small subset of osteoporotic women who have increased circulating parathyroid hormone levels [28–30,37].

It is evident that the role of the parathyroid glands and parathyroid hormone in osteoporosis is not completely understood. Just as osteoporosis is likely to be the end point of different processes in differing clinical situations, the pathogenetic role of parathyroid hormone is likely to differ as well. Each of the following hypotheses may hold true in certain situations, which have, as their end point, the bone loss characteristic of osteoporosis.

Secondary Hyperparathyroidism

The hypothesis that age-related osteoporosis is due to secondary hyperparathyroidism extends the physiological changes observed in aging and summarized earlier. With regard to parathyroid hormone, the concept implicates the normal age-related increase in parathyroid hormone as a pathophysiological state. The pathophysiology in this view is in fact the normal physiology of aging. With dysfunctional mechanisms of calcium absorption in the gastrointestinal tract, renal resistance to parathyroid hormone, and/or altered sensitivity of the parathyroid glands, parathyroid hormone levels rise to levels that maintain serum calcium levels at the expense of the skeleton. Riggs and Melton [38] have focused on this hypothesis as an explanation for "type II" or age-related osteoporosis. It is important to demonstrate, however, that in age-related osteoporosis, these so-called normal homeostatic adjustments are, in fact, abnormal and to distinguish those with age-related osteoporosis from similarly aged individuals who do not have osteoporosis. If all individuals experience this normal aging process, then what differentiates those with osteoporosis from those without?

In support of the idea that there are important differences from normal individuals in osteoporosis, studies of fractional calcium absorption and metabolic clearance have shown an even greater reduction in osteoporotic subjects [12–16]. Thus, a primary abnormality in the gastrointestinal tract (i.e., reduction in 1,25-dihydroxyvitamin D receptor number or binding affinity [18–20]) or alterations in vitamin D metabolism could account for the reduction in calcium absorption, ultimately leading to secondary hyperparathyroidism and bone loss.

Studies have also focused on the kidney as a site that could be implicated in the pathophysiological events associated with increasing parathyroid hormone levels. In osteoporosis, reductions in 1,25-dihydroxyvitamin D_3 could be due to a decreased renal responsiveness to parathyroid hormone. Early studies were hampered by the use of pharmacologic doses of parathyroid extract to test renal responsiveness. A similar rise in 1,25-dihydroxyvitamin D was observed in normal and osteoporotic individuals when high doses of parathyroid hormone were administered. Thus, under pharmacologic conditions, normal renal responsiveness could be demonstrated [39]. However, it remained possible that an abnormality in renal responsiveness existed at more physiologic doses of parathyroid hormone. Subsequently, studies from Tsai *et al.* [40] suggested that renal 1-α hydroxylase activity in response to parathyroid hormone decreases with advancing age, with a further impairment seen in those with osteoporosis. However, that study was confounded by differences in renal function among the two study groups, raising the possibility that the observed differences may not be specific to the osteoporotic process, but rather to differences in renal function. At more physiologic doses, Slovik *et al.* [41] demonstrated that osteoporotic women had blunted 1,25-dihydroxyvitamin D_3 responses to parathyroid hormone. However, interpretation of these results was confounded by the use of a young, nonosteoporotic control group. It was therefore not possible to know whether the differences in parathyroid hormone responsiveness were due to advancing age or to osteoporosis.

Thus, despite the attractiveness of the hypothesis that blunted parathyroid responsiveness in the kidney is a primary pathophysiological abnormality in age-related osteoporosis, no studies have yet clearly distinguished osteoporotic from normal age-matched subjects in this regard. It is clear that renal responsiveness to parathyroid hormone declines with age; it is not clear that this aging process is etiologically related to osteoporosis.

While most studies of altered vitamin D metabolism in osteoporosis have implicated a defect in 1,25-dihydroxyvitamin D_3, it remains possible that alterations in its metabolic precursor 25-hydroxyvitamin D could be a factor. Villereal *et al.* [42] found that 9.1% of a population of American women with osteoporosis had low 25-hydroxyvitamin D levels and secondary hyperparathyroidism. Increased parathyroid hormone levels correlated with a decrease in bone density in those patients.

Moreover, more recent studies have called further attention to the increasing detection of subclinical reductions in vitamin D levels in the United States [43]. Additionally, our understanding of normal vitamin D levels is being refined with the recognition that levels of 25-hydroxyvitamin D technically within normal limits (i.e., 9–52 ng/ml) but below 20 ng/ml are associated with physiological changes associated with vitamin D deficiency (i.e., reduced calcium absorption and increases in parathyroid hormone). Such widespread deficiencies in vitamin D in the population could be an important risk factor for the mechanisms that lead to age-related bone loss.

Parathyroid Gland Suppression (Secondary Hypoparathyroidism)

This hypothesis runs counter to most ideas implicating increases in parathyroid hormone in age-related osteoporosis. Instead of a secondary increase in parathyroid hormone, this hypothesis argues for a secondary suppression of parathyroid gland function. According to this concept, a process or agent, independent of parathyroid hormone, increases bone resorption and ultimately causes osteoporosis. According to this paradigm, with enhanced bone resorption, ionized calcium rises, which leads, in turn, to a suppression of parathyroid hormone and reduced intestinal calcium absorption (a secondary phenomenon in this model). With regard to the designation of Riggs and Melton [38] type I osteoporosis (postmenopausal osteoporosis) is most consistent with this hypothesis. The primary "event" in this kind of osteoporosis is estrogen deficiency. Studies have elucidated some of the local mechanisms in the skeleton that lead to bone loss associated with estrogen deficiency. None of these mechanisms invoke parathyroid hormone either directly or indirectly.

Interleukin-1, reportedly produced at an increased rate by activated monocytes from postmenopausal osteoporotic patients, is one possible agent to explain this phenomenon [44,45]. Interleukin-6 is another agent, which has also been implicated in the bone resorption of estrogen deficiency [46,47]. Other cytokines that stimulate bone resorption and could contribute to putative parathyroid gland suppression include transforming growth factor [48,49], tumor necrosis factor [50], lymphotoxin [50], and some of the prostaglandins [51–53].

Few studies have shown that parathyroid hormone is actually suppressed in the early years after menopause. Although careful studies comparing parathyroid hormone levels in early postmenopausal women with or without estrogen replacement have not been completed, the studies of Ebeling *et al.* [54] do provide some support for the concept that parathyroids are suppressed in osteoporosis. Comparison of parathyroid hormone and bone markers in normal and osteoporotic women showed the osteoporotic cohort to have lower parathyroid hormone levels and higher osteocalcin and hydroxypyridinium cross-link levels. These data are consistent with a nonparathyroid hormone-mediated increase in bone resorption, with a secondary suppression of parathyroid hormone.

Increased Skeletal Sensitivity to Parathyroid Hormone

Originally proposed by Heaney in 1965, this concept states that in osteoporosis, the skeleton is more sensitive to parathyroid hormone, so that more bone is resorbed in response to parathyroid hormone at any circulating level [28,34,55]. Support for this hypothesis came from histologic and histomorphometric data documenting increased bone resorption in the face of normal or low parathyroid hormone levels [28]. In addition, osteoporotic women had greater activation frequency (1.3% per year), a higher bone resorption rate (3.9% per year), and more cancellous bone loss (2.8% per year) than nonosteoporotic women for each picomole per liter increase in parathyroid hormone levels [28]. It is evident that there are many other processes that could be associated with enhanced skeletal turnover in postmenopausal women. The mere association of parathyroid hormone with these indices does not establish that parathyroid hormone is responsible for them. However, experience with primary hyperparathyroidism, a disorder that is clearly different from osteoporosis, does provide some insights in this regard. Most women with primary hyperparathyroidism are discovered within the first decade after menopause. It is intriguing to note that at this time the effects of estrogen to counter the actions of parathyroid hormone are eliminated by virtue of the estrogen deficiency state. Another indirect argument in favor of the enhanced sensitivity of parathyroid hormone when menopause ensues is from our experience in perimenopausal women with primary hyperparathyroidism who enter menopause. These women seem to be at greater risk for bone loss at this time without further increases in parathyroid hormone concentration [56]. Nevertheless, studies that measure bone markers do not support enhanced skeletal sensitivity to parathyroid hormone. As mentioned earlier, Tsai *et al.* [40,57] showed no difference between normal and osteoporotic individuals in response to pharmacologic doses of parathyroid hormone. Another study, using physiologic doses of parathyroid hormone, reached a similar conclusion [54].

Altered Parathyroid Gland Responsiveness

Most of the discussion so far has considered the parathyroid glands as being secondarily involved in the events associated with age-related osteoporosis. Both with regard to increasing and decreasing parathyroid gland function, the system is responding to abnormalities at the level of the gastrointestinal tract, the kidney, or vitamin D metabolism. A possible abnormality in calcium sensing by the parathyroid glands has been introduced as a possible means by which the parathyroid glands could be primarily (vs secondarily) involved in the events associated with age-related osteoporosis. This section covers in more detail evidence that supports a role for the parathyroid glands as possible "protectors" from the age-related changes in mineral metabolism that lead to osteoporosis. Instead of being proposed as a causative agent in the pathophysiology of osteoporosis, the parathyroids in these studies are viewed as protective. This concept is supported by the clear anabolic effects of parathyroid hormone that can be demonstrated at sites of cancellous bone (i.e., the lumbar spine).

One study that supports the protective role for the parathyroids in osteoporosis comes from the work of Silverberg *et al.* [58]. Using oral phosphate administration as a hypocalcemic stimulus, the effects of ensuing mild hypocalcemia on parathyroid hormone and calcitriol levels were studied [58]. Three groups were defined: postmenopausal healthy and osteoporotic women and young healthy individuals. Despite a similar increase in the inorganic phosphorus concentration in response to the oral phosphate challenge and a similar fall in serum calcium concentration among the groups, parathyroid hormone levels rose by a modest 43% in those with osteoporosis (a change similar to the 53% increase in young normal subjects), but were much less than the more marked 2.5-fold rise in circulating parathyroid hormone seen in the older control group. In those with osteoporosis, whose response was modest and similar to young normal subjects, 1,25-dihydroxyvitamin D levels fell by 50%, while levels were unchanged in young and older normal women. The latter appeared to require a greater parathyroid hormone stimulus than their younger counterparts to overcome the suppressive effects of phosphate on 1,25-dihydroxyvitamin D formation. Data support the existence of an age-related decline in the renal mechanism to generate 1,25-dihydroxyvitamin D. Nonosteoporotic postmenopausal women maintained their levels of 1,25-dihydroxyvitamin D only by mounting a more vigorous parathyroid hormone response to hypocalcemia than is required at a younger age. In osteoporosis, the age-appropriate rise in parathyroid hormone responsiveness is not seen. The results support the concept of abnormal parathyroid hormone responsiveness in osteoporosis, superimposed on a universal age-related decline in 1,25-dihydroxyvitamin D production.

In a study that assessed parathyroid gland function while avoiding potential confounding effects of phosphorus on 1,25-dihydroxyvitamin D metabolism [35], infusion of parathyroid hormone(1–34) at physiologic doses led to suppression of endogenous parathyroid hormone secretion. The extent of the response to parathyroid hormone infusion was indistinguishable among premenopausal and postmenopausal normal women, as well as untreated and estrogen replaced postmenopausal women with osteoporosis. However, for any given increment in serum calcium concentration, in response to parathyroid hormone, osteoporotic individuals showed less suppression of endogenous parathyroid hormone secretion as compared to healthy women. Age, or the menopause itself, did not seem to affect the result. The authors concluded that skeletal sensitivity to parathyroid hormone is not altered by aging or osteoporosis. Instead, in osteoporosis they postulate altered parathyroid gland responsiveness, with a change in the set point for hormone secretion. This is consistent with the blunted stimulatory response to hypocalcemia reported by Silverberg *et al.* [58].

PARATHYROID HORMONE AND ESTROGEN

Despite *in vitro* [59,60] evidence that estrogen plays a role in the control of parathyroid hormone secretion, *in vivo* data are not supportive [61,62]. Some [63] but not all [64,65] studies have supported the existence of estrogen receptors in parathyroid tissue. However, clinical observations support the idea of interactions between parathyroid hormone and estrogen as mentioned previously. Increased bone resorptive activity, a skeletal effect of parathyroid hormone, emerges in the menopause when estrogen deficiency develops. It has been postulated that estrogen deficiency potentiates parathyroid hormone-mediated bone loss in the postmenopausal period.

Menopause is associated with a state of negative calcium balance [66]. Decreased intestinal calcium absorption contributes to the negative balance. This abnormality is more pronounced in osteoporotic women than in normal women and can be reversed by estrogen replacement therapy. Data from Gallagher *et al.* [67] suggested that estrogen treatment increases calcium absorption in postmenopausal osteoporosis by increasing parathyroid hormone levels. The ensuing stimulation of renal 1-α hydroxylase activity due to parathyroid hormone would lead to a rise in 1,25-dihydroxyvitamin D and hence a positive effect on the gastrointestinal tract. An alternative explanation calls for a direct effect of estrogen on calcium absorption [68].

More recent studies have led to a revision of this formulation. Estrogen deficiency does seem to be associated with a small decrement in total and ionized serum calcium, which can be reversed by replacement therapy. The reported effect of this mild hypocalcemia on parathyroid hormone levels has been variable, with a decrease [61] or no change [62,69,70] in normal postmenopausal women and an increase [28,67] or no change [35] reported in osteoporotic individuals. Free as well as total 1,25-dihydroxyvitamin D and vitamin D-binding protein levels rise when normal postmenopausal women are given estrogen replacement [61]. Several studies have proposed that estrogen deficiency may alter the set point for parathyroid hormone stimulation by circulating calcium. Estrogen replacement reportedly leads to a decrease in the set point for parathyroid hormone secretion in normal women, whereas in osteoporotic women, Cosman *et al.* [35] also found blunted parathyroid gland sensitivity to circulating calcium. In addition, estrogen treatment of postmenopausal woman with osteoporosis leads to reduced bone resorptive (but not bone formative) activity in response to parathyroid hormone administration [71].

Distinctions between Early and Late Menopause Effects of Parathyroid Hormone

The interaction of estrogen and parathyroid hormone differs as women advance through menopause, just as the primacy of estrogen deficiency itself changes over time. It is therefore helpful to consider this interaction as it evolves from the early to the later postmenopausal years.

Early Menopause

The early postmenopausal period is characterized by rapid bone loss over the first 5–8 years. Estrogen deficiency rather than parathyroid hormone seems to play the primary role at this time. Prince *et al.* [71] found no difference in parathyroid hormone levels in age-matched pre- and postmenopausal women. Nor are parathyroid hormone levels of early postmenopausal women affected by their level of calcium intake [72]. The parathyroid gland in the early postmenopausal woman seems to respond to changes in mineral metabolism induced by the recent onset of estrogen deficiency.

There are several theories to explain the effect of estrogen and the response of parathyroid hormone in the early menopause. One view holds that estrogen deficiency is directly responsible for accelerated bone resorption, which induces a transient rise in serum ionized calcium levels. This, in turn, leads to a decrease in parathyroid hormone secretion, leading to normalization of serum calcium. These changes are reversed by estrogen replacement therapy, which is documented in the early postmenopausal years to increase parathyroid hormone levels [73–75].

Yet another view of the interaction of estrogen and parathyroid hormone in the early postmenopausal period holds that the primary effect of estrogen is at the level of the kidney [76–78]. Loss of the normal effect of estrogen to promote renal calcium conservation leads to hypercalciuria. The observed rise in parathyroid hormone and bone resorption would thus be a compensatory response. McKane *et al.* [74] attempted to distinguish between these two possibilities by examining the effect of estrogen replacement therapy in early postmenopause. Their data support a major effect of estrogen replacement to decrease bone resorption, with the increase in parathyroid hormone and, subsequently, in tubular reabsorption of calcium being secondary events.

On the whole, therefore, parathyroid hormone does not seem to play a primary role in the pathophysiological events that transpire at the time of menopause. Clearly, there are interactions, as noted, but the predominant effect on the skeleton appears to be related to estrogen deficiency and the concomitant local production of bone-resorbing cytokines. The most telling argument in this regard is the observed changes that actually occur in skeletal mass. In the early menopausal years, bone loss is characterized by reductions in cancellous bone, best typified by the lumbar spine. This is a site that is normally responsive to sex steroids where a deficiency leads to rapid loss. However, parathyroid hormone is not recognized to have major catabolic effects at cancellous bone unless the levels are very high and prolonged. In the setting of early menopause, therefore, if parathyroid hormone elevations were playing a major role, one would not expect to see reductions in cancellous bone. In fact, just the opposite occurs in postmenopausal women with primary hyperparathyroidism. Their cancellous skeleton is, in general, remarkably well preserved despite the estrogen deficiency state. In clinical trials, in fact, parathyroid hormone can be shown to be clearly anabolic at this site.

Late Postmenopause

Parathyroid hormone levels have, by this point, increased (see "Normal Aging" section). Circulating parathyroid hormone levels in this population are responsive to calcium supplementation [79–81] and to 1,25-dihydroxyvitamin D_3 administration [10]. As discussed in the section on "Normal Aging," the secondary hyperparathyroid state observed in these individuals may account for the continued bone loss of aging. However, data support a role for estrogen deficiency in the late postmenopausal woman as well [75]. Data from Khosla *et al.* [75] demonstrate that estrogen therapy in this group abolishes the age-related increase in parathyroid hormone. Furthermore, in postmenopausal women not receiving hormone therapy, serum estrone levels (representing residual estrogen status) were predictive of bone resorption markers. These authors hypothesize a continued role for estrogen deficiency late in menopause. At this point, they theorize, the effects of estrogen deficiency are no longer primarily to increase bone resorption, but may instead reflect an estrogen effect on calcium absorption, renal calcium conservation, or parathyroid gland secretory function [75].

The skeletal effects of aging can accommodate a role for parathyroid hormone in terms of the time sequence by which cortical bone (the appendicular skeleton of the arms and legs) eventually becomes involved in the osteoporotic process. This is not to say that cortical bone is not being lost in the early years of menopause, but that estrogen deficiency seems to target the cancellous skeleton preferentially in early phase. Over time, one sees more of the cortical skeleton eroded as bone turnover continues to increase and parathyroid hormone levels rise. This late increase in the parathyroid hormone due to the many possible mechanisms reviewed in this chapter could well account for the later erosions of cortical bone. It could also account for the slowing of cancellous bone loss.

SUMMARY

This chapter reviewed the potential role of parathyroid hormone in the processes associated with age-related bone loss. It is evident that there is much more to be learned about how parathyroid hormone serves as a potential catabolic or anabolic force in the events associated with osteoporosis. This book covers many other factors that are important for skeletal health and disease as age takes its toll on the struggle for a homeostatically normal bone balance. The reader is referred to these other chapters that together provide a more complete view of the panoply of factors and events that are associated with age-related bone loss.

Acknowledgment

Supported in part by NIH Grants NIDDK 32333, NIAMS 39191, and RR 00645.

References

1. Gallagher, J. C., Riggs, B. L., Jerpbak, C. M., and Arnaud, C. D. The effect of age on serum immunoreactive parathyroid hormone in normal and osteoporotic women. *J. Lab. Clin. Med.* **95,** 373–385 (1980).
2. Insogna, K. L., Lewis, A. M., Lipinski, B. A., Bryant, C., and Baran, D. T. Effect of age on serum immunoreactive parathyroid hormone and its biological effects. *J. Clin. Endocrinol. Metab.* **53,** 1072–1075 (1981).
3. Marcus, R., Madvig, P., and Young, G. Age-related changes in parathyroid hormone and parathyroid hormone action in normal humans. *J. Clin. Endocrinol. Metab.* **58,** 223–230 (1984).
4. Epstein, S., Bryce, G., Hinman, J. W., Miller, O. N., Riggs, B. L., Hui, S. L., and Johnston, C. C. Jr. The influence of age on bone mineral regulating hormones. *Bone* **7,** 421–425 (1986).
5. Orwoll, E. S., and Meier, D. E. Alterations in calcium, vitamin D and parathyroid hormone physiology in normal men with aging: Relationship to the development of senile osteopenia. *J. Clin. Endocrinol. Metab.* **63,** 1262–1269 (1986).
6. Endres, D. B., Morgan, C. H., Garry, P. J., and Omdahl, J. L. Age related changes in serum immunoreactive parathyroid hormone and its biological action in healthy men and women. *J. Clin. Endocrinol. Metab.* **655,** 724–731 (1987).
7. Gallagher, J. C., Kinyamu, H. K., Fowler, S. E., Dawson-Hughes, B., Dalsky, G. P., and Sherman, S. S. Calciotropic hormones and bone markers in the elderly. *J. Bone Miner. Res.* **13,** 475–482 (1998).
8. Forero, M. S., Klein, R. F., Nissenson, R. A., and Heath, H. Effect of age on circulating immunoreactive and bioactive PTH in women. *J. Bone Miner. Res.* **2,** 363–366 (1987).
9. Halloran, B. P., Lonergan, E. T., and Portale, A. A. Aging and renal responsiveness to PTH in healthy men. *J. Clin. Endocrinol. Metab.* **81,** 2192–2197 (1996).
10. Ledger, G. A., Burritt, M. F., Kao, P. C., O'Fallon, W. M., Riggs, B. L., and Khosla, S. Abnormalities of PTH secretion in elderly women are reversible by short term therapy with 1,25-dihydroxyvitamin D. *J. Clin. Endocrinol. Metab.* **79,** 211–216 (1994).
11. Minisola, S., Pacitti, M. T., Scarda, A., Rosso, R., Romagnoli, E., and Carnevale, V. Serum ionized calcium, PTH and related variables: effect of age and sex. *Bone Miner.* **23,** 183–193 (1993).
12. Bullamore, J., Gallagher, J., Wilkinson, R., Nordin, B., and Marshall, D. Effect of age on calcium absorption. *Lancet* **ii,** 535–537 (1970).
13. Gallagher, J., Riggs, B., Eisman, J., Hamstra, A., Arnaud, S., and DeLuca, H. Intestinal calcium absorption and serum vitamin D metabolites in normal subjects and osteoporotic patients. *J. Clin. Invest.* **66,** 729 (1979).
14. Caniggia, A., Gennari, C., Bianchi, V., and Guideri, R. Intestinal absorption of ^{47}calcium in senile osteoporosis. *Acta Med. Scan.* **173,** 613–617 (1963).
15. Szymendera, J., Heaney, R., and Saville, P. Intestinal calcium absorption: concurrent use of oral and intravenous tracers and calculation by the inverse convolution method. *J. Lab. Clin. Med.* **79,** 570–578 (1972).
16. Kinney, V., Tauxe, W., and Dearing, W. Isotopic tracer studies of intestinal calcium absorption. *J. Lab. Clin. Med.* **66,** 187–203 (1966).
17. Eastell, R., Yergey, A. L., Vieira, N., Cedar, S. L., Kumar, R., Riggs, B. L. Interrelationship among vitamin D metabolism, true calcium absorption, parathyroid function and age in women: evidence of an age-related resistance to 1,25(OH)2D action. *J. Bone Miner. Res.* **6,** 125–132 (1991).
18. Ebeling, P., Sandgren, M., DiMango, E., Lane, A., DeLuca, H., and Riggs, B. L. Evidence of an age-related decrease in intestinal responsiveness to vitamin D: relationship between serum 1,25-dihydroxyvitamin D and intestinal vitamin D receptor concentrations in normal women. *J. Clin. Endocrinol. Metab.* **75,** 176–182 (1992).
19. Gallagher, J. The pathogenesis of osteoporosis. *Bone Miner.* **9,** 215–227 (1990).
20. Francis, R., Peacock, M., Taylor, G., Storer, J., and Nordin, B. Calcium malabsorption in elderly women with vertebral fractures: evidence for resistance to the action of vitamin D metabolites on the bowel. *Clin. Sci.* **66,** 103–107 (1984).
21. Portale, A. A., Lonergan, E. T., Tanney, D. M., and Halloran, B. P. Aging alters calcium regulation of serum concentration of parathyroid hormone in healthy men. *Am. J. Physiol.* **272**(part I), E139–E146 (1997).
22. Gray, R. W. Evidence that somatomedians mediate the effect of hypophosphatemia to increase serum $1,25(OH)_2D$ levels in rats. *Endocrinology* **121,** 504–509 (1987).
23. Halloran, B. P., and Spencer, E. M. Dietary phosphorus and 1,25-dihydroxyvitamin D metabolism: Influence of insulin-like growth factor I. *Endocrinology* **123,** 1225–1230 (1988).
24. Menaa, C., Vrtovsnik, F., Friedlander, G., Corvol, M., and Garabedian, M. Insulin-like growth factor I, a unique calcium-dependent stimulator of 1,25-dihydroxyvitamin D production. *J. Biol. Chem.* **270,** 25461–25467 (1995).
25. Halloran, B. P., and Portale, A. A. Vitamin D metabolism: the effects of aging. *In* "Vitamin D" (Feldman, Glorieux, and Pike eds.), pp. 541–554. Academic Press, San Diego, 1997.

25a. Wong, M. S., Sriussadaporn, S., Tembe, V. A., and Favus, M. J. IGF-I increases renal 1,25(OH)2D3 biosynthesis during low-P diet in adult rats. *Am. J. Physiol.* F698–F703 (1997).

26. Dawson-Hughes, B. Regulation of PTH by dietary calcium and vitamin D. *In* "The Parathyroids" (Bilezikian, Levine, and Marcus, eds.), pp. 55–64. Raven Press, New York, 1994.
27. Uden, P., Halloran, B., Daly, R., Duh, Q. Y., and Clark, O. Set-point for PTH release increases with postmaturational aging in the rat. *Endocrinology* **131,** 2251–2256 (1992).
28. Riggs, B. L., Ryan, R., Wahner, H., *et al.* Serum concentration of estrogen, testosterone and gonadotropins in osteoporotic and non-osteoporotic postmenopausal women. *J. Clin. Endocrinol. Metab.* **36,** 1097–1099 (1973).
29. Gallagher, J., Riggs, B. L., Jerpbak, C., and Arnaud, C. The effect of age on serum immunoreactive parathyroid hormone in normal and osteoporotic women. *J. Lab. Clin. Med.* **95,** 373–385 (1980).
30. Teitelbaum, S., Rosenberg, E., Richardson, C., and Avioli, L. Histologic studies of bone from normocalcemic postmenopausal women with increased circulating parathyroid hormone levels. *J. Clin. Endocrinol. Metab.* **42,** 537–543 (1976).
31. Civitelli, R., Agnusdei, D., Nardi, P., *et al.* Effect of one year treatment with estrogens on bone mass, intestinal calcium absorption, and 25-dihydroxyvitamin D 1-alpha hydroxylase reserve in postmenopausal osteoporosis. *Calcif, Tissue Int.* **42,** 76–86 (1988).
32. Bouillon, R., Geusens, P., Dequeker, J., and DeMoor, P. Parathyroid function in primary osteoporosis. *Clin Sci.* **578,** 167–171 (1979).
33. Sorenson, O., Lumholtz, B., Lund, B., *et al.* Acute effects of parathyroid hormone on vitamin D metabolism in patients with the bone loss of aging. *J. Clin. Endocrinol. Metab.* **54,** 1258–1261 (1981).
34. Kotowicz, M., Klee, G., Kao, P., Hodgson, S., Cedel, S., Eriksen, E., Gonchoroff, D., Judd, H., and Riggs, B. L. Relationship between serum intact PTH and bone remodeling in Type I osteopo-

rosis: Evidence that skeletal sensitivity is increased. *Osteoporosis* **1,** 14–20 (1990).
35. Cosman, F., Shen, V., Herrington, B., and Lindsay, R. Response of the parathyroid gland to infusion of human parathyroid hormone(1-34). *J. Clin. Endocrinol. Metab.* **73,** 1345–1351 (1991).
36. Brown, R., Atson, J., Weeks, I., and Woodhead, J. Circulating intact parathyroid hormone measured by immunochemiluminometric assay. *J. Clin. Endocrinol. Metab.* **65,** 407–414 (1987).
37. Saphier, P., Stamp, T., Kelsey, C., and Loveridge, N. PTH bioactivity in osteoporosis. *Bone Miner.* **3,** 75–83 (1987).
38. Riggs, B. L., and Melton, L. Evidence for two distinct syndromes of involutional osteoporosis. *Am. J. Med.* **75,** 899–901 (1983).
39. Riggs, B. L., Hamstra, A., and DeLuca, H. Assessment of 25-hydroxyvitamin D 1-alpha hydroxylase reserve in postmenopausal osteoporosis by administration of parathyroid extract. *J. Clin. Endocrinol. Metab.* **53,** 833–835 (1981).
40. Tsai, K., Heath, H., Kumar, R., and Riggs, B. L. Impaired vitamin D metabolism with aging in women. *J. Clin. Invest.* **73,** 1668–1672 (1984).
41. Slovik, D. M., Adams, J. S., Neer, R. M., Holick, M. F., and Potts, J. T. Deficient production of 1,25-dihydroxyvitamin D in elderly osteoporotic patients. *N. Engl. J. Med.* **305,** 372–374 (1981).
42. Villareal, D., Civitelli, R., Chines, A., and Avioli, L. Subclinical vitamin D deficiency in postmenopausal women with low vertebral bone mass. *J. Clin. Endocrinol. Metab.* **72,** 628–634 (1991).
43. Finkelstein, J. Hypovitaminosis D in medical inpatients. *N. Engl. J. Med.* **338,** 773–783, 1998.
44. Pacifici, R., Rifas, L., Teitelbaum, S., *et al.* Spontaneous release of interleukin-1 from human blood monocytes reflects bone formation in idiopathic osteoporosis. *Proc. Natl. Acad. Sci. USA* **84,** 4616–4620 (1987).
45. Gowen, M., and Mundy, G. Actions of recombinant interleukin-1, interleukin-2 and interferon-gamma on bone resorption in vitro. *J. Immunol.* **136,** 2478–2482 (1986).
46. Jilka, R., G. H., Girasole, G., Passeri, G., Williams, D., Abrams, J., Boyce, B., Broxmeyer, H., and Manolagas, S. Increased osteoclast development after estrogen loss: mediation by interleukin-6. *Science* **257,** 88–91 (1992).
47. Roodman, G. D. Interleukin-6: an osteotropic factor? *J. Bone Miner. Res.* **7,** 475–478 (1992).
48. Bertolini, D., Nedwin, G., Bringman, T., Smith, D., and Mundy, G. Stimulation of bone resorption and inhibition of bone formation in vitro by human tumor necrosis factor. *Nature* **319,** 516–518 (1986).
49. Tashjian, A., Tice, J., and Sides, K. Biological activities of prostaglandin analogues and metabolites on bone in organ culture. *Nature* **266,** 645–647 (1977).
50. Raisz, L., Simmons, H., Sandberg, A., and Cannalis, E. Direct stimulation of bone resorption by epidermal growth factor. *Endocrinology* **107,** 270–273 (1980).
51. Dietrich, J., Goodson, J., and Raisz, L. Stimulation of bone resorption by various prostaglandins in organ culture. *Prostaglandins* **10,** 231–238 (1975).
52. Tashjian, A., and Levine, L. Epidermal growth factor stimulates prostaglandin production and bone resorption in cultured mouse calvaria. *Biochem. Biophys. Res. Commun.* **85,** 966–975 (1978).
53. Dewhirst, F. 6-Keto-prostaglandin E1-stimulated bone resorption in organ culture. *Calcif. Tissue Int.* **36,** 380–383 (1984).
54. Ebeling, P., Jones, J., Burritt, M., Duerson, C., Lane, A., Hassager, C., Kumar, R., and Riggs, B. Skeletal responsiveness to endogenous parathyroid hormone in postmenopausal osteoporosis. *J. Clin. Endocrinol. Metab.* **75,** 1033–1038 (1992).
55. Heaney, R. A unified concept of osteoporosis. *Am. J. Med.* **39,** 377–380 (1965).
56. Silverberg, S. J., Locker, F. G., Shane, E., Jacobs, T. P., Siris, E. S., and Bilezikian, J. P. The effect of the menopause on lumbar spine bone density in primary hyperparathyroidism. *J. Bone Miner. Res.* **11**(Suppl. 1), S486 (1996).
57. Tsai, K., Ebeling, P., and Riggs, B. Bone responsiveness to parathyroid hormone in normal and osteoporotic postmenopausal women. *J. Clin. Endocrinol. Metab.* **69,** 1024–1027 (1989).
58. Silverberg, S., Shane, E., de la Cruz, L., Segre, G., Clemens, T., and Bilezikian, J. Abnormalities in parathyroid hormone secretion and 1,25-dihydroxvitamin D_3 formation in women with osteoporosis. *N. Engl. J. Med.* **320,** 277–281 (1989).
59. Duarte, B., Hargis, G., and Kukreja, S. Effects of estradiol and progesterone on parathyroid hormone secretion from human parathyroid tissue. *J. Clin. Endocrinol. Metab.* **66,** 584–587 (1988).
60. Greenberg, C., Kukreja, S., Bowser, E., Hargis, G., Henderson, W., and Williams, G. Parathyroid hormone secretion: effect of estradiol and progesterone. *Metabolism* **36,** 151–154 (1987).
61. Stock, J., Coiderre, J., and Malette, L. Effects of a short course of estrogen on mineral metabolism in postmenopausal women. *J. Clin. Endocrinol. Metab.* **61,** 595–600 (1985).
62. Selby, P., Peacock, M., Barkworth, S., and Brown, W. Early effects of ethynyloestradiol and norethisterone treatment in postmenopausal women on bone resportion and calcium regulating hormones. *Clin. Sci.* **69,** 265–271 (1985).
63. Naveh-Many, T., Almongi, G., Livni, N., and Silver, J. Estrogen receptors and biologic response in rat parathyroid tissue and cells. *J. Clin. Invest.* **90,** 2434–2438 (1992).
64. Prince, R. L., MacLaughlin, D. T., Gaz, R. D., and Neer, R. M. Lack of evidence for estrogen receptors in human and bovine parathyroid tissue. *J. Clin. Endocrinol. Metab.* **72,** 1226–1228 (1991).
65. Saxe, A. W., Gibson, G. W., Russo, I. H., and Gimotty, P. Measurement of estrogen and progesterone receptors in abnormal human parathyroid tissue. *Calcif. Tissue Int.* **51,** 344–347 (1992).
66. Heaney, R., Recker, R., and Saville, P. Menopausal changes in calcium balance performance. *J. Lab. Clin. Med.* **92,** 953–963 (1978).
67. Gallagher, J., Riggs, B., and DeLuca, H. Effect of estrogen on calcium absorption and serum vitamin D metabolites in postmenopausal osteoporosis. *J. Clin. Endocrinol. Metab.* **51,** 1359–1364 (1980).
68. Gennari, C., Agnusdei, D., Nardi, P., and Civitelli, R. Estrogen preserves a normal intestinal responsiveness to 1,25-dihydroxyvitamin D in oophorectomized women. *J. Clin. Endocrinol. Metab.* **71,** 1288–1293 (1990).
69. Stevenson, J., Abeyasekera, G., Hillyard, C., *et al.* Calcitonin and the calcium regulating hormones in postmenopausal osteoporosis. *Lancet* **1,** 693–695 (1981).
70. Marshall, R., Selby, P., Chilvers, D., and Hodgkinson, A. The effect of ethinyl estradiol on calcium and bone metabolism in peri- and postmenopausal women. *Horm. Metab. Res.* **16,** 1359–1364 (1984).
71. Prince, R. L., Dick, L., Garcia-Webb, P., and Retallack, R. W. The effects of the menopause on calcitriol and parathyroid hormone: responses to a low dietary calcium stress test. *J. Clin. Endocrinol. Metab.* **70,** 119–1123 (1990).
72. Nilas, L., Christiansen, C., and Roabro, P. Calcium supplementation and postmenopausal bone loss. *Br. Med. J.* **289,** 1103–1106 (1985).
73. Gallagher, J. C., Riggs, B. L., and DeLuca, H. F. Effect of estrogen on calcium absorption and serum vitamin D metabolites in postmenopausal osteoporosis. *J. Clin. Endocrinol. Metab.* **51,** 1359–1364 (1980).

74. McKane, W. R., Khosla, S., Burritt, M. F., Kao, P. C., Wilson, D. M., Ory, S. J., and Riggs, L. Mechanism of renal calcium conservation with estrogen replacement therapy in women in early postmenopause. *J. Clin. Endocrinol. Metabol.* **80,** 3458–3464 (1995).
75. Khosla, S., Atkinson, E. F., Melton, L. J., and Riggs, B. L. Effects of age and estrogen status on serum PTH levels and biochemical markers of bone turnover in women. *J. Clin. Endocrinol. Metab.* **82,** 1522–1527 (1997).
76. Nordin, B. E. C., Need, A. G., Morris, H. A., Horowitz, M., and Robertson, W. G. Evidence for a renal calcium leak in postmenopausal women. *J. Clin. Endocrinol. Metab.* **72,** 401–407 (1991).
77. Adami, S., Gatti, D., Bertoldo, F., *et al.* The effects of menopause and estrogen replacement therapy on the renal handling of calcium. *Osteopor. Int.* **2,** 180–185 (1992).
78. Prince, R. L., Smith, M., Dick, I. M., *et al.* Prevention of postmenopausal osteoporosis. A comparative study of exercise, calcium supplementation, and hormone-replacement therapy. *N. Engl. J. Med.* **325,** 1189–1195 (1991).
79. Bikle, D. D., Herman, R. H., Hull, S., Hagler, L., Harris, D., and Halloran, B. Adaptive response of humans to changes in dietary calcium: relationship between vitamin D regulated intestinal function and serum 1,25-dihydroxyvitamin D levels. *Gastroenterology* **84,** 314–323 (1983).
80. Reid, I. R., Ames, R. W., Evans, M. C., Gamble, G. D., and Sharpe, S. J. Effect of calcium supplementation on bone loss in postmenopausal women. *N. Engl. J. Med.* **328,** 460–464 (1993).
81. Dawson-Hughes, B., Shapis, P., and Shipp, C. Dietary calcium intake and bone loss from the spine in healthy postmenopausal women. *Am. J. Clin. Nutr.* **46,** 685–687 (1987).

CHAPTER 17

Vitamin D

F. MICHAEL GLOTH, III Department of Geriatrics, Union Memorial Hospital and Johns Hopkins University School of Medicine, Baltimore, Maryland 21218

INTRODUCTION

Age-Associated Changes in Vitamin D

The role of vitamin D has long been recognized as vital to the growth and development of bone. While the lack of vitamin D may easily be considered as a cause of juvenile rickets, the impact of vitamin D extends beyond childhood and beyond bone. In fact, changes associated with aging may make the elderly population most susceptible to vitamin D deficiency and its consequences.

Vitamin D metabolism is illustrated in Fig. 1. Skin changes associated with aging reduce the amount of 7-dehydrocholesterol, the precursor to cholecalciferol (vitamin D_3), as well as its rate of conversion [1–4]. Absorption of dietary vitamin D is also reduced by as much as 40% in older individuals compared to younger ones [5]. The aging adult also has a reduction in the quantity and activity of the renal 1-α-hydroxylase, which affects the production of the most active metabolite of vitamin D, 1,25 dihydroxyvitamin D (calcitriol) [6–9].

Physiologic changes in vitamin D metabolism are not the only changes that affect the vitamin D status in older individuals. Reducing sun exposure for a variety of reasons, the increase in use of medications that may interfere with vitamin D metabolism, and the greater likelihood of comorbid conditions that can also interfere with vitamin D metabolism all contribute to a greater prevalence of vitamin D deficiency in older people [10–17].

SUNLIGHT

Lack of sunlight may be the determining factor for the development of vitamin D deficiency in the elderly [18–27]. A cross-sectional study from the United States that carefully controlled for diseases and medications that might confound an accurate assessment of vitamin D status demonstrated little problem with vitamin D status across the age span (see Fig. 2) [28]. However, in settings where subjects have not received adequate sunlight, the prevalence of vitamin D deficiency becomes quite high (see Fig. 3) [29,30]. Changes associated with aging alone are rarely substantial enough to result in low levels of vitamin D metabolites [28,31].

In the United States the average vitamin D intake is reportedly among the highest in the world [32,33]. However, even with a relatively high vitamin D intake, the vitamin D status of many of our elderly is likely to be low [13,34].

Despite average intakes of vitamin D in excess of twice the recommended dietary allowance (RDA) of *200 IU* per day, a third of elderly homebound (sunlight-deprived) subjects in one study had low vitamin D status with 25-hydroxyvitamin D levels <10 ng/ml (25 nmol/liter) [18]. At least 30% of sunlight-deprived, nursing-home subjects were reported to have vitamin D deficiency (defined as hypovitaminosis D accompanied by physiological or biochemical abnormalities) [30,35–37].

Risk Factors Understanding the prevalence of vitamin D deficiency in the United States is important, but of perhaps equal importance is understanding the risk factors and the usual clinical presentation for an elderly person in this country with a vitamin D deficit.

One risk factor is clearly sunlight deprivation, which has been associated with depleted vitamin D stores in the elderly [15,20,29]. Other factors that have been linked to vitamin D deficiency include a low intake of foods containing vitamin D, medications that impair vitamin D metabolism (e.g., phenytoin and phenobarbital), medical conditions that increase risk (e.g., partial gastrectomy, renal disease, severe hepatic disease, and malabsorption), obesity, hypocalcemia, and elevated alkaline phosphatase in the serum [1,38,39].

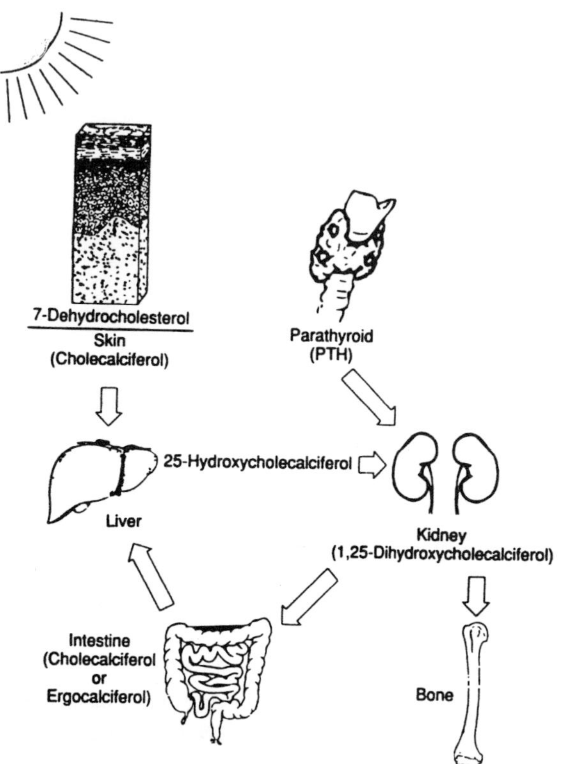

FIGURE 1 Abbreviated diagram of vitamin D metabolism. Vitamin D precursors in the dermis are influenced by ultraviolet light and temperature and are converted to cholecalciferol (vitamin D_3). Cholecalciferol (or ergocalciferol, vitamin D_2, in the case of some dietary sources absorbed in the gut) is carried by the bloodstream to the liver where hydroxylases act to stimulate conversion to 25-hydroxyvitamin D (calcidiol). These molecules are also carried in the bloodstream and, on reaching the kidney, are converted under the influence of α-hydroxylase and parathyroid hormone to the most active vitamin D metabolite, 1,25-dihydroxyvitamin D (calcitriol). 1,25-Dihydroxyvitamin D regulates calcium homeostasis primarily through the action on vitamin D receptors in the gut (calcium absorption) and the kidney (calcium excretion in the urine).

CONSEQUENCES OF VITAMIN D DEFICIENCY

Bone-Related Changes

Although osteomalacia is the most recognized skeletal consequence of vitamin D deficiency, other abnormalities in bone metabolism can occur [23,40,41]. Osteoporosis is often accompanied by, and may be more commonly exacerbated by, vitamin D deficiency, especially in the elderly and usually in the absence of osteomalacia [30]. Parathyroid hormone and the marker of bone formation, osteocalcin, are influenced by 25-hydroxyvitamin D and 1,25-dihydroxyvitamin D [10,17,42,43]. Secondary changes (secondary hyperparathyroidism in particular) related to low levels of vitamin D metabolites and calcium in the serum result in augmented bone resorption even in the absence of osteomalacia [1,44–47]. 25-Hydroxyvitamin D levels should be kept at least above 15 ng/ml (see Fig. 4) because levels below this concentration are associated with progressive increases in the parathyroid hormone (PTH) [30]. A relationship between bone mineral density and intact PTH in the setting of 25-hydroxyvitamin D and/or 1,25-dihydroxyvitamin D depletion and repletion, however, remains to be demonstrated in a controlled clinical trial.

The concept of "free" and protein-bound metabolites is important in many endocrine states. This concept may have similar importance for vitamin D status in the elderly. The effect of "free" 1,25-dihydroxyvitamin D on PTH, phosphorus, alkaline phosphatase, and calcium has been evaluated by Bouillon *et al.* [11] in 15 elderly subjects with mild to severe vitamin D deficiency over the course of repletion in comparison to controls. Studies by Bouillon *et al.* in Belgium, by Toss and Sörbo in Sweden, and by our group indicate that vitamin D-binding protein levels do not change with age nor with institutionalization unless there is evidence of protein-energy malnutrition [30,48,49]. These data imply currently available measures of vitamin D status, in particular 25-hydroxyvitamin D, should reflect vitamin D stores in a clinically relevant fashion. Except in the rarest cases, an assessment of "free" vitamin D metabolites will not contribute additional, worthwhile clinical information.

In vitro exposure of osteoblasts to 1,25-dihydroxyvitamin D in both human and animal experiments results in an increase in production of osteocalcin [50–55]. The majority of newly synthesized osteocalcin is incorporated into the bone matrix, while the remainder can be found in measurable quantities in the serum. Serum measurements of osteocalcin can aid in the appraisal of bone turnover [56,57].

The increase in bone turnover characteristic of an immobile, frail elderly population is related, in part, to low dietary calcium, reduced dietary vitamin D intake, and little or no sunlight contribution to vitamin D status. Such low dietary intakes can, for reasons mentioned earlier, be anticipated to be more frequent in community homebound subjects. Consequently, osteocalcin levels may become elevated. Although elevated levels of osteocalcin are common in the setting of vitamin D deficiency, transient further elevations are seen during the first 1–3 months of replacement [43,58]. Eventually, with correction of the vitamin D deficiency and the return of bone metabolism to normal, osteocalcin levels also return to normal.

The relationship between osteocalcin and parathyroid hormone *in vivo* also has not been clearly established. Reports from studies in the elderly have been inconsistent. Pietschmann *et al.* [59] reported a parallel

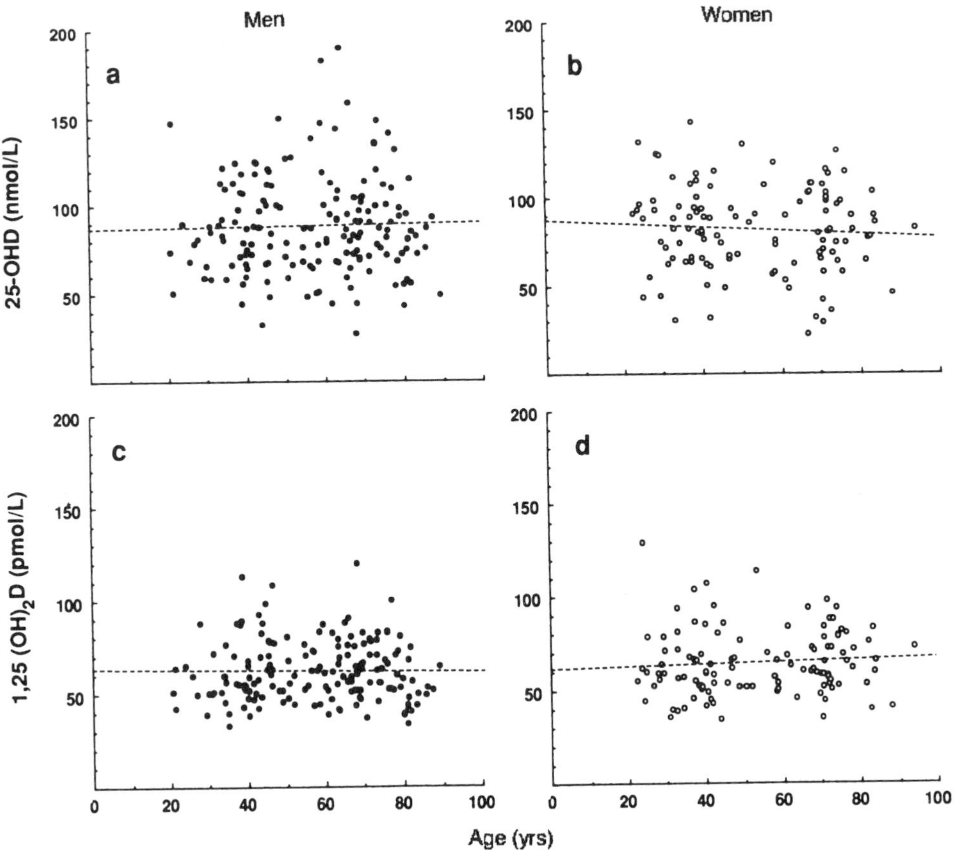

FIGURE 2 Stable vitamin D metabolites in the Baltimore Longitudinal Study on Aging across the age span (see Ref. 28).

increase in osteocalcin and parathyroid hormone, whereas Dandona *et al.* [60] reported no effect of parathyroid hormone on osteocalcin levels. Part of the inconsistency in these reports may be related to the timing of the osteocalcin measurement in the setting of vitamin D replacement (i.e., before or after a 3-month replacement period as noted earlier). Another important consideration is that different assays for osteocalcin have

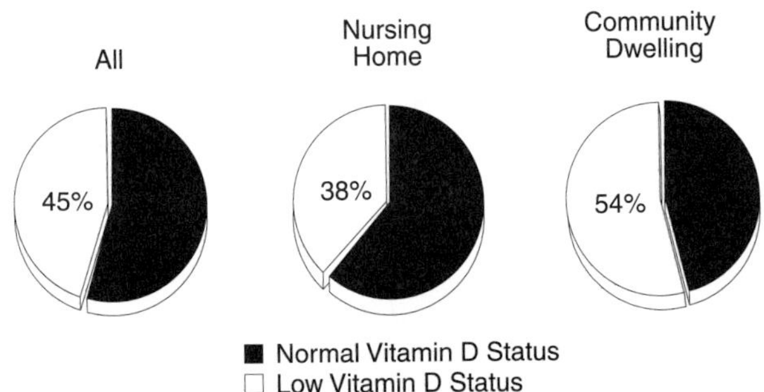

FIGURE 3 Prevalence of vitamin D deficiency (25-hydroxyvitamin D level less than 10 ng/ml) in two sunlight-deprived elderly groups. Adapted from Ref. 30.

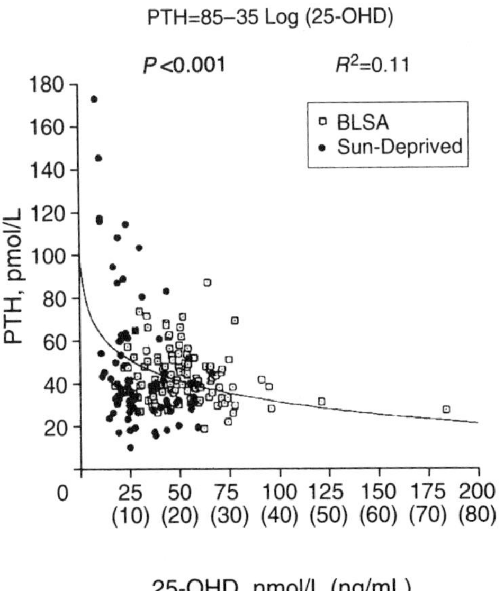

FIGURE 4 Parathyroid hormone vs 25-hydroxyvitamin D. Secondary hyperparathyroidism becomes evident when 25-hydroxyvitamin D levels exceed 15 ng/ml. Adapted from Ref. 30.

measured different fragments of the total molecule. Thus, some assays may reflect breakdown products related to resorption or be inordinately affected by renal function and altered clearance. Measurement of the intact molecule may help to resolve this issue.

Allelic variation in the vitamin D receptor locus has been demonstrated to have an association with bone turnover and overall bone density as well [61]. Vitamin D also acts by nongenomic intracellular actions and may play a role in calcium regulation involving calcium channel regulation [62]. The impact of nongenomic, intracellular mechanisms remains an area in need of further research.

Bone mineral density is associated with fracture risk, a relationship that has also been demonstrated for biomarkers of bone turnover *in vivo* [63]. Unfortunately, these observations have been made in populations that are active and mobile and relatively free of confounders that may exist in the elderly. For example, substantial osteophyte formation in the lumbar spine and aortic calcifications may raise anterior–posterior spine densitometry readings artifactually. Nevertheless, bone densitometry at other sites (e.g., hip) still may be a valuable source of information in these subjects. Some subjects still will not qualify for successful testing because of excessive obesity, contractures, and difficulties in physically moving some patients to a center to be studied. Standardization of bone densitometry in these older populations awaits further documentation.

Although the therapeutics of vitamin D deficiency are covered in detail in the Chapter 49, a few comments are worthy of mention here. One study from the United States showed that spine and total body bone mineral density measures could be positively influenced by vitamin D replacement therapy of 400 IU per day [64]. Although no correlation was given between serum vitamin D metabolites and either PTH or bone mineral density measures, subjects receiving vitamin D with calcium differed significantly from controls receiving calcium and placebo, who, by the end of winter, demonstrated higher PTH values and lower bone mineral density measures for total body and spine.

Chapuy *et al.* [65,66] have presented findings demonstrating the stabilization of bone mineral density in association with vitamin D (800 IU per day) and calcium supplementation compared to a loss of bone in a placebo control group. Foods are not supplemented with vitamin D in France and presumably these nursing home subjects included mostly vitamin D-deficient subjects. In that same study, early data also showed a decreased fracture rate in the cohort receiving vitamin D supplementation. In New Zealand, Tilyard *et al.* [67] demonstrated fracture reduction in association with $1,25(OH)_2D$ supplementation. Neither of these studies delineated risk factors for low vitamin D status. Also, neither study presented a relationship between vitamin D metabolite levels in the serum and bone density or fracture rates. Nevertheless, given the 14 billion dollars in health care costs associated with fractures yearly in the elderly, it behooves us to note the outcomes of such interventions with a potential to impact on the tremendous economic and caregiver burden of osteopenia [68,69]. Also of importance is the association between bone mineral density and fracture rates and the fact that over 50% of hip fracture patients do not return to baseline functional levels [70].

As mentioned earlier, osteomalacia is perhaps most commonly associated with vitamin D deficiency even if it is not the most prevelant clinical consequence of such a deficit. Chalmers *et al.* [71] reported on the clinical features of osteomalacia in a series of 37 cases (34 female) ranging in age between 39 and 89 years (mean age 72 years). Interestingly, in their series, 24% of cases had no radiologic (Looser's zones) or biochemical (exclusive of vitamin D metabolite measurements) evidence of osteomalacia and only upon biopsy was a diagnosis of osteomalacia made [68]. At the time of Chalmer's study, bone mineral density was not available. Whether bone mineral density measures would have been low in such subjects is open to speculation.

The use of clothing that screens out sunshine and the ingestion of foods that inhibit vitamin D absorption have been attributed to a severe lack of vitamin D in such groups [27,72–74].

Other Effects of Vitamin D Deficiency

Although vitamin D deficiency is most often associated with effects on bone, vitamin D receptors are found in many tissues. The effects of vitamin D deficiency thus extend well beyond the skeleton. Other sites include the brain, dermal capillaries, keratinocytes, macrophages, vascular smooth muscle cells, leukocytes, and the pancreas [75–81].

Muscle Weakness

Vitamin D deficiency has been associated with muscle weakness, limb pain, and impaired physical function [15,82,83]. In Chalmers' study describing osteomalacia, muscular weakness was described as

> *. . . a striking feature in several patients and produced a typical flat-footed, springless gait which one patient's family aptly described as "mother penguin's walk." Rising from a chair was difficult for those severely affected, and in one instance the patient was confined to bed by the severity of the weakness. Many patients who had not specifically complained of muscular weakness before*

treatment volunteered that they felt stronger and more vigorous after treatment than they had in years.

A cause and effect relationship between vitamin D deficiency and muscle weakness is supported by the fact that vitamin D receptors exist on muscle [84]. Birge and Haddad [85] have also provided evidence that 25-hydroxyvitamin D directly influences the intracellular accumulation of phosphate by muscle and offer this as an important role in the maintenance of muscle metabolism and function. Deficiency of vitamin D is associated with type II muscle fiber atrophy that requires 6–12 months after the initiation of vitamin D treatment to recover [84]. Although muscle strength has been reported by others to improve after vitamin D intake [68,69,86], the impact of changes in muscle strength on bone density has not been measured before or after treatment for vitamin D deficiency. Overall, this picture can be further complicated by hypophosphatemia or hyperparathyroidism, each of which can be associated with muscle weakness as well.

PAIN

Deep musculoskeletal limb pain, as well as neuropathy and hyperesthesia, has been associated with vitamin D deficiency with or without osteomalacia [23,69,81,87,88].

Pain and weakness can lead to functional disability, which may prevent a person from venturing outdoors [10,76]. This, in turn, exacerbates a poor vitamin D status by eliminating the exposure to sunlight, thus perpetuating the cycle (Fig. 1). Whether weakness and functional impairment are secondary to limb pain or can be independent outcomes of vitamin D deficiency in the pain-free frail elderly also need to be studied. A syndrome of hyperesthesia has been described in association with variably subnormal levels of vitamin D metabolites in the serum [80]. Immobility associated with pain also may be associated with less sunlight exposure and loss of bone.

FUNCTION

Vitamin D deficiency has also been associated with loss of function [89–92]. The study by Corless *et al.* [89] did not demonstrate a statistically significant change in function, but the authors themselves elaborated on potential problems with the study design. For example, the time course of the study was 8 weeks, much shorter than the time needed to complete muscle recovery of type II fiber atrophy from vitamin D deficiency [84]. Another study that assessed functional change with a vitamin D intervention by Sørensen and colleagues [90] showed improvement with treatment. In this study, "timed dressing" (time to put on stockings, vest, underpants, shirt, and frock) was measured and a significant decrease in time to dress occurred after treatment with 1,25-dihydroxyvitamin D. More recently, data were presented demonstrating an association between improvement in vitamin D status and function for frail homebound elderly [93]. Low vitamin D status and secondary hyperparathyroidism are also associated with muscle weakness as well as increased body sway [94,95].

While some studies have followed biochemical indices with vitamin D treatment in an elderly population, no study has ever followed parameters of vitamin D metabolism in conjunction with function, muscle strength, limb pain, and bone mineral density during replenishment with vitamin D in adults with a low vitamin D status [1,96]. It is reasonable to assume that a host of physical and biochemical factors associated with vitamin D deficiency may contribute to loss of bone.

OSTEOARTHRITIS

Vitamin D status has also been associated with the prevalence of osteoarthritis [97,98]. While the association has peaked interest, much work needs to be done to determine whether more severe osteoarthritis simply limits outdoor activity (and therefore sun exposure) or that there is indeed a causal relationship between the two through some other yet to be determined mechanism.

SEASONAL AFFECTIVE DISORDER

Data have also implicated a possible role for vitamin D deficiency in seasonal affective disorder [99]. A small study of 15 subjects with seasonal affective disorder demonstrated an improvement in vitamin D status and depressive symptoms with 100,000 IU of vitamin D when compared to light therapy.

Toxicity

Vitamin D status may affect bone loss at each end of the spectrum. While a lack of vitamin D has most often been associated with bone loss, vitamin D toxicity may have a similar consequence. At least one study has demonstrated an improvement in bone density with resolution of vitamin D toxicity [100]. This observation reinforces the concept that excessive vitamin D can be associated with bone resorption.

VITAMIN D REQUIREMENTS IN THE ELDERLY

Lack of Data

Without further data on the symptoms of vitamin D deficiency in an older population and the physiologic alterations related to such a deficiency, it is difficult to recommend a daily dietary intake for vitamin D. Much of the information used to arrive at a RDA of vitamin D in adults was extrapolated from studies of infantile rickets [101]. It is little wonder why no consensus exists for vitamin D intake in individuals over 65 years old [102,103]. Data suggest that the RDA is insufficient to maintain an adequate vitamin D status in elderly, sunlight-deprived subjects [10,20,34,74]. Evaluation of vitamin D intake without the confounding influence of sunlight would be necessary to determine the dietary amount to be recommended as a daily average. Although some studies have examined the nutritional intake of vitamin D [15,31,104–111], none have simultaneously measured vitamin D metabolites and related calciotropic parameters and followed these measures throughout replacement therapy. Moreover, assessments of the vitamin D content of ingested foods have often been crude and rather inaccurate. The Food and Nutrition Board has revised calcium and vitamin D recommendations based on age [112]. These improvements have been useful, with increasing amounts of vitamin D and calcium being recommended in older individuals, especially where lack of sunlight is a concern. Specific recommendations on vitamin D and calcium replacement are outlined in Chapter 49.

Type, Route, and Amount of Replenishment

Debate remains concerning the route and metabolite for vitamin D replacement in vitamin D deficiency. The patient with renal failure requires calcitriol [1,25-$(OH)_2$ vitamin D]. When to supplement is an issue as well. Recommending replacement in anyone with 25-hydroxyvitamin D (which reflects body stores of vitamin D) levels in the serum below 5 ng/ml may overlook subjects with secondary hyperparathyroidism, which may occur between 10 and 15 ng/ml of 25-hydroxyvitamin D [11,18,37].

Treatment recommendations range from 200 IU per day of vitamin D to doses in excess of 50,000 IU per day [22,84,105,113–120]. Megadose prescriptions of 50,000 to 100,000 IU of vitamin D per day place older subjects, in particular, at risk for vitamin D toxicity [121,122]. Lower doses, such as 100,000 IU of vitamin D every 3 months or 800–1600 IU of vitamin D per day, would be less expensive. Additional savings would be realized from fewer hypercalcemic events. Interestingly, some studies have looked at vitamin D replacement in subjects who were not vitamin D deficient at the onset. Such study designs provide little guidance for clinicians interested in the replacement of vitamin D for deficient subjects. The author's practice is to recommend 100,000 IU by mouth every 3 months in the setting of low vitamin D status. Because our patient population is relatively frail and visits occur about once every 3 months, the dosage can be administered in the office, thereby assuring compliance. Calcium supplementation remains important and must occur on a daily basis. In the institutional setting, it may be more reliable to administer 800–1600 IU per day by mouth. Evaluation of 25-hydroxyvitamin D status during that first year will be helpful in assessing status and monitoring compliance.

Vitamin D analogs have also been used, especially in Asia [123]. Reductions in hip fracture rates by as much as 70% with only 0.5–0.75 μg per/day of α-calcidol can be demonstrated [123,124].

Vitamin D Supplementation with or without Measuring Vitamin D Status

It could be argued that 25-hydroxyvitamin D levels should not be measured because of the relatively little cost and the high degree of safety in taking vitamin D as 800 IU per day (if sunlight deprived) or as 100,000 IU every 3–6 months. The cost of a vitamin D assay can be as high as $100. Given the exorbitant costs of hip fractures and the reduction in rates with a relatively inexpensive assessment and intervention, either decision would be cost effective. Replacement with or without testing should be decided on an individual basis incorporating other issues such as compliance, ease of administration, and risk of vitamin D deficiency.

SUMMARY

Because of changes that occur with aging, elderly individuals with any other risk factors for vitamin D deficiency are likely to have inadequate stores of this vitamin. The consequences of vitamin D deficiency are likely to be losses in bone mass, strength, function, and the acquisition of pain. Thus, vitamin D replacement may have a positive impact on the quality of life not only for patients, but also in the frail.

Many questions remain regarding screening, prevention, and treatment of vitamin D deficiency. Supplementation may be unnecessary in most healthy, ambulatory seniors. Excessive supplementation in this group may lead to vitamin D toxicity. Physician supervision of higher doses of vitamin D is important for this reason. While the argument can be made that the use of 1,25 dihydroxyvitamin D would have a reduction in the duration of symptoms from vitamin D intoxication should it occur, that metabolite is also more difficult to regulate and intoxication or actual resorption of bone at levels slightly higher than desired may be substantially more frequent.

Probably the most important role for supplementation is in homebound elderly who do not get adequate vitamin D from sunlight exposure. This population is at a particular risk of developing vitamin D deficiency [30]. Issues such as inadequate diet, physiologic changes with aging, polypharmacy, and diseases that interfere with vitamin D metabolism contribute to this risk. In such circumstances a recommendation of 800 IU per day is reasonable. An alternative to daily dosing is a single oral dose of 100,000 IU of vitamin D (ergocalciferol or cholecalciferol) every 3–6 months. A simple maneuver for geriatricians, who see many chronically ill patients with low vitamin D stores (who are likely to be seen in the office every 3–6 months), is to administer vitamin D during office visits. These dosing schedules have not been associated with toxicity and can be considered safe in the homebound (sunlight-deprived) elderly. Serum levels of 25-hydroxyvitamin D (the metabolite that best reflects vitamin D stores) and 1,25-dihydroxyvitamin D (the most active metabolite) can be measured but are expensive to follow frequently and it is not clear whether routinely following such levels is useful or cost effective.

In addition to the issues presented in this chapter, other roles for vitamin D are under investigation. The role of vitamin D in deterring some cancers, including prostate, breast, and colon, is currently being examined along with its use in treating psoriasis.

A high level of suspicion will lead to the necessary steps to remedy the common, treatable, and underappreciated problem of vitamin D deficiency.

References

1. Parfitt, A. M., Gallagher, J. C., Heaney, R. P., *et al.* Vitamin D and bone health in the elderly. *Am. J. Clin. Nutr.* **36,** 1014–1031 (1982).
2. Holick, M. F. Vitamin D synthesis by the aging skin. *In* "Nutrition and Aging," pp. 45–58. Academic Press, New York, 1986.
3. MacLaughlin, J., and Holick, M. F. Aging decreases the capacity of human skin to produce vitamin D. *J. Clin. Invest.* **76,** 1536–1538 (1985).
4. Holick, M. F., Matsuoka, L. Y., and Wortsman, J. Age, vitamin D, and solar ultraviolet. *Lancet* **ii,** 1104–1105 (1989).
5. Baragry, J. M., France, M. W., Corless, D., *et al.* Intestinal cholecalciferol absorption in the elderly and in younger adults. *Clin. Sci. Mol. Med.* **55,** 213–220 (1978).
6. Holick, M. F. Vitamin D and the kidney. *Kidney Intl.* **32,** 912–929 (1987).
7. Tsai, K. S., Heath, H., III, Kumar, R., and Riggs, B. L. Impaired vitamin D metabolism with aging in women. *J. Clin. Invest.* **73,** 1668–1672 (1984).
8. Riggs, L. B., Hamstra, A., and DeLuca, H. F. Assessment of 25-hydroxyvitamin D 1 alpha-hydroxylase reserve in postmenopausal osteoporosis by administration of parathyroid extract. *J. Clin. Endocrinol. Metab.* **53,** 833–835 (1981).
9. Sørensen, O. H., Lumholtz, B., Lund, B., *et al.* Acute effects of parathyroid hormone on vitamin D metabolism in patients with the bone loss of aging. *J. Clin. Endocrinol. Metab.* **54,** 1258–1261 (1982).
10. Bouillon, R. A., Auwerx, J. H., Lissens, W. D., and Pelemans, W. K. Vitamin D status in the elderly: Seasonal substrate deficiency causes 1,25-dihydroxycholecalciferol deficiency. *Am. J. Clin. Nutr.* **45,** 755–763 (1978).
11. Lips, P., Wiersinga, A., Van Ginkel, F. C., *et al.* The effect of vitamin D supplementation on vitamin D status and parathyroid function in elderly subjects. *J. Clin. Endocrinol. Metab.* **67**(4), 644–649 (1988).
12. Corless, D., Gupta, S. P., Sattar, D. A., Switala, S., and Boucher, B. J. Vitamin D status of residents of an old people's home and long-stay patients. *Gerontology* **24,** 350–355 (1979).
13. Omhdahl, J. L., Garry, P. J., Hunsaker, L. A., *et al.* Nutritional status in a healthy elderly population: Vitamin D. *Am. J. Clin. Nutr.* **36,** 1225–1233 (1982).
14. Baker, M. R., Peacock, M., and Nordin, B. E. C. The decline in vitamin D status with age. *Age Ageing* **9,** 249–252 (1980).
15. Aksnes, L., Rodland, O., and Arskog, D. Serum levels of vitamin D_3 in elderly and young adults. *Bone Miner.* **3,** 351–357 (1988).
16. Aksnes, L., Rϕdland, O., Odegaard, O. R., Bakke, K. J., and Aarskog, D. Serum levels of vitamin D metabolites in the elderly. *Acta Endocrinol.* **121,** 27–33 (1989).
17. Orwoll, E. S., and Meier, D. E. Alterations in calcium, vitamin D, and parathyroid hormone physiology in normal men with aging: Relationship to the development of senile osteopenia. *J. Clin. Endocrinol. Metab.* **63,** 1262–1269 (1986).
18. Gloth, F. M., III, Tobin, J. D., Sherman, S. S., and Hollis, B. W. Is the recommended daily allowance for vitamin D too low in the homebound elderly? *J. Am. Geriatr. Soc.* **39**(2), 137–141 (1991).
19. Stamp, T. C. B., Haddad, J. G., and Twigg, C. A. Comparison of oral 25-hydroxycholecalciferol, vitamin D and ultraviolet light as determinants for circulating 25-hydroxyvitamin D. *Lancet* **I,** 1341–1343 (1977).
20. Hodkinson, H. M., Round, P., Stanton, B. R., and Morgan, C. Sunlight, vitamin D and osteomalacia in the elderly. *Lancet* **I,** 910–912 (1973).
21. Egsmose, C., Lund, B., McNair, P., *et al.* Low serum levels of 25-hydroxyvitamin D and 1,25-dihydroxyvitamin D in institutionalized old people: Influence of solar exposure and vitamin D supplementation. *Age Ageing* **16,** 35–40 (1987).
22. Weisman, Y., Schen, R. J., Eisenberg, Z., Edelstein, S., and Harell, A. Inadequate status and impaired metabolism of vitamin D in the elderly. *Isr. J. Med. Sci.* **17,** 19–21 (1981).
23. Frame, B., and Parfitt, M. A. Osteomalacia: Current concepts. *Ann. Intern. Med.* **89,** 966–982 (1978).
24. Sem, S. W., Sjøen, R. J., Trygg, K., and Pedersen, J. I. Vitamin D status of two groups of elderly in Oslo: living in old people's homes and living in own homes. *Comp. Gerontol. A* **1,** 126–130 (1987).
25. Corless, D., Boucher, B. J., Beer, M., Gupta, S. P., and Cohen, R. D. Vitamin D status in long-stay geriatric patients. *Lancet* **I,** 1404–1406 (1975).
26. Vir, S. C., and Love, A. H. G. Vitamin D status of elderly at home and institutionalized in hospital. *J. Vit. Nutr. Res.* **48,** 123–130 (1978).
27. Quesada, J. M., Jans, I., Benito, P., Jimeniz, J. A., and Bouillon, R. Vitamin D status of elderly people in Spain. *Age Ageing* **18,** 392–397 (1989).

28. Sherman, S. S., Hollis, B. W., and Tobin, J. D. Vitamin D status and related parameters in a healthy population: The effects of age, sex, and season. *J. Clin. Endocrinol. Metab.* **71,** 405–413 (1990).
29. Corless, D., Gupta, S. P., Sattar, D. A., Switala, S., and Boucher, B. J. Vitamin D status of residents of an old people's home and long-stay patients. *Gerontology* **24,** 350–355 (1979).
30. Gloth, F. M., III, Gundberg, C. M., Hollis, B. W., Haddad, J. G., and Tobin, J. D. The prevalence of vitamin D deficiency in a cohort of homebound elderly subjects compared to a normative matched population in the United States. *JAMA* **274,** 1683–1686 (1995).
31. McKenna, M., Freaney, R., Keating, D., and Muldowney, F. P. The prevalence and management of vitamin D deficiency in an acute geriatric unit. *Irish Med. J.* **74**(11), 336–336 (1981).
32. McKenna, M. J., Freaney, R., Meade, A., and Muldowney, F. P. Hypovitaminosis D and elevated serum alkaline phosphatase in elderly Irish people. *Am. J. Clin. Nutr.* **41,** 101–109 (1985).
33. McKenna, M. J. Differences in vitamin D status between countries in young adults and the elderly. *Am. J. Med.* **93,** 69–77 (1992).
34. Haddad, J. Vitamin D: Solar rays, Milky Way, or both. [Ed.] *N. Engl. J. Med.* **326,** 1213 (1992).
35. McMurtry, C. T., Young, S. E., Adler, R. A., and Downs, R. W. Mild vitamin D deficiency and secondary hyperparathyroidism in nursing home patients receiving adequate dietary vitamin D. *J. Am. Geriatr. Soc.* **40,** 343–347 (1992).
36. O'Dowd, K. J., Clemens, T. L., Lindsay, R., and Kelsey, J. L. Vitamin D status of nursing home residents in the Northeastern United States. *Am. Soc. Bone Miner. Res.* S158 (1988). [Abstract 357]
37. Webb, A., Pillbeam, C., Hanafin, N., and Holick, M. An evaluation of the relative contributions of exposure to sunlight and of diet to the circulating concentrations of 25-hydroxyvitamin D in an elderly nursing home population in Boston. *Am. J. Clin. Nutr.* **51,** 1075–1081 (1990).
38. McKenna, J. M., Freaney, R., Casey, O. M., Towers, R. P., and Muldowney, F. P. Osteomalacia and osteoporosis: evaluation of a diagnostic index. *J. Clin. Pathol.* **36,** 245–252 (1983).
39. Liel, Y., Ulmer, E., Shary, J., Hollis, B. W., and Bell, N. H. Low circulating vitamin D in obesity. *Calcif. Tissue Int.* **43,** 199–201 (1988).
40. Hess, A. *In* "Rickets, including Osteomalacia and Tetany" (A. Hess, ed.), pp. 22–37. Lea & Febiger, Philadelphia, 1929.
41. Gloth, F. M., III, and Tobin, J. D. A review of vitamin D deficiency in the elderly: What we know and what we don't. *J. Am. Geriatr. Soc.* **43,** 822–828 (1995).
42. Gloth, F. M., III, Tobin, J. D., Sherman, S. S., Hollis, B. W., and Gundberg, C. Vitamin D repletion in sun-deprived elderly. *J. Bone Miner. Res.* **5**(Suppl 2); (1990). [Abstract 778]
43. Murphy, S., Khaw, K., Prentice, A., and Compston, J. Relationships between parathyroid hormone, 25-hydroxyvitamin D, and bone mineral density in elderly men. *Age Ageing* **22,** 198–204 (1993).
44. Holick, M. F. Vitamin D synthesis by the aging skin. *In* "Nutrition and Aging," pp. 45–58. Academic Press, New York, 1980.
45. Riggs, B. L. Nutritional factors in age-related osteoporosis. *In* "Nutrition and Aging," pp. 207–216, Academic Press, New York, 1980.
46. DeLuca, H. F. Significance of vitamin D in age-related bone disease. *In* "Nutrition and Aging," pp. 217–224. Academic Press, New York, 1980.
47. Orwoll, E. S., and Meier, D. E. Alterations in calcium, vitamin D, and parathyroid hormone physiology in normal men with aging: relationship to the development of senile osteopenia. *J. Clin. Endocrinol. Metab.* **63,** 1262–1269 (1986).
48. Bouillon, R., Van Assche, F. A., Van Baelen, H., Heyns, W., and De Moor, P. Influence of the vitamin D-binding protein on the serum concentration of 1,25-dihydroxyvitamin D_3. *J. Clin. Invest.* **67,** 589–596 (1981).
49. Toss, G., and Sörbo, B. Serum concentrations of 25-hydroxyvitamin D and vitamin D-binding protein in elderly people. *Acta Med. Scand.* **220,** 273–277 (1986).
50. Price, P. A., and Baukol, S. A. 1,25-Dihydroxyvitamin D_3 increases synthesis of the vitamin K-dependent bone protein by osteosarcoma cells. *J. Biol. Chem.* **255,** 11660–11663 (1980).
51. Pan, L. C., and Price, P. A. Effect of transcriptional inhibitors on the bone-Γ-carboxyglutamic acid protein response to 1,25 dihydroxyvitamin D_3 in osteosarcoma cells. *J. Biol. Chem.* **259,** 5844–5847 (1984).
52. Yoon, K., Rutledge, S. J. C., Buenaga, R. F., and Rodan, G. A. Characterization of the rat osteocalcin gene: stimulation of promoter activity by 1,25-dihydroxyvitamin D_3. *Biochemistry* **27,** 8521–8526 (1988).
53. Lian, J. B., Stewart, C., Puchacz, E., Mackowiak, Shalhoub, V., Collart, D., Zambetti, G., and Stein, G. Structure of the rat osteocalcin gene and regulation of vitamin D-dependent expression. *Proc. Natl. Acad. Sci. USA* **86,** 1143–1147 (1989).
54. Marie, P. J., Connes, D., Hott, M., Miravet, L. Comparative effects of a novel vitamin D analogue MC-903 and 1,25-dihydroxyvitamin D_3 on alkaline phosphatase, activity, osteocalcin and DNA synthesis by human osteoblastic cells in culture. *Bone* **11,** 171–179 (1990).
55. Morrison, N. A., Shine, J., Fragonas, J.-C., Verkest, V., McMenemy, M. L., and Eisman, J. A. 1,25-Dihydroxyvitamin D-responsive element and glucocorticoid repression in the osteocalcin gene. *Science* **246,** 1158–1161 (1989).
56. Gundberg, C. M., Cole, D. E. C., Lian, J. B., Reade, T. M., and Gallup, P. M. Serum osteocalcin in the treatment of inherited rickets with 1,25-dihydroxyvitamin D_3. *J. Clin. Endocrinol. Metab.* **56,** 1063–1067 (1983).
57. Eastell, R., Delmas, P. D., Hodgson, S. F., Eriksen, E. F., Mann, K. G., and Riggs, B. L. Bone formation rate in older normal women: concurrent assessment with bone histomorphometry calcium kinetics, and biochemical markers. *J. Clin. Endocrinol. Metab.* **67,** 741–748 (1988).
58. Guillemant, S., Guillemant, J., Feteanu, D., and Sebag-Lanoé, R. Effect of vitamin D_3 administration on serum 25-hydroxyvitamin D_3 1,25-dihydroxyvitamin D_3 and osteocalcin in vitamin D-deficient elderly people. *J. Steroid Biochem.* **33,** 1155–1159 (1989).
59. Pietschmann, P., Woloszczuk, W., and Pietschmann, H. Increased serum osteocalcin levels in elderly females with vitamin D deficiency. *Exp. Clin. Endocrinol.* **95**(2), 275–278 (1990).
60. Dandona, P., Menon, R. K., Shenoy, R., Houlder, S., Thomas, M., and Mallinson, W. J. W. Low 1,25-dihydroxyvitamin D, secondary hyperparathyroidism, and normal osteocalcin in elderly subjects. *J. Clin. Endocrinol. Metab.* **63,** 459–462 (1986).
61. Morrison, N. A., Qi, J. C., Tokita, A., Kelly, P. J., Crofts, L., Nguyen, T. V., Sambrook, P. N., and Eisman, J. A. Prediction of bone density from vitamin D receptor alleles. *Lancet* **367,** 284–287 (1994).
62. Barsony, J., McKoy, W., De Grange, D. A., Liberman, U. A., and Marx, S. J. Selective expression of a normal action of the 1,25-dihydroxyvitamin D3 receptor in human skin fibroblasts with hereditary severe defects in multiple actions of that receptor. *J. Clin. Invest.* **83,** 2093–2101 (1989).

63. Chesnut, C. H., III, McClung, M. R., Ensrud, K. E., *et al.* Alendronate treatment of the postmenopausal osteoporotic woman: effect of multiple dosages on bone mass and bone remodeling. *Am. J. Med.* **99,** 144–152 (1995).
64. Dawson-Hughes, B., Dallal, G. E., Krall, E. A., Harris, S., Sokoll, L. J., and Falconer, G. Effect of vitamin D supplementation on wintertime and overall bone loss in healthy postmenopausal women. *Ann Intern Med.* **115,** 505–512 (1991).
65. Chapuy, M. C., Arlot, M. E., Duboeuf, F., Brun, J., Crouzet, B., Arnaud, S., Delmas, P. D., and Meunier, P. J. Vitamin D_3 and calcium to prevent hip fractures in elderly women. *N. Engl. J. Med.* **327,** 1637–1642 (1992).
66. Chapuy, M. C., Arlot, M. E., Delmas, P. D., and Meunier, P. J. Effect of calcium and cholecalciferol treatment for three years on hip fractures in elderly women. *Br. Med. J.* **308,** 1081–1082 (1994).
67. Tilyard, M. W., Spears, G. F. S., Thomson, J., and Dovey, S. Treatment of postmenopausal osteoporosis with calcitriol or calcium. *N. Engl. J. Med.* **326,** 357–362 (1992).
68. Holbrook, T. L., Grazier, K., Kelsey, J. L., and Stauffer, R. N., "The Frequency of Occurrence, Impact and Cost of Selected Musculoskeletal Conditions in the United States." American Academy of Orthopedic Surgeons, Chicago, 1984.
69. Ray, N. F., *et al. J. Bone Miner. Res.* **12,** 24–35 (1997).
70. Cummings, S. R., Phillips, S. L., Wheat, M. E., *et al.* Recovery of function after hip fracture. *J. Am. Geriatr. Soc.* **36,** 801–806 (1988).
71. Chalmers, J., Conacher, W. D. H., Gardner, D. L., and Scott, P. J. Osteomalacia—a common disease in elderly women. *J. Bone Joint Surg.* **49B,** 403–423.
72. Weisman, Y., Schen, R. J., Eisenberg, Z., Edelstein, S., and Harell, A. Inadequate status and impaired metabolism of vitamin D in the elderly. *Isr. J. Med. Sci.* **17,** 19–21 (1981).
73. Meller, Y., Kestenbaum, R. S., Galinsky, D., and Shany, S. Seasonal variation in serum levels of vitamin D metabolites and parathormone in geriatric patients with fractures in southern Israel. *Isr. J. Med. Sci.* **22,** 8–11 (1986).
74. Quesada, J. M., Jans, I., Benito, P., Jimeniz, J. A., and Bouillon, R. Vitamin D status of elderly people in Spain. *Age Ageing* **18,** 392–397 (1989).
75. Pike, J. W., Goozle, L. L., and Haussler, M. R. Biochemical evidence for 1,25-dihydroxyvitamin D receptor macromolecules in parathyroid, pancreatic, pituitary, and placental tissues. *Life Sci.* **26,** 407–414 (1980).
76. Gelbard, H. A., Stern, P. H., and U'Prichard, D. C. 1 Alpha 25-hydroxyvitamin D3 nuclear receptors in pituitary. *Science* **209,** 1247–1249 (1980).
77. Merke, J., Milde, P., Lewicka, S., *et al.* Identification and regulation of 1,25-dihydroxyvitamin D3 receptor activity and biosynthesis of 1,25-dihydroxyvitamin D3: studies in cultured bovine aortic endothelial cells and human dermal capillaries. *J. Clin. Invest.* **83,** 1903–1915 (1989).
78. Barsony, J., McKoy, W., De Grange, D. A., Liberman, U. A., and Marx, S. J. Selective expression of a normal action of the 1,25-dihydroxyvitamin D3 receptor in human skin fibroblasts with hereditary severe defects in multiple actions of that receptor. *J. Clin. Invest.* **83,** 2093–2101 (1989).
79. Merke, J., Hofmann, W., Goldschmidt, D., and Ritz, E. Demonstration of 1,25-$(OH)_2 D_3$ receptors and action in vascular smooth muscle cells *in vitro. Calcif Tissue Int.* **41,** 112–114 (1987).
80. Provvedini, D. M., Tsoukas, C. D., Deftos, L. J., and Manolagas, S. C. 1,25-dihydroxyvitamin D3 receptor in human leukocytes. *Science* **221,** 1181–1183 (1983).
81. Pillai, S., Bikle, D. D., and Elias, P. M. 1,25-dihydroxyvitamin D production and receptor binding in human keratinocytes varies with differentiation. *J. Biol. Chem.* **263,** 5390–5395 (1988).
82. Skaria, J., Katiyar, B. C., Srivastava, T. P., and Dube, B. Myopathy and neuropathy associated with osteomalacia. *Acta Neurol. Scand.* **51,** 37 (1975).
83. Young, A., Edwards, R. H. T., Jones, D. A., *et al.* Quadriceps muscle strength and fibre size during the treatment of osteomalacia. *In* "Mechanical Factors and Skeleton" (I. A. F. Stokes and J. Stokes, eds.), pp. 137–145.
84. Simpson, R. U., Thomas, G. A., and Arnold, A. J. Identification of 1,25-dihydroxyvitamin D_3 receptors and activities on muscle. *J. Biol. Chem.* **260,** 8882–8891 (1985).
85. Birge, S. J., and Haddad, J. G. 25-hydroxycholecalciferol stimulation of muscle metabolism. *J. Clin. Invest.* **56,** 1100–1107 (1975).
86. Young, A., Edwards, R. H. T., Jones, D. A., *et al.* Quadriceps muscle strength and fibre size during the treatment of osteomalacia. *In* "Mechanical Factors and the Skeleton" (I. A. O. Stokes and J. Stokes, eds.), pp. 137–145.
87. Gloth, F. M., III, Lindsay, J. M., Zelesnick, L. B., and Greenough, W. B. III, "Can vitamin D deficiency produce an unusual pain syndrome?"*Arch. Intern. Med.* **151,** 1662–1664 (1991).
88. Huaux, J. P., Malghem, J., Maldague, B. *et al.* Reflex sympathetic dystrophy syndrome: an unusual mode of presentation of osteomalacia. *Arthritis Rheum.* **29,** 918–925 (1986).
89. Corless, D., Dawson, D., Fraser, F., Ellis, M., *et al.* Do vitamin D supplements improve the physical capabilities of elderly hospital patients. *Age Ageing* **14,** 76–84 (1985).
90. Sørensen, O. H., Lund, B. I., Saltin, B., Lund, B. J., Andersen, R. B., Hjorth, L., Melsen, F., and Mosekilde, L. Myopathy in bone loss of ageing: Improvement by treatment with 1α-hydroxycholecalciferol and calcium. *Clin Sci.* **56,** 157–161 (1979).
91. Benjamin, J. The Northwick Park ADL index. *Occup. Ther.* 301–306 (1976).
92. Sheikh, K., Smith, D. S., Meade, T. W., Goldenberg, E., Brennan, P., and Kinsella, G. Repeatability and validity of modified activities of daily living (ADL) index in studies of chronic disability. *Int. Rehabil. Med.* **1,** 51–58 (1979).
93. Gloth, F. M., III, Smith, C. E., Hollis, B. W., and Tobin, J. D. Vitamin D replenishment in a cohort of frail, vitamin D deficient elderly improves functional dynamics. *J. Am. Geriatr. Soc.* **43,** 1269–1271 (1995).
94. Begerow, B., Pfeifer, M., Pospeschill, M., Scholz, M., Hass, K., Schlotthauer, T., Makosch, S., Lazarescu, A. D., Pollaehne, W., and Minne, H. W. Vitamin-D-deficiency impairs muscle strength and body sway in patients with postmenopausal osteoporosis and increases risk of falling. *J. Bone Miner. Res.* **12**(Suppl. 1), S2–S18 (1997).
95. Bischoff, H., Urscheler, N., Binder, K., Vogt, P., Ehrsam, R., Vonthein, R., Perrig-Chiello, P., Perrig, W., Stähelin, H. B., Tyndall, A., and Theiler, R. Leg extension power and 1,25 $(OH)_2$ vitamin D in free-living elderly persons. *J. Bone Miner. Res.* **12**(Suppl. 1), S217 (1997).
96. MacLennan, W. J., and Hamilton, J. C. Vitamin D supplements and 25-hydroxyvitamin D concentrations in the elderly. *Br. Med. J.* **2,** 859–861 (1977).
97. Sambrook, P., and Nagantathan, V. What is the relationship between osteoarthritis and osteoporosis? *Clin Rheumatol.* **11,** 695–710 (1997).
98. Relationship of dietary intake and vitamin D to osteoarthritis. *Ann. Int. Med.* **125,** 353–359 (1996).
99. Gloth, F. M., III, and Adam, W. Treatment of seasonal affect disorder (SAD) with vitamin D vs full spectrum light. *J. Bone Miner. Res.* **12**(Suppl. 1), S217 (1997). [Abstract T460]
100. Adams, J. S., and Lee, G. Gains in bone mineral density with resolution of vitamin D intoxication. *Ann. Intern. Med.* **127,** 203–206 (1997).

101. Personal communication with Harold H. Harrison who performed much of the early vitamin D research with E. V. McCullom and participated in establishing the current RDA for vitamin D in the United States.
102. "National Academy of Science Recommended Dietary Allowances," 10th revised edition, pp. 95–96. The National Academy Press, Washington, DC, 1989.
103. Zheng, J. J., and Rosenberg, I. H. What is the nutritional status of the elderly? *Geriatrics* **44,** 57–64 (1989).
104. Barzel, U. S. Osteomalacia caused by vitamin D deficiency in the aged (letter). *Mayo Clin. Proc.* **61,** 303 (1986).
105. McGandy, R. B., Russell, R. M., Hartz, S. C., *et al.* Nutritional status survey of healthy non-institutionalized elderly: Energy and nutrient intakes from three-day diet records and nutrient supplements. *Nutr Res.* **6,** 785–798 (1986).
106. Sahyoun, N. R., Otradovec, C. L., Hartz, S. C., *et al.* Dietary intakes and biochemical indicators of nutritional status in an elderly, institutionalized population. *Am. J. Clin. Nutr.* **47,** 524–533 (1988).
107. Anwar, M. Nutritional hypovitaminosis-D and genesis of osteomalacia in the elderly. *J. Am. Ger. Soc.* **26,** 309–317 (1978).
108. Exton-Smith, A. N., Hodkinson, H. M., and Stanton, B. R. Nutrition and metabolic bone disease in old age. *Lancet* **ii,** 999–1001 (1966).
109. MacLeod, C. C., Judge, T. G., and Caird, F. I. Nutrition of the elderly at home II. Intakes of vitamins. *Age Ageing* **3,** 209–220 (1974).
110. Lonergan, M. E., Milne, J. B., Maule, M. M., and Williamson, J. A dietary survey of older people in Edinburgh. *Br. J. Nutr.* **34,** 517–527 (1975).
111. Somerville, P. J., Lien, J. W. K., and Kaye, M. The calcium and vitamin D status in an elderly female population and their response to administered supplemental vitamin D. *J. Gerontol.* **32,** 659–663 (1977).
112. "National Academy of Science Recommended Dietary Allowances," 10th revised edition, The National Academy Press, Washington, DC, 1997.
113. Matsuoka, M., Otsuka, H., Masuda, S., Okano, T., Kobayashi, T., Takeuchi, T., and Itokawa, Y. Changes in the concentrations of vitamin D and its metabolites in the plasma of healthy subjects orally given physiological doses of vitamin D_2 by multivitamin or vitamin preparations. *J. Nutr. Sci. Vitaminol.* **35,** 253–266 (1989).
114. Dunnigan, M., McIntosh, W., and Sumner, D. Vitamin D supplementation in the elderly. *In* "Abstracts of Fifth Workshop on Vitamin D," p. 403, 1982.
115. Honkanen, R., Alhava, E., Parviainen, M., Talasniemi, S., and Mönkkönen, R. The necessity and safety of calcium and vitamin D in the elderly. *J. Am. Geriatr. Soc.* **38,** 862–866 (1990).
116. Weisman, Y., Schen, R. J., Eisenberg, Z., *et al.* Single oral high dose vitamin D_3 prophylaxis in the elderly. *J. Am. Ger. Soc.* **34,** 515–518 (1986).
117. Matsuoka, M., Otsuka, H., Masuda, S., Okano, T., Kobayashi, T., Takeuchi, T., and Itokawa, Y. Changes in the concentrations of vitamin D and its metabolites in the plasma of healthy subjects orally given physiological doses of vitamin D_2 by multivitamin or vitamin preparations. *J. Nutr. Sci. Vitaminol.* **35,** 253–266 (1989).
118. Dunnigan, M., McIntosh, W., and Sumner, D. Vitamin D supplementation in the elderly. *In* "Abstracts of Fifth Workshop on Vitamin D, p. 403, 1982.
119. Honkanen, R., Alhava, E., Parviainen, M., Talasniemi, S., and Mönkkönen, R. The necessity and safety of calcium and vitamin D in the elderly. *J. Am. Geriatr. Soc.* **38,** 862–866 (1990).
120. Weisman, Y., Schen, R. J., Eisenberg, Z., *et al.* Single oral high dose vitamin D_3 prophylaxis in the elderly. *J. Am. Geriatr. Soc.* **34,** 515–518 (1986).
121. Paterson, C. R. Vitamin-D poisoning: survey of causes in 21 patients with hypercalcaemia. *Lancet* **I,** 1164–1165 (1980).
122. Davies, M., and Adams, P. H. The continuing risk of vitamin-D intoxication. *Lancet* **i,** 621–623 (1978).
123. Shiraki, M., Kushida, K., Yamazaki, K., Nagai, T., Inoue, T., and Orimo, H. Effects of 2 years' treatment of osteoporosis with 1alpha-hydroxyvitamin D_3 on bone mineral density and incidence of fracture: a placebo-controlled, double-blind prospective study. *Endocr. J.* **43,** 211–220 (1996).
124. Francis, R. M. Is there a differential response to alphacalcidiol and vitamin D in the treatment of osteoporosis? *Calcif Tissue Int.* **60,** 111–114 (1997).

CHAPTER 18

Cytokines and Prostaglandins in the Aging Skeleton

MARK C. HOROWITZ Department of Orthopaedics and Rehabilitation, Yale University School of Medicine, New Haven, Connecticut 06510

LAWRENCE G. RAISZ Department of Medicine, University of Connecticut Health Center, Farmington, Connecticut 06030

CYTOKINES AND THE AGING SKELETON

Skeletal Life

The skeleton is not fixed or stagnant, but rather it is a living organ that carries out multiple functions central to the survival of the organism. Bones develop, grow, and age in a relatively predictable manner. This pattern can be characterized by four distinct but contiguous stages. In the first stage, during early embryonic life, the patterning of bone is genetically determined and likely to be controlled by genes such as the hedgehog proteins, parathyroid hormone-related peptide, and the bone morphogenetic proteins (BMPs) and their regulatory molecules such as the BMP antagonist, noggin. As the embryo develops *in utero,* bone anlagen are formed by mesenchymal cell condensation. The differentiation of osteoblasts and their secretion of extracellular matrix proteins, which form the structure of new bone, is regulated by factors such as BMP and transforming growth factor β (TGFβ). These factors are intimately involved in osteoblast differentiation and are central to skeletal development [1]. The second stage encompasses the time *in utero* when the embryo has a complete set of fully shaped and mineralizing bones to the time when bones stop adding mass, sometime in the second or third decade of life in humans. This stage is characterized by rapid bone growth and modeling during which the individual attains peak bone mass. The opposing processes of bone resorption and bone formation, which are critical in maintaining bone homeostasis, greatly favor bone formation as bones grow and model to adult proportions. In humans the skeleton then enters the third stage, a long period (~20–30 years) in which bone resorption and bone formation are in approximate balance. Although the bone continues to turn over, the net change in bone mass is essentially zero and skeletal homeostasis is maintained. Population studies suggest a slight, gradual decline in skeletal mass during this period, but this is difficult to appreciate in individual subjects (see Chapter 15). For women, this decline accelerates with the onset of menopause. For men, "male menopause" occurs, but later in life. These latter two periods are characterized by a shift from the balance between bone resorption and formation to significantly favor increased resorption with associated bone loss.

Bone resorption and formation are complicated and highly regulated cellular processes. The circuitry of this regulation is not completely understood, but it is clear that one important aspect of this control is mediated by cytokines. Cytokines play an important role in the regulation of both osteoblast and osteoclast differentiation and function. As we age, bone mass is lost and this loss is associated with a significant increase in fractures and associated morbidity and mortality. Although complicated by specific pathologies like tumors and metabolic bone disease, age-related bone loss can be accounted for by at least two general mechanisms. First, the number of osteoblasts and their ability to make new bone appear to decrease with age, resulting in less new bone tissue. Second, the number of osteoclasts and their activity increase, resulting in accelerated bone loss. These two related mechanisms work in concert to weaken the skeleton. This section examines how cytokines regulate these two functions in the aging skeleton.

Bones and Fat: Here's the Skinny

It is generally agreed that the bone marrow, in addition to being the site of hematopoiesis and lymphopoiesis, also contains the cells that give rise to the mesenchymal cell lineage. This lineage includes the precursor cells that form bone (osteoblasts), fat (adipocytes), cartilage (chrondocytes), muscle (myocytes), support hematopoiesis (stromal cells) and connective tissue (fibroblasts) [2,3]. The prevailing model is that this lineage, like that of the hematopoietic cell lineage, arises from uncommitted pluripotent stem cells and passes through a series of discrete stages of differentiation, resulting in mature functional cells (Fig. 1). Progress along this pathway requires specific signals, some of which are cytokines and their cell surface expressed receptors. This lineage, like the hematopoietic lineage, is found in bone marrow and spleen in some species [4,5]. This maturation process continues throughout life, seeding new cells into their appropriate physical locations for continued maturation and eventual function. However, the proportions of the lineages change with age. Clinically, it is well known that marrow from newborns and young adults contains few adipocytes and is rich in erythropoietic activity. This tissue is often referred to as "red marrow." This marrow is also high in osteogenic potential [6]. As we get older the number and size of the adipocytes increase in a linear manner, resulting in "yellow marrow" [7,8]. Eventually 50% of the marrow cavity is filled with fat. In humans aged 0–60 years, a 50% reduction in proliferating bone cells was observed in the 0- to 30-year group; however, in the 30- to 60-year group, the proliferating cell number remained stable and similar [9]. These observations seen in humans have also been observed in other species. Marrow from older mice or rats contains fewer stromal stem cells than marrow from younger mice as measured by assays for fibroblast colony-forming units or numbers of bone nodules formed [10–12]. "Stromal stem cells" refer to the stem cell or early progenitor population, most often found in the bone marrow, which gives rise to the mesenchymal cell lineage, including osteoblasts, adipocytes, and stromal cells. The terms mesenchymal stem cell and stromal stem cell are often used interchangeably. In the SAMP6 mouse, which is a model for accelerated aging, low bone mineral density is associated with a decrease in osteoblastogenesis and a concomitant increase in the number of adipocytes [13,14]. These data suggest a causal relationship between the decrease in osteogenesis and the increase in adipogenesis with age. This relationship is further supported by the fact that osteoblasts and adipocytes appear to share a common progenitor [15,16]. However, controversy continues over whether osteoblasts and adipocytes are distinct or related lineages. The BMS2 murine stromal cell line spontaneously undergoes adipogenesis in fetal calf serum and this process can be accelerated by exposing the cells to hydrocortisone, indomethacin, and isobutyl methylxanthine

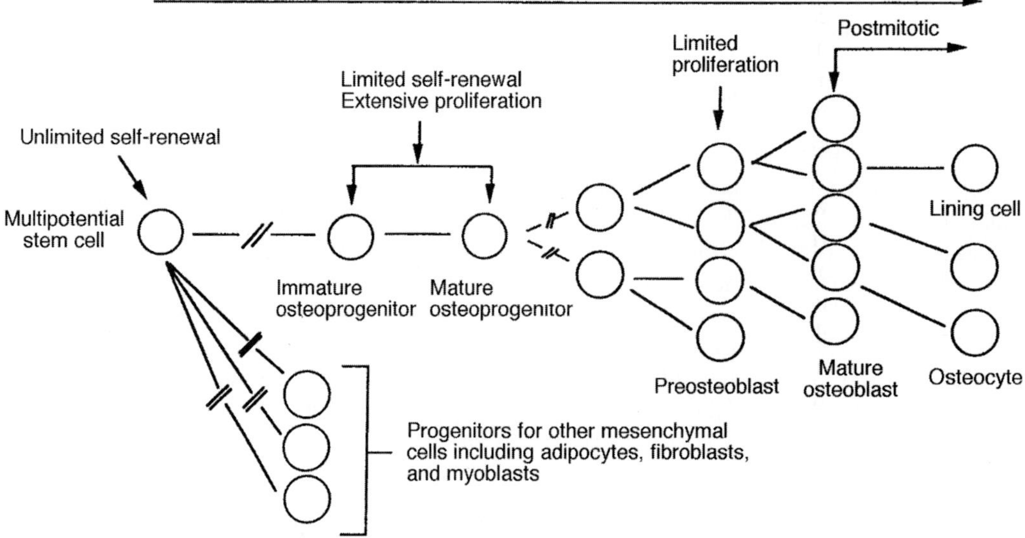

FIGURE 1 Postulated steps in the osteoblast lineage implying recognized stages of differentiation. Adapted from Aubin and Liu [136].

(IBMX) [17]. However, these cells may also express a number of osteoblastic markers, including alkaline phosphatase, osteopontin, type I collagen, and bone sialoprotein [18]. MG63 cells are a human transformed osteoblast-like cell line that can also exhibit an adipocytic phenotype [19]. Osteogenic cells derived from explants of adult human trabecular bone are capable of differentiating into adipocytes [20]. As with mouse cells, adipogenesis by human bone cells was stimulated by the addition of dexamethasone and IBMX. It is notable that dexamethasone is often found in media used to induce mouse osteoblast differentiation. Responsiveness to dexamethasone is another small, but possibly important, fact linking osteogenic and adipogenic cell types. In osteoporotic patients, increased marrow fat was correlated with decreased trabecular bone volume in a manner similar to the bone marrow of SAMP6 mice [21]. In addition, in *in vitro* studies of rat or mouse cells, osteoblastic markers decreased as adipogenic cell-specific markers increased [18,22]. These data suggest, and it is the authors' view, that these lineages arise from a common progenitor and that their phenotypes overlap at early stages of differentiation. This ancestry, combined with the retained plasticity of certain differentiation genes, would explain the bipotential phenotype of these cells.

The authors suggest, as others have, that cytokines play a role in this age-dependent shift in lineage expression. Members of the TGFβ super family (TGFβ-1 and BMPs 2, 4, and 7) have opposing effects on osteogenesis and adipogenesis. TGFβ and BMP in general are potent inducers of osteogenesis [23–25]. Although the concentration of TGFβ does have a biphasic effect on osteoblast proliferation and collagen synthesis, it is a potent inhibitor of adipogenesis [26,27]. Transgenic mice overexpressing a constitutively active human TGFβ-1 gene exhibited a severe reduction in body fat [28]. These data suggest that multimeric receptors for these growth factors (cytokines) are present and functional on cells in both osteoblastic and adipocytic lineages. Therefore, it is possible that differences in the downstream signaling pathways used by these two cytokines may alter the cellular differentiation pattern.

Two other groups of cytokines can regulate osteoblastic function and may also regulate the balance of osteogenic and adipogenic cells. Osteoblasts and adipocytes are sensitive to cytokines in the LIF/IL-6 family of cytokines [29,30]. These factors signal cells through ligand binding to a multichain receptor that includes the common signal transducing protein gp130 [31]. Of this family of factors, LIF, oncostatin-M, and IL-11 activate osteoblasts and are potent antiadipogenic agents [30,32]. Treatment of bone marrow from SAMP6 mice with indomethacin, which induces adipogenic differentiation, causes a marked induction of adipocytes as compared to control bone marrow. Addition of IL-11 to these cultures inhibits that differentiation [135]. IL-11 mRNA expression and secreted protein are reduced in the SAMP6 bone marrow cultures, suggesting that IL-11 is responsible for the increased adipogenesis. IL-6 also has antiadipogenic activity but does not directly activate osteoblasts. These cytokines have been shown to double alkaline phosphatase activity, a marker of osteoblastic cells, in the preadipocyte cell line BMS2 [30]. This is consistent with other reports showing that the *in vivo* administration of LIF or IL-6 is associated with loss of fat and induction of cachexia [33,34]. The other group of cytokines with regulatory activity are the proinflammatory agents IL-1 and TNFα. Both IL-1 and TNFα are adipogenic antagonists [27,35,36].

These data suggest that with age the adipogenic potential of bone marrow increases at the expense of its osteogenic potential. Part of this shift in lineage is caused by the positive or negative effects of specific cytokines, some of which have been identified. Many of these cytokines have potent activity on cells in both osteogenic and adipogenic lineages because these cells arise from a shared progenitor. The secretion and specific binding of these cytokines define part of the regulatory circuitry that controls the interactions between osteoblastic and adipocytic cells. The sensitivity of these interactions may be dependent on the stage of differentiation and may also control that differentiation.

Menopause: The End of a Good Thing (for Your Bones)

Deficiency in 17β-estradiol (E_2) caused by either menopause or ovariectomy results in accelerated bone loss. There is a significant decline in bone mass at menopause in many women; this is the major factor contributing to the high prevalence of disabling fractures in postmenopausal women. The pathologic bone loss associated with this condition can largely be prevented by early estrogen replacement therapy. However, the mechanism by which E_2 exerts its bone-sparing effect is likely to be multifaceted. Numerous studies now indicate that E_2 regulates the cytokine circuity that controls bone remodeling [37].

One of the first observations in this line of investigation demonstrated that peripheral blood monocytes (PBM) from both men and women with osteoporosis secreted elevated levels of IL-1 [38]. This observation was extended to show that PBM from either premenopausal or postmenopausal women with osteoporosis who were treated with estrogen and progesterone secreted less IL-1 than untreated postmenopausal women (both nonosteoporotic and osteoporotic) [39]. Additional data showed that PBM from ovariectomized premenopausal women, with reduced serum E_2 levels, constitutively secrete more IL-1 and TNFα and can be induced to secrete higher levels of granulocyte–macrophage colony-stimulating factor (GM-CSF) relative to age-matched controls [40]. Some ovariectomized women on estrogen replacement therapy following surgery showed a decrease in cytokine production with a concomitant reduction in bone resorption. In contrast, amounts of cytokines produced by PBM from ovariectomized women who received no estrogen therapy steadily increased, whereas women who underwent a hysterectomy without ovariectomy showed no change in either cytokine secretion or biochemical parameters of bone resorption. These data show that the loss of E_2, which accompanies menopause, allows PBM to secrete more IL-1 and TNFα and that E_2 inhibits IL-1 secretion. However, other studies have been unable to confirm some of these observations [41,42]. Bacterial lipopolysaccharide (LPS) is a potent inducer of IL-1 and TNFα secretion from monocytes and macrophages. Conditioned medium from PBM activated with LPS from ovariectomized women had greater bone-resorbing activity than similarly prepared conditioned medium from premenopausal or estrogen-treated postmenopausal women [43]. Use of neutralizing antibodies showed this activity to be caused by both IL-1 and TNFα. Whether the PBM results are an accurate reflection of events occurring in the bone marrow microenvironment remains controversial. This may be of particular importance because bone remodeling is highly regulated at the local level within the bone and bone marrow. To some degree this issue has been put to rest because similar responses have been reported for marrow-derived cells. A more direct approach has been to measure IL-1 in the serum of pre- and postmenopausal women. In one study, IL-1 levels were increased 30 days postovariectomy, but similar studies have failed to find a correlation between IL-1α, IL-β, or IL-1 receptor antagonist (IL-1ra) levels and measures of bone turnover in pre- and postmenopausal women or between osteoporotic and normal controls [44–46].

As mentioned previously, IL-1 and TNFα regulate bone cell differentiation and function in the marrow. Therefore, the ability of E_2 to regulate these cytokines is a likely mechanism for how E_2 exerts its effects on bone cell function. Elevated levels of bone active cytokines, including IL-1α, TNFα, PGE_2 (prostaglandin E_2), and GM-CSF, were reported in conditioned media of bone marrow cell cultures from postmenopausal women who had stopped E_2 replacement within 1 month before sampling as compared to conditioned media from premenopausal or late postmenopausal controls [47].

Studies with murine models shed some light on these mechanisms. Studies with cocultures of purified murine osteoclast precursors and stromal cells showed that stromal cells from ovariectomized mice induced more osteoclast formation than stromal cells from sham-operated animals [48]. Ovariectomy also increased the secretion of IL-1 and TNFα from the osteoclast precursors and increased M-CSF secretion from the stromal cells. This result has potentially added significance because of the essential role M-CSF plays in osteoclast development [49]. For direct assessment of the role of IL-1 in E_2-deficient bone remodeling, gene targeting was used to generate mice deficient in the type I receptor for IL-1 (IL-1R1) [50]. This receptor appears to mediate all known responses to IL-1 [51]. IL-1R1-deficient mice failed to lose bone mass following ovariectomy as compared to strain and age-matched controls. These data are clear in demonstrating that IL-1 is involved in the pathogenesis of bone loss due to estrogen deficiency.

Because the agents that induce IL-1 may also induce IL-1ra in equimolar concentrations, this natural antagonist regulates IL-1-induced bone loss. Bone loss in rats following ovariectomy was inhibited by the *in vivo* administration of IL-1ra [52]. Bone marrow cells from ovariectomized mice treated with IL-1ra had a decreased ability to generate osteoclasts *in vitro* [53]. Like that seen in humans, IL-1 bioactivity was increased in the conditioned media (CM) from bone marrow cells of ovariectomized mice [54,55]. Further, IL-1 levels in the CM were not changed by the ovariectomy. However, specific inhibitors of IL-α blocked the increased bioactivity of IL-1. These results suggest that it was the inhibitors of IL-1, and not the IL-1 itself, that were responsible for the change in IL-1 bioactivity following ovariectomy. It has been reported that E_2 increases the levels of mRNA for the type II receptor of IL-1 (IL-1R2) in both mouse bone marrow cells and human osteoclasts [56,57]. This receptor is found both on the cell surface or as a secreted protein [58]. IL-1 activity is decreased by the increased expression of IL-1R2 [59]. Therefore, changes in the levels of this antagonist may regulate some of the effects estrogen exerts on IL-1 activity in both the bone marrow and, subsequently, on remodeling.

In addition to IL-1, other bone-active cytokines are regulated by E_2 and may be involved in postmenopausal bone loss. TNFα, like IL-1, is a potent inducer of bone resorption, requires the presence of osteoblasts for its activity, and induces osteoblasts to secrete factors such as GM-CSF and IL-6, which induce the formation of osteoclasts from precursors. TNFα production by *in vitro* cultured human osteoblasts was shown to be modulated by E_2 in one study [60]. However, other investigators failed to find similar results in human osteoblast-like cells [61]. Like the *in vivo* effects of IL-1ra, treatment of mice with soluble TNF-binding protein, a specific inhibitor of TNF action, caused a marked reduction in the loss of bone following ovariectomy [62]. In a similar study, transgenic mice overexpressing the soluble TNF type I receptor were protected against bone loss following ovariectomy [63]. These data support the idea that IL-1 and TNFα are important mediators of the increased osteoclastic activity associated with the loss of E_2. This is consistent with other data showing IL-1 and TNFα to be potent inducers of osteoclastic bone resorption. The importance of TNF and TNF family members has been recognized with the identification of osteoclastogenesis inhibitory factor (OCIF) and osteoprotegrin (OPG), which have been shown to be identical proteins [64,65]. OPG is a member of the TNF receptor family. This protein lacks an apparent transmembrane domain and functions as a soluble inhibitory receptor. OPG suppresses bone resorption by inhibiting the terminal stages of osteoclast differentiation. The ligand for OPG, osteoclast differentiation factor (ODF), has also been identified [66]. ODF is a member of the TNF ligand family and is identical to TRANCE/RANKL. ODF is a membrane-bound protein and functions as a potent inducer of osteoclast formation. Presently no data are available on the effect of age on either of these proteins.

In a separate line of investigation, murine stromal cells, human bone cells, and rat and mouse osteoblast-like cell lines activated with IL-1 and TNFα all secreted IL-6 [67]. It is thought that the major effect of the osteoblast/stromal cell-derived IL-6 is its colony-stimulating activity, which functions to increase osteoclast precursors, resulting in increased numbers of mature cells [68]. The secretion of IL-6 induced in this way can be inhibited by treating the cells with E_2 and, to a lesser extent, with testosterone and progesterone. These experiments have been extended to show that testosterone inhibits IL-6 production from murine bone marrow stromal cells [69]. Loss of E_2 in ovariectomized mice led to an increase in colony-forming units for granulocytes and macrophages, enhanced osteoclast development *in vitro* in bone marrow cell cultures, and increased the number of osteoclasts *in vivo* [70]. As in previous experiments, these changes were inhibited by E_2 or an antibody to IL-6. These findings support the contention that osteoblast precursors, possibly in the form of marrow stromal cells, respond to the loss of E_2 by secreting IL-6, which then induces osteoclastogenesis. These studies further demonstrated that cytokine secretion by authentic bone cells can be downregulated by the addition of E_2, which is consistent with the expression of E_2 receptors by osteoblasts [71,72]. However, some studies have been unsuccessful in reproducing the inhibitory effect of E_2 on IL-6 secretion [61]. Additional reports indicated that neither E_2 nor progesterone inhibited IL-6 mRNA or protein levels induced by IL-1, TNFα, or IL-1 plus TNFα in normal human osteoblast-like cells and human marrow stromal cells [73]. In a model for the loss of E_2 that accompanies menopause, murine bone marrow cells and primary calvarial cells secreted more IL-6 following E_2 withdrawal [74]. Those data were substantiated by the observation that mice who were made IL-6 deficient by gene targeting did not have increased numbers of osteoclasts and were protected from bone loss following ovariectomy [75]. Those experiments have been difficult to reproduce, however, particularly with regard to whether the protective effect is sustained over time. Part of the problem in reproducing the observation may relate to the background strain of mice used for the homologous recombination.

The idea that the loss of E_2 is the only factor controlling the increase in IL-6 levels should be viewed with some skepticism. Bone marrow from patients undergoing hip replacement was used to analyze osteoclastogenesis and cytokine secretion. The formation of human osteoclast-like cells from these samples increased significantly with increasing age in both women and men [76]. This work has been extended to show that the constitutive secretion of IL-6 also increased with age [77]. In addition, cells from women receiving estrogen replacement therapy had significantly lower cytokine secretion than age-matched controls. In mice, serum IL-6 levels were shown to be elevated in aged mice [78]. Moreover, constitutive secretion of IL-6 could be detected in the conditioned medium of spleen cells from aged but not mature adults. It appears that IL-6 levels in both serum and conditioned medium from *in vitro* cultured cells increase with advancing age [45,77–80]. Both of these effects could be reversed by the administration of dehydroepiandrosterone (DHEA). DHEA is a steroid hormone (adrenal androgen) whose production declines with age [81,82]. In one report, increased IL-6 expression correlated with postmenopausal status in women; however, there was no effect on bone mineral density [83]. In a second report, elevated levels of IL-6 were correlated highly with age but not with menopausal status, serum estradiol concentration, or markers of bone turnover [45]. These data suggest that IL-6 levels increase by two mechanisms in the aging human skeleton. The first is a natural occurrence with aging, independent of the loss of sex steroids. The second mechanism is dependent on the loss of sex steroids. Alternatively, both mechanisms may be functional, one layered over the other. (Further information on this topic is contained in Chapter 15.) The age-dependent increase in IL-6 levels is in striking contrast to that of other cytokines. In humans and rodents there is a dramatic decline in $CD4^+$ T cells producing IL-2 and a decreased expression of IL-2 receptors [84,85,86]. IL-1 production by peritoneal macrophages from old vs young mice has also been reported to be reduced and this reduction could be partially restored by indomethacin treatment [87]. It is unknown whether this loss of IL-1 also occurs in bone. In light of these data and the fact that essentially all nucleated cells produce IL-6 either constitutively or following appropriate stimulation, IL-6 must be under extraordinary regulation, throughout the animal, that is different from other cytokines.

These findings and the observation that IL-6 has colony-stimulating activity point to the importance of IL-6 in osteoclast differentiation, particularly in animal models [88]. However, the relationship of increased levels of IL-6 to demonstrable changes in bone mineral density in humans remains controversial [45,83]. Whereas many of these studies suggest that a primary effect of E_2 is to modulate IL-6 secretion, previously described findings with IL-1, TNFα, and other factors indicate that E_2 exerts its influence on multiple cytokines. Furthermore, an increase in IL-6 secretion could also result from a primary effect of E_2 on IL-1 or TNFα production because both of them are potent inducers of IL-6 secretion. E_2 also appears to affect both the osteoclast precursor and the osteoblast/stromal cell, each of which respond independently [48].

An additional issue must be considered when assessing the role IL-6 plays in bone remodeling and its regulation by E_2. This refers to the role the IL-6 receptor (IL-6R) and its soluble form (sIL-6R) play in bone cell activation. The IL-6R is an 80-kDa glycoprotein (α subunit, gp80) required for ligand binding. In conjunction with the gp130 signaling subunit, a complete and active receptor is formed [89]. Although gp130 is expressed on normal stromal and osteoblastic cells, there is little evidence that the IL-6 receptor is similarly expressed. IL-6 does not directly induce tyrosine phosphorylation in primary mouse or human osteoblasts unless sIL-6R is added [90,91]. IL-6 also fails to directly induce osteoclast formation in coculture experiments [92,93]. This failure can be overcome by the addition of sIL-6R. In contrast, IL-11, OSM, or LIF, other members of the IL-6 family of cytokines that require gp130 for cell activation, all directly induce osteoclast formation in this system. At present there is little evidence to support the idea that IL-6 plays a significant role in normal bone cell differentiation and function. In fact, data indicate that IL-6 does play a role in the regulation of bone cell function during certain pathologic states, as discussed earlier, and in the aging process. As an example, the treatment of murine osteoblastic cells with dexamethasone induces a marked increase in IL-6 receptor expression [94]. Patients with untreated primary hyperparathyroidism had serum IL-6 levels 16-fold higher than controls [95]. Circulating levels of sIL-6R and TNF-α were also elevated and the elevation of IL-6 correlated with markers of bone resorption. Following successful parathyroid adenomectomy, each returned to the normal range. Circulating levels of sIL-6R were increased in ovariectomized women [96]. No increase was observed in women who had received a hysterectomy or an ovariectomy and supplemental E_2. Similar results have been reported for postmenopausal women as compared to premenopausal and perimenopausal women [97]. No difference in IL-6 levels was observed. In related work with murine models, E_2 or dihydrotestosterone decreased the abundance of mRNA for both the IL-6 receptor (gp80) and gp130 in osteoblastic/stromal cells [98]. Studies with a human IL-6 reporter construct cotransfected with an androgen receptor into HeLa cells, showed that DHEA inhibited the transcriptional activity of the IL-6 promoter [69]. Again, this suggests that the bone-sparing effect of this class of steroids may relate to their ability to regulate IL-6. Consistent with these reports, gp80 and gp130 mRNA from murine bone marrow cell cultures was increased following ovariectomy.

The important implications of these investigations are that the antiosteoporotic effect of E_2 may be explained by its fundamental ability to interact with bone cells and regulate the cytokine circuitry that controls bone remodeling (Fig. 2). In the E_2 replete state, the hormone functions as a governor to reduce cytokine production, thereby tempering the rate or extent of osteoclast formation and activity. This represents normal remodeling. In the E_2-deficient state, the governor is lost, allowing for increased cytokine secretion, leading to more osteoclast formation and increased bone resorption.

PROSTAGLANDINS AND THE AGING SKELETON

Introduction

While it seems likely that changes in skeletal prostaglandin production and/or response will play an important role in age-related bone loss, there is little evidence that directly bears on this question. There are reasons for expecting age-related effects: (1) prostaglandins are critical in the local regulation of bone turnover, including the response to mechanical forces, which is necessary to maintain skeletal strength and viability with age, and (2) prostaglandin production in bone is affected by both systemic and local regulators that are known to change with age such as parathyroid hormone and cytokines. This section provides a summary of the effects of prostaglandins on bone cells and the regulation of endogenous prostaglandin production in bone. Extensive reviews on

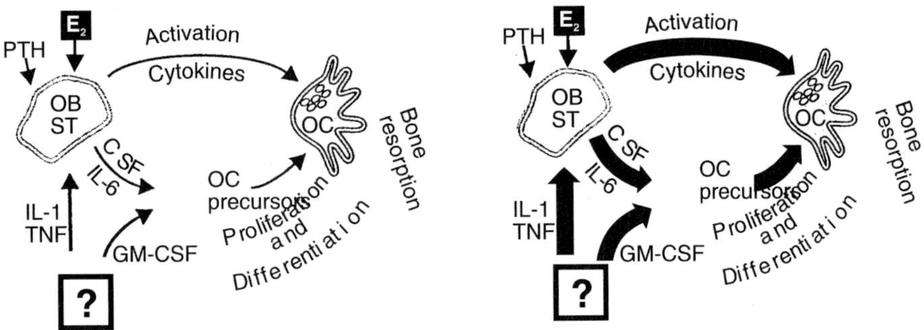

FIGURE 2 Estrogen regulates bone cell cytokines. (Left) Normal bone remodeling. With E_2 acting as an inhibitor, IL-1 and TNFα activate stromal cells or osteoblasts. The precise source of IL-1 and TNF is unknown. Possible sources include marrow macrophages or osteoclast precursors. The stromal cells or osteoblasts respond by secreting small amounts of IL-6 and CSF. (Right) Estrogen deficiency. In the E_2-deficient situation, osteoblasts and stromal cells secrete more IL-6, causing increased osteoclast differentiation and also secrete more cytokines that directly activate osteoclasts. IL-1 and TNF levels may also be increased. OB, osteoblasts; ST, stromal cells; OC, osteoclast; CSF, colony-stimulating factors.

this topic are available [99–101]. The limited data on age effects in bone cells and potentially relevant information on age-related changes in other cells will also be reviewed here.

Effects of Prostaglandins on Bone

The major effects of exogenous prostaglandins *in vivo* are to stimulate bone resorption and formation in rodents, dogs, and humans [101]. More complex biphasic responses can be found *in vitro* using multiple prostanoids and different cell models. Stimulation of bone resorption is predominantly a cyclic AMP-mediated effect of prostaglandins of the E series (PGE_2) acting through osteoblasts [102,103]. However, a direct effect on the monocyte-macrophage precursor lineage has also been suggested [104]. Prostaglandins stimulate bone formation by increasing the replication and differentiation of precursor cells [105]. However, in some cell culture systems an inhibition of cell replication has been seen with PGE_2, similar to that seen with fibroblasts and lymphocytes [106]. Moreover, the fully mature osteoblast prostaglandins, particularly of the F series, inhibit collagen synthesis [107]. These different effects are probably mediated by different receptors. Among the multiple receptors for prostaglandin E_2, the EP_2 and EP_4 receptors are known to increase cyclic AMP [108]. In addition, prostacyclin (IP) receptors can also increase cyclic AMP and may be present in bone. The inhibitory effect on collagen may be mediated by the prostaglandin F-selective (FP) receptor [107,109]. Thus, available data suggest that multiple receptors are expressed on osteoblasts and that this expression may change with differentiation.

Many factors regulate prostaglandin synthesis in bone, including systemic hormones, cytokines, growth factors, and mechanical forces. In addition, there is an autoamplification pathway whereby prostaglandins increase their own production [110]. Almost all of the regulation of prostaglandin synthesis in bone has been attributed to the inducible form of prostaglandin G/H synthase or cyclooxygenase (COX-2) [111,112]. However, additional regulation at the level of arachidonic acid release, which would then supply substrate to the constitutive cyclooxygenase (COX-1), probably occurs and may initiate rapid responses.

These stimuli for endogenous prostaglandin production are probably important in mediating changes in both resorption and formation. For example, the increases in bone resorption associated with inflammation and immobilization appear to be at least in part prostaglandin dependent [113,114]. A strong prostaglandin dependence has been demonstrated for the stimulation of bone formation by intermittent loading [115]. This response may be mediated by both prostacyclin and prostaglandin E_2 [116]. It seems likely that microdamage to skeletal tissues could also result in an increase in prostaglandin production, which could be important in initiating the remodeling response.

Age-Related Changes in Prostaglandins

The effects of aging of the cell or the organism on prostaglandin production or responsiveness in bone have not been examined adequately to make any conclusions. There are a few studies on bone cells. Aubin and associates [117] have examined the cyclic AMP response to prostaglandins in long-term cultures of fetal rat calvarial cells. The response to PGE_2 is maintained longer than the response to PTH and even increases transiently. However, the PGE_2 response does decrease with prolonged culture of these cells, even though responses to β-adrenergic agonists are maintained. This loss of responsiveness may pertain only to more differentiated osteoblastic cells. The ability of osteoblast precursors to respond to prostaglandins does appear to be maintained *in vivo* to the extent that there is a substantial increase in bone formation in older rats given injections of PGE_2 [118].

Evidence on the role of endogenous prostaglandins in maintaining bone turnover in older humans is limited. In an epidemiologic study, a slightly increased bone mass was observed in older individuals who habitually took aspirin or other nonsteroidal anti-inflammatory drugs (NSAIDs) [119]. However, the measurement of N-telopeptide cross-links as a marker of bone resorption showed no difference in aspirin and NSAID users vs controls [120]. Interpretation of any studies using NSAIDs is complex because prostaglandins stimulate both formation and resorption so that the net change in bone mass may be difficult to predict. Indeed, in animal models of osteoarthritis and in bone loss associated with immobilization, NSAIDs can inhibit the resorptive component but have little effect on the decrease in formation [121,122].

A review of some of the age-related changes in other cell types suggests how aging may affect prostaglandins in bone. Studies in other cell systems suggest that there may be a decreased responsiveness to prostaglandins in older cells. Both the production of cyclic AMP and the activation of the subsequent steps in the signal transduction pathway, such as phosphorylation of CREB, can decrease with cellular aging, i.e., after multiple passages in culture [123]. If this were to occur in the osteoblast precursor population, a decrease in the anabolic response to mechanical forces and other stimuli might be expected. However, increased prostaglandin production has been reported in aging skeletal muscle and in lung fibroblasts [124,125]. The decrease in cell-mediated immune responses that occur with aging has been attributed to an increase in prostaglandin production and the subsequent inhibition of mitogenesis in T cells [126,127]. An increased endogenous production of prostaglandins in macrophages may lead to enhanced osteoclastogenesis, in as much as treatment of cells of this lineage with prostaglandins enhances osteoclastogenesis *in vitro*. Changes in specific prostanoids have also been reported in various cell types. For example, after a prolonged culture of gingival fibroblasts there is a decrease in prostacyclin production and an increase in the production of prostaglandin F_{2a} [129]. Because prostaglandin F_{2a} both stimulates proliferation of osteoblasts [106] and inhibits collagen synthesis [107], it is difficult to predict how age-related changes in the type of prostaglandin produced might affect the adjacent skeletal tissues. Changes in prostaglandin production with age have also been described for endothelial cells and smooth muscle cells [130–133]. These are likely to decrease vascular reactivity and hence could diminish bone blood flow. Here again, a decreased production of prostacyclin and an increased production of prostaglandin F_{2a} have been reported.

If prostaglandin production and/or responsiveness changes in the aging skeleton, this information will be of great importance in improving our understanding of the pathogenesis and treatment of age-related bone loss. However, it will be extremely difficult to make the relevant measurements to determine these changes. Measuring prostaglandin production in bone is particularly difficult because these compounds are both lipid and water soluble and metabolized rapidly. It may be more appropriate to measure the levels of the enzymes responsible for prostaglandin production. Because both COX-1 and COX-2 are important in regulation, and arachidonate release through phospholipase, particularly phospholipase A_2, may also play a regulatory role, it would be appropriate to measure the levels of both mRNA and protein for all of these enzymes. There may also be some degree of regulation of the enzymes that convert the precursor, PGH_2, to different active prostanoids. These complexities are compounded by the fact that tissue samples obtained from bone are likely to have different cellular composition. It is not feasible to separate hematopoietic and fatty marrow and bone cells for biochemical analysis, but localization of enzymes to a specific cell type can be accomplished by immunocytochemistry or *in situ* hybridization.

In addition to such direct studies, a great deal could be learned by measuring the response of markers of bone formation and resorption to selective inhibitors of prostaglandins. COX-1 and COX-2 selective inhibitors are now available [134], and it will be important to examine their effects on bone remodeling in subjects with and without metabolic bone disease at different ages.

Acknowledgments

We thank Ms. Martha Altieri and Ms. Claudia McSwain for their careful review of the manuscript. We thank Ms. Lynn Limeburner for her careful preparation of this manuscript. We also thank Ms. Sarah Whitaker for her expertise in the preparation of the art work.

References

1. Ducy, P., Zhang, R., Geoffroy, V., Ridall, A., and Karsenty, G. Osf2/Cbfa1: A transcriptional activator of osteoblast differentiation. *Cell* **89,** 747–754 (1997).

2. Bianco, P., Bradbeer, J. N., Riminucci, M., and Boyde, A. Marrow stromal (Westen-Bainton) cells: Identification, morphometry, confocal imaging and changes in disease. *Bone* **14,** 315–320 (1993).
3. Caplan, A. I. The mesengenic process. *Clin. Plast. Surg.* **21,** 429–435 (1994).
4. Beresford, J. N. Osteogenic stem cells and the stromal system of bone and marrow. *Clin. Orthop. Rel. Res.* **240,** 270–280 (1989).
5. Grigoriadis, A. E., Heerche, J. N. M., and Aubin, J. E. Differentiation of muscle, fat, cartilage, and bone from progenitor cells present in bone-derived clonal cell populations: effect of dexamethasone. *J. Cell Biol.* **106,** 2139–2151 (1988).
6. Tavassoli, M., and Crosby, W. H. Bone marrow histogenesis: A comparison of fatty and red marrow. *Science* **169,** 291–293 (1970).
7. Rozman, C., Feliu, E., Berga, L., Reverter, J.-C., Climent, C., and Ferran, M.-J. Age related variations of fat tissue fraction in normal human bone marrow depend both on size and number of adipocytes. A serological study. *Exp. Hematol.* **17,** 34–37 (1989).
8. Gimble, J. M. The function of adipocytes in the bone stroma. *New Biol.* **2,** 304–312 (1990).
9. Fedarko, N. S., Vetter, U. K., Weistein, S., and Gehron-Roby, P. Age-related changes in hyaluron, proteoglycan, collagen and osteonectin synthesis in human bone cells. *J. Cell Physiol.* **151,** 215–227 (1992).
10. Jiang, D., Fei, R. G., Pendergass, W. R., and Wolf, N. S. An age-related reduction in the replicative capacity of two murine hematopoietic stroma cell types. *Exp. Hematol.* **20,** 1216–1222 (1992).
11. Egrise, D., Martin, A., Vienne, A., Neve, P., and Schoutens, A. The number of fibroblastic colonies formed from bone marrow is decreased and the *in vitro* proliferation rate of trabecular bone cells increased in aged rats. *Bone* **13,** 355–361 (1992).
12. Tsuiji, T., Hughes, F. J., McCulloch, C. A. G., and Melcher, A. H. Effects of donor age on osteogenic cells of rat bone marrow in vitro. *Mech. Ageing Dev.* **51,** 121–132 (1990).
13. Uchiyama, Y., Miyama, K., Kataginri, T., Yamaguchi, A., Takamori, H., Nakashima, K., Sato, T., and Suda, T. Adipose conversion is accelerated in bone marrow cells of congenitally osteoporotic SAMP6 mice. *J. Bone Miner. Res.* **9**(Suppl. 1), B365 (1994).
14. Jilka, R. L., Weinstein, R. S., Takahashi, K., Parfitt, A. M., and Manolagas, S. C. Linkage of decreased bone mass with impaired osteoblastogenesis in a murine model of accelerated senescence. *J. Clin. Invest.* **97,** 1732–1740 (1996).
15. Owen, M. E., and Friedenstein, A. J. Stromal stem cells: Marrow-derived osteogenic precursors. *In* "Cell and Molecular Biology of Vertabrate Hard Tissues," pp. 42–60. Ciba Foundation Symposium 136, Wiley, Cichester, UK, (1988).
16. Bennett, J. H., Joyner, C. J., Triffitt, J. T., and Owen, M. E. Adipocytic cells cultured from marrow have osteogenic potential. *J. Cell Sci.* **99,** 131–139 (1991).
17. Gimble, J. M., Dorheim, M.-A., Cheng, Q., Medina, K., Wang, C.-S., Jones, R., Koren, E., Pietrangeli, C. E., and Kincade, P. W. Adipogenesis in a murine bone marrow stromal cells line capable of supporting B lymphocyte growth and proliferation: Biochemical and molecular characterization. *Eur. J. Immunol.* **20,** 379–387 (1990).
18. Dorheim, M. A., Sullivan, M., Dadapani, V., Wu, X., Hudson, J., Segarini, P. R., Rosen, D. M., Aulthouse, A. L., and Gimble, J. M. Osteoblastic gene expression during adipogenesis in hematopoietic supporting murine bone marrow stromal cells. *J. Cell Physiol.* **154,** 317–328 (1993).
19. Nuttall, M. E., Olivera, D. L., and Gowen, M. Control of osteoblastic adipocyte differentiation in MG63 cells. *J. Bone Miner. Res.* **9**(Suppl. 1), A28 (1994).
20. Nuttall, M. E., Patton, A. J., Olivera, D. L., Nadeau, D. P., and Gowen, M. Human trabecular bone cells are able to express both osteoblastic and adipocytic phenotype: implications for osteopenic disorders. *J. Bone Miner. Res.* **13,** 371–382 (1998).
21. Meunier, P., Aaron, J., Edouard, C., and Vignon, G. Osteoporosis and the replacement of cell populations of the marrow by adipose tissue. A quantitative study of 84 iliac bone biopsies. *Clin. Orthop.* **80,** 147–154 (1971).
22. Beresford, J. N., Bennet, J. H., Devlin, C., Leboy, P. S., and Owen, M. E. Evidence for an inverse relationship between the differentiation of adipocytes and osteogenic cells in rat marrow stromal cells. *J. Cell Sci.* **102,** 341–351 (1992).
23. Gazit, D., Ebner, A. J., Kahn, A. J., and Derynck, R. Modulation of expression and cell surface binding of members of the transforming growth factor beta super-family during retinoic acid-induced osteoblastic differentiation of multipotential mesenchymal cells. *Mol. Endocrinol.* **7,** 189–198 (1993).
24. Centrella, M., Horowitz, M. C., Wozney, J. M., and McCarthy, T. L. Transforming growth factor-β gene family members and bone. *Endocr. Rev.* **15,** 27–39 (1994).
25. Richard, D. J., Sullivan, T. A., Shenker, B. J., Leboy, P. S., and Kazhdan, I. Induction of rapid osteoblast differentiation in rat bone marrow stromal cell cultures by dexamethasone and BMP-2. *Dev. Biol.* **161,** 218–228 (1994).
26. Centrella, M., McCarthy, T. L., and Canalis, E. Transforming growth factor beta is a bifunctional regulator of replication and collagen synthesis in osteoblast-enriched cell cultures from fetal rat calvariae. *J. Biol. Chem.* **262,** 2869–2874 (1987).
27. Gimble, J. M., Dorheim, M. A., Cheng, Q., Pekala, P., Enerback, S., Ellingsworth, L., Kincade, P. W., and Wang, C. S. Response of bone marrow stromal cells to adipogenic antagonists. *Mol. Cell Biol.* **9,** 4587–4595 (1989).
28. Clouthier, D. E., Comerford, S. A., and Hammer, R. E. Hepatic fibrosis, glomerulosclerosis, and a lipodystrophy-like syndrome in PEPCK-TGF-β1 transgenic mice. *J. Clin. Invest.* **100,** 2697–2713 (1997).
29. Jay, P. R., Centrella, M., Lorenzo, J., Bruce, A. G., and Horowitz, M. C. Oncostatin-M: A new bone active cytokine which activates osteoblasts and inhibits bone resorption. *Endocrinology* **137,** 1151–1158 (1996).
30. Gimble, J. M., Wanker, F., Wang, C. S., Bass, H., Wu, X., Kelly, K., Yancopoulos, G. D., and Hill, M. R. Regulation of bone marrow stromal cell differentiation by cytokines whose receptors share the gp130 protein. *J. Cell Biochem.* **54,** 122–133 (1994).
31. Horowitz, M. C., and Levy, J. B. The LIF/IL-6 subfamily of cytokines induce protein phosphorylation and signal transduction by non-receptor tyrosine kinases in human and murine osteoblasts. *Calcif. Tissue Int.* (Suppl. 1), **56,** S32–S34 (1995).
32. Kawashima, I., Ohsumi, J., Mita-Honjo, K., Shimoda-Takano, K., Ishikawa, H., Sakakibara, S., Miyadai, K., and Takguchi, Y. Molecular cloning of cDNA encoding adipogenesis inhibitory factor and identity with interleukin-11. *FEBS Lett.* **283,** 199–202 (1991).
33. Greenberg, A. S., Nordan, R. P., McIntosh, J., Calvo, J. C., Scow, R. O., and Jablons, D. Interleukin 6 reduces lipoprotein lipase activity in adipose tissue of mice *in vivo* and in 3T3-L1 adipocytes: A possible role for interleukin 6 in cancer cachexia. *Cancer Res.* **52,** 4113–4116 (1992).
34. Metcalf, D., and Gearing, D. P. Fetal syndrome in mice engrafted with cells producing high levels of the leukemia inhibitory factor. *Proc. Natl. Acad. Sci. USA* **86,** 5948–5952 (1989).
35. Delikat, S., Harris, R. J., and Galvani, D. W. IL-1β inhibits adipocyte formation in human long-term bone marrow culture. *Exp. Hematol.* **21,** 31–37 (1993).
36. Doerrler, W., Feingold, K. R., and Grunfeld, C. Cytokines induce catabolic effects in cultured adipocytes by multiple mechanisms. *Cytokine* **6,** 478–484 (1994).

37. Horowitz, M. C. Cytokines and estrogen in bone: anti-osteoporotic effects. *Science* **260,** 626–627 (1993).
38. Pacifici, R., Rifas, L., Teitelbaum, S., Slatopolsky, E., McCracken, R., Bergfeld, M., Lee, W., Avioli, L. V., and Peck, W. Spontaneous release of interleukin 1 from human monocytes reflects bone formation in idiopathic osteoporosis. *Proc. Natl. Acad. Sci. USA* **84,** 4616–4620 (1987).
39. Pacifici, R., Rifas, L., McCracken, R., Vered, I., McMurtry, C., Avioli, L. V., and Peck, W. Ovarian steroid treatment blocks a postmenopausal increase in blood monocyte interleukin 1 release. *Proc. Natl. Acad. Sci. USA* **86,** 2398–2402 (1989).
40. Pacifici, R., Brown, C., Puscheck, E., Friedrich, E., Slatopolsky, E., Maggio, D., McCracken, R., and Avioli, L. V. Effect of surgical menopause and estrogen replacement on cytokine release from blood mononuclear cells. *Proc. Natl. Acad. Sci. USA* **88,** 5134–5138 (1991).
41. Stock, J. L., Coderre, J. A., McDonald, B., and Rosenwasser, L. J. Effects of estrogen *in vivo* and *in vitro* on spontaneous interleukin-1 release by monocytes from postmenopausal women. *J. Clin. Endocrinol. Metab.* **68,** 364–368 (1989).
42. Hustmeyer, F. G., Walker, E., Xu, X. P., Girasole, G., Sakagami, Y., Peacock, M., and Manolagas, S. C. Cytokine production and surface antigen expression by peripherial blood mononuclear cells in postmenopausal osteoporosis. *J. Bone Miner. Res.* **8,** 1135–1141 (1993).
43. Cohen-Solal, M. E., Graulet, A. M., Denne, M. A., Gueris, J., Baylink, D., and De Vernejoul, M. C. Peripheral monocyte culture supernatants of menopausal women can induce bone resorption: Involvement of cytokines. *J. Clin. Endocrinol. Metab.* **77,** 1648–1653 (1993).
44. Fiore, C. E., Falcidia, E., Foti, R., Motta, M., and Tamburino, C. Differences in the time course of the effects of oophorectomy in women on parameters of bone metabolism and interleukin-1 levels in the circulation. *Bone Miner.* **20,** 79–85 (1994).
45. McKane, W. R., Khosla, S., Peterson, J. M., Egan, K., and Riggs, B. L. Circulating levels of cytokines that modulate bone resorption: effects of age and menopause in women. *J. Bone Miner. Res.* **9,** 1313–1318 (1994).
46. Khosla, S., Peterson, J. M., Egan, K., Jones, J. D., and Riggs, B. L. Circulating cytokine levels in osteoporotic and normal women. *J. Clin. Endocrinol. Metab.* **79,** 707–711 (1994).
47. Bismer, H., Diel, I., Ziegler, R., and Pfeilschifter, J. Increased cytokine secretion by human bone marrow cells after menopause or discontinuation of estrogen replacement. *J. Clin. Endocrinol. Metab.* **80,** 3351–3355 (1995).
48. Kimble, R. B., Srivastava, S., Ross, F. P., Matayoshi, A., and Pacifici, R. Estrogen deficiency increases the ability of stromal cells to support murine osteoclastogenesis via an interleukin-1 and tumor necrosis factor-mediated stimulation of macrophage colony-stimulating factor production. *J. Biol. Chem.* **271,** 28890–28897 (1996).
49. Tanaka, S., Takahashi, N., Udagawa, N., Tamura, T., Akatsu, T., Stanley, E. R., Kurokawa, T., and Suda, T. Macrophage colony-stimulating factor is indispensible for both proliferation and differentiation of osteoclast progenitors. *J. Clin. Invest.* **91,** 257–263 (1993).
50. Lorenzo, J. A., Naprta, A., Rao, Y., Alander, C., Glaccum, M., Widmer, M., Gronowicz, G., Kalinowski, J., and Pilbeam, C. C. Mice lacking the type I interleukin-1 receptor do not lose bone mass after ovariectomy. *Endocrinology* **139,** 3022–3025 (1998).
51. Sims, J. E., Gayle, M. A., Slack, J. L., Alderson, M. R., Bird, T. A., Giri, J. G., Collotta, F., Re, F., Mantovani, A., and Shanebeck, K. Interleukin-1 signaling occurs exclusively via the type I receptor. *Proc. Natl. Acad. Sci. USA* **90,** 6155–6159 (1993).
52. Kimble, R. B., Vannice, J. L., Bloedow, D. C., Thompson, R. C., Hopfer, W., Kung, V. T., Brownfield, C., and Pacific, R. Interleukin-1 receptor antagonist decreases bone loss and bone resorption in ovariectomized rats. *J. Clin. Invest.* **93,** 1959–1967 (1994).
53. Kitazawa, R., Kimble, R. B., Vannice, J. L., Kung, V. T., and Pacifici, R. Interleukin-1 receptor antagonist and tumor necrosis factor binding protein decrease osteoclast formation and bone resorption in ovariectomized mice. *J. Clin. Invest.* **94,** 2397–2406 (1994).
54. Miyaura, C., Kusano, K., Masuzawa, T., Chaki, O., Onoe, Y., Aoyagi, M., Sasaki, T., Tamura, T., Koishihara, Y., Ohsugi, and Suda, T. Endogenous bone-resorbing factors in estrogen deficiency: Cooperative effects of IL-1 and IL-6. *J. Bone Miner. Res.* **10,** 1356–1373 (1995).
55. Kawaguchi, H., Pilbeam, C. C., Vargas, S. J., Morse, E. E., Lorenzo, J. A., and Raisz, L. G. Ovariectomy enhances and estrogen replacement inhibits the activity of bone marrow factors that stimulate prostaglandin production in cultured mouse calvariae. *J. Clin. Invest.* **96,** 539–548 (1995).
56. Pilbeam, C., Rao, Y., Alander, C., Voznesensky, J., Okkada, Y., Sims, J. E., Raisz, L., and Lorenzo, J. Down regulation of mRNA expression for the "decoy" interleukin-1 receptor 2 by ovariectomy in mice. *J. Bone Miner. Res.* **12,** S433 (1997). [Abstract]
57. Sunyner, T., Lewis, J., and Osdoby, P. Estrogen decreases the steady state level of the IL-1 signaling receptor (Type I) while increasing those of the IL-1 decoy receptor (Type II) mRNAs in human osteoclast-like cells. *J. Bone Miner. Res.* **12,** S135 (1997). [Abstract]
58. Colotta, F., Dower, S. K., Sims, J. E., and Mantovani, A. The type II decoy receptor: a novel regulatory pathway for interleukin 1. *Immunol. Today* **15,** 562–566 (1994).
59. Re, F., Sironi, M., Muzio, M., Matteucci, C., Introna, S., Penton-Rol, G., Dower, S. K., Sims, J. E., Collotta, F., and Mantovani, A. Inhibition of interleukin-1 responsiveness by type II receptor gene transfer: A surface receptor with anti-interleukin-1 function. *J. Exp. Med.* **183,** 1841–1850 (1996).
60. Richard, D., Russell, G., and Gowen, M. Oestradiol inhibits the release of tumour necrosis factor but not interleukin 6 from adult human osteoblasts *in vitro. Osteoporos. Int.* **2,** 94–102 (1992).
61. Chaudhary, L. R., Spelsberg, T. C., and Riggs, B. L. Production of various cytokines by normal human osteoblast-like cells in response to interleukin-1β and tumor necrosis factor-α: Lack of regulation by 17β-estradiol. *Endocrinology* **130,** 2528–2534 (1992).
62. Kimble, R. B., Bain, S., and Pacifici, R. The functional block of TNF but not IL-6 prevents bone loss in ovariectomized mice. *J. Bone Miner. Res.* **12,** 935–941 (1997).
63. Ammann, P., Rizzoli, R., Bonjour, J. P., Bourrin, S., Meyer, J. M., Vassalli, P., and Garcia, I. Transgenic mice expressing soluble tumor necrosis factor-receptor are protected against bone loss caused by estrogen deficiency. *J. Clin. Invest.* **99,** 1699–1703 (1997).
64. Tsuda, E., Goto, M., Mochizuki, S.-I., Yano, K., Kobayashi, F., Morinaga, T., and Higashio, K. Isolation of a novel cytokine from human fibroblasts that specifically inhibits osteoclastogenesis. *Biochem. Biophys. Res. Commun.* **234,** 137–142 (1997).
65. Simonet, W. S., Lacey, D. L., Dunstan, C. R., Kelly, M., Chang, M.-S., Luthy, R., Nguyen, H. Q., Wooden, S., Bennett, L., Boone, T., Shimamoto, G., DeRose, M., Elliott, R., Colombero, A., Tan, H.-L., Trail, G., Sullivan, J., Davey, E., Bucay, N., Renshaw-Greeg, L., Hughes, T. M., Hill, D., Pattison, W., Campbell, P., Sander, S., Van, G., Tarpley, J., Derby, P., and Lee, R. Osteopro-

tegrin: A novel secreted protein involved in the regulation of bone density. *Cell* **89,** 309–319 (1997).

66. Yasuda, H., Shima, N., Nakagawa, N., Yamaguchi, K., Kinosaki, M., Mochizuki, S.-I., Tomoyasu, A., Yano, K., Goto, M., Murakami, A., Tsuda, E., Morinaga, T., Higashio, K., Udagawa, N., Takahashi, N., and Suda, T. Osteoclast differentiation factor is a ligand for osteoprotegrin/osteoclastogenesis inhibitory factor and is identical to TRANS/RANKL. *Proc. Natl. Acad. Sci. USA* **95,** 3597–3602 (1998).
67. Girasole, G., Jilka, R., L., Passeri, G., Boswell, S., Boder, G., Williams, D. C., and Manolagas, S. C. 17 beta-estradiol inhibits interleukin-6 production by bone marrow-derived stromal cells and osteoblasts *in vitro:* a potential mechanism for the antiosteoporotic effect of estrogens. *J. Clin. Invest.* **89,** 883–891 (1992).
68. Roodman, G. D. Interleukin-6: an osteotropic factor? *J. Bone Miner. Res.* **7,** 475–478 (1992).
69. Bellido, T., Jilka, R. L., Boyce, B. F., Girasole, G., Broxmeyer, H., Dalrymple, S. A., Murry, R., and Manolagas, S. C. Regulation of interleukin-6, osteoclastogenesis, and bone mass by androgens: The role of the androgen receptor. *J. Clin. Invest.* **95,** 2886–2895 (1995).
70. Jilka, R. L., Hangoc, G., Girasole, G., Passeri, G., Williams, D. C., Abrams, J. S., Boyce, B., Broxmeyer, H., and Manolagas, S. C. Increased osteoclast development after estrogen loss: Mediation by interleukin-6. *Science* **257,** 88–91 (1992).
71. Komm, B. S., Terpening, C. M., Benz, D. J., Graeme, K. A., Gallegos, A., Korc, M., Green, G. L., O'Malley, B. W., and Hausler, M. R. Estrogen binding, receptor mRNA, and biologic response in osteoblast-like osteosarcoma cells. *Science* **241,** 81–84 (1988).
72. Eriksen, E. F., Colvard, D. S., Berg, N. J., Graham, M. L., Mann, K. G., Spelsberg, T. C., and Riggs, B. L. Evidence of estrogen receptors in normal human osteoblast-like cells. *Science* **241,** 84–86 (1988).
73. Rifas, L., Kenney, J. S., Marcelli, M., Pacifici, R., Cheng, S.-L., Dawson, L. L., and Avioli, L. V. Production of interleukin-6 in human osteoblasts and human bone marrow stromal cells: evidence that induction by interleukin-1 and tumor necrosis factor-α is not regulated by ovarian steroids. *Endocrinology* **136,** 4056–4067 (1995).
74. Passeri, G., Girasole, G., Jilka, R. L., and Manolagas, S. C. Increased interleukin-6 production by murine bone marrow and bone cells after estrogen withdrawal. *Endocrinology* **133,** 822–828 (1993).
75. Poli, V., Balena, R., Fattori, E., Markatos, A., Yamamoto, M., Tanaka, H., Ciliberto, G., Roda, G. A., and Costantine, F. Interleukin-6 deficient mice are protected from bone loss caused by estrogen depletion. *EMBO J.* **13,** 1189–1196 (1994).
76. Glowacki, J. Influence of age on human marrow. *Calcif. Tissue Int.* **56**(Suppl. 1), S50–S51 (1995).
77. Cheleuitte, D., Mizuno, S., and Glowacki, J. *In vitro* secretion of cytokines by human bone marrow: Effects of age and estrogen status. *J. Clin. Endocrinol. Metab.* **83,** 2043–2051 (1998).
78. Daynes, R. A., Araneo, B. A., Ershler, W. B., Maloney, C., Li, G.-Z., and Ryu, S.-Y. Altered regulation of IL-6 production with normal aging. Possible linkage to the age-associated decline in dehydroepiandrosterone and its sulfated derivative. *J. Immunol.* **150,** 5219–5230 (1993).
79. Ershler, W. B., Sun, W. H., and Binkley, N. Interleukin-6 and aging: blood levels and mononuclear cell production increases with advancing age and *in vitro* production is modified by dietary restriction. *Lymphokine Cytokine Res.* **12,** 225–230 (1993).
80. Wei, J., Xu, H., Davies, J. L., and Hemming, G. P. Increase of plasma IL-6 concentration with age in healthy subjects. *Life Sci.* **51,** 1953 (1992).
81. Migeon, C. J., Keller, A. R., Lawrence, B., and Shepard, T. H. Dehydroepiandrosterone and androsterone levels in human plasma, effect of age and sex; day-to-day and diurnal variations. *J. Clin. Endocrinol. Metab.* **17,** 1051–1062 (1957).
82. Orentreich, N., Brind, J. L., Rizer, R. L., and Vogelman, J. N. Age changes and sex differences in serum dehydroepiandrosterone sulfate concentrations throughout adulthood. *J. Clin. Endocrinol. Metab.* **59,** 551–555 (1984).
83. Kania, D. M., Binkley, N., Checovich, M., Havighurst, T., Schilling, M., and Ershler, W. B. Elevated plasma levels of interleukin-6 in postmenopausal women do not correlate with bone density. *J. Am. Geriatr. Soc.* **43,** 236–239 (1995).
84. Nordin, A. A., and Collins, G. D. Limiting dilution analysis of alloreactive cytotoxic precursor cells in aging mice. *J. Immunol.* **131,** 2215–2218 (1983).
85. Negro, S., Hara, H., Miyata, S., Saiki, O., Tanaka, T., Yoshizaki, K., Igarashi, T., and Kishimoto, S. Mechanisms of age-related decline in antigen-specific T cell proliferative response: IL-2 receptor expression and recombinant IL-2 induced proliferative response of purified TAC-positive T cells. *Mech. Ageing Dev.* **36,** 223–241 (1986).
86. Thoman, M., and Weigle, W. O. Lymphokines and aging: interleukin-2 production and activity in aged animals. *J. Immunol.* **127,** 2102–2106 (1981).
87. Inamizu, T., Chang, M.-P., and Makinodan, T. Influence of age on the production and regulation of interleukin-1 in mice. *Immunology* **55,** 447–455 (1985).
88. Lowik, C. W. G. M., van der Pluijm, G., Bloys, H., Hoekman, K., Bijvoet, O. L. M., Aarden, L. A., and Pappoulos, S. E. Parathyroid hormone (PTH) and PTH-like protein (PLP) stimulate interleukin-6 production by osteogenic cells: A possible role of interleukin-6 in osteoclastogenesis. *Biochem. Biophys. Res. Commun.* **162,** 1546–1552 (1989).
89. Horowitz, M. C., and Lorenzo, J. A. Local regulators of bone: IL-1, TNF, lymphotoxin, interferon-γ, IL-8, IL-10, IL-4, the LIF/IL-6 family, and additional cytokines. *In* "Principles of Bone Biology" (J. P. Bilezikian, L. G. Raisz, and G. A. Rodan, eds.), pp. 687–700. Academic Press, San Diego, 1996.
90. Levy, J. B., Baron, R., and Horowitz, M. C. Oncostatin M induces signal transduction by non-receptor tyrosine kinases in primary osteoblasts. *J. Bone Min. Res.* **9,** S149 (1994). [Abstract]
91. Nishimura, R., Moriyama, K., Yasukawa, Mundy, G. R., and Yoneda, T. Combination of interleukin-6 and soluble interleukin-6 receptors induces differentiation and activation of JAK-STAT and MAP kinase pathways in MG-63 human osteoblastic cells. *J. Bone Miner. Res.* **13,** 777–785 (1998).
92. Tamura, T., Udagwa, N., Takahashi, N., Miyaura, C., Tanaka, S., Kisimoto, T., and Suda, T. Soluble interleukin-6 receptor triggers osteoclast formation by interleukin 6. *Proc. Natl. Acad. Sci. USA* **90,** 11924–11928 (1993).
93. Suda, T., Takahashi, N., and Martin, T. J. Modulation of osteoclast differentiation: Update 1995. *Endocr. Rev.* **4,** 266–270 (1995).
94. Udagawa, N., Takahashi, N., Katagiri, T., Tamura, T., Wada, S., Findlay, D. M., Martin, T. J., Hirota, H., Taga, T., Kishimoto, T., and Suda, T. Interleukin-6 induction of osteoclast differentiation depends on IL-6 receptors expressed on osteoblastic cells but not on osteoclastic progenitors. *J. Exp. Med.* **182,** 1461–1468 (1995).
95. Grey, A., Mitnick, M.-A., Shapses, S., Ellison, A., Gundberg, C., and Insogna, K. Circulating levels of interleukin-6 and tumor necrosis factor-α are elevated in primary hyperparathyroidism and correlate with markers of bone resorption—A clinical research center study. *J. Endocrinol. Metabol.* **81,** 3450–3454 (1996).

96. Girasole, G., Pedrazzoni, M., Giuliani, N., Passeri, G., and Passeri, M. Increased serum soluble interleukin-6 receptors levels are induced by ovariectomy, prevented by estrogen replacement and reversed by alendronate administration. *J. Bone Miner. Res.* **10,** S160 (1995). [Abstract]
97. Chen, J. T., Maruo, N., Kato, T., Hasumi, K., Ogata, E., Shiraki, M., and Morita, I. Serum levels of soluble interleukin 6 receptor, not interleukin 6, is correlated with bone resorption markers and lumber bone mineral density after menopause. *J. Bone Miner. Res.* **10,** S347 (1995). [Abstract]
98. Lin, S.-C., Yamate, T., Taguchi, Y., Borba, V. C., Girasole, G., O'Brien, C. A., Bellido, T., Abe, E., and Manolagas, S. C. Regulation of the gp80 and gp130 subunits of the IL-6 receptor by sex steroids in the murine bone marrow. *J. Clin. Invest.* **100,** 1980–1990 (1997).
99. Kawaguchi, H., Pilbeam, C. C., Harrison, J. R., and Raisz, L. G. The role of prostaglandins in the regulation of bone metabolism. *Clin. Orthopaed. Rel. Res.* **313,** 36–46 (1995).
100. Pilbeam, C. C., Harrison, J. R., and Raisz, L. G. Prostaglandins and bone metabolism. *In* "Principles of Bone Biology" (J. P. Bilezikian, L. G., Raisz, and G. A. Rodan, eds.), pp. 715–728. Academic Press, San Diego, 1996.
101. Jee, W. S., and Ma, Y. F. The *in vivo* anabolic actions of prostaglandins in bone. *Bone* **21,**(4), 297–304 (1997).
102. Kaji, H., Sugimoto, T., Kanatani, M., Fukase, M., Kumegawa, M., and Chihara, K. Prostaglandin E_2 stimulates osteoclast-like cell formation and bone-resorbing activity via osteoclasts: Role of cAMP-dependent protein kinase. *J. Bone Miner. Res.* **11**(1), 62–71 (1996).
103. Collins, D. A., and Chambers, T. J. Effect of prostaglandins E_1, E_2, and F_{2a} on osteoclast formation in mouse bone marrow cultures. *J. Bone Miner. Res.* **6,**(20), 157–164 (1991).
104. Collins, D. A., and Chambers, T. J. Prostaglandin E_2 promotes osteoclast formation in murine hematopoietic cultures through an action on hematopoietic cells. *J. Bone Miner. Res.* **7,**(5), 555–561 (1992).
105. Woodiel, F. N., Fall, P. M., and Raisz, L. G. Anabolic effects of prostaglandins in cultured fetal rat calvariae: Structure-activity relations and signal transduction pathway. *J. Bone Miner. Res.* **11**(9), 1249–1255 (1996).
106. Hakeda, Y., Harada, S., and Matsumoto, T. Prostaglandin F_{2a} stimulates proliferation of clonal osteoblastic MC3T3-E1 cells by up regulation of insulin-like growth factor-1 receptor. *J. Biol. Chem.* **266,** 21044–21050 (1991).
107. Fall, P. M., Breault, D. T., and Raisz, L. G. Inhibition of collagen synthesis by prostaglandins in the immortalized rat osteoblastic clonal cell line, Py1a: Structure activity relations and signal transduction mechanisms. *J. Bone Miner. Res.* **9,** 1935–1943 (1994).
108. Coleman, R. A., Smith, W. L., and Narumiya, S. International Union of Pharmacology classification of prostanoid receptors: Properties, distribution and structure of the receptors and their subtypes. *Pharmacol. Rev.* **46**(2), 205–209 (1994).
109. Nemoto, K., Bernecker, P. M., Pilbeam, C. C., and Raisz, L. G. Expression and regulation of prostaglandin F receptor mRNA in rodent osteoblastic cells. *Prostaglandins* **50**(5/6), 349–358 (1995).
110. Pilbeam, C. C., Raisz, L. G., Voznesensky, O., Alander, C. B., Delman, B. N., and Kawaguchi, H. Autoregulation of inducible prostaglandin G/H synthase in osteoblastic cells by prostaglandins. *J. Bone Miner. Res.* **10**(3), 406–414 (1995).
111. Kawaguchi, H., Nemoto, K., Raisz, L. G., Harrison, J. R., Voznesensky, O., Alander, C. B., and Pilbeam, C. C. Interleukin-4 inhibits prostaglandin G/H synthase-2 and cytosolic phospholipase A_2 induction in neonatal mouse parietal bone cultures. *J. Bone Miner. Res.* **11**(3), 358–366 (1996).
112. Pilbeam, C., Rao, Y., Voznesensky, O., Kawaguchi, H., Alander, C., Raisz, L. G., and Herschman, H. Transforming growth factor-b1 regulation of prostaglandin G/H synthase-2 expression in osteoblastic MC3T3-E1 cells. *Endocrinology* **138**(11), 4672–4682 (1997).
113. Boyce, B. F., Aufdemorte, T. B., Garrett, I. R., Yates, A. J. P., and Mundy, G. R. Effects of interleukin-1 on bone turnover in normal mice. *Endocrinology* **125**(3), 1142–1150 (1989).
114. Thompson, D. D., and Rodan, G. A. Indomethacin inhibition of tenotomy-induced bone resorption in rats. *J. Bone Miner. Res.* **3,** 409–414 (1988).
115. Chow, J. W., and Chambers, T. J. Indomethacin has distinct early and late actions on bone formation induced by mechanical stimulation. *Am. J. Physiol.* **267,** E287–E292 (1994).
116. Cheng, M. Z., Zaman, G., and Lanyon, L. E. Estrogen enhances the stimulation of bone collagen synthesis by loading and exogenous prostacyclin, but not prostaglandin E_2, in organ cultures of rat ulnae. *J. Bone Miner. Res.* **9**(6), 805–816.
117. Aubin, J. E., Tertinegg, I., Ber, R., and Heersche, J. N. Consistent patterns of changing hormone responsiveness during continuous culture of cloned rat calvaria cells. *J. Bone Miner. Res.* **3,** 333–339 (1988).
118. Lin, B. Y., Jee, W. S., Ma, Y., Ke, H. Z., Kimmel, D. B., and Li, X. J. Effects of prostaglandin E_2 and risedronate administration on cancellous bone in older female rats. *Bone* **15,** 489–496 (1994).
119. Bauer, D. C., Orwoll, E. S., Fox, K. M., Vogt, T. M., Lane, N. E., Hochber, M. C., Stone, K., and Nevitt, M. C. Aspirin and NSAID use in older women: Effect on bone mineral density and fracture disk: Study of Osteoporotic Fractures Research Group. *J. Bone Miner. Res.* **11,** 29–35 (1996).
120. Lane, N. E., Bauer, D. C., Nevitt, M. C., Pressman, A. R., and Cummings, S. R. Aspirin and nonsteroidal antiinflammatory drug use in elderly women: Effects on a marker of bone resorption: The study of Osteoporotic Fractures Research Group. *J. Rheumatol.* **24,** 1132–1136 (1997).
121. Boiskin, I., Epstein, S., Ismail, F., Fallon, M. D., and Levy, W. Long-term administration of prostaglandin inhibitors in vivo fail to influence cartilage and bone metabolism in the rat. *Bone Miner.* **4,** 27–36 (1988).
122. Aota, S., Nakamura, T., Suzuki, K., Tanaka, Y., Okazaki, Y., Segawa, Y., Miura, M., and Kikuchi, S. Effects of indomethacin administration on bone turnover and bone mass in adjuvant-inducted arthritis in rats. *Calcif. Tissue Int.* **59,** 385–391 (1996).
123. Chin, J., Okazaki, M., Frazier, J. S., Hu, Z. W., and Hoffman, B. B. Impaired cAMP-mediated gene expression and decrease cAMP response element protein in senescent cells. *Am. J. Physiol.* **271,** C362–C371 (1996).
124. Young, M. K., Bocek, R. M., Herrington, P. T., and Beatty, C. H. Aging: Effects on the prostaglandin production by skeletal muscle of male rhesus monkeys (*Macaca mulatta*). *Mech. Ageing Dev.* **16,** 345–353 (1981).
125. Polgar, P., and Taylor, L. Alterations in prostaglandin synthesis during senescence of human lung fibroblasts. *Mech. Ageing Dev.* **12,** 305–310 (1980).
126. Beharka, A. A., Wu, D., Han, S. N., and Meydani, S. N. Macrophage prostaglandin production contributes to the age-associated decrease T cell function which is reversed by the dietary antioxidant vitamin E. *Mech. Ageing Dev.* **93,** 59–77 (1997).
127. Hayek, M. G., Meydani, S. N., Meydani, M., and Blumberg, J. B. Age differences in eicosanoid production of mouse splenocytes: Effects of mitogen-induced T-cell proliferation. *J. Gerontol.* **49,** B197–207 (1994).

128. Hayek, M. G., Mura, C., Wu, D., Beharka, A. A., Sung, N. H., Paulson, K. P., Hwang, D., and Meydani, S. N. Enhanced expression of inducible cyclooxygenase with age in murine macrophages. *J. Immunol.* **159,** 2445–2451 (1997).
129. Takiguchi, H., Yamaguchi, M., Okamura, H., and Abiko, Y. Contribution of IL-1b to the enhancement of Campylobacter rectus lipopolysaccharide-stimulated PGE_2 production in old gingival fibroblasts *in vitro*. *Mech. Ageing Dev.* **98,** 75–90 (1997).
130. Hiremath, A. N., Pershe, R. A., Hoffman, B. B., and Blaschke, T. F. Comparison of age-related changes in prostaglandin E_1 and b-adrenergic responsiveness of vascular smooth muscle in adult males. *J. Gerontol.* **44,** M13–M17 (1989).
131. Takeuchi, K., Abe, K., Sato, M., Yasujima, M., Hagino, T., Fang, S., and Yoshinaga, K. Effect of *in vitro* aging on prostaglandin synthesis in cultured rat vascular smooth muscle cells. *Agents Actions* **22,** 49–54 (1987).
132. Chang, W. C., Murota, S. I., Nako, J., and Orimo, H. Age-related decrease in prostacyclin biosynthetic activity in rat aortic smooth muscle cells. *Biochim. Biophys. Acta* **620,** 159–166 (1980).
133. Lennon, E. A., and Poyser, N. L. Effect of age on vascular prostaglandin production in male and female rats. *Prostaglandins Leukot. Med.* **25,** 1–15 (1986).
134. Pilbeam, C. C., Fall, P. M., Alander, C. B., and Raisz, L. G. Differential effects of nonsteroidal anti-inflammatory drugs on constitutive and inducible prostaglandin G/H synthase in cultured bone cells. *J. Bone Miner. Res.* **12**(8), 1198–1203 (1997).
135. Kodama, Y., Takeuchi, Y., Suzawa, M., Fukumoto, S., Murayama, H., Yamato, H., Fujita, T., Kurokawa, T., Matsumoto, T. Reduced expression of interleukin-11 in bone marrow stromal cells of senescence-accelerated mice (SAMP6): Relationship to osteopenia with enhanced adipogenesis. *J. Bone Miner. Res.* **13,** 1370–1377 (1998).

CHAPTER 19

Role of Growth Hormone/Insulin-like Growth Factor Axis

SUBBURAMAN MOHAN AND DAVID J. BAYLINK

Mineral Metabolism, Jerry L Pettis Veterans' Administration Medical Center, Departments of Medicine, Biochemistry and Physiology, Loma Linda University, Loma Linda, California 92357

INTRODUCTION

Osteoporosis is a disease characterized by low bone mass and microarchitectural deterioration of bone tissue leading to enhanced bone fragility and a consequent increase in the fracture risk with age [1]. The pathogenesis of postmenopausal osteoporosis is not known in detail. During bone remodeling, which occurs throughout life, bone resorbed by osteoclasts is replaced by new bone formed by osteoblasts. This phenomenon is called the coupling of bone formation to bone resorption [2,3]. In osteoporosis, the rate of bone resorption is greater than the rate of bone formation, which results in net bone loss. If we understand the reasons why bone formation is impaired during aging, that knowledge could provide strategies for increasing bone formation and, thus, could lead to new treatments for this debilitating disease.

The amount of new bone formed at a given site is subject to regulation by the combined actions of systemic hormones, such as parathyroid hormone, estradiol, testosterone, vitamin D_3, and growth hormone (GH), and local growth factors, including cytokines and bone growth factors [2,3]. Of the various systemic hormones, it is well known that GH plays an important role in the regulation of postnatal skeletal growth [4–7]. The GH/insulin-like growth factor (IGF) axis has also been proposed to play an important role in the maintenance of adult bone mass. It is also known that the actions of GH on target tissues, including bone, are mediated largely via the IGF system, an important growth factor system in bone [4–7]. This chapter discusses the role of the GH/IGF axis in the regulation of bone formation, the pathophysiological changes in the GH/IGF axis during aging, and how these changes could potentially impair bone formation during aging.

ROLE OF GH/IGF AXIS IN THE REGULATION OF BONE FORMATION

GH Effects on Bone

It has long been known that excess GH clearly affects the structure and dynamics of bones of patients with acromegaly [8–10]. The most striking clinical features of acromegaly are due to the excessive growth of bone after closure of the epiphyseal growth plates. Total body bone mineral density is frequently increased in acromegaly with a greater increase in cortical bone than in trabecular bone [8–10]. In contrast to patients with acromegaly, adults with childhood-onset GH deficiency exhibit decreased bone mass and increased fracture incidence compared to age-matched controls [11]. In addition, children with GH receptor deficiency exhibit delayed skeletal maturation and substantially lower bone mineral density compared to age-matched control children [12]. Based on the findings that bone mass is increased in acromegaly and decreased in GH deficiency, it has been postulated that GH promotes bone formation to a greater extent than bone resorption at each remodeling site and, thus, results in positive bone balance.

Almost three decades ago, Harris and Heany [13] clearly demonstrated that GH administered to adult dogs led to a marked increase in bone mass. Isaksson and co-workers [14] have demonstrated that the unilateral administration of GH into the tibial epiphyseal growth plate of hypophysectomized rats stimulated bone growth on the injected side only. Subsequently, Baker *et al.* [15] have shown that osteoblast-specific overexpression of GH in transgenic mice is able to stimulate bone growth directly without significant systemic effects. In addition, the administration of human recombinant GH has been shown to maintain trabecular bone mass in primates rendered hypogonadal by a gonadotropin-releasing hormone analog [8–10]. Consistent with these data, several *in vitro* and *in vivo* studies have demonstrated that GH is important in the regulation of bone formation [4–7].

According to original somatomedin hypothesis, GH has been proposed to stimulate skeletal growth indirectly by stimulating the liver production of IGF-I to act in an endocrine manner to stimulate bone growth [16]. Subsequent studies, however, have shown that GH has direct actions on bone [17–21]. Based on the findings that osteoblasts contain GH receptors [22] and that GH treatment increases the production of IGF-I in rat osteoblast-like cells [19], it has been proposed that GH may exert its direct effects via GH receptors to stimulate the local production of IGF-I to act in an autocrine/paracrine manner. However, it is also possible that GH may have some intrinsic effects on osteoblasts not dependent on IGFs. Thus, the mechanism for the stimulatory effect of GH on bone formation is not yet fully understood.

The findings that bone resorption is increased in patients with acromegaly and that GH treatment increases serum levels of markers of both bone formation and bone resorption suggest an effect of GH on bone resorption [6,23]. In regard to the mechanisms for the stimulatory effect of GH on bone resorption, an *in vitro* study has shown that GH induces osteoclast differentiation and activates mature osteoclasts [24]. In addition, Swolin and Ohlsson [21] have shown that GH treatment increases interleukin-6 production in human osteoblast-like cells. Based on these findings and the findings that IGF-I exerts significant biological effects on osteoclasts (see later), it can be speculated that the effects of GH to increase bone resorption may be mediated via a GH-induced increase in IGF-I and interleukin-6 production in osteoblasts.

IGF System Effects on Bone

IGFs are unique regulators of bone formation in that they act both systemically and locally to regulate bone formation. Regarding the systemic IGF actions, several studies have shown that the systemic administration of IGF-I, which increases serum levels of IGF-I, causes a marked increase in bone formation in both animals and humans [3,25]. In addition, increases in serum levels of IGFs during GH therapy and during puberty correlate with increases in bone formation markers [6,26,27], emphasizing that circulating IGFs are potential regulators of bone formation. Regarding local IGF actions, it is noteworthy that IGFs are the most abundant factors stored in bone; moreover, they are the most abundant growth factors produced by osteoblast line cells in culture [28,29]. The finding that 50% of basal osteoblast cell proliferation can be blocked by inhibiting the actions of endogenously produced IGFs provides evidence that locally produced IGFs may contribute to basal bone cell proliferation *in vitro* [30]. Consistent with the hypothesis that IGFs are important stimulators of bone formation are the following findings: (1) Mice lacking functional IGF-I and IGF-II genes exhibit severe retardation of bone growth [31,32]. (2) A mouse strain, C3H/HeJ, with high bone mineral density has 30% greater serum and bone IGF-I levels compared to another mouse strain, C57BI/6J, with low bone mineral density [33]. (3) Several cross studies have shown a strong positive linear relationship between serum IGF-I and bone mineral density in postmenopausal women even after other experimental variables have been kept constant [34–36]. Thus, a large body of evidence suggests that the IGF system is an important growth factor system in bone.

Descriptive Features of the IGF System

Recent findings demonstrate that the local actions of IGFs in the bone microenvironment may be regulated by multiple components of the IGF regulatory system, including IGF-I, IGF-II, type I and type II IGF receptors, IGF-binding proteins (IGFBPs), and extracellular IGFBP proteases (Fig. 1). The different components of the IGF system in bone are briefly described below.

IGFs are the most abundant growth factors produced by osteoblasts. The production of IGFs by osteoblasts has been shown to be dependent on the skeletal site as well as the stage of osteoblast differentiation [37]. The expression of IGF-I, the predominant IGF produced in rat osteoblasts, is regulated by systemic hormones including GH, PTH (parathyroid hormone), and estradiol, as well as by local growth factors including TGFβ (transforming growth factor β), basic FGF (fibroblast growth factor), and interleukins [29]. The expression

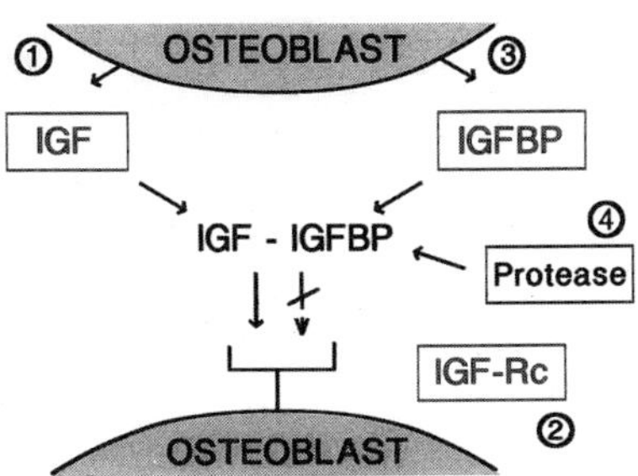

FIGURE 1 Components of the IGF system in bone. The activity of IGFs in the bone microenvironment is determined not only by (1) the synthesis of IGFs but also by (2) the presence of IGF receptors, (3) inhibitory and stimulatory IGFBPs, and (4) IGFBP proteases.

of IGF-II, the predominant IGF produced in human osteoblasts, is also regulated by both systemic (e.g., progesterone, glucocorticoid) and local (BMP-7, mechanical loading) factors [29,38]. In addition to osteoblasts, osteoclasts have also been shown to express mRNA for both IGF-I and IGF-II. It has been speculated that locally produced IGFs by osteoclasts and osteoblasts may act to regulate the coupled increase in bone formation in response to bone resorption. IGF actions in osteoblasts and osteoclasts are mediated through the binding of IGF peptides to specific plasma membrane receptors, namely type I IGF receptors. However, the binding of IGFs to signal-transducing IGF-I receptors is modified by the presence of IGF-binding proteins. Human osteoblasts in culture produce all six high-affinity IGFBPs known to date [29,39,40]. Studies on the regulation of IGFBP levels in the conditioned medium of osteoblasts derived from humans, rats, and mice demonstrate that a number of systemic and local factors influence the concentration of IGFBPs. For example, GH has been shown to increase the expression of IGFBP-3 and IGFBP-5 in rat osteoblasts and to decrease the production of IGFBP-4 in human osteoblasts [29,41]. One of the important regulators of IGFBP expression in osteoblasts is the IGF themselves [29,42]. IGFs increase levels of IGFBP-3 and IGFBP-5 and decrease levels of IGFBP-4 in the conditioned medium of osteoblasts. Based on these findings, two conclusions can be made: (1) IGFs may function to regulate IGFBPs and vice versa and (2) different mechanisms may regulate the amount of inhibitory IGFBP-4 and stimulatory IGFBP-5 in biological fluids.

The actions of IGFBPs in bone microenvironment in turn depend on IGFBP proteases, which are capable of cleaving IGFBPs into forms that have either significantly reduced or no affinity for IGFs [29,39,43]. Studies demonstrate that degradation of IGFBP by proteases may be as important as synthesis in determining IGFBP abundance in extracellular body fluids. Although IGFBP proteases produced by osteoblasts have not been characterized, studies to date reveal evidence that osteoblasts in culture produce, in addition to IGFBP specific proteases, other proteases (e.g., matrix metalloprotease, cathepsin D, plasmin) capable of degrading not only IGFBPs but also other proteins [29,39,43]. The findings that human osteoblasts in culture produce proteases capable of degrading one or more IGFBPs and that the production and/or activity of IGFBP proteases can be regulated by a number of osteoregulatory agents raise interesting possibilities for the involvement of IGFBP proteases in regulating the local actions of IGFs.

ACTIONS OF IGF SYSTEM COMPONENTS

IGFs are essential factors for longitudinal bone growth, as they stimulate proliferation and differentiation of chondrocytes in the epiphyseal plate [44]. IGFs also play an important role in trabecular and cortical bone formation in that they stimulate both proliferation and differentiation of osteoblasts [3]. IGF-I and IGF-II have been shown to increase alkaline phosphatase activity, osteocalcin production, and collagen synthesis in osteoblast line cells [3]. In addition, IGFs have been shown to decrease collagen degradation in osteoblasts [45]. Studies have also shown that IGF-I can selectively stimulate the transport of phosphate across the plasma membrane in some osteoblastic cell lines [46]. Besides the well-established effects of IGFs on osteoblasts, studies demonstrate that IGFs exert significant biological effects on osteoclasts, which include increase formation and survival rate of osteoclasts [47]. Consistent with these *in vitro* effects, several studies have shown that the administration of IGF-I causes an acute increase in both bone formation and bone resorption markers in serum [6,25]. Furthermore, studies have shown that low doses of IGF-I substantially increase bone formation activity and only slightly increase bone resorption activity in older women, thus suggesting that IGF-I therapy may represent an effective therapy to increase bone mass [6].

Studies demonstrate that the actions of IGFs in the bone microenvironment depend not only on the amount of IGFs produced, but also on the relative amounts and types of IGFBPs produced in the local bone microenvironment. Studies on the biological actions of IGFBPs in osteoblasts reveal that some IGFBPs inhibit (e.g., IGFBP-4 and IGFBP-6) whereas others stimulate (e.g., IGFBP-3 and IGFBP-5) IGF actions [39,48]. Studies on the molecular mechanisms by which IGFBPs mediate their effects on osteoblasts revealed that IGFBP-4 inhibits IGF action in osteoblasts by preventing the binding of IGF ligand to its membrane receptors. In contrast to

IGFBP-4, stimulatory IGFBP-5 has been shown to bind to cell surface as well as extracellular matrix proteins [39,49]. It has been proposed that the association of IGFBP-5 with proteins on cell surface or in the extracellular matrix results in an increase in the local concentration of IGFs in the vicinity of IGF receptors, thereby allowing IGF to bind to receptors.

In addition to modulating IGF actions, IGFBPs may also exert effects in an IGF-independent manner in various cell types [39,50]. Consistent with this idea, two reports provide evidence for the nuclear localization of IGFBP-3 [39]. In addition, IGFBP-5 contains the nuclear localization signal. Based on the findings that IGFBPs modulate IGF actions both in a positive and in a negative manner, it can be speculated that the balance between stimulatory and inhibitory classes of IGFBPs will determine the degree and extent of the IGF-induced cellular response in target tissues such as bone.

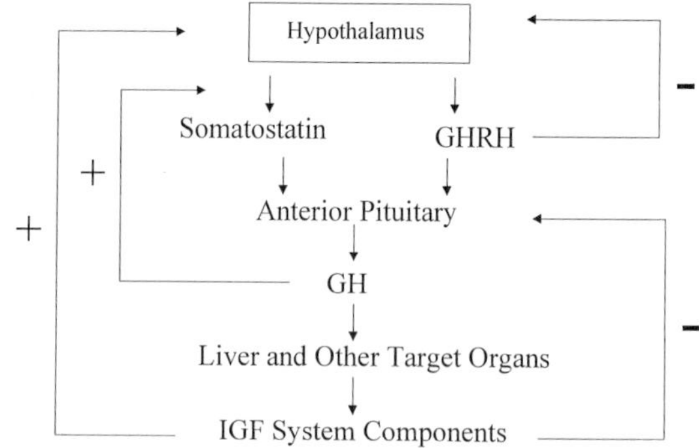

FIGURE 2 Relationships within the GH/IGF axis. GH secretion by the anterior pituitary is under the control of positive and negative signals, namely GHRH and somatostatin. Both GH and IGF-I may modulate hypothalamic secretion of GHRH and somatostatin. GH effects on target tissues are mediated in part via GH-induced changes in the production of IGF system components in liver and other target tissues.

AGE CHANGES IN GH SECRETION: POTENTIAL MECHANISMS

The two most important clinical changes in endocrine activity during aging involve the pancreas and the thyroid. The third endocrine system that gradually declines in activity during aging is the GH/IGF axis [51]. Maximal GH secretion occurs during puberty. After the age of 20 years, GH secretion declines approximately 14% per decade. For example, healthy boys secrete approximately 1–1.5 mg of GH daily, whereas healthy elderly men produce as little as 50–300 μg GH daily [51–54]. Thus, a remarkable 30-fold change in GH secretion can occur within the human life span. The first change that occurs with advancing age is in the reduction of GH secretion during the day, although the majority of GH is produced during sleep. With advancing age, the amount of GH secreted during sleep declines, and the number of GH secretory bursts and the amplitude and duration of the GH pulses also decrease. Although the decline in basal GH secretion with advances in age has been well established, it is not clear whether stimulated GH secretion declines with age. Studies on the peak GH response to the insulin tolerance test and GH-releasing hormone (GHRH) in young and elderly individuals have produced conflicting data [53].

Multiple elements appear to be involved in the pathophysiology of diminished GH secretion in aging humans [52,53,55,56]. The GH axis is under primary control by both a stimulating and an inhibiting hypothalamic peptidergic system, namely GHRH and somatostatin (Fig. 2). The pulsatile secretion of GH and the absolute amounts of GH stored and secreted are jointly coordinated by the regulated release of GHRH and somatostatin and the responsiveness of GH-secreting cells. Studies on the mechanism that contribute to the observed decline in GH secretion during aging support a view of combined GHRH and somatostain dysregulation caused by a decline in the GHRH stimulatory input and an increase in the somatostain inhibitory output [51].

The negative impact of age on the secretory activity of the hypothalamo-somatotrop axis appears to be mediated in part by the age-related decline in the production of sex steroid hormones. Based on the findings that the total and free testosterone concentrations in serum strongly correlated with the GH secretory burst mass and the daily GH production rate in boys during puberty, it has been speculated that testosterone is an important variable that controls GH secretion in men [57]. Furthermore, the administration of small doses of testosterone to prepubertal boys with isolated GnRH-LH deficiency has been shown to influence GH secretion. However, it remains unknown whether the effect of testosterone on the GHRH/somatostatin/GH/IGF-I axis is direct or whether testosterone is first converted to estrogen via aromatization and estrogen per se regulates feedback coordination within the GHRH/somatostain/GH/IGF axis in men. Although changes in gonadal function are interrelated with the decline in the GH/IGF axis, the molecular mechanisms by which androgens and estrogens regulate the hypothalamo-somatotrop unit remain unknown at the present time.

Other variables postulated to contribute to the age-related decline in GH secretion include changes in adiposity, a decrease in physical activity, aberrant sleep patterns, a poor nutritional status, an increased negative feedback by GH/IGF-I, and a diminished capacity of somatotrops to synthesize and store GH (Table

I). Of these variables, a large body of evidence demonstrates that a change in adiposity with advances in age is an important physiological variable that negatively regulates the secretory activity of the hypothalamus-somatotrop axis. In men, the dominant effect of body fat on GH secretion is evident even after controlling for androgen status. Based on the findings that visceral body fat content shows a strong negative correlation with daily GH secretion and that the amount of visceral fat deposition increases with age, it has been proposed that visceral fat is a major regulator of GH secretion [53]. In terms of the molecular signals responsible for mediating the effects of body fat on GH secretion, leptin has received much attention based on a number of findings: (1) Leptin levels are elevated in GH-deficient subjects and (2) leptin administration decreases GH secretion in fasting rats [58,59]. However, the role of leptin as a mediator of the effects of adiposity on GH secretion remains to be established.

Protein depletion and generalized malnutrition are two conditions that are often found in elderly men and women. The restriction of dietary nutrients adversely effects IGF-I synthesis and action at multiple steps, including decreased GH receptors, postreceptor defects in GH action, decreased steady-state levels of IGF-I mRNA, and attenuation of IGF-I action [60]. Exercise appears to be another potential confounding variable that could influence the output of the GH axis. Findings that high-intensity exercise causes an acute increase in GH secretion and that physical fitness as judged by maximal oxygen consumption rate shows strong positive correlation with mean 24-hr serum GH concentration [53,61] are consistent with a role of physical activity in regulating GH secretion. Further studies are needed to determine the extent to which changes in nutrition and exercise can influence the GH/IGF axis during aging.

Several findings suggest a negative feedback role for endogenous IGF-I in the control of GH secretion. First, exogenous IGF-I suppresses GH secretion in both animals and humans [62,63]. Second, serum concentrations of GH are elevated in conditions such as starvation/malnutrition and Laron-type dwarfism, in which plasma IGF-I concentrations are decreased as a result of GH resistance at the receptor or postreceptor level [60,64]. To evaluate if the increased endogenous IGF-I negative feedback is a causative factor in the age-associated decline in GH secretion, Chapman *et al.* [65] studied the effect of aging on the suppression of GH secretion by IGF-I in healthy young and older subjects. Based on the findings that the amount of GH suppression expressed in relation to increases in both total and free serum IGF-I concentrations was significantly less in the elderly subjects compared to the young subjects, these authors concluded that an increased sensitivity to endogenous IGF-I negative feedback is not a cause of the decline in GH secretion with increasing age.

The diminished capacity of somatotrops to synthesize and store GH with advancing age has been proposed to contribute to the age-related decline in GH secretion. However, studies using GH secretagogues suggest that this may not be the case. For example, long-acting derivatives of GHRH given daily subcutaneously for 14 days to healthy men 70 years old increased GH and IGF-I levels similar to the young adults [51]. In addition, nonpeptide analogs such as MK-677 and L-692,479 restored IGF-I secretion in the elderly to levels seen in young adults. Although these studies support the concept that pituitary somatotrops retain their ability to synthesize and secrete high levels of GH even in the elderly, further dose–response studies with GH secretagogues in a larger number of elderly subjects are needed, as only 35% of men over 60 years old were found to be GH deficient, as defined by IGF-I concentrations below the young adult normal range [66].

Based on the just-described discussion, it is obvious that complex mechanisms regulate the pulsatile secretion of GH and that the age-related decline in GH secretion is probably caused by confounding changes in sex steroid hormone concentrations, body composition, sleep pattern, nutrition, exercise, and other variables yet to be identified. It is important to identify the molecular mechanisms that contribute to the diminished GH secretion in aging humans in order for us to come up with suitable replacement therapies to correct the adverse changes in multiple organ systems that accrue as a result of the age-related decrease in GH secretion.

TABLE I Potential Causes for Age-Related Decline in GH Secretion

1. Decrease in the production of sex steroid hormones
2. Change in body composition—increase in adiposity
3. Decrease in physical activity
4. Aberrant sleep patterns
5. Poor nutritional status

AGE CHANGES IN IGF SYSTEM COMPONENTS: POTENTIAL MECHANISMS

In adult humans, IGFs circulate in serum in high abundance compared to other polypetide growth factors [39,50]. It has been speculated that circulating IGFs may provide a readily available reserve to act systemically in an endocrine manner. In addition to endocrine effects,

IGFs are involved in local regulation where IGFs produced by one cell type act in an autocrine or paracrine manner. IGFBPs have been proposed to play a role in modulating both endocrine and local actions of IGFs. The changes in IGF system components during aging in serum (endocrine actions) and bone (local actions) are described next.

Serum

An age-related decrease in serum IGF-I has been reported by several investigators [39]. The mean serum IGF-I level was 40% lower in the 41- to 60-year-old age group compared with a 23- to 40-year-old age group [67]. The decline in GH secretion appears to be one of the contributing factors for the age-related decline in serum IGF-I levels [51]. Several cross-sectional studies have demonstrated a strong linear relationship between serum IGF-I and bone mineral density (BMD) in postmenopausal women [33,39]. In addition, studies of GH-deficient patients have revealed that serum IGF-I concentrations closely correlate with reduced BMD and that GH replacement therapy increases both serum IGF-I and BMD [68]. These data suggest an important role for circulating IGF-I in the maintenance of adult bone mass.

Much less is known about the relationship between serum levels of IGF-II and BMD. One study found that serum levels of IGF-II showed a significant positive correlation with spinal BMD even when age was held constant [34]. These data, together with findings that IGF-II is produced in greater abundance than IGF-I by human osteoblasts, provide circumstantial evidence that circulating IGF-II may play an important role in the regulation of bone mass [69]. In addition, because both IGF-I and IGF-II mediate their biological effects by binding to the type I IGF receptor, most of the signaling in bone via the IGF-I receptor will be from IGF-II.

In serum, the majority of IGFs circulate as a 150- to 200-kDa complex, which consists of a 7.5-kDa IGF-I/IGF-II plus a 38- to 43-kDa IGFBP-3 and a 80- to 90-kDa acid labile subunit. This large molecular weight IGF complex acts as a reservoir, as it cannot cross the vascular endothelium. About 20–25% of IGFs exist as a 40- to 50-kDa complex by binding to one of the remaining five high-affinity IGFBPs [39]. These smaller molecular weight complexes can translocate across the vascular endothelium and, thus, this pool is bioavailable to the local tissues [39]. Each of the IGFBPs is important in the regulation of serum IGF levels and the bioavailability at the site of target tissues.

Serum levels of IGFBPs are altered with age; however, the magnitude and direction of change with age are different for the various IGFBPs [39]. Serum levels of IGFBP-1, IGFBP-2, and IGFBP-4 increase with age, whereas those of IGFBP-3 and IGFBP-5 decline with age. Although the mechanisms that cause the age-related changes in various IGFBPs remain unknown, the findings that serum levels of IGFBP-3 and IGFBP-5 correlate with serum levels of IGF-I, as well as with each other, suggest that serum levels of IGFBP-3 and IGFBP-5 may be GH dependent and that age-related changes in the serum levels of these two IGFBPs may be due, in part, to the age-related decline in GH secretion (Table II). Consistent with this hypothesis, we have found that GH treatment of GH-deficient adults increased serum levels of IGFBP-3 and IGFBP-5 to those levels seen in normal healthy adults [68]. In addition, treatment of healthy obese subjects with the GH secretagogue MK-677 increased serum IGFBP-5 levels by 44% after 2 weeks of treatment [70]. Further studies are needed to evaluate the extent to which changes in GH secretion contribute to the age-related changes in the levels of various IGF system components in the serum.

Age-related changes in IGFs and IGFBPs demonstrate that multiple deficits in the IGF system components occur as a consequence of aging (Table II). The underproduction of stimulatory IGF system components and the overproduction of inhibitory IGF system components could lead to an age-related decrease in the hormonal as well as local actions of the IGFs, all of which contribute to an impairment in the functions of various organs during aging.

Bone

The actions of IGFs at the local level depend on a number of factors, which include the amount of IGFs, the types and amounts of IGFBPs produced, the types and amounts of IGFBP proteases, and the responsiveness of the target cell to growth factor effect. The following section describes some of these variables shown to change with age.

TABLE II Changes in IGF System Component Levels in Serum during GH Deficiency and Aging

IGF system component	GH deficiency	Aging
IGF-I	Decrease	Decrease
IGF-II	Decrease	Decrease
IGFBP-1	Increase	Increase
IGFBP-2	Increase	Increase
IGFBP-3	Decrease	Decrease
IGFBP-4	Decrease	Increase
IGFBP-5	Decrease	Decrease

The concentration of IGF-I in human femoral cortical bone decline by 60% between 20 and 60 years of age [71]. Subsequent studies by Pfeilschifter *et al.* [72] have shown that the decline in skeletal IGF-I is more pronounced during the first half of life, but is not affected by menopause. These studies also showed that individuals with low IGF-I, on average, have a lower bone volume at the iliac crest than individuals with high IGF-I concentrations. Because IGFs do not appear to bind to either collagen or hydroxylapatite and because IGFBP-5 binds to both IGFs and hydroxylapatite with high affinity and, thus, may act to sequester IGFs in bone, the skeletal content of IGFBP-5 was assessed as a function of age [73]. It was found that the skeletal content of IGFBP-5 decreased by 28% between 20 and 60 years of age. In addition, the skeletal content of IGFBP-5, but not IGFBP-3, showed significant positive correlations with both IGF-I and IGF-II. These data, together with the findings that the age-related decrease in IGF-I varies depending on the skeletal site studied, suggest that the concentrations of IGFs in bone may be a reflection of osteoblast cell production and that bone cell production of IGFs declines with age [74]. The potential mechanisms that contribute to the age-related decline in the skeletal content of IGF-I remain to be established.

In addition to the age changes in the production of IGF system components, several studies have shown age-dependent decreases in osteoblastic responsiveness to IGF-I. Pfeilschifter *et al.* [75] have shown that osteoblasts from older donors require approximately 10-fold higher concentrations of IGF-I to yield comparable increases in DNA synthesis than cells from younger donors. D'Avis *et al.* [76] have shown that osteoblast-like cells derived from younger patients are more responsive to rhIGF-I than cells derived from older patients. In addition, these authors have shown an age-related decline in the synthesis of extracellular matrix components in response to IGF-I. Although it is not known whether the decrease in the responsiveness of osteoblasts to IGF-I is due to a deficiency in IGF-I receptors or to a deficiency in the postreceptor signaling pathway, these findings are consistent with the idea that a deficiency in both osteoblast cell production and responsiveness to growth factors may contribute to the age-related decline in bone formation.

MODEL OF AGE CHANGES IN THE GH/IGF AXIS AND THE AGE-RELATED IMPAIRMENT IN BONE FORMATION

Based on previously published findings from a number of laboratories, the authors have proposed a model to explain the mechanisms involved in age-related changes in the GH/IGF axis (Fig. 3). According to this model, the dysregulation of reduced GHRH secretion and/or action and increased somatostatin secretion and/or action appears to play a major role in the age-related decline in GH suppression by the pituitary. The factors that contribute to the age-related dysregulation of GHRH/somatostatin axis include a decline in sex steroid hormones, an increase in adiposity, a decrease in exercise, and changes in nutrition. The decline in GH secretion by the pituitary may also be due to a decrease in the number of pituitary somatotrops and/or the reduced ability of pituitary somatotrops to synthesize and store GH. Thus, multiple mechanisms appear to contribute to the remarkable decrease in GH secretion that accompanies aging [51,53].

Although GH exerts its effects on a number of organs, the liver represents one of the major target tissues for GH action. It is possible that there is an impairment in the GH-induced increase in IGF-I production in the liver that could contribute to the decline in IGF-I production with age. This would tend to decrease the endocrine actions of IGFs. GH has also important direct effects on other target tissues such as bone. The direct effects of GH on osteoblasts are mediated in part via a GH-induced increase in IGF-I production [19]. The age-related impairment in IGF-I production in bone in response to GH would tend to decrease the local actions of IGF-I. The molecular mechanisms that could contribute to the age-related impairment in IGF-I production in response to GH include a reduction in the number of GH receptors, a postreceptor signaling defect, and decreased IGF-I gene transcription. Although the decrease in the skeletal content of IGF-I is consistent with the possibility that there is an impairment in osteoblast cell production of IGF-I with age, the molecular mechanisms contributing to this deficiency remain unknown.

In addition to the decrease in IGF-I actions, evidence also demonstrates that the responsiveness of osteoblasts to IGF-I declines with age. It is not known what mechanisms contribute to the age-related resistance to the anabolic actions of IGF-I. In this regard, indirect evidence shows that the osteoblast cell production of inhibitory IGFBP-4 may increase with age (Fig. 4). This conclusion is based on the findings that serum levels of PTH, a major regulator of IGFBP-4 production in osteoblasts, increase with age and that serum levels of PTH correlate with serum levels of IGFBP-4 [77]. In addition to the increase in the osteoblast cell production of IGFBP-4, there is also indirect evidence that the osteoblast cell production of stimulatory IGFBP-5 may decrease with age (Fig. 4). This conclusion is based on the findings that serum levels of GH and IGFs, which increase IGFBP-5 expression in osteoblasts, decline with age and that serum levels of IGFBP-5 show significant positive correla-

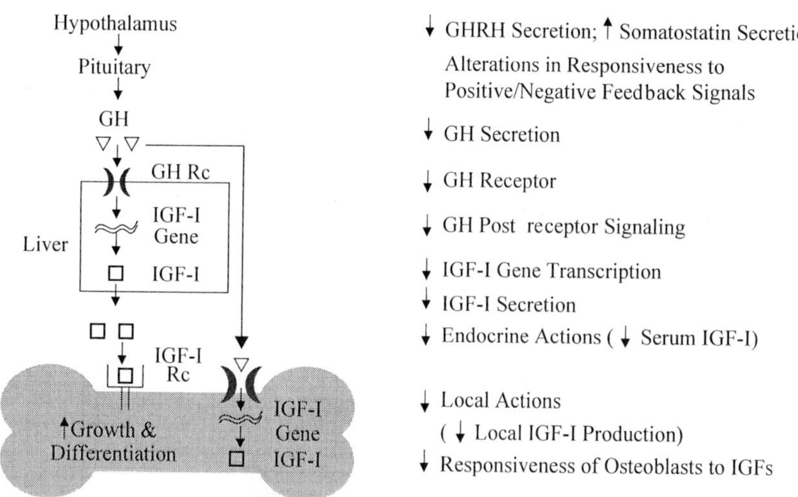

FIGURE 3 Schematic representation of potential mechanisms that could contribute to the age-related changes in the GH/IGF axis (see text for details). GH Rc, GH receptor; IGF-I Rc, IGF-I receptor.

tions with serum levels of IGF-I [78]. Consistent with this possibility, the authors have found that the skeletal content of IGFBP-5 declines with age [73]. Thus, the underproduction of stimulatory IGFBP-5 and the overproduction of inhibitory IGFBP-4 could contribute to the decreased responsiveness of osteoblasts with advances in age. The decrease in endocrine (serum) and local (bone) actions of IGFs, together with an increased resistance to IGF action in osteoblasts (may be mediated in part via changes in IGFBP production), could contribute to a decrease in osteoblast cell proliferation and a subsequent reduction in bone formation.

If the deficiency in the GH/IGF axis is a major contributor to the decline in the functional capacity of bone during aging, we should be able to correct it by GH or IGF-I treatment. GH administration in adults with a GH deficiency increased serum levels of IGF-I and IGFBP-5 to those observed in control individuals and increased bone mineral content significantly [68]. More recently, Bonjour *et al.* [79] have observed in undernourished

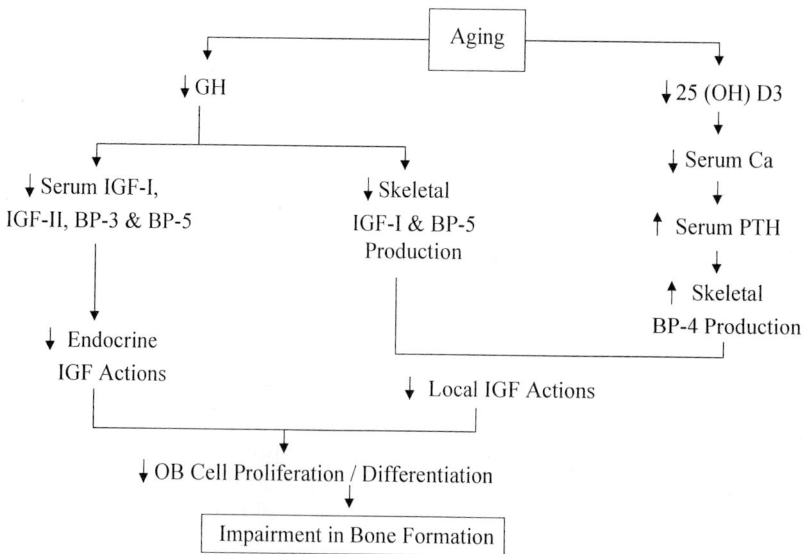

FIGURE 4 Schematic representation of age-related changes that could contribute to impairment in bone formation (see text for details). OB, osteoblast; 25(OH)D_3, 25-hydroxycholecalciferol.

elderly subjects that an increase in protein intake, from low to normal, caused a significantly greater gain in serum IGF-I and a decrease in dexoypyridinoline, a biochemical marker of bone resorption. In addition, protein supplementation resulted in attenuation of the decrease in proximal femur BMD seen at 1 year in the placebo group. Future long-term intervention studies with orally active GH secreting analogs, such as MK-677 or IGF-I in combination with a stimulatory IGFBP, are needed to evaluate the relative contribution of the GH/IGF axis to the bone loss seen in elderly men and women.

SUMMARY

Multiple deficits occur in the serum and bone levels of various IGF system components with advances in age. Although the potential mechanisms that contribute to these deficits are not fully understood, an age-related decline in GH secretion appears to be a major mechanism contributing to the IGF system deficit in the elderly. Although multiple elements, including changes in sex steroid hormone concentrations, body composition, sleep pattern, nutrition, and exercise, appear to be involved in the pathophysiology of diminished GH secretion in aging humans, further studies are needed to determine the potential contribution of each of these variables to the diminished GH secretion.

A number of *in vitro* and *in vivo* findings support a role for age-associated changes in the endocrine and local actions of IGFs in the pathogenesis of senile type II osteoporosis. Further intervention studies are needed to test the hypothesis that age-related bone loss is associated with a deficit in endocrine and local IGF actions.

Acknowledgment

This work was supported by funds from NIH (AR31062), Veterans Administration, and Loma Linda University School of Medicine.

References

1. Rodan, G. A., Raisz, L. G., and Bilezikian, J. P. Pathophysiology of osteoporosis. *In* "Principles of Bone Biology" (J. P. Bilezikian, L. G. Raisz, and G. A. Rodan, eds.), pp. 979–990. Academic Press, San Diego, 1996.
2. Mohan, S., and Baylink, D. J. Therapeutic potential of the TGFβ, BMP and FGF in the treatment of bone loss. *In* "Principles of Bone Biology" (J. P. Bilezikian, L. G. Raisz, and G. A. Rodan, eds.), pp. 1111–1123. Academic Press, San Diego, 1996.
3. Baylink, D. J., Finkelman, R. D., and Mohan, S. Growth factors to stimulate bone formation. [Review] *J. Bone Miner. Res.* **8**(Suppl. 2), S565–S572 (1993).
4. Canalis, E. Growth hormone, skeletal growth factors and osteoporosis. *Endocr. Pract.* **1,** 39–43 (1995).
5. Clark, R. Growth hormone and insulin-like growth factor 1: New endocrine therapies in cardiology. *Trends Cardiovasc. Med.* **7,** 264–268 (1997).
6. Marcus, R. Skeletal effects of growth hormone and IGF-I in adults. *Horm. Res.* **48,** 60–64 (1997).
7. Rosen, C. J. Growth hormone, insulin-like growth factors, and the senescent skeleton: Ponce de Leon's fountain revisited? *J. Cell. Biochem.* **56,** 348–356 (1994).
8. Bouillon, R. Growth hormone and bone. *Horm. Res.* **36,** 49–55 (1991).
9. Inzycchi, S. E., and Robbins, R. J. Effects of growth hormone on human bone biology. *J. Clin. Endocinol. Metab.* **79,** 691–694 (1994).
10. Slootweg, M. C. Growth hormone and bone. *Horm. Metab. Res.* **25,** 335–343 (1998).
11. Saggese, G., Baroncelli, G. I., Bertelloni, S., Cinequanta, L., and DiNero, G. Effects of long term treatment with growth hormone in bone and mineral development in children with growth hormone deficiency. *J. Pediatr.* **122,** 37–45 (1993).
12. Guevara-Aguirre, J., Vasconez, O., Martinez, V., Martinez, A. L., Rosenbloom, A. L., Diamond, F. B., Jr., Gargosky, S. E., Nonoshita, L., and Rosenfeld, R. G. A randomized, double blind, placebo-controlled trial on safety and efficacy of recombinant human insulin-like growth factor-I in children with growth hormone receptor deficiency. *J. Clin. Endocrinol. Metabol.* **80,** 1393–1398 (1995).
13. Harris, W. H., and Heaney, R. P. Effect of growth hormone on skeletal mass in adult dogs. *Nature* **223,** 403–404 (1969).
14. Isaksson, O. G. P., Lindahl, A., Nilsson, A., and Isagaard, J. Mechanism of the stimulatory effect of growth hormone on longitudinal bone growth. *Endocr. Rev.* **8,** 426–438 (1987).
15. Baker, A. R., Hollingshead, P. G., Pitts-Meek, S., Hansen, S., Taylor, R., and Stewart, T. A. Osteoblast-specific expression of growth hormone stimulates bone growth in transgenic mice. *Mol. Cell. Biol.* **12,** 5541–5547 (1992).
16. Daughaday, W. H., and Rotwein, P. Insulin-like growth factors I and II. Peptide, messenger ribonucleic acid and gene structures, serum and tissue concentrations. *Endocr. Rev.* **10,** 68–91 (1989).
17. Ernst, M., and Rodan, G. A. Increased activity of insulin-like growth factor (IGF) in osteoblastic cells in the presence of growth hormone (GH): positive correlation with the presence of GH-induced IGF binding protein BP-3. *Endocrinology* **127,** 807–814 (1990).
18. Schmid, C., Schlapfer, I., Peter, M., Boni-Schnetzler, M., Schwander, J., Zapf, J., and Froesch, E. R. Growth hormone and parathyroid hormone stimulate IGFBP-3 in rat osteoblasts. *Am. J. Physiol.* **267,** E226–E233 (1994).
19. Ernst, M., and Froesch, E. R. Growth hormone dependent stimulation of osteoblast-like cells in serum-free cultures via local synthesis of insulin-like growth factor-I. *Biochem. Biophys. Res. Commun.* **151,** 142–147 (1988).
20. Mohan, S., Strong, D. D., Lempert, U. G., Tremollieres, F., Wergedal, J. E., and Baylink, D. J. Studies on regulation of insulin-like growth factor binding protein (IGFBP)-3 and IGFBP-4 production in human bone cells. *Acta Endocrinol.* **127,** 555–564 (1992).
21. Swolin, D., and Ohlsson, C. Growth hormone increases interleukin-6 produced by human osteoblast-like cells. *J. Clin. Endocrinol. Metab.* **81,** 4329–4333 (1996).
22. Nilsson, A., Swolin, D., Enerback, S., and Ohlsson, C. Expression of functional growth hormone receptors in cultured human osteoblast-like cells. *J. Clin. Endocrinol. Metab.* **80,** 3483–3488 (1995).

23. Ghiron, L. J., Thompson, J. L., Holloway, L., Hintz, R. L., Butterfield, G. E., Hoffman, A. R., and Marcus, R. Effects of recombinant insulin-like growth factor I and growth hormone on bone turnover in elderly women. *J. Bone Miner. Res.* **10,** 1844–1852 (1995).
24. Nishiyama, K., Sugimoto, T., Kaji, H., Kantani, M., Kobayashi, T., and Chihara, K. Stimulatory effect of growth hormone on bone resorption and osteoclast differentiation. *Endocrinology* **137,** 35–41 (1996).
25. Rosen, C. J., and Donahue, L. R. Insulin-like growth factors: Potential therapeutic options for osteoporosis. *Trends Endocrinol. Metab.* **6,** 235–240 (1995).
26. Ono, T., Kanzaki, S., Seino, Y., Baylink, D. J., and Mohan, S. Growth hormone (GH) treatment of GH-deficient children increases serum levels of insulin-like growth factors (IGFs), IGF binding protein-3 and -5, and bone alkaline phosphatase isoenzyme. *J. Clin. Endocrinol. Metab.* **81,** 2111–2116 (1996).
27. Libanati, C., Srinivasan, N., Baylink, D. J., Lois, E., and Mohan, S. Skeletal size increases during Tanner stages II and III: association with a marked upregulation of the serum IGF system. *J. Bone Miner. Res.* **10,** S344. [Abstract]
28. Mohan, S., and Baylink, D. J. Bone growth factors. [Review] *Clin. Orthop. Related Res.* 30–48 (1991).
29. Conover, C. A. The role of insulin-like growth factors and binding proteins in bone cell biology. *In* "Principles of Bone Biology" (J. P. Bilezikian, and G. A. Rodan, eds.), pp. 607–618. Academic Press, San Diego, 1996.
30. Mohan, S., Bautista, C. M., Wergedal, J., and Baylink, D. J. Isolation of an inhibitory insulin-like growth factor (IGF) binding protein from bone cell-conditioned medium: a potential local regulator of IGF action. *Proc. Natl. Acad. Sci. USA* **86,** 8338–8342 (1989).
31. Liu, J.-P., Baker, J., Perkins, A. S., Robertson, E. J., and Efstratiadis, A. Mice carrying null mutations of the genes encoding insulin-like growth factor I (IGF-1) and type 1 IGF receptor (IGF1r). *Cell* **75,** 59–72 (1993).
32. Baker, J., Liu, J.-P., Robertson, E. J., and Efstratiadis, A. Role of insulin-like growth factors in embryonic and postnatal development. *Cell* **75,** 73–82 (1993).
33. Rosen, C. J., Dimai, H. P., Vereault, D., Donahue, L. R., Beamer, W. G., Farley, J., Linkhart, S., Linkhart, T., Mohan, S., and Baylink, D. J. Circulating and skeletal insulin-like growth factor-I (IGF-I) concentrations in two inbred strains of mice with different bone mineral densities. *Bone* **21,** 217–223 (1997).
34. Mohan, S., and Baylink, D. J. Development of a simple valid method for the complete removal of insulin-like growth factor (IGF)-binding proteins from IGFs in human serum and other biological fluids: comparison with acid-ethanol treatment and C18 Sep-Pak separation. *J. Clin. Endocrinol. Metab.* **80,** 637–647 (1995).
35. Sugimoto, T., Nishiyama, K., Kuribayashi, F., and Chihara, K. Serum levels of insulin-like growth factor (IGF) I, IGF-binding protein (IGFBP)-2, and IGFBP-3 in osteoporotic patients with and without spinal fractures. *J. Bone Miner. Res.* **12,** 1272–1279 (1997).
36. Romagnoli, E., Minisola, S., Carnevale, V., Rosso, R., Pacitti, M. T., Scarda, A., Scarnecchia, L., and Mazzuoli, G. Circulating levels of insulin-like growth factor binding protein 3 (IGFBP-3) and insulin-like growth factor I (IGF-I) in perimenopausal women. *Osteopor. Int.* **4,** 305–308 (1994).
37. Malpe, R., Baylink, D. J., Linkhart, T. A., Wergedal, J. E., and Mohan, S. Insulin-like growth factor (IGF)-I, -II, IGF binding proteins (IGFBP)-3, -4, and -5 levels in the conditioned media of normal human bone cells are skeletal site-dependent. *J. Bone Miner. Res.* **12,** 423–430.
38. Mohan, S. Insulin-like growth factor binding proteins in bone cell regulation. *Growth Regul.* **3,** 67–70 (1993).
39. Rajaram, S., Baylink, D. J., and Mohan, S. Insulin-like growth factor binding proteins in serum and other body fluids: Regulation and functions. *Endoc. Rev.* **18,** 801–831 (1997).
40. Canalis, E., Pash, J. M., and Verghese, S. Skeletal growth factors. *Crit. Rev. Euk. Gene Exp.* **3,** 155–166 (1993).
41. McCarthy, T. L., Casinghino, S., Centrella, M., and Canalis, E. Complex pattern of insulin-like growth factor binding protein expression in primary rat osteoblast enriched cultures: regulation by prostaglandin E2, growth hormone and the insulin-like growth factors. *J. Cell Physiol.* **160,** 163–175 (1994).
42. Mohan, S., Strong, D. D., Linkhart, T. A., and Baylink, D. J. Regulation and actions of insulin-like growth factor binding protein (IGFBP)-4 and IGFBP-5 in bone: physiological and clinical implications. *In* "The Insulin-like Growth Factors and Their Regulatory proteins" (R. C. Baxter, P. D. Gluckman, and R. G. Rosenfeld, eds.), pp. 205–215. Exerpta Medica, Amsterdam, 1994.
43. Conover, C. A. Insulin-like growth factor binding protein proteolysis in bone cell models. *Progr. Growth Factor Res.* **6,** 301–309 (1995).
44. Froesch, E. R., Schmid, C., Schwander, J., and Zapf, J. Actions of insulin-like growth factors. *Annu. Rev. Physiol.* **47,** 443–467 (1985).
45. Canalis, E., Rydziel, S., Delany, A. M., Varghese, S., and Jeffrey, J. J. Insulin-like growth factors inhibit interstitial collagenase synthesis in bone cell cultures. *Endocrinology* **136,** 1348–1354 (1995).
46. Caverzastio, J., Montessuit, C., and Bonjour, J. P. Stimulatory effect of insulin-like growth factor I on renal Pi transport and plasma 1,25-dihydroxyvitamin D3. *Endocrinology* **127,** 453–459 (1990).
47. Hou, P., Sato, T., Hofstetter, W., and Foged, N. T. Identification and characterization of the insulin-like growth factor I receptor in mature rabbit osteoclasts. *J. Bone Miner. Res.* **12,** 534–540 (1997).
48. Mohan, S., Nakao, Y., Honda, Y., Landale, E., Leser, U., Dony, C., Lang, K., and Baylink, D. J. Studies on the mechanisms by which insulin-like growth factor (IGF) binding protein-4 (IGFBP-4) and IGFBP-5 modulate IGF actions in bone cells. *J. Biol. Chem.* **270,** 20424–20431 (1995).
49. Jones, J. I., and Clemmons, D. R. Insulin-like growth factors and their binding proteins: biological actions. [Review] *Endocr. Rev.* **16,** 3–34 (1995).
50. Mohan, S., and Baylink, D. J. Editorial: Insulin-like growth (IGF)-binding proteins in serum: Do they have additional roles besides modulating the endocrine IGF actions. *J. Clin. Endocrinol. Metab.* **81,** 3817–3820 (1996).
51. Lamberts, S. W. J., van den Beld, A. W., and van der Lely, A.-J. The endocrinology of aging. *Science* **278,** 419–424 (1997).
52. Rosen, C. J., and Conover, C. Growth hormone insulin-like growth factor-I axis in aging: A summary of a National Institutes of Aging-sponsored symposium. *J. Clin. Endocrinol. Metab.* **82,** 3919–3922 (1997).
53. Veldhuis, J. D., Iranmanesh, A., and Wendland, M. Elements in pathophysiology of diminished growth hormone (GH) secretion in aging humans. *Endocrinology* **7,** 41–48 (1997).
54. Toogood, A. A., O'neill, P. A., and Shalet, S. M. Beyond the somatopause: Growth hormone deficiency in adults over the age of 60 years. *J. Clin. Endocinol. Metab.* **81,** 460–465 (1996).
55. Ho, K. Y., Evans, W. S., Blizzard, R. M., Veldhuis, J. D., Merriam, G. R., Samojlik, E., Furlanetto, R., Rogol, A. D., Kaiser, D. L., and Thorner, M. O. Effect of sex and age on the 24-hour profile of growth hormone secretion in man: Importance of endogenous

estradiol concentrations. *J. Clin. Endocinol. Metab.* **64,** 51–58 (1987).
56. Uberti, E. C., Amrosio, M. R., Cella, S. G., Margutti, A. R., Trasforini, G., Rigamonti, A. G., Petrone, E., and Muller, E. E. Defective hypothalamic growth hormone (GH)-releasing hormone activity may contribute to declining GH secretion with age in man. *J. Clin. Endocinol. Metab.* **82,** 2885–2888 (1997).
57. Veldhuis, J. D., Liem, A. Y., South, S., Weltman, A., Weltman, J., Clemmons, D. A., Abbott, R., Mulligan, T., Johnson, M. L., Pincus, S., Straume, M., and Iranmanesh, A. Differential impact of age, sex steroid hormones, and obesity on basal versus pulsatile growth hormone secretion in men as assayed in an ultrasensitive chemiluminescence assay. *J. Clin. Endocinol. Metab.* **80,** 3209–3222 (1995).
58. Carro, E., Senaris, R., Considine, R. V., Casanueva, F. F., and Dieguez, C. Regulation of *in vivo* growth hormone secretion by leptin. *Endocrinology* **138,** 2203–2206 (1997).
59. Fisker, S., Vahl, N., Hansen, T. B., Jorgensen, J.-O., Hagen, C., Orskov, H., and Christiansen, J. S. Serum leptin is increased in growth hormone-deficient adults: relationship to body composition and effects of placebo-controlled growth hormone therapy for 1 year. *Metab. Clin. Exp.* **47,** 812–817 (1997).
60. Underwood, L. E., Thissen, J. P., Lemozy, S., Ketelslegers, J. M., and Clemmons, D. R. Hormonal and nutritional regulation of IGF-I and its binding proteins. [Review] *Horm. Res.* **42,** 145–151 (1994).
61. Cappon, J., Brasel, J. A., Mohan, S., and Cooper, D. M. Effect of brief exercise on circulating insulin-like growth factor I. *J. Appl. Physiol.* **76,** 2490–2496 (1994).
62. Guler, H. P., Zapf, J., and Froesch, E. R. Short-term metabolic effects of recombinant human insulin-like growth factor I in healthy adults. *N. Engl. J. Med.* **317,** 137–140 (1987).
63. Bermann, M., Jaffer, C. A., Tsai, W., DeMott-Frieberg, R., and Barkan, A. L. Negative feedback regulation of pulsatile growth hormone secretion by insulin-like growth factor-I. Involvement of hypothalamic somatostain. *J. Clin. Invest.* **94,** 138–145 (1994).
64. Rosenfeld, R. G., Rosenbloom, A. L., and Guevara-Aguirre, J. Growth hormone (GH) insensitivity due to primary GH receptor deficiency. *Endocr. Rev.* **15,** 369–390 (1994).
65. Chapman, I. M., Hartman, M. L., Pezzoli, S. S., Harrell, F. E., Jr., Hintz, R. L., Alberti, K. G. M. M., and Thorner, M. O. Effect of aging on the sensitivity of growth hormone secretion to insulin-like growth factor-I negative feedback. *J. Clin. Endocrinol. Metab.* **82,** 2996–3004 (1997).
66. Rudman, D., Feller, A. G., Nagaraj, H. S. *et al.,* Effects of human growth hormone in men over 60 years old. *N. Engl. J. Med.* **323,** 1–6 (1990).
67. Mohan, S., Farley, J. R., and Baylink, D. J. Age-related changes in IGFBP-4 and IGFBP-5 levels in human serum and bone: Implications for bone loss with aging. *Progr. Growth Fact. Res.* **6,** 465–473 (1995).
68. Thoren, M., Hilding, A., Brismar, T., Magnusson, P., Degerblad, M., Larsson, L., Saaf, M., Baylink, D. J., and Mohan, S. Serum levels of insulin-like growth factor binding protein (IGFBP)-4 and -5 correlate with bone mineral density in growth hormone (GH) deficient adult and increase with GH replacement therapy. *J. Bone Miner. Res.* **13,** 891–899 (1998).
69. Mohan, S., and Baylink, D. J. Insulin-like growth factor system components and the coupling of bone formation to resorption. *Horm. Res.* **45,** 59–62 (1996).
70. Svensson, J., Ohlsson, C., Jansson, J.-O., Murphy, G., Wyss, D., Krupa, D., Cerchio, K., Polvino, W., Gertz, B., Baylink, D., Mohan, S., and Bengtsson, B.-A. Treatment with the oral growth hormone (GH) secretagogue MK-677 increases markers of bone formation and bone resorption in obese young males. *J. Bone Miner. Res.* **13,** 1158–1166 (1998).
71. Nicolas, V., Prewett, A., Bettica, P., Mohan, S., Finkelman, R. D., Baylink, D. J., and Farley, J. R. Age-related decreases in insulin-like growth factor I and transforming growth factor-beta in femoral cortical bone from both men and women: implications for bone loss with aging. [see comments] *J. Clin. Endocrin. Metab.* **78,** 1011–1016 (1994).
72. Pfeilschifter, J. IGF-I and the aging human skeleton: Evidence for a decline in tissue concentration and biological activity. "Working Group on Aging and the Human Skeleton," 3rd Annual Meeting, Cincinnati, OH, 1997. [Abstract]
73. Nicolas, V., Mohan, S., Honda, Y., Prewett, A., Finkelman, R. D., Baylink, D. J., and Farley, J. R. An age-related decrease in the concentration of insulin-like growth factor binding protein-5 in human cortical bone. *Calcif. Tissue Int.* **57,** 206–212 (1995).
74. Mohan, S., and Baylink, D. J. Serum insulin-like growth factor binding protein (IGFBP)-4 and IGFBP-5 levels in aging and age-associated diseases. *Endocrine* **7,** 87–91 (1997).
75. Pfeilschifter, J., Diel, I., Pilz, U., Brunotte, K., Naumann, A., and Ziegler, R. Mitogenic responsiveness of human bone cells *in vitro* to hormones and growth factors decrease with age. *J. Bone Miner. Res.* **8,** 707–717 (1993).
76. D'Avis, P. Y., Frazier, C. R., Shapiro, J. R., and Fedarko, N. S. Age-related changes in effects of insulin-like growth factor I on human osteoblast-like cells. *Biochem. J.* **324,** 753–760 (1997).
77. Honda, Y., Landale, E. C., Strong, D. D., Baylink, D. J., and Mohan, S. Recombinant synthesis of insulin-like growth factor-binding protein-4 (IGFBP-4): Development, validation, and application of a radioimmunoassay for IGFBP-4 in human serum and other biological fluids. *J. Clin. Endocrinol. Metab.* **81,** 1389–1396 (1996).
78. Mohan, S., Libanati, C., Dony, C., Lang, K., Srinivasan, N., and Baylink, D. J. Development, validation, and application of a radioimmunoassay for insulin-like growth factor binding protein-5 in human serum and other biological fluids. *J. Clin. Endocrinol. Metab.* **80,** 2638–2645 (1995).
79. Bonjour, J. P., Schurch, M.-A., Chevalley, T., Ammann, P., and Rizzoli, R. Protein intake, IGF-I and osteoporosis. *Osteopor. Int.* **7,** S36–S42 (1997).

CHAPTER 20

Other Pharmacologic Agents Influencing Bone Loss

PAULA H. STERN Department of Molecular Pharmacology and Biological Chemistry, Northwestern University Medical School, Chicago, Illinois
PETER LAKATOS Department of Medicine, Semmelweis University Medical School, Budapest, Hungary

INTRODUCTION

The major focus of this chapter is the question of whether aging makes bones more vulnerable to pharmacological agents that have been shown to cause bone loss and susceptibility to fracture. Included in this list of agents are glucocorticoids and other immunosuppressive drugs, thyroid hormones, anticonvulsants, and antimetabolites. We have also included some consideration of vitamin D analogs because they may be used to counteract the bone loss from anticonvulsants and the thiazide diuretics because they are another class of pharmacologic factors affecting bone. A concise answer to the question of whether the responses to all of these drugs are affected by aging would be that for the most part, this has not been systematically investigated, and further investigation is warranted. However, we can at least consider the likelihood that there will be differences, based not only on the effects of aging on bone, but on the indications for the use of the agents, whether pharmacokinetic factors that change with aging have an impact on these drugs and whether there are other general factors that could determine whether this is likely to be a consideration in the therapeutic use of the agents. Table I lists some relevant categories and the drugs that would fall into each.

GENERAL PHARMACOKINETIC ISSUES

Although the alterations in intestinal, hepatic, and renal function with aging and their influence on drug action have been rather extensively studied and reviewed [1,2], the influence of these changes on the effects of agents that adversely affect bone and calcium metabolism has not been thoroughly assessed. Thus, we can mainly enumerate some of the changes that occur with aging that could affect the actions of these drugs and speculate as to what their impact might be.

Absorption of nutrients as well as drugs can change with aging. In the older individual, there is a decrease in gastric parietal cell function. Gastric pH increases [3] and gastric emptying may slow [4]. There is a thinning or reduction in intestinal absorptive surface [5]. Possible changes in the absorption of the drugs of interest have not been systematically studied, although it is a general observation that the intestinal absorption of drugs that are absorbed by passive diffusion are relatively unaffected by aging [1]. However, efficiency in the absorption of calcium declines, which could theoretically affect the bone risks from agents such as glucocorticoids or anticonvulsants that affect calcium absorption directly or indirectly.

After the age of about 40 years, liver mass begins to decline. Phase I metabolic processes of hydroxylation and N-dealkylation decrease slightly with age, which can result in increased concentrations of anticonvulsants [6]. Total liver blood flow can decrease 40–50% in the elderly individual [7] and can be further decreased when there is congestive heart failure. Plasma albumin concentrations are reduced in the elderly [8], especially in those who are chronically ill or have poor nutrition. Both glomerular filtration rate and renal plasma flow decline with age [1]. The impact of these latter factors

TABLE I Characteristics of Drugs of Concern for the Aging Skeleton

1. Is the drug more or less likely to be used in older individuals?
Yes: glucocorticoids
2. Is the drug used chronically, resulting in the accumulation of effects over many years?
Yes: glucocorticoids, thyroid hormones, immunosuppressants, anticonvulsants
3. Is the dose of the drug often reduced in older individuals due to potential organ toxicity?
Yes: thyroid hormones (cardiotoxicity)
4. Are the active concentrations of the drug itself altered by pharmacokinetic factors that can change with aging, such as intestinal absorption, regional blood flow, drug metabolism, and renal excretion?
Yes: anticonvulsants
5. Does the drug produce its effects on bone by actions on systems that are altered during aging?
Calcium absorption: glucocorticoids, immunosuppressants
Vitamin D metabolism: anticonvulants
Parathyroid hormone secretion: glucocorticoids
Cytokine production: glucocorticoids, immunosuppressants, thyroid hormones (?)
6. Does the disorder for which the drug is being used increase the susceptibility of bone to agents that cause bone loss?
Possibly: rheumatoid arthritis (glucocorticoids, methotrexate); renal, hepatic disease requiring organ transplantation (glucocorticoids, immunosuppressive agents)

on the drugs under consideration is also not established. A final pharmacokinetic consideration is the possibility for drug interactions with agents that affect pharmacokinetic factors. Elderly patients may be chronically taking antacids, laxatives, analgesics, antihistamines, sedatives, and vitamins at greater frequency than younger individuals, which could have an impact on the pharmacokinetics of the agents affecting bone. In addition to pharmacokinetic factors, there may be differences in receptor number or affinity with increasing age [9]. However, these factors seem less critical than pharmacokinetic differences [10] and are certainly less well defined.

PHARMACOLOGIC AGENTS

Glucocorticoids

Glucocorticoids have marked effects on bone metabolism. With continued exposure of skeletal tissue to excessive amounts of these compounds, severe bone loss may result, leading to osteoporosis and consequently to increased fracture rate [11]. Changes in the aging bone include a growing number of microcracks and cement lines, increased cortical porosity, decreased mineralization of osteons, and change in collagen elasticity. There is no evidence showing a direct influence of glucocorticoids on these processes. However, there is a vast array of data indicating that changes occurring during glucocorticoid therapy may worsen the metabolic balance in the aging bone. Because bone loss is a frequent health problem of the elderly, glucocorticoids may further aggravate this situation. Whereas the exact mechanisms of involutional osteoporosis and glucocorticoid-induced bone loss are uncertain, recent investigations have led to some clues as to how these two pathological processes might interfere.

During aging, both intestinal absorption [12] and renal reabsorption [13] of calcium decrease. The inhibition of intestinal calcium transport is probably due to alterations in vitamin D metabolism. Parallel with declining renal function, a gradually decreasing 1α-hydroxylase activity has been observed, resulting in the decreased production of 1,25-dihydroxyvitamin D [14], although normal serum levels have been reported as well [15]. As a consequence of decreased intestinal calcium absorption, secondary hyperparathyroidism develops, which results in the deterioration of bone tissue. Reduced renal calcium reabsorption may be a consequence of estrogen deficiency in women [13]. All these processes contribute to the development of age-related osteoporosis.

Glucocorticoids enhance bone resorption by reducing intestinal calcium transport [16]. They oppose the effects of vitamin D, but the exact mechanism has not been established. Serum concentrations of vitamin D metabolites in patients receiving glucocorticoids are mostly normal [17,18], although some authors found reduced [19] or elevated [20] levels. A number of studies have found increased parathyroid hormone (PTH) levels during corticosteroid treatment [21,22]. This has not been confirmed by others [23,24]. A slight increase in PTH levels has been attributed to malabsorption of calcium in both the gastrointestinal tract and the renal tubule. There is substantial evidence for increased urinary calcium loss with long-term glucocorticoid therapy [23]. This is not necessarily accompanied by increases in other indices of bone resorption [23], suggesting that hypercalciuria in this case is attributable mainly to the altered renal handling of calcium. Tubular reabsorption of calcium was found to be reduced in those receiving glucocorticoids [25]. These actions of glucocorticoids can amplify the similar age-related physiological changes in calcium metabolism and add to the bone loss.

Interleukin (IL)-6 is a cytokine known to induce osteoclast recruitment and thus to play an important role in bone resorption [26]. IL-6 production increases with age, especially after menopause [27]. The stimulatory effect of glucocorticoids on bone resorption *in vivo* may involve the induction of IL-6 receptors in skeletal cells

[28], which could lead to more pronounced IL-6 effects in corticosteroid-treated subjects.

Bone formation decreases with aging. One of the reasons behind this phenomenon is the age-dependent reduction in bone anabolic growth factor production. Insulin-like growth factor (IGF) levels are inversely correlated with age [29]. Transforming growth factor (TGF)-β production is lower after menopause [30]. Glucocorticoid excess inhibits bone formation, as reflected by decreased serum osteocalcin levels [31]. This is a direct effect of glucocorticoids on cells of the osteoblastic lineage. Glucocorticoids and IGFs have opposite effects on bone formation. Glucocorticoids at high concentrations inhibit IGF-I synthesis in osteoblasts by a transcriptional mechanism [32]. A glucocorticoid-responsive region of the rat IGF-I exon 1 promoter has been identified [33]. The activity of IGFs is regulated by six IGF-binding proteins (BPs), which are all expressed by osteoblasts [34]. Glucocorticoids decrease the expression of IGFBP-3, -4, and -5 in these cells [35]. The inhibitory effect on the IGFBP-5 gene is mediated through a Myb consensus sequence [36]. IGFBP-5 stimulates bone cell growth and enhances the effects of IGF-I. Thus, reduced levels of IGFBP-5 in bone tissue may augment the inhibitory effect of glucocorticoids on bone formation. The observed decline in IGF production with aging may be further aggravated by these glucocorticoid-induced changes, leading to faster bone loss in the elderly.

TGF-β is also anabolic for the bone by stimulating osteoblast replication and differentiation, collagen synthesis and matrix apposition rates, as well as by inhibiting osteoclast function. Glucocorticoids do not interfere with the expression of TGF-β but promote the activation of its latent form by increasing the amount of proteases in bone [37]. Cortisol shifts the binding of TGF-β from its signal-transducing receptors to β-glycan [38]. As a result, cortisol inhibits the stimulatory effects of TGF-β on cell replication. Similar to the IGF/IGFBP system, negative changes in TGF-β production with aging and by glucocorticoids may be additive. Effects of glucocorticoids on local factors in bone are summarized in Table II.

Sex steroid production also decreases with aging, which has a major impact on bone metabolism. Patients on glucocorticoids develop hypogonadism [39]. High-dose glucocorticoid therapy is associated with oligomenorrhoea in women and a dose-dependent reduction in free testosterone levels in men [40]. This effect is probably mediated through an inhibition of gonadotropin secretion and a reduction in gonadotropin-binding sites. This effect of glucocorticoids on sex hormones may not be that important in the late menopause, but it could negatively affect bone status during perimenopause, when bone is more susceptible to deleterious effects.

TABLE II Effects of Glucocorticoids on Local Factors in Bone

IGF-I transcription ↓
IGF-II receptor transcription ↓
IGFBP-3, -4, -5 expression ↓
IGFBP-6 transcription ↑
TGF-β activation ↑
TGF-β binding to β-glycan ↑
IL-6 receptors ↑

As can be seen, the (patho)physiological changes are similar during aging and glucocorticoid treatment. Changes in calciotropic hormone profiles, together with glucocorticoid administration, serve to weaken the aging skeleton. Subtle metabolic changes in bone tissue may become apparent with the use of steroids. Morris *et al.* [41] have shown that corticosteroid-treated postmenopausal women with vertebral fractures have significantly lower intestinal calcium absorption than their corticosteroid-treated controls who have not fractured. This indicates that impaired calcium absorption contributes to the development of clinically significant osteoporosis. Laan *et al.* [42] found that postmenopausal women with rheumatoid arthritis who were treated with prednisone had twice as many fractures as patients not receiving the drug. According to the available evidence, the underlying disease does not influence the susceptibility to glucocorticoid-induced bone loss [43]. However, the disease for which the steroid is used may itself be associated with bone loss, such as in the case of rheumatoid arthritis and inflammatory bowel disease. The increased incidence of fractures in postmenopausal patients might be due to the altered bone metabolism around menopause.

Other Immunosuppressive Agents and Antimetabolites

Deleterious effects on bone are induced by other immunosuppressive agents and antimetabolites. Immunosuppressive agents such as cyclosporine and tacrolimus and antimetabolites such as methotrexate have therapeutic applications in combination with glucocorticoids or as replacements for glucocorticoids. Nonsteroid immunosuppressive agents are widely used to prevent rejection after organ transplantation and have been used for the treatment of rheumatoid arthritis and other disorders of immunoregulation. The syndrome of transplantation osteoporosis [44] is a recognized clinical problem, although the relative roles of glucocorticoids, the nonsteroidal protein phosphatase inhibitory agents such as cyclosporine, given to reduce exposure to glucocorticoids, and the underlying disease still remain to be sorted out. The mechanism of action of cyclosporine and tacrolimus in the T lymphocyte is through the inhibition of the phosphatase calcineurin, resulting in the failure of the regulatory protein, nuclear factor-activated T cells (NFAT), to form activating transcriptional complexes, which are involved in the synthesis of a number of cytokines, including interleukin-2 [45]. In a placebo-controlled study, low cyclosporine was found to improve the condition of patients with rheumatoid arthritis [46], probably due to reductions in the production of inflammatory cytokines that can cause bone loss. It is also unclear whether the same molecular mechanism by which cyclosporine and tacrolimus affect the cells of the immune system applies in bone cells and whether the same gene products are involved. In *in vitro* models, cyclosporine inhibits bone loss from a range of agents [47] and inhibits osteoclast formation in marrow cultures [48]. In *in vivo* studies in rats, cyclosporine induces a high turnover osteopenia, which is not seen in an immunodeficient rat model [49]. Newer immunosuppressive agents with different mechanisms of action [50] could prove to be less deleterious to bone. The possibility should be considered that changes in the immune response with aging [51] might result in altered skeletal responses to the immunosuppressive agents.

The antimetabolite methotrexate has caused severe osteopenia in patients treated with high-dose, short-term intravenous therapy for osteosarcoma [52]. A similar methotrexate osteopathy has been described in patients given long-term, low-dose methotrexate for psoriasis and rheumatoid arthritis [53]. In a group of patients with rheumatoid arthritis who became resistant to methotrexate, there was a decline in bone mineral density that was reversed when the inflammation was controlled by cyclosporine [54]. When human bone-derived osteoblasts were treated with methotrexate, there was an inhibition of cell proliferation, although alkaline phosphatase was unaffected [55].

Thyroid Hormones

Triiodothyronine (T3) is a critical regulator of skeletal development and function. Thyroid hormones are used in replacement therapy for hypothyroidism, such as after thyroidectomy and in autoimmune thyroiditis. Thyroid hormones are also used as suppressive therapy for toxic nodular goiter and after surgery for differentiated thyroid cancers to suppress thyroid-stimulating hormone (TSH). In addition, some patients may have taken excess thyroid hormones inappropriately, such as for weight loss or as a tonic. Excessive T3, whether for replacement or suppression, is associated with decreased bone density [56,57], and postmenopausal women overtreated with levothyroxin are particularly at risk [58]. Histomorphometric analyses show increases in both osteoblastic and osteoclastic activity and loss of cortical trabecular bone volume [59]. Biochemical markers also provide evidence of increased turnover with thyroid hormone treatment. Pyridinoline and hydroxypyridinoline cross-link excretion is elevated [60,61], as are alkaline phosphatase and osteocalcin [62]. Consistent with histomorphometric findings, there are greater increases in resorption markers than formation markers, suggesting an imbalance between resorption and formation, leading to bone loss [61].

A particularly critical issue is the question of what amounts of exogenously administered thyroid hormones increase the risk of bone loss, especially among individuals already at risk for osteoporotic fractures from other causes. The literature reveals highly diverse findings, with a number of studies showing decreased bone density and accelerated bone turnover in patients treated with T4 [e.g., 63,64] and a large number finding no evidence of bone loss [e.g., 65,66] even in older patients; more extensive references are cited in an earlier review [67]. In addition to higher doses of T3 [68], factors that have been found to increase susceptibility to bone loss with thyroid hormone treatment include increasing age [69] and postmenopausal status [70,71] when coupled with a previous history of thyrotoxicosis. A low dietary calcium intake may contribute to the risk of T4-induced bone loss [58]. Treatments reported to be protective include estrogen [68], androgen [72], and bisphosphonates [73]. The recovery of bone loss in hyperthyroid patients following antithyroid treatment has been inconsistent, but may be achieved more readily in younger individuals [74,75]. Although the use of highly sensitive TSH assays may help guide T3 dosage [76], it is likely that the problem will persist, especially in high-risk individuals.

Despite the clinical importance of the effects of T3 on bone, very little is known about the molecular mechanism by which this occurs. The osteoblast appears to be the critical target cell for T3 action in bone, as T3 fails to activate isolated osteoclasts to resorb in the absence of osteoblasts [77,78]. Rodent osteoblastic cell lines have been shown to express both T3Rα1 and T3Rβ1 receptor isoforms [79]. T3 potentiates the IL-1β-stimulated production of IL-6 in bone [80] and in human osteosarcoma cells (MG-63) [81]. IL-6 and IL-6 soluble receptor were found to be higher in hyperthyroid patients [81]. Circulating IL-6 is higher in hyperthyroid (Graves disease and toxic nodular goiter) than in euthyroid premenopausal women [82]. Monocytes from the patients with Graves disease or toxic nodular goiter had elevated IL-6 production compared with controls [82]. These results all suggest that IL-6 could play a role in T3-stimulated bone loss. There is evidence that IL-6 increases with age in both women [27] and men [83]. Whether this may be increased further by thyroid hormone excess needs to be determined.

T3 has direct actions on IGF-I production in bone [84–86]. An increase in IGF-I mRNA is seen in MC3T3-E1 cells treated with T3 [86]. The effect on IGF-I is biphasic and supraphysiologic concentrations of T3 have lesser effects [85]. The ability of T3 to increase IGF-I could be important in T3 effects to promote bone formation during development and may also function as a protective mechanism against bone loss. This protection may decline with aging. Several studies have revealed a decline in IGF-I [29,87], with aging. There are also alterations in the relative concentrations of IGF-binding proteins (increased IGFBP-1,-3, and -4 and decreased IGFBP-5) with aging [87,88], which could result in a diminished effectiveness of IGF-I. Thyroid hormone itself affects IGFBP concentrations that could inhibit effects of IGF-I [84,89]. Postmenopausal women with hyperthyroidism and severe bone loss did not show the elevation of IGF-I observed in premenopausal hyperthyroid women, and the latter group had less severe bone loss [90]. Effects of T3 on local factors in bone are summarized in Table III.

Anticonvulsants

Anticonvulsants can induce the hepatic enzymes that lead to the inactivation of vitamin D [91], and the syndrome of anticonvulsant-induced bone loss is a dose- and time-dependent side effect of this class of drugs. Hypocalcemia and elevated osteoblastic activity may occur in patients undergoing long-term anticonvulsant therapy, and calcitriol treatment may be required [92]. With long-term anticonvulsant therapy, there may also be an imbalance between resorption and formation, with excessive resorption [93]. Even if negative effects on bone balance are detected, withdrawing the anticonvulsant therapy may not be an option, as it may be essential for preventing seizures. With aging, there are several factors that limit vitamin D production and could have a potential impact on the deleterious effects of anticonvulsants on bone. Lower than normal 25-hydroxyvitamin D concentrations have been found in about 20% of elderly subjects in North America and Europe [94–96]. Moreover, half of this 20% appears resistant to cholecalciferol and may require an active analog to stimulate calcium absorption and to decrease PTH and bone turnover [97,98]. Renal function declines with age. The major rate-limiting step in the production of 1,25-dihydroxyvitamin D, 1 α-hydroxylation in the kidney, decreases with age as well [97]. This change may be the cause of the apparent vitamin D resistance in the elderly, although an age-related decrease in intestinal responsiveness to vitamin D has also been reported [99]. However, active vitamin D analogs decrease PTH in the elderly better than in young adults [100]; with this mechanism the effects of active vitamin D analogs could be more beneficial in the elderly.

TABLE III Effects of Thyroid Hormones on Local Factors in Bone

IGF-I transcription ↑
IGF-I expression ↑, ↓
IGF-I receptor transcription ↑
IGFBP-2, IGFBP-3, IGFBP-4 expression ↑
IL-6 transcription and expression potentiated

Thiazide Diuretics

Thiazide diuretics may decrease the fracture rate in the elderly population [101]. The mechanism of action of these drugs is presumably the reduction of urinary calcium excretion and thus the suppression of PTH. Preventing the hypercalciuria and secondary hyperparathyroidism frequently observed in the elderly could serve as an explanation for the effectiveness of thiazides in reducing the fracture rate in the elderly. A seasonal beneficial effect of thiazides to reduce bone loss, associated with decreased PTH and 1,25-dihydroxyvitamin D, has been observed [102]. Direct effects of thiazides on human osteoblastic cells have also been described [103], suggesting that the beneficial effects of these agents could derive from direct actions on bone in addition to their renal actions.

SUMMARY

Despite the importance of the question, there is as yet little definitive information on the influence of age on the deleterious and beneficial effects of pharmacologic agents on bone. However, various changes in physiological processes and in bone itself with aging would lead to the prediction that there would be alterations in the response to these drugs in the elderly individual. One final consideration is that treatment regimens could interact with the normal homeostatic processes, including the established diurnal rhythms in calcemic hormones and bone metabolism [104]. Gender-related differences in some of these rhythms have been described in elderly individuals [105]. Also, many hormonal diurnal rhythms flatten with age, which has been suggested to result from an inability of target cells to upregulate after their downregulation [106]. The impact of these modulations on the action of drugs affecting bone could have consequences for the aging skeleton.

References

1. Schmucker, D. L. Aging and drug disposition: an update. *Pharmacol. Rev.* **37,** 133–148 (1985).
2. Turner, N., Scarpace, P. J., and Lowenthal, D. T. Geriatric pharmacology: basic and clinical considerations. *Annu. Rev. Pharmacol. Toxicol.* **32,** 271–302 (1992).
3. Kekki, M., Samloff, I., Ihamaki, T., Varis, K., and Siurala, M. Age- and sex-related behavior of gastric acid secretion at the population level. *Scand. J. Gastroenterol.* **17,** 737–743 (1982).
4. Evans, M., Triggs, E., Cheung, M., Broe, G., and Creasy, H. Gastric emptying rate in the elderly: implications for drug therapy. *J. Am. Geriatr. Soc.* **29,** 201–205 (1982).
5. Warren, P., Pepperman, M., and Montgomery, R. Age changes in the small intestinal mucosa. *Lancet* **2,** 849–850 (1978).
6. Houghton, G., Richens, A., and Keighton, M. Effects of age, height, weight and sex on serum phenytoin concentration in epileptic patients. *Br. J. Clin. Pharmacol.* **2,** 251–256 (1975).
7. Greenblatt, D., Sellers, E., and Shader, R. Drug disposition in old age. *N. Engl. J. Med.* **306,** 1081–1087 (1982).
8. Wallace, S., Whiting, B., and Runcie, J. Factors affecting drug-binding in plasma of elderly patients. *Br. J. Clin. Pharmacol.* **3,** 327–330 (1976).
9. Roth, G. Hormone receptor changes during adulthood and senescence: significance for aging research. *Fed. Proc.* **38,** 1910–1914 (1979).
10. Reidenberg, M. Drugs in the elderly. *Bull. N.Y. Acad. Med.* **56,** 287–294 (1980).
11. Michel, B. A., Bloch, D. A., and Fries, J. F. Predictors of fractures in early rheumatoid arthritis. *J. Rheumatol.* **18,** 804–808 (1991).
12. Wemeau, J. L. Calciotropic hormones and aging. *Horm. Res.* **43,** 76–79 (1995).
13. Nordin, B. E., Horowitz, M., Need, A., and Morris, H. A. Renal leak of calcium in postmenopausal osteoporosis. *Clin. Endocrinol. Oxf.* **41,** 41–45 (1994).
14. Tsai, K. S., Heath, H., Kumar, R., and Riggs, B. L. Impaired vitamin D metabolism with aging in women. Possible role in pathogenesis of senile osteoporosis. *J. Clin. Invest.* **73,** 1668–1672 (1984).
15. Francis, R. M., Peacock, M., Taylor, G. A., Storer, J. H., and Nordin, B. E. Calcium malabsorption in elderly women with vertebral fractures: evidence for resistance to the action of vitamin D metabolites on the bowel. *Clin. Sci.* **66,** 103–107 (1984).
16. Nordin, B. E. C., Marshal, D. H., Francis, R. M., and Crilly, R. G. The effects of sex steroid and cortocosteroid hormones on bone. *J. Steroid Biochem.* **15,** 171–174 (1981).
17. Reid, I. R., Chapman, G. E., Fraser, T. R. C., Davies, A. D., Surus, A. S., Meyer, J., Huq, N. L., and Ibbertson, H. K. Low serum osteocalcin levels in glucocorticoid-treated asthmatics. *J. Clin. Endocrinol. Metab.* **62,** 378–388 (1986).
18. Seeman, E., Kumar, R., Hunder, G. G., Scott, M., and Heath, H. Production, degradation and circulating levels of 1,25-dihydroxyvitamin D in health and in chronic glucocorticoid excess. *J. Clin. Invest.* **66,** 664–669 (1980).
19. Chesney, R. W., Mazess, R. B., Hamstra, A. J., DeLuca, H. F., and OReagan, S. Reduction of serum-1,25-dihydroxyvitamin-D3 in children receiving glucocorticoids. *Lancet* **2,** 1123–1125 (1978).
20. Nielsen, H. K., Charles, P., and Mosekilde, L. The effect of single oral doses of prednisone on the circadian rhythm of serum osteocalcin in normal subjects. *J. Clin. Endocrinol. Metab.* **67,** 1025–1030 (1988).
21. Fucik, R. F., Kukreja, S. C., Hargis, G. K., Bowser, E. N., and Henderson, W. J. Effects of glucocorticoids on function of the parathyroid glands in man. *J. Clin. Endocrinol. Metab.* **40,** 152–185 (1975).
22. Suzuki, Y., Ichikawa, Y., Saito, E., and Homma, M. Importance of increased urinary calcium excretion in the development of secondary hyperparathyroidism of patients under glucocorticoid therapy. *Metabolism* **32,** 151–156 (1983).
23. Gray, R. E. S., Doherty, S. M., Galloway, J., Coulton, L., and Broe, D. M. A double-blind study of deflazacort and prednisone in patients with chronic inflammatory disorders. *Arthr. Rheum.* **34,** 287–295 (1991).
24. Prummel, M. F., Wiersinga, W. M., Lips, P., Sanders, G. T. B., and Sauerwein, H. P. The course of biochemical parameters of bone turnover during treatment with corticosteroids. *J. Clin. Endocrinol. Metab.* **72,** 382–386 (1991).
25. Reid, I. R., and Ibbertson, H. K. Evidence for decreased tubular reabsorption of calcium in glucocorticoid-treated asthmatics. *Horm. Res.* **27,** 200–204 (1987).
26. Jilka, R. L., Hangoc, G., Girasole, G., Passeri, G., Williams, D. C., Abrams, J. S., Boyce, B., Broxmeyer, H., and Manolagas, S. C. Increased osteoclast development after estrogen loss: mediation by interleukin-6. *Science* **257,** 88–91 (1992).
27. Cohen, H. J., Pieper, C. F., Harris, T., Rao, K. M., and Currie, M. S. The association of plasma IL-6 levels with functional disability in community dwelling elderly. *J. Gerontol.* **52,** 201–208 (1997).
28. Geisterfer, M., Richards, C. D., and Gauldie, J. Cytocines oncostatin M and interleukin 1 regulate the expression of the IL-6 receptor (gp80,gp130). *Cytokine* **7,** 503–509 (1995).
29. Ho, K. K., OSullivan, A. J., Weissberger, A. J., and Kelly, J. J. Sex steroid regulation of growth hormone secretion and action. *Horm. Res.* **45,** 67–73 (1996).
30. Marie, P. Growth factors and bone formation in osteoporosis: roles for IGF-1 and TGF-beta. *Rev. Rheum. Engl. Ed.* **64,** 44–53 (1997).
31. Peretz, A., Praet, J. P., Bosson, D., Rozenberg, S., and Bourdoux, P. Serum osteocalcin in the assessment of corticosteroid induced osteoporosis. Effect of long and short term corticosteroid treatment. *J. Rheumatol.* **16,** 363–367 (1989).
32. McCarthy, T., Centrella, M., and Canalis, E. Cortisol inhibits the synthesis of insulin-like growth factor-I in skeletal cells. *Endocrinology* **126,** 1569–1575 (1990).
33. Delamy, A. M., and Canalis, E. Transcriptional repression of insulin-like growth factor I by glucocorticoids in rat bone cells. *Endocrinology* **136,** 4776–4781 (1995).
34. Rechler, M. M. Insulin-like growth factor binding proteins. *Vitam. Horm.* **47,** 1–114 (1993).
35. Okazaki, R., Riggs, B. L., and Conover, C. A. Glucocorticoid regulation of insulin-like growth factor-binding protein expression in normal human osteoblast-like cells. *Endocrinology* **134,** 126–132 (1994).
36. Gabbitas, B., Pash, J. M., Delany, A. M., and Canalis, E. Cortisol inhibits the synthesis of insulin-like growth factor binding protein-5 in bone cell cultures by transcriptional mechanisms. *J. Biol. Chem.* **271,** 9033–9038 (1996).

37. Oursler, M. J., Riggs, B. L., and Spelsberg, T. C. Glucocorticoid-induced activation of latent transforming growth factor-β by normal human osteoblast-like cells. *Endocrinology* **133,** 2187–2196 (1993).
38. Centrella, M., McCarthy, T. L., and Canalis, E. Glucocorticoid regulation of transforming growth factor $\beta 1$ (TGF-$\beta 1$) activity and binding in osteoblast-enriched cultures from fetal rat bone. *Mol. Cell. Biol.* **11,** 4490–4496 (1991).
39. Lukert, B. P., and Raisz, L. G. Glucocorticoid-induced osteoporosis: pathogenesis and management. *Ann. Intern. Med.* **112,** 352–364 (1990).
40. MacAdams, M. R., White, R. H., and Chipps, B. E. Reduction of serum testosterone levels during chronic glucocorticoid therapy. *Ann. Intern. Med.* **104,** 648–651 (1986).
41. Morris, H. A., Need, A. G., OLoughlin, P. D., Horowitz, M., and Bridges, A. Malabsorption of calcium in corticosteroid-induced osteoporosis. *Calcif. Tissue Intl.* **46,** 305–308 (1990).
42. Laan, R. F., van Riel, P. L., van Erning, L. J., Lemmens, J. A., Ruijs, S. H., and van de Putte, L. B. Vertebral osteoporosis in rheumatoid arthritis patients: effect of low dose prednisone therapy. *Br. J. Rheumatol.* **31,** 91–96 (1992).
43. Reid, I. R., and Heap, S. W. Determinants of vertebral mineral density in patients receiving long-term glucocorticoid therapy. *Arch. Int. Med.* **150,** 2545–2548 (1990).
44. Epstein, S., and Shane, E. Transplantation Osteoporosis. *In* "Osteoporosis" (R. Marcus, D. Feldman, and J. Kelsey, eds.), pp. 947–957. Academic Press, San Diego, 1996.
45. Crabtree, G. R., and Clipstone, N. A. Signal transmission between the plasma membrane and nucleus of T lymphocytes. *Annu. Rev. Biochem.* **63,** 1045–1083 (1994).
46. Tugwell, P., Bombardier, C. Gent, M., Bennett, K. J., Bensen, W. G., Carette, S., Chalmers, A., Esdaile, J. M., Klinkoff, A. V., Kraag, G. R., Ludwin, D., and Roberts, R. S. Low-dose cyclosporine vs. placebo in patients with rheumatoid arthritis. *Lancet* **335,** 1051–1055 (1990).
47. Klaushofer, K., Hoffmann, O., Stewart, P. J., Czerwenka, E., Koller, K., Peterlik, M., and Stern, P. H. Cyclosporine A inhibits bone resorption in cultured neonatal mouse calvaria. *J. Pharmacol. Exp. Therap.* **243,** 584–590 (1987).
48. Orcel, P., Denne, M. A., and de Vernejoul, M. C. Cyclosporine A *in vitro* decreases bone resorption, osteoclast formation, and the fusion of cells of the monocyte macrophage lineage. *Endocrinology* **128,** 1638–1646 (1991).
49. Buchinsky, F. J., Ma, Y., Mann, G. N., Rucinski, B., Bryer, H. P., Romero, D. F., Jee, W. S., and Epstein, S. T lymphocytes play a critical role in the development of cyclosporine A-induced osteopenia. *Endocrinology* **137,** 2278–2285 (1996).
50. Suthanthiran, M., Morris, R. E., and Strom, T. B. Immunosuppressants: cellular and molecular mechanisms of action. *Am. J. Kidney Dis.* **28,** 159–172 (1996).
51. Hausman, P. B., and Weksler, M. E. Changes in the immune response with age. *In* "Handbook of the Biology of Aging" (C. E. Finch and E. L. Schneider, eds.), 2nd Ed., pp. 414–432, Academic Press, San Diego, 1985.
52. Ecklund, K., Laor, T., Goorin, A. M., Connolly, L. P., and Jaramillo, D. Methotrexate osteopathy in patients with osteosarcoma. *Radiology* **202,** 543–547 (1997).
53. Zonneveld, I. M., Bakker, W. K., Dijkstra, P. F., Bos, J. D., van Soesbergen, R. M., and Dinant, H. J. Methotrexate osteopathy in long-term, low-dose methotrexate treatment for psoriasis and rheumatoid arthritis. *Arch. Dermatol.* **132,** 184–187 (1996).
54. Ferraccioli, G., Casatta, L., and Bartoli, E. Increase of bone mineral density and anabolic variables in patients with rheumatoid arthritis resistant to methotrexate after cyclosporine A therapy. *J. Rheumatol.* **23,** 1539–1542 (1996).
55. van der Veen, M. J., Scheve, B. A., van Roy, J. L., Damen, C. A., Lefeber, F. P., and Bijlsma, J. W. *In vitro* effects of methotrexate on human articular cartilage and bone-derived osteoblasts. *Br. J. Rheumatol.* **35,** 342–349 (1996).
56. Riggs, B. L., and Melton, J. L. Involutional osteoporosis. *N. Engl. J. Med.* **314,** 1676–1686 (1986).
57. Baran, D. T., and Braverman, L. E. Thyroid hormones and bone. *J. Clin. Endocrinol. Metab.* **72,** 1182–1183 (1991).
58. Kung, A. W. C., Lorentz, T., and Tam, S. Thyroxine suppressive therapy decreases bone mineral density in post-menopausal women. *Clin. Endocrinol.* **39,** 535–540 (1983).
59. Mosekilde, L., and Melsen, F. A tetracycline-based histomorphometric evaluation of bone resorption and bone turnover in hyperthyroidism and hyperparathyroidism. *Acta Med. Scand.* **204,** 97–102 (1978).
60. Harvey, R. D., McHardy, K. C., Reid, I. W., Patterson, F., and Bewsher, P. D. Measurement of bone collagen degradation in hyperthyroidism and during thyroxine replacement therapy using pyridinium crosslinks as specific urinary markers. *J. Clin. Endocrinol. Metab.* **72,** 1189–1194 (1991).
61. Guarnero, P., Vassy, V., Bertholin, A., Riou, J. P., and Delmas, P. D. Markers of bone turnover in hyperthyroidism and the effects of treatment. *J. Clin. Endocrinol. Metab.* **78,** 955–959 (1994).
62. Martinez, M. E., Harranz, L., dePedro, C., and Pallardo, D. F. Osteocalcin levels in patients with hyper- and hypothyroidism. *Horm. Metab. Res.* **18,** 212–214 (1986).
63. Fallon, M. D., Perry, H. M., III, Bergfeld, M., Droke, D., Teitelbaum, S. L., and Avioli, L. V. Exogenous hyperthyroidism due to L-thyroxin treatment. *Arch. Intern. Med.* **143,** 442–444 (1983).
64. Coindre, J.-M., David, J.-P., Rivieve, L., Goussot, J.-F., Roger, P., deMascarel, A., and Meunier, P. J. Bone loss in hypothyroidism with hormone replacement. *Arch. Intern. Med.* **146,** 48–53 (1986).
65. Fujiyama, K., Kiriyama, T., Ito, M., Kimura, H., Ashizawa, K., Tsuruta, M., Nagayama, Y., Villadolid, M. C., Yokoyama, N., and Nagataki, S. Suppressive doses of thyroxine do not accelerate age-related bone loss in late postmenopausal women. *Thyroid* **5,** 13–17 (1995).
66. Bauer, D. C., Nevitt, M. C., Ettinger, B., and Stone, K. Low thyrotropin levels are not associated with bone loss in older women—a prospective study. *J. Clin. Endocrinol. Metab.* **82,** 2931–2936 (1997).
67. Stern, P. H. Thyroid hormone and bone. *In* "Principles of Bone Biology" (J. P. Bilezekian, L. G. Raisz, and G. A. Rodan, eds.), pp. 521–532, Academic Press, San Diego, 1996.
68. Schneider, D. L., Barrett-Connor, E. L., and Morton, D. J. Thyroid hormone use and bone mineral density in elderly women—effects of estrogen. *J. Am. Med. Assoc.* **271,** 1245–1249 (1994).
69. Duncan, W. E., Chang, A., Solomon, B., and Wartofsky, L. Influence of clinical characteristics and parameters associated with thyroid hormone therapy on the bone mineral density of women treated with thyroid hormone. *Thyroid* **4,** 183–190 (1994).
70. Stepan, J. J., and Limanova, Z. Biochemical assessment of bone loss in patients on long-term thyroid hormone treatment. *Bone Miner.* **17,** 377–388 (1992).
71. Franklyn, J., Betteridge, J., Holder, R., Daykin, J., Lilley, J., and Sheppard, M. Bone mineral density in thyroxine treated females with or without a previous history of thyrotoxicosis. *Clin. Endocrinol.* **41,** 425–432 (1994).
72. Lakatos, P., Hollo, I., and Horvath, C. Severe postmenopausal osteoporosis and thyroid hormones. *Arch. Intl. Med.* **146,** 1859–1863 (1986).
73. Rosen, H. N., Moses, A. C., Gundberg, C., Kung, V. T., Seyedin, S. M., Chen, T., Holick, M., and Greenspan, S. L. Therapy with

parenteral pamidronate prevents thyroid hormone-induced bone turnover in humans. *J. Clin. Endocrinol. Metab.* **77,** 664–669 (1993).

74. Fraser, S. A., Anderson, J. B., Smith, D. A., and Wilson, G. M. Osteoporosis and fractures following thyrotoxicosis. *Lancet* **1,** 981–983 (1971).
75. Saggese, G., Bertelloni, S., and Baroncelli, G. I. Bone mineralization and calcitropic hormones in children with hyperthyroidism. Effects of methimazole therapy. *J. Endocrinol. Invest.* **13,** 587–592 (1990).
76. Wartofsky, L. Use of sensitive TSH assay to determine optimal thyroid hormone therapy and avoid osteoporosis. *Annu. Rev. Med.* **42,** 341–345 (1991).
77. Allain, T. J., Chambers, T. J., Flanagan, A. M., and Mcgregor, A. M. Tri-Iodothyronine stimulates rat osteoclastic bone resorption by an indirect effect. *J. Endocrinol.* **133,** 327–331 (1992).
78. Britto, J. M., Fenton, A. J., Holloway, W. R., and Nicholson, G. C. Osteoblasts mediate thyroid hormone stimulation of osteoclastic bone resorption. *Endocrinology* **134,** 169–176 (1994).
79. Williams, G. R., Bland, R., and Sheppard, M. C. Characterization of thyroid hormone (T3) receptors in three osteosarcoma cell lines of distinct osteoblast phenotype: interactions among T3, vitamin D3, and retinoid signalling. *Endocrinology* **135,** 2375–2385 (1994).
80. Tarjan, G., and Stern, P. H. Triiodothyronine potentiates the stimulatory effects of interleukin-1-beta on bone resorption and medium interleukin-6 content in fetal rat limb bone cultures. *J. Bone Miner. Res.* **10,** 1321–1326 (1995).
81. Salvi, M., Girasole, G., Pedrazzoni, M., Passeri, M., Giuliani, N., Minelli, R., Braverman, L. E., and Roti, E. Increased serum concentrations of interleukin-6 (IL-6) and soluble IL-6 receptor in patients with Graves' disease. *J. Clin. Endocrinol. Metab.* **81,** 976–979 (1997).
82. Lakatos, P., Foldes, J., Horvath, C., Kiss, L., Tatrai, A., Takacs, I., Tarjan, G., and Stern, P. H. Serum IL-6 and bone metabolism in patients with thyroid function disorders. *J. Clin. Endocrinol. Metab.* **82,** 81 (1997).
83. Wei, J., Xu, H., Davies, J. L., and Hemmings, G. P. Increase of plasma IL-6 concentration with age in healthy subjects. *Life Sci.* **51,** 1953–1956 (1992).
84. Schmid, C., Schlapfer, I., Futo, E., Waldvogel, M., Schwander, J., Zapf, J., and Froesch, E. R. Triiodothyronine (T3) stimulates insulin-like growth factor (IGF)-1 and IGF binding protein (IGFBP)-2 production by rat osteoblasts *in vitro. Acta Endocrinol.* **126,** 467–473 (1992).
85. Lakatos, P., Caplice, M. D., Khanna, V., and Stern, P. H. Thyroid hormones increase insulin-like growth factor-I content in the medium of rat bone tissue. *J. Bone Miner. Res.* **8,** 1475–1481 (1993).
86. Varga, F., Rumpler, M., and Klaushofer, K. Thyroid hormones increase insulin-like growth factor mRNA levels in the clonal osteoblastic cell line MC3T3-E1. *FEBS Lett.* **345,** 67–70 (1994).
87. Benbasset, C. A., Maki, K. C., and Unterman, T. G. Circulating levels of insulin-like growth factor (IGF) binding protein-1 and -3 in aging men: relationships to insulin, glucose, IGF, and dehydroepiandrosterone sulfate levels and anthropometric measures. *J. Clin. Endocrinol. Metab.* **82,** 1484–1491 (1997).
88. Mohan, S., Farley, J. R., and Baylink, D. J. Age-related changes in IGFBP-4 and IGFBP-5 levels in human serum and bone: implications for bone loss with aging. *Prog. Growth Fact. Res.* **6,** 465–473 (1995).
89. Glantschnig, H., Varga, F., and Klaushofer, K. Thyroid hormone and retinoic acid induce the synthesis of insulin-like growth factor-binding protein-4 in mouse osteoblastic cells. *Endocrinology* **137,** 281–286 (1996).
90. Foldes, J., Lakatos, P., Zsadanyi, J., and Horvath, C. Decreased serum IGF-I and dehydroepiandrosterone sulphate may be risk factors for the development of reduced bone mass in postmenopausal women with endogenous subclinical hyperthyroidism. *Eur. J. Endocrinol.* **136,** 277–281 (1997).
91. Hahn, T. J., Birge, S. J., Scharp, C. R., and Avioli, L. V. Phenobarbital-induced alterations in vitamin D metabolism. *J. Clin. Invest.* **51,** 741–748 (1972).
92. Ohishi, T., Kushida, K., Takahashi, M., Kawana, K., Inoue, T., and Yagi, K. Analysis of urinary pyridinoline and deoxypyridinoline in patients undergoing long-term anticonvulsant drug therapy. *Eur. Neurol.* **36,** 300–302 (1996).
93. Alderman, C. P., and Hill, C. L. Abnormal bone mineral metabolism after long-term anticonvulsant treatment. *Ann. Pharmacother.* **28,** 47–48 (1997).
94. Jacques, P. F., Felson, D. T., Tucker, K. L., Mahnken, B., Wilson, P., Rosenberg, I. H., and Rush, D. Plasma 25-hydroxyvitamin D and its determinants in an elderly population sample. *Am. J. Clin. Nutr.* **66,** 929–936 (1997).
95. Bettica, P., Bevilacqua, M., Vago, T., and Norbiato, G. High prevalence of vitamin D deficiency among free-living postmenopausal women in Northern Italy. *J. Bone. Miner. Res.* **12,** 218 (1997).
96. Schmidt-Gayk, H., Bouillon, R., and Roth, H. J. Measurement of vitamin D and its metabolites (calcidiol and calcitriol) and their clinical significance. *Scand. J. Clin. Lab. Invest.* **57,** 35–45 (1997).
97. Chapuy, M. C., Preziosi, P., Maamer, M., Arnaud, S., Galan, P., Hercberg, S., and Menuiner, P. J. Prevelance of vitamin D insufficiency in an adult normal population. *Osteopor. Intl.* **7,** 439–443 (1997).
98. Francis, R. M., Boyle, I. T., Moniz, C., Sutcliffe, A. M., Davis, B. S., Beastall, G. H., Cowan, R. A., and Downes, N. A comparison of the effects of alfacalcidol treatment and vitamin D2 supplementation on calcium absorption in elderly women with vertebral fractures. *Osteopor. Intl.* **6,** 284–290 (1996).
99. Francis, R. M. Is there a differential response to alfacalcidol and vitamin D in the treatment of osteoporosis? *Calcif. Tissue Intl.* **60,** 111–114 (1997).
100. Ebeling, P. R., Sandgren, M. E., DiMagno, E. P., Lane, A. W., DeLuca, H. F., and Riggs, B. L. Evidence of an age-related decrease in intestinal responsiveness to vitamin D: relationship between serum 1,25-dihydroxyvitamin D3 and intestinal vitamin D receptor concentrations in normal women. *J. Clin. Endocrinol. Metab.* **75,** 176–182 (1992).
101. Jones, G., Nguyen, T., Sambrook, P. N., and Eisman, J. A. Thiazide diuretics and fractures: can meta-analysis help? *J. Bone Miner. Res.* **10,** 106–111 (1995).
102. Dawson-Hughes, B., and Harris, S. Thiazides and seasonal bone changes in healthy postmenopausal women. *Bone Miner.* **21,** 41–51 (1993).
103. Aubin, R., Menard, P., and Lajeunesse, D. Selective effect of thiazides on the human osteoblast-like cell line MG-63. *Kidney Intl.* **50,** 1476–1482 (1996).
104. Blumsohn, A., Herrington, K., Hannon, R. A., Shao, P., Eyre, D. R., and Eastell, R. The effect of calcium supplementation on the circadian rhythm of bone resorption. *J. Clin. Endocrinol. Metab.* **79,** 730–735 (1994).
105. Greenspan, S. L., Drezner-Pollack, R., Parker, R. A., London, D., and Ferguson, L. Diurnal variation of bone mineral turnover in elderly men and women. *Calcif. Tissue Intl.* **60,** 419–423 (1997).
106. MacGibbon, M. F. Aging as upregulation failure. *Med. Hypoth.* **46,** 523–527 (1996).

CHAPTER 21

Nutritional Mechanisms of Age-Related Bone Loss

JOHN J. B. ANDERSON Department of Nutrition, Schools of Public Health and Medicine, University of North Carolina, Chapel Hill, North Carolina 21599

INTRODUCTION TO NUTRIENT-INDUCED OSTEOPENIA

The emphasis in this chapter is on environmental, i.e., nutritional, contributions to age-related bone loss and the maintenance of bone tissue by the elderly. The occurrence of low bone mass (osteopenia) and osteoporosis late in life has become commonplace in the late 20th century because of greater numbers of elderly in the population—an estimated 15% over 60 years of age—and declines in intakes of bone-promoting nutrients. The ready availability of high-quality foods has provided a supply of nutrients in technologically advanced nations that have been, in part, responsible for the advancing age of the US population, but as physical activities decline among the elderly, so does total energy consumption. The intakes of all other nutrients decrease as energy intake falls. The plight of the elderly, then, is that they have difficulty consuming the many micronutrients from foods in amounts needed to maintain bone health. The logical answer is to recommend supplements balanced with respect to all micronutrients for the support of bone health. Issues related to calcium and vitamin D are covered in other chapters.

This chapter focuses on the micronutrients that are needed to maintain bone mineral content (BMC) and bone mineral density (BMD) late in life rather than on the energy-providing macronutrients (carbohydrates, fats, and proteins).

EXCESSIVE ANIMAL PROTEIN INTAKE

High intakes of animal protein contribute to increased urinary calcium excretion [1,2], whereas the calciuric effect of plant proteins, especially soy protein, is much smaller [3,4]. Normally, protein is considered to be essential for healthy bone maintenance, but the conclusions of numerous reports of experimental findings support the contention that excessive intakes of total protein, assuming that a large proportion is from animal sources, relative to the recommended intakes for each gender (of the order of 50 to 60 g per day), increase the urinary loss of calcium [5]. One group of investigators has even suggested that the high protein intakes of Western nations is responsible for the high rates of osteoporosis [6]. Longer studies are needed to verify these acute and short-term results.

Animal proteins are much more acid producing than plant proteins because of their higher levels of specific amino acids containing sulfur and phosphate groups [5]. The result of an increase in net acid excretion is an increase in urinary calcium, as shown in numerous dietary studies [7]. Vegetarians typically have urinary pH values near neutrality, whereas omnivores have pH values in the range of 4 to 6. This mechanism has been suggested as one way that the vegetarian diet may act to protect bone health.

EXCESSIVE SODIUM INTAKE AND INADEQUATE POTASSIUM INTAKE

High intakes of sodium also contribute to increased urinary calcium excretion [8]. In both human subjects [9,10] and experimental animals [11], convincing data on sodium-induced hypercalciuria have been shown. The pervasive use of high sodium has adverse effects on skeletal tissue, especially when calcium intakes are low. The mechanism by which bone tissue is lost is considered to be via an indirect elevation of parathyroid hormone (PTH) when the serum calcium ionic concentration is slightly reduced following renal calcium losses.

In contrast to a high sodium intake, potassium has been shown to improve calcium balance in postmenopausal women [12]. Following a 14-day period of administration of potassium bicarbonate, the improved calcium status of the subjects was credited to enhanced buffering by the bicarbonate to counter the acidogenic diets, typical of meat-eating individuals.

Potassium itself may also be beneficial to bone health. An epidemiologic study using the Framingham Heart Study population found that adequate potassium intake, derived primarily from plant sources, supports BMD maintenance better than inadequate potassium intake [13].

The role that acid per se plays in stimulating bone resorption has not been adequately appreciated, despite strong evidence derived from experimental animal and human investigations [5]. An important conclusion derived from these studies is that more plant sources and fewer animal foods should be consumed for the conservation of bone, as long as calcium intakes are sufficient.

INADEQUACIES OF OTHER NUTRIENTS

Several other micronutrients with essential roles in bone tissue, may also be inadequate in the diets of the elderly. They are vitamin K, vitamin C, vitamin A, magnesium, boron, and other trace minerals. Less research has been conducted on these micronutrients compared to calcium, phosphorus, and vitamin D, but they nevertheless are essential for bone health. Balanced dietary intakes should provide adequate amounts of all of these nutrients if energy intake is adequate. If total energy consumption, however, is not at least 1200 kcal per day, many elderly subjects, mainly females, will develop insufficiencies first and then deficiencies in one or more of these micronutrients. It has not been so easy to identify suboptimal intakes of other micronutrients because of the multiple variables that require a complexity of experimental designs. One type of approach has been to supplement one experimental group with several trace minerals at a time and compare the changes in bone measurements after a year to a group that receives only a placebo (or a placebo containing calcium) (see later). For example, Strause *et al.* [14] supplemented an elderly group of subjects with three trace minerals plus calcium and compared their bone measurements to those of a control group receiving only calcium.

Inadequate Vitamin K Intake

Vitamin K is required for the production of at least three different proteins of bone matrix, including osteocalcin. The action of vitamin K is to modify the protein molecules, after translation, by adding carboxyl groups to specific glutamate residues in the peptide chain. Undercarboxylated osteocalcin is considered to be a risk factor for fractures [15,16]. Except for supplements, vitamin K is only obtained from vegetable sources, particularly dark greens and legumes. Because so many North Americans consume far fewer servings of vegetables than recommended (minimum of three per day), it is easy to see why so many have inadequate intakes of vitamin K [17]. Individuals who consume more servings of dark greens and other good sources of vitamin K are suggested to be at lower risk of fractures [18,19].

Supplementation studies using vitamin K have been undertaken. For example, the administration of a large amount of vitamin K for 12 months resulted in improved BMD and bone markers [20]. In another study, fast bone losers during the postmenopause benefit in terms of significantly reduced urinary calcium losses from vitamin K supplementation [21].

Inadequate Vitamin C Intake

Vitamin C (ascorbic acid) is required for collagen (type I) modification in bone tissue. This molecular change is posttranslational, as is true for the vitamin K action on several matrix proteins of bone tissue, but in collagen, the changes include hydroxylations of proline and lysine residues in all three strands of the triple helix. Many animal studies have clearly established the essential role of vitamin C in the development of healthy bones. Animals on diets deficient in ascorbic acid develop severely compromised matrix structures [22]. In addition to vitamin C, iron is also required for the hydroxylation steps that lead to mature collagen. The amount of vitamin C needed to maintain bone health has not been established, but it has been suggested from studies of bone markers of collagen turnover that the current recommended dietary allowance (RDA) of 60 mg per day is sufficient. More studies are needed to establish the optimal vitamin C intake for bone health.

Inadequate Vitamin A Intake

Vitamin A is essential for bone growth and development, primarily for the differentiation of bone cells, osteoblasts and osteoclasts, that carry out the functions of bone formation and bone resorption, respectively. Several epidemiologic studies support an important role for dietary sources of vitamin A (β-carotene) in bone tissue, but little evidence from experimental models has been generated.

Inadequate Magnesium Intake

An epidemiologic study of older subjects in the Framingham Heart Study suggested that a lower magnesium intake was reported in male and female subjects with low BMD of the greater trochanter of the proximal femur compared to those with greater BMD [13]. Other findings from human trials [23] and observational studies [24], although limited, suggest that higher magnesium consumption or supplement use improves skeletal measurements and perhaps reduces fracture risk. It is not established yet whether individuals taking a combination supplement of calcium and vitamin D will have a negative impact on magnesium status.

Inadequate Boron Intake

So little is known about the role of boron in bone formation or resorption that a plausible mechanism cannot be proposed. It would seem almost impossible for an individual to develop boron deficiency because of its widespread abundance in foods and also as a contaminant in foods. Because boron is a "bone seeker" in the body, it probably accumulates in the skeleton with age. Although much has been written about this element in the popular press, only limited scientific evidence for an essential role of boron in human bone development or maintenance has been published [25]. Studies using rats have shown that both vertebral strength and compression are increased following boron treatment in the diet for 12 weeks [26].

Inadequate Intakes of Other Trace Minerals

Only one major investigation has examined the effect of a mixture of trace minerals (along with calcium) on changes in BMD over a period of a year [14]. Significant improvement in vertebral BMD was found, but it is unclear whether the gains were from calcium, the trace minerals, or both. Further investigations are warranted to sort out the beneficial nutrients.

EXCESSIVE FLUORIDE INGESTION

Although very uncommon in the United States and most nations with municipal water supplies, occasional cases of flouride overingestion have been reported by the CDC or in the dental literature because of the consumption of high fluoride well water. Because fluoride accumulation in the skeleton is age related, the elderly who have been consuming fluoridated water throughout their lives may already have a significant load. Because of the high avidity of the skeleton for fluoride ions, a positive balance occurs throughout life. Treatment of fluorosis or less severe aspects of this condition requires administering a daily calcium phosphate supplement (1000 mg of elemental calcium) to form healthy new bone and to stimulate the removal of fluoride from blood and skeletal tissues by renal and other routes.

Newly formulated fluoride supplements for the treatment of osteoporosis have yielded promising results in trials of postmenopausal women [27,28], but they have not yet been approved by the FDA for use.

BONE-RELATED FOOD ISSUES OF THE ELDERLY IN TECHNOLOGICALLY ADVANCED NATIONS

In the United States and most highly technological nations over the last five decades, the food supply has been modified in many important ways, most of them for good, but a few for bad. Many foods are highly processed with numerous additives and fortificants (nutrients) placed in them, as well as other components, such as dietary fiber, removed. The two major nutritional concerns raised here, namely the excessive use of salt or sodium and phosphate salts in many foods in the marketplace, are quite relevant to the aging skeleton. A third concern, i.e., excessive animal protein consumption, has been covered in an earlier section.

Western Food Supply—Highly Processed, Fast Foods, Snack Foods, and Soft Drinks: High Phosphate and High Sodium

Many fast foods and convenience or snack foods are high in salt or other sodium salts that are used by the food industry both to preserve foods and to provide the salt taste consumers crave. Over the last two decades, food producers have reduced the quantities of salt used in practically all foods, but consumers can still ingest excessive amounts by consuming the highly processed foods rather than unprocessed or lightly processed foods. Label reading, especially the ingredients list and Nutrition Facts, is important for consumers because the labels give a quick estimate of the percent of sodium of the daily value (PDV) and of the rank order of sodium or salt in the ingredients list. (This list is prepared in decreasing order by quantity of each ingredient in the food.) Excessive sodium consumption not only compromises calcium conservation and bone health [8], but excessive sodium, especially from sodium-processed foods, has also become an established risk factor for hypertension.

In addition to sodium, many processed foods and cola-type beverages have significant amounts of phosphate salts added to them. These phosphate additives have several useful functions in foods, but they add up in terms of extra amounts of phosphates in the diet. This increased commercial application has had a major impact on phosphate intake in the United States over the last few decades [29]. Even the processing of dairy foods, such as cheese slices and puffed cheeses, involves the use of phosphate additives. The total intake of phosphates from foods and beverages may have an adverse effect on both the calcium-to-phosphate ratio and bone health (see earlier chapters). Therefore, phosphorus intakes from foods, both natural and processed, can tip the balance with respect to calcium in an unhealthy direction [30].

Nutrient Fortification

Calcium-fortified foods, such as orange juice, bread, and other grain products, have been beneficial, in general, in increasing calcium intake. Because excessive calcium intake from all sources (foods and supplements), however, may interfere with the intestinal absorption of a few divalent cations (iron and zinc), it would be prudent to be certain that the upper limit of safety of calcium, estimated to be 2500 mg a day, not be exceeded. Several essential nutrients in supplements in addition to calcium, when consumed at approximately 100% of the U.S. RDA, may also be beneficial to bone health.

Multiple Nutrient Supplementation: Vitamins and Minerals

The use of a daily supplement may improve the intakes of many nutrients and it should provide each nutrient at approximately 100% of the U.S. RDA, but not higher unless prescribed by a physician. The reason for caution on the upper limits of amounts of micronutrients is because of the potential adverse interactions between two or more nutrients that typically depress the absorption or utilization of one nutrient (see earlier discussion).

Several commercial bone-promoting formulas, containing many of the nutrients mentioned herein, have been developed for the support of skeletal health. A few of these bone-related products are now available for consumers and others can be expected in the future. Attention needs to be paid to the amounts of the nutrients in these preparations before making recommendations to patients.

INTAKE RECOMMENDATIONS FOR BONE HEALTH

The Food and Nutrition Board of the Institute of Medicine and of the National Academy of Sciences has issued new recommendations for intakes of calcium, phosphate, fluoride, and vitamin D for populations in the United States and Canada [31]. These recommendations are currently our best guide to consumers in support of assuring intakes that should support the healthy development and maintenance of bone tissue across the life cycle. Recommendations for nutrient intakes that support bone health of the population beyond 50 years of age are listed in Table I. Additional recommendations for other essential nutrients related to the health of other organ systems of older age groups will be released within the next couple of years.

A concern among some nutrition experts is that the adequate intakes for calcium are, in general, set too high. Reasons for this concern revolve around the imprecise estimates of calcium requirements at various stages of the life cycle. Calcium has been clearly established as a threshold nutrient, and additional amounts of calcium beyond the threshold apparently have little effect on calcium retention or functional end points, such as BMD. Another concern relates to the potential adverse effects of excessive calcium intakes on the absorption and utilization of other divalent cations in the diet, an area of investigation that has received only limited attention by researchers.

Common foods that contain sufficient amounts of these nutrients to meet the recommendations are listed in Table II. Because of shortfalls in the intakes of several of these bone-promoting micronutrients—calcium, vitamin D, and others—by the U.S. population, nutrition education about the selection of foods and consumption of healthy diets containing these foods needs to be greatly expanded. A predominate message from dietary

TABLE I Recommended Intakes of Nutrients Required for Bone Development and Maintenance

Age (years)	Calcium (mg/day AI[a])	Phosphorus (mg/day RDA[b])	Magnesium (mg/day RDA)		Vitamin D (μg/day AI)	Fluoride (mg/day AI)	
1–3	500	460	80		5	0.7	
4–8	800	500	130		5	1.1	
			M	F		M	F
9–13	1300	1250	240	240	5	2.0	2.0
14–18	1300	1250	410	360	5	3.2	2.9
19–30	1000	700	400	310	5	3.8	3.1
31–50	1000	700	420	320	5	3.8	3.1
51–70	1200	700	420	320	10	3.8	3.1
>70	1200	700	420	320	15	3.8	3.1

[a] Adequate intake.
[b] Recommended dietary allowance.

surveys of Americans, including NHANES, is that more servings of vegetables and fruits need to be consumed each day to obtain at least the recommended minimum of five. Five servings or more a day should provide adequate amounts of potassium, magnesium, several B vitamins, and vitamins A (or β-carotene), C, and K. In addition, low-fat fortified dairy foods provide calcium, vitamins D and A, and several B vitamins. Fish foods also improve the diet by providing vitamin D, vitamin A, polyunsaturated fatty acids, and several essential trace minerals.

Another benefit derived from eating plant foods that are not generally available from supplements is the ingestion of many phytomolecules that are not classified as nutrients. These phytomolecules may play important roles in the health of several organ systems, including bone. Two examples are the diverse dietary fiber molecules and the phytoestrogens. Specific phytoestrogens found in soy foods, namely genistein and related isoflavones, may act on osteoblasts to improve bone mass, as demonstrated in experimental animal models [32] and one human investigation [33].

TABLE II Common Foods That Supply Good Amounts of Nutrients Required for the Development and Maintenance of Healthy Skeletal Tissues

Nutrient[a]	Common foods
Calcium	Dairy, tofu (calcium-set), dark greens, fortified orange juice and other foods
Phosphorus	Practically all foods except natural oils
Magnesium	Dark greens
Vitamin D	Fish, fish oils, fortified dairy
Fluoride	Seafoods of all kinds, tea, wine
Potassium	Fruits and vegetables, meats
Vitamin C	Fruits and vegetables, fortified drinks and other foods
Vitamin A	Fruits and vegetables, fortified dairy and other foods
Vitamin K	Dark greens, legumes

[a] Many of the nutrients can also be found in fortified breakfast cereals.

SUMMARY

A balanced selection of foods is recommended for each day, but a large percentage of the elderly population fail to achieve this balance, especially in the consumption of bone-related nutrients from plant sources such as cereals, vegetables, and fruits, as well as from dairy products. This failure is an age-old problem, but the solution for it is not simply the recommendation of taking a multinutrient supplement. Excessive reliance on supplements does not typically provide the nonnutrient phytochemical molecules that are so rich in plant sources. Many other plant molecules may also have health-promoting effects on human skeletal tissue, but prospective studies of elderly human subjects are currently in progress.

A balance of nutrient intake also implies getting the appropriate proportions of calcium and phosphate, and of sodium and potassium, so that imbalances do not contribute to calcium and bone losses. Other nutrients in excess, notably the acid-forming proteins from animal foods, may also contribute to losses of calcium and bone mineral. Typically, the nutrients consumed in excess, phosphate, sodium, and even animal protein, exert their adverse effects on calcium and bone metabolism through elevations in PTH.

Recommended intakes for bone health generated by the Food and Nutrition Board of the Institute of Medicine, plus the food guide pyramid should be used in guiding elderly patients. It is recommended that registered dietitians be consulted for difficult cases.

Acknowledgments

Appreciation for the careful reading and assistance in the preparation of this manuscript is expressed to Drs. Sanford C. Garner, Martin Kohlmeier, and Svein U. Toverud.

References

1. Schuette, S. A., and Linkswiler, H. M. Effects of Ca and P metabolism in humans by adding meat, meat plus milk, or purified proteins plus Ca and P to a low protein diet. *J. Nutr.* **112,** 338–349 (1982).
2. Lutz, J. Calcium balance and acid-base status of women as affected by increased protein intake and by sodium bicarbonate ingestion. *J. Nutr.* **39,** 281–288 (1984).
3. Anderson, J. J. B., Thomsen, K., and Christiansen, C. High protein meals, insular hormones and urinary calcium excretion in human subjects. *In* "Osteoporosis 1987" (C. Christiansen, J. S. Johansen, and B. J. Riis, eds.), pp. 240–245. Osteopress ApS, Copenhagen, 1987.
4. Kerstetter, J. E., and Allen, L. H. Dietary protein increases urinary calcium. *J. Nutr.* **120,** 134–136 (1990).
5. Barzel, U. S. The skeleton as an ion exchange system: Implications for the role of acid–base imbalance in the genesis of osteoporosis. *J. Bone Miner. Res.* **10,** 1431–1436 (1995).
6. Abelow, B. J., Holford, T. R., and Insogna, K. L. Cross-cultural association between dietary animal protein and hip fracture: A hypothesis. *Calcif. Tissue Int.* **150,** 14–19 (1992).
7. Lemann, J., Jr., Pleuss, J. A., and Gray, R. W. Potassium causes calcium retention in healthy adults. *J. Nutr.* **123,** 1623–1626 (1993).
8. Massey, L. K., and Whiting, S. J. Dietary salt, urinary calcium, and bone loss. *J. Bone Miner. Res.* **11,** 731–736 (1996).
9. Nordin, B. E. C., Need, A. G., Morris, H. A., and Horowitz, M. The nature and significance of the relationship between urinary sodium and urinary calcium in women. *J. Nutr.* **123,** 1615–1622 (1993).
10. Nordin, B. E. C., and Need, A. G. The effect of sodium on calcium requirement. *In* "Advances in Nutritional Research" (H. H. Draper, ed.), Vol. 9, pp. 209–230. Plenum Press, New York, 1994.
11. Goulding, A., and Gold, E. Effects of dietary NaCl supplementation on bone synthesis of hydroxyproline, urinary hydroxyproline excretion and bone ^{45}Ca uptake in the rat. *Hormone Metabol. Res.* **20,** 743–745 (1988).
12. Sebastian, A., Harris, S. T., Ottaway, J. H., Todd, K. M., and Morris, R. C., Jr. Improved mineral balance and skeletal metabolism in postmenopausal women treated with potassium bicarbonate. *N. Engl. J. Med.* **330,** 1776–1781 (1994).
13. Tucker, K. L., Hannan, M. T., Chen, H., Cupples, L. A., Wilson, P. W. F., and Kiel, D. P. Potassium, magnesium, and fruit and vegetable intakes are associated with greater bone mineral density in older men and women. *Am. J. Clin. Nutr.,* in press.
14. Strause, L., Saltman, P., Smith, K. T., Bracker, M., and Andon, M. B. Spinal bone loss in postmenopausal women supplemented with calcium and trace minerals. *J. Nutr.* **124,** 1060–1064 (1994).
15. Szulc, P., Chapuy, M. C., Meunier, P. J., and Delmas, P. D. Serum undercarboxylated osteocalcin is a marker of the risk of hip fracture: A three year follow-up study. *Bone* **18,** 487–488 (1996).
16. Vergnaud, P., Garnero, P., Meunier, P. J., Breart, G., Kamihagi, K., and Delmas, P. D. Undercarboxylated osteocalcin measured with a specific immunoassay predicts hip fracture in elderly women: The EPIDOS Study. *J. Clin. Endocrinol. Metab.* **82,** 719–724 (1997).
17. Kohlmeier, M., Gartis, S., and Anderson, J. J. B. Vitamin K: A vegetarian promoter of bone health. *Veg. Nutr.* **1,** 53–57 (1997).
18. Kohlmeier, M., Saupe, J., Shearer, M. J., Schaefer, K., and Asmus, G. Bone health of adult hemodialysis patients is related to vitamin K status. *Kidney Intl.* **51,** 1218–1221 (1997).
19. Kohlmeier, M., Saupe, J., Schaefer, K., and Asmus, G. Bone fracture history and prospective bone fracture risk of hemodialysis patients are related to apolipoprotein E genotype. *Calcif. Tissue Int.,* in press.
20. Orimo, H., Fujita, T., Onomura, T., Kushida, K., and Shiraki, M. Clinical evaluation of Ea-0167 (menetetranone) in the treatment of osteoporosis—Phase III double blind multicenter comparative study with alfacalcidiol. *Clin. Eval.* **20,** 45–100 (1992).
21. Knapen, M. H. J., Kon-Siong, G. J., Hamulyák, K., and Vermeer, C. Vitamin K-induced changes in markers for osteoblast activity and urinary calcium loss. *Calcif. Tissue Int.* **53,** 81–85 (1993).
22. Kipp, D. E., Grey, C. E., McElvain, M. E., Kimmel, D. B., Robinson, R. G., and Lukert, B. P. Long-term low ascorbic acid intake reduces bone mass in guinea pigs. *J. Nutr.* **126,** 2044–2049 (1996).
23. Stendig-Lindberg, G., Tepper, R., and Leichter, I. Trabecular bone density in a two-year controlled trial of peroral magnesium in osteoporosis. *Magn. Res.* **6,** 155–163 (1993).
24. Gullestad, L., Nes, M., Ronneberg, R., Midtvedt, K., Falch, D., and Kjekshus, J. Magnesium status in healthy free-living Norwegians. *J. Am. Coll. Nutr.* **13,** 45–50 (1994).
25. Nielsen, F. H., Gallagher, S. K., Johnson, L. K., and Nielsen, E. J. Boron enhances and mimics some effects of estrogen therapy in postmenopausal women. *J. Trace Elements Exp. Med.* **5,** 237–246 (1992).
26. Chapin, R. E., Ku, W. W., Kenney, M. A., McCoy, H., Gladen, B., Wine, R. N., Wilson, R., and Elwell, M. R. The effects of dietary boron on bone strength in rats. *Fundam. Appl. Toxicol.* **35,** 205–215 (1997).
27. Pak, C. Y. C., Sakhaee, K., Piziak, V., Peterson, R. D., Breslau, N. A., Boyd, P., Poindexter, J. R., Herzog, J., Heard-Sakhaee, A., Haynes, S., Adams-Huet, B., and Reisch, J. S. Slow-release sodium fluoride in the management of postmenopausal osteoporosis: A randomized controlled trial. *Ann. Intern. Med.* **120,** 625–632 (1994).
28. Pak, C. Y. C., Sakhaee, K., Adams-Huet, B., Piziak, V., Peterson, R. D., and Poindexter, J. R. Treatment of postmenopausal osteoporosis with slow-release sodium fluoride: Final report of a randomized control trial. *Ann. Intern. Med.* **123,** 401–408 (1995).
29. Calvo, M. S., and Park, Y. K. *J. Nutr.* **126,** 11685–11805 (1996).
30. Anderson, J. J. B. *In* "The Cambridge World History of Food and Nutrition" (K. F. Kiple, ed.), Cambridge Univ. Press, New York, in press.
31. Food and Nutrition Board, Institute of Medicine, National Research Council, "Dietary Reference Intakes." National Academy Press, Washington, DC, 1998.
32. Anderson, J. J. B., Ambrose, W. W., and Garner, S. C. Biphasic effects of genistein on bone tissue in the ovariectomized, lactating rat model. *Proc. Soc. Exp. Biol. Med.* **217,** 345–350 (1998).
33. Potter, S. M., Baum, J. A., Teng, H., Stillman, R. J., and Erdman, J. W., Jr. Soy protein and isoflavones: Their effects on blood lipids and bone density in postmenopausal women. *Am. J. Clin. Nutr.* **68**(Suppl), 1375S–1379S (1998).

Part IV

Quantifiable Manifestations of Age-Related Bone Loss

CHAPTER 22

Racial/Ethnic Influences on Risk of Osteoporosis

DOROTHY A. NELSON Department of Internal Medicine, Wayne State University School of Medicine, Detroit, Michigan 48201

MARIE LUZ VILLA Department of Medicine, University of Washington School of Medicine, Mercer Island, Washington 98040

INTRODUCTION

Race and Ethnicity

"Ethnicity" and "race" appear interchangeably in many publications. "Race" in the United States reflects the belief that there are several (i.e., a limited number) of genetically characterized human groups. This is exemplified by the list used by the U.S. census: White/Caucasian, Black/African American, Native American/American Indian, Alaskan native/Eskimo/Aleut, Asian/Pacific Islander, or other (Spanish or Hispanic origin is asked separately). Most investigators recognize, however, that distinct racial lines may not be drawn due to a significant genetic admixture that has occurred over time. Furthermore, population geneticists such as physical anthropologists believe that human biologic variability can usually be explained within an evolutionary framework of adaptations over time in a particular environment. The result of this is that the frequency of any trait or set of traits has a continuous and fluctuating (i.e., "clinal") distribution over space. Because environments have changed and continue to change and because populations move and interbreed, it would be difficult, if not impossible, to identify discrete subgroups of the human species that are meaningful biologically.

Factors that reflect cultural, religious, dietary, geographic, and other differences among major geographic groups ("races") comprise another category, known as ethnicity, that results in innumerable subgroups [1]. In fact, ethnicity plays an important role in disease prevalence even within races. For example, Hispanic whites show different trends in disease incidence compared to non-Hispanic whites (an ethnic dichotomization of the "White/Caucasian" category specific to the Americas). Mexican-Americans have a two- to fivefold greater risk of developing noninsulin-dependent diabetes mellitus (NIDDM) than the majority of the U.S. population [2].

Limitations of Using Arbitrary Categories in Medical Research

Lack of ethnic definition of study groups affects the general applicability of data. For example, a study reporting hip fracture rates of "Asians" is almost certainly not specific enough to determine a Korean woman's risk of suffering a hip fracture. Ethnic-specific data would be more valuable than a broad, racial summarization because bone mineral densities (BMD) and fracture rates vary among countries, as well as within ethnic subgroups. In a study comparing the average BMD of Japanese, Korean, and Taiwanese women, the Taiwanese had consistently greater BMD at the lumbar spine at almost every age [3]. In a study of African American and white children by Nelson and Barondess [4], a large subgroup of the whites considered themselves Chaldean, an Iraqi ethnic group. The Chaldean children's whole body bone mass was significantly higher than non-Chaldean white children and was not different from the subjects who considered themselves black. Because Middle Easterners are included in the U.S. census category "White/Caucasian," such a difference would not be expected a priori and would affect the results of the study if the Chaldeans were analyzed together with other white children.

The environment in which a member of a given population is born and raised also affects his/her risk for osteoporotic fracture [5]. This is illustrated by the wide range of hip fracture incidence for elderly Japanese women (from 450 to 1011 per 100,000 person-years/year) [6], depending on their region of origin. This variability may be due in part to the phenomenon known as "acculturation," or the degree to which an ethnic group assimilates the language, habits, and cultural values of the country or area to which it migrates [7–9]. Thus, a higher acculturation score means greater adoption of the dominant culture of a region. The degree of acculturation may also affect dietary and life-style habits of people inhabiting a given region for many years: for example, African Americans preserve many distinct customs and dietary habits when moving to regions outside the southern United States [10]. Returning to the example of ethnic differences in the incidence of diabetes, the prevalence of NIDDM varies within Hispanic ethnic groups, depending on degree of acculturation: for Mexican Americans, the rate of NIDDM decreases with increasing acculturation [11].

Sometimes acculturation may serve as a proxy for factors that affect the observed disease frequency but are themselves not easily measured. For instance, variations in calcium intake and physical activity during pubertal growth may influence differences in the attainment of peak bone mass. It is difficult to assess these factors retrospectively (in older age groups) because of the substantial inaccuracy of recall. If, in addition, the study group originated in another country or was reared under very different cultural conditions than the group for which the tool was validated, even greater measurement error may be introduced. Because the assessment of ethnicity and acculturation helps to describe disease occurrence among populations, such an approach to discovering reasons for observed differences in fracture rates is essential. For this reason, as well as the pitfalls associated with "race" described earlier, we will use "ethnic" instead of "racial" in most of the contexts that follow.

Ethnic Influences on Risk for Osteoporosis

Many factors affect the risk of developing osteoporosis or suffering nontraumatic hip fracture, although low bone mass is the major contributing factor. Age is an independent predictor of fracture risk, and family history, falls, bone geometry, and exposure to certain medications are other important contributors [12–16]. It is not clear that all populations are similarly characterized with respect to these and other variables relating to calcium intake, vitamin D levels, physical activity, body weight, and so on. Most purported risk factors were established from studies of non-Hispanic whites. It seems intuitive that most people should respond similarly to elements such as medication use, reproductive hormone status, and physical activity. However, some evidence shows that other factors such as calcium metabolism, bone mass, and body composition may have different effects from one racial or ethnic group to the next.

FACTORS AFFECTING BONE MASS

Ethnicity and Bone Mass

The term bone mass can refer to a variety of measurements, including bone mineral content (BMC in g), areal bone mineral density (BMD in g/cm^2), and volumetric or true bone density (BMD in g/cm^3). The degree of ethnic differences in bone mass reported by various investigators varies with the measurement used as well as with other factors. African Americans have significantly greater areal BMD than non-Hispanic whites [17–21], which is thought to contribute to their lower rate of osteoporosis and fracture. It is not well understood whether such differences in bone mass exist at birth or develop at some point thereafter. Most studies based on absorptiometry (SPA, DEXA) found a higher bone mass (bone mineral content or areal bone "density") throughout childhood [22–27]. Some studies of true bone density (g/cm^3), based on QCT, found no distinction in skeletal status between black and white children [28,29]. For example, Gilsanz and colleagues [29] examined bone mineral density in black and non-Hispanic white children at different stages of sexual development and found that significant differences did not occur until late puberty. However, Kleerekoper *et al.* [19] have shown that volumetric BMD measured by QCT is 40% higher in African American compared with white women. This is considerably greater than the 5–15% difference in areal BMD generally reported for African American versus white adults.

It has been suggested that the higher bone mass seen in North American blacks stems in part from genetic factors. This is logical because nearly 80% of bone mass is genetically determined [30,31]. However, U.S. blacks' gene pool is very heterogeneous and is the result of much admixture over several centuries. It might be assumed that any population of African origin would have a high bone mass similar to African Americans, but this has not been borne out. Investigations of blacks in South Africa [17,32–34] and Gambia [35] do not support this theory, inasmuch as their bone mass does not exceed that of age-matched African whites. These data illustrate the difficulty in generalizing about a "racial" group, when ethnic gradations in bone mass within people of African descent obviously exist, with further differences introduced by acculturation in areas to which black Africans migrated.

Another interesting issue that arises from studies of non-American blacks is that despite having a bone mass similar to whites, African blacks have a relatively low fracture risk [17,32]. Other paradoxical examples are that Hispanics have hip fracture incidence rates comparable to those of African Americans, yet have bone mass values closer to those of non-Hispanic whites [36,37], and Asian populations demonstrate a similar relationship [38–40]. One South American ethnic group in Vilcabamba, Ecuador, enjoys an extremely low rate of hip fracture despite bone mineral density values much lower than that of non-Hispanic whites [41]. Bone mass therefore may not be the factor that best predicts fracture risk in all ethnic groups other than non-Hispanic whites and blacks in the United States. This may render recent World Health Organization guidelines for diagnosis of osteoporosis [42] only narrowly applicable.

Bone Turnover

Risk for osteoporotic fracture depends not only on the mass of bone, but its quality as well. Bone architecture is an essential component of skeletal strength, which may be affected by the rate and efficiency of bone turnover. This, in turn, is affected by reproductive hormone status, body composition, vitamin D and calcium nutriture, and physical activity.

There have been a few studies of bone turnover in blacks compared with whites. It has been suggested that lower bone turnover in black adults may partially explain their greater lifelong bone mass and lower fracture risk than non-Hispanic whites. Two studies found biochemical evidence that blacks have lower rates of bone turnover than non-Hispanic whites [19,43]. In addition, Weinstein and Bell [44] demonstrated histomorphometrically that the mean rate of bone formation in American blacks appears to be about 35% that of non-Hispanic whites. However, studies comparing South Africans suggested higher bone turnover in blacks, which was proposed to lead to fewer fractures because of better trabecular bone quality and less skeletal fragility [45,46]. These contrasting studies again highlight the pitfalls associated with assuming that subgroups (such as geographically different populations) of a "racial" group will be biologically similar.

A series of articles by Parfitt's group [47–49] has illuminated some of the effects of ethnicity on the structure and geometry, remodeling and turnover, and mineralization indices of iliac bone. In studies of 35 African American and 109 white women, they found that African Americans had more cancellous and cortical bone than whites due to both thicker trabeculae and thicker cortices, but that both groups showed a reduction in the amount and structure of bone as the result of age or menopause [47]. They also reported that the geometric mean bone formation rate on the combined total surface was 25% lower in African Americans than in whites and that serum osteocalcin was lower by about 15% in blacks, but that bone-specific alkaline phosphatase was not different [48]. Finally, the ratio of mineralizing surface to osteoid surface was about 25% lower in African Americans than in whites on all surfaces; that finding indicates a slower terminal mineralization. Their overall conclusion was that most, if not all, ethnic differences observed in bone cell function could be the result of differences in bone accumulation during growth: a higher bone mass would result in less fatigue damage and less need for repair by directed bone remodeling [49].

No studies have directly compared bone turnover of Asians, blacks, and whites, but it appears that the reported normal values for circulating osteocalcin in Japanese women are lower than those of non-Hispanic white women [50,51]. However, Polynesians and whites do not manifest different serum concentrations of osteocalcin or parathyroid hormone (PTH) or urinary excretion of hydroxyproline, despite significant differences in BMD [52]. In one study of young Mexican American and non-Hispanic whites, osteocalcin levels did not differ significantly between the two groups despite differences in 25-hydroxyvitamin D and PTH values [53].

Differences in reproductive hormone status may contribute to ethnic variation in bone turnover, skeletal quality, and subsequent fracture risk. Androgens and estrogens contribute positively and independently to attainment of peak bone mass [54,55], and adult bone loss often stems from the increased bone turnover associated with decreased levels of reproductive hormones [50]. Furthermore, serum unbound sex steroid concentrations are lower in women with hip fracture than in controls [56]. Gilsanz and colleagues [29] found that black–white differences in bone mass develop during late stages of puberty, perhaps related to differences in serum sex hormone levels. Bone loss in Japanese women appears to be greatest in the early postmenopausal period, but subsequently declines at rates similar to those for non-Hispanic whites [50,57]. In a large study of postmenopausal women conducted in the northeast region of the United States, ethnicity and serum estrone levels contributed independently to observed black–white differences in bone mass [58]. Serum estrone was significantly higher in African Americans, but ethnic differences in estrone disappeared when analyses were adjusted for obesity (as determined by body mass index ≥ 27.3 kg/m^2).

Body Size and Composition

Body size appears to be an independent contributor to variance in BMD in most studies. Therefore, use of a mathematical correction for differences in densitometric bone size [59] from one population to another might correct for differences in body habitus and may shed some light on the seeming discrepancies between bone mass and fracture risk across ethnic groups. In a multisite study of hormone replacement and its effects on bone mass in postmenopausal women, it was noted that although African Americans had the highest measured bone mass, when adjustments were made for bone size, the ethnic differences in bone density were significantly attenuated [20]. Despite the widely accepted axiom that Asians have lower bone mass than non-Hispanic whites, a comparison of closely matched non-Hispanic white and Chinese women found slightly higher bone mass in the Chinese when height and weight (and theoretically differences in bone size) were controlled [60]. Data suggest that differences in bone accumulation in multiethnic teenagers may predominantly reflect bone size [61].

Body weight contributes heavily to the maintenance of bone density, and thinness is an important risk factor for hip fracture in African American, white, and Asian women [62–64]. However, it appears that both fat and lean body mass contribute to preservation of the skeleton [65,66], perhaps due in part to peripheral aromatization of androgen to estrogen that occurs in adipose tissue and skeletal muscle [56,66,67]. Serum estrone levels relate positively to the degree of obesity, and bone mass correlates positively with body weight in both black and white women [68]. However, differences in body weight do not explain the differences in bone mass between these groups [69]. Epidemiologic studies indicate that African American women are classified as overweight twice as frequently as non-Hispanic white women [70], but that differences in body mass index (BMI) do not develop until after adolescence (of note, that is about the time differences in bone mass become apparent as well). Obesity classification typically depends on self-report of weight and height, with subsequent computation of BMI. Obesity is defined as BMI ≥ 27.3 kg/m^2 [71]. This definition is based on statistics from the second National Health and Nutrition Examination Survey (NHANES II), using the 85th percentile of BMI for 20- to 29-year-old non-Hispanic whites as an obesity cutoff point. Application of this definition for obesity has not been race or ethnicity adjusted in the majority of studies. Lopez and Mâsse [72] compared anthropometric data from NHANES II to that acquired during the 1982–1984 Hispanic Health and Nutrition Examination Survey (HHANES). They found that use of the NHANES II obesity cutoff consistently labeled 12–14% more Puerto Rican and Mexican American women as obese than if ethnicity-specific cutoff data from HHANES were used [72]. Cuban American women's BMIs reflected those of NHANES II data; thus the use of an "Hispanic"-specific cutoff is meaningless because there are differences in height and weight distribution among the Hispanic ethnic groups.

The optimal formula for a body mass index, which is conventionally expressed as weight/height^2, varies among populations. If the purpose of using a weight for height index is to minimize the effect of height on body mass, then one approach to identifying an appropriate index is to find the exponent for the denominator that minimizes the correlation between weight and height (such that $r = 0$) in a given population [73]. Kleerekoper *et al.* [74] applied this approach to 201 white and 77 African American postmenopausal women participating in a longitudinal study of bone mass and biochemical markers of bone remodeling [74]. The African American women had a significantly greater BMI based on the conventional formula. However, the formula that best provided a height-free measure of weight was different for the white [weight (kg)/height(m)$^{1.17}$] and African American women [weight(kg)/height(m)$^{1.30}$]. When BMI was calculated using these population-specific formulae, there was no significant difference between the two groups, suggesting that these African American women were not more "obese." This underscores the need to consider population-specific approaches to studying human biologic phenomena.

Although BMI is often used to estimate the degree of obesity, body composition is much more complex. The simplest model uses bone, fat, and lean body mass as the three major components. Because bone and lean body mass are closely related [75], it stands to reason that groups with increased muscle mass, such as African Americans and Polynesians [52,76], will have higher bone mass. Therefore, total body weight will be greater in those with higher bone mass, not necessarily because of obesity but also due to the contribution of bone and muscle weight. Body composition comparisons made between African American and non-Hispanic white adults demonstrate consistently greater muscle and bone mass in the former [77,78], which again underscores the importance of using ethnicity-specific reference populations when interpreting body habitus data.

Calcium Nutrition and Calcium Metabolism

Calcium intake affects the attainment of peak bone mass as well as the ability to preserve skeletal calcium throughout life [79]. In an early study, Matkovic and colleagues demonstrated that hip fracture rates differed significantly in two regions of Croatia with divergent levels of dietary calcium intake [80] and concluded that these differences were due to differences in the attainment of peak bone mass. Gradations in bone mass related to calcium intake are also observed in other ethnic groups. In an excellent dietary study of Chinese women with similar ethnic backgrounds, Hu and collaborators [81] demonstrated a wide range in BMD depending on dietary calcium intake [81]. In that group, although the women with a higher calcium intake had higher BMD, the rate of bone loss with age was not affected by dietary calcium, supporting the hypothesis that the differences in bone mass observed in older women were realized earlier in life. Calcium nutriture may contribute to differences in the bone mass of Japanese and Japanese American groups as well [82,83], and calcium supplementation has been shown to reduce bone loss in elderly Chinese women [84].

Ethnic differences in the absorption and excretion of calcium may affect overall calcium balance. One study conducted under conditions of severe calcium restriction found African Americans to have low vitamin D levels and compensatory hypersecretion of parathyroid hormone [51]. It was proposed that these conditions could maximize urinary retention of calcium and theoretically contribute to greater bone mass. Another study that provided adequate dietary calcium found no evidence of an alteration in the vitamin D endocrine system [85]. However, despite a lack of ethnic differences in dietary calcium and vitamin D intake, it was found that African Americans had significantly lower urinary calcium excretion and that calcium excretion was inversely related to radial BMD. Kleerekoper *et al.* [19] reported statistically significant differences in calciotropic hormones and biochemical markers of bone remodeling in a group of 112 African American and 250 white women aged 55–75. Parathyroid hormone levels and 1,25-vitamin D were higher in African Americans, and 25-vitamin D, osteocalcin, hydroxyproline, and bone specific alkaline phosphatase were lower in African American compared to white women ($P < 0.05$). These data may suggest possible resistance to the skeletal actions of PTH in African Americans [19].

Vitamin D Exposure

Hypovitaminosis D, when present in non-Hispanic white populations, predicts low bone mass and increased risk for hip fractures [86,87]. A similar relationship is seen among inhabitants of Hong Kong, where hypovitaminosis D appears as a common problem in elders with hip fracture [88]. In this group, subclinical vitamin D deficiency is also associated with muscle weakness and an increased risk of falling. Studies conducted in Japan note a marked beneficial effect on BMD and spinal fracture rate in patients treated with vitamin D [89]. It appears, therefore, that individuals from divergent ethnic backgrounds respond similarly to the influence of circulating 25-hydroxyvitamin D (25OHD).

There are regional differences in vitamin D levels that are attributable to differences in the level of solar radiation, individuals' exposure to sunlight, and skin color. Differences in skin pigmentation reflect an evolutionary adaptation to solar radiation, according to one theory, so those living closer to the equator would have greater amounts of skin pigment in order to reduce the risk of hypervitaminosis D and/or other adverse conditions [90]. Conversely, those living in higher latitudes would have fairer skin in order to make sufficient amounts of vitamin D. Data suggest that there is a difference in the gradient of skin color south of the equator compared with north of the equator [91]; this would suggest that factors other than solar radiation affect skin pigmentation.

Some investigators find that individuals with high and low skin pigmentation possess similar 25OHD synthetic abilities in response to ultraviolet exposure [92]. Other suggest or propose that increased pigment reduces the capacity of skin to synthesize vitamin D [51,53,93]. Data presented in abstract form showed a high prevalence of inadequate vitamin D nutriture in a group of elderly Mexican American women, but this was related to vitamin D exposure rather than skin pigmentation [94]. Matsuoka and colleagues [95], in a multiracial/ethnic study of the relationship between skin pigment and cutaneous synthesis of vitamin D, found that increased skin pigmentation had a photoprotective effect but did not impair adequate formation of vitamin D. A comparison of African blacks and whites living in Zaire or Belgium found no racial differences when the study was conducted in Zaire [96]. However, evaluation of respective groups in Belgium demonstrated lower vitamin D levels in blacks, with an inverse relationship noted between serum 25OHD and length of stay in Belgium [96]. It is possible that at northern latitudes, life-style habits such as avoidance of sun-seeking behavior, and a low intake of vitamin D fortified foods, will result in lower levels of circulating 25OHD. This manifests itself in the protective response of mild secondary hyperparathyroidism reported by some investigators [97].

Vitamin D Receptor Gene

In 1992, Morrison *et al.* [98] reported that allelic variation in several polymorphisms at the vitamin D receptor (VDR) gene locus could be used to predict bone turnover (specifically, osteocalcin) and later reported an association with bone mass in a large group of white Australian women [98]. In a second study, *Bsm*I restriction fragment length polymorphism (RFLP) genotypes were characterized by significant differences in mean bone density such that the "bb" genotype had the highest bone mass, "BB" the lowest, and the heterozygote was intermediate [99]. Attempts to corroborate these findings in other populations have yielded variable results, as well as investigations of other RFLPs.

Investigations of the VDR in U.S. populations have included mainly white women but some have included other ethnic groups, including African Americans [100–104] and Mexican Americans [105]. Results of these are somewhat contradictory, as discussed later, which may reflect ethnic and/or environmental differences in the genotype frequencies as well as on the expression of the VDR. Outside the United States, data from a study of Japanese women suggest an association between VDR gene polymorphisms and both BMD and the rate of postmenopausal bone loss [106].

Fleet *et al.* [101] reported no significant ethnic difference in genotype distribution in 83 white and 72 African American women aged 20–40. There was also no significant interaction of ethnicity and genotype on BMD of the femoral neck and lumbar spine [101], although there was a significant relationship between genotypes and bone density in the group as a whole. Harris *et al.* [102], using a start codon polymorphism detected with the endonuclease *Fok*I, found black/white differences in its distribution among premenopausal women. They suggest that this polymorphism appears to influence peak bone density and that ethnic differences in the genotype frequencies may help explain some of the ethnic difference in femoral neck BMD. Nelson *et al.* drew a similar conclusion using the *Bsm*I polymorphism, reporting a significant difference in genotype distribution between groups of 19 African American and 23 white premenopausal women, as well as a significantly higher mean whole body bone mass in the bb genotype in the groups combined [103,104]. It was striking that the BB, or low bone mass genotype, was absent among the African American women. Their data suggest that ethnic differences in the distribution of the *Bsm*I genotypes may help explain observed ethnic difference in whole body bone mass in younger adult women. Zmuda *et al.* [100] investigated three VDR gene polymorphisms (*Bsm*I, *Apa*I, and *Taq*I), bone turnover, and rates of bone loss in older African American women. They did not find an association between VDR gene polymorphisms and BMD or indices of bone turnover in this group. McClure *et al.* [105] studied these three RFLPs in postmenopausal Mexican American women and did not find significant associations with BMD, but there were trends suggesting that a larger sample size may reveal such associations. It appears that the age ranges of the subjects and the sample sizes of different studies may account for some of the apparently contradictory findings.

Spotila *et al.* [107] reported a cross-sectional study of 48 men, 56 premenopausal women, and 80 postmenopausal women comprising three different sets of European ethnic groups: southern, eastern, and western European. They found ethnic/regional differences in the frequencies of the genotypes ($P = 0.048$) as well as in spine BMD in the men and the premenopausal women ($P < 0.05$). However, they found no effect of VDR genotype on BMD in any of the groups.

Although much of the literature since Morrison *et al.* first reported their VDR results has been negative, several investigators have suggested that there may be linkage of this RFLP with other genes that control bone and mineral metabolism. Such genes may affect intestinal calcium transport [100] or absorption [108] or other influences on bone mass. The VDR itself may modify the effect of vitamin D levels on bone turnover [109,110], and some studies have indicated that an increased calcium intake may modify the effect of the VDR genotype on the rate of bone loss [111,112].

Physical Activity and Other Life-Style Factors

Physical activity benefits the skeleton and health in general throughout all stages of life and is a life-style habit subject to great variation among different groups. Despite various cultural values and attitudes toward physical activity throughout life, its beneficial effect on bone mass appears ubiquitous. Ethnic differences in bone mass and fracture risk related to physical activity habits are seen in studies from Sweden [5], Japan [113], and Hawaii [114]. Although multicultural studies concerning type of physical activity and accretion of bone density are lacking, it would be valuable to determine whether culturally determined activities during adolescence affect lifetime risk for fracture. It could be that habitual activities or work during youth affect adult bone mass and possibly skeletal structure. In a study of prepubertal children, Nelson *et al.* [4] found that Chaldean (an Iraqi ethnic group) and black children had significantly greater bone mass than white children in a suburb of Detroit and that the Chaldean children paradoxically were less physically active than the other two groups. However, they had a larger body size and greater fat mass, suggesting that relative sedentism in these prepubertal children may temporarily enhance bone mass through a greater body mass. As discussed earlier body size is a significant predictor of bone mass in adults.

Physical activity and its effects on muscle strength, balance, and coordination are of benefit to the skeleton by reducing the risk and effects of falling in adults. Another life-style factor that may be important is smoking, which is thought to reduce calcium absorption [115], and heavy smokers appear to have lower bone mineral density than light smokers or nonsmokers [116]. Elderly Japanese American men who smoke have significantly faster rates of bone loss than those who do not [117], but the relationship among smoking, bone mass, race, and ethnicity has not been widely studied.

BONE GEOMETRY

Bone mineral density predicts fracture risk, but there is considerable overlap of BMD in hip fracture cases and white controls. Also, as noted previously, there is considerable variation in fracture risk among ethnic groups with similar BMD values. Thus, there must be factors other than bone mass that affect risk for osteoporotic fracture. Analysis of data collected in a large study of osteoporotic fracture suggests that a simple geometric measurement of femoral size, the hip axis length (HAL), is related to hip fracture risk [16]. In this study, longer HAL was associated with an increased risk of hip fracture; fracture cases had an average HAL of 6.9 ± 0.4 and controls 6.7 ± 0.4 cm ($p = 0.0001$). Two ethnic groups with lower risk for hip fracture than non-Hispanic whites also have shorter HALs: African Americans have a HAL of 6.4 ± 0.4 and Asian Americans 6.3 ± 0.3 cm [118]. Additionally, the HAL of Mexican American women, an ethnic group with a relatively low risk for hip fracture, averages 6.3 ± 0.3 cm [36], a value similar to that of African Americans and Asian Americans and significantly less than that of non-Hispanic Whites. A study comparing Japanese and white differences in geometric properties of the femoral neck demonstrated an association between low fracture risk and short femoral neck [119], substantiating the importance of considering bone geometric properties when evaluating fracture risk across ethnic groups. Data suggest that differences in hip axis length appear to be attenuated in American teenage multiethnic groups as opposed to populations living in countries of origin [61]. (Further discussion of bone geometry can be found in Chapter 10.) Other geometric measures include cross-sectional geometry using DEXA data, gross morphometry based on radiogrammetry, and grading of trabecular patterns such as the Singh index [120–126].

ETHNIC DIFFERENCES IN RATES OF HIP FRACTURE

Broad conclusions can be drawn regarding differences in hip fracture incidence rates for members of different ethnic groups. Age- and sex-adjusted incidence rates of hip fracture in blacks, Hispanic and non-Hispanic whites, Asians, or Pacific Islanders are available from many sources [6,127–157] (see Table I). However, many authors do not give detailed information about the racial and ethnic backgrounds of groups studied. As a result, data presented here include differences in the *use* of ethnic and racial categories.

Because few studies prior to 1980 were conducted in groups other than non-Hispanic whites, our discussion will be largely focused on studies conducted in the 1980s. Non-Hispanic whites show the greatest hip fracture incidence rates of any ethnic group, particularly in northern Europe and North America. Studies in the United States demonstrate that hip fracture incidence in Asian Americans is intermediate to those of non-Hispanic whites and blacks. Although the number of studies in Hispanics is small, estimates of hip fracture incidence in this group are close to (and in some cases lower than) rates among black Americans [130,131]. Hip fracture incidence among black South Africans was reported to be very low in a study conducted between 1950 and 1964 [133], but there are no more recent studies in African populations.

Studies conducted in racially mixed populations using the same methods for ascertaining hip fractures in all groups are particularly valuable for making inferences about ethnic differences in hip fracture incidence [127–131,136]. Most of these studies have been conducted in the United States and consistently indicate higher rates among non-Hispanic whites than among other ethnic groups. In a study conducted in Bexar County, Texas, the age- and sex-adjusted hip fracture incidence was lowest in blacks and highest in non-Hispanic whites, with intermediate rates for Hispanics [131]. In contrast, Silverman and Madison [130] found that the age- and sex-adjusted incidence of hip fracture in California was lower among Hispanic whites than among all other groups, including non-Hispanic whites, blacks, and Asians. A study comparing hip fracture incidence among native Japanese, Japanese American, and non-Hispanic whites [6] reported the lowest rates among Japanese Americans and the highest rates among non-Hispanic whites.

Increasing age is an established risk factor for hip fracture in all groups. A useful review of differences in age-specific incidence rates of hip fracture among ethnic groups is provided by Villa and Nelson [158]. Although

Table I Age-Adjusted Rates[a] of Hip Fracture per 100,000 Population for Females, Males, and Total by Ethnic Group and Year of Study[b]

Ethnic group	Site (reference)	Years of study	Female	Male	Total	Female : male
Blacks	United States [127]	1986–1989	214	179	200	1.2
	Maryland [128]	1979–1988	345	191	283	1.8
	United States [129]	1984–1985	344	235	300	1.5
	California [130]	1983–1984	241	153	202	1.6
	Texas [131]	1980	243	13	141	18.7
	United States [132]	1974–1979	174	108	137	1.6
	Johannesburg, South Africa [133]	1950–1964	26	20	23	1.3
Hispanics[c]	California [130]	1983–1984	219	97	165	2.3
	Texas [131]	1980	305	128	227	2.4
Asians	Tottori, Japan [134]	1986–1987	227	79	163	2.9
	Hong Kong [135]	1985	389	196	304	2.0
	Okinawa, Japan [6]	1984–1985	325	86	219	3.8
	California [130]	1983–1984	383	116	265	3.3
	Hawaii [6]	1979–1981	224	66	153	3.4
	New Zealand [136]	1973–1976	212	121	172	1.8
	Hong Kong [137]	1965–1967	179	113	150	1.6
	Singapore [138]	1955–1962	83	111	95	0.7
Caucasians[d]	United States [127]	1986–1989	968	396	738	2.4
	Maryland, [128]	1979–1988	950	358	712	2.7
	Sweden [139]	1985	714	268	517	2.7
	United States [129]	1984–1985	845	350	645	2.4
	Canada [140]	1976–1985	788	307	595	2.6
	California [130]	1983–1984	617	215	439	2.9
	Norway [141]	1983–1984	737	298	543	2.5
	Oxford, England [142]	1983	603	114	392	5.3
	United States [143]	1970–1983	705	244	506	2.9
	Minnesota [6]	1978–1982	613	285	468	2.2
	Hawaii [6]	1979–1981	645	205	451	3.1
	Alicante, Spain [144]	1974–1984	90	57	75	1.6
	Sweden [145]	1972–1981	714	319	540	2.2
	Sweden [146]	1972–1981	730	581	664	1.3
	Finland [147]	1980	432	199	329	2.2
	Dundee, Scotland [148]	1980	550	—	—	—
	Sweden [149]	1980	984	338	705	2.9
	Texas [131]	1980	593	223	430	2.7
	Oslo, Norway [150]	1978–1979	850	329	620	2.6
	Edin, Scotland [151]	1978–1979	529	174	376	3.0
	United States [132],	1974–1979	422	151	285	2.8
	Funen, Denmark [152]	1973–1979	4863	200	2804	24.3
	Yorkshire, United Kingdom [153]	1973–1977	310	102	218	3.0
	New Zealand [136]	1973–1976	466	139	321	3.4
	Rochester [154]	1965–1974	559	191	396	2.9
	Finland [147]	1970	377	142	273	2.7
	Kuopio, Finland [155]	1968	280	107	204	2.6
	Jerusalem, Israel [156]	1957–1966	355	168	272	2.1
	Malmo, Sweden [157]	1950–1960	468	153	329	3.1

[a] Rates were age and gender adjusted to the 1990 U.S. non-Hispanic Caucasian population.
[b] From Villa and Nelson [158].
[c] Hispanic Caucasians.
[d] Non-Hispanic Caucasians.

hip fracture incidence increases with age in all ethnic groups, the increase occurs earlier in non-Hispanic white populations than in black, Asian, and Hispanic populations [159]. Studies conducted in non-Hispanic white populations report higher rates of hip fracture among men than women before 50 years of age, whereas women have higher rates than men after age 50. Environmental factors such as diet, level of physical activity, frequency of cigarette smoking, and use of hormonal medications may explain some of the differences in hip fracture incidence observed among ethnic groups.

SUMMARY

The wide ranges in bone mass and in the incidence of osteoporotic fracture observed across ethnic groups and geographic regions confirm that many factors enter into the determination of osteoporosis risk. Interethnic studies that include a wide variety may help elucidate possible etiologies in the pathogenesis of osteoporosis. In order to best delineate these factors, investigators must explore contributions from the genetic, environmental, and cultural milieu that characterize different groups of people. Bone mass, in and of itself, may not best predict fracture risk in all groups. Variables such as rates of bone turnover, bone geometry, calcium intake and metabolism, vitamin D status, body composition, and life-style factors all contribute to fracture risk, reflecting the rich diversity and flexibility in adaptation that is peculiar to the human species.

References

1. Villa, M. L. Cultural determinants of skeletal health: The need to consider both race and ethnicity in bone research. *J. Bone Miner. Res.* **9,** 1329–1332 (1994).
2. Hanis, C. L., Ferrell, R. E., Barton, S. A., Aguilar, L., Garza-Ibarra, A., Tulloch, B. R., Garcia, C. A., and Schull, W. J. Diabetes among Mexican Americans in Starr County, Texas. *Am. J. Epidemiol.* **118,** 659–672 (1983).
3. Sugimoto, T., Tsutsumi, M., Fujii, Y., Kawakatsu, M., Negishi, H., Lee, M. C., Tsai, K. S., Fukase, M., and Fujita, T. Comparison of bone mineral content among Japanese, Koreans, and Taiwanese assessed by dual-photon absorptiometry. *J. Bone Miner. Res.* **7,** 153–159 (1992).
4. Nelson, D. A., and Barondess, D. A. Whole body bone, fat and lean mass in children: comparison of three ethnic groups. *Am. J. Phys. Anthropol.* **103,** 157–162 (1997).
5. Jónsson, B., Gärdsell, P., Johnell, O., Sernbo, I., and Gullberg, B. Life-Style and different fracture prevalence: A cross-sectional population-based study. *Calcif. Tissue Int.* **52,** 425–433 (1993).
6. Ross, P. D., Norimatsu, H., Davis, J. W., Yano, K., Wasnich, R. D., Fujiwara, S., Hosoda, Y., and Melton, L. A comparison of hip fracture incidence among native Japanese, Japanese Americans, and American Caucasians. *Am. J. Epidemiol.* **133,** 801–809 (1991).
7. Anderson, J., Moeschberger, M., Chen, M. J., Kunn, P., Wewers, M. E., and Guthrie, R. An acculturation scale for Southeast Asians. *Soc. Psychiatr. Psychiatr Epidemiol.* **28,** 134–141 (1993).
8. Cuellar, I., Harris, L. C., and Jasso, R. An acculturation scale for Mexican-American normal and clinical populations. *Hispanic J. Behav. Sci.* **2,** 199–217 (1980).
9. Hazuda, H. P., Stern, M. P., and Haffner, S. M. Acculturation and assimilation among Mexican Americans: Scales and population-based data. *Soc. Sci. Q.* **69,** 687–706 (1988).
10. Jerome, N. W. Diet and acculturation. *In* "Nutritional Anthropology: Contemporary Approaches to Diet and Culture" (N. W. Herome, R. F. Kandel, and G. H. Pelto, eds.), pp. 275–325, Redgrave, 1980.
11. Hazuda, H. P., Haffner, S. M., Stern, M. P., and Eifler, C. W. Effects of acculturation and socioeconomic status on obesity and diabetes in Mexican Americans. *Am. J. Epidemiol.* **128,** 1289–1301 (1988).
12. Ross, P. D., Wasnich, R. D., and Vogel, J. M. Detection of prefracture spinal osteoporosis using bone mineral absorptiometry. *J. Bone Miner. Res.* **3,** 1–11 (1988).
13. Stanley, H. L., Schmitt, B. P., Poses, R. M., and Deiss, W. P. Does hypogonadism contribute to the occurrence of minimal trauma hip fracture in elderly men? *J. Am. Geriatr. Soc.* **39,** 766–771 (1991).
14. Cummings, S. R., Kelsey, J. L., Nevitt, M. C., and O'Dowd, K. J. Epidemiology of osteoporosis and osteoporotic fractures. *Epidemiol. Rev.* **7,** 178–207 (1985).
15. Raisz, L. G. Local and systemic factors in the pathogenesis of osteoporosis. *N. Engl. J. Med.* **318,** 818–828 (1988).
16. Faulkner, K. G., Cummings, S. R., Black, D., Palermo, L., Glüer, C.-C., and Genant, H. K. Simple measurement of femoral geometry predicts hip fracture: The study of osteoporotic fractures. *J. Bone Miner. Res.* **8,** 1211–1217 (1993).
17. Solomon, L. Bone density in aging Caucasian and African populations. *Lancet* **2,** 1326–1330 (1979).
18. Luckey, M. M., Meier, D. E., Mandeli, J. P., DaCosta, M. C., Hubbard, M. L., and Goldsmith, S. J. Radial and vertebral bone density in white and black women: Evidence for racial differences in premenopausal bone homeostasis. *J. Clin. Endocrinol. Metab.* **69,** 762–770 (1989).
19. Kleerekoper, M., Nelson, D. A., Peterson, E. L., Flynn, M. J., Pawluszka, A. S. Jacobsen, G., and Wilson, P. Reference data for bone mass, calciotropic hormones, and biochemical markers of bone remodeling in older (55–75) postmenopausal white and black women. *J. Bone Miner. Res.* **9,** 1267–1276 (1994).
20. Marcus, R., Greendale, G., Blunt, B. A., Bush, T. L., Sherman, S., Sherwin, R., Wahner, H., and Wells, B. Correlates of bone mineral density in the Postmenopausal Estrogen/Progestin Interventions Trials. *J. Bone Miner. Res.* 1467–1476 (1994).
21. Liel, Y., Edwards, J., Shary, J., Spicer, K. M., Gordon, L., and Bell, N. H. The effects of race and body habitus on bone mineral density of the radius, hip, and spine in premenopausal women. *J. Clin. Endocrinol. Metab.* **66,** 1247–1250 (1988).
22. Li, J. Y., Specker, B. L., Ho, M. L., and Tsang, R. C. Bone mineral content in black and white children 1 to 6 years of age. Early appearance of race and sex differences. *Am. J. Dis. Child.* **143,** 1346–1349 (1989).
23. Bell, N. H., Shary, J., Stevens, J., Garza, M., Gordon, L., and Edwards, J. Demonstration that bone mass is greater in black than in white children. *J. Bone Miner. Res.* **6,** 719–723 (1991).
24. McCormick, D. P., Ponder, S. W., Fawcett, H. D., and Palmer, J. L. Spinal bone mineral density in 335 normal and obese children and adolescents: Evidence for ethnic and sex differences. *J. Bone Miner. Res.* **6,** 507–513 (1991).
25. Laraque, D., Arena, L., Karp, J., and Gruskay, D. Bone mineral content in black pre-schoolers: Normative data using single photon absorptiometry. *Pediatr. Radiol.* **20,** 461–463 (1990).
26. Garn, S. M., Sandusky, S. T., Nagy, J. M., and McCann, M. B. Advanced skeleton development in low-income and Negro children. *J. Pediatr.* **80,** 965–969 (1972).
27. Nelson, D. A., Simpson, P. M., Johnson, C. C., Barondess, D. A., and Kleerekoper, M. The accumulation of whole body

skeletal mass in third- and fourth-grade children: effects of age, sex, ethnicity, and body composition. *Bone* **20,** 73–78 (1997).

28. Southard, R. N., Morris, J. D., Mahan, J. D., Hayes, J. R., Torch, M. A., Sommer, A., and Zipf, W. B. Bone Mass in healthy children: Measurement with quantitative DXA. *Radiology* **179,** 735–738 (1991).
29. Gilsanz, V., Roe, T. F., Mora, S., Costin, G., and Goodman, W. G. Changes in vertebral bone density in black girls and white girls during childhood and puberty. *N. Engl. J. Med.* **325,** 1597–1600 (1991).
30. Kelly, P. J., Eisman, J. A., and Sambrook, P. N. Interaction of genetic and environmental influences on peak bone density. *Osteopor. Int.* **1,** 56–60 (1990).
31. Pocock, N. A., Eisman, J. A., Hopper, J. L., Yeates, M. G., Sambrook, P. N., and Eberl, S. Genetic determinants of bone mass in adults: a twin study. *J. Clin. Invest.* **80,** 706–710 (1987).
32. Daniels, E. D., Pettifor, J. M., Schnitzler, C. M., Russell, S. W., and Patel, D. N. Ethnic differences in bone density in female South African nurses. *J. Bone Miner. Res.* **10,** 359–67 (1995).
33. Daniels, E. D., Pettifor, J. M., Schnitzler, C. M., Moodley, G. P., and Zachen, D. Differences in mineral homeostasis, volumetric bone mass and femoral neck axis length in black and white South African women. *Osteopor. Int.* **7,** 105–112 (1997).
34. Patel, D. N., Pettifor, J. M., Becker, P. J., Grieve, C., and Leschner, K. The effect of ethnic group on appendicular bone mass in children. *J. Bone Miner. Res.* **7,** 263–272 (1992).
35. Prentice, A., Laskey, M. A., Shaw, J., Cole, T. J., and Fraser, D. R. Bone mineral content of Gambian and British children aged 0–36 months. *Bone Miner.* **10,** 211–224 (1990).
36. Villa, M. L., Marcus, R., Delay, R. R., and Kelsey, J. L. Factors contributing to skeletal health of postmenopausal Mexican-American women. *J. Bone Miner. Res.* **10,** 1233–1242 (1995).
37. Looker, A. C., Wahner, H. W., Dunn, W. L., Calvo, M. S., Harris, T. B., Heyse, S. P., Johnston, C. C., Jr., and Lindsay, R. L. Proximal femur bone mineral levels of U.S. adults. *Osteopor. Int.* **5,** 389–409 (1996).
38. Russell-Aulet, M., Wang, J., Thornton, J., Colt, E. W., and Pierson, R. J. Bone mineral density and mass by total body dual-photon absorptiometry in normal white and Asian men. *J. Bone Miner. Res.* **6,** 1109–1113 (1991).
39. Yano, K., Wasnich, R. D., Vogel, J. M., and Heilbrun, L. K. Bone mineral measurements among middle-aged and elderly Japanese residents in Hawaii. *Am. J. Epidemiol.* **119,** 751–764 (1984).
40. Hagiwara, S., Miki, T., Nishizawa, Y., Ochi, H., Onoyama, and Morii, H. Quantification of bone mineral content using dual-photon absorptiometry in a normal Japanese population. *J. Bone Miner. Res.* **4,** 217–222 (1989).
41. Mazess, R. B. Bone mineral in Vilcabamba, Ecuador. *Am. J. Roentgenol.* **130,** 671–674 (1978).
42. Kanis, J. A., Melton, L. J., III, Christiansen, C., Johnston, C. C., and Khaltaev, N. The diagnosis of osteoporosis. *J. Bone Miner. Res.* **9,** 1137–1141 (1994).
43. Meier, D. E., Luckey, M. M., Wallenstein, S., Lapinski, R. H., and Catherwood, B. Racial differences in pre- and postmenopausal bone homeostasis: Association with bone density. *J. Bone Miner. Res.* **7,** 1181–1189 (1992).
44. Weinstein, R. S., and Bell, N. H. Diminished rates of bone formation in normal Black adults. *N. Engl. J. Med.* **319,** 1698–1701 (1988).
45. Schnitzler, C. M. Bone quality: A determinant for certain risk factors for bone fragility. *Calcif. Tissue Int.* **53,** S27–S31 (1993).
46. Schnitzler, C. M., Pettifor, J. M., Mesquita, J. M., Bird, M. D., Schnaid, E., and Smyth, A. E. Histomorphometry of iliac crest bone in 346 normal black and white South African adults. *Bone Miner.* **10,** 183–199 (1990).
47. Han, Z.-H., Palnitkar, S., Nelson, D., Rao, D. S., and Parfitt, A. M. Effect of ethnicity and age or menopause on the structure and geometry of iliac bone. *J. Bone Miner. Res.* **11,** 1967–1975 (1996).
48. Han, Z.-H., Palnitkar, S., Rao, D. S., Nelson, D., and Parfitt, A. M. Effects of ethnicity and age or menopause on the remodeling and turnover of iliac bone: implications for mechanisms of bone loss. *J. Bone Miner. Res.* **12,** 498–508 (1997).
49. Parfitt, A. M., Han, Z.-H., Palnitkar, S., Rao, D. S., Shih, M.-S., and Nelson, D. Effects of ethnicity and age or menopause on osteoblast function, bone mineralization and osteoid accumulation in iliac bone. *J. Bone Miner. Res.* **12,** 1864–1873 (1997).
50. Hagino, H., Yamamoto, K., Teshima, R., Kishimoto, H., and Kagawa, T. Radial bone mineral changes in pre- and postmenopausal healthy Japanese women: Cross-sectional and longitudinal studies. *J. Bone Miner. Res.* **7,** 147–152 (1992).
51. Bell, N. H., Greene, A., Epstein, S., Oexman, M. J., Shaw, S., and Shary, J. Evidence for alteration of the vitamin D endocrine system in Blacks. *J. Clin. Invest.* **76,** 470–473 (1985).
52. Reid, I. R., Cullen, S., Schooler, B. A., Livingston, N. E., and Evans, M. C. Calcitropic hormone levels in Polynesians: Evidence against their role in interracial differences in bone mass. *J. Clin. Endocrinol. Metab.* **70,** 1452–1456 (1990).
53. Reasner, C., Dunn, J. F., Fetchick, D. A., Liel, Y., Hollis, B. W., Epstein, S., Shary, J., Mundy, G. R., and Bell, N. H. Alteration of vitamin D metabolism in Mexican-Americans. *J. Bone Miner. Res.* **5,** 13–17 (1990).
54. Buchanan, J. R., Myers, C. A., Lloyd, T., Leuenberger, P., and Demers, L. M. Determinants of peak trabecular bone density in women: The role of androgens, estrogen, and exercise. *J. Bone Miner. Res.* **3,** 673–680 (1988).
55. Finkelstein, J. S., Neer, R. M., Biller, B. M. K., Crawford, J. D., and Klibanski, A. Osteopenia in men with a history of delayed puberty. *N. Engl. J. Med.* **326,** 600–604 (1992).
56. Davidson, B. J., Ross, R. K., Paganini-Hill, A., Hammond, G. D., Siiteri, P. K., and Judd, H. L. Total and free estrogens and androgens in postmenopausal women with hip fractures. *J. Clin. Endocrinol. Metab.* **54,** 115–120 (1982).
57. Kin, K., Kushida, K., Yamazaki, K., Okamoto, S., and Inoue, T. Bone mineral density of the spine in normal Japanese subjects using dual-energy X-ray absorptiometry: Effect of obesity and menopausal status. *Calcif. Tissue Int.* **49,** 101–106 (1991).
58. Cauley, J. A., Gutai, J. P., Kuller, L. H., Scott, J., and Nevitt, M. C. Black-white differences in serum sex hormones and bone mineral density. *Am. J. Epidemol.* **139,** 1035–1046 (1994).
59. Katzman, D. K., Bachrach, L. K., Carter, D. R., and Marcus, R. Clinical and anthropometric correlates of bone mineral acquisition in healthy adolescent girls. *J. Clin. Endocrinol. Metab.* **73,** 1332–1339 (1991).
60. Russell-Aulet, M., Wang, J., Thornton, J. C., Colt, E. W., and Pierson, R. J. Bone mineral density and mass in a cross-sectional study of white and Asian women. *J. Bone Miner. Res.* **8,** 575–582 (1993).
61. Wang, M. C., Aguirre, M., Bhudhikanok, G. S., Kendall, C. G., Marcus, R., and Bachrach, L. K. Bone mass and hip axis length in healthy Asian, Black, Hispanic, and White American youths. *J. Bone Miner. Res.* **12,** 1922–1935 (1997).
62. Grisso, J. A., Kelsey, J. L., Strom, B. L., O'Brien, L. A., Maislin, G., LaPann, K., Samelson, L., and Hoffman, S. Risk factors for hip fracture in Black women. *N. Engl. J. Med.* **330,** 1555–1559 (1994).

63. Lau, E. M., Woo, J., Leung, P. C., and Swaminthan, R. Low bone mineral density, grip strength and skinfold thickness are important risk factors for hip fracture in Hong Kong Chinese. *Osteopor. Int.* **3,** 66–70 (1993).
64. Pruzansky, M. W., Turano, M., Luckey, M., and Senie, R. Low body weight as a risk factor for hip fracture in both black and white women. *J. Orthop. Res.* **7,** 192–197 (1989).
65. Reid, I. R., Plank, L. D., and Evans, M. C. Fat mass is an important determinant of whole body bone density in premenopausal women but not in men. *J. Clin. Endocrinol. Metab.* **75,** 779–782 (1992).
66. Aloia, J. F., McGowan, D. M., Vaswani, A. N., Ross, P., and Cohn, S. H. Relationship of menopause to skeletal and muscle mass. *Am. J. Clin. Nutr.* **53,** 1378–1383 (1991).
67. Matsumine, H., Hirato, K., Yanaihara, T., Tamada, T., and Yoshida, M. Aromatization by skeletal muscle. *J. Clin. Endocrinol. Metab.* **63,** 717–720 (1986).
68. DeSimone, D. P., Stevens, J., Edwards, J., Shary, J., Gordon, J., and Bell, N. H. Influence of body habitus and race on bone mineral density of the midradius, hip, and spine in aging women. *J. Bone Miner. Res.* **4,** 827–830 (1989).
69. Nelson, D. A., Kleerekoper, M., and Parfitt, A. M. Bone Mass skin color and body size among black and white women. *Bone Miner.* **4,** 257–264 (1988).
70. Kumanyika, S. Obesity in Black women. *Epidemiol. Rev.* **9,** 31–51 (1987).
71. Department of Health and Human Services Publication 87–1688, "Anthropometric Reference Data and Prevalence of Overweight, United States, 1976–1980." National Center for Health Statistics, Washington, DC, 1987.
72. López, L. M., and Masse, B. Comparison of body mass indexes and cutoff points for estimating the prevalence of overweight in Hispanic women. *J. Am. Diet Assoc.* **92,** 1343–1347 (1992).
73. Lee, J., Kolonel, L. N., and Hinds, M. W. Relative merits of the weight-corrected-for height indices. *Am. J. Clin. Nutr.* **34,** 2521–29 (1981).
74. Kleerekoper, M., Nelson, D. A., Peterson, E. L., Wilson, P. S., Jacobsen, G., and Longcope, C. Body composition and gonadal steroids in older white and black women. *J. Endocrinol. Metab.* **79,** 775–779 (1994).
75. Ellis, K. J., and Cohn, S. H. Correlation between skeletal calcium mass and muscle mass in man. *J. Appl. Physiol.* **38,** 455–460 (1975).
76. Cohn, S. H., Abesamis, C., Zanzi, I., Aloia, J. F., Yasumura, S., and Ellis, K. J. Body elemental composition: Comparison between black and white adults. *Am. J. Physiol.* **232,** E419–E422 (1997).
77. Côté, K. D., and Adams, W. C. Effect of bone density on body composition estimates in young adult black and white women. *Med. Sci. Sports Exercise* **25,** 290–296 (1993).
78. Ortiz, O., Russell, M., Daley, T. L., Baumgartner, R. N., Waki, M., Lichtman, S., Wang, J., Pierson, R. J., and Heymsfield, S. B. Differences in skeletal muscle and bone mineral mass between black and white females and their relevance to estimates of body composition. *Am. J. Clin. Nutr.* **55,** 8–13 (1992).
79. Heaney, R. P. Calcium, bone health and osteoporosis. *In* "Bone and Mineral Research" (W. A. Peck, ed.), pp. 255–301. Elsevier Science, New York, 1986.
80. Matkovic, V., Kostial, K., Simonovic, I., Buzina, R., Brodarec, A., and Nordin, B. E. C. Bone status and fracture rates in two regions of Yugoslavia. *Am. J. Clin. Nutr.* **32,** 540–549 (1979).
81. Hux, J. F., Zhao, X. H., Jia, J. B., Parpia, B., and Campbell, T. C. Dietary calcium and bone density among middle-aged and elderly women in China. *Am. J. Clin. Nutr.* **58,** 219–227 (1993).
82. Fujita, T., Okamoto, Y., Tomita, T., Sakagami, Y., Ota, K., and Ohata, M. Calcium metabolism in aging inhabitants of mountain versus seacoast communities *J. Am. Geriatr. Soc.* **25,** 254–258 (1977).
83. Yano, K., Heilbrun, L. K., Wasnich, R. D., Hankin, J. J., and Vogel, J. M. The relationship between diet and bone mineral content of multiple skeletal sites in elderly Japanese-American men and women living in Hawaii. *Am. J. Clin. Nutr.* **42,** 877–888 (1985).
84. Lau, E. M. C., Woo, J., Leung, P. C., Swaminathan, R., and Leung, D. The effects of calcium supplementation and exercise on bone density in elderly Chinese women. *Osteopor. Int.* **2,** 168–173 (1992).
85. Meier, D. E., Luckey, M. M., Wallenstein, S., Clemens, T. L., Orwoll, E. S., and Waslien, C. I. Calcium, vitamin D, and parathyroid hormone status in young white and black women: Association with racial differences in bone mass. *J. Clin. Endocrinol. Metab.* **72,** 703–710 (1991).
86. Villareal, D. T., Civitelli, R., Chines, A., and Avioli, L. V., Subclinical vitamin D deficiency in postmenopausal women with low vertebral bone mass. *J. Clin. Endocrinol. Metab.* **72,** 628–634 (1991).
87. Chapuy, M. C., Arlot, M. E., Duboeuf, F., Brun, J., Crouzet, B., Arnaud, S., Delmas, P. D., and Meunier, P. J. Vitamin D_3 and calcium to prevent hip fractures in elderly women. *N. Engl. J. Med.* **327,** 1637–1642 (1992).
88. Pun, K. K., Wong, F. H. W., Wang, C., Lau, P., Ho, W. M., Pun, W. K., Chow, S. P., Cheng, C. L., Leong, J. C. Y., and Young, R. T. T. Vitamin D status among patients with fractured neck of femur in Hong Kong. *Bone* **11,** 365–368 (1990).
89. Fujita, T. Studies of osteoporosis in Japan. *Metabolism* **39,** 39–42 (1990).
90. Robins, A. H., "Biological Perspectives on Human Pigmentation." Cambridge Studies in Biological Anthropology 7. Cambridge Univ. Press, New York, 1991.
91. Relethford, J. H. Hemispheric difference in human skin color. *Am. J. Phys. Anthropol.* **104,** 449–457 (1998).
92. Brazerol, W. F., McPhee, A. J., Mimouni, F., Specker, B. L., and Tsang, R. C. Serial ultraviolet B exposure and serum 25-hydroxyvitamin D response in young adult American Blacks and Whites: No racial differences. *J. Am. Coll. Nutr.* **7,** 111–118 (1988).
93. Clemens, T. L., Henderson, S. L., Adams, J. S., and Holick, M. F. Increased skin pigment reduces the capacity of skin to synthesis vitamin D3. *Lancet* **1,** 74–76 (1982).
94. Villa, M., Kelsey, J., Chen, J., and Marcus, R. Skin pigmentation does not affect vitamin D status in community-dwelling Mexican-American women. *J. Bone Miner. Res.* **9,** S418 (1994). [Abstract].
95. Matsuoka, L. Y., Wortsman, J., Haddad, J. G., Kolm, P. and Hollis, B. W. Racial pigmentation and the cutaneous synthesis of vitamin D. *Arch. Dermatol.* **127,** 536–538 (1991).
96. M'Buyamba-Kabangu, J. R., Fagard, R., Lijnen, R., Bouillon, R., Lissens, W., and Amery, A. Calcium, vitamin D-endocrine system, and parathyroid hormone in black and white males. *Calcif. Tissue Int.* **41,** 70–74 (1987).
97. Perry, H. M. I., Miller, D. K., Morley, J. E., Horowitz, M., Kaiser, F. E., Perry, H. M. J., Jensen, J., Bentley, J., Boyd, S., and Krawnzel, D. A preliminary report of vitamin D and calcium metabolism in older African Americans. *J. Am. Geriatr Soc.* **40,** 612–616 (1993).
98. Morrison, N. A., Yeoman, R., Kelly, P. J., and Eisman, J. A. Contribution of trans-acting factor alleles to normal physiological variability: Vitamin D receptor gene polymorphisms and

circulating osteocalcin. *Proc. Natl. Acad. Sci. USA* **89,** 6665–6669 (1992).

99. Morrison, N. A., Qi, J. C., Tokita, A., Kelly, P. J., Crofts, L., Nguyen, T. V., Sambrook, P. N., and Eisman, J. A. Prediction of bone density from vitamin D receptor alleles. *Nature* **367,** 284–287 (1994).
100. Zmuda, J. M., Cauley, J. A., Danielson, M. E., Wolf, R. L., and Ferrell, R. E. Vitamin D receptor gene polymorphisms, bone turnover, and rates of bone loss in older African-American women. *J. Bone Miner. Res.* **12,** 1446–1452 (1997).
101. Fleet, J. C., Harris, S. S., Wood, R. J., and Dawson-Hughes, B. The *Bsm*1 vitamin D receptor restriction fragment length polymorphism (BB) predicts low bone density in premenopausal black and white women. *J. Bone Miner. Res.* **10,** 985–990 (1995).
102. Harris, S. S., Eccleshall, T. R., Gross, C., Dawson-Hughes, B., and Feldman, D. The vitamin D receptor start codon polymorphism (*Fok*I) and bone mineral density in premenopausal American black and white women. *J. Bone Miner. Res.* **12,** 1043–1048 (1997).
103. Nelson, D. A., Wooley, P., Davis, P., Morrison, N., Eisman, J., and Kleerekoper, M. Ethnic differences in vitamin D receptor gene frequencies and bone mass in children and adults. *In* "Proceedings of 10th International Congress of Endocrinology" San Francisco, 1996.
104. Davis, P. J., Nelson, D., Kleerekoper, M., Morrison, N., Eisman, J., and Wooley, P. H. Ethnic variations influence the association of polymorphisms in the vitamin D receptor gene and bone mass in adults. *Arthritis Rheum.* **39**(Suppl.), S123 (1996).
105. McClure, L., Eccleshall, T. R., Gross, C., Villa, M. L., Lin, N., Ramaswamy, V., Kohlmeier, L., Kelsey, J. L., Marcus, R., and Feldman, D. Vitamin D receptor polymorphisms, bone mineral density, and bone metabolism in postmenopausal Mexican-American women. *J. Bone Miner. Res.* **12,** 234–240 (1997).
106. Yamagata, Z., Miyamura, T., Lijima, S., Asaka, A., Sasaki, M., Kato, J., and Koizumi, K. Vitamin D receptor gene polymorphism and bone mineral density in healthy Japanese women. *Lancet* **344,** 1027 (1994).
107. Spotila, L. D., Caminis, J., Johnston, R., Shimoya, K. S., O'Connor, M. P. O., Prockop, D. J., Tenenhouse, A., and Tenenhouse, H. S. Vitamin D receptor genotype is not associated with bone mineral density in three ethnic/regional groups. *Calcif. Tissue Int.* **59,** 235–237 (1996).
108. Kiel, D. P., Myers, R. H., Cupples, L. A., Kong, X. F., Zhu, X. H., Ordovas, J., Schaefer, E. J., Felson, D. T., Rush, D., Wilson, P. W. F., Eisman, J. A., and Holick, M. F. The *Bsm*I Vitamin D receptor restriction fragment length polymorphism (bb) influences the effect of calcium intake on bone mineral density. *J. Bone Miner. Res.* **12,** 1049–1057 (1997).
109. Graafmans, W. C., Lips, P., Ooms, M. E., van Leeuwen, J. P. T. M., Pols, H. A. P., and Uitterlinden, A. G. The effect of vitamin D supplementation on the bone mineral density of the femoral neck is associated with vitamin D receptor genotype. *J. Bone Miner. Res.* **12,** 1241–1245 (1997).
110. Jorgensen, H. L., Scholler, J., Sand, J. C., Bjuring, M., Hassager, C., and Christiansen, C. Relationship of common allelic variation at the vitamin D receptor locus to bone mineral density and bone turnover. *Br. J. Obstet. Gynecol.* **103**(Suppl. 13), 28–31 (1996).
111. Krall, E. A., Parry, P., Lichter, J. B., and Dawson-Hughes, B. Vitamin D receptor alleles and rates of bone loss: influence of years since menopause and calcium intake. *J. Bone Miner. Res.* **10,** 978–984 (1995).
112. Ferrari, S., Rizzoli, R., Chevalley, T., Slosman, D., Eisman, J. A., and Bonjour, J. P. Vitamin-D-receptor gene polymorphisms and change in lumbar spine bone mineral density. *Lancet* **345,** 423–424 (1995).
113. Hirota, T., Nara, M., Ohguri, M., Manago, E., and Hirota, K. Effect of diet and lifestyle on bone mass in Asian young women. *Am. J. Clin. Nutr.* **55,** 1168–1173 (1992).
114. Ross, P. D., Orimo, H., Wasnich, R. D., Vogel, J. M., MacLean, C. J., Davis, J. W., and Nomura, A. Methodological issues in comparing genetic and environmental influences on bone mass. *Bone Miner.* **7,** 67–77 (1989).
115. Krall, E. A., and Dawson-Hughes, B. Smoking and bone loss among postmenopausal women. *J. Bone Miner. Res.* **6,** 331–338 (1991).
116. Slemenda, C. W., Hui, S. L., Longcope, C., and Johnston, C. J. Cigarette smoking, obesity, and bone mass. *J. Bone Miner. Res.* **4,** 737–741 (1989).
117. Davis, J. W., Ross, P. D., Vogel, J. M., and Wasnich, R. D. Effects of smoking and alcohol on the rates of bone loss among elderly Japanese-American men. *J. Bone Miner. Res.* **7,** S138 (1992). [Abstract].
118. Cummings, S. R., Cauley, J. A., Palermo, L., Ross, P. D., Wasnich, R. D., Black, D., and Faulkner, K. G. Racial differences in hip axis length might explain racial differences in rates of hip fracture. *Osteopor. Int.* **4,** 226–229 (1994).
119. Nakamura, T., Turner, C. H., Yoshikawa, T., Slemenda, C. W., Peacock, M., Burr, D. B., Mizuno, Y., Orima, H., Ouchi, Y., and Johnston, C. C. I. Do variations in hip geometry explain differences in hip fracture risk between Japanese and White Americans? *J. Bone Miner. Res.* **9,** 1071–1076 (1994).
120. Beck, T. J., Ruff, C. B., Warden, K. E., *et al.* Predicting femoral neck strength from bone mineral data: A structural approach. *Invest. Rad.* **25,** 6–18 (1990).
121. Beck, T. J., Ruff, C. B., Scott, W. W., Plato, C. C., Tobin, J. D., and Quan, C. A. Sex differences in geometry of the femoral neck with aging: A structural analysis of bone mineral data. *Calcif. Tissue Int.* **50,** 24–29 (1992).
122. Yoshikawa, T., Turner, C. H., Peacock, M., Slemenda, C. W., Weaver, C. M., Teegarden, D., Markwardt, P., and Burr, D. B. Geometric structure of the femoral neck measured using dual-energy x-ray absorptiometry. *J. Bone Miner. Res.* **9,** 1053–1064 (1994).
123. Horsman, A., Nordin, C., Simpson, M., *et al.* Cortical and trabecular bone status in elderly women with femoral neck fracture. *Clin.Orthop.* **166,** 143–151 (1982).
124. Gluer, C.-C., Cummings, S. R., Pressman, A., Li, J., Gluer, K., Faulkner, K. G., Grampp, S., and Genant, H. K. Prediction of hip fractures from pelvic radiographs: The Study of Osteoporotic Fractures. *J. Bone Miner. Res.* **9,** 671–677 (1994).
125. Theobald, T. M., Cauley, J. A., Gluer, C. C., Bunker, C. H., Ukoli, F. A. M., and Genant, H. K. Black–White differences in hip geometry. *Osteopor. Int.* **8,** 61–67 (1998).
126. Singh, M., Nagrath, A. R., Maini, P. S., and Rohtak, M. S. Changes in trabecular pattern of the upper end of the femur as an index of osteoporosis. *J. Bone Joint Surg.* **52,** 457–467 (1970).
127. Baron, J. A., Barrett, J., Malenka, D., Fisher, E., Kniffin, W., Bubolz, T., and Tosteson, T. Racial differences in fracture risk. *Epidemiology* **5,** 42–47 (1994).
128. Fisher, E. S., Baron, J. A., Malenka, D. J., Barrett, J. A., Kniffin, W. D., Whaley, F. S., and Bubolz, T. A. Hip fracture incidence and mortality in New England. *Epidemiology* **2,** 116–122 (1991).
129. Hinton, R. Y., and Smith, G. S. The association of age, race and sex with the location of proximal femoral fractures in the elderly. *J. Bone Joint Surg. Am.* **75,** 752–759 (1993).
130. Silverman, S. L., and Madison, R. E. Decreased incidence of hip fracture in Hispanics, Asians, and Blacks: California Hospital Discharge Data. *Am. J. Public Health* **78,** 1482–1483 (1988).

131. Bauer, R. L. Ethnic differences in hip fracture: A reduced incidence in Mexican Americans. *Am. J. Epidemiol.* **127,** 145–149 (1988).
132. Farmer, M. E., White, L. R., Brody, J. A., and Bailey, K. R. Race and sex differences in hip fracture incidence. *Am. J. Public Health* **74,** 1374–1380 (1984).
133. Solomon, L. Osteoporosis and fracture of the femoral neck in the South African Bantu. *J. Bone Joint Surg.* **50B,** 2–11 (1968).
134. Hagino, H., Yamamoto, K., Teshima, R., Kishimoto, H., Kuranobu, K., and Nakamura, T. The incidence of fractures of the proximal femur and the distal radius in Tottori prefecture, Japan. *Arch. Orthop. Trauma Surg.* **109,** 43–44 (1990).
135. Lau, E. M. C., Cooper, C., Wickham, C., Donnan, S., and Barker, D. J. P. Hip fracture in Hong Kong and Britain. *Int. J. Epidemiol.* **19,** 1119–1121 (1990).
136. Stott, S., Gray, D. H., and Stevenson, W. The incidence of femoral neck fractures in New Zealand. *N. Zeal. Med. J.* **91,** 6–9 (1980).
137. Chalmers, J., and Ho, K. C. Geographical variations in senile osteoporosis: the association with physical activity. *J. Bone Joint Surg.* **52B,** 667–675 (1970).
138. Wong, P. C. N. Fracture epidemiology in a mixed southeastern Asian community (Singapore). *Clin. Orthop.* **45,** 55–61 (1966).
139. Nilsson, R., Lofman, O., Berglund, K., Larson, L., and Toss, G. Increased hip fracture incidence in the county of Ostergotland, Sweden, 1940–1986, with forecasts up to the year 2000: an epidemiological study. *Int. J. Epidemiol.* **20,** 1018–1024 (1991).
140. Ray, W. A., Griffin, M. R., West, R., Strand, L., and Melton, L. J., III. Incidence of hip fracture in Saskatchewan, Canada, 1976–1985. *Am. J. Epidemiol.* **131,** 502–509 (1990).
141. Finsen, V., and Benum, P. Changing incidence of hip fractures in rural and urban areas of central Norway. *Clin. Orthop. Rel. Res.* **218,** 104–110 (1987).
142. Boyce, W. J., and Vessey, P. M. Rising incidence of fracture in the proximal femur. *Lancet* **1,** 150–151 (1985).
143. Rodriguez, J. G., Sattin, R. W., and Waxweiler, R. J. Incidence of hip fractures, United States, 1970–1983. *Am. J. Prev. Med.* **5,** 175–181 (1989).
144. Lizaur-Utrilla, A., Orts, P., SanchezDelCampo, F., Barrio, A. A., and Gutierrez-Carbonell, P. Epidemiology of trochanteric fractures of the femur in Alicante, Spain, 1974–1982. *Clin. Orthop. Rel. Res.* **218,** 24–31 (1987).
145. Hedlund, R., Lindgren, U., and Ahlbom, A. Age- and sex-specific incidence of femoral neck and trochanteric fractures. *Clin. Orthop. Rel. Res.* **222,** 132–139 (1987).
146. Hedlund, R., Ahlbom, A., and Lindgren, U. Hip fracture incidence in Stockholm 1972–1981. *Acta Orthop. Scand.* **57,** 30–34 (1985).
147. Luthje, P. Incidence of hip fracture in Finland: A forecast for 1990. *Acta Orthop. Scand.* **56,** 223–225 (1985).
148. Swanson, A. J. G., and Murdoch, G. Fractured neck of femur: pattern of incidence and implications. *Acta Orthop. Scand.* **54,** 348–355 (1983).
149. Elabdien, B. S. Z., Olerud, S., Karlstrom, G., and Smedby, B. Rising incidence of hip fracture in Uppsala, 1965–1980. *Acta Orthop. Scand.* **55,** 284–289 (1984).
150. Falch, J. A., Ilebekk, A., and Slungaard, U. Epidemiology of hip fractures in Norway. *Acta Orthop. Scand.* **56,** 12–16 (1985).
151. Currie, A. L., Reid, D. M., and Brown, N. An epidemiological study of fracture of the neck of femur. *Health Bull.* **44,** 143–148 (1986).
152. Frandsen, P. E., and Kruse, T. Hip fractures in the county of Funen, Denmark: Implications of demographic aging and changes in incidence rates. *Acta Orthop. Scand.* **54,** 681–686 (1983).
153. Baker, M. R. An investigation into secular trends in the incidence of femoral neck fracture using hospital activity analysis. *Public Health* **94,** 368–374 (1980).
154. Gallagher, J. C., Melton, L. J., III, Riggs, B. L., and Bergstrath, E. Epidemiology of fractures of the proximal femur in Rochester, Minnesota. *Clin. Orthop. Rel. Res.* **150,** 163–171 (1980).
155. Alhava, E. M., and Puittinen, J. Fractures of the upper end of the femur as an index of senile osteoporosis in Finland. *Ann. Clin. Res.* **5,** 398–403 (1973).
156. Levine, S., Makin, M., Menczel, J., Robin, G., Naor, E., and Steinbert, R. Incidence of fractures of the proximal end of the femur in Jerusalem. A study of ethnic factors. *J. Bone Joint Surg.* **52,** 1193–1202 (1970).
157. Alffram, P. A. An epidemiologic study of cervical and trochanteric fractures of the femur in an urban population. *Acta Orthop. Scand Suppl* **65,** 101–109 (1964).
158. Villa, M. L., and Nelson, L. Race, Ethnicity, and Osteoporosis. *In* "Osteoporosis" (R. Marcus, D. Feldman, and J. Kelsey, eds.), pp. 435–447. Academic Press, San Diego, 1996.
159. Maggi, S., Kelsey, J. L., Litvak, J., and Heyse, S. P. Incidence of hip fractures in the elderly: A cross-national analysis. *Osteopor. Int.* **1,** 232–241 (1991).

CHAPTER 23

Histomorphometric Manifestations of Age-Related Bone Loss

JULIET COMPSTON School of Clinical Medicine, University of Cambridge, Cambridge, United Kingdom

INTRODUCTION

The bone loss that occurs during a normal lifetime can be visualized readily on macroscopic examination of individual bones or radiographic images. Early studies, both qualitative and quantitative, detailed changes in cortical and cancellous bone mass and structure using these relatively simple approaches, providing valuable information about the effects of aging on the skeleton [1–5]. These have subsequently been extended by the application of histomorphometric techniques that enable definition of the changes in bone remodeling responsible for bone loss. In addition, the development of more sophisticated analyses of bone structure has provided new insights into the effects of age-related bone loss on the architecture of cancellous bone and the impact of these changes on bone strength and fracture risk.

Normal Bone Structure

Cortical or compact bone forms approximately 90% of the skeleton and is found mainly in the shafts of long bones and surfaces of flat bones. Trabecular or cancellous bone is found predominantly at the ends of long bones and inner parts of flat bones and is composed of interconnecting plates and bars within which lies the bone marrow. The extracellular matrix of bone is composed predominantly of type 1 collagen, the fibers of which adopt a preferential orientation in the adult human skeleton, resulting in the formation of lamellar bone. In cortical bone, these lamellae are arranged concentrically around the Haversian systems, whereas in cancellous bone, they are parallel to one another.

BONE REMODELING AND TURNOVER

In the normal adult human skeleton, the mechanical integrity of bone is preserved by the process of bone remodeling, in which old bone is removed and replaced with new bone. Remodeling occurs around Haversian systems in cortical bone and on the cancellous bone surface; a quantum of bone is removed by osteoclasts and, in the cavity thus created, osteoid synthesized by osteoblasts is laid down and subsequently mineralized (Fig. 1). The temporal sequence of events is always that of resorption followed by formation (coupling) and, at least in the young adult skeleton, the amounts of bone resorbed and formed are quantitatively similar (balance). During the process of remodeling, the site is referred to as a bone remodeling unit; the completed packet of bone that results from the remodeling process is known as a bone structural unit. In the human skeleton, the time taken for completion of the bone remodeling cycle is 3–6 months, most of which is occupied by bone formation.

The process by which the bone surface is prepared for remodeling is known as activation. It is believed to involve retraction of the lining cells on the quiescent bone surface and removal of the thin, collagen-containing membrane covering the bone surface, thereby exposing mineralized bone for osteoclastic attack. Although the mechanisms by which these steps

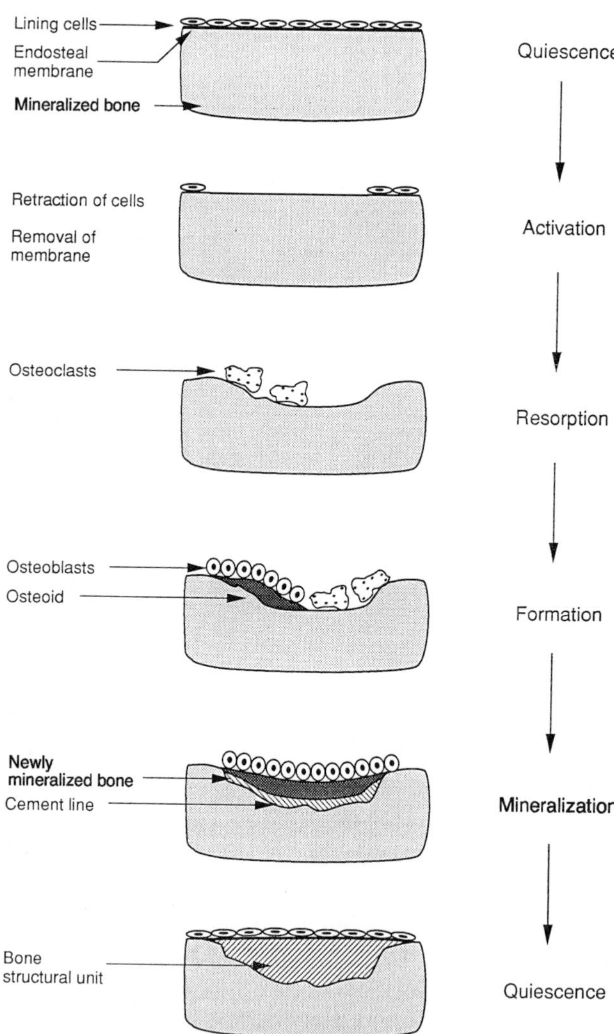

FIGURE 1 Schematic representation of cancellous bone remodeling. Reprinted with permission from Compston, J. E. Bone morphology: quality, quantity and strength. *In* "Oestrogen Deficiency: Causes and Consequences" (R. W. Shaw, ed.), Advances in Reproductive Endocrinology, Vol. 8, pp. 63–84. Parthenon, United Kingdom, 1996.

are achieved have not been defined clearly, collagenase and possibly other metalloproteinases synthesized by osteoblasts may play a role in digestion of the endosteal membrane. The factors that determine the site of activation of bone remodeling have not been established; the distribution of remodeling units on the bone surface is unlikely to be random, but rather determined by mechanical stresses acting in a site-specific manner.

MECHANISMS OF BONE LOSS

Two possible mechanisms of bone loss exist at a cellular level: increased activation frequency and remodeling imbalance (Fig. 2). An increase in activation frequency leads to increased bone turnover at the tissue level as a result of a greater number of remodeling units on the bone surface. It is potentially reversible as, provided that remodeling balance is maintained, the resorption cavities will eventually be filled with new bone. In theory, an increase in bone turnover may be due to increased activation or to increased osteoclast number or activity. Remodeling imbalance describes changes at the level of the individual bone remodeling unit, in which the amount of bone formed is less than that resorbed, due to an increase in the amount resorbed, a decrease in the amount formed, or a combination of the two. Once the remodeling sequence has been completed, this form of bone loss is irreversible, at least in terms of that remodeling unit. In practice, increased bone turnover and remodeling imbalance often coexist.

EFFECTS OF BONE LOSS ON BONE STRUCTURE

In cancellous bone, the changes in architecture depend to some extent on the cellular mechanisms of bone loss discussed earlier (Fig. 3) [6]. Increased activation frequency, particularly if accompanied by increased erosion depth, will result in trabecular penetration and erosion, leading to reduced connectivity of the cancellous bone structure. A remodeling imbalance due to decreased bone formation favors trabecular thinning, although as this progresses, the chances of trabecular penetration increase; these structural changes are thus to some extent interdependent. Although both trabecular thinning and penetration are associated with a reduction

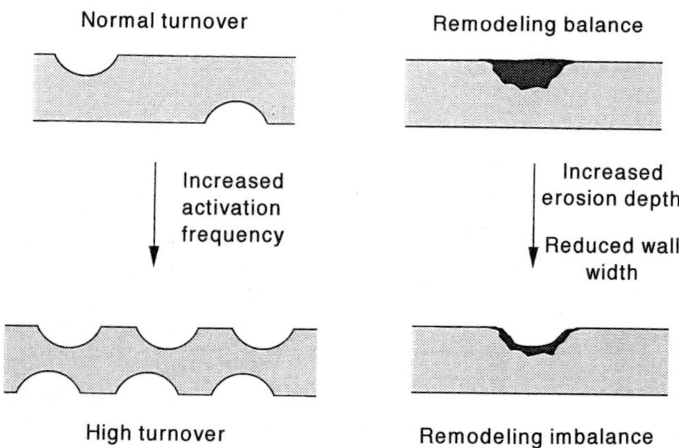

FIGURE 2 Mechanisms of bone loss. Reprinted with permission from Compston, J. E. Bone morphology: quality, quantity and strength. *In* "Oestrogen Deficiency: Causes and Consequences" (R. W. Shaw, ed.), Advances in Reproductive Endocrinology, Vol. 8, pp. 63–84. Parthenon, United Kingdom, 1996.

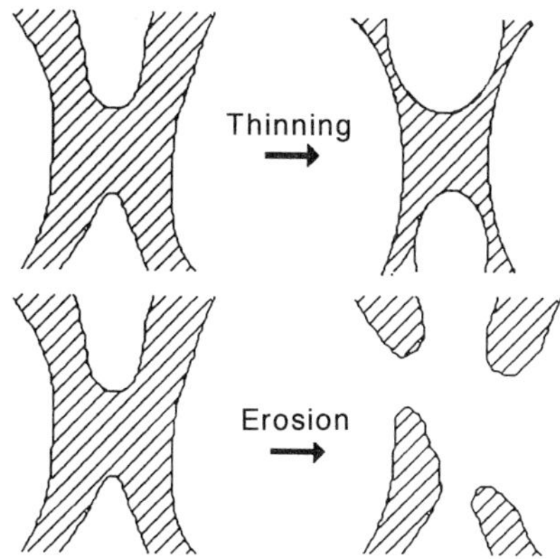

FIGURE 3 Structural changes in cancellous bone associated with bone loss. Reprinted with permission from Compston, J. E. Osteoporosis, corticosteroids and inflammatory bowel disease. *In* "Alimentary Pharmacology and Therapeutics," Vol. 9, pp. 237–250. Blackwell Scientific Press, Oxford, 1995.

in bone strength, the latter has greater adverse mechanical effects for any given level of bone mass.

Bone loss in cortical bone may be due to an increase in cortical porosity or to a reduction in cortical width; the latter results from increased endosteal bone resorption and leads to trabecularization of the endocortical surface. Because periosteal appositional growth occurs throughout life, age-related changes in cortical width will depend on the relative magnitude of changes at the periosteal and endosteal surfaces.

HISTOMORPHOMETRIC ASSESSMENT OF AGE-RELATED BONE LOSS IN HUMANS

Examination of the changes in bone remodeling and structure associated with aging has been made both from autopsy and biopsy samples of bone. Both of these approaches have limitations. Autopsy samples for such studies are often obtained from individuals who have suffered sudden death, based on the rationale that they are likely to have been healthy up to the moment of death; however, it is possible that such subjects are inherently less healthy than their surviving counterparts because of factors such as drug and alcohol abuse, cigarette smoking, and undetected disease, all of which may affect bone. This contention is supported by the finding of lower cancellous bone volume and trabecular width in autopsy bone samples than in biopsies obtained from age- and sex-matched controls [6]. Second, because tetracycline labeling cannot be administered prior to obtaining the bone sample in such cases, only static indices of bone remodeling can be assessed. The latter problem can be overcome in biopsies from healthy volunteers; however, these subjects may not be representative of the general population and the number of samples is limited by ethical constraints and unwillingness on the part of the majority of healthy people to undergo the procedure of bone biopsy. Finally, for obvious reasons, data from both autopsy and biopsy studies are cross-sectional and may be confounded by cohort effects and, in the case of biopsy studies, survivor bias.

Notwithstanding these limitations, much knowledge has been gained about the changes in bone remodeling and structure associated with aging, which has contributed to our understanding of the pathophysiology of osteoporosis and the mechanisms by which therapeutic interventions affect bone. Improvements in bone histomorphometric techniques, notably the use of sophisticated computerized systems and the development of new approaches to the assessment of cancellous bone structure, have enabled significant advances to be made in this area.

TECHNIQUES AND LIMITATIONS OF BONE HISTOMORPHOMETRY

Bone histomorphometry is generally applied to histological sections, which provide a two-dimensional representation of a three-dimensional structure. Using certain assumptions, two-dimensional values can be converted to three-dimensional units; in practice, values may be expressed in either terms. The use of manual techniques, using grids and graticules, has largely been superseded by interactive computerized systems that are faster, more operator friendly, and enable complex measurements to be made. The theoretical basis, methodology, and nomenclature of bone histomorphometry have been described in detail in a number of publications [7,8].

Some limitations of bone histomorphometry should be recognized. These reflect both imperfections in the measurement techniques and the variability in bone remodeling and structure throughout the skeleton. Measurement variance results from a number of factors, including inter- and intraobserver variation, sampling variation, and methodological issues such as the staining method and magnification used in sections undergoing measurement and the criteria chosen for corticomedullary differentiation [9]. There are variations in bone remodeling and cancellous structure at different skeletal sites, and changes at one site may not necessarily reflect those occurring elsewhere. Finally, some of the key processes in bone remodeling can at present only be assessed indirectly; these include activation frequency, bone resorption rates, and remodeling periods [10]. The accurate assessment of remodeling balance is also problematic, largely because of difficulties associated with the measurement of completed erosion depth.

HISTOMORPHOMETRIC ASSESSMENT OF BONE TURNOVER

The administration of two, time-spaced tetracycline doses prior to bone biopsy enables dynamic indices of bone formation to be measured directly and also allows indirect calculation of bone resorption rates and activation frequency [11]. Tetracycline binds to calcium at actively forming bone surfaces and fluoresces on unstained sections viewed under blue light (Fig. 4). Measurement of the separation and surface extent of the two labels provides information about the bone formation rate at both the cellular and the tissue level; the calculation from these of other derived indices, such as activation frequency, relies on the assumptions that bone remodeling is in a steady state and that resorption and formation are coupled in time and space.

In the absence of tetracycline labeling, assessment of bone turnover has to be made from the surface extent of osteoid and of resorption. The latter may be unreliable as the presence of resorption cavities per se does not necessarily indicate active resorption, but may rather reflect the failure of osteoblasts to synthesize and mineralize bone matrix in these cavities.

HISTOMORPHOMETRIC ASSESSMENT OF REMODELING BALANCE

Accurate assessment of remodeling balance requires the measurement of completed erosion depth and mean wall width, the latter reflecting the mean width of the completed bone structural unit. Both of these measurements present a number of problems that, at present, preclude the determination of remodeling balance.

Problems associated with the assessment of erosion depth include difficulties associated with the accurate identification of erosion cavities and the differentiation of those cavities in which resorption has been completed from those in which the resorptive process is ongoing or has become arrested [12]. Approaches to the measurement of erosion depth include counting of eroded lamellae, with or without morphological identification of cell types specifically associated with different stages of resorption [13,14], and measurement of the mean depth of cavities after computerized or manual reconstruction of the eroded bone surface [15]. Neither of these methods is ideal; the latter approach provides information about cavities at all stages of resorption and thus cannot generate a value for completed erosion depth.

The measurement of mean wall width requires identification of the cement line, which forms the inner boundary of the completed bone structural unit; this is not always easy but is facilitated by the use of polarized light or stains such as thionin or toluidine blue. The large variation in reported normal values between centers emphasizes not only this difficulty but probably also differences in sampling procedures [10]. In addition, bone structural units formed recently or in the past cannot be differentiated, so that the effects of the aging process are likely to be underestimated. Uncompleted bone structural units with a thin covering of osteoid can be presumed to reflect current or recent remodeling

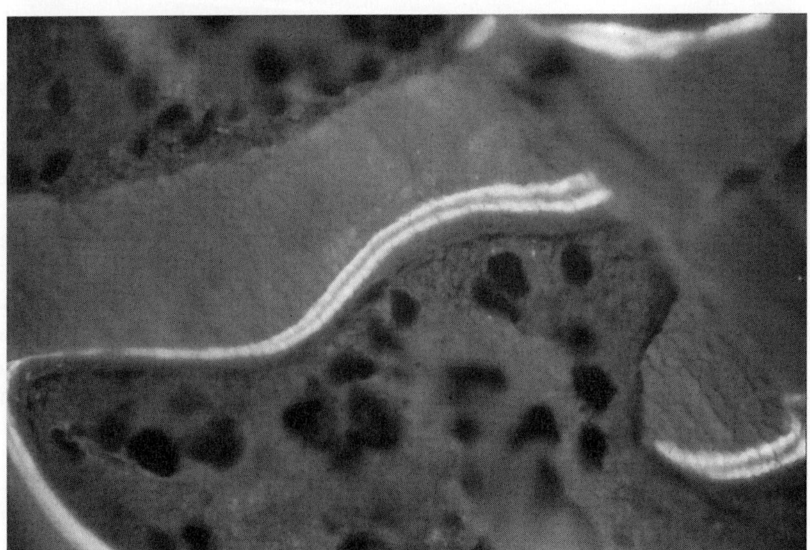

FIGURE 4 Undecalcified section of iliac crest bone showing double fluorescent tetracycline labels. The section is unstained and viewed under blue light.

activity [16]; however, the number of such units in any one sample is likely to be extremely small.

HISTOMORPHOMETRIC ASSESSMENT OF MINERALIZATION

Tetracycline labeling prior to biopsy is essential for the accurate assessment of mineralization. Using double labeling, the mineral apposition rate is calculated as the distance between the two labels divided by the time (days) between the administration of the two labels. Defective mineralization is associated with the accumulation of osteoid, resulting in an increase in osteoid seam width, which, together with a prolonged mineralization lag time, constitutes the histomorphometric definition of osteomalacia. In the absence of tetracycline labeling, calcification fronts can be demonstrated using stains such as toluidine blue or thionin, but dynamic indices of mineralization cannot be assessed using this approach.

ASSESSMENT OF CANCELLOUS BONE STRUCTURE

A number of methods for the assessment of cancellous bone structure have been described. These provide information about trabecular size and shape, connectivity, and anisotropy. Two-dimensional approaches, which include the measurement of trabecular width and number [17], strut analysis [18], star volume [19], and trabecular bone pattern factor [20], provide only indirect information about connectivity, although several lines of evidence support the contention that these measurements are representative of three-dimensional structure. Three-dimensional images of bone can be generated by techniques such as reconstruction of serial sections, scanning and stereomicroscopy, computed tomography, and magnetic resonance imaging; from these images, indices of cancellous structure, including connectivity, can be assessed directly.

AGE-RELATED CHANGES IN CANCELLOUS AND CORTICAL BONE

Many histomorphometric studies have documented a significant age-related decrease in cancellous bone volume in the iliac crest and in vertebrae, ribs, and sternal bone [4,21–31]. These changes affect both men and women; because of the cross-sectional nature of the studies and the relatively small numbers within each age group, it is difficult to obtain accurate information about the onset and rates of bone loss, although, in general, bone loss in both sexes appears to commence around the fifth or sixth decade of life and to continue thereafter into old age. Some of the larger studies have also shown significantly greater rates of loss in women after the age of 50 or so when compared to their male counterparts [24,28]. Subsequently, bone densitometric techniques have largely confirmed these findings and provided more detail about differential rates of bone loss in different parts of the skeleton.

Histomorphometric data on cortical bone loss associated with aging are more sparse. In a study of cortical bone samples obtained from the femoral midshaft, Thompson [32] reported a significant age-related decrease in cortical thickness in females; in men, a similar but nonsignificant trend was observed. Accompanying this age-related decrease in cortical thickness were significant increases in Haversian canal area and number in both sexes, indicating increased cortical porosity [32,33]. Quantitatively, however, thinning of the cortices was the most important factor contributing to age-related bone loss, with increased intracortical porosity playing a relatively minor role. Radiogrammetric studies have demonstrated clearly that the age-related reduction in cortical thickness results from endocortical bone loss, the amount of which exceeds periosteal bone apposition [5,34]. Melsen *et al.* [28] also reported an age-related reduction in cortical thickness in both sexes, although an increase in cortical porosity was seen only in women.

AGE-RELATED CHANGES IN BONE TURNOVER

In the majority of histomorphometric studies in normal subjects, double tetracycline labeling has not been used and information about bone turnover has thus been derived from static indices such as the surface extent of osteoid, resorption cavities, and osteoblasts. In some studies, a significant age-related increase in osteoid surface has been demonstrated [21,30], but others have failed to show any significant changes [28,35]. These differences may partly reflect the sample sizes in different studies and variations in the measurement techniques; in addition, geographical variations in the prevalence of vitamin D deficiency and secondary hyperparathyroidism in the elderly, resulting in increased bone turnover, may also account for some of the observed differences. Significant age-related changes in eroded surface have generally not been demonstrated, although some studies have reported a tendency toward an increase in the later decades of life. However, Croucher *et al.* [36] reported a significant age-related increase in eroded surface in a group of 41 healthy subjects (20 male), and in another study of 36 healthy subjects, mainly male, there was a significant age-related increase in the active resorption surface [14], defined as the surface extent of cells identified as osteoclasts using tartrate-resistant acid phosphatase (TRAP) staining.

Measurement of bone turnover in tetracycline-labeled biopsies has generated conflicting results. An inverse correlation in females between the bone formation rate at tissue level and age was reported by Melsen and Mosekilde [37] in a group of 29 women aged 19–56 years, whereas others have been unable to demonstrate any significant change with age. However, Eastell *et al.* [38] reported significantly higher values in a group of 11 women aged 55–73 years when compared to younger women aged 30–41 years and, in the study of Vedi *et al.* [39], there was a trend for values to increase in women in the sixth and seventh decades of life. In cortical bone of the iliac crest, Brockstedt *et al.* [40] reported an increase in activation frequency in women after menopause.

The lack of firm evidence for age-related changes in bone turnover in histomorphometric studies contrasts with results obtained from kinetic and biochemical measurements, which indicate an age-related increase in bone turnover, particularly in women at the time of menopause, and emphasize some of the limitations of both existing studies and bone histomorphometry. In particular, the small sample sizes, lack of prospective data, and large measurement variance are likely to contribute to the apparent inability of histomorphometric assessment to demonstrate well-documented age-related changes in bone turnover.

AGE-RELATED CHANGES IN MINERALIZATION

Because accurate assessment of indices of mineralization requires double tetracycline labeling prior to biopsy, histomorphometric data in normal subjects are sparse. However, unlike bone turnover, which can be assessed by nonhistomorphometric approaches, the dynamics of osteoid formation and mineralization can only be dissected by bone histomorphometry. In view of the postulated importance of vitamin D deficiency in age-related bone loss, at least in some populations, and the inability of bone densitometric techniques to distinguish between bone loss due to osteoporosis and osteomalacia, the investigation of age-related changes in mineralization is of considerable importance.

In the small number of studies in which it has been assessed in normal subjects, the mineral apposition rate in cancellous bone has not shown any significant age-related change, nor have significant changes been observed either in mineralization lag time or osteoid maturation period. Consistent with this finding, no age-related changes in osteoid seam width have been reported, indicating that even in populations in which a high prevalence of vitamin D deficiency has been documented, defective mineralization resulting in osteomalacia is rare. In rib cortical bone, however, an age-associated reduction in the mineral apposition rate has been described; because osteoid seam width did not change, this implies a quantitatively similar decrease in the osteoid apposition rate [41].

AGE-RELATED CHANGES IN REMODELING BALANCE

One of the best established age-related changes in cancellous bone is the reduction in wall width, which occurs in both men and women and appears to start around the fifth or sixth decade of life [42]. The reported magnitude of change varies between studies, but Vedi *et al.* [39] reported a reduction of approximately one-third between young adulthood and the seventh and eighth decades of life (Fig. 5). This decrease in wall width reflects a reduction in bone formation rate at the level of the basic multicellular unit and thus a decrease in osteoblast activity and/or life span; the lack of any significant age-related change in σ_f, the formation period, indicates that reduced activity is the predominant factor. Changes in cortical bone are less well documented; in one study, no age-related decline in wall

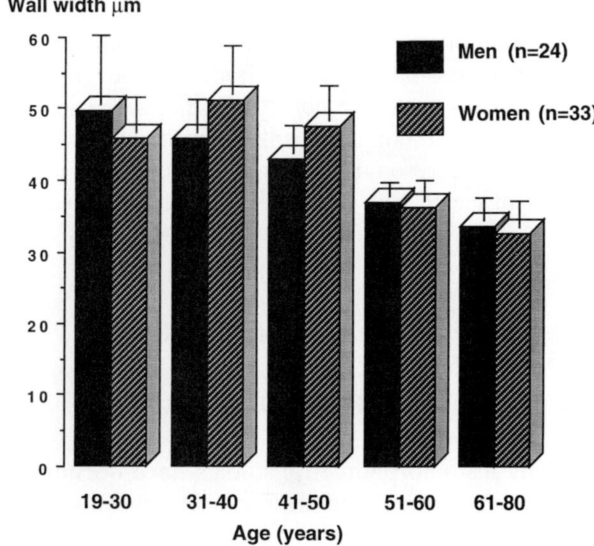

FIGURE 5 Age-related changes in mean wall width in healthy subjects. Data from Vedi *et al.* [39], shown as mean ± SD. A significant decrease is seen in both sexes ($p < 0.01$).

width in rib cortical bone was found [43], whereas a slight decrease was reported in corticoendosteal bone in the rib [44] and, in iliac crest cortical bone, a significant age-related decrease was demonstrated in women, but not in men [40].

Age-related changes in the other component of remodeling balance, namely erosion cavity depth, are less certain. Eriksen *et al.* [45], using the method of counting the number of eroded lamellae adjacent to resorption cavities containing preosteoblastic cells (and therefore presumably assessing the completed erosion depth), demonstrated a significant negative correlation between cavity depth and age in both men and women; however, statistical significance was not achieved with analysis of variance. Using a similar technique, Palle *et al.* [14] reported a significantly lower erosion depth in elderly women and elderly men when compared to a younger group. Croucher *et al.* [36], using the method described by Garrahan *et al.* [15] in which the eroded surface is reconstructed using a computerized technique and indices of erosion cavity size are then measured directly, were unable to demonstrate any significant correlation between erosion cavity size and age. However, this approach includes resorption cavities at all stages of completion, including those in which resorption has been arrested [12], possibly accounting for the different results obtained in this study.

Although these data collectively indicate that there is either no change or a small decrease in erosion cavity depth in cancellous bone with age, other lines of evidence indicate that an increase in erosion depth may play an important role in postmenopausal bone loss. In particular, the rapid and significant disruption of cancellous bone architecture induced by gonadotrophin-releasing hormone analogue therapy in premenopausal women would be consistent with this hypothesis [46]. It is thus possible that menopausal bone loss is associated with a transient increase in erosion depth, which, in combination with reduced wall width and increased bone turnover, leads to rapid structural deterioration and reduced connectivity in cancellous bone. These changes in remodeling balance may account, at least in part, for the different structural alterations accompanying cancellous bone loss in men and women, as there is no evidence that increased erosion depth occurs at any stage of age-related bone loss in men.

Histomorphometric data on age-related changes in healthy subjects from the studies of Vedi *et al.* [30,39] are shown in Tables I and II.

AGE-RELATED CHANGES IN CANCELLOUS BONE STRUCTURE

Qualitative studies of the changes in cancellous bone architecture that occur during aging have described changes in trabecular size and shape, connectivity, and anisotropy at a number of skeletal sites, particularly the iliac crest and vertebrae. The marked heterogeneity of cancellous structure throughout the skeleton makes generalization about age-related changes problematic and emphasizes the dangers of extrapolating between

TABLE I Normative Histomorphometric Data in Females

Parameter	19–30 yr	31–40 yr	41–50 yr	51–60 yr	61–80 yr
(n = 6)	(n – 5)	(n = 6)^a	(n = 6)^b	(n = 10)^c	
BV/TV%	25.9(3.1)	27.7(5.5)	29.6(2.1)	23.9(4.5)	19.8(3.9)
OV/BV%	2.4(1.4)	2.7(2.4)	2.3(1.3)	3.1(1.9)	4.7(1.9)
OS/BS%	13.1(5.9)	17.7(11.5)	14.5(7.8)	21.2(11.3)	35.0(12.1)
ES/BS%	2.15(0.36)	1.84(0.92)	1.78(1.03)	1.76(0.83)	1.66(0.66)
MS/BS%	9.4(1.8)	8.1(3.4)	8.1(4.2)	13.0(6.7)	14.8(8.1)
O.Th μm	5.4(1.9)	3.9(1.6)	5.8(1.1)	5.8(1.6)	5.8(2.3)
W. Th μm	45.7(4.9)	51.2(6.6)	47.5(4.9)	36.1(2.9)	32.5(3.6)
MAR μm/d	0.59(0.06)	0.60(0.12)	0.61(0.09)	0.61(0.10)	0.54(0.07)
Mlt days	12.2(6.2)	16.5(11.8)	20.7(8.7)	21.2(19.6)	29.6(13.5)
BFR $\mu m^3/\mu m^2$/day	0.056(0.013)	0.060(0.022)	0.051(0.031)	0.084(0.045)	0.081(0.043)

Note. Results are expressed as mean (SD). Data obtained from references 66 and 67. MS/BS was calculated as the double plus half the single tetracycline-labeled surface.

^{a} n = 4 for dynamic variables

^{b} n = 5 for dynamic variables

^{c} n = 9 for dynamic variables

TABLE II Normative Histomorphometric Data in Males

Parameter (n = 6)	19–30 yr (n − 3)	31–40 yr (n = 6)	41–50 yr (n = 3)	51–60 yr (n = 6)	61–80 yr
BV/TV%	31.3(6.4)	22.2(3.9)	26.9(7.1)	23.0(5.5)	21.4(2.6)
OV/BV%	1.6(0.8)	4.1(1.6)	2.8(0.9)	3.1(0.9)	5.6(3.6)
OS/BS%	10.0(5.3)	28.3(7.8)	26.3(6.0)	20.0(7.0)	34.8(15.7)
ES/BS%	2.84(1.27)	1.69(0.62)	1.68(0.32)	1.77(0.68)	1.91(0.42)
MS/BS%	9.9(4.0)	13.5(8.4)	8.7(7.0)	8.8(1.5)	9.2(5.1)
O.Th μm	8.3(3.0)	6.1(1.3)	6.9(2.9)	6.2(2.0)	6.6(2.8)
W. Th μm	49.7(9.6)	45.9(4.4)	42.8(4.0)	36.9(2.0)	33.4(3.3)
MAR μm/d	0.67(0.07)	0.60(0.10)	0.55(0.10)	0.57(0.13)	0.53(0.05)
Mlt days	10.5(1.9)	28.5(14.6)	36.1(6.2)	34.7(40.8)	49.1(28.1)
BFR $\mu m^3/\mu m^2$/day	0.066(0.006)	0.079(0.049)	0.047(0.005)	0.051(0.015)	0.045(0.023)

Note. Results are expressed as mean (SD). Data obtained from references 66 and 67. MS/BS was calculated as the double plus half the single tetracycline-labeled surface.

different skeletal sites. Even within individual bones, such as the iliac crest or a vertebra, there may be significant variations in structure [47]; nonetheless, overall there is evidence of similarity between the iliac crest and spine in terms of age-related structural changes [48].

Earlier studies in which quantitative approaches were adopted focused mainly on measurements or calculations of trabecular width, spacing, and number in iliac crest cancellous bone [17,35,49–53]. The majority of these have reported an age-related reduction in trabecular width (Fig. 6), although this has not always been statistically significant; some studies have not demonstrated any age-related change in women, whereas an age-related reduction has been a consistent finding in men. These reported differences may partly reflect the variety of methods used to assess mean trabecular width and differences in the selection and number of subjects examined. Increased trabecular spacing has been reported consistently in women, whereas in men, no change or only a small decrease has been observed. Taken together, these data indicate that trabecular thinning is the predominant change in men and presumably results mainly from a remodeling imbalance; in contrast, disruption of cancellous bone structure is more prominent in women, with a reduction in trabecular continuity and a loss of whole trabeculae. The latter changes are likely to result from a combination of increased bone turnover and increased erosion depth, particularly around the time of menopause. However, trabecular thinning probably also occurs in women as a result of increased bone turnover and remodeling imbalance; a possible explanation for the absence, in some studies, of any age-related change in trabecular width is the preferential removal of thin trabeculae by osteoclasts [50]. In vertebral bone, several studies have demonstrated a preferential thinning and loss of horizontal trabeculae.

More sophisticated methods of structural analysis have been applied to the study of age-related bone loss. Using strut analysis, which is based on the identification of nodes or junctions, termini, and topologically defined struts (trabeculae), a significant age-related reduction in the number of nodes was demonstrated in both sexes, indicating decreasing connectivity with age; in women,

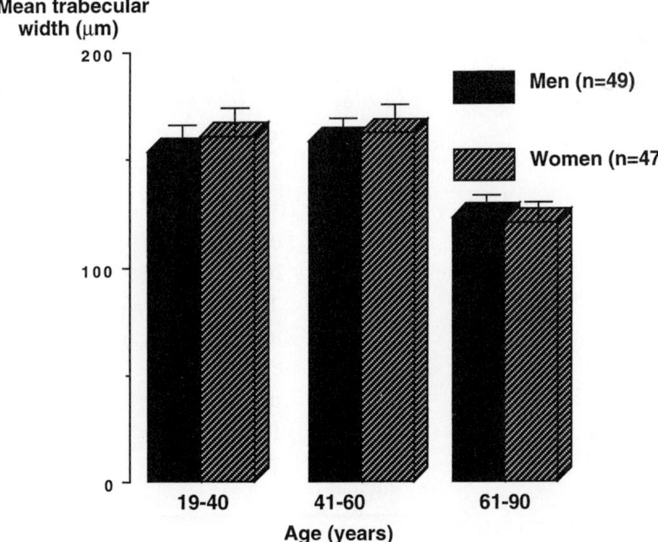

FIGURE 6 Age-related changes in mean trabecular width in healthy subjects. Data from Mellish *et al.* [53], shown as the mean ± SE. The decrease is statistically significant in males ($p < 0.02$) but not in females.

there was also a significant reduction in the node-to-terminus ratio and in the node-to-node strut length, which are both related positively to connectivity [54]. These data are consistent with the contention that loss of trabeculae is the main structural consequence of age-related bone loss in women; in men, some loss of connectivity also occurs with aging, but to a lesser extent than in women.

Similar results have also been obtained using the trabecular bone pattern factor (TBPF) to assess cancellous bone architecture. This method is based on the principle that convex structures are indicative of a poorly connected architecture, whereas the reverse is true for concave structures. In a study of 192 autopsy samples obtained from men and women over a large age range, Hahn *et al.* [20] demonstrated a significant age-related increase in TBPF in women, indicating increasing loss of connectivity after the age of 50 years or so; however, no change was observed in men. Using the marrow star volume as a measure of connectivity of cancellous bone, Vesterby [19] reported a significant age-related increase (implying reduced connectivity) in both vertebral and iliac crest bone in a small group of autopsy samples. In vertebral bone, this increase was significantly greater for women than men. However, using a similar approach to estimate trabecular thickness, no relationship with age could be demonstrated.

In summary, the majority of studies have demonstrated an age-related reduction in trabecular width in men and, to a lesser extent, in women. Indirect estimates of connectivity indicate that the degree of structural disruption is considerably greater in women than in men. Age-related changes in anisotropy and trabecular shape have been less well characterized and are likely to show large variations between different skeletal sites.

MICROFRACTURES

Microfractures may occur in cortical or cancellous bone and are believed to represent fatigue damage. They may act as a stimulus for bone remodeling, and it is generally assumed that failure of an appropriate response is associated with increased bone fragility, although a relationship between microdamage and mechanical strength has not been demonstrated directly. Microcallus formation is often seen close to intertrabecular nodes, suggesting that microfractures are caused by mechanical loading.

Microdamage has been shown to increase with age, both in cortical and in cancellous bone, and is seen more commonly in women than in men [55,56]. In one study, it was found to be significantly greater in the proximal femur than in the midshaft of the tibia [56]. In vertebral bone, microfractures tend to be grouped in the upper and lower thirds of each vertebral body adjacent to the end plates and are seen most commonly on vertical trabeculae [57].

RELATIONSHIP OF PRIMARY OSTEOPOROSIS TO AGE-RELATED BONE LOSS

Age-related bone loss is a normal phenomenon, in that it affects all people, but only a proportion of the elderly develop osteoporosis. The question therefore arises of whether the changes in bone remodeling and structure responsible for age-related bone loss and primary osteoporosis are qualitatively different or whether osteoporosis is a manifestation of biological aging, those who are affected simply having "older bones" than their sex- and age-matched counterparts. Specific differences in the cellular pathophysiology of bone loss associated with aging and osteoporosis have not been demonstrated, but this may reflect the lack of prospective histomorphometric data rather than absence of a true difference.

If osteoporosis is a specific disease process, it might be expected that the changes in cancellous bone structure, which reflect cellular mechanisms of bone loss, would differ between patients with established osteoporosis and the healthy aging population. Two studies have reported greater disruption of cancellous bone structure in patients with vertebral fracture when compared to control subjects matched for cancellous bone area, suggesting that osteoporosis differs qualitatively from age-related bone loss [58,59]. However, in a study of 35 patients with primary osteoporosis and 41 normal subjects, Croucher *et al.* [60] demonstrated that, after correction for cancellous bone area, the changes in cancellous structure in osteoporotic patients were not significantly different from those found in the control group. These results are consistent with the hypothesis that osteoporosis is a consequence of greater biological aging rather than a separate disease process and support other lines of evidence indicating that low bone mass is associated with increased mortality from causes other than osteoporotic fracture.

References

1. Jowsey, J. Age changes in human bone. *Clin. Orthop.* **17,** 210–217 (1960).
2. Trotter, M., Brewman, G. E., and Peterson, K. K. Densities of bones of white and negro skeletons. *J. Bone Joint Surg.* **42A,** 50–58 (1960).

3. Meema, H. E. The occurrence of cortical bone atrophy in old age and in osteoporosis. *J. Can. Assoc. Radiol.* **13,** 27–32 (1962).
4. Atkinson, P. J. Variation in trabecular structure of vertebrae with age. *Calcif. Tissue Res.* **1,** 24–32 (1967).
5. Garn, S. M. "The Earlier Gain and the Later Loss of Cortical Bone." Charles C. Thomas, Springfield, IL, 1970.
6. Compston, J. E., Mellish, R. W. E., Croucher, P., Newcombe, R., and Garrahan, N. J. Structural mechanisms of trabecular bone loss in man. *Bone Miner.* **6,** 339–350 (1989).
7. Parfitt, A. M., Drezner, M. K., Glorieux, F. H., Kanis, J. A., Malluche, H., Meunier, P. J., Ott, S. M., and Recker, R. R. Bone histomorphometry. Standardisation of nomenclature, symbols and units. *J. Bone Miner. Res.* **2,** 595–610 (1987).
8. Compston, J. E. Bone Histomorphometry. *In* "Vitamin D" (D. Feldman, F. H. Glorieux, and J. W. Pike, eds.), pp. 573–586. Academic Press, San Diego, 1997.
9. Wright, C. D. P., Vedi, S., Garrahan, N. J., Stanton, M., Duffy, S. W., and Compston, J. E. Combined inter-observer and inter-method variation in bone histomorphometry. *Bone* **13,** 205–208 (1992).
10. Compston, J. E., and Croucher, P. I. Histomorphometric assessment of trabecular bone remodelling in osteoporosis. *Bone Miner.* **14,** 91–102 (1991).
11. Frost, H. M. Tetracycline based histological analysis of bone remodeling. *Calcif. Tissue Res.* **33,** 199–204 (1981).
12. Croucher, P. I., Gilks, W. R., and Compston, J. E. Evidence for interrupted bone resorption in human iliac cancellous bone. *J. Bone Miner. Res.* **10,** 1537–1543 (1995).
13. Eriksen, E. F., Melsen, F., and Mosekilde, L. Reconstruction of the resorptive site in iliac trabecular bone: a kinetic model for bone resorption in 20 normal individuals. *Metab. Bone Dis. Rel. Res.* **5,** 235–242 (1984).
14. Palle, S., Chappard, D., Vico, L., Riffat, G., and Alexandre, C. Evaluation of osteoclastic population in iliac crest biopsies from 36 normal subjects: a histoenzymologic and histomorphometric study. *J. Bone Miner. Res.* **4,** 501–506 (1989).
15. Garrahan, N. J., Croucher, P. I., and Compston, J. E. A computerised technique for the quantitative assessment of resorption cavities in trabecular bone. *Bone* **11,** 241–246 (1990).
16. Kragstrup, J., Melsen, F., and Mosekilde, L. Thickness of bone formed at remodeling sites in normal human iliac trabecular bone: variations with age and sex. *Metab. Bone Dis. Rel. Res.* **5,** 17–21 (1983).
17. Parfitt, A. M., Mathews, C. H. E., Villanueva, A. R., Kleerekoper, M., Frame, B., and Rao, D. S. Relationships between surface volume and thickness of iliac trabecular bone in ageing and in osteoporosis. Implications for the microanatomic and cellular mechanisms of bone loss. *J. Clin. Invest.* **72,** 1396–1409 (1983).
18. Garrahan, N. J., Mellish, R. W. E., and Compston, J. E. A new method for the two-dimensional analysis of bone structure in human iliac crest biopsies. *J. Microsc.* **142,** 341–349 (1986).
19. Vesterby, A. Star volume of marrow space and trabeculae in iliac crest: sampling procedure and correlation to star volume of first lumbar vertebra. *Bone* **11,** 149–155 (1990).
20. Hahn, M., Vogel, M., Pompesius-Kempa, M., and Delling, G. Trabecular bone pattern factor—A new parameter for simple quantification of bone microarchitecture. *Bone* **13,** 327–330 (1992).
21. Bordier, P. J., Matrajt, H., Miravet, L., and Hioco, D. Mésure histologique de la masse et de la résorption des travées osseuses. *Pathol. Biol.* **12,** 1238–1243 (1964).
22. Schenk, R. K., Merz, W. A., and Muller, J. A quantitative histological study on bone resorption in human cancellous bone. *Acta Anat.* **74,** 44–53 (1969).
23. Arnold, J. S., Bartley, M. H., Tont, S. A., and Jenkins, D. P. Skeletal changes in ageing and disease. *Clin. Orthop.* **49,** 17–38 (1966).
24. Courpron, P. Données histologiques quantitatives sur le vieillissement osseux humain. Thesis, Lyon University, 1972.
25. Delling, G. Age-related bone changes. *Curr. Top. Pathol.* **58,** 117–147 (1973).
26. Meunier, P., Courpron, P., Edouard, C., Bernard, J., Bringuier, J., and Vignon, G. Physiological senile involution and pathological rarefaction of bone. *Clin. Endocrinol. Metab.* **2,** 239–256 (1973).
27. Giroux, J. M., Courpron, P., and Meunier, P. J. Histomorphometrie de l'osteopénie physiologique sénile. Master's Thesis, Lyon University, 1975.
28. Melsen, F., Melsen, B., Mosekilde, L., and Bergmann, S. Histomorphometric analysis of normal bone from the iliac crest. *Acta Pathol. Microbiol. Scand. A* **86,** 70–81 (1978).
29. Malluche, H. M., Meyer, W., Sherman, D., and Massry, S. G. Quantitative bone histology in 84 normal American subjects. *Calcif. Tissue Int.* **34,** 449–455 (1982).
30. Vedi, S., Compston, J. E., Webb, A., and Tighe, J. R. Histomorphometric analysis of bone biopsies from the iliac crest of normal British subjects. *Metab. Bone Dis. Rel. Res.* **4,** 231–236 (1982).
31. Ballanti, P., Bonucci, E., Rocca, C. D., Milani, S., LoCascio, V., and Imbimbo, B. Bone histomorphometric reference values in 88 normal Italian subjects. *Bone Miner.* **11,** 187–197 (1990).
32. Thompson, D. D. Age changes in bone mineralization, cortical thickness, and Haversian canal area. *Calcif. Tissue Int.* **31,** 5–11 (1980).
33. Atkinson, P. J. Quantitative analysis in cortical bone. *Nature* **201,** 373–375 (1964).
34. Carlson, D. S., Armelagos, G. J., and Van Gerven, D. P. Patterns of age-related cortical bone loss (osteoporosis) within the femoral diaphysis. *Hum. Biol.* **48,** 295–314 (1976).
35. Merz, W. A., and Schenk, R. K. Quantitative structural analysis of human cancellous bone. *Acta Anat.* **75,** 54–66 (1970).
36. Croucher, P. I., Garrahan, N. J., Mellish, R. W. E., and Compston, J. E. Age-related changes in resorption cavity characteristics in human trabecular bone. *Osteopor. Int.* **1,** 257–261 (1991).
37. Melsen, F., and Mosekilde, L. Tetracycline double-labelling of iliac trabecular bone in 41 normal adults. *Calcif. Tissue Res.* **26,** 99–102 (1978).
38. Eastell, R., Delmas, P. D., Hodgson, S. F., Eriksen, E. F., Mann, K. G., and Riggs, B. L. Bone formation rate in older normal women; concurrent assessment with bone histomorphometry, calcium kinetics and biochemical markers. *J. Clin. Endocrinol. Metab.* **67,** 741–748 (1988).
39. Vedi, S., Compston, J. E., Webb, A., and Tighe, J. R. Histomorphometric analysis of dynamic parameters of trabecular bone formation in the iliac crest of normal British subjects. *Metab. Bone Dis. Rel. Res.* **5,** 69–74 (1982).
40. Brockstedt, H., Kassem, M., Eriksen, E. F., Mosekilde, L., and Melsen, F. Age and sex-related changes in iliac cortical bone mass and remodeling. *Bone* **14,** 681–691 (1993).
41. Taylor, T. C., Epker, B. N., and Frost, H. M. The appositional rate of haversian and endosteal bone formation measured in tetracycline labeled human ribs. *J. Lab. Clin. Med.* **67,** 633–639 (1966).
42. Lips, P., Courpron, P., and Meunier, P. J. Mean wall thickness of trabecular bone packets in the human iliac crest: changes with age. *Calcif. Tissue Res.* **26,** 13–17 (1978).
43. Frost, H. M. Mean formation time of human osteons. *Can. J. Biochem. Physiol.* **41,** 1307–1310 (1963).
44. Jett, S., Wu, K., and Frost, H. M. Tetracycline-based histological measurement of cortical endosteal bone formation in normal and osteoporotic rib. *Henry Ford Hosp. Med. J.* **15,** 325–344 (1967).

45. Eriksen, E. F., Mosekilde, L., and Melsen, F. Trabecular bone resorption depth decreases with age: differences between normal males and females. *Bone* **6,** 141–146 (1985).
46. Compston, J. E., Yamaguchi, K., Croucher, P. I., Garrahan, N. J., Lindsay, P. C., and Shaw, R. W. The effects of gonadotrophin-releasing hormone agonists on iliac crest cancellous bone structure in women with endometriosis. *Bone* **16,** 261–267 (1995).
47. Amling, M., Herden, S., Pösl, M., Hahn, M., Ritzel, H., and Delling, G. Heterogeneity of the skeleton: comparison of the trabecular microarchitecture of the spine, the iliac crest, the femur and the calcaneus. *J. Bone Miner. Res.* **11,** 36–45 (1996).
48. Dempster, D. W., Ferguson-Pell, M. W., Mellish, R. W. E., Cochran, G. V. B., Xie, F., Fey, C., Horbert, W., Parisien, M., and Lindsay, R. Relationships between bone structure in the iliac crest and bone structure and strength in the lumbar spine. *Osteopor. Int.* **3,** 90–96 (1993).
49. Wakamatsu, E., and Sissons, H. A. The cancellous bone of the iliac crest. *Calcif. Tissue Res.* **4,** 147–161 (1969).
50. Aaron, J. E., Makins, N. B., Sagreiya, K. The microanatomy of trabecular bone loss in normal ageing men and women. *Clin. Orthop. Rel. Res.* **215,** 260–271 (1987).
51. Weinstein, R. S., and Hutson, M. S. Decreased trabecular width and increased trabecular spacing contribute to bone loss with aging. *Bone* **8,** 127–142 (1987).
52. Birkenhager-Frenkel, D. H., Courpron, P., Hüpscher, E. A., Clermonts, E., Coutinho, M. F., Schmitz, P. I. M., and Meunier, P. J. Age-related changes in cancellous bone structure. A two-dimensional study in the transiliac and iliac crest biopsy sites. *Bone Miner.* **4,** 197–216 (1988).
53. Mellish, R. W. E., Garrahan, N. J., and Compston, J. E. Age-related changes in trabecular width and spacing in human iliac crest biopsies. *Bone Miner.* **6,** 331–338 (1989).
54. Compston, J. E., Mellish, R. W. E., and Garrahan, N. J. Age-related changes in iliac crest trabecular microanatomic bone structure in man. *Bone* **8,** 289–292 (1987).
55. Hahn, M., Vogel, M., Amling, M., Ritzel, H., and Delling, G. Microcallus formation of the cancellous bone: a quantitative analysis of the human spine. *J. Bone Miner. Res.* **10,** 1410–1416 (1995).
56. Norman, T. L., and Wang, Z. Microdamage of human cortical bone: incidence and morphology in long bones. *Bone* **20,** 375–379 (1997).
57. Mosekilde, L. Consequences of the remodelling process for vertebral trabecular bone structure: a scanning electron microscopy study (uncoupling of unloaded structures). *Bone Miner.* **10,** 13–35 (1990).
58. Kleerekoper, M., Villanueva, A. R., Stanciu, J., Rao, D. S., and Parfitt, A. M. The role of three-dimensional trabecular microstructure in the pathogenesis of vertebral compression fractures. *Calcif. Tissue Int.* **37,** 594–597 (1985).
59. Recker, R. R., Smith, R. T., and Kimmel, D. B. Loss of trabecular connectivity in osteoporosis demonstrated with independent methods. *Bone* **13,** A28 (1992).
60. Croucher, P. I., Garrahan, N. J., and Compston, J. E. Structural mechanisms of trabecular bone loss in primary osteoporosis: specific disease mechanism or early ageing? *Bone Miner.* **25,** 111–121 (1994).

CHAPTER 24

Densitometric Manifestations in Age-Related Bone Loss

CARLOS A. MAUTALEN AND BEATRIZ OLIVERI
Sección Osteopatías Médicas, Hospital de Clínicas, University of Buenos Aires, Buenos Aires, Argentina

INTRODUCTION

The modern development of bone densitometry as a practical, clinical tool began at the University of Wisconsin, in the 1970's. The initial technique—single photon absorptiometry (SPA)—used a low-energy radionuclide source in order to measure a bone of the peripheral skeleton. A narrow beam of radiation produced by a monoenergetic radionuclide source (Iodine-125 at 28 keV or Americium-241 at 60 keV) was detected with a highly collimated scintillation detector coupled to a single-channel analyzer. A narrow beam was passed across the area of interest, usually the distal third of the radius. Only peripheral sites could be measured because a constant tissue thickness had to be maintained using a water bath. Measurements required 5 to 10 min with a precision error of approximately 2%.

In the 1980s, the SPA approach was improved by dual-photon absorptiometry (DPA). The new technique used a dual-energy radioisotope (Gadolinium-153 utilizing radiation at two different energies: 44- and 100-keV). DPA allowed measurement of the axial skeleton, spine and femur, as well as the total body. Since the advent of dual-energy technology, bone densitometry has become widely used for research and clinical assessment of patients with metabolic bone diseases.

During the last decade, X-rays have replaced radioisotopes as the source of the dual energy sources. The new technique of dual-energy X-ray absorptiometry (DXA) has the advantage of being more reproducible, a shorter measurement time, and greater stability of the energy source.

The physical basis of densitometry is the differential attenuation of radiation by bone mineral from the soft tissues that surround the bone. The SPA technique assumes that the soft tissue around the bone has a constant thickness. To achieve a constant thickness, a flexible cuff containing water is placed around the forearm, tightly pressed between two plates. With the DPA or DXA techniques, attenuation of the higher energy determines the tissue thickness, whereas the lower energy assesses by subtraction the amount of bone mineral, thus allowing measurement of specific skeletal sites.

Total body scans can be done in approximately 10 to 15 min using DXA. They provide not only bone mineral density (BMD) of the total skeleton and its subregions but also a very accurate measurement of soft tissue composition (fat and lean tissue).

Bone densitometry provides essentially two measurements: bone mineral content (BMC, in grams) and bone area (in cm^2). BMC/area is called bone mineral density (in g/cm^2). BMD is strongly correlated with bone strength and is therefore a powerful indicator of fracture risk. Bone densitometry, now a widely used, essential element in clinical evaluation, can (1) assess the skeletal status of patients with different metabolic bone diseases, (2) monitor the effect of the disease itself or its treatment on the bone, and (3) establish the risk for future osteoporotic fractures. The subject has been reviewed [1–3].

Other Techniques of Bone Mass Measurement

Quantitative computed tomography (QCT) provides a volumetric measurement of bone density in the vertebral body. Different from DXA, it distinguishes between cortical and cancellous bone. QCT is particularly useful in older individuals (>65 years old) in whom osteophytes and sclerotic facets could complicate conventional AP spine measurements by DXA.

Ultrasound (US) has been an investigational tool for over 20 years, but only in the past decade has its clinical applicability been actively pursued. US measurements may reflect elements of bone quality as well as bone density. The bone areas frequently evaluated by US are (a) the calcaneous (a load-bearing bone composed almost exclusively of cancellous bone); (b) the tibia; predominantly cortical bone; and (c) the patella, predominantly trabecular bone with a structure similar to the vertebral body.

US measurements include (a) speed of sound (SOS), in meters per second, which represents the velocity of ultrasound transmission through the bone. This index, which is influenced by elasticity and density, tends to correlate well with the measurement of bone mineral density. (b) Broad band ultrasound attenuation (BUA), expressed in decibels per megahertz, is indirectly reflective of bone architecture, suggesting that it is influenced not only by density but also by bone quantity, spacing, and orientation. It represents an interaction of ultrasound waves with the medium in which they are propagated, resulting in a loss of energy. (c) An index called *stiffness* is a combination of BUA and SOS and gives similar weighting. A review of ultrasound for the evaluation of bone has been published [4].

Basis of the Present Review

A large number of studies have evaluated the impact of age on bone mass. A comprehensive review of these studies is difficult because of major differences in methods and experimental approaches. Among these confounders are:

(a) Type of study: Cross-sectional vs longitudinal.
(b) Areas measured: radius vs lumbar spine vs proximal femur vs total skeleton and subgrouping within specified areas (e.g., Ward's space in the hip).
(c) The instrument: SPA, DPA, DXA, ultrasound, and QCT.
(d) Studies also differ itself with respect to the population tested by sex, race, and inclusion/exclusion criteria.
(e) Analyses differ greatly, some expressing the data as rate of change whereas others focus on absolute or percentage change from a given baseline.

In general, different cross-sectional or longitudinal studies expressing the impact of age as a percentage of bone loss from peak bone mass (PBM) have been reviewed. A separate analysis has been made according to the sex, area of bone, and type of evaluation (DXA, QCT, or ultrasound). Since it has been claimed that both absolute values and rate of bone loss differ according to the particular DXA equipment [5], the type of densitometer has been recorded in the different tables. However, this latter point, namely the influence of a particular densitometer is probably small in comparison to the much larger changes that occur over time. The authors here, therefore, calculated an "estimated mean change" based on the average loss reported. In general, a remarkably similar effect of age on bone loss has been observed in the vast majority of the studies.

Finally, a major factor of bone loss in women, is estrogen deficiency as the time of menopause. All bone areas, especially those with predominantly cancellous bone, sustain an accelerated period of bone loss during the first decade after the onset of menopause. The topic has been reviewed extensively [6]. In this chapter, the major emphasis is placed on the integral analysis of bone loss that occurs from peak bone mass, attained during the third to fourth decade of life to very old age.

Initial Estimations of the Effect of Age on Bone Densitometry

In 1970, Garn published a classical study [7] in which he determined the effect of age on bone using micrometric radiology of the metacarpal bones. After PBM was attained, continuous expansion of the external diameter of the metacarpal bones, as well as postmenopausal expansion of the internal medullary diameter, was observed. The latter exceeded the former so that cortical thickness started to decline in normal women after the sixth decade.

A few years later, with the availability of SPA, several investigators studied the differences in midradius bone mass between patients with osteoporosis and a control population. The design of this study included a large population of control subjects of both sexes [8]. It was observed that BMD of men was higher than that of women and that the rate of age related bone loss was faster in women than in men [9–11].

EFFECT OF AGING ON THE VERTEBRAL SKELETON

Women: Anterior–Posterior Projection

Since bone densitometry of the axial skeleton became available in the early 1980s, several studies were designed to note changes in BMD at different ages [12–15]. Initial approaches employed radioactive isotopes as a source, principally Gadolinium-153. However, in the late 1980s, DXA technology permitted many more subjects to be studied more quickly and with greater precision and accuracy [16].

Table I reviews values reported in the literature from different studies of normal Caucasian women from Europe, the United States, and South America [17–22]. The age-related changes are remarkably similar. As expected, peak BMD of the lumbar spine (AP projection) was maintained during the third and fourth decades. In the fifth decade (40–50 years), a small decrease (average 3% with a range of 2 to 4%) is observed. Because approximately 12% of women enter menopause before 45 years of age and because the failure to produce estrogen has a profound impact on bone mass, the very small average percentage bone loss during decade may be influenced by the inclusion of these early postmenopausal women.

From the sixth to eighth decade, the effect of aging on BMD of the AP lumbar spine is clearly evident. The decline averaged 11% (range: 9 to 18%) at 55 years, 18% (range: 13 to 24%) at age 65, and 21% (range: 16 to 25%) at age 75. This average loss of BMD of 20% from peak bone mass to the eighth decade observed in six different studies is very similar to the average loss of 18.3% reported in a multicenter study of a large number of normal women in France [23]. Average values are depicted in Fig. 1.

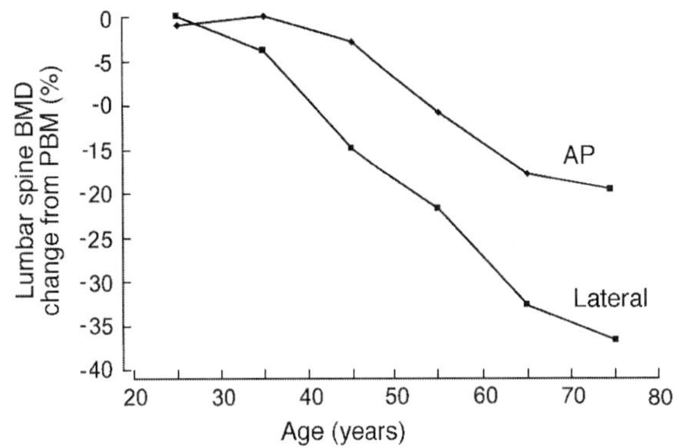

FIGURE 1 Average bone mineral density (BMD) change from peak bone mass (PBM) of the lumbar spine in anteroposterior (AP) or lateral view in women (Tables I and II).

Women: Lateral Projection

Few studies have determined normal BMD values of the lateral spine in women from 20 to 80 years of age (Table II). The differences among these reports are somewhat larger, probably due to technical factors and the smaller number of observations [21,22,24]. All studies concurred with peak bone mass becoming established between 20 and 30 years of age. A small reduction is seen during the following decade (average 4%, range 1 to 9%). By the next decade, similar to data from the AP studies, BMD has fallen significantly below peak bone mass (average: 16%; range 10 to 22%). Again, women who have lost ovarian function by a premature menopause may influence the average loss at this time, but it is also likely that cancellous bone loss has begun to occur at a young age. From the sixth decade, BMD loss becomes much more appreciable, with an average loss of 22% at age 55, 33% at age 65, and 37% at age 75.

Figure 1 illustrates the greater loss over time when lateral density is employed. This is probably due to two

TABLE I Bone Mineral Density of the Lumbar Spine (Anteroposterior) in Normal Women[a]

								Estimated mean
Reference	[17]	[18]	[19]	[20]	[21]	[21]	[22]	
Equipment	QDR	QDR	QDR	QDR	DPX	DPX	DPX	
Country	United States	Spain	Sweden	Germany	United States	Europe	Argentina	
Average PBM (g/cm^2)	1.05	1.04	1.04	1.07	1.23	1.21	1.19	
20–29	0	−1	−1	−2	−2	−1	0	−1
30–39	0	0	0	0	0	0	−1	0
40–49	−4	−4	−2	−2	−3	−3	−4	−3
50–59	−11	−11	−18	−9	−10	−9	−10	−11
60–69	−18	−19	−24	−16	−17	−13	−16	−18
70–79	−25	−22	−19	−16	−21	−20	−23	−21

[a] Average percentage difference from peak bone mass (PBM) per decade.

TABLE II Bone Mineral Density of the Lumbar Spine (Lateral) in Normal Women[a]

					Estimated mean
Reference	[24]	[21]	[21]	[22]	
Equipment	DPX	DPX	DPX	DPX	
Country	United States	United States	Europe	Argentina	
Average PBM (g/cm^2)	0.76	0.77	0.84	0.85	
20–30	0	0	0	0	0
30–40	−1	−1	−9	−9	−4
40–50	−12	−10	−22	−22	−16
50–60	−16	−15	−31	−31	−22
60–70	−31	−31	−36	−36	−33
70–80	−35	−35	−36	−36	−37

[a] Average percentage difference from peak bone mass (PBM) per decade.

factors. In the lateral projection, more cancellous bone is detected, an area that is more vulnerable to the effects of estrogen deficiency. Second, with age, osteophytes form and subject the AP measurement to that artifact, which would tend to underestimate the extent to which bone loss is occurring.

Longitudinal studies

At least two longitudinal studies have attempted to monitor bone loss of the lumbar spine in women over 60 years of age [25,26]. In contrast to cross-sectional studies of the spine, both studies have failed to appreciate the expected age-related bone loss in AP projection. The variation around the mean was very large, at least in part due to the error of the measurement. The failure to see any loss of bone mass at the lumbar spine (compared with 1% per year at the proximal femur—vide infra) suggests again that osteoarthritic changes of the spine cause a spurious compensation for the true bone loss that is probably occurring.

Men

Table III shows the results of five different cross-sectional studies of bone mass in the lumbar spine of men [17,18,20,21]. Similar to women, peak bone mass is maintained through age 50, with only a 5–6% reduction in the fourth decade (40–50). In contrast to women, who experience a much greater rate of bone loss after 50, men show only modest reductions, thereafter. The only exception is that of a normal male Japanese population in which a large 17% reduction was observed between 70 and 80. In that study, however, the number of observation was small (n = 38).

Studies of bone mass in the lateral projection in men are limited to that of Barelon *et al.* in which a 22% diminution of the BMD from the third to the eight decade was observed. That some group showed a 38% loss in women over this same period of time (21).

Longitudinal studies in men are also limited to one in a Caucasian population [26]. A comparison of cross-sectional data between men and women shows that bone loss occurs over time in both sexes with the expected greater reduction in women after menopause (Fig. 2).

EFFECT OF AGING ON THE PROXIMAL FEMUR

Women

Several cross-sectional studies with the older dual-photon technology (Gadolinium-153) as provided early information on age-related bone loss at the proximal femur [13–15,27–30]. With the new DXA technology, eight different studies on different Caucasian populations from Spain, Germany, Sweden, the United Kingdom, Argentina, and the United States are summarized in Table IV [17–22,31–33]. Peak bone mass of the femoral neck is reached during the third decade.

During the following two decades, small average losses of 3 to 5% are seen. However, it is noteworthy that there is wide discrepancy among the studies over this time period. Differences range from no change [19] to losses of BMD up to 8% [17,22]. The studies show a more uniform loss of bone after the age of 50. At an average age of 55, the mean reduction is 13% (range: 11–15%). At an average age of 65, the mean reduction is 19% (range: 17–22%); at 75, the mean reduction is 25% (range: 21–29%).

TABLE III Bone Mineral Density of the Lumbar Spine (Anteroposterior) in Normal Men[a]

						Estimated mean
Reference	[17]	[18]	[20]	[21]	[21]	
Equipment	QDR	QDR	QDR	DPX	DPX	
Country	United States	Spain	Germany	United States	Japan	
Average PBM (g/cm^2)	1.11	1.04	1.09	1.25	1.2	
20–30	0	0	0	0	0	0
30–40	0	−2	−5	−3	0	−2
40–50	−2	−3	−8	−6	−6	−6
50–60	−5	−5	−6	−7	−8	−6
60–70	−8	−5	−7	−6	−9	−7
70–80	−10	−10	−4	−6	−17	−9

[a] Average percentage difference from peak bone mass (PBM) per decade.

Other regions of the hip, besides the femoral neck, have received less attention. A summary of some of these observations [19,21,24,31] is that Ward's area appears to sustain more rapid and severe bone loss than the femoral neck. In fact, a loss of BMD at this level averages ~12% at age 45. Supporting these findings, the multicenter French study [23] disclosed a loss of ~11.2% at age 50 in this area. In fact, the only statistically significant sites of premenopausal bone mass were registered at Ward's triangle and the lateral view of the spine [23]. Bone loss at the trochanter appears to be less than either the femoral neck or Ward's triangle (Fig. 3).

In the four cross-sectional studies of women over 80 [34–37], a continuous and unabated bone loss persists at all areas: femoral neck, Ward's triangle, trochanter and total hip.

Longitudinal Studies

The most interesting data on the effect of age on the BMD of the proximal femur come from two longitudinal studies. Jones *et al.* [26] observed an average bone loss of the femoral neck of 0.96% year in a large group of women over 60 years with an average age of 71 years. Data suggested that the rate of bone loss increased with advancing age. An even more comprehensive study was reported by Ensrud *et al.* [38] on a large cohort of women from 65 to over 85 years of age. They found that the average loss of BMD at the femoral neck, ~0.35% year at 65 years of age, gradually increases to reach a rate of loss of ~1.0% year after age 85. Similar results were observed over Ward's triangle, trochanteric region, total hip, and calcaneous (Fig. 4).

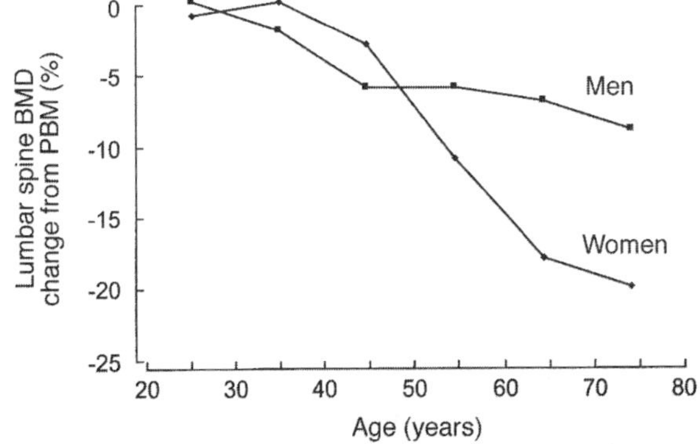

FIGURE 2 Average bone mineral density (BMD) change from peak bone mass (PBM) of the lumbar spine (anteroposterior view) in men and women (Tables I and III).

Effect of Age on Bone Mineral Content, Bone Area, and BMD of the Proximal Femur

Densitometric studies have confirmed the classical observation of Smith and Walker [39] on the expansion of the outer diameter of the femur with age. The meticulous study of Looker *et al.* [31] reports in detail the changes observed at all areas of the proximal femur. At the femoral neck, there is an enlargement in area of ~6 to 8% from the third to the eighth decade. Due to the expansion of area, the results of the BMD overestimates the bone loss compared to the determination of BMC. For example, at age 65 the respective changes were: BMC, −15%; BMD, −20%; and bone area, 8% (Fig. 5). These findings are similar to those observed over the trochanter and total proximal femur.

Men

Very few studies on age-related changes in femoral BMD have been published [15,17,18,21]. Apparently there is some loss from the third to the fifth decade

Table IV Bone Mineral Density of the Femoral Neck in Normal Women[a]

Reference	[17]	[18]	[19]	[31]	[22]	[21]	[32]	[33]	Estimated mean
Equipment	QDR	QDR	QDR	QDR	DPX	DPX	DPX	DPX	
Country	United States	Spain	Sweden	United States	Argentina	United States	United Kingdom	Sweden	
Average PBM (g/cm^2)	0.89	0.84	0.81	0.85	0.99	1	1.01	1.01	
20–30	0	0	0	0	0	0	0	0	0
30–40	−3	−4	0	−2	−7	−1	−1	−6	−3
40–50	−8	−4	−1	−5	−8	−6	−6	−2	−5
50–60	−14	−12	−15	−14	−12	−12	−12	−12	−13
60–70	−22	−17	−20	−20	−17	−19	−18	−22	−19
70–80	−29	−26	−23	−28	−21	−25	−23	−27	−25
80+	−35			−33					

[a] Average percentage from peak bone mass (PBM) per decade.

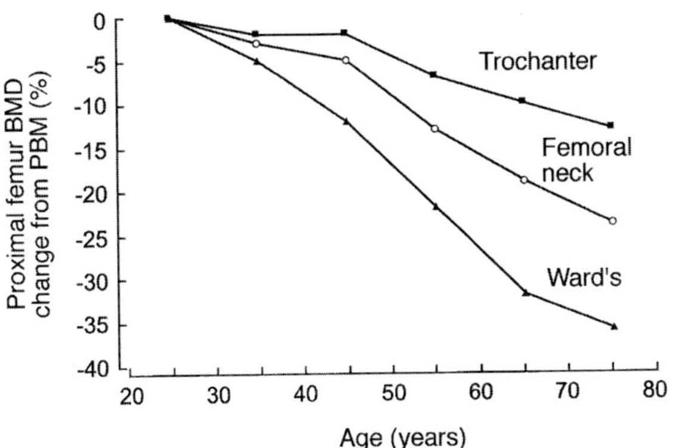

FIGURE 3 Average bone mineral density (BMD) change from peak bone mass (PBM) at different areas of the proximal femur, trochanter, neck, and Ward's in women.

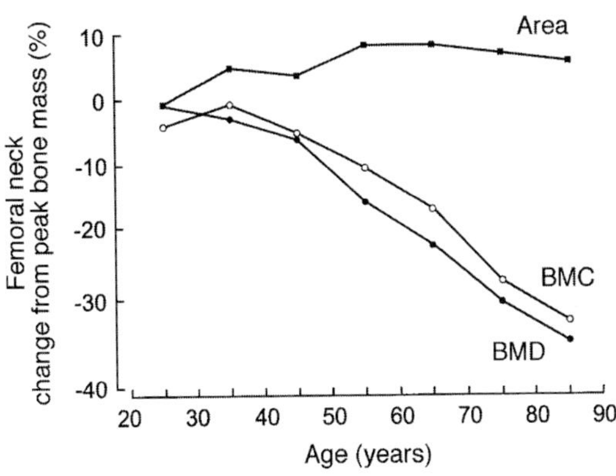

FIGURE 5 Average change with age of bone mineral content (BMC), bone area, and bone mineral density (BMD) of the femoral neck in white women. Adapted from Looker *et al.* [31].

(~9 to 11%). Then, diminution of bone mass continues without any overt acceleration. As in the case of women, the impact is greatest at Ward's triangle (−35% diminution from PBM) than the femoral neck (−22%) or the trochanter (−11%) [15].

Two studies conducted in large cohorts from age 55 to 90 disclosed that bone loss at this age is almost double in women compared to men. In one study, femoral neck BMD diminished 17% in women and 8% in men, while at the level of Ward's triangle the loss was 23% in women and 12% in men [35]. Similar findings were reported in a study in the United States: at the femoral neck the changes were −29% in women and −9% in men; results at Ward's triangle were −30 and −14%, respectively [36].

A longitudinal study determined that the femoral neck annual bone loss in men and women over 60 years of age was slightly lower in men. The respective results were 0.82 and 0.96% per year, respectively [26]. The rate of decrease was greater with advancing age supporting similar findings in women [38].

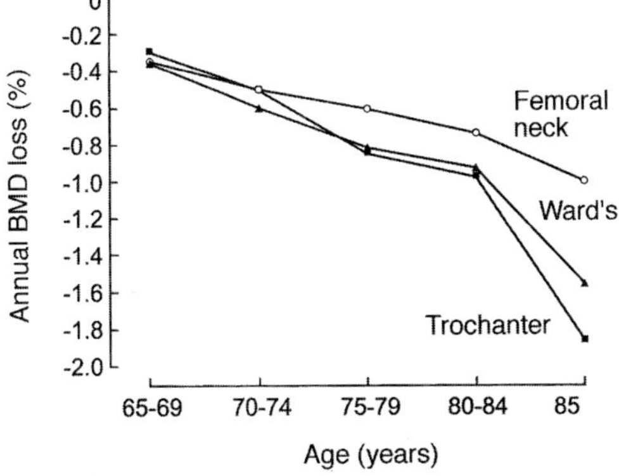

FIGURE 4 Average annual bone mineral density (BMD) loss with age at different areas of the proximal femur in women. Adapted from Ensrud *et al.* [38].

EFFECT OF AGING ON TOTAL SKELETON BONE MINERAL DENSITY

Women

Table V shows values for total skeleton peak bone mass in normal Caucasian women from Europe, the United States, and South America [21,40,41]. Most of the cross-sectional studies reported in the literature have found the highest values in the fourth decade, between 30 and 39 years of age [21,40,42], indicating that skeletal mineral accrual continues into that decade (20 to 29 years). Different results were reported in a 1-year longitudinal study of in 20- to 35-year-old healthy women and men. This study found appreciable gains over this period, even when the study population was divided into 5-year intervals. These results suggest that total skeleton peak bone mass, similar to individual sites, is reached by the third decade [43].

Most of the studies have found no significant loss of total skeletal mass in premenopausal women. Between 35 and 45 years of age, an average nonsignificant decline of 3% (range 0 to 5%) [21,40–42] was observed. Starting in the sixth decade, the effect of age on BMD of total skeleton is evident. The average decline is 5% (range: 4 to 7%) at age 55; 10% (range: 9 to 12%) at age 65; and 14% (range: 11 to 17%) at age 75. The cumulative loss from 30 to 80 years in a multicenter study reported by Arlot *et al.* [23] was approximately 15%, very similar to the average loss in the studies shown in Table V.

Men

Peak bone mass in Caucasian men was found in the third decade, followed by small declines averaging only 2% until the seventh decade. Average values indicate a

TABLE V Bone Mineral Density of the Total Skeleton in Normal Women[a]

Reference	[40]	[41]	[21]	[21]	Estimated mean
Equipment	XR26	DPX	DPX	DPX	
Country	Spain	Argentina	United States	Europe	
Average PBM (g/cm^2)	1.16	1.12	1.15	1.13	
20–29	−6	0	−2	−2	−3
30–39	0	−1	0	0	0
40–49	−5	−3	−3	0	−3
50–59	−7	−4	−6	−5	−5
60–69	−12	−9	−10	−9	−10
70–79	−17	−13	−13	−16	−15

[a] Average percentage difference from peak bone mass (PBM) per decade.

loss of 7% (range: 6–8%) and 8% (range: 6–11%) in the eighth and ninth decades, respectively [21,44].

Other Skeletal Sites

DXA permits evaluation of subregions such as arms, legs, spine, trunk, skull, and pelvis in addition to the more conventional sites summarized earlier.

Figure 6 shows changes in BMD, both in terms of total skeletal density and its subregions, in a group of Caucasian women and men [21]. Overall, men display a lower rate of bone loss at all sites compared to women. Total skeleton and its subregions lose bone mass in women after 45–50 years, coinciding with the onset of menopause. The decline in the different subregions varies among different studies [21,40,41,45]. In general, however, the extent of reduction appears to be greater over the axial skeleton—trunk and pelvis—and the legs than the arms and skull.

Effect of Aging on Body Composition in Women

DXA methodology also permits facile and precise assessment of lean and fat body mass. The percentage of fat body mass in women increases progressively from the age of 20 to 70–74 after which it tends to decrease [46]. Fat mass is lower in premenopausal as compared to healthy postmenopausal women (11–12%) and increases mainly in the first years of postmenopause [21,47]. Conversely, lean mass is maintained with slight variations throughout the premenopausal period and begins to decrease slowly after the onset of menopause, reaching cumulative reductions of 8% to 11% in the ninth decade [46–48]. Osteoporotic women have lower fat body mass than control women, but no apparent difference in their lean body mass [47,49].

EFFECT OF AGE ON ULTRASOUND VALUES

Women

Studies to evaluate the effect of aging on bone mass as assessed by ultrasound technology (US) have mainly been carried out in cross-sectional studies. A summary

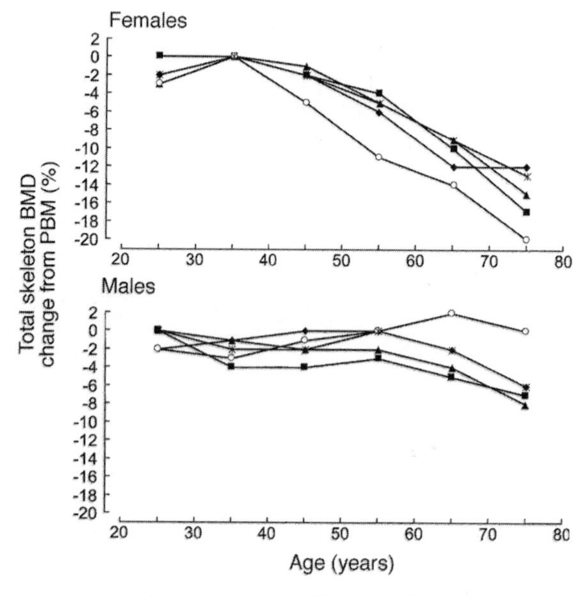

FIGURE 6 Average bone mineral density (BMD) age-related changes from peak bone mass (PBM) of the total skeleton and subregions in women and men. Adapted from Barden *et al.* [21].

TABLE VI BUA and SOS Ultrasound Measurements in Normal Women (Achilles Equipment)[a]

				Estimated average				Estimated average
Reference	[50]	[51]	[52]		[50]	[51]	[52]	
Country	Japan	Argentina	United Kingdom		Japan	Argentina	United Kingdom	
	BUA[b]	BUA	BUA[b]		SOS	SOS	SOS	
PV	113	123	118		1562	1567	1550	
20–29	0	0	0	0	0	0	0	0
30–39	0	−3	−3	−1	−1	−1	−1	−1
40–49	0	−8	−3	−4	−1	−2	−2	−2
50–59	−6	−8	−6	−7	−3	−2	−3	−3
60–69	−9	−10	−11	−11	−3	−3	−3	−4
70–79	−10	−13	−21	−15	−3	−4	−6	−5

[a] Average percentage of loss from peak values (PV) per decade.
[b] Recalculated from the 5-year interval reported in the study.

of data of bone ultrasound attenuation (BUA) and of speed of sound (SOS) provided by these studies [50–52] is presented in Table VI. Most of the studies refer the highest SOS, BUA and stiffness index values for the age range 20 to 29 years [50–54]. In most cases no significant changes are observed between 20 and 39 years of age but US values decrease gradually thereafter.

BUA diminution from peak values at the average age of 45 years is ~4% (range: 0 to −8%), continues to decline, reaching 7% at the sixth decade (range: 6–10%): 11% of the seventh decade (range: 9–12%): and 15% at 75 years (range: 10−−21%). A similar tendency but with smaller percentage diminution due to the smaller range of useful values was observed on the effect of age on SOS.

One of the studies performed in elderly women with an average age of 86 years (range 70 to 88) showed that SOS and stiffness index values continue to decrease at this old age [55]. Determinations of tibia cortical US reveal approximately 7% diminution of SOS between the age of 20 and 89 [56].

Several studies have focused on changes in US parameters in women with respect to the timing of menopause. Until menopause, no changes were observed [54,57–59]. Soon after menopause, however, loss is already apparent within 2 years [60] and as expected, the annual rate of loss in US values is more marked in the first 5 years menopausal years [61].

The few longitudinal studies that have used this technique [55,62,63] concur with cross-sectional data, indicating a greater loss during the early menopausal years, especially regarding SOS and stiffness [62]. In fact, the percentage of losses in these two indices is higher by 1.5 to 4.5 fold in longitudinal studies [62,63] than in cross-sectional studies.

Changes in Ultrasound Values in Men

Although US studies in men are scarce [63,64], it is noteworthy that a study carried out in Japan on both males and females [64] found higher US absolute values in men but a similar percentage of age-related loss in both sexes. In this study, the average loss between the ages of 20 and 70 was between 4 and 5% for SOS, 12 and 10% for BUA, and 30 and 28% for stiffness in women and men, respectively (Fig. 7), despite the higher percentage loss in women than in men when evaluation is conducted by densitometry.

One longitudinal study of US performed in a Caucasian population [63] also showed similar rates of diminution in SOS and stiffness in both women and men after 55 years. In both sexes, but especially in men, the rate of loss in these two parameters tended to increase with age.

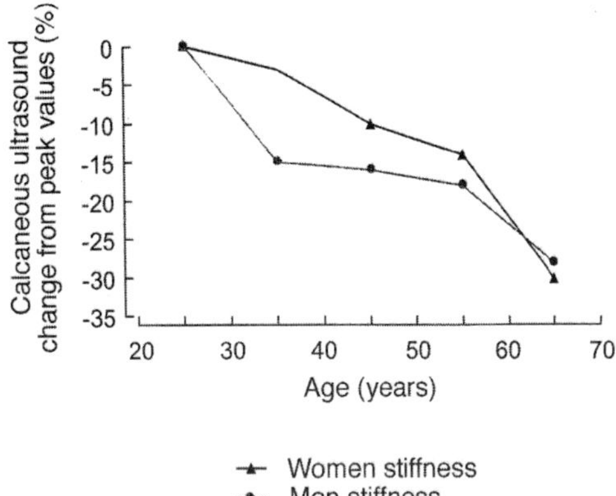

FIGURE 7 Average age-related changes in "stiffness" ultrasound in women (▲) and men (●). Adapted from Takeda *et al.* [64].

EFFECT OF AGING ON BONE MINERAL DENSITY BY QCT

Vertebral Mineral Density

Table VII shows the effect of age on vertebral bone density in Caucasian and Japanese populations [65]. PBM is set at 20–29 years. In the Caucasian population the average loss in the fourth decade is 4%. At the age of 57 the average loss is 35% and continues to decline to 42 and 49% in the seventh and eighth decades, respectively.

It is noteworthy that the decline in the Japanese population was substantially greater compared to the Caucasian population. This difference is seen in all age groups and is particularly pronounced in older age groups, reaching around a 59% loss of vertebral trabecular bone in the seventh decade versus an average 39% in Caucasians and a 72% loss in the female Japanese population above 70 years of age versus 49% in Caucasians. Other studies on Caucasian population [66,67] have observed similar age-related losses in vertebral bone density as the one reported by Ito *et al.* [65].

Cross-sectional studies in women have shown that the main factor affecting the diminution of cancellous bone density is the length of menopause rather than age [68]. As noted earlier, measurements in women with 25 years of menopausal life show as much as an approximately 35–40% reduction. Some studies have shown that the majority of the total reduction observed occurs within the first 5 years of a menopause [68].

TABLE VII QCT Vertebral Bone Mineral Density of Lumbar Vertebrae in Normal Women[a]

Average PBM(g/cm^2)	United States	Japan
	185	169
20–24	0	0
25–29	0	−9
30–34	−2	−7
35–39	−4	−14
40–44	−5	−17
45–49	−14	−28
50–54	−26	−42
55–59	−35	−52
60–64	−39	−59
65–68	−42	−63
70–74	−49	−72

[a] Average percentage difference from peak bone mass (PBM). From Ito *et al.* [65].

Effect of Aging in Peripheral Bone Evaluated by QCT (pQCT)

As is the case for central measurements by QCT, pQCT measures true dimensional density (i.e., three-dimensional, volumetric density) and distinguishes between cortical and cancellous bone density in the peripheral skeleton. Most of the studies have been carried out in radius [69–73]. Advances in pQCT methodology have enabled separate assessment of compact bone density (CBD) in the diaphysis and of trabecular bone (TBD) in a distal site.

In women [71], TBD of the radius diminishes by 28% between 20 and 70 years of age. Cortical bone density however, changes much less so throughout this period.

Bone mineral content and the density of cancellous bone (e.g., ultradistal radius) and cortical bone (e.g., proximal radius) [72] are subject to differences in forces associated with aging. Comparison of values for premenopausal women and for those in the age range of >70 years revealed that the ultradistal cancellous area was higher by 35% in the older group, with no variation in bone mineral content, thus resulting in ~28% loss of bone mineral density. The proximal cortical area diminished 13% and BMC decreased 20%, leading to a 9% loss in BMD (Fig. 8).

Other studies using pQCT at the radial site have differentiated two types of loss: a self-limiting component related to menopause that accounts for approximately 15% of bone (mainly cancellous) and a more continuous component that starts at age 55 and proceeds (mainly cortical) at an approximate rate of 1% per year [73].

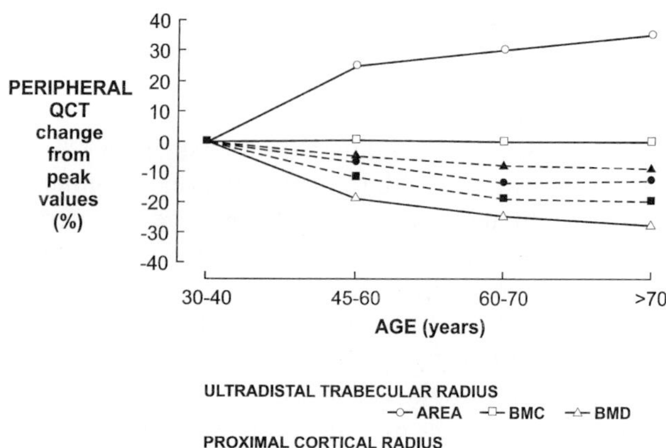

FIGURE 8 Age-related changes of bone mineral content (BMC), bone area, and bone mineral density (BMD) in ultradistal trabecular radius and proximal cortical radius. Adapted from Gatti *et al.* [72].

SUMMARY

This chapter has considered the various methodologies by which bone density is monitored and data revealing the universal loss of bone mass associated with aging. Several questions result from this review.

Onset of Age-Related Bone Loss in Normal Women

There is little doubt that at predominantly cancellous sites, bone loss starts as early as the fourth decade of life. The average differences between ages 25 and 45 indicate a diminution in BMD of ~16% in the lateral view of the spine, ~17% in the QCT assessment of the trabecular vertebral tissue, and ~12% at the Ward's area of the proximal femur. Some of this early loss may be perceived as early as the third decade but it is more evident between 30 and 40.

However, the changes that occur before menopause at other skeletal sites are relatively minor and statistically insignificant. Average BMD diminution from 25 to 45 years of age ranged between ~3% at the AP view of the lumbar spine and total skeleton and ~5% at the femoral neck. However, the study of Looker *et al.* [31] is of great interest because BMC increases from age 25 to 35 and the diminution of the BMD is due primarily to an increase in area. It seems therefore that what is taking place during this pre-menopausal period is a redistribution of bone tissue. Similar studies of total skeleton or AP spine could contribute further to understanding of these skeletal changes before menopause. Based on available data a partial conclusion at this time suggests that there is little or no bone loss at cortical sites before menopause. Whatever minor changes do occur could be due to the redistribution of bone tissue or to the inclusion of women with premature menopause within the control groups.

Bone Loss from Menopause to the Later Years

The abrupt loss in estrogen production after menopause induces a marked loss of bone that affects all areas and types of bones. Al least during the first decade after menopause changes in bone mass are more related significantly to the estrogen deficiency than to chronological age. However, is very important to point out that bone loss continues throughout life and may even accelerate at old age.

Cross-sectional studies disclose that bone loss is probably still more pronounced at the cancellous than at the cortical compartment. From age 45 to 75 the changes were ~−21% at the lateral spine and ~−31% by QCT of the vertebral bodies against losses of ~17% at AP view of the lumbar spine, ~−19% at femoral neck, and −11% at the total skeleton. Total skeletal, loss however, results from greater loss over the legs, trunk, and pelvis and to a lesser extent loss over the arms and head.

The average total BMD at the level of the lumbar spine by DXA does not diminish after 65 to 70 years of age due to the fact that osteoarthritic changes around the vertebral bodies compensate the true bone loss that occurs over the trabecular and cortical components of the bone.

Longitudinal studies at the proximal femur have been of great significance, especially considering the clinical relevance of this area as a site of hip fracture. Two studies concur that BMD loss increases with age [26,38]. In fact, the absolute and relative loss of bone more than doubles between 65 and 85 years of age. A reason for this observation relates to the fact that as bone trabeculae thin with age, they are more likely to become disconnected followed by rapid resorption of biomechanically not longer useful bone. In addition, a more rapid rate of trabeculation of the endosteal surface of the cortex would diminish the latter and increase the quantity of the more vulnerable cancellous bone.

Bone Loss in Men

Data available are rather scarce in comparison to the studies performed in women. However, review of the available data suggests that bone loss is minimal in men between 25 and 45 years. Average losses are ~5% at the AP spine and ~10% at the femoral neck. These observations suggest an early loss of axial cancellous bone in men not too different from that observed in women [74]. Well-conducted longitudinal studies could clarify this point.

Bone loss has been observed at older ages at the proximal femur and total skeleton. The rate of bone loss at all sites is approximately half the rate of bone loss observed in women after menopause.

The difference of bone loss rates between men and women appears to be less pronounced in longitudinal studies [26], but the rate of loss is still greater in women. However, it should be emphasized that, similar to the observations made in women, bone loss continues indefinitely in men and that the rate increases with advancing age, at least over the proximal femur [26].

An interesting observation is that the effect of age by ultrasound measurement appears to be similar in men and women. Because bone mass diminishes more rapidly in women, a similar effect might be expected by ultrasound detection. Further studies should clarify this point. If confirmed, it could indicate that despite a greater preservation of total bone mass, the quality and structure of bone or whatever else is detected by ultrasound deteriorates in both sexes.

References

1. Genant, H. K., Lang, T. F., Engelke, K., Fuerst, T., Gluer, C. C., Majumdar, S., and Jergas, M. Advances in the noninvasive assessment of bone density, quality, and structure. *Calcif, Tissue Int.* **59,** S10–S15 (1996).
2. Miller, P. D., Bonnick, S. L., and Rosen, C. J. Clinical utility of bone mass measurements in adults: consensus of an international panel. *Semin. Arthritis Rheum.* **25,** 361–372 (1996).
3. Mazess, R. Bone densitometry. *In* "Textbook of Nuclear Medicine" (M. A. Wilson, ed.), pp. 279–285. Lippincott-Raven, Philadelphia, 1998.
4. Gluer, Claus-C. Quantitative ultrasound techniques for the assessment of osteoporosis: Expert agreement of current status. *J. Bone Miner. Res.* **12,** 1280–1288 (1997).
5. Peel, N. F. A., and Eastell, R. Comparison of rates of bone loss from the spine measured using two manufacturer's densitometers. *J. Bone Miner. Res.* **10,** 1796–1801 (1995).
6. Gallagher, J. C., Goldgar, D., and Moy, A. Total bone calcium in normal women: effect of age and menopause status. *J. Bone Miner. Res.* **2,** 491–496 (1987).
7. Garn, S., "The Earlier Gain and the Later Loss of Cortical Bone in Nutritional Perspective." Charles Thomas, Springfield, IL, 1970.
8. Mazess, R. B., ed. *In* "Proceedings of the Fourth International Conference on Bone Measurement." Washington U.S. Department of Health and Human Services, Publication No. (NIH) 80, 1980.
9. Ringe Von, J. D., Rehpenning, W., and Kuhlencordt, F. Physiologische Aenderung des Mineralgehalts von Radius und Ulna in Abbangigkeit von Lebensalter und Geschlecht. *Fortschr. Rontgenstr.* **126,** 376 (1977).
10. Mazess, R. B., and Cameron, J. R. Bone mineral content in normal U.S. whites. *In* "International Conference on Bone Mineral Measurement" R. B. Mazess, (ed.), Washington U.S. Department of Health, Education, and Welfare, Publication No. (NIH) **75,** 1974.
11. Mautalen, C., Tau C., Casco, C., and Fromm, G. Contenido mineral oseo en la población normal de Buenos Aires. *Medicina* **44,** 356–360 (1984).
12. Hansson, and Roos, B. Age changes in the bone mineral of the lumbar spine in normal women. *Calcif. Tissue Int.* **38,** 249–251 (1986).
13. Pocock, N., Eisman, J., Mazess, R., Sambrook, P., Yeates, M., and Freund, J. Bone mineral density in Australia compared with the United States. *J. Bone Miner. Res.* **3,** 601–604 (1988).
14. Mautalen, C., Rubin, Z., Vega, E., Ghiringhelli, G., and Fromm, G. Densidad mineral de la columna lumbar y femur proximal en mujeres normales de Buenos Aires. *Medicina* **50,** 25–29 (1990).
15. Mazess, R., Barden, H., Drinka, P., Bauwens, S., Orwoll, E., and Bell, N. Influence of age and body weight on spine and femur bone mineral density in U.S. white men. *J. Bone Miner. Res.* **5,** 645–652 (1990).
16. Jergas, M., and Genant, H. K. Lateral dual x-ray absorptiometry of the lumbar spine: current status. *Bone* **20,** 311–314 (1997).
17. Favus, M. S., ed. Bone density reference data (for QDR systems). *In* "Primer on the Metabolic Bone Diseases and Disorders of Mineral Metabolism," p. 463. Lippincott-Raven, 1996.
18. Diaz Curiel, M., Carrasco de la Peña, J., Honorato Perez, J., Perez Cano, R., Rapado, A., and Ruiz Martinez, I. Study of bone mineral density in lumbar spine and femoral neck in a Spanish population. *Osteopor. Int.* **7,** 59–64 (1997).
19. Lofman, O., Larsson, L., Ross, I., Toss, G., and Berglund, K. Bone mineral density in normal Swedish women. *Bone* **20,** 167–174 (1997).
20. Lehmann, R., Wapniarz, M., Randerath, O., Kvasnicka, H., John, W., Reincke, M., Kutnar, S., Klein, K., and Allolio, B. Dual-energy X-ray absorptiometry at the lumbar spine in German men and women: A cross-sectional study. *Calcif. Tissue Int.* **56,** 350–354 (1995).
21. (a) Barden, H., Mazess, R. B., Hanson, J., and Kamau, K. Bone mineral density of the spine and femur in normal U.S. white females. *J. Bone Miner. Res.* **12**(Suppl. 1), S248 (1997). (b) Lunar News, August, p. 10, 1997.
22. Vega, E., Bagur, A., and Mautalen, C. Densidad mineral osea en mujeres osteoporóticas y normales de Buenos Aires. *Medicina* **53,** 211–216 (1993).
23. Arlot, M., Sornay-Rendu, Garnero, P., Vey-Marty, B., and Delmas, P. Apparent pre- and postmenopausal bone loss evaluated by DXA at different skeletal sites in women: the OFELY cohort. *J. Bone Miner. Res.* **12,** 683–690 (1997).
24. Mazess, R., Barden, H., Eberle, R., and Denton, M. Age changes of spine density in posterior–anterior and lateral projections in normal women. *Calcif. Tissue Int.* **56,** 201–205 (1995).
25. Greenspan, S., Maitland, L., Myers, E., Krasnow, M., and Kido, T. Femoral bone loss progresses with age: A longitudinal study in women over age 65. *J. Bone Miner. Res.* **9,** 1959–1965 (1994).
26. Jones, G., Nguyen, T., Sambrook, P., Kelly, P., and Eisman, J. Progressive loss of bone in the femoral neck in elderly people: longitudinal findings from the Dubbo osteoporosis epidemiology study. *Br. Med. J.* **309,** 691–695 (1994).
27. Mazess, R., Barden, H., Ettinger, M., Johnston, C., Dawson-Hughes, B., Baran, D., Powell, M., and Notelovitz, M. Spine and femur density using dual-photon absorptiometry in US white women. *Bone Mineral* **2,** 211–219 (1987).
28. Schaadt, O., and Bohr, H. Different trends of age-related diminution of bone mineral content in the lumbar spine, femoral neck, and femoral shaft in women. *Calcif. Tissue Int.* **42,** 71–76 (1988).
29. Mautalen, C., Vega, E., Ghiringhelli, G., and Fromm, G. Bone diminution of osteoporotic females at different skeletal sites. *Calcif. Tissue Int.* **46,** 217–221 (1990).
30. Hannan, M., Felson, D., and Anderson, J. Bone mineral density in elderly men and women: results from the Framingham osteoporosis study. *J. Bone Miner. Res.* **7,** 547–553 (1992).
31. Looker, A. C., Wahner, H. W., Dunn, W. L., Calvo, M. S., Harris, T. B., Heyse, S. P., Johnston C. C., Jr., and Lindsay, R. L. Proximal femur bone mineral levels of US adults. *Osteopor. Int.* **5,** 389–409 (1995).
32. Truscott, J. G., Simpson, D., and Fordham, J. N. *In* "Compilation of National Bone Densitometry Reference Data" (E. F. J., Ring, C. M., Elvins, and A. K. Bhalla, eds.), pp. 77–78. British Institute of Radiology, Bath, UK, 1996.
33. Karlsson, M. K., Gardsell, P., Johnell, O., Nilsson, B. E., Akesson, K., and Obrant, K. J. Bone mineral normative data in Malmo, Sweden. *Acta Orthop. Scand.* **64,** 168–172 (1993).
34. Looker, A., Johnston, C., Wahner, H., Dunn, W., Calvo, M., Harris, T., Heyse, S., and Lindsay, R. Prevalence of low femoral bone density in older U.S. women from NHANES III. *J. Bone Miner. Res.* **10,** 796–802 (1995).

35. Burger, H., Van Daele, P., Algra, D., Van den Ouweland, F., Grobbee, D., Hofman, A., van Kuijik, C., Schutte, H., Birkenhager, J., and Pols, H. The association between age and bone mineral density in men and women aged 55 years and over: The Rotterdam study. *Bone Mineral* **25,** 1–13 (1994).
36. Blunt, B., Klauber, M., Barrett-Connor, E., and Edelstein, S. Sex differences in bone mineral density in 1653 men and women in the sixth through tenth decades of life: The Rancho Bernardo study. *J. Bone Miner. Res.* **9,** 1333–1338 (1994).
37. Steiger, P., Cumming, S., Black, D., Spencer, N., and Genant, H. Age-related decrements in bone mineral density in women over 65. *J. Bone Miner. Res.* **7,** 625–632 (1992).
38. Ensrud, K., Palermo, L., Black, D., Cauley, J., Jergas, M., Orwoll, E., Nevitt, M., Fox, K., and Cummings, S. Hip and calcaneal bone loss increase with advancing age: Longitudinal results from the study of osteoporotic fractures. *J. Bone Miner. Res.* **10,** 1778–1787 (1995).
39. Smith, R. W., Jr., and Walker, R. R. Femoral expansion in aging women: Implications for osteoporosis and fractures. *Science* **145,** 156–157 (1966).
40. Rico, H., Revilla, M., Villa, L., and Alvarez de Buergo, M. Age-related differences in total and regional bone mass: a cross-sectional study with DXA in 429 normal women. *Osteopor. Int.* **3,** 154–159 (1993).
41. Bagur, A., Vega, E., and Mautalen, C. Discrimination of total body bone mineral density measured by Dexa in vertebral osteoporosis. *Calcif. Tissue Int.* **56,** 263–267 (1995).
42. Nuti, R., and Martini, G. Measurements of bone mineral density by DXA total body absorptiometry in different skeletal sites in postmenopausal osteoporosis. *Bone* **13,** 173–178 (1992).
43. Slosman, D. O., Rizzoli, R., Pichard, C., Donath, A., and Bonjour, J.-P. Longitudinal measurement of regional and whole body bone mass in young healthy adults. *Osteopor. Int.* **4,** 185–190 (1994).
44. Nuti, R., Martini, G., and Gennari, C. Age-related changes of whole skeleton and body composition in healthy men. *Calcif. Tissue Int.* **57,** 336–339 (1995).
45. Nuti, R., and Martini, G. Effects of age and menopause on bone density of entire skeleton in healthy and osteoporotic women. *Osteopor. Int.* **3,** 59–65 (1993).
46. Khosla, S., Atkinson, E., Riggs, B. L., and Melton, L. J., III Relationship between body composition and bone mass in women. *J. Bone Miner. Res.* **11,** 857–863 (1996).
47. Martini, G., Valenti, R., Giovani, S., and Nuti, R. Age-related changes in body composition of healthy and osteoporotic women. *Maturitas* **27,** 25–33 (1997).
48. Tsunenari, T., Tsutsumi, M., Ohno, K., Yamamoto, Y., Kawakatsu, M., Shimogaki, K., Negishi, H., Sugimoto, T., Fukase, M., and Fujita, T. Age- and gender-related changes in body composition in Japanese subjects. *J. Bone Miner. Res.* **8,** 397–402 (1993).
49. Mautalen, C., Bagur, A., Vega, E., and Gonzalez, D. Composición corporal en mujeres normales y osteoporóticas. *Medicina* (*Buenos Aires*) **56,** 29–34 (1996).
50. Yamazaki, K., Kushida, K., Ohmura, A., Sano, M., and Inoue, T. Ultrasound bone densitometry of the os calcis in Japanese women. *Osteopor. Int.* **4,** 220–225 (1994).
51. Mautalen, C., Vega, E., Gonzalez, D., Carrilero, P., Otaño, A., and Silberman, F. Ultrasound and dual x-ray absorptiometry densitometry in women with hip fracture. *Calcif. Tissue Int.* **57,** 165–168 (1995).
52. Truscott, J. Reference data for ultrasonic bone measurement: variation with age in 2087 caucasian women aged 16-93 years. *Br. J. Radiol.* **70,** 1010–1016 (1997).
53. Schott, A., Hans, D., Sornay-Rendu, E., Delmas, P., and Meunier, P. Ultrasound measurements on Os calcis: precision on age-related changes in a normal female population. *Osteopor. Int.* **3,** 249–254 (1993).
54. Damilakis, J., Dretaiks, E., and Gourtsoyiannis, C. Ultrasound attenuation of the calcanus in the female population: normative data. *Calcif. Tissue Int.* **51,** 180–183 (1992).
55. Krieg, M., Tiebuaud, D., and Burckhardt, P. Quantitative ultrasound of bone in institutionalized elderly women: a cross-sectional and longitudinal study. *Osteopor. Int.* **6,** 189–195 (1996).
56. Vega, E., Wittich, A., Mautalen, C., Carrilero, P., Otaño Sahores, A., and Silberman, F. Tibial ultrasound velocity in normal and hip fracture women. *Calcif. Tissue Int.* in press.
57. Rosenthall, L., Caminis, J., and Tenenhouse, A. Correlation of ultrasound velocity in the tibial cortex, calcaneal ultrasonography, and bone mineral densitometry of the spine and femur. *Calcif. Tissue Int.* **58,** 415–418 (1996).
58. Funck, C., Wuster, Chr., Alenfeld, F., Pereira-Lima, J., Tritz, T., Meeder, P., Gotz, M., and Ziegler. Ultrasound velocity of the tibia in normal German women and hip fracture patients. *Calcif. Tissue Int.* **58,** 390–394 (1996).
59. Lechman, R., Wapniarz, M., Kvasnicka, M., Klein, K., and Allolio, B. Velocity of ultrasound at the Patella: Influence of age, menopause and estrogen replacement therapy. *Osteopor. Int.* **3,** 308–313 (1993).
60. Kawana, K., Kushida, K., Takahashi, M., Ohishi, T., Denda, M., Yamazaki, K., and Inoue, T. The effect of menopause on biochemical markers and ultrasound densitometry in healthy females. *Calcif. Tissue Int.* **55,** 420–425 (1994).
61. Herd, R., Blake, G., Ramalingam, T., Miller, C., Ryan, P., and Fogelman, I. Measurements of postmenopausal bone loss with a new contact ultrasound system. *Calcif. Tissue Int.* **53,** 153–157 (1993).
62. Schott, A., Hans, D., Garnero, P., Sornay-Rendu, E., Delmas, P., and Meunier, P. Age-related changes in Os calcis ultrasonic indices: a 2-year prospective study. *Osteopor. Int.* **5,** 478–483 (1995).
63. van Daele, P. L. A., Burger, H., De Laet, C. E. D. H., Hofman, A., and Grobbee, D. E. Longitudinal changes in ultrasound parameters of the calcaneus. *Osteopor. Int.* **7,** 207–212 (1997).
64. Takeda, N., Miyake, M., Kita, S., Tomomitsu, T., and Fukunaga, M. Sex and age patterns of quantitative ultrasound densitometry of the calcaneous in normal Japanese subjects. *Calcif. Tissue Int.* **59,** 84–88 (1996).
65. Ito, M., Lang, T. F., Jergas, M., Ohki, M., Takada, M., Nakamura, T., Hayashi, K., and Genant, H. K. Spinal trabecular bone loss and fracture in American and Japanese women. *Calcif. Tissue Int.* **61,** 123–128 (1997).
66. Laval-Jeantet, A. M., Miravet, L., Bergot, C., De Vernejoul, M. C., Kuntz, D., and Laval-Jeantet, M. Tomodensitometric vertebrale quantitative. *J. Radiol.* **68,** 495–502 (1987).
67. Sandor, T., Felsenberg, D., Kalender, W., Clain, A., and Brown, E. Compact and trabecular components of the spine using quantitative computed tomography. *Calcif. Tissue Int.* **50,** 502–506 (1992).
68. Nordin, C., Need, A., Bridges, A., and Horowitz, M. Relative contributions of years since menopause, age, and weight to vertebral density in postmenopausal women. *J. Clin. Endocrinol. Metab.* **74,** 20–23 (1992).
69. Boonen, S., Cheng, X., Nijs, J., Nicholson, P., Verbeke, G., Lesaffre, E., Aerssens, J., and Dequeker, J. Factors associated with cortical and trabecular bone loss as quantified by peripheral computed tomography (pQCT) at the ultradistal radius in aging women. *Calcif. Tissue Int.* **60,** 164–170 (1997).

70. Butz, S., Wuster, C., Scheidt-Nave, C., Gotz, M., and Ziegler, R. Forearm BMD as measured by peripheral quantitative computed tomography (pQCT) in a German reference population. *Osteopor. Int.* **4,** 179–184 (1994).
71. Ruegsegger, P., Durand, E., and Dambacher, M. Differential effects of aging and disease on trabecular and compact bone density of the radius. *Bone* **12,** 99–105 (1991).
72. Gatti, D., Rossini, M., Zamberlan, N., Braga, V., Fracassi, E., and Adami, S. Effect of aging on trabecular and compact bone components of proximal and ultradistal radius. *Osteopor. Int.* **6,** 355–360 (1996).
73. Nordin, B., Need, A. G., Chatterton B. E., Horowitz, M., and Morris, H. A. Relative contributions of age and years since menopause to postmenopausal bone loss. *J. Clin. Endocrinol. Metab.* **70,** 83–88 (1990).
74. Mazess, R. B. On aging bone loss. *Clin Orthop.* **165,** 239–252 (1982).

Biochemical Dynamics

MARKUS J. SEIBEL Department of Medicine, Division of Endocrinology and Metabolism, University of Heidelberg, 69115 Heidelberg, Germany

SIMON P. ROBINS Skeletal Research Unit, Rowett Research Institute, Bucksburn, Aberdeen AB 21 9SB, United Kingdom

CAREN M. GUNDBERG Department of Orthopedics and Rehabilitation, Yale University School of Medicine, New Haven, Connecticut 06520

INTRODUCTION

Because of profound changes in the age structure of Western industrialized countries, disorders of connective tissue, bone, and mineral metabolism have become more relevant in everyday clinical practice. Consequently, the interest in and the need for effective measures to be used in the screening, diagnosis, and follow-up of such pathologies have grown markedly. Laboratory techniques such as biochemical markers of bone metabolism, together with clinical and imaging techniques, play an important role in the assessment and differential diagnosis of metabolic bone disease.

In recent years, the isolation and characterization of cellular and extracellular components of the skeletal matrix have resulted in the development of biochemical markers that specifically reflect either bone formation or bone resorption. These new biochemical indices have greatly enriched the spectrum of analytes used in the assessment of skeletal pathologies. Apart from serum total alkaline phosphatase (sTAP), which is routinely available from any laboratory, a host of other markers, such as the bone-specific isozymes of alkaline phosphatase (sBAP), osteocalcin (sOC), and the collagen propeptides, are now being used to assess bone formation rates. All of these parameters exhibit a significantly higher degree of tissue specificity than sTAP. Bone resorption, formerly assessable only by the measurement of urinary calcium and hydroxyproline, may now be detected more effectively by a number of new serum and urine markers. Among these, the pyridinium crosslinks and their peptide-based derivatives are presently considered the most specific markers of bone resorption.

Bone is a metabolically active tissue and undergoes continuous turnover and remodeling. These processes rely largely on the activity of two major types of cells and their precursors, namely osteoblasts and osteoclasts. Accordingly, bone remodeling is achieved by two counter-acting processes, bone formation and bone resorption. Both processes are usually summarized under the term of bone turnover. Under normal conditions, bone formation and bone resorption are coupled to each other, and the long-term maintenance of skeletal balance is achieved through the intricate action of systemic hormones and local mediators. In contrast, metabolic bone diseases, states of increased or decreased mobility, and certain therapeutic interventions are characterized by more or less pronounced imbalances between the rate of bone formation and of bone resorption. The long-term result of imbalances in bone turnover (i.e., changes in bone mass) is usually assessed using densitometric techniques. In contrast, the value of bone biomarkers lies in the detection of the metabolic imbalance itself and in the classification of low or high, decreased or increased bone turnover. Static bone mass and dynamic bone turnover are thus two complementary parameters that contribute specifically to the assessment of skeletal homeostasis and to the diagnosis of bone disease. Bone densitometry and laboratory tests should therefore not be viewed as opposing methodologies but always used in conjunction to complement each other.

Biochemical markers of bone turnover are noninvasive, comparatively inexpensive, and, when applied and interpreted correctly, helpful tools in the assessment of metabolic bone disease, therapeutic efficacy, and patient compliance. Although the various serum and urinary markers of bone turnover include both cellular-derived enzymes and nonenzymatic peptides, they are usually classified according to the metabolic process they are considered to reflect. For clinical purposes, therefore, markers of bone formation (Table I) are distinguished from indices of bone resorption (Table II). It should be kept in mind, however, that some of these compounds may reflect, at least to a some degree, both bone formation and bone resorption. Second, most if not all of these markers are present in tissues other than bone and may therefore be influenced by nonskeletal processes as well. Third, changes in biochemical markers of bone turnover are usually not disease specific, but reflect alterations in skeletal metabolism independently of the underlying cause.

Attempts to derive a "balance" index by combining measurements of bone formation and of bone resorption have been disappointing, probably because of disparities caused by the temporal differences between the formative and the resorptive events in bone remodeling. The major use of biochemical markers of bone turnover is therefore the detection of changes in bone metabolism, with the notion in mind that high rates of bone turnover are often associated with an imbalance in bone metabolism and with accelerated bone loss.

BIOCHEMICAL MARKERS OF BONE FORMATION

Osteocalcin

Biochemistry

Osteocalcin is a small protein synthesized by mature osteoblasts, odontoblasts, and hypertrophic chondrocytes. It is characterized by the presence of three residues of the calcium-binding amino acid, γ-carboxyglutamic acid (Gla). Vitamin K is required for the addition of a second γ-carboxyl group to the side chain of specific glutamate residues, resulting in the production of Gla residues in the newly synthesized protein. This reaction, which is inhibited by warfarin, is identical to that responsible for the activation of the vitamin-K dependent blood coagulation factors [1]. Two major structural features of osteocalcin are (1) the "Gla helix," a compact Ca^{2+}-dependent helical conformation in which the Gla residues project the Ca-binding sites into the same plane, thereby facilitating adsorption to hydroxyapatite, and (2) the COOH-terminal β sheet, a locus for potential interaction with cellular receptors and extracellular proteins [2]. Although it is one of the most abundant noncollagenous proteins in bone, the biological function of osteocalcin has not been precisely defined. Early studies of the appearance of osteocalcin in embryonic bone tissue demonstrated that osteocalcin synthesis occurred coincident with the onset of mineralization and that it increased in concert with hydroxyapatite deposition during the period of skeletal growth [3–5].

Gene targeting has produced a mouse in which the osteocalcin gene has been "knocked out." Preliminary characterization of the animals shows the bones to be normal in young mice, but with age there is a progressive development of increased cortical and trabecular thickness, decreased articular cartilage, and an increased load to failure [6]. Further characterization of these animals will determine if in fact osteocalcin is involved with some aspect of bone remodeling and whether these changes are due to events related to the deposition of osteocalcin into the bone matrix or are cell-mediated events that depend on osteocalcin.

Table I Biomarkers of Bone Formation

Marker (abbreviation)	Tissue of origin	Specimen	Method	Specificity
Total alkaline phosphatase (AP; TAP)	Bone Liver Intestine Kidney (placenta)	Serum	Colorimetric	In healthy adults, 1:1 ratio between liver/biliary system and bone-derived enzyme
Bone-specific AP (BAP)	Bone	Serum	Colorimetric Electrophoretic Precipitation IRMA Activity immunoassay	Specific product of osteoblasts. In some assays, cross-reactivity with liver isoenzyme
Osteocalcin (OC, BGP)	Bone (platelets ?)	Serum	RIA ELISA	Specific product of osteoblasts. Many immunoreactive forms are in blood, some may be derived from bone resorption
Carboxy-terminal propeptide of type I procollagen (PICP)	Bone (soft tissue, skin)	Serum	RIA ELISA	Major product of osteoblasts and fibroblasts
Amino-terminal propeptide of type I procollagen (PINP)	Bone (soft tissue, skin)	Serum	RIA ELISA	Major product of osteoblasts and fibroblasts

TABLE II Biomarkers of Bone Resorption

Marker (abbreviation)	Tissue of origin	Specimen	Method	Specificity
Hydroxyproline, (HYP; OHP)	Bone Cartilage Soft tissue Skin, blood	Urine	Colorimetric HPLC	All fibrillar collagens and collagenous proteins, include C1q and elastin. Present in newly synthesized and mature collagen
Pyridinoline (PYD)	Bone Cartilage Tendon Blood vessels	Urine	HPLC ELISA	Collagens, with highest concentrations in cartilage and bone. Absent from skin. Present in mature collagen only
Deoxypyridinoline (DPD)	Bone Dentin	Urine Serum	HPLC ELISA RIA	Collagens, with highest concentration in bone. Absent from cartilage or skin. Present in mature collagen only
Carboxy-terminal cross-linked telopeptide of type I collagen (ICTP)	Bone Skin	Serum	RIA ELISA	Collagen type I, with highest contribution probably from bone
Amino-terminal telopeptide of type I collagen (NTx)	Bone Skin	Urine Serum	ELISA	Collagen type I, with highest contribution probably from bone
Carboxy-terminal telopeptide of type I collagen (CTx)	Bone Skin	Urine Serum	ELISA RIA	Collagen type I, with highest contribution probably from bone. Assayed as isoaspartyl and nonisomerized forms
Galactosyl-hydroxylysine (GHL; Gal-Hyl)	Bone Soft tissue Skin	Urine	HPLC	Collagens and collagenous proteins. High proportion of GHL in skeletal collagens compared with other tissues
Tartrate-resistant acid phosphatase (TRAP)	Bone Blood	Plasma Serum	Colorimetric ELISA	Osteoclasts Platelets Erythrocytes
Bone sialoprotein (BSP)	Bone Hypertrophic cartilage	Serum	RIA	Osteoblasts Osteoclasts (?) Bone matrix

MEASUREMENT

Osteocalcin is primarily deposited in the extracellular matrix of bone, but a small amount enters the blood. Serum osteocalcin is a sensitive and specific marker of osteoblastic activity and its serum level reflects the rate of bone formation [7]. The first osteocalcin assays were competitive radioimmunoassays using bovine osteocalcin, purified to homogeneity, as antigen and assay reagents [8,9]. Newer methods use purified human osteocalcin for antibody production and for radioimmunoassays (RIA) or two-site ELISAs. There are several commercial kits for human osteocalcin. However, there is considerable inconsistency when comparing values from these various assays and wide variations are reported in control and patient populations [10,11].

Various fragments of osteocalcin can be found in blood [12–16]. Commercial and research assay variability may be the result of differences in the ability of the various antibodies to recognize these fragments. Epitope specificity and the degree of reactivity with multiple circulating forms of the protein are often unknown. Several laboratories have developed two-site immunoassays with the intention of measuring only the intact molecule [17–23]. However, a rapid loss of immunoreactivity is observed with these assays when samples are left at room temperature for a few hours.

A new generation of assays is based on studies showing that intact osteocalcin is degraded to a large N-terminal midmolecule fragment encompassing residues 1–43. Data suggest that the intact molecule represents only about one-third of the circulating osteocalcin immunoreactivity. One-third consists of the large N-terminal midmolecule fragment and another third by several other smaller fragments [14]. The large N-terminal midmolecule fragment is thought to be generated by proteolysis in the circulation or during sample processing and storage. However, evidence shows that the osteoblast can be another source of this fragment. Nevertheless, whether this fragment is derived from processing by the osteoblast or degradation in the circulation, its measurement appears to provide a more comprehensive picture of osteocalcin biosynthesis. With this assay, the apparent instability of osteocalcin in the circulation and during sample handling is eliminated [24–26].

The remaining fragments have not been fully characterized. Data indicate that there are smaller N-terminal immunoreactive species of osteocalcin in serum in addition to a larger midmolecule fragment [27,28]. They are in greatest abundance in normal children, in patients with osteoporosis, and in hyperparathyroidism, suggesting that these immunoreactive species are produced in a high turnover state. Some have suggested that these are the products of osteoclastic resorption of bone. Further evidence for this possibility comes from the study of Salo *et al.,* who cultured osteoclasts on bovine bone. Using a commercial polyclonal antibody to bovine osteocalcin, they detected immunoreactive material liberated from resorption lacunae [29]. In other studies, osteocalcin was shown to be a substrate for osteoclastic enzymes [30]. Cathepsins D, L, and H can degrade human osteocalcin to fragments and these were recognized by several commercial kits that employed a single-antibody RIA [31,32]. Thus, circulating osteocalcin may be derived from osteoblastic synthesis, osteoclastic dissolution of bone, or proteolysis in the circulation or extraosseous sites.

Alkaline Phosphatase

Biochemistry

Alkaline phosphatase (AP) belongs to a large group of proteins that are anchored to glycosyl-phosphatidylinositol (GPI) moieties on the extracellular surface of cell membranes [33]. As such, it is expressed and functions on the outside of the cell. The enzyme is a tetramer when membrane bound, but circulates as a dimer [34]. Phospholipase C or D (which is abundant in plasma) potentially converts the membrane-bound form to the soluble circulating form [35,36]. Total alkaline phosphatase in serum includes several isoforms. Elevated values result from increased activity in intestine, spleen, kidney, placental, liver, bone, or expression by tumors [37]. Four gene loci code for AP: the three tissue-specific genes that encode the intestine, mature placenta, and germ cell enzymes and the tissue-nonspecific (tns) gene that is expressed in numerous tissues (including bone, liver, kidney, and early placenta). Tissue-nonspecific APs are the products of a single gene [38], but tissue-specific differences are found in their electrophoretic mobility, stability to heat, and sensitivity to a variety of chemical inhibitors. These differences are due to variations in their carbohydrate side chains and degree of sialation [39]. Altered glycosylated forms are also present in disease states, particularly in malignancy, and the tumor-producing forms can mimic the bone form [40]. Extracts of human bone from neonates and patients with Paget's disease or osteosarcoma demonstrate a range of glycosylation patterns; this raises the question of immunological heterogeneity even in the bone isoform [40,41].

An essential role for the alkaline phosphatase enzyme in bone mineralization is evidenced by the disease hypophosphatasia, a rare inherited autosomal recessive disorder of osteogenesis characterized by the defective mineralization of bones and teeth. The biochemical hallmark of the disease is deficient tns-alkaline phosphatase activity. No metabolic consequences in liver or kidney have been identified and the activity of the tissue-specific isoenzymes is normal [42].

Methods

The usefulness of AP as a marker of bone activity depends on the ability to quantitatively distinguish the activity of the bone isoform from that of other tissues. Because the two most common sources of elevated alkaline phosphatase levels are liver and bone, a number of techniques have been developed that rely on these differences to distinguish between bone and liver isoforms. These include heat denaturation, chemical inhibition of selective activity, gel electrophoresis, precipitation by wheat germ lectin, and immunoassays.

The heat denaturation method is based on the gradation in heat stability at 56°C of the AP enzymes found in serum, which ranges from placental (completely heat stable) to liver AP, which has intermediate stability (half life of 7.6 ± 1.5 min), and bone AP, which is very labile (half life of 1.9 ± 0.4 min). When activity in heated serum is 20% or less of that in unheated serum, AP is attributed to the bone enzyme, whereas the heat-stable activity of 25–55% is attributed to the liver enzyme. Liver and bone AP can be separated sufficiently by polyacrylamide gel electrophoresis to allow visual assessment of their relative proportions, but these methods are tedious and there is often overlap between the two, making precise quantitation difficult. Several methods have used selective inhibition to improve the separation [43,44].

Newer methods use wheat germ lectin, which binds to *N*-acetylglucosamine and sialic acid residues, to separate liver and bone AP [45–47]. Based on their different glycosylation patterns, wheat germ lectin selectively binds the bone form. This method effectively predicts bone mineralization rates as determined by ^{47}Ca kinetics [48]. Increased activity is found in patients with high bone turnover disorders when wheat germ lectin precipitation is used [49,50]. Two commercial kits are currently available that use monoclonal antibodies with preference for the bone isoform [51,52]. One assay, an IRMA, measures the mass of the enzyme, whereas the other measures the activity of the antibody-bound enzyme. Cross-reactivity with the liver isoform ranges from 8 to 16% with these kits [52,53]. Consequently, in patients with significant elevations in total AP (more than twice the upper limit of normal), cross-reactivity between bone and liver may lead to falsely elevated increases in skeletal alkaline phosphatase with immunoassay and lectin kits [54–56].

Procollagen Peptides

All collagens contain molecular domains of triple-helical conformation. The newly translated polypeptide, a pre-pro-α chain, includes a signal sequence and amino (N)- and carboxyl (C)-terminal propeptide extensions [57]. During collagen synthesis, intramolecular disulfide bonds form among the three carboxyl propeptides and guide helical formation. Specific endopeptidases cleave the procollagen molecule at precise sites in each chain, first at the amino terminus and then at the carboxyl terminus. Type I collagen propeptides are produced not only by bone but by other tissues that synthesize type I collagen: skin, gingiva, heart valve, dentin, cornea, fibrocartilage, and tendon. Procollagen type I carboxy-terminal propeptide (PICP), with a molecular mass of 117 kDa, is a trimeric globular glycoprotein with asparagine-linked carbohydrate units [58]. PICP, stabilized by disulfide bonds, circulates as a single molecule. It has a serum half-life of 6–8 min and is cleared in the liver endothelial cells by the mannose-6-phosphate receptor [59]. The procollagen type I amino-terminal propeptide (PINP), a 70-kDa globular protein, contains an internal region of 17 contiguous GLY-X-Y triplets containing proline and hydroxyproline in the same proportion as the collagen molecule [60]. PINP can be cleared from the circulation by the scavenger receptor of liver endothelial cells.

Assays for the measurement of PICP are based on polyclonal antiserum made against purified collagen isolated from human skin or lung fibroblast cultures [61–63]. None of the assays eliminate the potential contribution to circulating PICP from soft tissue synthesis of type I collagen. The rate of turnover of collagen in bone is faster than in other tissues and therefore changes in PICP are assumed to reflect changes primarily in bone collagen synthesis. However, a number of studies have questioned the specificity of PICP for bone [64–66].

BIOCHEMICAL MARKERS OF BONE RESORPTION

Most resorption markers are based on the measurement of specific components or fragments of bone collagen, a sound strategy as collagen type I comprises about 90% of the protein matrix of bone. In contrast to bone formation assays, most resorption markers are based on measurements in urine, although several serum assays have been developed recently. Serum assays have some clear advantages over urine-based measurements in obviating the need for creatinine corrections and in allowing more direct comparisons of the rates of bone resorption and formation. Attempts to derive a "balance" index by combining the two measurements have, however, been disappointing, probably because of disparities caused by the temporal differences between the formative and the resorptive events in bone remodeling [67,68].

Hydroxyproline

Although urinary hydroxyproline was the archetypal bone resorption marker for many years [69], this assay has now been largely replaced by collagen cross-link-related assays. The main disadvantages of urinary hydroxyproline are the lack of specificity for bone, the dependence on an adequate dietary control to avoid the contributions of exogenous hydroxyproline, the high level (about 90%) of metabolism of hydroxyproline in the liver, and the contributions of hydroxyproline from the degradation of newly synthesized collagen. In situations where there are very high rates of bone turnover, such as in Paget's disease of bone, urinary hydroxyproline provides an adequate bone marker because a large proportion of urinary hydroxyproline is derived from bone collagen. The lack of specificity for this marker arises for more subtle changes in resorption rates, and it has been estimated that only about 50% of urinary hydroxyproline is normally derived from bone resorption [70].

Galactosylhydroxylysine

The formation of both galactosylhydroxylysine (GHL) and glucosyl-galactosylhydroxylysine is an intracellular event during procollagen synthesis. Early analytical studies showed that the monosaccharide predominated in bone collagen whereas the disaccharide was more prevalent in skin collagen as well as in collagen-like proteins such as C1q [71]. The monosaccharide, GHL, therefore appears to be relatively specific for bone, and the renal conversion of the disaccharide to GHL that was shown in rats does not occur in humans [72]. Initial studies of the glycosides showed that these compounds were essentially not metabolized and that contributions from dietary sources were much less than for hydroxyproline [73]. As GHL is the product of an intracellular modification, it is possible that the degradation of newly synthesized collagen may contribute to the rate of excretion. For many cell types, there appears to be a basal level of lysosome-mediated intracellular procollagen degradation of about 15%, but this may rise to as much as 40% in certain circumstances [74]. At present, however, there is no direct evidence that excretion of GHL is affected significantly by this phenomenon.

Moro and colleagues [75] developed an HPLC method for the analysis of GHL in urine that requires no preliminary fractionation of the sample, but involves a dansylation step followed by separation using a reversed-phase column. This assay generally shows good correlations with other resorption markers [76], but the lack of a direct immunoassay for GHL has probably limited its wider clinical application.

Pyridinium Cross-links

Following the initial characterization of pyridinoline [77], the potential value of this trifunctional collagen cross-link as a marker was suggested by the discovery that the compound could be detected and quantified in urine [78,79]. The development of a reversed-phase HPLC separation [80] facilitated the analysis of tissue hydrolysates for both pyridinoline (PYD), also referred to as hydroxylysyl pyridinoline (HP), and deoxypyridinoline (DPD), an analog derived from a lysyl residue in the collagen helix [81], giving rise to the alternative nomenclature of lysyl pyridinoline (LP). Inclusion of a prefractionation step using cellulose partition chromatography facilitated analysis by HPLC of both cross-links in hydrolyzed urine samples [82], a procedure that was later automated [83]. An alternative automated assay applicable to both urine and serum samples has been described [84].

Cross-link markers provide advantages over urinary hydroxyproline in several respects. First, the lack of any significant dietary contribution to their excretion [85] means that no special dietary restrictions are necessary. Because the cross-links are formed only at the final stages of fibril formation, the cross-links indicate degradation of only mature, functional tissue and are unaffected by the degradation of newly synthesized collagen. Another important consideration is that of tissue specificity. PYD has been shown to have a much wider tissue distribution than DPD [80,86], although both cross-links are absent from dermal tissue, which represents a major body pool of collagen. Initially it appeared that DPD was present only in mineralized tissues, but it is now known to be present in cardiovascular tissue, intramuscular collagen, and some ligaments. These findings do not, however, contradict the original suggestion that DPD should be considered a bone-specific marker since the pool size of the tissue and its turnover rate have to be taken into account in addition to the concentration in tissue. On this basis, the very low metabolic turnover rates of the soft tissues in which DPD has been detected makes their likely contribution to urinary DPD negligible. This view is supported experimentally by the close correlation observed between bone resorption rates determined by DPD excretion and by radioisotopic exchange [87]. Most analyses of urinary cross-links were initially performed using acid hydrolysates to liberate all peptide-bound and other conjugated forms. Direct analysis of urine by HPLC combined with prefractionation on cellulose indicated that 40–50% of the cross-links were free [88,89]. A further analysis of urine from several groups of patients with disorders associated with increased bone resorption revealed that mean proportions of free cross-link relative to the total amounts were similar for each group. This indicated that similar information about bone resorption could be obtained by the direct analysis of urine without the time-consuming hydrolysis step. These results also suggested the possible application of direct immunoassays for the cross-links, and a number of ELISA systems have been reported [90–92].

Telopeptide Assays

Several assays have been described that are based on the measurement of peptides associated with the cross-link regions in collagen rather than measuring the cross-links themselves. The cross-links are derived from (hydroxy)lysine residues present in both the N- and the C-terminal telopeptides that are converted to aldehydes by lysyl oxidase. Assays based on measurements of peptides derived from both ends of the collagen type I molecule have been described.

The ICTP assay refers to measurement of a component from the collagen type I C-terminal telopeptide [93]. Antibodies were raised against a cross-link-containing, 8.5-kDa peptide partially purified from a bacterial collagenase digest of human bone collagen. Although the peptide contained pyridinium cross-links, other forms of cross-link were also detected, and antibody recognition is not dependent on the form of cross-link present. ICTP is a serum assay that appears to be more sensitive to changes in bone resorption brought about by pathological processes than to alterations associated with normal remodeling.

An assay based on a cross-linked peptide from the N-terminal telopeptide of collagen type I, referred to as NTx, was developed using a monoclonal antibody raised against a peptide isolated from urine of a patient with Paget's disease of bone [94]. The ELISA was shown to react with several pyridinium cross-link-containing peptides in urine, although the pyridinium cross-link was not essential for reactivity. Sequences from the $\alpha2$ chain telopeptide were essential for antibody recognition, but the presence of these cross-linked species may not confer specificity for bone as skin collagen peptides showed the same molar reactivity with the NTx assay [95]. The NTx assay therefore appears to measure collagen type I degradation products. Because the antibody does not react with the linear telopeptide sequences, this assay is unlikely to detect the degradation of newly formed collagen. As a urinary measurement, the NTx assay has been applied to a wide range of clinical samples. The assay has been developed for use in serum, and preliminary data showed clinical utility in monitoring decreased bone resorption in patients with Paget's disease treated with bisphosphonates [96].

By raising polyclonal antibodies against a synthetic, linear octapeptide that contained the cross-linking site of the C-terminal telopeptide of collagen I, Bonde and colleagues [97] developed a urinary assay (referred to as CTx) that would recognize degradation products of all cross-link forms of this collagen. Subsequent analysis has shown that the assay (termed "cross-laps") in fact recognized only a form of the peptide containing an isoaspartyl (or β-aspartyl) peptide bond [98]. The transformation of aspartyl to isoaspartyl residues in proteins is well known and, for extracellular proteins, the process is thought to be time dependent as well as a function of the particular environment of the susceptible bond. The interpretation of results from this assay is therefore complex without knowledge of the rate of isomerization that occurs in the collagen type I of bone and other tissues. A CTx assay based on a monoclonal antibody directed against the nonisomerized form of the octapeptide sequence derived from the C-terminal telopeptide cross-linking site has been described [99]. This assay is referred to as α-CTx to distinguish it from the measurement of the isomerized form of peptide, which is known as β-CTx. The availability of these two forms of assays has allowed their application to studies of the changes in α-CTx/β-CTx ratio as a novel marker of alterations in the bone turnover rate. Thus, the urinary ratio was found to be elevated in patients with Paget's disease of bone with increased amounts of the nonisomerized material in woven bone [100]; this ratio decreased rapidly in response to bisphosphonate therapy [101].

A serum β-CTx assay has been developed, although it is not based on the same immunochemistry used for the urinary assay. For the serum assay, a polyclonal antiserum raised against collagenase-digested collagen type I was used with the conjugated isomerized C-terminal octapeptide attached to the ELISA plate providing the required specificity [102].

Comparison of Cross-link-Related Assays

It is clear that both the measurement of urinary pyridinium cross-links and the various forms of telopeptide assays overcome most of the disadvantages of urinary hydroxyproline. Generally, results for free pyridinium cross-link measurements and the telopeptide assays correlate closely. Thus, there may be little disparity in the specificity for bone resorption. However, one situation in which differences between the assays have been observed is the response to bisphosphonate treatment, where much larger changes in NTx and CTx values were observed compared with the changes in free DPD [103]. In another study, the proportion of free DPD in urine was shown to increase in patients during a 4-week treatment with bisphosphonate [104]. It is likely, therefore, that some treatments for high bone resorption states not only affect true bone resorption but also the patterns of free cross-links and peptides released into urine. These effects may be at the osteoclast level in bone or at other sites of the body, such as liver or kidney [95,103]. These considerations serve to emphasize that a better understanding of the degradative metabolism of bone matrix is necessary before the cross-link-related assays can be fully evaluated.

Tartrate-Resistant Acid Phosphatase

Of the many isoenzymes of acid phosphatase, tartrate-resistant acid phosphatase (TRAP) synthesized and secreted by osteoclasts presents an attractive potential serum marker of the bone resorption rate. Although initially analyzed by kinetic methods, interference by other acid phosphatase isoenzymes caused problems despite the application of more specific substrates for the osteoclastic enzyme [105]. Immunoassays for the TRAP enzyme protein have been developed using an antiserum raised against material isolated from the spleen of a patient with hairy cell leukemia [106] or against TRAP isolated from human cord plasma [107]. The latter assay showed good correlation between immunoreactivity and enzyme activity, little cross-reaction with acid phosphatases from nonosteoclastic sources, and a 70% decrease in serum TRAP in postmenopausal women after 3–6 months of estrogen replacement therapy.

Bone Sialoprotein

Bone sialoprotein (BSP) is one of the most abundant noncollagenous, glycosylated phosphoproteins in bone, having a molecular mass of about 80 kDa, of which approximately 34 kDa is core protein. BSP is synthesized by osteoblasts and certain osteoclastic cell lines and appears to have important functions in bone mineralization processes and in integrin-mediated cell–matrix interactions. Development of an immunoassay established a normal range for serum concentrations of BSP and showed that increased immunoreactive protein was present in serum from patients with metabolic and malignant bone disease [108,109]. Interestingly, comparison of the BSP results with other markers of bone metabolism suggested that the immunoassay primarily reflected processes associated with bone resorption [108]. The reason for this association is unclear but further knowledge of the function of BSP in bone will help to resolve this question.

EFFECTS OF NORMAL AGING ON BONE TURNOVER

Changes in Bone Formation Markers during Normal Aging

It is generally accepted that the accelerated rate of bone loss that occurs after menopause is due to increased rates of turnover. Studies using bone-specific markers, however, have suggested that increased bone turnover is also responsible for the slow phase of bone loss in elderly women. In adults, osteocalcin levels are relatively stable but start to rise in men after the age of 60. Several studies in women show a significant rise with menopause [110–116]. This increase significantly correlated with an increase in the bone turnover rate assessed by bone histomorphometry and calcium kinetics [117].

For alkaline phosphatase, the ratio of bone to liver activity in healthy adults is approximately 1:1. Total AP activity is greater in men than in women between the ages of 20 and 50. In both genders total alkaline phosphatase increases after the age of 50 [40,118,119]. Substantial increases have been observed in bone-specific alkaline phosphatase with age and menopause in normal women. Eastell *et al.* [48] reported a 73% increase in bone AP in older women compared to women in their third and fourth decade of life. Another study found bone AP to be increased by 77% in women within 10 years of menopause [53]. Total and bone-specific AP are highly correlated in normal subjects [56].

PICP values decline with age in men but increase in women [64]. Two studies found a slight but insignificant increase in PICP after menopause [120,121], but other studies found no change [63]. In a direct comparison, Garnero *et al.* [122] measured intact osteocalcin, bone-specific alkaline phosphatase, and PICP in 653 women. They found that menopause induced a 37 and 52% increase in osteocalcin and BSAP, respectively. These markers remained elevated in those women with the lowest bone density up to 40 years after menopause. PICP values did not change in this study.

Changes in Bone Resorption Markers during Normal Aging

Several studies of pyridinium cross-link excretion have revealed progressive increases with age for both men and women, with marked increases in women after menopause [91,123–125]. Similar trends were evident for both free cross-links and the total fraction determined after hydrolysis. A study of the concentrations of pyridinium cross-links in bone at different ages showed that there were no significant changes throughout adult life, at least up to the 7th decade [126]. Thus, the observed changes in pyridinium cross-link excretion appear to correspond to real increases in bone resorption with age.

The mean increase in serum ICTP between groups of premenopausal and postmenopausal women was found to be relatively small (>20%), much less than the corresponding changes in PYD and DPD [127]. In a major study of the changes in urinary excretion of the telopeptide resorption markers through menopause, the differences between premenopausal and early (<10 years) postmenopausal groups was 80 and 97% for CTx and NTx assays, respectively, with intermediate values in the perimenopausal group [122]. This study also showed statistically significant decreases in CTx and NTx excretion between early and late (>10 years) postmenopausal groups, although this difference was abolished after correction of the values for total body bone mineral content. The conclusions of this study were that the bone resorption markers play an increasingly important role with time after menopause as a determinant of bone mass [122]. Treatment of elderly women with estrogen was shown to decrease resorption markers [128], and a more recent study found that the resorption markers, DPD and NTx, were normalized to premenopausal levels by long-term estrogen therapy, associated with a correction of secondary hyperparathyroidism [129]. These results suggest that the increased bone turnover in elderly women may be viewed as a late consequence of estrogen deficiency rather than an aging phenomenon.

BIOCHEMICAL DYNAMICS OF BONE TURNOVER IN POSTMENOPAUSAL AND AGE-RELATED OSTEOPOROSIS

As stated earlier, diseases of the locomotor system, particularly osteoporosis, are of increasing medical and socioeconomic importance. The development of more effective techniques for screening, diagnosis, prevention, and therapeutic follow-up of metabolic bone diseases is therefore of interest from more than a purely medical perspective. The development of new biochemical markers of bone metabolism has generated a substantial amount of data on all of these issues. When used in combination with clinical data and imaging techniques, these parameters permit a comprehensive and noninvasive evaluation of the skeletal status. Biochemical markers of bone metabolism may therefore be used

- to predict future bone loss and hip fractures in larger cohorts
- to evaluate the current state of bone turnover in individual patients
- to identify individuals at risk for osteoporosis
- to select therapy for individual patients
- to predict the therapeutic response in individual patients
- to monitor therapeutic response and efficacy in, and compliance of individual patients.

For an initial clinical diagnosis of osteoporosis, none of the biochemical markers of bone turnover has proved useful as a single determination [125,130,131]. As with bone density measurements, a broad overlap between healthy and diseased populations is observed. This observation, however, does not devalue the use of biochemical markers per se, but rather is the expected answer to an oversimplified approach, i.e., no diagnosis is ever made on the basis of a single laboratory measurement.

Nevertheless, once the diagnosis of osteoporotic bone disease is made, biochemical markers of bone metabolism are useful tools in further work-up, particularly in identifying patients with high rates of bone turnover. Thus, patients with accelerated bone turnover not only lose bone at a faster rate, but also carry a significantly higher risk of hip fractures. Much like bone density measurements, bone biomarkers are indicators of *risk* rather than of the disease itself (see later). Furthermore, patients with high bone turnover appear to benefit from antiresorptive treatments more than subjects with low or normal rates of bone metabolism. The measurement of bone turnover, i.e., the quantitative assessment of bone formation and of bone resorption by specific biochemical markers, may therefore not only be useful in therapeutic decision making, but can also help to reduce *costs* by identifying those individuals who may not respond well to treatment. Finally, bone markers are of clinical relevance in monitoring both the disease itself and therapeutic efficacy. Future uses may also include the measurement of bone biomakers to improve patient compliance. However, the development of new "bone markers" to improve primary diagnostics and screening is still a specified research goal.

Biochemical Markers of Bone Metabolism and the Prediction of Future Bone Loss and Fracture Risk

PREDICTION OF BONE LOSS

Bone mass, rates of bone loss, and the risk of osteoporotic fractures are closely related to each other. Thus, low bone mass and rapid bone loss have both been shown to be independent predictors of future fracture risk [132–137]. The rate of bone loss is determined by a number of factors, one of which appears to be the rate of bone turnover. In fact, an abundance of research data now suggests that increased rates of bone turnover are associated with accelerated bone loss. Earlier observations demonstrated that both bone formation and bone resorption increase shortly after natural menopause, a phase that in most women is also associated with a significantly accelerated bone loss. Similar observations have been made in ovariectomized, premenopausal women and in castrated men [138,139]. The withdrawal of endogenous sex steroid induces both high bone turnover and rapid bone loss. Markers of bone metabolism return to premenopausal levels a few months after the implementation of hormone replacement therapy (HRT) [131,140,141], a therapy known to inhibit postmenopausal bone loss. However, whereas previous histomorphometric data suggested that bone turnover returns to normal or subnormal levels even without HRT approximately 10 years after menopause [142,143], newer biochemical studies show that high rates of bone turnover are sustained throughout life in most postmenopausal women [122,125,144–146].

A number of cross-sectional studies in early and late postmenopausal women showed that bone mass is negatively correlated with markers of both bone resorption and bone formation [122,125,146–153]. Although the highest correlations were observed between resorption markers and total bone mineral density (TBMD), associations were usually lower but still significant when calculated for individual sites of measurements (i.e., spine, hip, radius). This difference is due to the fact that biochemical markers of bone turnover reflect metabolic changes of the entire skeleton and not of specific skeletal sites. Markers of bone resorption (hydroxyproline, collagen type I cross-links) usually show a stronger correlation with bone mass measurements and therefore appear to be better predictors of bone loss than markers of bone formation (e.g., osteocalcin, alkaline phosphatase). In most studies, the inverse correlation between bone metabolism and bone loss increases with the time after menopause. Thus, in women more than 20 years after menopause, up to 52% of the variance in BMD could be explained by changes in bone turnover. These relationships are much less pronounced, yet are still present in early postmenopausal women, but seem absent in premenopausal women [122].

Most longitudinal studies, both of retrospective and prospective design, support the notion that individuals with high rates of bone turnover are at risk to lose bone at a faster rate than subjects with normal or low bone turnover [154–165]. Following a small group of early postmenopausal women, previous investigations demonstrated that the combined measurement of serum total alkaline phosphatase, osteocalcin, fasting urinary calcium, hydroxyproline, or deoxypyridinoline can predict 60–70% of the variability in measured bone loss [154,155,166]. These studies also showed that the correlation between baseline markers of bone turnover and the subsequent rate of postmenopausal bone loss is consistent over a period of at least 12 years [135,155]. Similar but less optimistic estimates were reported by other groups using different combinations [161,162]. For example, Dresner-Pollak *et al.* [161] showed that urinary NTX, serum osteocalcin, and serum parathyroid hormone together explained 43% of the variability of bone loss at the total hip in elderly women. Using single marker measurements instead of combinations, similar results were reported for a number of markers of both bone formation and resorption and in a variety of skeletal sites (lumbar, hip, radius). Again, markers of bone resorption seemed to be stronger predictors of future bone loss than markers of bone formation, and correlations were stronger in elderly than in younger women [158,159,162,165]. Following 354 women for a mean interval of 13 years, Ross and Knowlton [165] showed a continuous relationship between the measured levels of various bone biomarkers and the risk of rapid bone loss at the calcaneus. Thus, the odds of rapid bone loss (i.e., >2.2% per year) increased approximately twice for each standard deviation increase in serum bone-specific alkaline phosphatase, serum osteocalcin, urinary free pyridinoline, or deoxypyridinoline [165] (Fig. 1). In a study of 227 early postmenopausal women treated with either

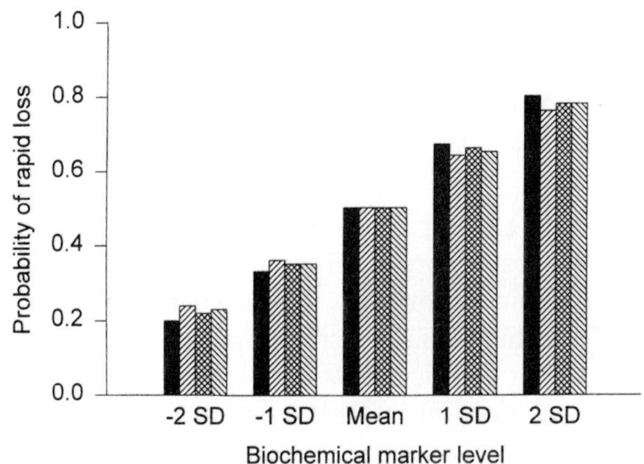

FIGURE 1 Probability of rapid bone loss as a function of biochemical marker levels. At each level, bars from left (filled) to right (hatched) represent the following markers: bone-specific alkaline phosphatase (BAP), osteocalcin (OC), deoxypyridinoline (DPD), and pyridinoline (PYD). For more details, see text. From Ross and Knowlton [165], with permission.

calcium alone or HRT plus calcium, Chesnut *et al.* [163] and Rosen *et al.* [164] showed that women with high baseline rates of bone resorption were at a higher risk of losing bone than women with normal turnover rates. The authors calculated that a woman with high baseline values of urinary NTX (>67 units) had a 17.3 times higher risk of future bone loss if not treated with HRT [163].

Rather contrasting results were reported by Keen *et al.* [167], who in a 4-year prospective study did not detect any correlation between rates of bone turnover and changes in lumbar or hip BMD. Finally, other groups [162,168] argue that due to the high degree of variability in urinary markers of bone turnover, predicting either bone density or changes therein for an individual patient from a single marker measurement may not be possible.

Although there is now increasing evidence that bone turnover is a strong predictor of future bone loss under certain conditions, no final consensus has been reached about whether these markers can be used to identify high-risk patients, i.e., "fast bone losers." More long-term studies are needed to prove that a "fast loser" will remain so for the rest of his or her life. In addition, the interpretation of biochemical markers clearly depends on the timing of the sample with respect to the interval since menopause, as rates of loss are greater in the immediate, postmenopausal period. Finally, it is not clear whether a combination of markers or a single marker will gain the highest predictive results. Clearly, the measurement of bone markers does not substitute for bone mass measurement, the latter giving, at this time, the most useful information about fracture risk. However, there is little doubt that with the development of new and/or more precise assays, the combined use of BMD and marker measurements will become the standard in individual risk assessment.

PREDICTION OF FRACTURES

Bone mass, evaluated by BMD measurements, is not the only determinant of skeletal fractures. Other factors, such as trabecular connectivity, the number of bone-remodeling sites, or other determinants of skeletal microarchitecture, may all contribute to the mechanical stability of bone. However, trabecular connectivity, which may decrease as the result of high bone turnover and bone resorption, is not necessarily reflected in bone mass measurements. Therefore, bone turnover (and markers thereof) may be independent predictors of fracture risk.

A reanalysis of data from several clinical trials suggested that vertebral fracture rates in placebo-treated osteoporotic women increase as a direct function of either increased bone turnover or decreased vertebral BMD [169]. Thus, at a given level of vertebral BMD, the rate of vertebral fractures increases with the rate of bone turnover. When bone turnover is normal, however, the main determinant of vertebral fractures is vertebral BMD [169].

In a large, prospective and population-based sample of the EVOS study, van Daele and co-workers [170] were the first to show that increased urinary levels of both total and free pyridinium cross-links in women more than 75 years of age are associated with an increased risk of hip fracture. For example, the relative risk per standard deviation increase in free DPD as determined by HPLC was 3.0 (95% confidence interval 1.3–8.6). Interestingly, part of this association appeared to be related to disability at baseline. However, when the data set was corrected for disability, a relative risk of 1.9 (95% confidence interval 0.6–5.6) remained. Furthermore, later analyses of the same study revealed that *low* serum osteocalcin concentrations were also associated with an increased risk of hip fracture (odds ratio: 3.1; 95% confidence interval: 1.0–9.2; HAP Pols, personal communication). In another prospective study, low serum levels of both the carboxy-terminal propeptide and the telopeptide of type I collagen were associated with an increased risk of hip fracture, independent of age and BMD (170) (Fig. 2).

Similar results have been published for a larger number of elderly subjects (n = 120) recruited from the EPIDOS study [172]. Interestingly, the relative risks as defined by either BMD or marker measurements were not only similar, but the combined measurement of hip bone density and of bone resorption markers predicted future hip fractures better than the determination of either bone density or bone markers alone. In other words, in older postmenopausal women, the relative

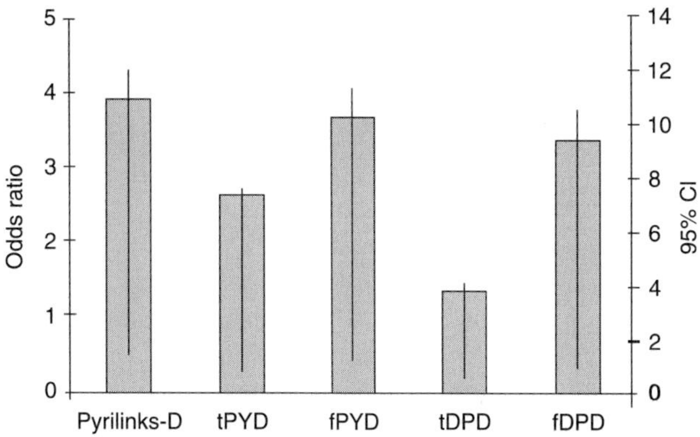

FIGURE 2 Relationship between bone markers and odds ratios for fracture risk: the Rotterdam study. Bars indicate odds ratio, vertical lines the 95% confidence interval (95% CI). Results are shown for urinary-free immunoreactive deoxypyridinoline (Pyrilinks-D, measured by ELISA) and for urinary total pyridinoline (tPYD) and deoxypyridinoline (tDPD), as well as for urinary-free pyridinoline (fPYD) and deoxypyridinoline (fDPD) as measured by HPLC. For more details, see text. Courtesy of Dr. P. van Daele and Professor Huibert Pols, Rotterdam, The Netherlands.

risk of fracture seems to be highest in individuals with both low bone mass and high rates of bone resorption.

A nested case control study from the same group later suggested that levels of serum undercarboxylated osteocalcin (ucOC), but not of total osteocalcin, were predictive of future hip fractures (odds ratio 2.0; 95% confidence interval: 1.2–3.2) [173]. Although serum levels of ucOC showed a significant negative correlation with bone mineral density (BMD), adjustment for BMD did not change the odds ratios significantly. Adjustment for a factor related to risk of falling (gait speed) also did not change the predictive value of ucOC. Again, when BMD (lowest quartile) and serum ucOC (highest quartile) were considered together, the odds ratio increased to 5.5 (confidence interval: 2.7–11.2).

These data supplement and extend previous reports from the same group, which suggested that increased serum levels of ucOC are predictive of hip fractures in elderly, institutionalized women [149,174,175]. These earlier results, however, may merely indicate an association between poor nutritional status and hip fracture risk among institutionalized subjects and not a general biological mechanism possibly relevant to a more representative sampling of the population (see Chapter 20). The significance of vitamin K deficiency to the undercarboxylation of osteocalcin had been demonstrated earlier by Price and Kaneda [176], and subsequent clinical studies showed that overt vitamin K deficiency may lead to a disproportionate increase in ucOC in the circulation [177,178]. Additionally, vitamin K_2 levels have been shown to be lower in women with osteoporotic fractures than in healthy individuals [179]. Although the measurement of ucOC may be useful in providing an integrated assessment of the factors that are responsible for the γ-carboxylation of osteocalcin, such as vitamin K and D, the underlying biochemical mechanisms by which ucOC could be associated with impaired bone metabolism are, as yet, unknown. Analysis of osteocalcin in bone samples from a relatively small number of patients with osteoporosis has shown negligible differences in the proportion of ucOC compared with bone specimens from healthy controls [180]. The lower affinity of the undercarboxylated protein for bone mineral may also serve to diminish its relative importance in influencing bone metabolism. Alternatively, OC-deficient, transgenic mice show enhanced bone formation [6], which suggests an inhibitory function of osteocalcin on osteoblast activity.

Nevertheless, data from large epidemiological studies now indicate that an increase in the rate of bone resorption may be predictive of future fracture risk in healthy women beyond the age of 70. Furthermore, measurements of components such as ucOC may provide information even more useful than the simple quantification of bone turnover because they begin to address the issue of mechanisms of bone loss. If these results are confirmed, certain marker components may become useful tools in the assessment of fracture risk for individuals. Combined with the assessment of BMD and of risk factors such as family history, hip axis length, disability, and postural integrity, markers of bone turnover will not only help to identify the patients at risk but also to define thresholds and timing of intervention strategies.

Biochemical Markers of Bone Metabolism in Osteoporosis

Osteoporosis is a heterogeneous disease. It is therefore not surprising that in untreated patients with either overt postmenopausal or age-related osteoporosis, rates of bone turnover tend to vary over a wide range. Although most cross-sectional studies show accelerated bone turnover in a certain proportion of postmenopausal osteoporotic women, there is usually a broad overlap between diseased and healthy populations [67,105,131,181–185] (Fig. 3). In this context, it is important to keep in mind that research studies usually include highly selective patient populations, which may not always represent the clinical setting. Using a population-based data set, and therefore avoiding this selection bias, the authors have previously shown that none of the major biochemical markers of bone turnover provide sufficient diagnostic information to be useful in the screening for vertebral osteopenia or osteoporosis [125]. However, another population-based study showed that

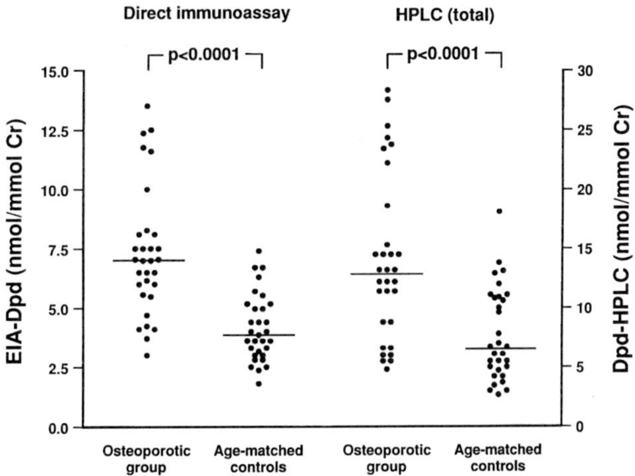

FIGURE 3 Urinary deoxypyridinoline in patients with vertebral osteoporosis and age-matched healthy controls. Note the wide overlap between the two groups.

urinary levels of NTX could discriminate between older individuals with normal hip bone density (T score $\leq$ -1 SD), osteopenia (T score > -1.0 and < -2.5 SD), and osteoporosis (T score ≥ -2.5 SD) [153]. Again, this association did not hold true for men at the level of the spine.

In a retrospective population-based study, Akesson and co-workers [186–188] demonstrated that previous fractures were associated with abnormal bone turnover. After adjustment for age and BMD, women with fractures occurring within 6 years prior to the study were characterized by lower serum levels of OC and PICP, but normal rates of bone resorption. In another investigation, the same authors found decreased serum levels of OC and elevated urinary concentrations of collagen cross-links in elderly women at the time of admission for a newly sustained hip fracture [186]. Taken together, these data suggest that a long-term imbalance of bone metabolism, namely decreased bone formation and normal or increased bone resorption, may lead to increased fragility. Together with the fact that high bone turnover may be sustained for long periods and bone loss may increase with age, these findings may provide a rationale for designing more effective intervention strategies. However, other factors such as age, medication, immobilization, and the fracture itself [189,190] do influence bone metabolism and therefore need to be considered in the interpretation of biochemical data and their use in individual patients.

Biochemical Markers of Bone Metabolism and Therapeutic Monitoring

The range of treatments for osteoporosis matches the heterogeneity of the disease. Ideally, treatment of the patient with osteoporosis should be tailored to the individual, taking into account age, sex, mobility and disability, comorbidity, life expectancy, and a number of other relevant factors. Under certain conditions, the dynamics of bone turnover, namely the rates of bone formation and of bone resorption, also appear to be important determinants of therapeutic efficacy and response.

SELECTION OF THERAPY AND PRETREATMENT PREDICTION OF THERAPEUTIC RESPONSE

From a theoretical point of view, it is conceivable that intervention strategies may differ between patients with accelerated, normal, or even low bone turnover at the time of diagnosis. Thus, a patient presenting with high rates of bone resorption may benefit from antiresorptive therapy, whereas in the same individual with low bone turnover a stimulator of bone formation may yield better long-term results. It was therefore hypothesized that pretreatment levels of biochemical markers of bone metabolism may be helpful in guiding the selection of therapy for individual patients.

In an early study, Civitelli *et al.* [191] showed that in osteoporotic patients treated with subcutaneous calcitonin, increases in lumbar BMD were much greater in individuals with high baseline rates of bone turnover than in those with low rates of bone formation and resorption (Fig. 4). Similar results were later reported by others [192,193], although more recent studies with

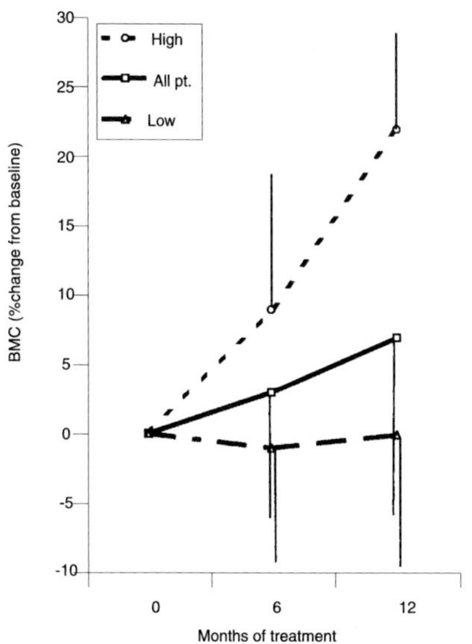

FIGURE 4 Change in bone mineral density (lumbar spine) during 1 year of treatment with subcutaneous calcitonin. The magnitude of change depends on the rate of bone turnover at baseline. Subjects with a high bone turnover show a more pronounced response than the total group or individuals with low rates of bone turnover. Modified after Civitelli *et al.* [191]. Similar patterns (although not as pronounced) have been seen in patients treated with hormone replacement therapy, but not with bisphosphonates.

bisphosphonates suggest that patients respond to treatment independently of their pretherapeutic turnover rates [182]. However, no data exist that compare the various antiresorptive agents in similar populations.

Riggs and associates [169] demonstrated that depending on the baseline rate of bone turnover, both an increase in vertebral BMD and a decrease in bone turnover are equally effective in reducing vertebral fractures in osteoporotic women. Thus, in patients with high levels of bone turnover, estrogen (i.e., antiresorptive) treatment and normalization of bone metabolism resulted in a decrease in vertebral fractures, independent of changes in vertebral BMD. In contrast, when bone turnover was normal, changes in lumbar BMD remained the main determinant of therapeutic efficacy. In women treated with nontoxic levels of fluorides, lumbar BMD and fracture rates were inversely related to each other. Therefore, it was concluded that bone-forming agents, such as fluorides, act by directly increasing BMD and vertebral strength, whereas inhibitors of bone resorption prevent fractures mainly through the reduction of bone turnover. These results not only support the concept that, under certain conditions, biochemical markers are predictors of future fracture risk, but also provide a rationale for the use of bone markers in the selection of therapy and in the prediction of therapeutic response.

Prospective studies in early postmenopausal women seem to substantiate this concept further. In 227 women treated with either calcium alone or a combination of HRT plus calcium, Chesnut *et al.* [163] and Rosen *et al.* [164] demonstrated that individuals within the highest quartile for baseline measures of bone turnover also experienced the greatest gain in BMD after 6 and 12 months of treatment with HRT and calcium. In this study, baseline urinary NTX and serum OC showed the highest predictive values for a change in spinal BMD after 1 year of either HRT or calcium. In reverse, those women showing a gain in BMD after 1 year of HRT had significantly higher baseline rates of bone resorption (as determined by urinary NTX) than nonresponders or subjects losing bone during HRT [164]. This observation is in agreement with the hypothesis that the rate of bone turnover influences the likelihood of vertebral fractures only if accelerated [169].

In contrast, Stevenson *et al.* [194], in a 3-year prospective study on the effect of HRT on spine and hip BMD, were unable to distinguish between responders and nonresponders by means of either baseline or follow-up measures of bone turnover. Both groups showed the same pretreatment values of bone formation and resorption, and the change in bone markers in response to HRT was identical in the affected and unaffected groups [194].

In total, there is increasing evidence of a relationship between bone turnover at baseline and BMD response to antiresorptive treatment. Patients with markedly accelerated rates of bone formation or of bone resorption appear to benefit more from either calcitonin or HRT than those with normal or low rates of bone turnover. In the former, markers of bone metabolism may be used to select therapy and predict therapeutic response. So far, however, no such relationship has been established for other antiresorptive agents, including certain bisphosphonates and vitamin D. Moreover, the relationship between bone turnover and therapeutic response seems to hold true only for patients with clearly accelerated rates of bone turnover. Clinical experience shows that the majority of patients with osteoporosis show normal or moderately elevated bone turnover. In this group, biomarkers of bone formation and resorption are still valid measures of pretreatment bone turnover and thus important in further monitoring. However, their clinical value must be questioned with respect to the prediction of response and therefore for the selection of therapy.

THERAPEUTIC AND DISEASE MONITORING

Therapeutic and disease monitoring is certainly the most relevant area for the clinical use of biochemical markers of bone metabolism. This specifically includes (i) monitoring of therapeutic efficacy, (ii) within-treatment prediction of therapeutic response, (iii) monitoring of patient compliance, and (iv) follow-up of the natural course of the disease.

Serial measurements of bone density are the standard approach to monitor spontaneous bone loss and therapeutic efficacy and, in many studies, changes in bone mass are the primary end point. Although not a truly static parameter, bone mass changes slowly, however, and a therapeutic effect is usually not detectable before 12 to 24 months of treatment. This delay is not only due to the slow dynamics of bone remodeling itself, but also to a disadvantageous change: the precision ratio of bone mass measurements over short periods. In other words, within a year of treatment, comparatively small changes in bone density are contrasted by relatively high precision errors, therefore rendering bone mass measurements unsuitable for the early assessment of therapeutic effects or spontaneous bone loss. In contrast, biochemical markers of bone metabolism usually react rapidly to therapeutic interventions, and significant effects are often seen within 6 to 8 weeks of therapy. For example, treatment with subcutaneous calcitonin [195–202] or intravenous bisphosphonates [182,203–205] leads to a significant reduction in the levels of resorption markers as early as 48 to 72 hr after the first injection (Fig. 5). Hormone replacement therapy has been shown to result in a 50–100% decrease in markers of bone turnover within 3 to 4 months of treatment [128,206–208] Although biochemical bone markers generally exhibit a high degree of variability (both technically and biologically), their change:precision ratio compares favorably to bone mass measurements, as far as the short-term monitoring of therapeutic effects is concerned.

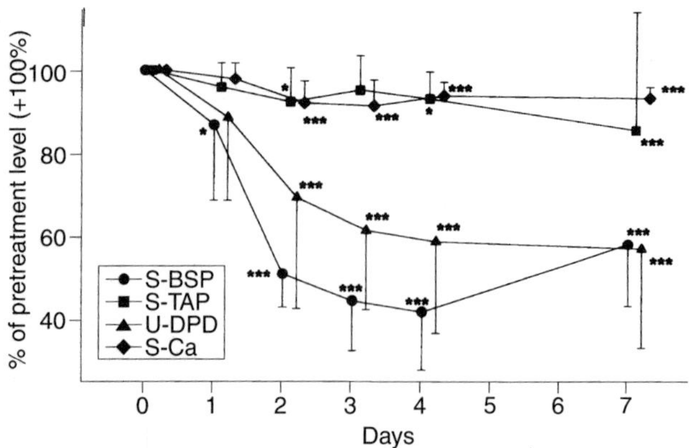

FIGURE 5 Change in markers of bone turnover after 2 mg of intraveneous ibandronate. S-BSP, serum bone sialoprotein; S-TAP, serum total alkaline phosphatase; U-DPD, urinary deoxypyridinoline; S-Ca, serum calcium. P versus baseline, *<0.05, ***<0.001. From Seibel *et al.* [205], with permission.

Biochemical markers of bone metabolism therefore appear to be ideal tools in evaluating therapeutic effects after a relatively short period. Currently, most recommendations suggest the measurement of bone biomarkers shortly before and 3–6 months after treatment is implemented. These recommendations are based on the observation that most biomarkers will react within this time frame, but also on novel findings suggesting that the therapeutically induced change in bone turnover predicts the efficacy of an antiresorptive agent in terms of BMD at a later time point. Thus, a number of studies have shown that the magnitude of the change in bone markers at 3, 4, or 6 months of treatment with HRT or bisphosphonates ($\Delta t_1 - t_0$) correlates directly with the increase in BMD after 12 or 24 months of treatment [163,164,209]. In a prospective study, patients with the most pronounced change in biomarkers after 6 months of HRT also showed the highest gain in BMD after 1 year of treatment [164]. A somewhat weaker inverse correlation between changes in bone biomarkers and spinal/hip BMD was also reported for early postmenopausal women treated with HRT and Vitamin D [141].

Taken together, these data suggest that serial measurements of bone biomarkers soon after the initiation of therapy may be helpful in deciding whether or not a patient responds to a specific treatment regimen. As bone resorption markers appear to respond to potent bisphosphonates, irrespective of baseline rates of bone turnover, it has also been suggested that these indices may serve as a measure of patient compliance. In the case of nonresponsiveness or noncompliance, a repeated measurement of bone turnover could save medication-related costs that would otherwise accumulate over a period of 1 or 2 years. However, it should also be noted that none of these concepts has been confirmed in prospective clinical trials so far. Moreover, no general scientific consensus has been reached, as yet, on the use of biomarkers in the follow-up of osteoporotic patients. In fact, some national guidelines totally ignore these tools at the present time.

In contrast to these clinical limitations, biochemical markers of bone turnover play an important and essential role within the research setting. An abundance of experimental, preclinical, and clinical studies have demonstrated that markers of bone formation and resorption are valid tools in the assessment of the skeletal response to a great variety of influences. For example, markers of bone turnover may reflect changes in bone metabolism induced by oophorectomy [138, 210–213], physical exercise [214,215], immobilization [216,217], alcoholism [218–224], vitamin D deficiency [225], or chronic starving [226,227], as well as the pharmacological effects of glucocorticosteroids [228–237], androgens [238–240], parathyroid hormone [241–250], gonadotropin-releasing hormone agonists [251–253], warfarin [254–256], growth hormone, or insulin-like growth factors [257–258]. Although these just-mentioned studies represent only a small selection of the available literature, they all demonstrate that biomarkers of bone turnover are extremely helpful tools in evaluating the physiology and pathophysiology of bone metabolism and in elucidating the pathogenesis of bone disease.

SUMMARY

With the increasing importance of diseases of the locomotor system, the development of more effective techniques for the screening, diagnosis, and prevention of metabolic bone diseases has become a relevant issue. This is particularly true when considering the recent advent of novel preventive and therapeutic strategies for age-related bone loss and their impact on the cost effectiveness of national health systems.

When used in combination with clinical data and imaging techniques, biochemical markers of bone metabolism permit a comprehensive and noninvasive evaluation of the skeletal status. These parameters may therefore be used

- to predict future bone loss and hip fractures in larger cohorts
- to evaluate the current state of bone turnover in individual patients
- to identify individuals at risk for osteoporosis
- to select therapy for individual patients
- to predict the therapeutic response in individual patients
- to monitor therapeutic response and efficacy in, and compliance of, individual patients.

As far as the initial clinical diagnosis of osteoporosis is concerned, none of the biochemical markers of bone turnover has proven useful as a single determination. As with bone density measurements, a broad overlap between healthy and diseased populations is observed.

Nevertheless, once the diagnosis of osteoporotic bone disease is made, biochemical markers of bone metabolism are useful tools in further work-up, particularly in identifying patients with high rates of bone turnover. Thus, patients with accelerated bone turnover not only lose bone at a faster rate, but also carry a significantly higher risk of hip fractures. Much like bone density measurements, bone biomarkers are indicators of *risk* rather than of the disease itself. Furthermore, patients with high bone turnover appear to benefit from antiresorptive treatments more than subjects with low or normal bone metabolism. The measurement of bone formation and bone resorption may therefore not only be useful in therapeutic decision making but can also help reduce costs by identifying those individuals who may not respond well to treatment. Finally, bone markers are of clinical relevance in monitoring both the disease itself and therapeutic efficacy. Future uses may also include the measurement of bone biomarkers to improve patient compliance. However, the development of new "bone markers" to improve primary diagnostics and screening is still a specified research goal.

Acknowledgments

MJS thanks Dr. P. van Daele and Professor H. Pols for providing Fig. 2 and for the productive and enjoyable collaboration over the years. MJS also thanks Dr. H. W. Woitge, Dr. Y. Li, and Dr. H. Oberwittler for their continuous support. SPR thanks the Scottish Office Agriculture, Environment, and Fisheries Department for support.

References

1. Gallop, P. M., Lian, J. B., and Hauschka, P. V. Carboxylated calcium binding proteins and vitamin K. *N. Eng. J. Med.* **302,** 1460–1466 (1980).
2. Hauschka, P. V., and Carr, S. A. Calcium-dependent alpha-helical structure in osteocalcin. *Biochemistry* **21,** 2538–2547 (1982).
3. Hauschka, P. V., and Reid, M. L. Timed appearance of a calcium-binding protein containing g-carboxyglutamic acid in developing chick bone. *Dev. Biol.* **65,** 426–434 (1978).

4. Lian, J. B., Roufosse, A. H., Reit, B., and Glimcher, M. J. Concentrations of osteocalcin and phosphoprotein as a function of mineral content and age in cortical bone. *Calcif. Tissue Int.* **34,** S82–S87 (1982).
5. Owen, T. A., Aronow, M., Shalhoub, V., Barone, L. M., Wilming, L., Tassinari, M. S., Kennedy, M. B., Pockwinse, S., Lian, J. B., and Stein, G. S. Progressive development of the rat osteoblast phenotype *in vitro:* reciprocal relationships in expression of genes associated with osteoblast proliferation and differentiation during formation of the bone extracellular matrix. *J. Cell. Physiol.* **143,** 420–430 (1990).
6. Ducy, P., Desbois, C., Boycem, B., Pinero, G., Story, B., Dunstan, C., Smith, E., Bonadio, J., Goldstein, S., Gundberg, C., Bradley, A., and Karsenty, G. Increased bone formation in osteocalcin-deficient mice. *Nature* **382,** 448–452 (1996).
7. Hauschka, P. V., Lian, J. B., Cole, D. E., and Gundberg, C. Osteocalcin and matrix Gla protein: vitamin K-dependent proteins in bone. *Physiol. Rev.* **69,** 990–1047 (1989).
8. Gundberg, C. M., Hauschka, P. V., Lian, J. B., and Gallop, P. M. Osteocalcin: Isolation, characterization and detection. *In* "Methods in Enzymology" (K. Moldave, eds.), 516–544. Academic Press, New York, 1984.
9. Price, P. A., and Nishimoto, S. K. Radioimmunoassay for the vitamin K-dependent protein of bone and its discovery in plasma. *Proc. Natl. Acad. Sci. USA* **77,** 2234–2238 (1980).
10. Delmas, P. D., Christiansen, C., Mann, K. G., and Price, P. A. Bone Gla protein (osteocalcin) assay standardization report. *J. Bone Min. Res.* **5,** 5–10 (1990).
11. Masters, P. W., Jones, R. G., Purves, D. A., Cooper, E. H., and Cooney, J. M. Commercial assays for serum osteocalcin give clinically discordant result. *Clin. Chem.* **40,** 358–363 (1994).
12. Power, M. J., Gosling, J. P., and Fottrell, P. F. Radioimmunoassay of osteocalcin with polyclonal and monoclonal antibodies. *Clin. Chem.* **35,** 1408–1415 (1989).
13. Gundberg, C. M., and Weinstein, R. S. Multiple immunoreactive forms of osteocalcin in uremic serum. *J. Clin. Invest.* **77,** 1762–1767 (1986).
14. Garnero, P., Grimaux, M., Seguin, P., and Delmas, P. D. Characterization of immunoreactive forms of human osteocalcin generated *in vivo* and *in vitro. J. Bone Min. Res.* **9,** 255–264 (1994).
15. Taylor, A. K., Linkhart, S., Mohan, S., Christenson, R. A., Singer, F. R., and Baylink, D. J. Multiple osteocalcin fragments in human urine and serum as detected by a midmolecule osteocalcin radioimmunoassay. *J. Clin. Endocrinol. Metab.* **70,** 467–472 (1990).
16. Tracy, R. P., Andrianorivo, A., Riggs, B. L., and Mann, K. G. Comparison of monoclonal and polyclonal antibody-based immunoassays for osteocalcin: a study of sources of variation in assay results. *J. Bone Min. Res.* **5,** 451–461 (1990).
17. Garnero, P., Grimaux, M., Demiaux, B., Preaudat, C., Seguin, P., and Delmas, P. D. Measurement of serum osteocalcin with a human-specific two-site immunoradiometric assay. *J. Bone Min. Res.* **7,** 1389–1398 (1992).
18. Jaouhari, J., Schiele, F., Dragacci, S., Tarallo, P., Siest, J.-P., Henny, J., and Siest, G. Avidin-biotin enzyme immunoassay of osteocalcin in serum or plasma. *Clin. Chem.* **38,** 1968–1974 (1992).
19. Hosoda, K., Eguchi, H., Nakamoto, T., Kubota, T., Honda, H., Jindai, S., Hasegawa, R., Kiyoki, M., Yamaji, T., and Shiraki, M. Sandwich immunoassay for intact human osteocalcin. *Clin. Chem.* **38,** 2233–2238 (1992).
20. Monaghan, D. A., Power, M. J., and Fottrell, P. F. Sandwich enzyme immunoassay of osteocalcin in serum with use of an antibody against human osteocalcin. *Clin. Chem.* **39,** 942–947 (1993).
21. Parviainen, M., Kuronen, I., Kokko, H., Lakaniemi, M., Savolainen, K., and Mononen, I. Two-site enzyme immunoassay for measuring intact human osteocalcin in serum. *Bone Min. Res.* **9,** 347–354 (1994).
22. Kuronen, I., Kokko, H., and Parviainen, M. Production of monoclonal and polyclonal antibodies against human osteocalcin sequences and development of a two-site ELISA for intact human osteocalcin. *J. Immunol. Methods* **163,** 223–240 (1993).
23. Deftos, L. J., Wolfert, R. L., Hill, C. S., and Burton, D. W. Two-site assays of bone Gla protein (osteocalcin) demonstrate immunochemical heterogeneity of the intact molecule. *Clin. Chem.* **38,** 2318–2321 (1992).
24. Diego, E. M. D., Guerrero, R., and de la Piedra. Six osteocalcin assays compared. *Clin. Chem.* **40,** 2071–2077 (1994).
25. Dumon, J. C., Wantier, H., Mathieu, J., Body, J. J. Technical and clinical validation of a new immunoradiometric assay for human osteocalcin. *Eur. J. Endocrinol.* **135,** 231–237 (1996).
26. Rosenquist, C., Quist, P., Bjarnason, N., and Christiansen, C. Measurement of a more stable region of osteocalcin in serum by ELISA with two monoclonal antibodies. *Clin. Chem.* **41,** 1439–1445 (1995).
27. Chen, J. T., Hosoda, K., Hasumi, K., Ogata, E., and Shiraki, M. Serum N-terminal osteocalcin is a good indicator for estimating responders to hormone replacement therapy in postmenopausal women. *J. Bone Min. Res.* **11,** 1784–1792 (1996).
28. Gorai, L., Hosoda, K., Taguchi, Y., Chacki, O., Nakavama, M., Yoh, K., Yamaii, T., and Minaguchi, H. A heterogeneity in serum osteocalcin N-terminal fragments in Paget's disease: A comparison with other biochemical indices in pre- and post-menopause. *J. Bone Min. Res.* **12**(S1), T678 (1997).
29. Salo, J., Lehenkari, P., Mulari, M., Metsikk, K., and Väänänen, H. K. Removal of osteoclast bone resorption products by transcytosis. *Science* **276,** 270–273 (1997).
30. Page, A. E., Hayman, A. R., Andersson, L. M. B., Chambers, T. J., and Warburton, M. J. Degradation of bone matrix proteins by osteoclast cathepsins. *J. Biochem.* **25,** 545–550 (1993).
31. Baumgrass, R., Williamson, M. K., and Price, P. A. Identification of peptide fragments generated by digestion of bovine and human osteocalcin with the lysosomal proteinases cathepsin B, D, L, H, and S. *J. Bone Min. Res.* **12,** 447–455 (1997).
32. Baumgrass, R., Felsenberg, D., and Price P. A. The cross-reactivities of cathepsin generated bone GLA protein-fragments in different immunoassays. *J. Bone Min. Res.* **10,** S339 (1995).
33. Low, M. G., and Saltiel, A. R. Structural and functional roles of glycosyl-phosphatidylinositol in membranes. *Science* **239,** 268–275 (1988).
34. Stinson, R. A., and Hamilton, B. A. Human liver plasma membranes contain an enzyme activity that removes membrane anchor from alkaline phosphatase and converts it to a plasma-like form. *Clin. Biochem.* **27,** 49–55 (1994).
35. Low, M. G., and Huang, K. S. Factors affecting the ability of glycosylphosphatidylinositol-specific phospholipase D to degrade the membrane anchors of cell surface proteins. *Biochem. J.* **279,** 483–493 (1991).
36. Li, J. Y., Hollfelder, K., Huang, K. S., and Low, M. G. Structural features of GPI-specific phospholipase D revealed by proteolytic fragmentation and Ca^{2+} binding studies. *Biol. Chem.* **269,** 28963–28971 (1994).
37. Crofton, P. S. Biochemistry of alkaline phosphatase isoenzymes. *CRC Crit. Rev. Clin. Lab. Sci.,* 161–194 (1982).
38. Harris, H. The human alkaline phosphatases: what we know and what we don't know. *Clin. Chim. Acta* **186,** 133–150 (1989).
39. Van Hoof, V. O., and DeBroe, M. E. Interpretation and clinical significance of alkaline phosphatase isoenzyme patterns. *Crit. Rev. Clin. Lab. Sci.* **31,** 197–293 (1994).

40. Van Hoof, V. O., Holyaerts, M. F., Geryl, H., Van Mullem, M., Lepoutre, L. G., and De Broe, M. E. Age and sex distribution of alkaline phosphatase isoenzymes by agarose electrophoresis. *Clin. Chem.* **36,** 875–878 (1990).
41. Koyama, I., Miura, M., Matsuzaki, H., Sakagishi, Y., and Komoda, T. Sugar-chain heterogeneity of human alkaline phosphatases: differences between normal and tumour-associated isozymes. *Am. J. Dis. Child.* **139,** 736–740 (1985).
42. Whyte, M. P. Hypophosphatasia and the role of alkaline phosphatase in skeletal mineralization. *Endocr. Rev.* **15,** 439–461 (1994).
43. Chamberlain, B., Buttery, J., and Pannall, P. A simple electrophoretic method for separating elevated liver and bone alkaline phosphatase isoenzymes in plasma after neuraminidase treatment. *Clin. Chim. Acta* **208,** 219–224 (1992).
44. Mazda, T., and Gyure, W. L. Assay of alkaline phosphatase isoenzymes by a convenient precipitation and inhibition methodology. *Chem. Pharm. Bull.* **36,** 1814–1818 (1988).
45. Rosalki, S. B., and Foo, A. Y. Two new methods for separating and quantifying bone and liver alkaline phosphatase isoenzymes in plasma. *Clin. Chem.* **30,** 1182–1186 (1984).
46. Behr, W., and Barnert, J. Quantification of bone alkaline phosphatase in serum by precipitation with wheat-germ lectin: a simplified method and its clinical plausibility. *Clin. Chem.* **32,** 1960–1966 (1986).
47. Sorenson, S. Wheat-germ agglutinin method for measuring bone and liver isoenzymes of alkaline phosphatase assessed in postmenopausal osteoporosis. *Clin. Chem.* **34,** 1636–1640 (1988).
48. Eastell, R., Delmas, P. D., Hodgson, S. F., Eriksen, E. F., Mann, K. G., and Riggs, B. Bone formation rate in older normal women: concurrent assessment with bone histomorphometry, calcium kinetics, and biochemical markers. *J. Clin. Endocrinol. Metab.* **67,** 741–748 (1988).
49. Crofton, P. M. Wheat-germ lectin affinity electrophoresis for alkaline phosphatase isoforms in children: age-dependent reference ranges and changes in liver and bone disease. *Clin. Chem.* **38,** 663–670 (1992).
50. Leung, K., Fung, K., Sher, A., Li, C., and Lee, K. Plasma bone-specific alkaline phosphatase as an indicator of osteoblastic activity. *J. Bone Joint Surg.* **75B,** 288–292 (1993).
51. Hill, C. S., and Wolfert, R. L. The preparation of monoclonal antibodies which react preferentially with human bone alkaline phosphatase and not liver alkaline phosphatase. *Clin. Chin. Acta* **186,** 315–320 (1989).
52. Gomez, B., Jr., Ardakani, S., Ju, J., Jenkins, D., Cerelli, M. J., Daniloff, G. Y., and Kung, V. T. Monoclonal antibody assay for measuring bone-specific alkaline phosphatase activity in serum. *Clin. Chem.* **41,** 1560–1566 (1995).
53. Garnero, P., and Delmas, P. D. Assessment of the serum levels of bone alkaline phosphatase with a new immunoradiometric assay in patients with metabolic bone disease. *J. Clin. Endocrinol. Metab.* **77,** 1046–1053 (1993).
54. Langlois, M. R., Delanghe, J. R., Kaufman, J. M., De Buyzere, M. L., Van Hoecke, M. J., and Leroux-Roels, G. G. Posttranslational heterogeneity of bone alkaline phosphatase in metabolic bone disease. *Eur. J. Clin. Chem. Clin. Biochem.* **32,** 675–680 (1994).
55. Martin, M., Van Hoof, V. Couttenye, M., Prove, A., and Blokx, P. Analytical and clinical evaluation of a method to quantify bone alkaline phosphatase, a marker of osteoblastic activity. *Anticancer Res.* **17,** 3167–70 (1997).
56. Woitge, H., Seibel, M. J., and Ziegler, R. Comparison of total and bone-specific alkaline phosphatase in patients with nonskeletal disorders or metabolic bone disease. *Clin. Chem.* **42,** 1796–1804 (1996).
57. Robey, P. G., Fisher, L. W., Young, M. F., and Termine, J. D. The biochemistry of bone. *In* "Osteoporosis: Etiology, Diagnosis and Management" (B. L. Riggs and L. J. Melton III, eds.), pp. 95–109. Raven Press, New York, 1988.
58. Olsen, B. R., Guzman, N. A., Engel, J., Condit, C., and Aase, S. Purification and characterization of a peptide from the carboxy-terminal region of chick tendon procollagen type I. *Biochemistry* **16,** 3030–3036 (1977).
59. Smedsrod, B., Melkko, J., Risteli, L., and Risteli, J. Circulating C-terminal propetide of type I procollagen is cleared mainly via the mannose receptor in liver endothelial cells. *Biochem. J.* **271,** 345–350 (1990).
60. Kivirikko, K. I., and Myllyla, R. Biosynthesis of the collagens. *In* "Extracellular Matrix Biochemistry" (K. A. Piez and A. H. Reddi, eds.), pp. 83–119. Elsevier, New York, 1984.
61. Melkko, J., Niemi, S., Risteli, L., and Risteli, J. Radioimmunassay of the carboxyterminal propetide of human type I procollagen. *Clin. Chem.* **36,** 1328–1332 (1990).
62. Taubman, M. B., Goldberg, B., and Sherr, C. Radioimmunoassay for human procollagen. *Science* **186,** 1115–1117 (1974).
63. Pedersen, B. J., and Bonde, M. Purification of human procollagen type I carboxyl-terminal propeptide cleaved as *in vivo* from procollagen and used to calibrate a radioimmunassay of the propeptide. *Clin. Chem.* **40,** 811–816 (1994).
64. Ebeling, P. R., Peterson, J. M., and Riggs, B. L. Utility of type I procollagen propeptide assays for assessing abnormalities in metabolic bone diseases. *J. Bone. Miner. Res.* **7,** 1243–1250 (1992).
65. Minisola, S., Romagnoli, E., Scarnecchia, L., Rosso, R., Pacitti, M. T., Scarda, A., and Mazzuoli, G. Serum carboxy-terminal propetide of human type I procollagen in patients with primary hyperparathyroidism: studies in basal conditions and after parathyroid surgery. *Eur. J. Endocrinol.* **130,** 587–591 (1994).
66. Charles, P., Mosekilde, L., Risteli, L., Risteli, J., and Eriksen, E. F. Assessment of bone remodeling using biochemical indicators of type I collagen synthesis and degradation: relation to calcium kinetics. *Bone Miner.* **24,** 81–94 (1994).
67. Eastell, R., Robins, S., Colwell, T., Assiri, A., Riggs, B., and Russell, R. Evaluation of bone turnover in type I osteoporosis using biochemical markers specific for both bone formation and bone resorption. *Osteoporos. Int.* **3,** 255–260 (1993).
68. Lotz, J., Steeger, D., Hafner, G., Ehrenthal, W., Heine, J., and Prellwitz, W. Biochemical bone markers compared with bone density measurement by dual energy X-ray absorptiometry. *Calcif. Tissue Int.* **57,** 253–257 (1995).
69. Kivirikko, K. I. Urinary excretion of hydroxyproline in health and disease. *Int. Rev. Connect. Tissue Res.* **5,** 93–163 (1970).
70. Deacon, A. C., Hulme, P., Hesp, R., Green, J. R., Tellez, M., and Reeve, J. Estimation of whole body bone resorption rate: a comparison of urinary total hydroxyproline excretion with two radioisotopic tracer methods in osteoporosis. *Clin. Chim. Acta* **166,** 297–306 (1987).
71. Krane, S. M., Kantrowitz, F. G., Byrne, M., Pinnell, S. R., and Singer, F. R. Urinary excretion of hydroxylysine and its glycosides as an index of collagen degradation. *J. Clin. Invest.* **59,** 819–827 (1977).
72. Moro, L., Noris-Suarez, K., Michalsky, M., Romanello, M., and de Bernard, B. The glycosides of hydroxylysine are final products of collagen degradation in humans. *Biochim. Biophys. Acta* **1156,** 288–290 (1993).
73. Segrest, J. P., and Cunningham, L. W. Variations in human urinary O-hydroxylysyl glycoside levels and their relationship to collagen metabolism. *J. Clin. Invest.* **49,** 1497–1509 (1970).

74. Bienkowski, R. Intracellular degradation of newly synthesized collagen. *Collagen Rel. Res.* **4,** 399–412 (1984).
75. Moro, L., Modricky, C., Rovis, L., and DeBernard, B. Determination of galactosyl hydroxylysine in urine as a means for the identification of osteoporotic women. *Bone Miner.* **3,** 271–276 (1988).
76. Bettica, P., Moro, L., Robins, S. P., Taylor, A. K., Talbot, J., Singer, F. R., and Baylink, D. J. The comparative performance of urinary bone resorption markers: galactosyl hydroxylysine, pyridinium crosslinks, hydroxyproline. *Clin. Chem.* **38,** 2313–2318 (1992).
77. Fujimoto, D., Moriguchi, T., Ishida, T., and Hayashi, H. The structure of pyridinoline, a collagen crosslink. *Biochem. Biophys. Res. Commun.* **84,** 52–57 (1978).
78. Gunja-Smith, Z., and Boucek, R. J. Collagen crosslink components in human urine. *Biochem. J.* **197,** 759–762 (1981).
79. Robins, S. P. An enzyme-linked immunoassay for the collagen crosslink, pyridinoline. *Biochem. J.* **207,** 617–620 (1982).
80. Eyre, D. R., Koob, T. J., and VanNess, K. P. Quantitation of hydroxypyridinium crosslinks in collagen by high-performance liquid chromatography. *Anal. Biochem.* **137,** 380–388 (1984).
81. Ogawa, T., Ono, T., Tsuda, M., and Kawanashi, Y. A novel fluor in insoluble collagen: a crosslinking molecule in collagen molecule. *Biochem. Biophys. Res. Commun.* **107,** 1252–1257.
82. Black, D., Duncan, A., and Robins, S. P. Quantitative analysis of the pyridinium crosslinks of collagen in urine using ion-paired reversed-phase high-performance liquid chromatography. *Anal. Biochem.* **169,** 197–203 (1988).
83. Pratt, D. A., Daniloff, Y., Duncan, A., and Robins, S. P. Automated analysis of the pyridinium crosslinks of collagen in tissue and urine using solid-phase extraction and reversed-phase high-performance liquid chromatography. *Anal. Biochem.* **207,** 168–175 (1992).
84. James, I. T., and Perrett, D. Automated on-line solid-phase extraction and high-performance liquid chromatographic analysis of total and free pyridinium crosslinks in serum. *J. Chromatogr. A.* **79,** 159–166 (1998).
85. Colwell, A., Russell, R., and Eastell, R. Factors affecting the assay of urinary 3-hydroxy pyridinium crosslinks of collagen as markers of bone resorption. *Eur. J. Clin. Invest.* **23,** 341–349 (1993).
86. Seibel, M. J., Robins, S. P., and Bilezikian, J. P. Urinary pyridinium crosslinks of collagen: specific markers of bone resorption in metabolic bone disease. *Trends Endocrinol. Metab.* **3,** 263–270 (1992).
87. Eastell, R., Colwell, A., Hampton, L., and Reeve, J. Biochemical markers of bone resorption compared with estimates of bone resorption from radiotracer kinetic studies in osteoporosis. *J. Bone Miner. Res.* **12,** 59–65 (1997).
88. Robins, S. P., Duncan, A., and Riggs, B. L. Direct measurement of free hydroxy-pyridinium crosslinks of collagen in urine as new markers of bone resorption in osteoporosis. *In* "Osteoporosis" (C. Christiansen and K. Overgaard, eds.), pp. 465–468. Osteopress ApS, Copenhagen, 1990.
89. Abbiati, G., Bartucci, F., Longoni, A., Fincato, G., Galimberti, S., Rigoldi, M., and Castiglioni, C. Monitoring of free and total urinary pyridinoline and deoxypyridinoline in healthy volunteers: sample relationships between 24-h and fasting early morning urine concentrations. *Bone Miner.* **21,** 9–19 (1993).
90. Seyedin, S. M., Kung, V. T., Daniloff, Y. N., Hesley, R. P., Gomez, B., Nielsen, L. A., and Rosen, H. N. Z. R. F. Immunoassay for urinary pyridinoline: the new marker of bone resorption. *J. Bone Miner. Res.* **8,** 635–641 (1993).
91. Robins, S. P., Woitge, H., Hesley, R., Ju, J., Seyedin, S., and Seibel, M. J. Direct, enzyme-linked immunoassay for urinary deoxypyridinoline as a specific marker for measuring bone resorption. *J. Bone Miner. Res.* **9,** 1643–1649 (1994).
92. Gomez, B., Ardakani, S., Evans, B., Merrell, L., Jenkins, D., and Kung, V. Monoclonal antibody assay for free urinary pyridinium cross-links. *Clin. Chem.* **42,** 1168–1175 (1996).
93. Risteli, J., Elomaa, I., Niemi, S., Novamo, A., and Risteli, L. Radioimmunoassay for the pyridinoline cross-linked carboxy-terminal telopeptide of type I collagen: a new serum marker of bone collagen degradation. *Clin. Chem.* **39,** 635–640 (1993).
94. Hanson, D. A., Weis, M. A., Bollen, A. M., Maslan, S. L., Singer, F. R., and Eyre, D. R. A specific immunoassay for monitoring human bone resorption: quantitation of type I collagen cross-linked N-telopeptides in urine. *J. Bone Miner. Res.* **7,** 1251–1258 (1992).
95. Robins, S. P. Collagen crosslinks in metabolic bone disease. *Acta Orthop. Scand. Suppl.* **266,** 171–175 (1995).
96. Clemens, J. D., Herrick, M. V., Singer, F. R., Eyre, D. R. Evidence that serum NTx (collagen-type I N-telopeptides) can act as an immunochemical marker of bone resorption. *Clin. Chem.* **43,** 2058–2063 (1997).
97. Bonde, M. Q. P., Fidelius, C., Riis, B. J., and Christiansen, C. Immunoassay for quantifying type I degradation products in urine evaluated. *Clin. Chem.* **40,** 2022–2025 (1994).
98. Fledelius, C., Johnsen, A. H., Cloos, P. A. C., Bonde, M., and Qvist, P. Characterization of urinary degradation products derived from type I collagen. Identification of a beta-isomerized Asp-Gly sequence within the C-terminal telopeptide (alpha1) region. *J. Biol. Chem.* **272,** 9755–9763 (1997).
99. Bonde, M., Fledelius, C., Qvist, P., and Christiansen, C. Coated-tube radioimmunoassay for C-telopeptides of type I collagen to assess bone resorption. *Clin. Chem.* **42,** 1639–1644 (1996).
100. Garnero, P., Fledelius, C., Gineyts, E., Serre, C. M., Vignot, E., and Delmas, P. D. Decreased beta-isomerization of the c-terminal telopeptide of type i collagen alpha 1 chain in Paget's disease of bone. *J. Bone Miner. Res.* **12,** 1407–1415 (1997).
101. Garnero, P., Gineyts, E., Schaffer, A. V., Seaman, J., and Delmas, P. D. Measurement of urinary excretion of nonisomerized and beta-isomerized forms of type I collagen breakdown products to monitor the effects of the bisphosphonate zoledronate in Paget's disease. *Arthritis Rheum.* **41,** 354–360 (1998).
102. Bonde, M., Garnero, P., Fledelius, C., Qvist, P., Delmas, P. D., and Christiansen, C. Measurement of bone degradation products in serum using antibodies reactive with an isomerized form of an 8 amino acid sequence of the C-telopeptide of type I collagen. *J. Bone Miner. Res.* **12,** 1028–1034 (1997).
103. Garnero, P., Gineyts, E., Arbault, P., Christiansen, C., and Delmas, P. D. Different effects of bisphosphonate and estrogen therapy on free and peptide-bound bone cross-links excretion. *J. Bone Miner. Res.* **10,** 641–649 (1995).
104. Tobias, J., Laversuch, C., Wilson, N., and Robins, S. Neridronate preferentially suppresses the urinary excretion of peptide-bound deoxypyridinoline in postmenopausal women. *Calcif. Tissue Int.* **59,** 407–409 (1996).
105. Rico, H., and Villa, L. Serum tartrate-resistant acid phosphatase (TRAP) as a biochemical marker of bone remodeling. *Calcif. Tissue Int.* **52,** 149–150 (1993).
106. Kraenzlin, M. E., Lau, K. H., Liang, L., Freeman, T. K., Singer, F. R., Stepan, J., and Baylink, D. J. Development of an immunoassay for human serum osteoclastic tartrate-resistant acid phosphatase. *J. Clin. Endocrinol. Metab.* **71,** 442–451 (1990).
107. Cheung, C., Panesar, N., Haines, C., Masarei, J., and Swaminathan, R. Immunoassay of a tartrate-resistant acid phosphatase in serum. *Clin. Chem.* **41,** 679–686 (1995).

108. Seibel, M., Woitge, H., Pecherstorfer, M., Karmatschek, M., Horn, E., Ludwig, H., Armbruster, F., and Ziegler, R. Serum immunoreactive bone sialoprotein as a new marker of bone turnover in metabolic and malignant bone disease. *J. Clin. Endocrinol. Metab.* **81,** 3289–3294 (1996).
109. Karmatschek, M., Maier, I., Seibel, M. J., Woitge, H. W., Ziegler, R., and Ambruster, F. P. Improved purification of human bone sialoprotein and development of a homologous radioimmunoassay. *Clin. Chem.* **43,** 2076–2082 (1997).
110. Cantatore, F., Carrozzo, M., Magli, D., D'Amore, M., and Pipitone, V. Serum osteocalcin levels in normal humans of different sex and age. *Panminerva. Med.* **30,** 23–25 (1988).
111. Catherwood, B., Marcus, R., Madvig, P., and Cheung, A. Determinants of bone gamma-carboxyglutamic acid-containing protein in plasma of healthy aging subjects. *Bone* **6,** 9–13 (1985).
112. Delmas, P. D., Stenner, D., Wahner, H. W., Mann, K. G., and Riggs, B. L. Increase in serum bone g-carboxyglutamic acid protein with aging in women. *J. Clin. Invest.* **71,** 1316–1321 (1983).
113. Epstein, S., McClintock, R., Bryce, G., Poser, J., Johnston, C. C., Jr., and Hui, S. Differences in serum bone Gla protein with age and sex. *Lancet* **11,** 307–310 (1984).
114. Galli, M., and Caniggia, M. Osteocalcin in normal adult humans of different sex and age. *Horm. Metab. Res.* **17,** 165–166 (1984).
115. Tarallo, P., Henny, J., Fournier, B., and Seist, B. Plasma osteocalcin: biological variations and reference limits. *Scand. J. Clin. Lab. Invest.* **50,** 649–655 (1990).
116. Johansen, J. S., Thomsen, K., and Christiansen, C. Plasma bone Gla protein concentrations in healthy adults. Dependence on sex, age, and glomerular filtration. *Scand. J. Clin. Lab. Invest.* **47,** 345–350 (1987).
117. Nilas, L., and Christiansen, C. Bone mass and its relationship to age and the menopause. *J. Clin. Endocrinol. Metab.* **65,** 697–702 (1987).
118. Schiele, F., Henny, J., Hitz, J., Peiticlerc, C., Gueguen, R., and Siest, G. Total bone and liver alkaline phosphatases in plasma: biological variations and reference limits. *Clin. Chem.* **29,** 634–641 (1983).
119. Tietz, N. W., Wekstein, D. R., Shuey, D. F., and Brauer, G. A. A two-year longitudinal reference range study for selected enzymes in a population more than 60 years of age. *J. Am. Geriatr. Soc.* **32,** 563–570 (1984).
120. Sgherzi, M., Fabbri, G., Bonati, M., Maietta, Latessa, A., Segre, A., De Vita, D., De Leo, V., Genazzani, A., Petraglia, F., and Genazzani, A. Episodic changes of serume procollagen type I carboxy-terminal propeptide levels in fertile and postmenopausal women. *Gynecol. Obstet. Invest.* **38,** 60–64 (1994).
121. Hassager, C., Fabbri-Mabelli, G., and Christiansen, C. The effect of the menopause and hormone replacement therapy on serum carboxyl-terminal propeptide of type I collagen. *Osteoporos. Int.* **3,** 50–52 (1993).
122. Garnero, P., Sornay-Rendu, E., Chapuy, M-C., and Delmas, P. D. Increased bone turnover in late postmenopausal women is a major determinant of osteoporosis. *J. Bone Min. Res.* **11,** 337–349 (1996).
123. Beardsworth, L. J., Eyre, D. R., and Dickson, I. R. Changes with age in the urinary excretion of lysyl- and hydroxylysylpyridinoline, two new markers of bone collagen turnover. *J. Bone Miner. Res.* **5,** 671 (1990).
124. Eastell, R., Simmons, P. S., Colwell, A., Assiri, A. M. A., Burritts, M. F., Russell, R. G. G., and Riggs, B. L. Nyctohemeral changes in bone turnover assessed by serum bone Gla-protein concentration and urinary deoxypyridinoline excretion: effects of growth and ageing. *Clin. Sci.* **83,** 375–382 (1992).
125. Seibel, M., Woitge, H., Scheidt, N. C., Leidig, B. G., Duncan, A., Nicol, P., Ziegler, R., and Robins, S. Urinary hydroxypyridinium crosslinks of collagen in population-based screening for overt vertebral osteoporosis: results of a pilot study. *J. Bone Miner. Res.* **9,** 1433–1440 (1994).
126. Eyre, D. R., Dickson, I. R., and VanNess, K. P. Collagen crosslinking in human bone and cartilage: age-related changes in the content of mature hydroxypyridinium residues. *Biochem. J.* **252,** 495–500 (1988).
127. Hassager, C., Risteli, J., Risteli, L., and Christiansen, C. Effect of the menopause and hormone replacement therapy on the carboxy-terminal pyridinoline cross-linked telopeptide of type I collagen. *Osteoporos. Int.* **4,** 349–352 (1994).
128. Prestwood, K., Pilbeam, C., Burleson, J., Woodiel, F., Delmas, P., Deftos, L., and Raisz, L. The short-term effects of conjugated estrogen on bone turnover in older women. *J. Clin. Endocrinol. Metab.* **79,** 366–371 (1994).
129. McKane, W., Khosla, S., Risteli, J., Robins, S., Muhs, J., and Riggs, B. Role of estrogen deficiency in pathogenesis of secondary hyperparathyroidism and increased bone resorption in elderly women. *Proc. Assoc. Am. Physic.* **109,** 174–180 (1997).
130. McLarren, A. M., Hordon, L. D., Bird, H. A., and Robins, S. P. Urinary excretion of pyridinium crosslinks of collagen in patients with osteoporosis and the effects of bone fracture. *Ann. Rheum. Dis.* **51,** 648–651 (1992).
131. Seibel, M. J., Cosman, F., Shen, V., Ratcliffe, A., and Lindsay, R. Urinary hydroxy-pyridinium crosslinks of collagen as markers of bone resorption and estrogen efficacy in postmenopausal osteoporosis. *J. Bone Miner. Res.* **8,** 881–889 (1993).
132. Hui, S. L., Slemenda, C. W., and Johnston, C. C. The contribution of bone loss to postmenopausal osteoporosis. *Osteopor. Int.* **1,** 30–34 (1990).
133. Seeley, D. G., Browner, W. S., Nevitt, M. C., Genant, H. K., Scott, J. C., and Cummings, S. R. Which fractures are associated with low appendicular bone mass in elderly women? *Ann. Intern. Med.* **115,** 837–842 (1991).
134. Cummings, S. R., Black, D. M., and Navic, M. C. Appendicular bone density and age predict hip fracture in women. *J. Am. Med. Soc.* **263,** 665–668 (1990).
135. Hansen, M. Assessment of age and risk factors on bone density and bone turnover in healthy premenopausal women. *Osteopor. Int.* **4,** 123–128 (1994).
136. Ensrud, K. E., Palermo, L., Black, D. M., Cauley, J., Jergas, M., Orwoll, E. S., Nevitt, M. C., Fox, K. M., and Cummings, S. R. Hip and calcaneal bone loss increase with advancing age: Longitudinal results from the study of osteoporotic fractures. *J. Bone Miner. Res.* **10,** 1778–1787 (1995).
137. Gardsell, P., Johnell, O., and Nilsson, B. E. The predictive value of bone loss for fragility in women: A longitudinal study over 15 years. *Calcif. Tissue Int.* **49,** 90–94 (1991).
138. Stepan, J. J., Pospichal, J., Presl, J., and Pacovsky, V. Bone loss and biochemical indices of bone remodeling in surgically induced postmenopausal women. *Bone* **8,** 279–284 (1987).
139. Stepan, J. J., Presl, J., Broulik, P., and Pacovsky, V. Serum osteocalcin levels and bone alkaline phosphatase isoenzyme after oophorectomy and in primary hyperparathyroidism. *J. Clin. Endocrinol. Metab.* **64,** 1079–1082 (1987).
140. Hassager, C., Colwell, A., Assiri, A. M. A., Eastell, R., Russell, R. G. G., and Christiansen, C. Effect of menopause and hormone replacement therapy on urinary excretion of pyridinium crosslinks: a longitudinal and cross-sectional study. *Clin. Endocrinol.* **37,** 45–50 (1992).
141. Heikkinen, A. M., Parvianen, M., Niskanen, L., Komulainen, M., Tuppurainen, M. T., Kröger, H., and Saarikoski, S. Biochemical bone markers and bone mineral density during postmenopausal

hormone replacement therapy with and without vitamin D3: A prospective, controlled, randomized study. *J. Clin. Endocrinol. Metab.* **82,** 2476–2482 (1997).
142. Lips, P., Courpron, P., and Meunier, P. J. Mean wall thickness of trabecular bone packets in the human iliac crest: changes with age. *Calcif. Tissue Res.* **26,** 13–17 (1978).
143. Parfitt, A. M. The coupling of bone formation to bone resorption: A critical analysis of the concept and of its relevance to the pathogenesis of osteoporosis. *Metab. Bone Dis. Rel. Res.* **4,** 1–12 (1982).
144. Ledger, G. A., Burritt, M. F., Kao, P. C., O'Fallon, W. M., Riggs, B. L., and Khosla, S. Role of parathyroid hormone in mediating nocturnal and age-related increases in bone resorption. *J. Clin. Endocrinol. Metab.* **80,** 3304–3310 (1995).
145. Koshla, S., Atkinson, E. J., Melton, L. J., III, and Riggs, B. L. Effects of age and estrogen status on serum parathyroid hormone levels and biochemical markers of bone turnover in women: a population based study. *J. Clin. Endocrinol. Metab.* **82,** 1522–1527 (1997).
146. Melton, L. J., Khosla, S., Atkinson, E. J., O'Fallon, W. M., and Riggs, B. L. Relationship of bone fractures to bone density and fractures. *J. Bone Miner. Res.* **12,** 1083–1091 (1997).
147. Scarneggia, L., Minisola, S., Pacitti, M. T., Carnevale, V., Romagnoli, E., Rosso, R., and Mazzuoli, G. F. Clinical usefulness of serum tartrate-resistant acid phosphatase activity determination to evaluate bone turnover. *Scand. J. Clin. Lab. Invest.* **51,** 517–524 (1991).
148. Sherman, S. S., Tobin, J. D., Hollis, B. W., Gundberg, C. M., Roy, T. A., and Plato, C. C. Biochemical parameters associated with low bone density in healthy men and women. *J. Bone Miner. Res.* **7,** 1123–1130 (1992).
149. Szulc, P., Arlot, M., Chapuy, M. C., Duboeuf, F., Meunier, P. J., and Delmas, P. D. Serum undercarboxylated osteocalcin correlates with hip bone mineral density in elderly women. *J. Bone Miner. Res.* **9,** 1591–1595 (1994).
150. Ebeling, P. R., Atley, L. M., Guthrie, J. R., Burger, H. G., Dennerstein, L., Hopper, J. L., and Wark, J. D. Bone turnover markers and bone density across the menopausal transition. *J. Clin. Endocrinol. Metab.* **81,** 3366–3371 (1996).
151. Ravn, P., Rix, M., Andreassen, H., Clemmesen, B., Bidstrup, M., and Gunnes, M. High bone turnover is associated with low bone mass and spinal fracture in postmenopausal women. *Calcif. Tissue Int.* **60,** 255–260 (1997).
152. Krall, E. A., Dawson-Hughes, B., Hirst, K., Gallagher, J. C., Sherman, S. S., and Dalsky, G. Bone mineral density and biochemical markers of bone turnover in healthy elderly men and women. *J. Gerontol. A Biol. Sci. Med. Sci.* **52,** M61–M67 (1997).
153. Schneider, D. L., and Barrett-Connor, E. L. Urinary N-telopeptide levels discriminate normal, osteopenic, and osteoporotic bone mineral density. *Arch. Intern. Med.* **157,** 1241–1245 (1997).
154. Christiansen, C., Riis, B. J., and Rodboro, P. Prediction of rapid bone loss in postmenopausal women. *Lancet* **1,** 1105–1108 (1987).
155. Christiansen, C., Riis, B. J., and Rodbro, P. Screening procedure for women at risk of developing postmenopausal osteoporosis. *Osteopor. Int.* **1,** 35–40 (1990).
156. Slemenda, C., Hui, S. L., and Longcope, C. Sex steroids and bone mass. *J. Clin. Invest.* **80,** 1261–1269 (1987).
157. Johansen, J. S., Riss, B. J., Delmas, P. D., and Christiansen, C. Plasma BGP: an indicator of spontaneous bone loss and effect of estrogen treatment in postmenopausal women. *Eur. J. Clin. Invest.* **18,** 191–195 (1988).
158. Mole, P. A., Walkinshaw, M. H., Robins, S. P., and Paterson, C. R. Can urinary pyridinium crosslinks and urinary oestrogens predict bone mass and rate of bone loss after the menopause. *Eur. J. Clin. Invest.* **22,** 767–771 (1992).
159. Miura, H., Yamamoto, I., Yuu, I., Kigami, Y., Ohta, T., Yamamura, Y., Ohnaka, Y., and Morita, R. Estimation of bone mineral density and bone loss by means of bone metabolic markers in postmenopausal women. *Endocrin. J.* **42,** 797–802 (1995).
160. Reeve, J., Pearson, J., Mitchell, A., *et al.* Evolution of spinal bone loss and biochemical markers of bone remodeling after menopause in normal women. *Calcif. Tissue Int.* **57,** 105–110 (1995).
161. Dresner-Pollak, R., Seibel, M. J., Greenspan, S., *et al.* Biochemical markers of bone turnover reflect femoral bone loss in elderly women. *Calcif. Tissue Int.* **59,** 328–333 (1996).
162. Cosman, F., Nieves, J., Wilkinson, C., Schnering, D., Shen, V., and Lindsay, R. Bone density change and biochemical indices of skeletal turnover. *Calcif. Tissue Int.* **58,** 236–243 (1996).
163. Chesnut, C. H,. III, Bell, N. H., Clark, G. S., Drinkwater, B. L., English, S. C., Johnston, C. C., Notelovitz, M., Rosen, C., Cain, D. F., Flessland, K. A., and Mallinak, N. J. S. Hormone replacement therapy in postmenopausal women: Urinary N-telopeptide of type I collagen monitors therapeutic effect and predicts response of bone mineral density. *Am. J. Med.* **102,** 29–37 (1997).
164. Rosen, C., Chesnut, C. H., III, and Mallinak, N. J. S. The predictive value of biochemical markers of bone turnover for bone mineral density in early postmenopausal women treated with hormone replacement or calcium supplementation. *J. Clin. Endocrinol. Metab.* **82,** 1904–1910 (1997).
165. Ross, P. D., and Knowlton, W. Rapid bone loss is associated with increased levels of biochemical markers. *J. Bone Miner. Res.* **13,** 297–302 (1998).
166. Uebelhart, D., Schlemmer, A., Johansen, J. S., Gineyts, E., Christiansen, C., and Delmas, P. D. Effect of menopause and hormone replacement therapy on the urinary excretion of pyridinium crosslinks. *J. Clin. Endocrinol. Metab.* **72,** 367–373 (1991).
167. Keen, R. W., Nguyen, T., Sobnack, R., Perry, L. A., Thompson, P. W., and Spector, T. D. Can biochemical markers predict bone loss at the hip and spine?: a 4-year prospective study of 141 early postmenopausal women. *Osteopor. Int.* **6,** 399–406 (1996).
168. Bluhmson, A., and Eastell, R. Prediction of bone loss in postmenopausal women. *Eur. J. Clin. Invest.* **22,** 764–766 (1992).
169. Riggs, B. L., Melton, L. J., III, and O'fallon, W. M. Drug therapy for vertebral fractures in osteoporosis: Evidence that decreases in bone turnover and increases in bone mass both determine antifracture efficacy. *Bone* **18,** 197S–201S (1996).
170. van Daele, P. L., Seibel, M. J., Burger, H., Hofman, A., Grobbee, D. E., van Leeuwen, J. P., Birkenhäger, J. C., and Pols, H. A. P. Case control analysis of bone resorption markers, disability and hip fracture risk: the Rotterdam study. *Br. Med. J.* **312,** 482–483 (1996).
171. Akesson, K., Ljunghall, S., Jonsson, B., *et al.* Assessment of biochemical markers of bone metabolism in relation to the occurrence of fracture: A retrospective and prospective population-based study in women. *J. Bone Miner. Res.* **10,** 1823–1829 (1995).
172. Garnero, P., Hausherr, E., Chapuy, M. C., Marcelli, C., Grandjean, H., Muller, C., Cormier, C., Breard, G., Meunier, P., and Delmas, P. D. Markers of bone resorption predict hip fractures in elderly women. *J. Bone Miner. Res.* **11,** 1531–1538 (1996).
173. Vergnaud, P., Garnero, P., Meunier, P., *et al.* Undercarboxylated osteocalcin measured with a specific immunoassay predicts hip fracture in elderly women. *Clin. Endocrinol. Metab.* **82,** 719–724 (1997).
174. Szulc, P., Chapuy, M.-C., Meunier, P., and Delmas, P. Serum undercarboxylated osteocalcin is a marker of the risk of hip fracture in elderly women. *J. Clin. Invest.* **91,** 1769–1774 (1993).

175. Szulc, P., Chapuy, M. C., Meunier, P., and Delmas, P. Serum undercarboxylated osteocalcin is a marker of the risk of hip fracture: a three year follow-up study. *Bone* **18,** 487–488 (1996).
176. Price, P. A., and Kaneda, Y. Vitamin D counteracts the effect of warfarin in liver but not in bone. *Thromb. Res.* **46,** 121–131 (1987).
177. Knapen, M. H., Manulyak, K., and Vermeer, C. The effect of vitamin K supplementation on circulating osteocalcin and urinary calcium excretion. *Ann. Intern. Med.* **111,** 1001–1005 (1989).
178. Plantalech, L., Guillaumont, M., Vergnaud, P., *et al.* Impairment of gamma carboxylation of circulating osteocalcin (bone Gla protein) in elderly women. *J. Bone Miner. Res.* **6,** 1211–1216 (1991).
179. Hodges, S. J., Pilkington, M., Stamp, T. C. H., *et al.* Depressed levels of circulating menaquinones in patients with osteoporotic fractures of the spine and femoral neck. *Bone* **12,** 387–389 (1991).
180. Cairns, J. R., and Price, P. A. Direct demonstration that the vitamin K-dependent bone Gla protein is incompletely γ-carboxylated in humans. *J. Bone Miner. Res.* **9,** 1989–1997 (1994).
181. Charles, P., Hasling, C., Risteli, L., Risteli, J., Mosekilde, L., and Eriksen, E. Assessment of bone formation by biochemical markers in metabolic bone disease: separation between osteoblastic activity at the cell and tissue level. *Calcif. Tissue Int.* **51,** 406–411 (1992).
182. Garnero, P., Shih, W. J., Gineyts, E., Karpf, D. B., and Delmas, P. D. Comparison of new biochemical markers of bone turnover in late postmenopausal osteoporotic women in response to alendronate treatment. *J. Clin. Endocrinol. Metab.* **79,** 1693–1700 (1994).
183. Kushida, K., Takahashi, M., Kawana, K., and Inoue, T. Comparison of markers for bone formation and resorption in premenopausal and postmenopausal subjects and osteoporosis patients. *J. Clin. Endocrinol. Metab.* **80,** 2447–2450 (1995).
184. Cheung, C. K., Panesar, N. S., Lau, E., Woo, J., and Swaminathan, R. Increased bone resorption and decreased bone formation in Chinese patients with hip fracture. *Calcif. Tissue Int.* **56,** 347–349 (1995).
185. Gonelli, S., Cepollaro, C., Montagnani, A., *et al.* Bone alkaline phosphatase measured with a new immunoradiometric assay in patients with metabolic bone disease. *Eur. J. Clin. Invest.* **26,** 391–396 (1996).
186. Akesson, K., Ljunghall, S., Gardsell, P., Sernbo, I., and Obrant, K. J. Serum osteocalcin and fracture susceptibility in elderly women. *Calcif. Tissue Int.* **53,** 86–90 (1993).
187. Akesson, K., Vergnaud, P., Gineyts, E., Delmas, P. D., and Obrant, K. J. Impairment of bone turnover in elderly women with hip fracture. *Calcif. Tissue Int.* **53,** 162–169 (1993).
188. Akesson, K., Vergnaud, P., Delmas, P. D., and Obrant, K. J. Serum osteocalcin increases during fracture healing in elderly women with hip fracture. *Bone* **6,** 427–430 (1995).
189. Obrant, K. J., Merle, B., Bejui, J., and Delmas, P. D. Serum bone-gla protein after fracture. *Clin. Orthop.* **258,** 300–303 (1990).
190. Mallmin, H., Ljunghall, S., and Larsson, K. Biochemical markers of bone metabolism in patients with fracture of the distal forearm. *Clin. Orthop.* **295,** 259–263 (1993).
191. Civitelli, R., Gonnelli, S., Zacchei, F., Bigazzi, S., Vattimo, A., Avioli, L. V., and Gennari, C. Bone turnover in postmenopausal osteoporosis. *J. Clin. Invest.* **82,** 1268–1274 (1988).
192. Overgaard, K., Hansen, M. A., Nielsen, V. H., Riis, B. J., and Christiansen, C. Discontinous calcitonin treatment of established osteoporosis. Effects of withdrawal and treatment. *Am. J. Med.* **89,** 1–6 (1990).
193. Nielsen, N. M., Von der Recke, P., Hansen, M. A., Overgaard, K., and Christensen, C. Estimation of the effect of salmon calcitonin in established osteoporosis by biochemical bone markers. *Calcif. Tissue Int.* **55,** 8–11 (1994).
194. Stevenson, J. C., Hillard, T. C., Lees, B., Whitcroft, S. I., Ellerington, M. C., and Whitehead, M. I. Postmenopausal bone loss: does HRT always work? *Int. J. Fertil. Menopausal. Stud.* **38**(Suppl. 2), 88–91 (1993).
195. Stein, B., Takizawa, M., Katz, I. *et al.* Salmon calcitonin prevents cyclosporin A induced high turnover bone loss. *Endocrinology* **129,** 92–98 (1991).
196. Tsakalakos, N., Magiasis, B., Tsekoura, M., and Lyritis, G. The effect of short term calcitonin administration on biochemical bone markers with acute immobilization following hip fracture. *Osteopor. Int.* **3,** 337–340 (1993).
197. Arrigoni, M., Abbiati, G., Negroni, M., *et al.* Acute effects of salmon calcitonin on bone biomarkers in normal subjects: A placebo controlled study. *J. Bone Miner. Res.* **13**(Suppl. 1), S193 (1993).
198. Kollerup, G., Hermann, A., Brixen, K., Lindblad, B., Mosekilde, L., and Sorensen, O. Effects of salmon calcitonin suppositories on bone mass and turnover in established osteoporosis. *Calcif. Tissue Int.* **54,** 12–15 (1994).
199. Abbiati, G., Arrigoni, M., Frignani, S., Longoni, A., Bartucci, F., and Castiglioni, C. Effect of salmon calcitonin on deoxypyridinoline (Dpyr) urinary excretion in healthy volunteers. *Calcif. Tissue Int.* **55,** 346–348 (1994).
200. Adami, S., Passeri, M., Ortolani, S. *et al.* Effects of oral alendronate and intranasal salmon calcitonin on bone mass and biochemical markers of bone turnover in postmenopausal women with osteoporosis. *Bone* **17,** 383–390 (1995).
201. Lyritis, G. P., Magiasis, B., and Tsakalakos, N. Prevention of bone loss in early nonsurgical and nonosteoporotic high turnover patients with salmon calcitonin: the role of biochemical bone markers in monitoring high turnover patients under calcitonin treatment. *Calcif. Tissue Int.* **56,** 38–41 (1995).
202. Kraenzlin, M. E., Seibel, M. J., Trechsel, U., Boerlin, V., Azria, M., Kraenzlin, C. A., and Hass, H. G. The effect of intranasal salmon calcitonin on postmenopausal bone turnover: evidence for maximal effect after 8 weeks of continous treatment. *Calcif. Tissue Int.* **58,** 216–220 (1996).
203. Ongphiphadhanakul, B., Jenis, L. G., Braverman, L. E., Alex, S., Stein, G. S., Lian, J. B., and Baran, D. T. Etidronate inhibits the thyroid hormone-induced bone loss in rats assessed by bone mineral density and messenger ribonucleic acid markers of osteoblast and osteoclast function. *Endocrinology* **133,** 2502–2507 (1993).
204. Pedrazzoni, M., Alfano, F. S., Gatti, C., *et al.* Acute effects of bisphosphonates on new and traditional markers of bone resorption. *Calcif. Tissue Int.* **57,** 25–29 (1995).
205. Seibel, M. J., Woitge, H. W., Pecherstorfer, M., Karmatschek, M., Horn, E., Ludwig, M., Armbruster, F. P., and Ziegler, R. Serum immunoreactive bone sialoprotein as a new marker of bone turnover in metabolic and malignant bone disease. *J. Clin. Endocrinol. Metab* **81,** 3289–3294 (1996).
206. Horowitz, M., Wishart, J. M., Need, A. G., Morris, H. A., and Nordin, B. E. Effects of norethisterone on bone related biochemical variables and forearm bone mineral in post-menopausal osteoporosis. *Clin. Endocrinol. Oxf.* **39,** 649–655 (1993).
207. Cosman, F., Nieves, J., Shen, V., and Lindsay, R. Oral 1,25-dihydroxyvitamin D administration in osteoporotic women: effects of estrogen therapy. *Bone Miner. Res.* **10,** 594–600 (1995).
208. Gambacciani, M., Spinetti, A., Cappagli, B., *et al.* Hormone replacement therapy in perimenopausal women with a low dose oral contraceptive preparation: Effects on bone mineral density and metabolism. *Maturitas* **19,** 125–131 (1994).

209. Riis, B. J., Overgaard, K., and Christiansen, C. Biochemical markers of bone turnover to monitor the bone response to postmenopausal hormone replacement therapy. *Osteopor. Int.* **5,** 276–280 (1995).
210. Yasuda, M., Kurabayashi, T., Yamamoto, Y., Fujimaki, T., Oda, K., and Tanaka, K. Effect of hormone replacement therapy on bone and lipid metabolism in women oophorectomized for the treatment of gynecologic malignancies. *Int. J. Gynecol. Obstet.* **47,** 151–156 (1994).
211. Hashimoto, K., Nozaki, M., Yokoyama, M., Sano, M., and Nakano, H. Urinary excretion of pyridinium crosslinks of collagen in oophorectomized women as markers for bone resorption. *Maturitas* **18,** 135–142 (1994).
212. Hashimoto, K., Nozaki, M., Inoue, Y., Sano, M., and Nakano, H. The chronological change of vertebral bone loss following oophorectomy using dual energy X-ray absorptiometry: The correlation with specific markers of bone metabolism. *Maturitas* **22,** 185–191 (1995).
213. Gaumet, N., Seibel, M. J., Coxam, V., Davicco, M. J., Lebecque, P., and Barlet, J. P. Influence of ovarectomy and estradiol treatment on calcium homeostasis during ageing in rats. *Arch. Physiol. Biochem.* **105,** 1–10 (1997).
214. Virtanen, P., Viitasalo, J. T., Vuori, J., Vaananen, K., and Takala, T. E. Effect of concentric exercise on serum muscle and collagen markers. *J. Appl. Physiol.* **75,** 1272–1277 (1993).
215. Woitge, H. W., Friedman, B., Suttner, S., Farahmand, I., Müller, M., Schmidt-Gayk, H., Bärtsch, P., Ziegler, R., and Seibel, M. J. Effect of aerobic and anaerobic physical training markers of bone metabolism. *J. Bone Mineral Res.* **13**(12), 1797–1804 (1998).
216. Yamauchi, M., Young, D. R., Chandler, G. S., and Mechanic, G. L. Cross-linking and new bone collagen synthesis in immobilized and recovering primate osteoporosis. *Bone* **9,** 415–421 (1988).
217. Tuukkanen, J., Jalovaara, P., and Vaananen, K. Calcitonin treatment of immobilization osteoporosis in rats. *Acta Physiol. Scand.* **141,** 119–124 (1991).
218. Preedy, V. R., Sherwood, R. A., Akpoguma, C. I., and Black, D. The urinary excretion of the collagen degradation markers pyridinoline and deoxypyridinoline in an experimental rat model of alcoholic bone disease. *Alcohol* **26,** 191–198 (1991).
219. Laitinen, K., Lamberg-Allardt, C., Tunninen, R., Karonen, S. L., Ylikahri, R., and Valimaki, M. Effects of 3 weeks' moderate alcohol intake on bone and mineral metabolism in normal men. *Bone Miner.* **13,** 139–151 (1991).
220. Laitinen, K., Lamberg-Allardt, C., Tunninen, R., Harkonen, M., and Valimaki, M. Bone mineral density and abstention-induced changes in bone and mineral metabolism in noncirrhotic male alcoholics. *Am. J. Med.* **93,** 642–650 (1992).
221. Laitinen, K., Karkkainen, M., Lalla, M., Lamberg-Allardt, C., Tunninen, R., Tahtela, R., and Valimaki, M. Is alcohol an osteoporosis-inducing agent for young and middle-aged women? *Metabolism* **42,** 875–881 (1993).
222. Lindholm, J., Steiniche, T., Rasmussen, E., Thamsborg, G., Nielsen, I. O., Brockstedt-Rasmussen, H., Storm, T., Hyldstrup, L., and Schou, C. Bone disorder in men with chronic alcoholism: a reversible disease? *J. Clin. Endocrinol. Metab.* **73,** 118–124 (1991).
223. Pepersack, T., Fuss, M., Otero, J., Bergmann, P., Valsamis, J., and Corvilain, J. Longitudinal study of bone metabolism after ethanol withdrawal in alcoholic patients. *J. Bone Miner. Res.* **7,** 383–387 (1992).
224. Nyquist, F., Ljunghall, S., Berglund, M., and Obrant, K. Biochemical markers of bone metabolism after short and long time ethanol withdrawal in alcoholics. *Bone* **19,** 51–54 (1996).
225. Meunier, P. Prevention of hip fractures by correcting calcium and vitamin D insufficiencies in elderly people. *Scand. J. Rheumatol.* **103,** S75–S78 (1996).
226. Klibanski, A., Biller, B. M., Schoenfeld, D. A., Herzog, D. B., and Saxe, V. C. The effects of estrogen administration on trabecular bone loss in young women with anorexia nervosa. *Clin. Endocrinol. Metab.* **80,** 898–904 (1995).
227. Zipfel, S., Seibel, M. J., Herzog, W., Woitge, H. W., and Ziegler, R. Bone turnover in anorexia nervosa. *Clin. Lab.,* in press.
228. Prummel, M. F., Wiersinga, W. M., Lips, P., *et al.* The course of biochemical parameters of bone turnover during treatment with corticosteroids. *J. Clin. Endocrinol. Metab.* **72,** 382–386 (1991).
229. Bijlsma, J. W., Lems, W. F., Gerrits, M. I., Jacobs, J. W., van Vugt, R. M., and vanRijn, H. J. Effect of high-dose corticosteroid pulse therapy on (markers of) bone formation and resorption in rheumatoid arthritis. *Calcif. Tissue Int.* **56,** 500–506 (1995).
230. Kerstjens, H. A. M., Postma, D. S., van Doormaal, J. J., *et al.* Effects of short term and long term treatment with inhaled corticosteroids on bone metabolism in patients with airways obstruction. *Thorax* **49,** 652–656 (1994).
231. Meeran, K., Hattersley, A., Burrin, J., Shiner, R., and Ibbertson, K. Oral and inhaled corticosteroids reduce bone formation as shown by plasma osteocalcin levels. *Am. J. Respir. CritCare Med.* **151,** 333–336 (1995).
232. Valero, M. A., Leon, M., Ruiz Valdepenas, M. P., Larrodera, L., Lopez, M. B., Papapietro, K., Jara, A., and Hawkins, F. Bone density and turnover in Addison's disease: effect of glucocorticoid treatment. *Bone Miner.* **26,** 9–17 (1994).
233. Hall, G. M., Spector, T. D., and Delmas, P. D. Markers of bone metabolism in postmenopausal women with rheumatoid arthritis. Effects of corticosteroids and hormone replacement therapy. *Arthritis Rheum.* **38,** 902–906 (1995).
234. King, C. S., Weir, E. C., Gundberg, C. W., Fox, J., and Insogna, K. L. Effects of continuous glucocorticoid infusion on bone metabolism in the rat. *Calcif. Tissue Int.* **59,** 184–191 (1996).
235. Montecucco, C., Baldi, F., Fortina, A., *et al.* Serum osteocalcin (bone Gla-protein) following corticosteroid therapy in postmenopausal women with rheumatoid arthritis. Comparison of the effect of prednisone and deflazacort. *Clin. Rheumatol.* **7,** 366–371 (1988).
236. Ekenstam, E., Stalenheim, G., and Hallgren, R. The acute effect of high dose corticosteroid treatment on serum osteocalcin. *Metabolism* **37,** 141–144 (1988).
237. Peretz, A., Praet, J. P., Bosson, D., Rozenberg, S., and Bourdoux, P. Serum osteocalcin in the assessment of corticosteroid induced osteoporosis. Effect of long and short term corticosteroid treatment. *J. Rheumatol.* **16,** 363–367 (1989).
238. Hassager, C., Jensen, L. T., Johansen, J. S., Riis, B. J., Melkko, J., Podenphant, J., Risteli, L., Christiansen, C., and Risteli, J. The carboxy-terminal propeptide of type I procollagen in serum as a marker of bone formation: the effect of nandrolone decanoate and female sex hormones. *Metabolism* **40,** 205–208 (1991).
239. Wang, C., Eyre, D. R., Clark, R., Kleinberg, D., Newman, C., Iranmanesh, A., *et al.* Sublingual testosterone replacement improves muscle mass and strength, decreases bone resorption, and increases bone formation markers in hypogonadal men—a clinical research center study. *J. Clin. Endocrinol. Metab.* **81,** 3654–3662 (1996).
240. Anderson, F. H., Francis, R. M., Peaston, R. T., and Wastell, H. J. Androgen supplementation in eugonadal men: effects of six months' treatment on markers of bone formation and resorption. *J. Bone Miner. Res.* **12,** 472–478 (1997).
241. Hock, J. M., Fonseca, J., Gunness-Hey, M., Kemp, B. E., and Martin, T. J. Comparison of the anabolic effects of synthetic

parathyroid hormone related protein 1-34 and PTH 1-34 on bone in rats. *Endocrinology* **125,** 2022–2027 (1989).

242. Liu, C., and Kalu, D. N. Human parathyroid hormone (1-34) prevents bone loss and augments bone formation in sexually mature ovariectomized rats. *J. Bone Miner. Res.* **5,** 973–982 (1990).
243. Brahm, H., Ljunggren, O., Larsson, K., Lindh, E., and Ljunghall, S. Effects of infusion of parathyroid hormone and primary hype-Iparathyroidism on formation and breakdown of type I collagen. *Calcif. Tissue Int.* **55,** 412–416 (1994).
244. Cheng, P.-T., Aye, L. M., Vieth, R., and Mÿller, K. Cyclical parathyroid hormone and estrogen treatment of osteopenic ovariectomized adult rats. *J. Bone Miner. Res.* **9**(Suppl. 1), S201 (1994).
245. Finkelstein, J. S., Klibanski, A., Schaefer, E. H., Hornstein, M. D., Schiff, I., and Neer, R. M. Parathyroid hormone for the prevention of bone loss induced by estrogen deficiency. *N. Engl. J. Med.* **331,** 1618–1623 (1994).
246. Gundberg, C. M., Fawzi, M. I., Clough, M. E., and Calvo, M. S. A comparison of the effects of parathyroid hormone and parathyroid hormone-related protein on osteocalcin in the rat. *J. Bone Miner. Res.* **10,** 903–909 (1995).
247. Sone, T., Fukunaga, M., Ono, S., and Nishiyama, T. A small dose of human parathyroid hormone (1-34) increased bone mass in the lumbar vertebrae in patients with senile osteoporosis. *Miner. Electrolyte Metab.* **21,** 232–235 (1995).
248. Delmas, P. D., Vergnaud, P., Arlot, M. E., Pastoureau, P., Meunier, P. J., and Nilssen, M. H. L. The anabolic effect of human PTH (1-34) on bone formation is blunted when bone resorption is inhibited by the bisphosphonate tiludronate—Is activated resorption a prerequisite for the *in vivo* effect of PTH on formation in a remodeling system? *Bone* **16,** 603–610 (1995).
249. Hodsman, A. B., Fraher, L. J., Watson, P. H., Ostbye, T., Stitt, L. W., *et al.* A randomized control trial to compare the efficacy of cyclical parathyroid hormone versus cyclical parathyroid hormone and sequential calcitonin to improve bone mass in postmenopausal women with osteoporosis. *J. Clin. Endocrinol. Metab.* **82,** 620–628 (1996).
250. Cosman, F., Shen, V., Herrington, B. S., Fang, X., Seibel, M. J., Ratcliffe, A., and Lindsay, R. Estrogen protection against bone resorbing effects of parathyroid hormone infusion. Assessment by use of biochemical markers. *Ann. Int. Med.* **118,** 337–343 (1993).
251. Saggese, G., Bertelloni, S., Baroncelli, G. I., Di Nero, G., and Battini, R. Growth velocity and serum aminoterminal propeptide of type III procollagen in precocious puberty during gonadotropin-releasing hormone analogue treatment. *Acta Paediatr* **82,** 261–266 (1993).
252. Hertel, N. T., Stoltenberg, M., Juul, A., *et al.* Serum concentrations of type I and III procollagen propeptides in healthy children and girls with central precocious puberty during treatment with gonadotropin-releasing hormone analog and cyproterone acetate. *J. Clin. Endocrinol. Metab.* **76,** 924–927 (1993).
253. Seibel, M. J., Woitge, H. W., Parviz, M., Sillem, M., Kiesel, L., Pfeilschifter, J., Runnebaum, B., and Ziegler, R. Medrogestone prevents accelerated bone turnover in GnRH analogue treated endometriosis. *Clin. Lab.* **42,** 1075–1078 (1996).
254. Price, P. A., and Williamson, M. K. Effects of warfarin on bone. *J. Biol. Chem.* **256,** 12754–12758 (1981).
255. Lian, J. B., Tassinari, M., and Glowacki, J. Resorption of implanted bone prepared from normal and warfarin-treated rats. *J. Clin. Invest.* **73,** 1223–1226 (1984).
256. Philip, W. J. U., Martin, J. C., Richardson, J. M., Reid, D. M., Webster, J., and Douglas, A. S. Decreased axial and peripheral bone density in patients taking long-term warfarin. *Q. J. Med.* **88,** 635–640 (1995).
257. Valk, N. K., Erdtsieck, R. J., Algra, D., Lamberts, S. W. J., and Pols, H. A. P. Combined treatment of growth hormone and the bisphosphonate pamidronate, versus treatment with GH alone, in GH-deficient adults: The effects on renal phosphate handling, bone turnover and bone mineral mass. *Clin. Endocrinol. (Oxf.)* **43,** 317–324 (1995).
258. Ghiron, L. J., Thompson, J. L., Holloway, L., *et al.* Effects of recombinant insulin-like growth factor-I and growth hormone on bone turnover in elderly women. *J. Bone Miner. Res.* **10,** 1844–1852 (1995).

Biomechanical Measurements in Age-Related Bone Loss

DAVID B. BURR[*,†] AND CHARLES H. TURNER[†,‡]
Departments of *Anatomy, †Orthopedic Surgery, and ‡Mechanical Engineering, Biomechanics and Biomaterials Research Center, Indiana University School of Medicine, Indianapolis, Indiana 46202

INTRODUCTION

Our skeletons become more fragile as we age [1]. This occurs in both cancellous and cortical bone, and in both women and men [2], although the rapid changes in men begin about 20 years later than comparable changes in women. Increasing fragility may occur for a variety of reasons: increased porosity consequent to bone loss [3]; hypermineralization of the tissue matrix as a result of the slowing of bone turnover and replacement [4]; changes in the nature, organization, or cross-linking of collagenous and noncollagenous proteins [5,6]; or the accumulation of unrepaired microdamage [7], among others. These aging changes make the skeleton less able to withstand the impact forces that are generated when an individual falls and increase the risk of fracture. Not all of the mechanical properties of bone change equally with age, and it is worthwhile to explore the nature of the mechanical changes as a basis for assessing the reasons for the increased risk of fracture in older adults.

BIOMECHANICAL MEASUREMENTS AND CONCEPTS

To fully understand the nature of the biomechanical changes that occur with age, it is necessary to distinguish between changes that affect the mechanical properties of a whole bone as a structure and those that affect the mechanical properties of the bony tissue [8]. Structurally, the mechanical properties of a bone are largely determined by the amount of bone present. This can be measured histomorphometrically from biopsies or after death as bone volume or its inverse, porosity. It can also be measured less invasively using radiologic and bone densitometric techniques, as bone mineral content or apparent density. The structural strength of a bone is also dependent on the location of the bone with respect to some loading axis, such that a bone with a larger outer diameter may be stronger than a bone that is smaller, even though each has exactly the same bone volume. Any aspect of a bone's geometry that changes with age will affect the mechanical properties of the bone as a structure. Trabecular bone architecture and connectivity are aspects of cancellous bone that contribute to the structural properties of the bone.

The properties of bone tissue are also important to its mechanical integrity. The material properties of bone are primarily dependent on the nature of its macromolecular constituents, collagen and mineral. This includes not only the amount of collagen and mineral, but aspects of its cross-linking, or mineral maturity and size.

At the structural level, the relationship between the load applied to a bone and its deformation is defined by the *load–deformation curve.* The load–deformation curve is a measure of the amount of load required to produce a unit deformation; it is dependent on both the properties of the tissue and the geometry of the bone. The load–deformation curve can be divided into two portions that are separated by the *yield point.* This is the point on the curve where the deformation of the bone is not fully recoverable when the load is released. In this portion of the curve, a small increase in load will cause a relatively large deformation in the bone. Before the yield point, the bone deforms linearly as load increases and will return to its original shape when the load is removed; this is called *elastic deformation.* The slope of this linear part of the load–deformation curve is the *structural stiffness* (or *rigidity*) of the bone. After the yield point, deformation is *plastic,* meaning that damage to the structure is permanent and the structure will not recover its original shape. Because the yield point separates the elastic from the plastic portions of the load–deformation curve, elastic deformation is sometimes called *preyield deformation,* while plastic deformation is termed *postyield deformation.* The *energy* required to fracture bone is an important mechanical property that is defined as the area under the load–deformation curve, sometimes called *work of fracture.*

To determine only the properties of the material, it is necessary to adjust for the effects of geometry. This can be done by converting load to stress (defined as load/area) and deformation to strain (defined as a percentage change in length), creating a *stress–strain curve* (Fig. 1). The stress–strain curve defines the relationship between measures of load and deformation that have been normalized for area (stress) or for the original length of the bone (strain); it defines the amount of strain required to generate a unit of stress in the bone tissue. The same features defined on the load–deformation curve can be defined on the stress–strain curve, but these features are related to the stiffness or strength of the bone tissue, independent of geometry. Thus, the slope of the linear

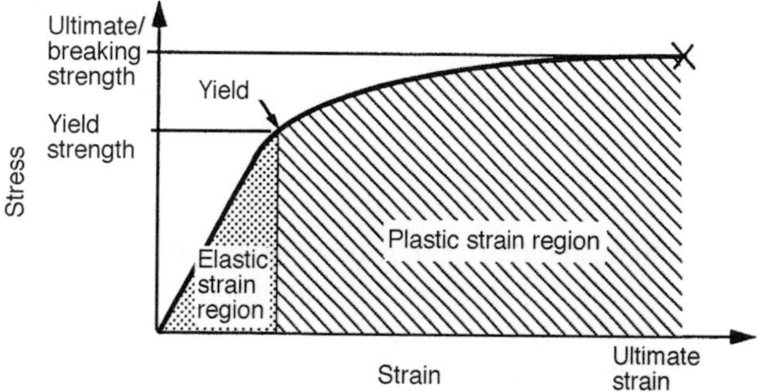

FIGURE 1 Stress–strain curve. The elastic strain energy is separated from the plastic strain energy by the yield point, the point at which irreversible damage occurs in the bone. The ultimate or breaking strength marks the stress and strain magnitudes of fractures. In bone, the ultimate strength and breaking strength generally are coincident. The strength of bone can be measured either from the yield point (yield strength) or at the point of fracture (ultimate strength) and can be measured either in units of stress or strain. Adapted from *Bone,* vol. 14, C. H. Turner and D. B. Burr, Basic biomechanical measurements of bone: A tutorial, pp. 595–608, 1993 with permission from Elsevier Science.

part of the stress–strain curve is material stiffness, often referred to as the *elastic* (*or Young's*) *modulus.* A comparison of preyield and postyield areas of the stress-strain curve can provide a lot of information about the propensity of the bone tissue toward damage and the nature of the mechanisms of its failure. A material that sustains little postyield strain before fracture is *brittle,* whereas one that sustains much postyield strain is considered *ductile.*

The stress achieved at yield, when permanent damage is sustained within the bone, is one measure of bone strength. Another measure of strength is the maximum stress achieved before failure. This is called the *ultimate stress,* and for bone is generally the same as its breaking strength.

Toughness is important in bone biomechanics because a tough bone will be more resistant to fracture, even though it may yield at a lower stress and be considered, by that measure, weaker. Toughness can be evaluated in several different ways, but one value of toughness, *the modulus of toughness,* can be measured as the area under the stress–strain curve (in units of N-m/m^3 or Joules/m^3). As the units indicate, this is a volumetric measurement of toughness. The stress intensity factor K_{Ic} (in N/m or Joules/m^2) is a planar measure of fracture toughness that indicates how easily cracks initiate or grow in a tissue. Although these are measurements of different aspects of bone quality, they tend to follow similar trends in the way that they change with age.

Measurements of the structural and material properties of bone (Table I) are generally made using servo-hydraulic testing equipment. Structural measurements can be made from whole bone specimens, uncorrected for geometry, but measurements of the material properties of bone tissue generally require utilizing standardized test specimens that are machined into specific shapes. Standardized specimens are also required for measurements of fracture mechanics (fracture toughness) properties of bone. In addition, elasticity can be measured using quantitative ultrasonic instruments or an acoustic microscope.

MECHANICAL STRENGTH OF BONE DECLINES WITH AGE

There is a massive literature showing that the mechanical properties of bone decline as one ages [10–12]. The precise amount of the decline in mechanical strength and stiffness depends on many factors, including biological ones (e.g., the kind of bone, its porosity, mineralization, extent of collagen cross-linking, or the location from which it was taken) as well as mechanical ones (e.g., the kind and mode of mechanical test performed or the magnitude and rate of loading). Extrapo-

TABLE I Types of Mechanical Tests[a]

Test	Measurement	Specimen
Extrinsic properties		
Bending test	Ultimate force, stiffness, work to failure	Whole bone
Torsional test	Shear fracture force, stiffness, work to failure	Whole bone
Compressive test	Ultimate compressive force, stiffness, work to failure	Vertebral body
Tensile test	Ultimate tensile force, stiffness, work to failure	Whole bone
Shearing test	Neck strength, stiffness, work to failure	Femoral neck
Quantitative ultrasound	Acoustic velocity (elastic modulus/density)	Calcaneus (*in vivo*)
Intrinsic properties		
Bending test	Bending strength, elastic modulus, toughness	Standardized (machined) beam
Torsional test	Shear strength, shear modulus, toughness	Standardized cylinder or dumbbell-shaped specimen
Compressive test	Compressive strength, elastic modulus, toughness	Standardized block or dumbbell-shaped specimen
Tensile test	Tensile strength, elastic modulus, toughness	Dumbbell-shaped specimen
Pure shear test	Shear strength	Arcan, Iosipescu standardized specimens
Acoustic wave propagation	Acoustic velocity (elastic modulus/density)	Block (~500 μm thick)
Micromechanical tests	Strength, elastic modulus, toughness	Trabecular tissue
Other properties		
Fatigue test	Number of loading cycles to failure, rate of stiffness loss	Whole bone or machined specimens
Fracture mechanics	Crack propagation and failure mechanisms (stress intensity factor, strain energy release rate, crack velocity)	Notched and machined beam

[a] There are several kinds of testing apparatuses. Generally, servo-hydraulic testing equipment is used. However, quantitative ultrasound uses a clinical ultrasonic instrument, and measurements of acoustic wave propagation for intrinsic properties utilize an acoustic microscope.

lation from more recent studies [13,14] supports earlier studies [10,15,16] by showing that the decline in strength after age 35 is in the range of 2–5% per decade for cortical bone tissue. The amount of energy absorbed prior to bone fracture for comparable sites declines slightly more over the same age range, perhaps 7–12% per decade [13–15]. The decline in trabecular bone strength is faster, between 8 and 10% per decade [17–19].

Much of the decline in mechanical properties is attributed to the loss of bone that occurs postmenopausally in women [20]. However, even small changes in bone density/volume that occur as people age can translate into larger and more significant changes in structural mechanical properties [21], leading some to speculate that the age-related decrease in bone strength can occur independently of the decline in bone mass [22]. For femoral cortical bone, a 2.6% decline in density results in a 20% loss of strength [21]. The density of the vertebral body (measured by ash content) declines 35–40% between the ages of 20 and 80 years in both men and women, causing a decrease in lumbar vertebral body strength (measured as maximum load prior to failure) of 60–65% [18]. Only slightly greater losses of density (48–50%) can result in a 75–80% reduction of vertebral strength. Other mechanical properties such as stiffness and energy absorption capacity of the vertebrae also decline more with age than bone mass [17,23–25]. Similar relationships occur at other skeletal sites: a 48% decrease in apparent density in the cancellous bone from the distal femur is associated with a 68–75% decline in compressive strength between the ages of 20–100 years. The slight density reduction results in larger strength reductions because of the nonlinear relationship between bone density and strength, first pointed out by Carter and Hayes [26], and later reinforced by others [19,27,28]. Even for the same bone mass, however, the risk of fracture increases exponentially with age [29]. This suggests that there are factors other than bone density that are important to bone's mechanical strength.

One of these factors may be architectural. Although bone mineral density (BMD) is correlated highly with vertebral ultimate stress in both men ($r^2 = 0.88$) and women ($r^2 = 0.67$), the addition of a texture parameter to BMD accounts for an additional 9% of the variation in strength in female vertebrae ($r^2 = 0.76$; $p < 0.001$) [30]. It is notable that texture analysis does not contribute additional information to the prediction of male vertebral strength over BMD alone. The reasons for this are unclear, but may have to do with differences in trabecular bone volumes in men and women's vertebrae [31].

The anisotropy of vertebral trabecular bone, defined as the ratio of strength in vertical and horizontal directions [32], changes significantly over the 20- to 80-year range, indicative of the loss of horizontally oriented trabeculae that may contribute to overall strength by acting as supporting struts that prevent trabecular buckling (Fig. 2) [33,34]. Anisotropy of trabecular structure contributes significantly to the modulus and strength of bone, independently of bone volume or mass [22,35]. Trabecular orientation, in combination with density, may account for up to 94% of the variability in the elastic properties of bone [35,36].

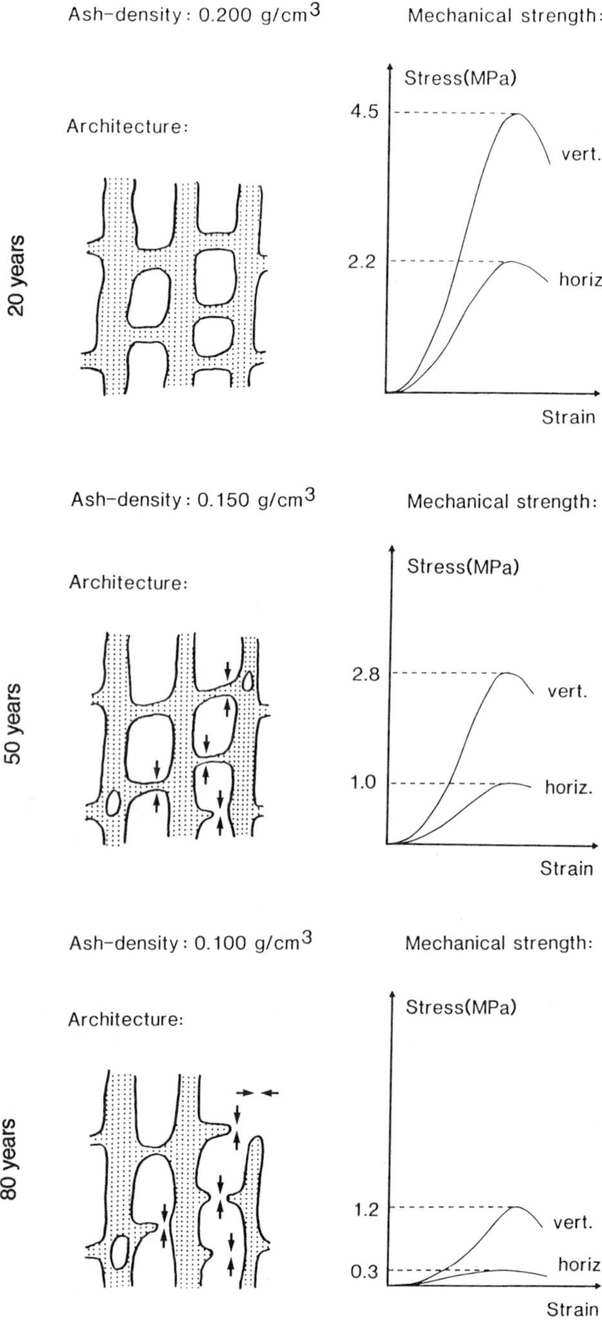

FIGURE 2 The loss of horizontal trabeculae that occurs with age reduces the mechanical strength of vertebral trabecular bone, both in horizontal and in vertical directions. Note that the 50% reduction in ash density results in greater than 50% decrease in strength. Reprinted with permission from Mosekilde [24].

Connectivity of trabeculae is different from the orientation of trabeculae. Theoretically, anisotropy can be associated with either a high degree or a low degree of connectivity. Connectivity is not independent of bone mass [35,37], however, and does not explain significantly more of the variation in mechanical strength than bone mass alone [19,38]. Studies that demonstrate strong correlations between trabecular thickness, for instance, and bone strength [39] without correcting for the covariate of bone volume may provide a skewed view of the importance that connectivity plays in overall bone strength. These relationships have been studied primarily in bone from nonosteopenic people. The same relationships may not hold true for osteoporotic bone, in which connectivity declines and anisotropy increases with age [24,25]. Correlations of the strength of osteopenic/osteoporotic bone with bone volume and connectivity are sorely needed.

The loss of biomechanical competence does not occur in only weight-bearing areas of the body. Similar declines in mechanical strength can be found from biopsies of the iliac crest [32]. This demonstrates that the loss of strength with age is part of a generalized systemic decline in mechanical properties, regardless of the need for mechanical strength.

QUALITY OF BONE TISSUE DETERIORATES WITH AGE

Bone from elderly women may be inherently more fragile than bone from younger women [9]. The bending stiffness of the ulna decreases significantly in women between the ages of 23 and 53 years, signaling a decline in the material properties of bone tissue that is independent of bone mineral density [40,41]. In *ex vivo* mechanical tests in which cyclic loads were applied to bone from older women (72 ± 6 years) and young women (26 ± 6 years), Courtney *et al.* [42] found that a unit decrease in elastic modulus in bone from the elderly women was associated with greater microstructural damage than the same modulus degradation in the younger women's bone. Cracks initiated in bone from older women grow at a greater rate than those in bone from younger donors [42].

This indicates that differences between younger and older bone are related most strongly to the postyield behavior of bone, i.e., differences in the amount of plastic deformation that the bone tissue can tolerate before complete fracture (Fig. 1). These changes in the postyield behavior of bone with age are probably due to the initiation and growth of microcracks in the tissue

[42–44] that accumulate with age at both cancellous and cortical sites and in both men and women [42,45,46]. Age-related changes in the elastic modulus or stiffness of cortical bone, but not cancellous bone, are smaller than changes in its plastic behavior (Table II) [13]. Decreased tensile plastic deformation, characterized by smaller ultimate strain (Fig. 1) [47–49] and decreased work to fracture [9,49] in bone from older individuals, has been reported several times [16,50] and can probably be attributed to the slower bone turnover and increased mean tissue age of older bone [51] or to molecular changes in either the organic [5,6,52–55] or the inorganic [4,56–59] bone matrix [60]. They are probably not caused entirely by the increased porosity that accompanies bone loss with aging [61]. The age-related reduction in the ability of bone to absorb energy prior to failure is clinically important in making osteoporotic bone more prone to failure from any impact load, such as one resulting from a fall. The loss of energy absorption capability, therefore, may be a primary factor increasing the risk of fracture in older women with low bone mass.

Older bone is more highly mineralized than younger bone, accounting for the tendency of bone from older individuals with higher material density to be weaker than those with lower material density, independent of porosity or volume [16,23,61,62]. Reports using infrared spectrometry [56,57] suggest that larger crystals are present in the bone of older, osteoporotic women and that this increased crystallinity itself could impair the mechanical properties of the tissue. More highly mineralized and more highly crystalline bone may permit earlier crack initiation by decreasing the amount of plastic deformation that can occur before ultimate failure. In older bone, increased porosity contributes to the effects of hypermineralization in that there is a smaller proportion of new, less mineralized but more ductile bone. This increases the contribution of the older hypermineralized tissue to bone's mechanical properties and reduces significantly the amount of energy the bone can absorb on impact. The effects of mineralization and porosity explain the observation that older bone has more damage than younger bone [42,45,46] and that older bone is more susceptible to damage at any given load level. These relationships explain the increased fragility of older bone because the bone can sustain very little post-yield strain before fracture, i.e., it becomes more brittle.

Changes in the morphology of the mineral crystal with age may contribute to increasing brittleness. Although the size of the apatite crystal itself may change very little [58], the normally elongated crystals may become more spherical in older, osteoporotic women and men [59]. It has been hypothesized that this can change the local stress distributions in the tissue and alter its load-bearing mechanical properties [59]. The precise effect of such changes in the mineral crystal on the mechanical properties of bone, however, is not known.

Because the differences in mechanical properties are a function of processes that occur during plastic deformation, rather than during elastic deformation, it should not be surprising that tensile and compressive elastic moduli of cortical bone, or of cancellous bone at the tissue level, do not change very much with age [16]. The increased tissue mineralization that occurs with age combined with the decreased integrity of collagen provide a trade-off that results in little overall change in the elastic modulus of the tissue. The change in elastic modulus with age is to some extent bone and mode specific. For example, neither the compressive or tensile modulus of the femur nor the tensile modulus of the tibia change much with age, but the compressive modulus of the tibia declines by about 5% per decade [16]. Likewise, it is difficult to identify any consistent differences in tensile modulus in specimens from normal and osteoporotic individuals [16]. Acoustic velocity measurements of elasticity (Table I) made either *in vivo* [63] or *ex vivo*

TABLE II Changes in Elastic Properties and Energy Absorption of Human Femur with Age[a]

Age (years)	Elastic modulus (Gpa)	Δ, previous decade (%)	Ultimate strain ($\mu\epsilon$)	Δ, previous decade (%)	Energy absorption (MN/m^2)	Δ, previous decade (%)
20–29	17.0 (2.24)		34,000 (6700)		3.85 (1.10)	
30–39	17.6 (0.28)	+3.53	32,000 (9200)	−5.88	3.55 (0.98)	−7.79
40–49	17.7 (4.45)	+0.57	30,000 (4000)	−6.25	3.19 (0.53)	−10.14
50–59	16.6 (1.74)	−6.21	28,000 (5900)	−6.67	2.84 (0.61)	−10.97
60–69	17.1 (2.21)	+3.01	25,000 (5500)	−10.71	2.65 (0.78)	−6.69
70–79	16.3 (1.78)	−4.68	25,000 (6000)	−0.00	2.57 (0.68)	−3.02
80–89	15.6 (0.71)	−4.29	24,000 (2100)	−4.00	2.23 (0.12)	−13.23
Overall Δ (%)		−8.24		−29.41		−42.08

[a] Data from Ref. [16]. Data expressed as mean (SD).

[64] in pre- and postmenopausal normal women and in age-matched osteoporotic women have not demonstrated any consistent relationship between elastic properties and the putative strength of bone.

FRACTURE TOUGHNESS OF HUMAN BONE DECLINES WITH AGE

Fracture toughness, as defined previously and measured in N/m or Joules/m^2, is a measure of how easily cracks can initiate or grow in the tissue. Tough materials have the ability to sustain large amounts of damage without failure. Bone that is highly mineralized and highly crystalline will tend not to sustain much damage before failure and will not be very tough. Consequently, highly mineralized bone will sustain little plastic deformation prior to failure, which is evident in the significantly decreased impact energy absorption and work to fracture that occurs in bone with a higher mineral content [9,65].

The age-related difference in postyield behavior of bone is indicative of a material that can no longer prevent the growth and coalescence of damage caused by physical forces. The fragility caused by changes in the nature of its mineralization may be one reason for decreased fracture toughness in older men and women [14,66] Fig. 3, Table III). In younger people, bone remodeling serves as a means to keep mineral "young" and available for calcium homeostasis. In older people, however, remodeling does not function as efficiently to remove *and* replace the more mature mineral. Although it seems paradoxical, bone mineral content can decrease at the same time that the mineralization of bone matrix is increasing, for reasons described previously. Consequently, although mineral content decreases with age, the remaining bone tends to be older. Thus there is a higher fraction of more mineralized bone, which increases the fragility of the tissue [4].

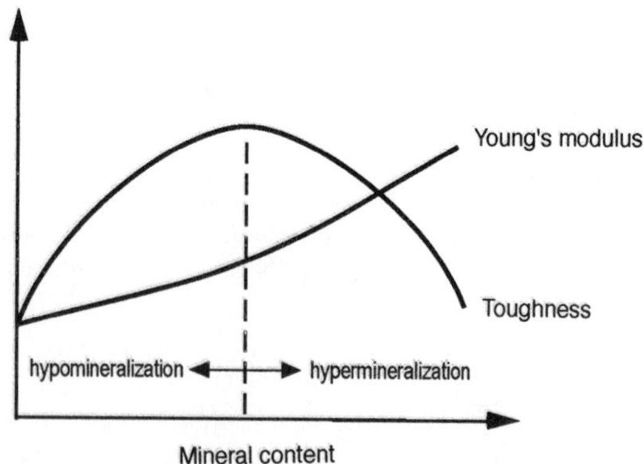

FIGURE 3 The modulus of toughness, a measure of the energy that can be sustained before failure, is reduced by either hyper- or hypomineralization of the bone tissue. Even though higher mineralization will increase Young's modulus even at very high levels of mineral content, there appears to be an optimum range of mineralization to maximum bone toughness. Adapted from a concept presented by Wainwright *et al.* [91].

There may be other reasons for reduced fracture toughness with age as well (Table III). The increased bone turnover that occurs at menopause in women has the effect both of reducing bone volume, which will decrease strength, and of increasing porosity, which may have effects on toughness that are independent of the simple decline in bone volume. Greater porosity is associated with greater water content in bone, and greater water content alone is associated with reduced bone toughness in tension and shear independent of volumetric changes. In this sense, bone has the worst of two worlds: not only does the mineralized matrix become more brittle with age, but the reduced bone volume and increased water that are the consequence of a stimulated remodeling system contribute independently to impair the ability of bone to sustain damage prior to failure.

Increased bone turnover has several other deleterious effects on the bone's mechanical properties, and toughness, apart from its effect on bone mass. It can be shown that the effects of Haversian canals and resorption spaces in bone become increasingly significant when the rate of load/strain is increased [67]. The greater number of porosities in bone that accompany the aging process will significantly reduce the impact energy-absorbing capabilities of bone independently of the reduction in bone mass. This can exacerbate the effects of any trauma, such as falling. Beyond this, the large number of resorption cavities in older bone, which are a function of both the increased turnover and the longer period required to fill the resorbed area with new bone, will have an additional stress concentrating effect because of the geometry of the resorption lacunae within them. Depending on the geometry and the orientation of the cavity with respect to the principal stresses [68], the resorption lacunae can intensify the local stress field to the point that the threshold for failure is reached. This may be an additional factor contributing to the reduction in fracture toughness with age.

The decrease in fracture toughness in older people is indicative of a change in the quality of bone tissue with age. This change in material property of aging bone may partly explain the observation that fracture risk in older people is greater than predicted by the loss of bone mass alone [29]. There is a component of bone fragility that accompanies aging and that is independent of bone mass, and this fragility can be detected by a change in fracture toughness.

The modulus of toughness [the area under the stress-strain curve (Fig. 1)] is a measure of the amount of

TABLE III Features of Bone Tissue That Reduce Strength and Fracture Toughness

Feature	Effect				Cause/example
	Modulus	Ultimate strain	Ultimate stress	Toughness	
Poorly mineralized bone	⇓	⇑	⇓	⇓	Osteomalacia
Hypermineralized bone	⇑	⇓	⇑	⇓	Reduced turnover Increased mean tissue age
Increased crystallinity; Δ morphology of apatite crystal	⇑	⇓	?	⇓	Reduced turnover Increased mean tissue age Fluoride accumulation[b]
Porosity; increased osteon population density (cortical bone)	⇓	⇒	⇓	⇓	Increased turnover Resorption lacunae
Reduced bone volume (trabecular bone)	⇓	⇒	⇓	⇓	Increased activation frequency Altered resorption/formation balance
Denaturation of collagen molecule[a]	⇓	⇓	⇓	⇓	Unclear
Debonding of mineral/collagen[a]	⇓	⇑	⇓	⇓	Fluoride accumulation[b,c]

[a] From Refs. [52,53,89, and 90].
[b] From Ref. [93].
[c] From Ref. [89].

energy required to cause fracture. Bone toughness measured in this way from quasi-static tests largely confirms the results of the fracture mechanics approach [9,16]. Currey *et al.* [9] attributed this reduced toughness to the higher mineral content of the bone tissue from older individuals because it is known that more highly mineralized bone is able to absorb less energy prior to failure, even though it is stiffer and more rigid (Fig. 3). The toughness of hypomineralized bone is also compromised. There is clearly a range of mineralization within which toughness is maximized, and deviations from this optimum will reduce fracture toughness.

FATIGUE PROPERTIES OF BONE DECREASE WITH AGE

Although bone becomes less tough and more brittle with age, there is little information about how these changes affect the number of loading cycles bone can withstand before it fractures. This property of bone is called its fatigue life. Fatigue properties can be measured in a variety of ways, including the rate at which bone loses strength and stiffness in response to repeated bouts of cyclic loading. With the possible exception of the impact energy imparted by falling or other trauma, bone *in vivo* is generally not loaded monotonically by large single loads, although that is the way many *in vitro* tests are performed. It would be useful to know something about the change in the fatigue properties, or fatigue life, of older bone, but little of this information exists in the current literature. We can infer, given the decline in fracture toughness in older bone, that its fatigue life will be affected negatively by aging as well, but experimental validation of this concept is weak. Zioupos *et al.* [69] reported reduced fatigue strength of bone from older women, which they attributed to the increased porosity and reduced bone mineral content of the tissue.

AGE-RELATED STRUCTURAL COMPENSATIONS FOR REDUCED MECHANICAL STRENGTH

The deterioration in bone's material properties that occur as men and women age can be partially or wholly offset by structural changes that increase bone's biomechanical competence. This can occur even in the face of significant losses of bone from the trabecular or endocortical envelopes. From a mechanical standpoint, small amounts of bone apposed to the periosteal surface of a long bone [70–72] or to the cortical shell of a vertebra (which is loaded in bending rather than pure compression [73]) can offset the negative biomechanical consequences that occur consequent to losses of large amounts of trabecular or endocortical bone [74]. Even the small amount of bone in the cortical shell of the lumbar vertebrae contributes 20–60% of its peak strength [75–77], and thus additions of small amounts of bone to this skeletal envelope can improve strength quite significantly.

The mechanical strength of any bone is defined by its geometry and material properties; only the latter depend on mineral content. The distribution of bone around the marrow cavity has a significant effect of the bone's strength that can be independent of mineral content. Consequently, noninvasive measures of bone mineral content or density, without knowledge of the distribution of material, provide an incomplete picture of bone strength and fracture risk at any given location.

The distribution of material within a cross section of bone is defined by the cross-sectional moment of inertia (or the second moment of the area), which can be mathematically defined as the sum of the squared distances of each unit of area from a given loading axis (Fig. 4). The cross-sectional moment of inertia is proportional to the bending rigidity of the bone and can therefore be used as one measure of bone strength even when mechanical testing cannot be done. The sum of the area moments of inertia in any two perpendicular planes define a similar parameter, the polar moment of inertia, which is proportional to the torsional rigidity of the bone. From this definition, it is clear that if the loading axis passes through the marrow cavity, bone along the periosteal surface, which is furthest from the marrow cavity, will have the most positive biomechanical influence. The bending and torsional rigidity of the bone can increase exponentially by additions of bone to the periosteal surface, even when the absolute bone volume and bone mineral density have decreased significantly (Fig. 5). This emphasizes the im-

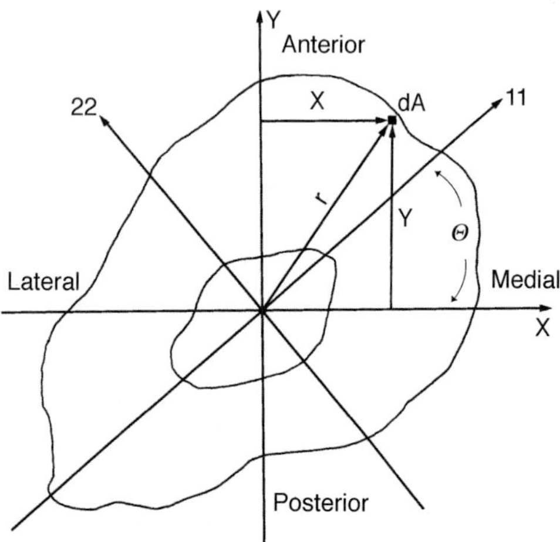

FIGURE 4 Cross-sectional moments of inertia are calculated as the sum of all units of bone area (dA) and their squared distances from some axis (the neutral axis) about which bending occurs. The 11 and 22 axes indicate the directions associated with the principal moments of inertia, i.e., the axes about which the maximum and minimum bending rigidity would occur. θ defines the angle between the axes of greatest and least inertial moment and the anatomical axes. Cross-sectional moments of inertia are a measure of the distribution of material within a cross section of bone and are proportional to the bending rigidity of the bone. Reprinted from *J. Biomech.,* vol. 13, G. J. Miller and W. W. Purkey, Jr., The geometric properties of paired human tibiae, pp. 1–8, 1980 with permission from Elsevier Science.

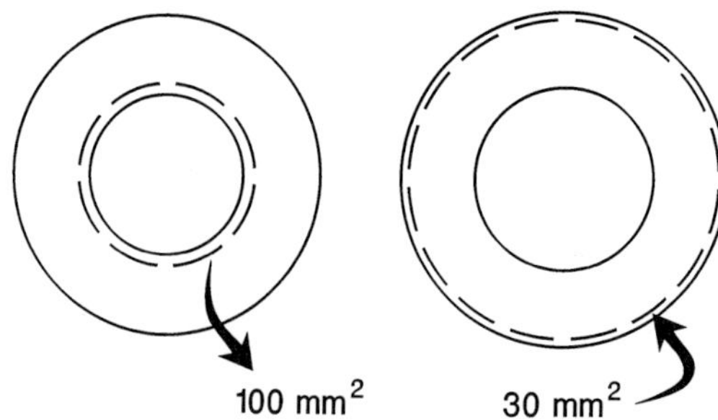

FIGURE 5 Two idealized long bone cross sections. The section on the left represents a younger person's bone and that on the right represents an older person's bone following loss of bone from the endocortical surface and subsequent periosteal bone apposition. Despite the fact that 100 units of area were removed from the endocortical surface, and only 30 units were added back onto the periosteal surface, the sections have equal resistance to bending. Reprinted from Martin and Burr [12].

portance of knowing the distribution of tissue within a bone that may be at risk for fracture. Although bone mineral content may decline with age, the force required to break the bone may not decrease.

Periosteal apposition of bone with age serves a biomechanically important function by compensating for reduced tissue properties (or reduced bone volume) in men [71], but this compensation is not sufficient to offset the larger losses of bone that occur in modern populations of women [70,78,79]. In women, femoral bending strength estimated from density data and cross-sectional geometry shows an increase in strength in women to about the age of 35, after which strength steadily declines into old age [2,10,16,70]. The same changes occur in aging men, but do not begin until age 60 in the metacarpals, and age 80 in the humerus and femur [71]. This is also true for the femoral neck. Although women lose bone at the rate of 4% per decade at this site before menopause, the cross-sectional moment of inertia is maintained. Postmenopausally, however, the increased rate of loss (7% per decade) is not compensated and results in estimated femoral neck stresses that are 4–12% higher than in younger women [80].

Similar periosteal compensations have been shown for the vertebral body in males but not in females [24]. An age-related decrease in the thickness of the vertebral cortical shell [81] is compensated in men by significant increases in vertebral body diameter [77,82,83], on the order of 25–30% [18]. This partially offsets the increased vertical stress on the vertebral body that occurs as a consequence of trabecular bone loss. Compressive strength is strongly correlated to cortical thickness *and* trabecular volume ($r^2 > 0.80$). Increases in diameter are particularly large in American blacks [82].

The failure in women to adequately compensate for tissue loss is probably due to excessive endocortical resorption rather than to any gender difference in periosteal apposition. Periosteal expansion with age has been demonstrated many times in both men and women [12]. However, the exact nature of the failure to compensate may be population or bone specific. Ruff and Hayes [84] found no gender differences in endocortical resorption, but did detect a failure of periosteal expansion in women. Burr and Martin [72] also failed to observe any periosteal expansion in the radius of women between the ages of 39 and 90. However, periosteal expansion of the femoral cortex in women has been reported many times [70,85].

These relationships could also be size related. As one might expect if apposition of bone to the periosteal surface is mechanically mediated, men or women with larger bones have less periosteal apposition and greater endocortical resorption than those with smaller bones [86]. Because men on average have larger bones, they may be able to compensate for the loss of bone tissue with smaller additions subperiosteally. The evidence that men may lose just as much bone as women do in the long bones [86] and in the cancellous bone of the spine [87] suggests this as one possible explanation.

Porosity gradients in aging bone reflect these biomechanical influences. The endocortical surface of bone is typically more porous than the periosteal, and the circumferential addition of new bone periosteally is primary bone and not very porous. The porosity along the endocortical surface of bone has less of a negative effect on bone strength than would that same porosity if it were found closer to the periosteal surface. Moreover, it can be shown that porosity is greatest along the axis of greatest geometric resistance to bending in the femur [88]. Consequently, it would appear that periosteal expansion occurs preferentially along those axes where bone is being lost.

SUMMARY

Several important changes occur in the biomechanical properties of bone during the aging process:

1. The loss of a small amount of bone has profound effects on the reduction in mechanical strength and toughness.
2. Bone tissue from older people is inherently less tough and more fragile than that from younger people. It is less capable of sustaining damage before failure.
3. The deterioration of the material properties of bone are largely related to changes in the amount and crystallinity of the mineral, which affect the plastic deformation of the bone tissue more than its Young's modulus. This means that bone becomes more brittle and fails earlier than it would otherwise for a given bone mass.
4. Measures of tissue elasticity are not the best measures of bone quality. The postyield behavior of bone may be a better indicator of bone quality.
5. There is little information regarding the effects of aging on fatigue life in bone, even though bone is loaded cyclically throughout life. The small amount of data that exist suggest that aging reduces the fatigue life of bone.
6. Structurally, bones attempt to compensate both for the loss of volume and for the change in material properties through apposition of bone periosteally. This geometric adaptation maximizes strength with a minimum amount of material.
7. Although the mechanical properties of bone decline overall as a consequence of normal aging processes, the most clinically important message from biomechanical measurements of bone properties is that the bone's ability to absorb energy is reduced significantly. This seriously impairs its ability to sustain impact loads of any great magnitude and emphasizes the importance of averting falls to prevent bone fracture.

References

1. Sherman, S., Heaney, R. P., Parfitt, A. M. Hadley, E. C., and Dutta, C. NIA Workshop on aging and bone quality. *Calcif. Tissue Int.* **54**(Suppl. 1), S1–S180 (1993).
2. Martin, R. B. Aging and strength of bone as a structural material. *Calcif. Tissue Int.* **53**(Suppl. 1), S34–S40 (1993).
3. Martin, R. B. Porosity and specific surface of bone. *CRC Crit. Rev. Bioeng.* **10,** 179–222 (1984).
4. Grynpas, M. Age and disease-related changes in the mineral of bone. *Calcif. Tissue Int.* **53**(Suppl. 1), S57–S64 (1993).
5. Bailey, A. J., Wotton, S. F., Sims, T. J., and Thompson, P. W. Biochemical changes in the collagen of human osteoporotic bone matrix. *Connect. Tissue Res.* **29,** 119–132 (1993).
6. Danielsen, C. C., Mosekilde, Li., Bollerslev, J., and Mosekilde, Le. Thermal stability of cortical bone collagen in relation to age in normal individuals and in individuals with osteoporosis. *Bone* **15,** 91–96 (1994).
7. Burr, D. B., Forwood, M. R., Fyhrie, D. P., Martin, R. B., Schaffler, M. B., and Turner, C. H. Bone microdamage and skeletal fragility in osteoporotic and stress fractures. *J. Bone Miner. Res.* **12,** 6–15 (1997).
8. Turner, C. H., and Burr, D. B. Basic biomechanical measurements of bone: A tutorial. *Bone* **14,** 595–608 (1993).
9. Currey, J. D., Brear, K., and Zioupos, P. The effects of ageing and changes in mineral content in degrading the toughness of human femora. *J. Biomech.* **29,** 257–260 (1996).
10. Yamada, H., "Strength of Biological Materials." The Williams and Wilkins Co., Baltimore, 1970.
11. Evans, F. G., "Mechanical Properties of Bone." C. C. Thomas, Springfield, IL, 1973.
12. Martin, R. B., and Burr, D. B., "Structure, Function, and Adaptation of Compact Bone." Raven Press, New York, 1989.

13. McCalden R. W., McGeough, J. A., Barker, M. B., and Court-Brown, C. M. Age-related changes in the tensile properties of cortical bone. *J. Bone Joint Surg.* **75A,** 1193–1205 (1993).
14. Zioupos, P., and Currey, J. D. Changes in the stiffness, strength and toughness of human cortical bone with age. *Bone* **22,** 57–66 (1998).
15. Melick, R. A., and Miller, D. R. Variations of tensile strength of human cortical bone with age. *Science* **30,** 243–248 (1998).
16. Burstein, A. H., Reilly, D. T., and Martens, M. Aging of bone tissue: Mechanical properties. *J. Bone Joint Surg.* **58A,** 82–86 (1976).
17. Mosekilde, Li., Mosekilde, Le., and Danielsen, C. C. Biomechanical competence of vertebral trabecular bone in relation to ash density and age in normal individuals. *Bone* **8,** 79–85 (1987).
18. Mosekilde, Li., and Mosekilde, Le. Sex differences in age-related changes in vertebral body size, density and biomechanical competence in normal individuals. *Bone* **11,** 67–73 (1990).
19. McCalden, R. W., McGeough, J. A., and Court-Brown, C. M. Age-related changes in the compressive strength of cancellous bone. *J. Bone Joint Surg.* **79A,** 421–427 (1997).
20. Smith, C. B., and Smith, D. A. Relations between age, mineral density and mechanical properties of human femoral compacta. *Acta Orthop. Scand.* **47,** 496–502 (1976).
21. Wall, J. C., Chatterji, S. K., and Jeffery, J. W. Age-related changes in the density and tensile strength of human femoral cortical bone. *Calcif. Tissue Int.* **27,** 105–108 (1979).
22. Turner, C. H. Age, bone material properties and bone strength. *Calcif. Tissue Int.* **53**(Suppl. 1), S32–S33 (1993).
23. Currey, J. D. Changes in impact energy absorption of bone with age. *J. Biomech.* **12,** 459–469 (1979).
24. Mosekilde, Li. Normal age-related changes in bone mass, structure, and strength—consequences of the remodeling process. *Danish Med. Bull.* **40,** 65–83 (1993).
25. Mosekilde, Li. Vertebral structure and strength in vivo and in vitro. *Calcif. Tissue Int.* **53**(Suppl. 1), S121–S126 (1993).
26. Carter, D. R., and Hayes, W. C. The compressive behavior of bone as a two phase porous structure. *J. Bone Joint. Surg.* **59A,** 954–962 (1977).
27. Schaffler, M. B., and Burr, D. B. Stiffness of compact bone: Effects of porosity and density. *J. Biomech.* **21,** 13–16 (1988).
28. Rice, J. C., Cowin, S. C., and Bowman, J. A. On the dependence of the elasticity and strength of cancellous bone on apparent density. *J. Biomech.* **21,** 155–168 (1988).
29. Hui, S. L., Slemenda, C. W., and Johnston, C. C. Age and bone mass as predictors of fracture in a prospective study. *J. Clin. Invest.* **81,** 1804–1809 (1988).
30. Veenland, J. F., Link, T. M., Monermann, W., Meier, N., Grashuis, J. L., and Gelsema, E. S. Unraveling the role of structure and density in determining vertebral bone strength. *Calcif. Tissue Int.* **61,** 474–479 (1997).
31. Nottestad, S. Y., Baumel, J. J., Kimmel, D. B., Recker, R. R., and Heaney, R. P. The proportion of trabecular bone in human vertebrae. *J. Bone Miner. Res.* **2,** 221–229 (1987).
32. Mosekilde, Li., Viidik, A., and Mosekilde, Le. Correlation between the compressive strength of iliac and vertebral trabecular bone in normal individuals. *Bone* **6,** 291–295 (1985).
33. Mosekilde, Li. Sex differences in age-related loss of vertebral trabecular bone mass and structure—biomechanical consequences. *Bone* **10,** 425–432 (1989).
34. Jensen, K. S., Mosekilde, Li., and Mosekilde, Le. A model of vertebral trabecular bone architecture and its mechanical properties. *Bone* **11,** 417–423 (1990).
35. Goldstein, S. A., Goulet, R., and McCubbrey, D. Measurement and significance of three-dimensional architecture of the mechanical integrity of trabecular bone. *Calif. Tissue Int.* **53**(Suppl. 1), S127–S133 (1993).
36. Keaveny, T. M., and Hayes, W. C. A 20-year perspective on the mechanical properties of trabecular bone. *Trans. ASME* **115,** 534–542 (1993).
37. Compston, J. E. Connectivity of cancellous bone: Assessment and mechanical implications. *Bone* **5,** 463–466 (1994).
38. Snyder, B. D., "Anisotropic Structure-Property Relations for Trabecular Bone." Ph.D. thesis, University of Pennsylvania, Philadelphia, 1991.
39. Dempster, D. W., Ferguson-Pell, M. W., Mellish, R. W. E., Cochran, G. V. B., Xie, F., Fey, C., Horbert, W., Parisien, M., and Lindsay, R. Relationship between bone structure in the iliac crest and bone structure and strength in the lumbar spine. *Osteopor. Int.* **3,** 90–96 (1993).
40. McCabe, F., Zhou, L.-J., Steele, C. R., and Marcus, R. Noninvasive assessment of ulnar bending stiffness in women. *J. Bone Miner. Res.* **6,** 53–59 (1991).
41. Kann, P., Graeben, S., and Beyer, J. Age-dependence of bone material quality shown by the measurement of frequency of resonance in the ulna. *Calcif. Tissue Int.* **54,** 96–100 (1994).
42. Courtney, A. C., Hayes, W. C., and Gibson, L. J. Age-related differences in post-yield damage in human cortical bone. Experiment and model. *J. Biomech.* **29,** 1463–1471 (1996).
43. Currey, J. D. Biocomposites: micromechanics of biological hard tissues. *Curr. Opin. Solid State Mater. Sci.* **1,** 440–445 (1996).
44. Burr, D. B., Turner, C. H., Naick, P., Forwood, M. R., Ambrosius, W., Hasan M. S., and Pidaparti, R. Does microdamage accumulation affect the mechanical properties of bone? *J. Biomech.* **31,** 337–345 (1998).
45. Schaffler, M. B., Choi, K., and Milgrom, C. Aging and bone matrix microdamage accumulation in human compact bone. *Bone* **17,** 521–525 (1995).
46. Mori, S., Harruff, R., Ambrosius, W., and Burr, D. B. Trabecular bone volume and microdamage accumulation in the femoral heads of women with and without femoral neck fractures. *Bone* **21,** 521–526 (1997).
47. Lindahl, O., and Lindgren, A. G. Cortical bone in man. II. Variation in tensile strength with age and sex. *Acta Orthop. Scand.* **38,** 141–147 (1967).
48. Lindahl, O., and Lindgren, A. G. Cortical bone in man. III. Variation of compressive strength with age and sex. *Acta Orthop. Scand.* **39,** 129–135 (1968).
49. Currey, J. D. Physical characteristics affecting the tensile failure properties of compact bone. *J. Biomech.* **23,** 837–844 (1990).
50. Currey, J. D., and Butler, G. The mechanical properties of bone tissue in children. *J. Bone Joint Surg.* **57A,** 810–814 (1975).
51. Birkenhäger-Frenkel, D. H., and Nigg, A. L. Age-related bone loss as reflected by changes of interstitial bone thickness. *Calcif. Tissue Int.* **52**(Suppl. 1), S60 (1993).
52. Wang, X., Bank, R. A., Tekoppele, J. M., Athanasiou, K. A., and Agrawal, C. M. Relationship between bone mechanical properties and collagen denaturation. *In* "Proc. 17th Southern Biomedical Engineering Conference," p. 111. San Antonio, TX, 1998.
53. Wang, X., Athanasiou, K. A., Agrawal, C. M. Contribution of collagen to bone mechanical properties. *In* "Proc. 17th Southern Biomedical Engineering Conference," p. 112. San Antonio, TX, 1998.
54. Oxlund, H., Mosekilde, Li., and Ørtoft, G. Reduced concentration of collagen reducible cross links in human trabecular bone with respect to age and osteoporosis. *Bone* **19,** 479–484 (1996).
55. Mehta, S. S., Orhan, K. Öz, and Antich, P. P. Bone elasticity and ultrasound velocity are affected by subtle changes in the organic matrix. *J. Bone Miner. Res.* **13,** 114–121 (1998).

56. Paschalis, E. P., Betts, F., diCarlo, E., Mendelsohn, R., and Boskey, A. L. FTIR microspectroscopic analysis of normal human cortical and trabecular bone. *Calcif. Tissue Int.* **61,** 480–486 (1997).
57. Paschalis, E. P., Betts, F., diCarlo, E., Mendelsohn, R., and Boskey, A. L. FTIR microspectroscopic analysis of human iliac crest biopsies from untreated osteoporotic bone. *Calcif. Tissue Int.* **61,** 487–492 (1997).
58. Simmons, E. D., Jr., Pritzker, K. P. H., and Grynpas, M. D. Age-related changes in the human femoral cortex. *J. Orthop. Res.* **9,** 155–167 (1991).
59. Mongiorgi, R., Romagnoli, R., Olmi, and Moroni, A. Mineral alterations in senile osteoporosis. *Biomaterials* **4,** 192–196 (1983).
60. Bätge, B., Diebold, J., Bodo, M., Fehm, H. L., and Müller, P. K. Evidence for bone matrix alterations in osteoporosis. *In* "Current Research in Osteoporosis and Bone Mineral Measurement II" (E. F. J., Ring, ed.,), p. 3. British Institute of Radiology, London, 1992.
61. Dickenson, R. P., Hutton, W. C., and Stott, J. R. R. The mechanical properties of bone in osteoporosis. *J. Bone Joint Surg.* **63B,** 233–238 (1981).
62. Currey, J. D. The mechanical properties of bone. *Clin. Orthop. Rel. Res.* **73,** 210–231 (1970).
63. Antich, P. P., Pak, C. Y. C., Gonzales, J., Anderson, J. Sakhaee, K., and Rubin, C. Measurement of intrinsic bone quality *in vivo* by reflection ultrasound: Correction of impaired quality with slow-release sodium fluoride and calcium citrate. *J. Bone Miner. Res.* **8,** 301–311 (1993).
64. Hasegawa, K., Turner, C. H., Recker, R. R., Wu, E., and Burr, D. B. Elastic properties of osteoporotic bone measured by scanning acoustic microscopy. *Bone* **16,** 85–90 (1995).
65. Currey, J. D. The effects of strain rate, reconstruction and mineral content on some mechanical properties of bovine bone. *J. Biomech.* **8,** 81–86 (1975).
66. Norman, T. L., Nivargikar S. V., and Burr, D. B. Resistance to crack growth in human cortical bone is greater in shear than in tension. *J. Biomech.* **29,** 1023–1031 (1996).
67. Cartwright, A. G. The effect of histological variation on the tensile strength of cortical bone. *Biomed. Eng.* **10,** 442–446 (1975).
68. Currey, J. D. Stress concentrations in bone. *J. Microscop. Sci.* **103,** 111–133 (1962).
69. Zioupos, P., Wang, X. T., and Currey, J. D. Experimental and theoretical quantification of the development of damage in fatigue tests of bone and antler. *J. Biomech.* **8,** 989–1002 (1996).
70. Martin, R. B., and Atkinson, P. J. Age and sex-related changes in the structure and strength of the human femoral shaft. *J. Biomech.* **10,** 223–231 (1977).
71. Martin, R. B., Pickett, J. C., and Zinaich, S. Studies of skeletal remodeling in aging men. *Clin. Orthop. Rel. Res.* **149,** 268–282 (1980).
72. Burr, D. B., and Martin, R. B. The effects of composition, structure and age on the torsional properties of the human radius. *J. Biomech.* **16,** 603–608 (1983).
73. Burr, D. B., Yang, K. H., Haley, M, and Wang, H.-C. Morphological changes and stress redistribution in osteoporotic spine. *In* "Spinal Disorders in Growth and Aging" (H. E. Takahashi, ed.), pp, 127–147. Springer-Verlag, Tokyo, 1995.
74. Carter, D. R., and Spengler, D. M. Mechanical properties and composition of cortical bone. *Clin. Orthop. Rel. Res.* **135,** 192–217 (1978).
75. Rockoff, S. D., Sweet, E., and Bleustein, J. The relative contribution of trabecular and cortical bone to the strength of human lumbar vertebrae. *Calcif Tissue Res.* **3,** 163–175 (1969).
76. Yoganandan, N., Myklebust, J. B., Cusick, J. F., Wilson, C. R., and Sances, A., Jr. Functional biomechanics of the thoracolumbar vertebral cortex. *Clin. Biomech.* **3,** 11–18 (1988).
77. Mosekilde, Li., and Mosekilde, Le. Normal vertebral body size and compressive strength: Relations to age and to vertebral and iliac trabecular bone compressive strength. *Bone* **7,** 207–212 (1986).
78. Van Gerven, D. P., Armelagos, G. J., and Bartley, M. H., Jr. Roentogenographic and direct measurement of cortical involution in a prehistoric Mississippian population. *Am. J. Phys. Anthropol.* **31,** 23–38 (1969).
79. Carlson, D. S., Armelagos, G. J., and Van Gerven, D. P. Patterns of age-related cortical bone loss (osteoporosis) within the femoral diaphysis. *Hum. Biol.* **48,** 295–314 (1976).
80. Beck, T. J., Ruff, C. B., and Bissessur, K. Age-related changes in female femoral neck geometry. Implications for bone strength. *Calcif. Tissue Int.* **53**(Suppl. 1), S41–S46 (1993).
81. Vesterby, A., Mosekilde Li, Gunderson, H. J. G., Melsen, F., Mosekilde, Le., Holme, K., and Sorensen, S. Biologically meaningful determinants of the *in vitro* strength of lumbar vertebrae. *Bone* **12,** 219–224 (1991).
82. Ericksen, M. F. Aging in the lumbar spine. III. L5. *Am. J. Phys. Anthropol.* **48,** 247–250 (1978).
83. Pesch, H. J., Scharf, H. P., Lauer, G., and Seibold, H. Der Altersabhängige Verbundabbau der Lendenwirbelkörper. *Virch. Arch. Pathol. Anat. Histol.* **386,** 21–41 (1980).
84. Ruff, C. B., and Hayes, W. C. Sex differences in age-related remodeling of the femur and tibia. *J. Orthop. Res.* **6,** 886–896 (1988).
85. Smith, R. W., Jr., and Walker, R. R. Femoral expansion in aging women: Implications for osteoporosis and fractures. *Science* **145,** 156–157 (1964).
86. Garn, S. M., Sullivan, T. V., Decker, S. A., Larkin, F. A., and Hawthorne, V. M. Continuing bone expansion and increasing bone loss over a two-decade period in men and women from a total community sample. *Am. J. Hum. Biol.* **4,** 57–67 (1992).
87. Kalender, W. A., Felsenberg, D., Louis, O., Lopez, P., Klotz, E., Osteaux, M., and Fraga, J. Reference values for trabecular and cortical vertebral bone density in single- and dual-energy quantitative computed tomography. *Eur. J. Radiol.* **9,** 75–80 (1989).
88. Lazenby, R. Porosity-geometry interaction in the conservation of bone strength. *J. Biomech.* **19,** 257–258 (1986).
89. Walsh, W. R., and Guzelsu, N. Electrokinetic behavior of intact wet bone: Compartmental model. *J. Orthop. Res.,* **9,** 683–692 (1991).
90. Catanese, J., III, and Keaveny, T. M. Role of collagen and hydroxyapatite in the mechanical behavior of bone tissue. *J. Bone Miner. Res.* **11**(Suppl. 1), S295 (1996).
91. Wainwright, S. A., Biggs, W. D., Currey, J. D., and Gosline, J. M., "Mechanical Design in Organisms." Princeton University Press, Princeton, NJ, 1976.
92. Burr, D. B., Piotrowski, G., and Miller, G. J. Structural strength of the macaque femur. *Am. J. Phys. Anthropol.* **54,** 305–319 (1981).
93. Turner, C. H., Garetto, L. P., Dunipace, A. J., Zhang, W., Wilson, M. E., Grynpas, M. D., Chachra, D., McClintock, R., Peacock, M., Stookey, G. K. Fluoride treatment increased serum IGF-1, bone turnover, and bone mass, but not bone strength, in rabbits. *Calcif. Tissue Int.* **61,** 77–83.

PART V

Fractures: A Consequence of the Aging Skeleton

CHAPTER 27

Application of Biomechanics to the Aging Human Skeleton

MARY L. BOUXSEIN Orthopedic Biomechanics Laboratory, Beth Israel Deaconess Medical Center and Harvard Medical School, Boston, Massachusetts, 02215

INTRODUCTION

One of the most dramatic consequences of the aging of the human skeleton is the exponential increase in fracture incidence with age [1]. In the United States alone, there are over 1.5 million age-related fractures annually with associated medical expenditures of nearly $14 billion [2,3]. Moreover, based on current demographic trends, this number is projected to double or triple in the next 50 years due to the "graying" of the population [4]. Interventions to reduce fracture incidence are called for and, to be effective, these interventions must be based on a sound understanding of the etiology of fractures.

From a biomechanics viewpoint, fractures of any type are due to a structural failure of the bone. This failure occurs when the forces applied to the bone exceed its load-bearing capacity. The load-bearing capacity of a bone depends primarily on the material that comprises the bone (and its corresponding mechanical behavior), the geometry of the bone (its size, shape, and distribution of bone mass), and the specific loading conditions (Fig. 1). Thus it is clear that factors related to the forces applied to the bone, as well as to its load-bearing capacity, are important determinants of fracture risk. To apply these concepts to the study of fracture risk, Hayes and colleagues [5] introduced a term called the "factor of risk." The factor of risk, Φ, is defined as the ratio of the load delivered to a bone (*applied load*) to the load-bearing capacity of that bone (*failure load*):

$$\Phi = \text{applied load/failure load}$$

When the factor of risk is low ($\Phi \ll 1$), the forces applied to the bone are much lower than those required to fracture it, and the bone is at low risk of fracture. However, when the factor of risk is high ($\Phi \gg 1$), fracture of the bone is predicted to occur. A high factor of risk can occur either when the bone is very weak and its load-bearing capacity is compromised or when very high loads, such as those resulting from trauma, are applied to the bone. In the aging skeleton, it is likely that the coupling of a weak bone with an increased incidence of traumatic loading leads to the dramatic rise in fracture incidence with age.

To apply the factor of risk concept in studies of hip or vertebral fracture, the loads applied to the bone of interest and the corresponding load required to fracture the bone must be identified. For example, the majority of hip fractures are associated with a fall. Therefore, to compute the factor of risk for hip fracture due to a fall, information about the loads applied to the femur during a fall and about the load-bearing capacity of the femur in a fall configuration is required. While this approach is relatively easy to conceive, in practice it is difficult to apply. There are few data describing the magnitude and direction of loads applied to the skeleton during activities of daily living and even fewer data describing the loads engendered during traumatic events, such as a trip, slip, or fall. Moreover, due to the complex morphology of the skeleton and associated muscle and tendon attachments, it is difficult to design a laboratory study that mimics the loading environment encountered by the bone *in vivo*. Therefore, it is challenging to determine the load-bearing capacity of skeletal elements un-

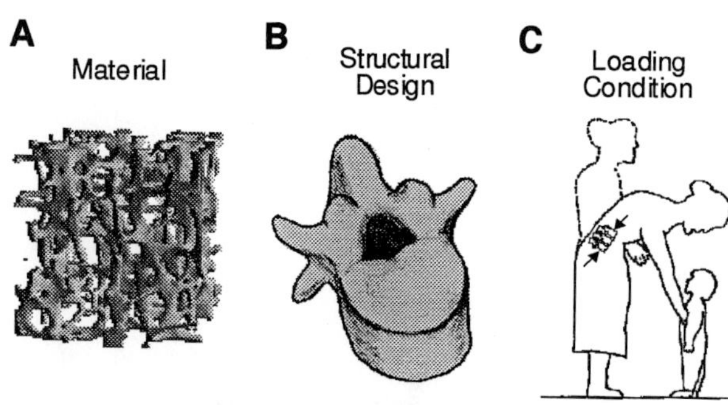

FIGURE 1 Characteristics of the spine that determine the capacity to carry load: The trabecular bone (left), the design and organization of the vertebral body (middle), and the loading conditions, which are illustrated as lifting, but could be any loading action (right). With permission from Myers and Wilson [115].

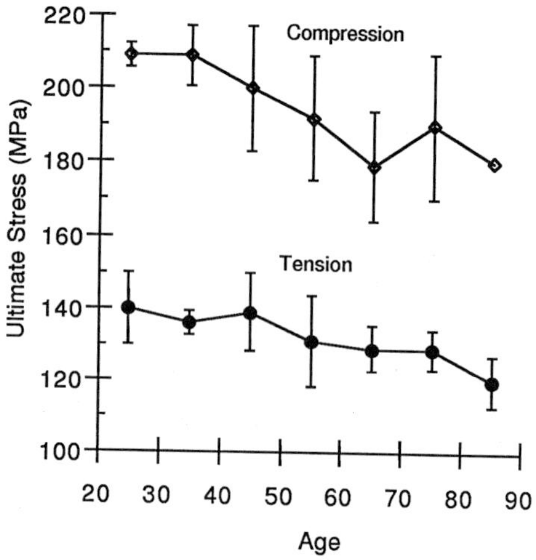

FIGURE 2 Age-related changes in the ultimate stress of human femoral cortical bone in tension and compression (error bars represent 1 SD). The mean change per decade is −2.1% for tension and −2.5% for compression. These data indicate that femoral cortical bone becomes weaker with age. Data from Burstein *et al.* [6].

der realistic loading conditions. Despite these uncertainties and limitations, rough estimates of the factor of risk for hip and vertebral fracture can be computed using data from laboratory investigations. These estimates may provide insights into the complex roles of loading severity and skeletal fragility in the etiology of age-related fractures.

The remainder of this chapter will discuss, from a biomechanics viewpoint, the age-related changes in the skeleton that influence fracture risk of the hip and spine. Changes in the material properties of trabecular and cortical bone will be reviewed, as will changes in femoral and vertebral geometry and load-bearing capacity. Finally, the concept of the factor of risk will be applied to hip and vertebral fractures.

AGE-RELATED CHANGES IN THE MECHANICAL PROPERTIES OF BONE AS A MATERIAL

The mechanical properties of cortical [6–13] and trabecular bone [14–20] decline with age in both men and women. In human cortical bone, after age 20, the elastic modulus decreases 2% per decade [6,13] (Fig. 2), while the ultimate strength declines 2–5% per decade [6,12,13]. In addition, the incurred deformation and energy absorbed before fracture decrease 5–12% per decade [6,12,13], suggesting that bone becomes more brittle and less tough with increasing age. Moreover, the energy required to fracture a cortical bone specimen under *impact* loading decreases threefold between the ages of 3 and 90 [21]. These changes in the elastic and ultimate properties of cortical bone are likely the result of porosity increases with age. McCalden and colleagues [12] found that age was correlated strongly with porosity ($r = -0.73$), and that porosity explained over 75% of the variability in cortical bone strength. In summary, age-related changes in cortical bone lead to a weaker, more brittle material.

Human trabecular bone also exhibits an age-related decline in material properties [15–20,22–25]. Aging is characterized by a decline in the apparent density of trabecular bone. It appears that the *amount* of bone is reduced and therefore the integrity of the trabecular network is compromised, but that the remaining bone is histologically normal. Previous studies have shown that the strength of trabecular bone is proportional to the square of the apparent density [26–29]. Therefore, a decline in apparent density is predicted to cause an even greater decline in mechanical strength.

In support of this, Mosekilde and colleagues [19] found that the apparent density of vertebral trabecular bone decreases approximately 50% from age 20 to 80 (−9% per decade), whereas the mechanical properties (compressive elastic modulus, strength, and energy absorption) decrease 75–80% in the same time period (−12 to 15% per decade) (Table I). In trabecular bone of the proximal tibia, an age-related decline in apparent density of 25% is accompanied by a 30–40% reduction in compressive strength and energy absorption properties [20]. Direct age-related changes in the material properties of trabecular bone from other anatomical sites, such as the proximal femur, distal radius, or calcaneus, have not been reported. However, there are strong correlations between the material properties at these sites and apparent density [30–36], which declines with age.

In trabecular bone specimens from the iliac crest that were matched in pairs for density, compressive strength

TABLE I Age-Related Changes in Vertically Oriented Trabecular Bone Specimens Compressed in Either the Vertical or the Horizontal Direction[a]

	Specimens compressed in vertical direction		Specimens compressed in horizontal direction	
	% per decade	Correlation with age (r)	% per decade	Correlation with age (r)
Ash density	−9	−0.85[b]	−9	not reported
Ultimate stress	−12.8	−0.79[c]	−15.5	−0.87[c]
Elastic modulus	−13.5	−0.83[c]	−15.9	−0.83[c]
Energy to failure	−14	−0.75[c]	−15.2	−0.88[c]
Ultimate strain	+4	0.45[b]	+3.1	0.30[d]

[a] The mean percent change per decade and the linear correlation with age are presented. Specimens were taken from 42 persons, aged 15 to 87. Data from Mosekilde *et al.* [19].
[b] $P < 0.01$.
[c] $P < 0.001$.
[d] $0.05 < P < 0.06$.

was approximately 40% lower in specimens from older donors (>60 years) compared with younger donors (<40 years) [22]. These data indicate that the mechanical behavior of trabecular bone is not only a function of apparent density, but is dependent on other factors, such as trabecular architecture [28,29,37,38]. Trabecular architecture is characterized by the thickness, number, and separation of the individual trabecular elements, as well as the extent to which these elements are interconnected. Changes in trabecular architecture accompany the age-related declines in bone density. Trabecular number and thickness decline with decreasing density, whereas trabecular separation increases [23,24,39,40].

Because changes in trabecular architecture are often strongly intercorrelated, it is difficult to discern the relative effect on bone strength of reductions in trabecular number vs trabecular thickness for both vertically and horizontally oriented trabecular struts. To address this issue, Silva and Gibson [41] developed a two-dimensional model of vertebral trabecular bone to simulate the effects of age-related changes in trabecular microstructure. They found that reductions in the *number* of trabeculae decreased bone strength two to five times more than reductions in trabecular thickness that resulted in an identical decrease in bone density. For example, removing longitudinally oriented *trabecular elements* to create a 10% reduction in density resulted in a 70% reduction in bone strength. In contrast, reducing *trabecular thickness* to achieve a 10% reduction in density resulted in only a 20% reduction in strength. This study implies that it is important to maintain trabecular number in order to preserve bone strength with aging. Consequently, therapies designed to counter age-related declines in bone strength should strive to maintain or restore the number of trabeculae rather than just increasing the thickness of existing trabecular struts.

Other factors may influence age-related changes in the mechanical behavior of bone, including the histologic structure (primary vs osteonal bone), the collagen content and orientation of collagen fibers, the number and composition of cement lines, and the presence of fatigue microdamage and microfractures [42–50]. For example, an increase in osteonal remodeling (and the subsequent increase in the number of cement lines) reduces the strength of the bone for single load applications. However, the cement lines act as deterrents to crack proliferation, possibly improving the mechanical behavior of bone under repetitive loading conditions [51].

Burr and colleagues [50] reviewed the potential role of skeletal microdamage in age-related fractures. They suggested that microdamage due to repetitive loading of bone likely initiates at the level of the collagen fiber or below and may include collagen fiber–matrix debonding, disruption of the mineral–collagen aggregate, and failure of the collagen fiber itself. They hypothesized that the accumulation and coalescence of these small defects eventually leads to microcracks that are visible under light microscopy. Although the relationship between existing microcracks and bone mechanical properties has not been established *in vivo,* investigators have shown that damage accumulation in devitalized bone leads to a decrease in bone strength [45,52]. Thus, the accumulation of microdamage *in vivo* may contribute to the increased fragility of the aging skeleton.

Microcracks occur naturally in human specimens from several anatomic locations, including trabecular bone from the femoral head and vertebral body, as well as cortical bone from the femoral and tibial diaphyses [49,53–57]. It appears that the incidence of microcracks increases with age, probably in an exponential fashion, and that after age 40, microdamage accumulates faster in women than in men [54,56] (Fig. 3). For instance, Mori and colleagues [53] reported that the density of microcracks in the femoral head of older women is more than double the density seen in younger women. In addition, they observed an inverse, nonlinear relationship between microcrack density and trabecular bone area, indicating that microcracks accumulate more rapidly as bone mass decreases. Similar evidence for a nonlinear relationship between microcrack density and trabecular bone area has been reported for vertebral trabecular bone specimens [55]. Thus, the accumulation of microdamage *in vivo* may contribute to the increased fragility of the aging skeleton.

AGE-RELATED CHANGES IN BONE GEOMETRY

Age-related changes in the material properties of bone tissue are frequently accompanied by a redistribution of the cortical and trabecular bone material. It is likely that the structural rearrangement of bone tissue is driven by "preprogrammed" behavior of the endosteal and periosteal bone cells as well as the local mechanical loading environment and biochemical signals [51,58]. Hence, the adaptation pattern depends on age, gender, skeletal site, physical activity patterns, and expression (local and systemic) of cytokines and growth factors.

The general pattern of adaptation in the appendicular skeleton includes endosteal resorption and periosteal apposition of bone tissue (Fig. 4). Thus, the diameter of the bone increases, but the thickness of the cortex decreases. This redistribution of bone tissue away from the center of the bone allows the bone to better resist

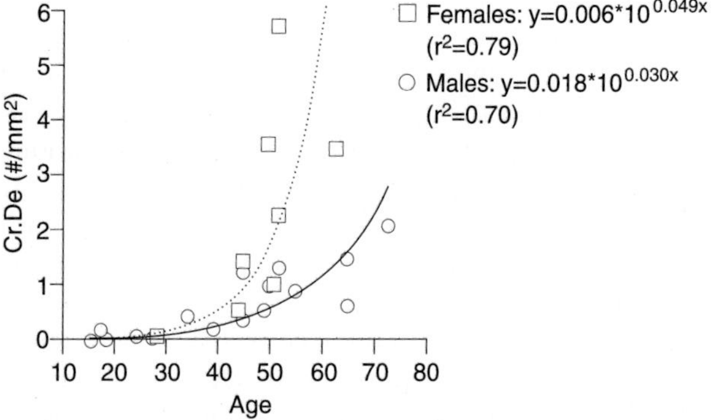

FIGURE 3 Bone microcrack density vs age. There is an exponential increase in microdamage accumulation in the femoral cortex in both men and women after the age of 40 years. Damage accumulation occurs about twice as rapidly in women as in men. From Burr *et al.* [50]. Reproduced from J. Bone Miner. Res. 1997;12:6–15 with permission of the American Society for Bone and Mineral Research.

bending and torsional loads. Resistance to bending and torsional loading is particularly important, as the highest stresses in the appendicular skeleton are due to these loading modes [51]. The most efficient design for resisting bending and torsional loads involves distributing the material far from the neutral axis of bending or torsion (generally the center of the bone). The distribution of mass about the center of a structural element is described quantitatively by the area moment of inertia (see Chapter 26). For example, consider three circular bars, each composed of the same material (Fig. 5). The resistance of each bar to tensile and compressive loads is directly proportional to the cross-sectional area. However, the resistance to bending and torsional loads is influenced not only by how much bone (i.e., the cross-sectional area), but also by how it is distributed. Therefore, the structural capacity of bar C in bending or torsion is twice that of bar A due to its greater moment of inertia.

Some studies indicate that both men and women exhibit endosteal resorption accompanied by periosteal expansion [59–63], whereas others report that women undergo geometric changes that lead to decreased bone strength [64–68]. Smith and Walker [63] studied femoral radiographs of 2030 women aged 45 to 90 and reported that periosteal diameter and cortical cross-sectional area (assuming a circular cross section) both increased approximately 11% in 35 years. Furthermore, the section modulus (an indicator of the resistance to bending loads) increased 32% in the same time period.

In contrast, Ruff and Hayes [68], using direct assessment of cadaveric femurs and tibiae from 75 Caucasian adults, reported that although both men and women undergo endosteal resorption and medullary expansion with age, only men show subperiosteal expansion and bone apposition at the femoral diaphysis. They reported that, in men, cortical area is nearly constant and moments of inertia increase slightly with age. In women, however, both cortical area and moments of inertia decrease with age. The authors concluded, therefore, that in this sample from modern humans, only men exhibit bone remodeling patterns that would compensate for the age-related decline in bone material properties.

Age-related changes in bone shape and size have been observed not only at diaphyseal sites, but also at the vertebral body and femoral neck. However, age-related changes at these latter sites are much smaller than those seen at diaphyseal sites. In a study of 338 skeletons from the Smithsonian Institution, Ericksen [69] found that the transverse breadths of the L3 and L4 vertebrae increase slightly with increasing age in both men and women. Using indirect measurements, Mosekilde and Mosekilde [16] also found that, in men, the cross-sectional area of lumbar vertebrae is only very weakly associated with age ($r^2 = 0.11$), increasing approximately 25–30% from age

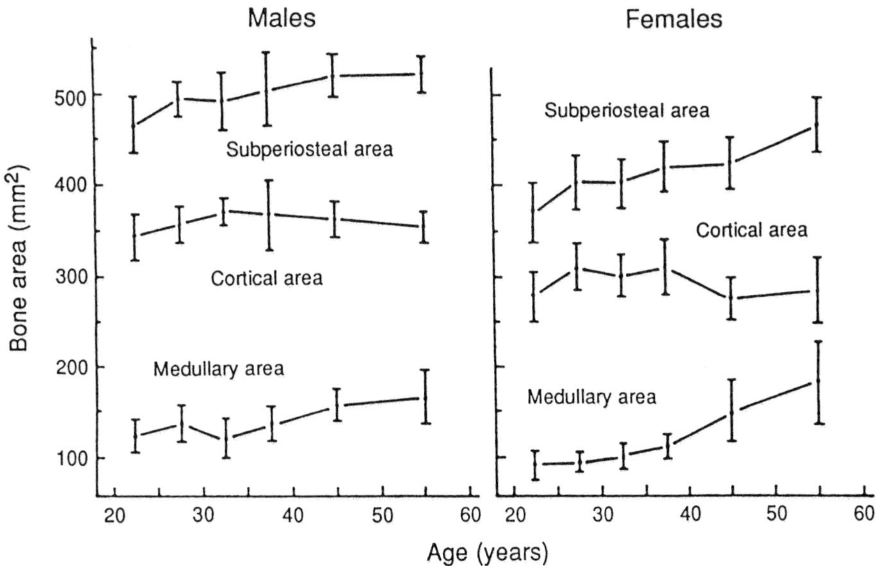

FIGURE 4 Age-related changes in the femoral midshaft demonstrating periosteal expansion and endosteal resorption. Data represent the mean ± 2 SE. Reprinted with permission from Ruff and Hayes [61]. Copyright 1982 American Association for the Advancement of Science.

20 to 90. In women, however, there was no age-related change in vertebral cross-sectional area.

Based on methodology originally presented by Martin and Burr [70], techniques have been developed to assess femoral geometry from X-ray absorptiometry exams, thereby allowing *in vivo* assessment of bone structure [64,71–74]. Investigators have used these methods to investigate race- [73] and sex-based [64,72,74] differences in femoral geometry.

For instance, Beck and colleagues [64] studied the cross-sectional relationship between femoral neck geometry and age in 1044 women, age 18–89. In women under age 50, femoral neck bone mineral density (BMD) decreased on average 4% per decade with no observable changes in femoral neck geometry. In women over age 50, femoral neck BMD declined 2.5 times faster than in the younger group (on average 7% per decade). However, in contrast to the younger group, the older women also showed changes in femoral geometry wherein the cross-sectional area and cross-sectional moment of inertia of the femoral neck declined approximately 7 and 5% per decade, respectively. These data suggest that after menopause, women lose bone mass at an accelerated rate, but that unlike men [72], they do not exhibit changes in femoral geometry that would compensate for this loss. As a result, in women, the stress in the femoral neck during walking is predicted to increase from 25 to 40% from age 50–80. In another study, however, there were no age-related changes in the moment of inertia of the femoral neck in either men or women [74].

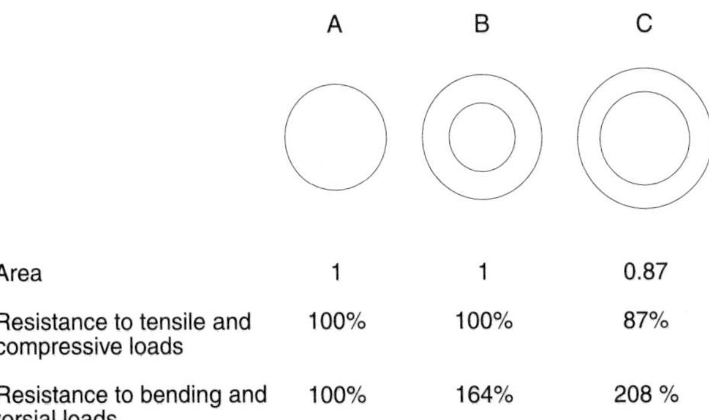

FIGURE 5 The influence of cross-sectional geometry on the structural strength of circular structures. From Bouxsein *et al.* [154].

As can be seen from the results of the previous studies, the sex-specific nature of age-related changes in skeletal structure remains controversial. The discrepancies in findings related to sex-specific bone adaptation patterns may be attributed to several factors. Most importantly, most of these studies use a cross-sectional design, thereby possibly introducing secular changes that confound data and eliminate the possibility of a causal relationship with age. In addition, differences in methodology (direct vs *in vivo* measurements), subject populations (archaeological vs modern human specimens), and measurement site (femoral shaft vs femoral neck) likely contribute to the conflicting findings. Thus, it appears that women may have a reduced capacity to alter their bone geometry in order to preserve bone strength with aging compared to men. However, the extent to which this reduced capacity contributes to the increased fracture risk observed in women is unknown.

BIOMECHANICS OF HIP FRACTURES

Recall that the "biomechanics" view of fractures states that a fracture occurs when the loads applied to the bone exceed its load-bearing capacity. Therefore, to study the etiology of hip fractures, it is important first to identify what event(s) is associated with hip fractures and then to determine the loads that are applied to the bone during that event and what the load-bearing capacity of the femur is during that loading situation. It is estimated that over 90% of hip fractures in the elderly are associated with a fall [75,76]. Thus, studies of the etiology of hip fractures are complicated by the need to examine risk factors for falls, as well as risk factors for fracture. In addition, given that fewer than 2% of falls in the elderly result in a hip fracture [77–79], investigations of hip fracture etiology must also distinguish factors related to "high-risk" falls that result in fracture. Therefore, this section reviews clinical and laboratory studies related to factors influencing the loads applied to the femur during a fall and the load-bearing capacity of the femur in a fall configuration.

Loads Applied to the Femur during a Fall

A fall can be defined as a sudden, unexpected event that results in a person coming to rest on a horizontal surface [80,81]. A fall can be further characterized by several phases: (1) an instability phase resulting in fall initiation, (2) a descent phase, (3) an impact phase, and (4) a post impact phase during which the faller comes to rest [80]. The definition of "fall severity" is more difficult. From a biomechanical perspective, fall severity can be described by the *magnitude* and *direction* of the load applied to the hip and by the *impact site*. From a clinical perspective, Cummings and Nevitt [82] suggest that a high-risk fall includes: (1) impact on or near the hip, (2) lack of active protective mechanisms such as an outstretched arm to break the fall, and (3) insufficient energy absorption by local soft tissues. Thus, by these criteria, a high-risk fall could transmit a force to the proximal femur that exceeds the force required to fracture the hip.

A few surveillance studies have been conducted to more fully characterize falls as they relate to hip fracture [78,80,83,84]. Among nursing home residents, falling to the side and impacting the hip or side of the leg increased the risk of hip fracture approximately 20-fold relative to falling in any other direction [80]. An increase in the potential energy content of the fall, computed from fall height and body mass, was also associated with an increased risk for fracture. Similar results were reported in a nested case-control analysis of the Study of Osteoporotic Fractures cohort, a large, prospective study in community-dwelling women [84]. Women who suffered a hip fracture were more likely to have fallen sideways or straight down and to have landed on or near the hip than women who fell and did not suffer fracture [84]. Thus, these surveillance studies have identified several factors that are related to the "severity" of a fall in terms of hip fracture risk. From these data, it is clear that a fall to the side represents a particularly risky event.

Several laboratory investigations have been conducted to further study the characteristics of sideways falls. In a study of the descent phase of sideways falls, van den Kroonenberg and colleagues [85] estimated the impact velocities and energies that may occur during falls from standing height, the effect of muscle activity on these impact velocities, and insights into the high-risk nature of sideways falls. Six young, healthy adults (age 19–30) were asked to fall sideways, as naturally as possible, onto a thick gymnastics mattress. To investigate the effect of muscle activity on fall dynamics, subjects were instructed to fall either as relaxed as they could or to fall naturally, using the musculature of the trunk and upper extremity as they would in a reflex-mediated fall. To investigate potential protective mechanisms, subjects were instructed to try to break the fall with their arm during some falls. The vertical velocity at impact with the floor ranged between 2.1 and 4.8 m/sec. The impact velocity was 7% lower in relaxed than in muscle-active falls, a finding attributed to the observation that hip impact occurs close to the feet in the muscle-relaxed case. Despite instructions to break the fall with an outstretched arm, only two of six subjects were able to do so (Fig. 6). In the remaining subjects, hip impact occurred first, followed by impact of the arm or hand. Finally, the authors found that, in these young adults, approximately 70% of the total energy available is dissipated during the descent phase of a sideways fall from standing height. This energy dissipation is likely due to muscle activity and the stiffness and damping characteristics of the hip and knee joints. It is likely that with age, the ability to dissipate this energy during a fall will decrease, and therefore it may be that elderly individuals will "fall harder" than young adults.

The forces applied to the proximal femur during a sideways fall depend not only on the dynamics of the *descent phase* of the fall, but also on characteristics of the *impact phase* of the fall. Robinovitch and colleagues [86–90] have conducted a series of experiments to study the potential roles of trochanteric soft tissues, muscle contraction, and body configuration in determining the load applied to the femur during a sideways fall with impact to the greater trochanter. In these experiments,

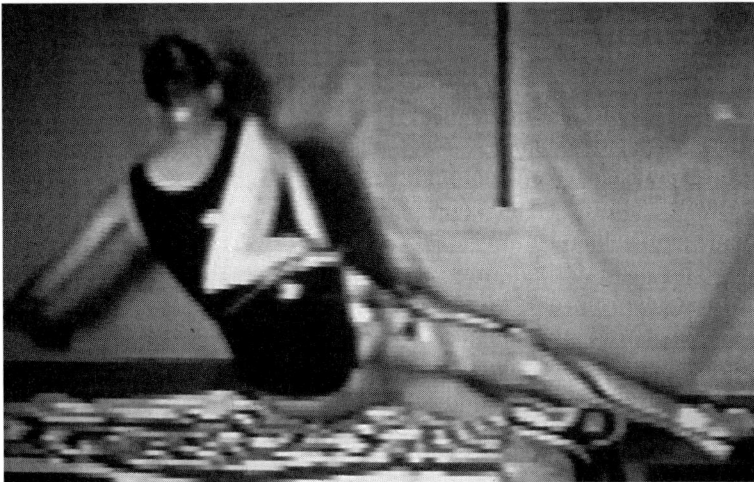

FIGURE 6 Example of a sideways fall onto a thick gymnastics mattress. Despite instructions to break the fall with the hand, only two of six subjects were able to do so. In the other subjects, hip impact occurred first, thus providing insight into the high-risk nature of sideways falls. With permission from van den Kroonenberg *et al.* [85], with permission from Elsevier Science.

they used a "pelvis release" system (Fig. 7) in which a small force is applied to the lateral aspect of the hip and the dynamic response of the body is measured [86]. This system allows impact forces from falls to be predicted with reasonable accuracy from the body's response to safe, simulated collisions [87]. They found that during a sideways fall with impact to the greater trochanter, only about 15% of the total impact force is distributed to structures peripheral to the hip, whereas the remainder of the force is delivered along a load path directly in line with the hip [88]. In addition, for the same body mass and height, sideways falls with the trunk

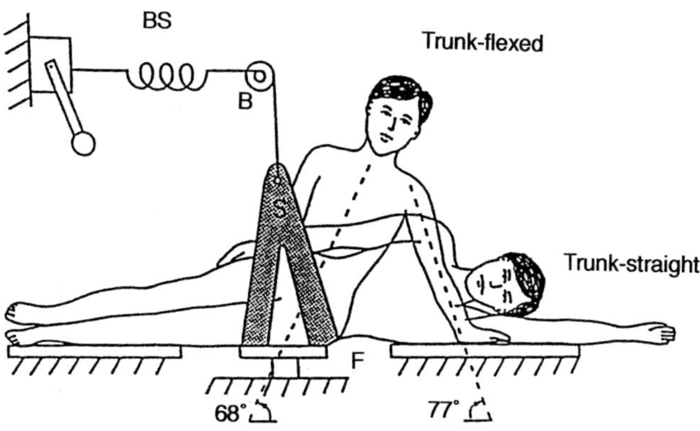

FIGURE 7 Schematic diagram of the setup used for "pelvis release" experiments. The subject's pelvis was supported by the sling, raised a small amount, and then released onto the force platform, which recorded the body's dynamic response. Experiments were conducted in two body configurations: in the trunk-straight and trunk-flexed positions to determine the effect of trunk position on fall impact dynamics. Reprinted with permission from Robinovitch *et al.* [88]. Copyright 1998 Biomedical Engineering Society.

in a more upright position are predicted to result in greater impact forces on the proximal femur than falls where the trunk is more horizontal at impact.

To study the force attenuation and energy absorption properties of the soft tissues overlying the greater trochanter, we obtained tissue samples from nine cadavers, positioned them over a surrogate proximal femur and pelvis, and subjected them to a typical impact load associated with a sideways fall [90]. For a constant impact energy, trochanteric soft tissue thickness was strongly negatively correlated with the peak femoral impact force ($r^2 = 0.91$), such that the force applied to the femur decreased approximately 70 N per 1 mm increase in tissue thickness. However, the force attenuation due to trochanteric soft tissues alone is likely insufficient to prevent hip fracture in falls where an elderly person lands directly on the hip [90]. These findings suggest that trochanteric padding systems may be an effective means of reducing the load applied to the femur during a fall.

Finally, van den Kroonenberg *et al.* [91] developed a series of biomechanical models to estimate peak impact forces delivered to the proximal femur during a sideways fall from standing height. The models incorporated stiffness and damping parameters from the "pelvis-release" experiments [86–88], and the models' behavior was compared with previous observations of the dynamics of voluntary sideways falls [85]. Using the most accurate model, peak impact forces applied to the greater trochanter ranged from 2900 to 4260 N for the 5th to 95th percentile woman, based on weight and height. Thus, these findings support the idea that "the bigger they are, the harder they fall" [92]. Given an individual's height and weight, these models can be used to estimate femoral impact forces associated with a sideways fall.

Load-Bearing Capacity of the Proximal Femur

As mentioned previously, several factors contribute to the load-bearing capacity of the proximal femur, including its intrinsic material properties as well as the total amount (size) and spatial distribution (shape) of the bone tissue. Because the mechanical properties of both cortical and trabecular bone are strongly related to bone density, many have hypothesized that age-related bone loss is a primary contributor to the steep increase in hip fracture incidence with age. In support of this hypothesis, strong evidence from prospective clinical studies shows that low BMD, measured both at the hip and at other sites, is a risk factor for hip fracture [93–96]. Furthermore, case-control studies of elderly fallers have reported that low bone mineral density of the hip is a risk factor for hip fracture that is independent of fall characteristics [83,84].

Initially, laboratory studies evaluating the load-bearing capacity of the proximal femur used a configuration designed to simulate the single-leg stance phase of gait [71,97–101]. The loads required to fracture the femur in the stance phase of gait ranged from approximately 1000 to 13,000 N. These studies demonstrated a strong relationship between the load required to fracture the femur in this stance configuration and noninvasive measurements of bone geometry and bone mineral density or content.

More recent studies have evaluated the load-bearing capacity of the proximal femur in a configuration designed to simulate a sideways fall with impact to the greater trochanter [102–107]. Courtney and colleagues [103,104] studied the effect of age and loading rate on the failure load of the proximal femur in the fall configuration. At a slow loading rate (2 mm/sec), they found that femurs from young individuals (age 17–51) were more than twice as strong as femurs from older individuals (age 59–83) (Fig. 8). At high loading rates (100 mm/sec), such as might be expected during a fall, femurs from both young and older individuals were approximately 20% stronger than at the slower loading rate [104]. However, femurs from the younger group were still approximately 80% stronger than those from the older group. This difference in load-bearing capacity between younger and older groups was explained almost completely by lower bone mineral density in the older group.

In addition to age and loading rate, femoral geometry also influences the load-bearing capacity of the proximal

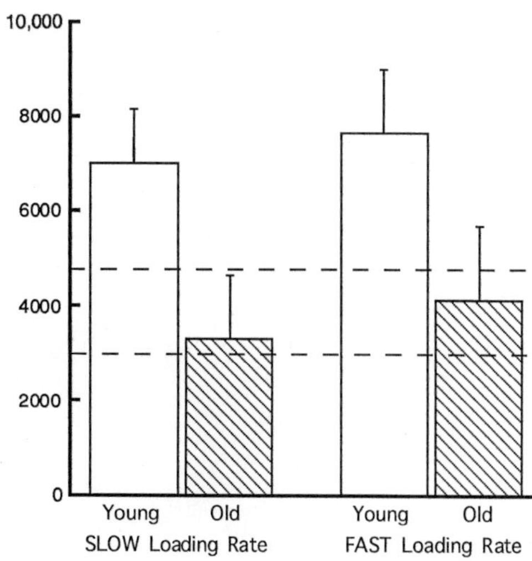

FIGURE 8 Mean failure loads for cadaveric proximal femurs from young and elderly donors tested in a sideways fall configuration at slow and fast loading rates. For each loading rate, femurs from the younger individuals were 80–100% stronger than femurs from the older individuals. Data from Courtney *et al.* [103,104], with permission.

femur. The relationship between femoral geometry and load-bearing capacity is not unexpected. Because the load-bearing capacity is a *structural* property (see Chapter 26), it is influenced by the size of the specimen. Therefore, as expected, femoral neck area, neck width, and neck axis length are all positively correlated (r^2 = 0.21–0.79) with femoral failure loads [103,105,107]. It is interesting to note that the positive correlation between femoral neck length and femoral strength appears to contradict findings from clinical studies, where a longer hip axis length (HAL) is associated with a greater risk of hip fracture [108]. This discrepancy may be attributed to the differences in the portion of hip anatomy that is included in the *in vitro* measurements (neck axis length only) vs *in vivo* measurements (neck axis length plus acetabular thickness). Some evidence suggests that is the "acetabular thickness" portion of the measurement that is associated with fracture risk, not the "femoral neck length" portion [109]. Additional laboratory studies are required to understand the complex relationship between hip geometry and fracture risk.

Although it is important to understand what factors influence the load-bearing capacity of the femur in the laboratory environment, it is also critical to develop techniques that can be used clinically to predict femoral strength. Several studies have confirmed that noninvasive assessments of bone mineral density and geometry using dual-energy X-ray absorptiometry (DXA) or quantitative computed tomography (QCT) are correlated strongly to the load-bearing capacity of human cadaveric femurs. Femoral bone mineral content and density explain over 80% of the variation in the load-bearing capacity of the proximal femur [103,105,107] (Fig. 9).

In summary, the load-bearing capacity of cadaveric proximal femurs ranges from approximately 800 to 10,000 N and is influenced, at least in part, by femoral bone mineral density, femoral geometry, loading direction, and loading rate. At a given moment, an individual's bone density and geometry are constant, although they can certainly change with age or therapeutic intervention. However, other factors, such as loading direction and loading rate that are influenced by the characteristics of the fall, may significantly influence fracture risk.

Factor of Risk for Hip Fracture

The concept of a factor of risk for fracture (introduced in the introduction) suggests that low BMD is not the only indicator of risk, but rather that the loads applied to the bone must also be considered. Two case-control studies have demonstrated the importance of both fall severity and bone mineral density as risk factors for hip fracture [83,84]. Nevitt and Cummings [84], in a nested case-control analysis of the Study of Osteoporotic Fractures cohort, studied 130 women who fell and suffered a hip fracture and a consecutive sample of 467 women who fell and did not fracture. They reported that among those who fell on or near their hip, those who fell sideways or straight down were at increased risk for hip fracture (odds ratio = 4.3), whereas those who fell backwards were less likely to suffer a hip fracture (odds ratio = 0.2). Furthermore, low BMD at the femoral neck (odds ratio = 2.6 for a 1 SD decrease) or calcaneus (odds ratio = 2.4 for a 1 SD decrease) strongly increased the risk of fracture among those who fell on or near the hip. Greenspan and co-workers [83] reported similar findings in a study of 149 community-dwelling men and women, including 72 cases who fell and suffered a hip fracture and 77 control subjects who fell and did not fracture. In these elderly fallers, they showed that independent risk factors for hip fracture included characteristics related to fall severity, low bone mineral density at the hip, and body habitus (Table II).

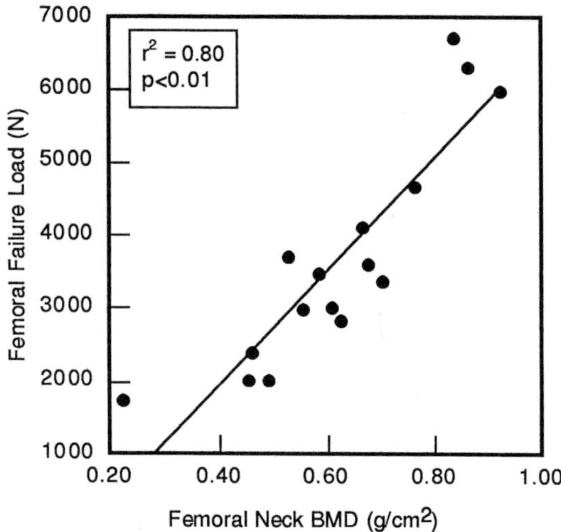

FIGURE 9 Bone mineral density of the femoral neck vs femoral failure load of cadaveric proximal femurs. Femurs were tested to failure in a configuration designed to simulate a sideways fall with impact to the greater trochanter. With permission from Bouxsein *et al.* [105].

Clinical studies provide valuable information about the independent contributions of fall severity and skeletal fragility to hip fracture risk. However, further insight may be achieved by considering a "factor of risk" for hip fracture. The previous two sections have described how laboratory techniques can be used to develop and validate methods for estimating the loads applied to the femur and the load-bearing capacity of the femur from data that can be acquired in a clinical setting. Thus, these findings can be used to estimate the factor of risk for hip fracture due to a sideways fall from standing height.

Myers and co-workers [110] applied the factor of risk concept in a case-control study of elderly fallers. The numerator of the factor of risk, the applied load, was estimated from previous studies of the descent and impact phases of a sideways fall with impact to the lateral aspect of the hip [85–88,91]. Each individuals' body height and weight was used as input parameters for the model to estimate the impact force delivered to the proximal femur during a sideways fall from standing height. The denominator of the factor of risk, the load-bearing capacity of the proximal femur, was determined from linear regressions between noninvasive bone den-

TABLE II Multiple Logistic Regression Analysis of Factors Associated with Hip Fracture in Community-Dwelling Men and Women Who Fell[a]

Factor	Adjusted odds ratio	95% confidence interval	P
Fall to the side	5.7	2.3–14	<0.001
Femoral neck BMD (g/cm^2)[b]	2.7	1.6–4.6	<0.001
Potential energy of fall (Joules)[c]	2.8	1.5–5.2	<0.001
Body mass index (kg/m^2)[b]	2.2	1.2–3.8	0.003

[a] Data from Greenspan *et al.* [83].
[b] Calculated for a decrease of 1 SD.
[c] Calculated for an increase of 1 SD.

sitometry and femoral failure loads in a fall configuration [105]. For each subject, femoral bone mineral density was assessed by DXA and then used to estimate the femoral failure load. There was a strong association between the factor of risk and hip fracture in these elderly fallers, with the odds of hip fracture increasing by 5.1 for a 1 SD increase in the factor of risk (95% confidence interval: 2.9, 9.2) (Fig. 10). In comparison, the odds ratio for a 1 SD decrease in femoral BMD was 2.0 (95% confidence interval: 1.4, 2.6).

BIOMECHANICS OF VERTEBRAL FRACTURES

Investigations of the etiology and biomechanics of vertebral fractures are particularly difficult, as the precise definition of a vertebral fracture remains controversial [111,112]. Vertebral fractures are often characterized by subtle deformities and reductions in height. In addition, many fractures that are identified by radiographic review are asymptomatic [113], further complicating the interpretation of many studies. Thus, in contrast to the growing recognition of the importance of bone fragility and fall severity in the etiology of hip fractures, the role of spinal loading in the etiology of age-related vertebral fractures has received relatively little attention [114,115]. As loads are applied to the spine during nearly every activity of daily living, it is important to distinguish which of these activities (and the resulting loads on the spine) are associated with vertebral fractures to try to understand the loading environment that leads to vertebral fractures.

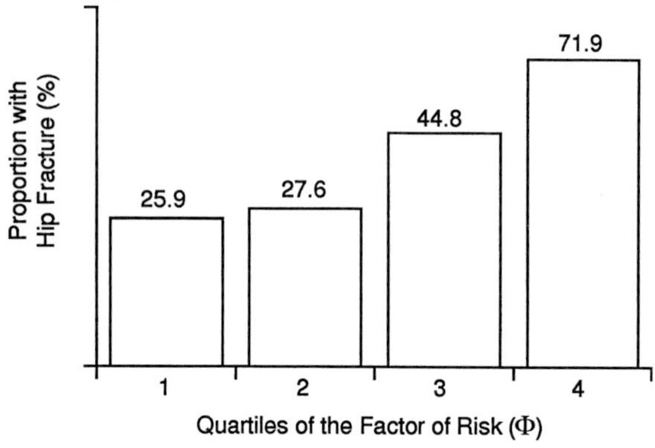

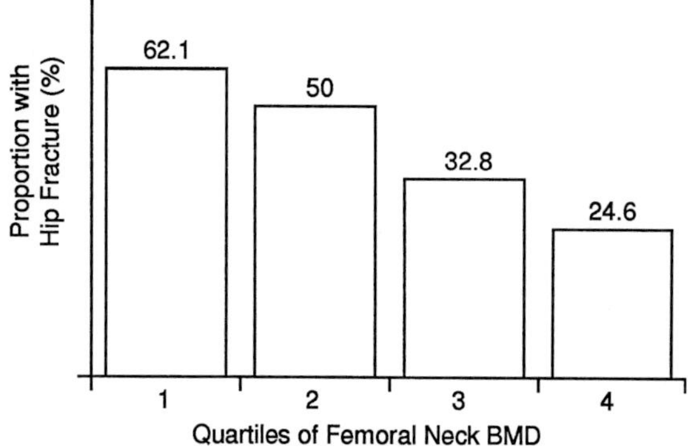

FIGURE 10 Proportion of subjects with hip fracture in each quartile of the factor of risk for hip fracture (top) and femoral neck BMD (bottom). Data from Myers *et al.* [110].

Loads Applied to the Spine

A few observational studies have attempted to identify the activities surrounding the onset of a vertebral fracture. These investigators have reviewed medical records or interviewed patients to assess the "degree of trauma" associated with vertebral fractures [113,116–118]. Cooper *et al.* [113] reviewed medical records from a 5-year period to determine the circumstances associated with "clinically diagnosed" vertebral fractures in a population-based sample of 341 Rochester, Minnesota, residents. In their study, a specific loading event was reported for approximately 50% of the total fractures. In contrast to the commonly held belief that lifting plays a major role in the development of vertebral fractures, relatively few of the fractures were associated with lifting. Excluding fractures that were diagnosed incidentally, only 10% of fractures were associated with "lifting a heavy object," whereas nearly 40% were associated with falling. In a hospital-based study, Myers *et al.* [119] interviewed patients after diagnosis of a vertebral fracture, with respect to their activity at the time of fracture. Their results indicate that nearly 50% of acute, symptomatic vertebral fractures in individuals over age 60 are associated with a fall, whereas 20% are associated with "controlled" activities, such as bending, lifting, and reaching. Most of the remainder of the patients could not identify a specific activity at the time of fracture. Therefore, determining the forces on the spine during controlled activities and falls may improve our understanding of the biomechanics of vertebral fractures.

Although it is impossible to measure the loads on the vertebral bodies *in vivo,* investigators have used kinematic analysis, electromyographic measurements, and biomechanical modeling to estimate the loads on the lumbar spine during various activities [120–123]. The models use optimization techniques to estimate the trunk muscle forces and compressive forces on the spine during various tasks and have been verified by comparing predicted compressive spine loads and muscle activity with direct measurements of intradiscal pressure

[123–126] and myoelectric trunk muscle activity [120,121,123,127–129].

These models were originally developed to study the potential origins and mechanisms of low-back pain and injury in working adults. Therefore, they are generally based on anthropometric data from young, healthy adults and are limited to estimating the vertebral forces in the lumbar region. However, Wilson [130] has extended these models to include the mid- and lower thoracic spine and incorporated geometric properties of the trunk using computed tomography (CT) scans of older individuals. Using this model, they computed the compressive forces applied to the T8, T11, and L2 vertebrae during various activities for a woman who weighed 65 kg and was 1.6 m tall (mean values from a cohort of 120 women aged 65 yrs or older [131]). The estimated forces to the spine ranged from approximately 400 to 2100 N for typical activities. From these estimates, it is clear that everyday activities, such as rising from a chair or bending over and picking up a full grocery bag, can generate high forces on the spine.

There are currently few biomechanicals models designed to estimate the load on the spine during falls. However, based on data from a study of the dynamics of backwards falls [132] and from the previously described "pelvis-release" experiments [86], Myers and Wilson [115] estimated that the impact force on the pelvis due to a backward fall would be approximately 2000–2500 N. This impact force would be expected to be dissipated somewhat before reaching the thoracolumbar spine. Research projects are currently underway to further characterize the loads applied to the spine during falls in order to better our understanding of the circumstances surrounding acute vertebral fractures.

Load-Bearing Capacity of Vertebrae

As in other skeletal structures, the load-bearing capacity of a vertebra is determined by its instrinsic material properties, as well as its overall geometry and shape. The vertebral body is characterized by a central core of trabecular bone surrounded by a thin covering of condensed trabecular bone (often referred to as a "cortical shell") [133,134]. In the spine, compressive loads are transferred from the intervertebral discs to adjacent vertebral bodies. Therefore, age-related changes in the properties of the intervertebral disc, the vertebral centrum, and the vertebral shell can each influence the load-bearing capacity of vertebrae. For instance, the thickness of the outer shell decreases from approximately 400–500 μm at age 20–40, to 200–300 μm at age 70–80, and to 120–150 μm in osteoporotic individuals [135]. The relative contributions of the vertebral centrum and shell to overall vertebral strength remain controversial. It is suggested that the vertebral shell may account for 10–30% of vertebral strength in healthy individuals and, due to decreased bone mass in the trabecular centrum, from 50 to 90% in osteoporotic persons [134–139].

A number of laboratory investigations have been conducted to relate the load-bearing capacity of human lumbar and thoracic vertebrae to age, bone density, and vertebral geometry [14,18,138,140–150]. The load-bearing capacity of thoracolumbar vertebrae is reduced from a value of 8000–10,000 N at age 20–30 to 1000–2000 N by age 70–80 [135,151]. In severely osteoporotic individuals, the load-bearing capacity may be even less [147].

The load-bearing capacity of human vertebrae is strongly correlated with noninvasive estimates of vertebral bone density and geometry, with approximately 50–80% of the variance in load-bearing capacity explained by parameters measured noninvasively [18,138,141–150]. For example, strong correlations have been reported between bone density and vertebral cross-sectional area assessed by QCT and vertebral failure loads [143,144]. In addition, several investigators have reported strong correlations between bone mineral density, assessed by DXA, and vertebral strength [147,148,150]. For example, Moro *et al.* [147] found that lumbar bone mineral density assessed by DXA correlates strongly with the compressive failure load and energy to failure of both L2 and T11 vertebrae (Fig. 11). The standard error of the estimate for predicting vertebral failure load from lumbar BMD was 527 N (25% of the mean failure load) for T11 and 733 N (28% of the mean failure load) for L2.

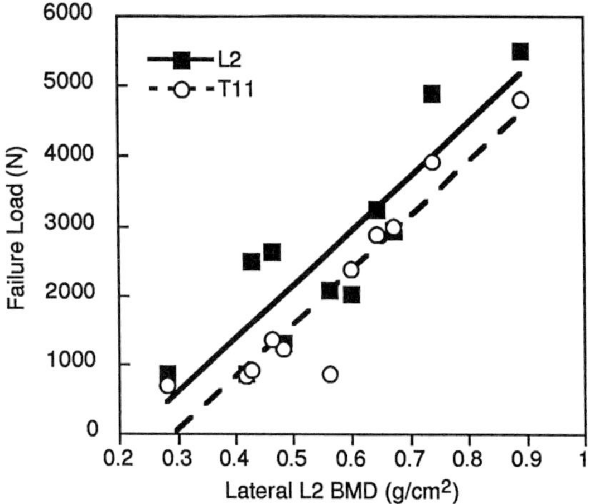

FIGURE 11 Linear relationship between lumbar BMD and compressive failure loads of T11 and L2 vertebrae as reported by Moro *et al.* [147]. The correlation coefficients between lumbar BMD and failure loads of T11 and L2 were r = 0.94 ($P < 0.001$) and r = 0.89 ($P < 0.001$), respectively.

Thus, it appears that noninvasive assessments of bone mass and bone mineral density provide a reasonable estimate of the failure loads of cadaveric vertebrae subjected to controlled compression tests in the laboratory. It remains to be seen whether BMD or other bone density parameters can predict the strength of vertebrae subjected to loading conditions that may more closely resemble the mechanical environment *in vivo,* such as falling or compression combined with forward flexion or compression combined with lateral bleeding.

Factor of Risk for Vertebral Fractures

Although it has not been demonstrated clearly by clinical surveillance studies, it seems reasonable to suggest that, similar to hip fractures, both bone fragility and skeletal loading are important factors in the etiology of vertebral fractures [152]. To investigate the potential roles of bone fragility and spinal loading, Myers and Wilson [115] estimated a factor of risk for vertebral fractures for various activities of daily living (Fig. 12). As before, the factor of risk was defined as the ratio between load applied to the bone and its load-bearing capacity for a given loading event. They estimated the numerator of the factor of risk (i.e., the applied load) using predictions of compressive loading in the spine from the model developed by Wilson [130]. The denominator of the factor of risk (i.e., the failure load) was estimated from linear regressions between lumbar BMD and the compressive failure load of cadaveric vertebrae [147].

Their predictions of the factor of risk indicate that osteopenic individuals may perform many activities wherein their factor of risk for vertebral fracture is close to or greater than one, suggesting that they are at high risk for fracture. Individuals with *extremely low* bone mineral density may be at risk for vertebral fracture during simple activities such as tying one's shoes or opening a window. Individuals with low bone mineral density (still in the osteopenic range) may be at risk for vertebral fracture when lifting groceries out of the car or picking up a toddler. These examples illustrate the need for strategies to prevent vertebral fractures, such as reducing spinal loading by avoiding certain "high-risk" activities.

SUMMARY

This chapter emphasized the concept that age-related fractures represent a structural failure whereby the

BMD (g/cm2)	0.3	0.4	0.5	0.6	0.7	0.8	0.9
Get up from sitting	1.5	0.6	0.4	0.3	0.2	0.2	0.2
Lift 15 kg knees straight	2.6	1.1	0.7	0.5	0.4	0.3	0.3
Lift 15 kg w/ deep knee bend	2.1	0.9	0.6	0.4	0.3	0.3	0.2
Lift 30 kg knees straight	3.7	1.5	1.0	0.7	0.6	0.5	0.4
Lift 30 kg w/ deep knee bend	3.0	1.3	0.8	0.6	0.5	0.4	0.3
Open window w/ 50 N of force	1.1	0.5	0.3	0.2	0.2	0.1	0.1
Open window w/ 100 N of force	1.4	0.6	0.4	0.3	0.2	0.2	0.2
Tie shoes sitting down	1.4	0.6	0.4	0.3	0.2	0.2	0.2

FIGURE 12 Factor of risk for vertebral fracture for eight common activities as a function of lumbar bone mineral density. The numerator of the factor of risk was determined from models of spine loading at L2 for an elderly woman of average height and weight. The denominator was determined on the basis of regression analysis between lateral lumbar BMD and the load-bearing capacity of the L2 vertebra. Values for lateral BMD cover a wide range and got down to very low values. The T score (number of standard deviations from the mean value for BMD in young women) is approximately +1 for a BMD = 0.9 g/cm^2 and −5 for BMD = 0.4 g/cm^2. The factor of risk is predicted to be greater than or close to 1 for low BMD values (shaded area). With permission from Myers and Wilson [115].

forces applied to the bone exceed its load-bearing capacity. Viewing fractures in this manner, it is clear that studies of their etiology must include factors that influence skeletal fragility or its load-bearing capacity, as well as those that influence the forces that are applied to the skeleton.

The load-bearing capacity of a skeletal structure is determined by its intrinsic material properties as well as the total amount (size) and spatial distribution (shape) of the bone tissue. Considerable evidence indicates that the material properties of both cortical and trabecular bone decrease with increasing age in both men and women. This decrease in material properties is likely due, in part, to age-related reductions in bone mass, as the elastic modulus and strength of trabecular bone are related to density by a squared relationship. Therefore, small changes in bone density can dramatically influence bone material properties. These decrements in bone density and material properties may be partially offset by geometric rearrangement of the bone tissue, particularly in the long bones, that helps to preserve the bone's ability to resist bending and torsional loads.

Estimates of the forces applied to the proximal femur during a sideways fall range from 2900 to 4260 N for the 5th to 95th percentile woman based on height and weight. Factors that influence the load applied to the femur include, but are not limited to, fall height, fall direction, body habitus, muscle activity, and trochanteric soft tissue thickness. In comparison, estimates of the load required to fracture the elderly cadaveric femur in a configuration simulating a sideways fall range from 800 to 10,000 N. This femoral failure load is influenced by femoral bone mineral content and density, femoral geometry, and the direction and rate of the applied load.

In contrast to hip fractures, little is known about the combined roles of spinal loading and skeletal fragility in the etiology of vertebral fractures. In contrast to previously held beliefs that vertebral fractures are caused primarily by bending and lifting activities, evidence shows that falls may play a significant role in the etiology of vertebral fractures. Thus, future studies should incorporate assessments of fall severity in order to determine the characteristics of falls associated with vertebral fracture. In addition, models to estimate the loads applied to the spine during a fall should be developed. Mathematical models used to estimate the forces generated in the spine during bending and lifting activities indicate that compressive forces generated in the lower thoracic and upper lumbar spine range from approximately 400 to 2100 N. A comparison of these loads with predicted vertebral strengths suggests that activities of daily living may place the elderly, osteopenic person at high risk for vertebral fracture.

To date, investigators have focused primarily on methods to prevent bone loss and to restore bone to the osteopenic skeleton. However, alternative approaches for fracture prevention that are directed at reducing the loads applied to the skeleton may prove to be both effective and cost efficient. For example, trochanteric padding systems designed to reduce the load applied to the hip during a fall have shown great potential for reducing fracture risk [89,153]. Vertebral fracture incidence may be reduced by teaching high-risk patients to avoid activities that generate high loads on the spine, thereby putting them at increased risk for fracture. Clearly, identification of these high-risk activities is critical to the success of this approach for preventing fractures. Ultimately, fracture prevention may be best achieved by an educational program designed to limit high-risk activities in conjunction with interventions targeted at increasing bone mass and reducing loads applied to the skeleton during traumatic events.

References

1. Cooper, C., and Melton, L. Epidemiology of osteoporosis. *Trends Endocrinol. Metab.* **3,** 224–229 (1992).
2. Ray, N. F., Chan, J., Thamer, M., and Melton, L. Medical expenditures for the treatment of osteoporotic fracture in the United States in 1995: Report from the National Osteoporosis Foundation. *J. Bone Miner. Res.* **12,** 24–35 (1997).
3. Praemer, A., Furner, S., and Rice, D., "Musculoskeletal Conditions in the United States." American Academy of Orthopeadic Surgeons, Park Ridge, IL, 1992.
4. Cooper, C., Campion, G., and Melton, L. J. Hip fractures in the elderly: a world-wide projection. *Osteopor. Int.* **2,** 285–289 (1992).
5. Hayes, W., Piazza, S., and Zysset, P. Biomechanics of fracture risk prediction of the hip and spine by quantitative computed tomography. *In* "Radiologic Clinics of North America" (D. I., Rosenthal, ed.), pp. 1–18. Saunders, Philadelphia, 1991.
6. Burstein, A., Reilly, D., and Martens, M. Aging of bone tissue: mechanical properties. *J. Bone Joint Surg.* **58A,** 82–86 (1976).
7. Currey, J. The mechanical consequences of variation in the mineral content of bone. *J. Biomech.* **2,** 1–11 (1969).
8. Lindahl, O., and Lindgren, A. Cortical bone in man. II. Variation in tensile strength with age and sex. *Acta Orthop. Scand.* **38,** 141–147 (1967).
9. Melick, R., and Miller, D. Variations of tensil strength of human cortical bone with age. *Clin. Sci.* **30,** 243–248 (1996).
10. Smith, C., and Smith, D. Relations between age, mineral density and mechanical properties of human femoral compacta. *Acta Orthop. Scand.* **47,** 496–502 (1976).
11. Wall, J. C., Chatterji, S. K., and Jeffery, J. W. Age-related changes in the density and tensile strength of human femoral cortical bone. *Calcif. Tissue Int.* **27,** 105–108 (1979).
12. McCalden, R., McGeough, J., Barker, M., and Court-Brown, C. Age-related changes in the tensile properties of cortical bone. *J. Bone Joint Surg.* **75A,** 1193–1205 (1993).
13. Zioupos, P., and Currey, J. Changes in the stiffness, strength, and toughness of human cortical bone with age. *Bone* **22,** 57–66 (1998).

14. Bell, G. H., Dunbar, O., and Beck, J. S. Variations in strength of vertebrae with age and their relation to osteoporosis. *Calcif. Tissue Res.* **1,** 75–86 (1967).
15. Mosekilde, L., and Mosekilde, L. Normal vertebral body size and compressive strength: relations to age and to vertebral and iliac trabecular bone compressive strength. *Bone* **7,** 207–212 (1986).
16. Mosekilde, L., and Mosekilde, L. Sex differences in age-related changes in vertebral body size, density and biomechanical competence in normal individuals. *Bone* **11,** 67–73 (1990).
17. Weaver, J., and Chalmers, J. Cancellous bone: its strength and changes with ageing and an evaluation of some methods for measuring its mineral content. *J. Bone Joint Surg.* **48A,** 289–299 (1966).
18. Mosekilde, L., Viidik, A., and Mosekilde, L. Correlation between the compressive strength of iliac and vertebral trabecular bone in normal individuals. *Bone* **6,** 291–295 (1985).
19. Mosekilde, L., Mosekilde, L., and Danielson, C. C. Biomechanical competance of vertebral trabecular bone in relation of ash density and age in normal individuals. *Bone* **8,** 79–85 (1987).
20. Ding, M., Dalstra, M., Danielsen, C., Kabel, J., Hvid, I., and Linde, F. Age variations in the properties of human tibial trabecular bone. *J. Bone Joint Surg.* **79B,** 995–1002 (1997).
21. Currey, J. D. Changes in the impact energy absorption of bone with age. *J. Biomech.* **12,** 459–469 (1979).
22. Britton, J. M., and Davie, M. W. J. Mechanical properties of bone from iliac crest and relationship to L5 vertebral bone. *Bone* **11,** 21–28 (1990).
23. Mosekilde, L. Age-related changes in vertebral trabecular bone architecture—assessed by a new method. *Bone* **9,** 247–250 (1988).
24. Mosekilde, L. Sex differences in age-related loss of vertebral trabecular bone mass and structure—biomechanical consequences. *Bone* **10,** 425–432 (1989).
25. Lindahl, O. Mechanical properties of dried defatted spongy bone. *Acta Orthop. Scand.* **47,** 11–19 (1976).
26. Carter, D. R., and Hayes, W. C. Bone compressive strength: the influence of density and strain rate. *Science* **194,** 1174–1176 (1976).
27. Carter, D. R., and Hayes, W. C. The compressive behavior of bone as a two-phase porous structure. *J. Bone Joint Surg.* **59A,** 954–962 (1977).
28. Keaveny, T. M., and Hayes, W. C. A 20-year perspective on the mechanical properties of trabecular bone. *J. Biomech. Eng.* **115,** 534–542 (1993).
29. Rice, J. C., Cowin, S. C., and Bowman, J. A. On the dependence of the elasticity and strength of cancellous bone on apparent density. *J. Biomech.* **21,** 155–168 (1988).
30. Esses, S. I., Lotz, J. C., and Hayes, W. C. Biomechanical properties of the proximal femur determined in vitro by single-energy quantitative computed tomography. *J. Bone Miner. Res.* **4,** 715–722 (1989).
31. Hvid, I., Bentzen, S., Linde, F., Losekilde, L., and Pongsoipetch, B. X-ray quantitative computed tomography: the relations to physical properties of proximal tibial trabecular bone specimens. *J. Biomech.* **22,** 837–844 (1989).
32. Goulet, R., Goldstein, S., Ciarelli, M., Kuhn, J., Brown, M., and Feldkamp, L. The relationship between the structural and orthogonal compressive properties of trabecular bone. *J. Biomech.* **27,** 375–389 (1994).
33. Linde, F., Hvid, I., and Pongosoipetch, B. Energy absorptive properties of human trabecular bone specimens during axial compression. *J. Orthop. Res.* **7,** 432–439 (1989).
34. Lotz, J., Gerhart, T., and Hayes, W. Mechanical properties of trabecular bone from the proximal femur: a quantitative CT study. *J. Comp. Assist. Tomogr.* **14,** 107–113 (1990).
35. Keyak, J., Lee, I., and Skinner, H. Correlations between orthogonal mechanical properties and density of trabecular bone: use of different densitometric measures. *J. Biomed. Mater. Res.* **28,** 1329–1336 (1994).
36. Martens, M., Van Audekerchke, R., Delport, P., De Meester, P., and Mulier, J. The mechanical characteristics of cancellous bone at the upper femoral region. *J. Biomech.* **16,** 971–983 (1983).
37. Gibson, L. The mechanical behaviour of cancellous bone. *J. Biomech.* **18,** 317–328 (1985).
38. Compston, J. Connectivity of cancellous bone: assessment and mechanical implications. *Bone* **15,** 463–466 (1994).
39. Snyder, B. D., Piazza, S., Edwards, W. T., and Hayes, W. C. Role of trabecular morphology in the etiology of age-related vertebral fractures. *Calcif. Tissue Int.* **53,** S14–S22 (1993).
40. Bergot, C., Laval-Jeantet, A., Prêteux, F., and Meunier, A. Measurement of anisotropic vertebral trabecular bone loss during aging by quantitative image analysis. *Calcif. Tissue, Int.* **43,** 143–149 (1988).
41. Silva, M., and Gibson, L. Modeling the mechanical behavior of vertebral bone: effects of age-related changes in microstructure. *Bone* **21,** 191–199 (1997).
42. Burr, D. B., Schaffler, M. B., and Frederickson, R. G. Composition of the cement line and its possible mechanical role as a local interface in human compact bone. *J. Biomech.* **21,** 939–945 (1988).
43. Burstein, A., Zika, J., Heiple, K., and Klein, L. Contribution of collagen and mineral to the elastic-plastic properties of bone. *J. Bone Joint. Surg.* **57,** 956–961 (1975).
44. Carando, S., Portigliatti Barbos, M., Ascenzi, A., and Boyde, A. Orientation of collagen in human tibial and fibular shafts and possible correlation with mechanical properties. *Bone* **10,** 139–142 (1989).
45. Carter, D. R., and Hayes, W. C. Compact bone fatigue damage—I. Residual strength and stiffness. *J. Biomech.* **10,** 325–337 (1977).
46. Evans, F., and Vincintelli, R. Relations of the compressive properties of human cortical bone to histological structure and calcification. *J. Biomech.* **7,** 1–10 (1974).
47. Katz, J., and Meunier, A. The elastic anisotropy of bone. *J. Biomech.* **20,** 1063–1070 (1987).
48. Martin, R., and Ishida, J. The relative effects of collagen fiber orientation, porosity, density, and mineralization on bone strength. *J. Biomech.* **22,** 419–426 (1989).
49. Schaffler, M. B., Choi, K., and Milgrom, C. Microcracks and aging in human femoral compact bone. *Trans. Orthop. Res. Soc.* **19,** 190 (1994).
50. Burr, D., Forwood, M., Fyhrie, D., Martin, R., Schaffler, M., and Turner, C. Bone microdamage and skeletal fragility in osteoporotic and stress fractures. *J. Bone Miner. Res.* **12,** 6–15 (1997).
51. Martin, R. Aging and strength of bone as a structural material. *Calcif. Tissue Int.* **53**(Suppl. 1), S34–S40 (1993).
52. Hoshaw, S., Cody, D., Saad, A., and Fhyrie, D. Decrease in canine proximal femoral ultimate strength and stiffness due to fatigue damage. *J. Biomech.* **30,** 323–329 (1997).
53. Mori, S., Harruf, R., Ambrosius, W., and Burr, D. Trabecular bone volume and microdamage accumulation in the femoral heads of women with and without femora neck fractures. *Bone* **21,** 521–526 (1997).
54. Schaffler, M., Choi, and Milgrom, C. Aging and matrix microdamage accumulation in human compact bone. *Bone* **17,** 521–525 (1995).

55. Wenzel, T., Schaffler, M., and Fyhrie, D. In vivo trabecular microcracks in human vertebral bone. *Bone* **19,** 89–95 (1996).
56. Norman, T., and Wang, Z. Microdamage of human cortical bone: incidence and morphology in long bones. *Bone* **20,** 375–379 (1997).
57. Courtney, A., Hayes, W., and Gibson, L. Age-related differences in post-yield damage in human cortical bone. Experiment and model. *J. Biomech.* **29,** 1463–1471 (1996).
58. van der Meulen, M. C. H., Beaupré, G. S., and Carter, D. R. Mechanobiologic influences in long bone cross-sectional growth. *Bone* **14,** 635–642 (1993).
59. Bouxsein, M., Myburgh, K., van der Meulen, M., Lindenberger, E., and Marcus, R. Age-related differences in cross-sectional geometry of the forearm bones in healthy women. *Calcif. Tissue Int.* **54,** 113–118 (1994).
60. Garn, S., Rohmann, C., Wagner, B., and Ascoli, W. Continuing bone growth throughout life: a general phenomenon. *Am. J. Phys. Anthrop.* **26,** 313–318 (1967).
61. Ruff, C., and Hayes, W. Subperiosteal expansion and cortical remodeling of the human femur and tibia with aging. *Science* **217,** 945–947 (1982).
62. Ruff, C., and Hayes, W. Cross-sectional geometry of Pecos Pueblo femora and tibiae—A biomechanical investigation: I. Method and general patterns of variation. *Am. J. Phys. Anthropol.* **60,** 359–381 (1983).
63. Smith, R., and Walker, R. Femoral expansion in aging women: implications for osteoporosis and fractures. *Science* **145,** 156–157 (1964).
64. Beck, T., Ruff, C., and Bissessur, K. Age-related changes in female femoral neck geometry: Implications for bone strength. *Calcif. Tissue Int.* **53**(Suppl. 1), S41–S46 (1993).
65. Burr, D., and Martin, R. The effects of composition, structure and age on the torsional properties of the human radius. *J. Biomech.* **16,** 603–608 (1983).
66. Martin, R., and Atkinson, P. Age and sex-related changes in the structure and strength of the human femoral shaft. *J. Biomech.* **10,** 223–231 (1977).
67. Meema, H. Cortical bone atrophy and osteoporosis as a manifestation of aging. *Am. J. Roentgenol. Radium Ther. Nuclear Med.* **89,** 1287–1295 (1963).
68. Ruff, D., and Hayes, W. Sex differences in age-related remodeling of the femur and tibia. *J. Orthop. Res.* **6,** 886–896 (1988).
69. Ericksen, M. F. Some aspects of aging in the lumbar spine. *Am. J. Phys. Anthrop.* **45,** 575–580 (1976).
70. Martin, R. B., and Burr, D. B. Non-invasive measurement of long bone cross-sectional moment of inertia by photon absorptiometry. *J. Biomech.* **17,** 195–201 (1984).
71. Beck, T. J., Ruff, C. B., Warden, K. E., Scott, W. W., and Rao, G. U. Predicting femoral neck strength from bone mineral data. *Invest. Radiol.* **25,** 6–18 (1990).
72. Beck, T., Ruff, C., Scott, W., Jr., Plato, C., Tobin, J., and Quan, C. Sex differences in geometry of the femoral neck with aging: a structural analysis of bone mineral data. *Calcif. Tissue Int.* **50,** 24–29 (1992).
73. Nakamura, T., *et al.* Do variations in hip geometry explain differences in hip fracture risk between Japanese and white Americans? *J. Bone Miner. Res.* **9,** 1071–1076 (1994).
74. Yoshikawa, T., *et al.* Geometric structure of the femoral neck measured using dual-energy x-ray absorptiometry. *J. Bone Miner. Res.* **9,** 1053–1064 (1994).
75. Cummings, S., *et al.* Appendicular bone density and age predict hip fractures in women. *JAMA* **263,** 665–668 (1990).
76. Grisso, J. A., *et al.* Risk factors for falls as a cause of hip fracture in women. *N. Engl. J. Med.* **324,** 1326–1331 (1991).
77. Michelson, J., Myers, A., Jinnah, R., Cox, Q., and Van Natta, M. Epidemiology of hip fractures among the elderly. Risk factors for fracture type. *Clin. Orthop. Rel. Res.* **311,** 129–135 (1995).
78. Nevitt, M. C., Cummings, S. R., and Hudes, E. S. Risk factors for injurious falls: a prospective study. *J. Gerontol.* **46,** M164–M170 (1991).
79. Tinetti, M. Factors associated with serious injury during falls among elderly persons living in the community. *J. Am. Geriatr. Soc.* **35,** 644–648 (1987).
80. Hayes, W., Myers, E., Morris, J. N., Yett, H. S., and Lipsitz, L. A. Impact near the hip dominates fracture risk in elderly nursing home residents who fall. *Calcif. Tissue Int.* **52,** 192–198 (1993).
81. Sattin, R. Falls among older persons. *Annu. Rev. Publ. Health* **13,** 489–508 (1992).
82. Cummings, S., and Nevitt, M. A hypothesis: the causes of hip fracture. *J. Gerontol.* **44,** M107–M111 (1989).
83. Greenspan, S. L., Myers, E. R., Maitland, L. A., Resnick, N. M., and Hayes, W. C. Fall severity and bone mineral density as risk factors for hip fracture in ambulatory elderly. *JAMA* **217,** 128–133 (1994).
84. Nevitt, M. C., and Cummings, S. R. Type of fall and risk of hip and wrist fractures: The study of osteoporotic fractures. *J. Am. Geriatr. Soc.* **41,** 1226–1234 (1993).
85. van den Kroonenberg, A., Hayes, W., and McMahon, T. Hip impact velocities and body configurations for experimental falls from standing height. *J. Biomech.* **29,** 807–811 (1996).
86. Robinovitch, S., Hayes, W., and McMahon, T. Prediction of femoral impact forces in falls on the hip. *J. Biomech. Eng.* **113,** 366–374 (1991).
87. Robinovitch, S., Hayes, W., and McMahon, T. Predicting the impact response of a nonlinear, single-degree-of-freedom shock-absorbing system from the measured step response. *J. Biomech. Eng.* **119,** 221–227 (1997).
88. Robinovitch, S., Hayes, W., and McMahon, T. Distribution of contact force during impact to the hip. *Ann. Biomed. Engl.* **25,** 499–508 (1997).
89. Robinovitch, S., Hayes, W., and McMahon, T. Energy-shunting hip padding system attenuates femoral impact force in a simulated fall. *J. Biomech. Eng.* **117,** 409–413 (1995).
90. Robinovitch, S., McMahon, T., and Hayes, W. Force attenuation in trochanteric soft tissues during impact from a fall. *J. Orthop. Res.* **13,** 956–962 (1995).
91. van den Kroonenberg, A., Hayes, W., and McMahon, T. Dynamic models for sideways falls from standing height. *J. Biomech. Eng.* **117,** 309–318 (1995).
92. Hemenway, D., Azrael, D., Rimm, E., Feskanich, D., and Willett, W. Risk factors for hip fracture in US men aged 40 through 75 years. *Am. J. Public Health* **84,** 1843–1845 (1994).
93. Cummings, S. R., *et al.* Bone density at various sites for prediction of hip fractures. *Lancet* **341,** 72–75 (1993).
94. Nevitt, M., Johnell, O., Black, D., Ensrud, K., Genant, H., and Cummings, S. Bone mineral density predicts non-spine fractures in very elderly women. *Osteopor. Int.* **4,** 325–331 (1994).
95. Ross, P. D., Davis, J. W., and Wasnich, R. D. A critical review of bone mass and the risk of fractures in osteoporosis. *Calcif. Tissue Int.* **46,** 149–161 (1990).
96. Hans, D., *et al.* Ultrasonographic heel measurements to predict hip fracture in elderly women: the EPIDOS prospective study. *Lancet* **348,** 511–514 (1996).
97. Dalén, N., Hellström, L., and Jacobson, B. Bone mineral content and mechanical strength of the femoral neck. *Acta Orthrop. Scand.,* **47,** 503–508 (1976).

98. Leichter, I., *et al.* The relation between bone density, mineral content, and mechanical strength in the femoral neck. *Clin. Orthop. Rel. Res.* **163,** 272–281 (1982).
99. Mizrahi, J., Margulies, J. Y., Leichter, I., and Deutsch, D. Fracture of the human femoral neck: Effect of density of the cancellous core. *J. Biomed. Eng.* **6,** 56–62 (1984).
100. Sartoris, D. J., Sonner, F. G., Kosek, J., Gies, A., and Carter, D. R. Dual-energy projection radiography in the evaluation of femoral neck strength, density, and mineralization. *Invest. Radiol.* **20,** 476–485 (1985).
101. Alho, A., Husby, T., and Høiseth, A. Bone mineral content and mechanical strength—an *ex vivo* study on human femora at autopsy. *Clin. Orthop. Rel. Res.,* **227,** 292–297 (1988).
102. Lotz, J., and Hayes, W. The use of quantitative computed tomography to estimate risk of fracture of the hip from falls. *J. Bone Joint Surg.* **72A,** 689–700 (1990).
103. Courtney, A., Wachtel, E. F., Myers, E. R., and Hayes, W. C. Age-related reductions in the strength of the femur tested in a fall loading configuration. *J. Bone Joint Surg.* **77,** 387–395 (1995).
104. Courtney, A., Wachtel, E. F., Myers, E. R., and Hayes, W. C. Effects of loading rate on the strength of the proximal femur. *Calcif. Tissue Int.* **55,** 53–58 (1994).
105. Bouxsein, M., Courtney, A., and Hayes, W. Ultrasound and densitometry of the calcaneus correlate with the failure loads of cadaveric femurs. *Calcif. Tissue Int.* **56,** 99–103 (1995).
106. Pinilla, T., Boardman, K., Bouxsein, M., Myers, E., and Hayes, W. Differences in loading direction from a fall can reduce the failure load of the proximal femur as much as age-related bone loss. *Trans. Orthop. Res. Soc.* **20,** 239 (1995).
107. Cheng, X., *et al.* Assessment of the strength of proximal femur in vitro: Relationship to femoral bone mineral density and femoral geometry. *Bone* **20,** 213–218 (1997).
108. Faulkner, K. G., Cummings, S. R., Black, D., Palermo, L., Glüer, C. C., and Genant, H. K. Simple measurement of femoral geometry predicts hip fracture: The study of osteoporotic fracture. *J. Bone Miner. Res.* **8,** 1211–1217 (1993).
109. Glüer, C. C., *et al.* Prediction of hip fractures from pelvic radiographs: The study of osteoporotic fractures. *J. Bone Miner. Res.* **9,** 671–677 (1994).
110. Myers, E. R., Robinovitch, S. N., Greenspan, S. L., and Hayes, W. C. Factor of risk is associated with frequency of hip fracture in a case-control study. *Trans. Orthop. Res. Soc.* **19,** 526 (1994).
111. O'Neill, T., *et al.* Variation in vertebral height ratios in population studies. *J. Bone Miner. Res.* **9,** 1895–1907 (1994).
112. Kleerekoper, M., and Nelson, D. Vertebral fracture or vertebral deformity? *Calcif. Tissue Int.* **50,** 5–6 (1992).
113. Cooper, C., Atkinson, E., O'Fallon, W., and Melton, L. Incidence of clinically diagnosed vertebral fractures: a population-based study in Rochester, Minnesota, 1985–1989. *J. Bone Miner. Res.* **7,** 221–227 (1992).
114. Nevitt, M. C. Epidemiology of Osteoporosis. *In* "Rheumatic Disease Clinics of North America: Osteoporosis" (N. E. Lane, ed.), pp. 535–560. Saunders, Philadelphia, 1994.
115. Myers, E., and Wilson, S. Biomechanics of osteoporosis and vertebral fractures. *Spine* **22,** 25S–31S (1997).
116. Bengnér, U., Johnell, O., and Redlund-Johnell, I. Changes in incidence and prevalence of vertebral fractures during 30 years. *Calcif. Tissue Int.* **42,** 293–296 (1988).
117. Patel, U., Skingle, S., Campbell, G., Crisp, A., and Boyle, I. Clinical profile of acute vertebral compression fractures in osteoporosis. *Br. J. Rheumatol.* **30,** 418–421 (1991).
118. Santavirta, S., Konttinen, Y., Heliövaara, M., Knekt, P., Lüthje, P., and Aromaa, A. Determinants of osteoporotic thoracic vertebral fracture. *Acta Orthop. Scand.* **63,** 198–202 (1992).
119. Myers, E., Wilson, S., and Greenspan, S. Vertebral fractures in the elderly occur with falling and bending. *J. Bone Miner. Res.* **11,** S355 (1996).
120. Andersson, G. B. J., Örtengren, R., and Schultz, A. Analysis and measurement of the loads on the lumbar spine during work at a table. *J. Biomech.* **13,** 513–520 (1980).
121. Schultz, A. B., Andersson, G. B. J., Haderspeck, K., Örtengren, R., Nordin, M., and Björk, R. Analysis and measurement of lumbar trunk loads in tasks involving bends and twists. *J. Biomech.* **15,** 669–675 (1982).
122. Schultz, A. B., and Andersson, G. B. J. Analysis of loads on the lumbar spine. *Spine* **6,** 76–82 (1981).
123. Schultz, A., Andersson G., Ortengren, R., Haderspeck, K., and Nachemson, A. Loads on the lumbar spine. Validation of a biomechanical analysis by measurements of intradiscal pressures and myoelectric signals. *J. Bone Joint Surg.* **64A,** 713–720 (1982).
124. Jäger, M., and Luttmann, A. Biomechanical analysis and assessment of lumbar stress during load lifting using a dynamic 19-segment human model. *Ergonomics* **32,** 93–112 (1989).
125. Nachemson, A., and Elfström, G. Intravital dynamic pressure measurements in lumbar discs. *Scand. J. Rehab. Med.* Suppl. 1, 3–40 (1970).
126. Nachemson, A. L. The lumbar spine–An orthopaedic challenge. *Spine* **1,** 59–69 (1976).
127. Cholewicki, J., McGill, S., and Norman, R. Comparison of muscle forces and joint load from an optimization and EMG assisted lumbar spine model: Towards development of a hybrid approach. *J. Biomech.* **28,** 321–331 (1995).
128. Schultz, A., Andersson, G. B. J., Örtengren, R., Björk, R., and Nordin, M. Analysis and quantitative myoelectric measurements of loads on the lumbar spine when holding weights in standing postures. *Spine* **7,** 390–397 (1982).
129. Yettram, A., and Jackman, M. Equilibrium analysis for the forces in the human spinal column and its musculature. *Spine* **5,** 402–411 (1980).
130. Wilson, S., "Development of a Model to Predict the Compressive Forces on the Spine Associated with Age-Related Vertebral Fractures." Massachusetts Institute of Technology, 1994.
131. Greenspan, S., Maitland-Ramsey, L., and Myers, E. Classification of osteoporosis in the elderly is dependent on site-specific analysis. *Calcif. Tissue Int.* **58,** 409–414 (1996).
132. van den Kroonenberg, A., Wilson, S., Myers, E., Hayes, W., and McMahon, T. Impact velocities and body configurations for backward falls from standing height. *J. Biomech.,* submitted for publication.
133. Mosekilde, L., and Mosekilde, L. Vertebral structure and strength *in vivo* and *in vitro. Calcif. Tissue Int.* **53,** S121–S126 (1993).
134. Silva, M., Keaveny, T., and Hayes, W. Load sharing between the shell and centrun in the lumbar vertebral body. *Spine* **22,** 140–150 (1997).
135. Mosekilde, L. Osteoporosis—Mechanisms and Models. *In* "Anabolic Treatments for Osteoporosis" (J. Whitfield and P. Morley, eds.), pp. 31–58. CRC Press, Boca Raton, FL, 1998.
136. Faulkner, K., Cann, C., and Hasedawa, B. Effect of bone distribution on vertebral strength: Assessment with a patient-specific nonlinear finite element analysis. *Radiology* **179,** 669–674 (1991).
137. Rockoff, S. D., Sweet, E., and Bleustein, J. The relative contribution of trabecular and cortical bone to the strength of human lumbar vertebrae. *Calcif. Tissue Res.,* **3,** 163–175 (1969).
138. McBroom, R. J., Hayes, W. C., Edwards, W. T., Goldberg, R. P., and White, A. A. Prediction of vertebral body compressive fracture using quantitative computed tomography. *J. Bone Joint Surg.* **67A,** 1206–1214 (1985).

139. Yoganandan, N., Myklebust, J., Cusick, J., Wilson, C., and Sances, A. Functional biomechanics of the thoracolumbar vertebral cortex. *Clin. Biomech.* **3,** 11–18 (1988).
140. Bartley, M. H., Arnold, J. S., Haslam, R. K., and Jee, W. S. S. The relationship of bone strength and bone quantity in health, disease, and aging. *J. Gerontol.* **21,** 517–521 (1966).
141. Biggemann, M., Hilweg, D., Seidel, S., Horst, M., and Brinckmann, P. Risk of vertebral insufficiency fractures in relation to compressive strength predicted by quantitative computed tomography. *Eur. J. Radiol.* **13,** 6–10 (1991).
142. Biggemann, M., Hilweg, D., and Brinckmann, P. Prediction of the compressive strength of vertebral bodies of the lumbar spine by quantitative computed tomography. *Skeletal Radiol.* **17,** 264–269 (1988).
143. Brinckmann, P., Biggeman, M., and Hilweg, D. Prediction of the compressive strength of human lumbar vertebrae. *Clin. Biomech.* **4,** S1–S27 (1989).
144. Cody, D., Goldstein, S., Flynn, M., and Brown, E. Correlations between vertebral regional bone mineral density (rBMD) and whole bone fracture load. *Spine* **16,** 146–154 (1991).
145. Eriksson, S. A., Isberg, B. O., and Lindgren, J. U. Prediction of vertebral strength by dual photon absorptiometry and quantitative computed tomography. *Calcif. Tissue Int.* **44,** 243–250 (1989).
146. Hansson, T., Roos, B., and Nachemson, A. The bone mineral content and ultimate compressive strength of lumbar vertebrae. *Spine* **5,** 46–55 (1980).
147. Moro, M., Hecker, A. T., Bouxsein, M. L., and Myers, E. R. Failure load of thoracic vertebrae correlates with lumbar bone mineral density measured by DXA. *Calcif. Tissue Int.* **56,** 206–209 (1995).
148. Myers, B., Arbogast, K., Lobaugh, B., Harper, K., Richardson, W., and Drezner, M. Improved assessment of lumbar vertebral body strength using supine lateral dual-energy x-ray absorptiometry. *J. Bone Miner. Res.* **9,** 687–693 (1994).
149. Vesterby, A., *et al.* Biologically meaningful determinants of the *in vitro* strength of lumbar vertebrae. *Bone* **12,** 219–224 (1991).
150. Tabensky, A., Williams, J., DeLuca, V., Briganti, E., and Seeman, E. Bone mass, areal, and volumetric bone density are equally accurate, sensitive, and specific surrogates of the breaking strength of the vertebral body. An *in vitro* study. *J. Bone Miner. Res.* **11,** 1981–1988 (1996).
151. Biggeman, M., and Brinckman, P. Biomechanics of osteoporotic vertebral fractures. *In* "Vertebral Fracture in Osteoporosis" (H. Genant, M. Jergas, and C. van Kuijk, eds.), pp. 21–34. Osteoporosis Research Group, University of California, San Francisco, 1995.
152. Hayes, W. C. Biomechanics of cortical and trabecular bone: implications for assessment of fracture risk. *In* "Basic Orthopaedic Biomechanics" (V. C. Mow and W. C. Hayes, eds.), pp. 93–142. Raven Press, New York, 1991.
153. Lauritzen, J., Petersen, M., and Lund, B. Effect of external hip protectors on hip fractures. *Lancet* **341,** 11–13 (1993).
154. Bouxsein, M., Myers, E., and Hayes, W. Biomechanics of Age-Related Fractures. *In* "Osteoporosis" (R. Marcus, D. Feldman, and J. Kelsey, eds.), pp. 373–393. Academic Press, San Diego, 1996.

CHAPTER 28

What Is a Fragility Fracture?

RICHARD D. WASNICH Hawaii Osteoporosis Center, Honolulu, Hawaii 96814

The consequential outcome of osteoporosis is fragility fracture. Because any bone may fracture with sufficient trauma, it becomes necessary to estimate the severity of trauma in order to define fragility fracture. In some situations, this distinction is easy. A fall from a tree or an automobile accident are clear examples of violent fractures resulting from major trauma. At the other extreme, spontaneous fractures, most commonly involving the spine and hip, occur without trauma and represent the ultimate "fragility" fracture. The difficulty involves the estimation of "low trauma."

It might appear to be an academic exercise to classify trauma so precisely. Indeed it is not academic. The presence of a fragility fracture in a patient is the strongest, known risk factor for future fractures [1,2]. Correct categorization of fragility fractures identifies patients with severe osteoporosis, in whom intervention is most indicated. Correct classification of fragility fractures is important for another reason. Both clinical and epidemiologic studies of osteoporosis are based on the presence of fragility fractures. If fractures resulting from severe trauma were to be misclassified as fragility fractures, it would compromise the results of such studies.

TRAUMA CATEGORIZATION

In the longitudinal Hawaii Osteoporosis Study (HOS), incident fractures were categorized according to the following trauma severities:

1. *Spontaneous,* defined as no trauma. An example is a vertebral fracture occurring without a fall or other trauma.
2. *Mild or moderate,* defined as a fall from a standing level (or less) to the ground, or an equivalent degree of trauma. The classic Colles' fracture, occurring from a fall forward on an outstretched hand, is an example.
3. *Indeterminate* trauma described those incidents that did not fall clearly into one of the other categories. An example might be a fall against the side of a sink, breaking a rib. If the force of the fall were sufficient, normal ribs might fail in this situation. Other examples include: "I broke my toe when I kicked the door." "I slipped on the last stair step and fell down two steps, on my side." "I slipped on the ice and went airborne before hitting the ground." Clearly it is not always possible to accurately estimate the degree of force involved in these fractures. They might best be considered suspicious of a low trauma fracture, but indeterminate. It is in these situations where bone density measurements may be the most helpful, particularly if the values are very high or very low.
4. *Severe* trauma, defined as a violent event that would be expected to result in fracture, even in a younger, normal person. A fall from a height of 8 feet or an auto accident are examples.

BONE DENSITY CATEGORIZATION

When the degree of trauma is indeterminate, the presence of other risk factors, particularly low bone density, may increase the probability that a true fragility fracture has occurred. If bone mineral density (BMD) is very high, say 1 or 2 standard deviations (SD) above the mean for age 30, the fracture is less likely to represent a fragility fracture. If BMD is more than 2 or 2.5 SD below the young mean, the probability that the fracture resulted from fragility is increased.

However, considerable caution must be employed in the use of simple, BMD cutoff levels. For example, a

BMD T score of -1.0 has a wholly different meaning in a 40-year-old woman as compared to an 80 year old. Because there is an approximate doubling of fracture risk with each decade of age (independent of bone density), the 80 year old has a 16-fold greater risk of fracture than the 40 year old with an identical bone density. Therefore, "osteopenia" by World Health Organization (WHO) criteria may be more properly interpreted as osteoporosis in an 80-year-old woman whose fracture resulted from "moderate" trauma. The younger woman with "osteopenia" may have a higher *future* risk than the 80 year old, but her *current* risk is so low that only fractures resulting from either grade 1 or 2 trauma should be interpreted as fragility fractures. Figure 1 illustrates how greatly two women of different ages may differ in terms of both current and future risk. There are other pitfalls inherent in the use of discrete BMD cutoffs, as proposed by the WHO. First, the WHO guidelines suggest that a "diagnosis" of osteoporosis can be made by bone density alone; that is not true. Bone density is a risk factor, not a diagnostic test. A patient who presents with a nonviolent vertebral fracture and *normal* bone density has a *higher* risk of future vertebral fracture than a patient with low bone density, but no vertebral fracture [1,2].

Also, low bone density is a manifestation of diseases other than osteoporosis, and these disease processes (such as hyperparathyroidism and osteomalacia) must be excluded by appropriate laboratory evaluation. Finally, T scores are a measure of "relative" risk, e.g., relative to a hypothetical "normal" BMD represented by "healthy," 30-year-old women. Unfortunately, this reference value itself varies according to geographic area, ethnicity, sex, and study; major changes in this "reference" value have already occurred, resulting in formerly "osteoporotic" patients suddenly being reclassified as nonosteoporotic, solely because of a change in the hypothetical "normal, reference" value.

Bone density in a Caucasian has the same meaning as bone density in a Japanese American. In fact, a given bone density level in a man relates to the same *absolute* fracture rate as it does in a woman [3]. Thus, rather than having an infinite number of reference populations, and a different "diagnostic" bone density level in every country and for every ethnic group, the solution is to translate bone density levels directly into fracture probabilities (Fig. 2). These fracture rates can then be expressed as 1-year, 5-year, or lifetime probabilities of fracture. The other advantage of this approach is that other risk factors, such as prevalent fractures, age, and bone turnover, can be directly incorporated into the estimate of absolute fracture risk. Thus a woman with existing fractures and high bone turnover will have a much higher, absolute fracture risk than another woman without these risk factors, even though their bone density levels are identical.

FRACTURE CLASSIFICATION

Vertebral fractures are the most common osteoporotic fracture, with an earlier age of onset than hip

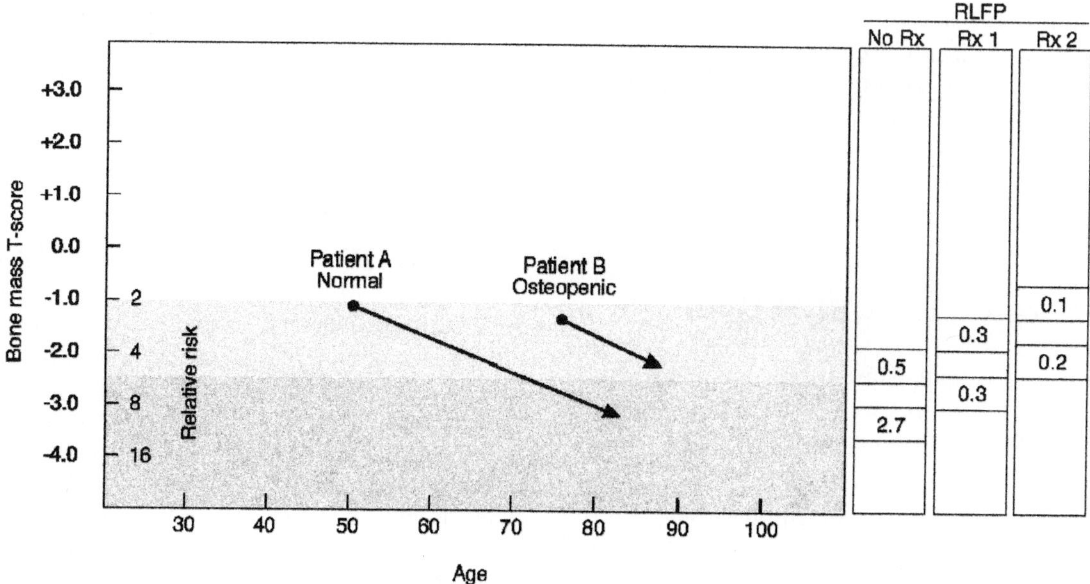

FIGURE 1 WHO classification of osteoporosis based on bone density T scores. The light-gray area denotes women with osteopenia and the dark-gray area, osteoporosis. This represents current fracture risk. An approach to future cumulative fracture risk has been incorporated into a standardized risk report, which is based on RLFP.

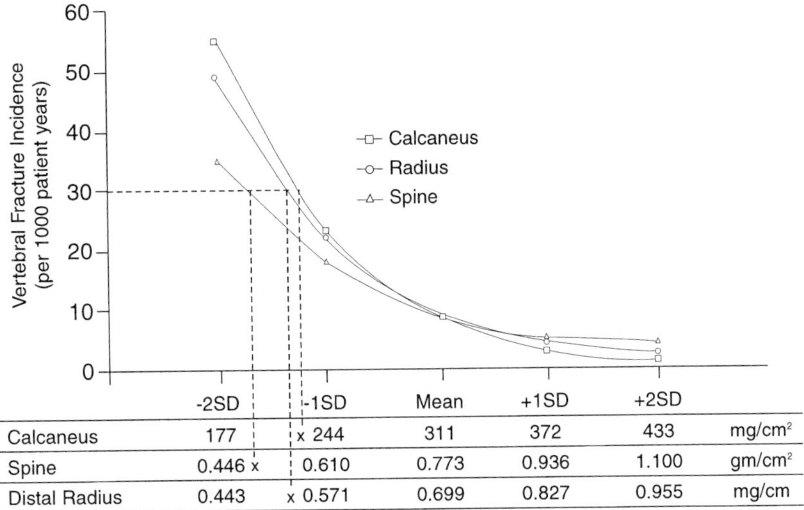

	-2SD	-1SD	Mean	+1SD	+2SD	
Calcaneus	177	x 244	311	372	433	mg/cm²
Spine	0.446 x	0.610	0.773	0.936	1.100	gm/cm²
Distal Radius	0.443	x 0.571	0.699	0.827	0.955	mg/cm

FIGURE 2 Vertebral fracture incidence versus bone mineral density (BMD) levels at three skeletal sites. Correct interpretation of the BMD results renders all BMD measurement sites equal. A vertebral fracture rate of 30 per 1000 patient years corresponds to slightly different relative BMD levels (as expressed by *T* scores), but all BMD sites yield the same information, e.g., absolute fracture incidence rates. It is incorrect to consecrate one BMD *T* score as the gold standard and to criticize other sites because they yield different *T* scores.

fractures. The study of vertebral fractures has been hampered by the absence of a consensus regarding the radiographic definition of vertebral fracture. Unlike long bone fractures, which are usually evident radiographically as a distinct break or cleft in the bone, vertebral fractures are represented by a continuous range of vertebral deformations. The fact that more than one-half of vertebral fractures are not clinically recognized further complicates the issue.

Traditionally, vertebral fracture diagnosis has been based on visual interpretation of the radiograph, and fractures have been classified as crush, wedge, or end plate (Fig. 3). When prior radiographs are available, the diagnosis of a new fracture is less problematic. Generally, a height reduction of more than 15–20%, compared to the prior radiograph, is adequate for the clinical diagnosis of a new vertebral fracture. Borderline changes can often be resolved by bone scintigraphy, if the fracture is recent. Borderline deformations are also more likely to be true, osteoporotic fractures if the patient also has low bone density. Although more quantitative and complex, analytic approaches are useful for research studies, the previous definitions are sufficiently adequate for clinical purposes.

Nonvertebral fractures occur at numerous skeletal sites. The frequency of distal radius fractures (Colles' fracture) increases rapidly after menopause and should serve as the clinical indication of severe osteoporosis. In the past, many such patients had the fracture treated, but were not actively treated for their underlying osteoporosis. Such patients should receive appropriate evaluation and differential diagnosis, including bone density measurements. They should then be considered for more aggressive management, meaning pharmacological agents in addition to life-style and dietary advice.

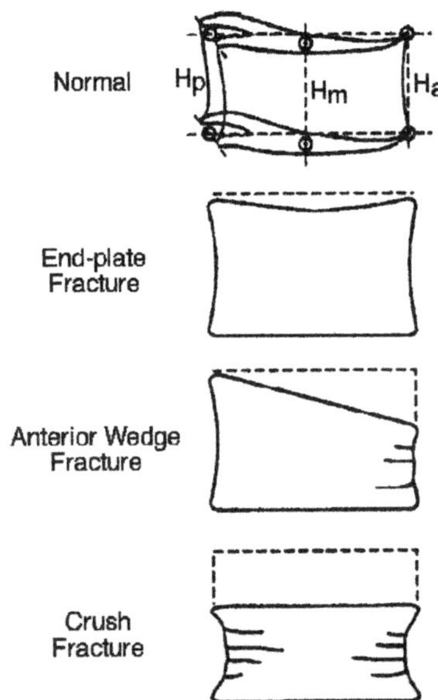

FIGURE 3 Vertebral morphometry measurements are typically based on placement of six points that define the anterior (H_a), middle (H_m), and posterior (H_p) heights of the vertebral body. Crush, wedge, and end plate fractures are illustrated.

Fractures of the proximal humerus are another consequence of falls forward on the outstretched hand. Unlike fractures of the shaft or distal humerus, proximal humerus fractures increase with age; three-fourths occur in women.

Most hip fractures occur at either the femoral neck (cervical fractures) or between the trochanteric processes (intertrochanteric fractures) (Fig. 4). Intertrochanteric fractures usually result from a fall, whereas femoral neck fractures often occur with little or no apparent trauma. Some of these patients present only with pain and no history of a fall. The radiograph may not show a distinct fracture line, and bone scintigraphy may be helpful in establishing the diagnosis of occult femoral neck fractures.

Seeley *et al.* [4] investigated a variety of other nonvertebral fracture sites and their association with low bone density. Except for fractures of face, fingers, patella, and elbow, all other fractures were associated with low bone density and therefore are presumptive osteoporotic in etiology (Table I).

TABLE I Comparison of Methods for Classifying a Type of Fracture Associated with Low Bone Mass

Fracture type	Bone mass[a]	Classified by minimal/moderate trauma[b]	Age[c]
Humerus	+	+	+
Hip	+	+	+
Vertebral	+	+	+
Pelvic	+	+	+
Wrist	+	+	–
Rib	+	+	–
Leg	+	+	–
Hand	+	+	–
Foot	+	–	–
Toe	+	–	–
Clavicle	+	–	–
Patella	–	+	+
Ankle	–	+	–
Elbow	–	+	–
Face	–	+	–
Finger	–	–	–

[a] Based on significant ($p < 0.05$) relation with at least two measures of appendicular bone mass.

[b] More than 50% of fractures at the site preceded by fall from standing height or less, or spontaneous.

[c] Based on significant ($p < 0.05$) relation with age.

PROGNOSTIC IMPLICATIONS OF A FRAGILITY FRACTURE

Patients who present with a fracture or who have a history of a nonviolent fracture have a much higher risk for subsequent fractures than comparable patients without fractures. The relationship is not only independent of bone density, but stronger than bone density. Hence a careful fracture history is an essential component of a patient's evaluation and risk assessment.

This interrelationship of fractures exists for all of the major, osteoporotic fracture sites that have been studied. Gardsell [5] first reported that hip, vertebral, and wrist fractures increased the risk of subsequent nonvertebral fractures. The HOS found that women with a single, existing vertebral fracture at initial examination had a nearly 3-fold increased risk of subsequent fractures, independent of bone density [1]. Women with two or more vertebral fractures had a 7- to 9-fold increased risk of another vertebral fracture. Of interest was the fact that women with one vertebral fracture *and* low bone density (lowest tertile) had a 25-fold increased risk of future vertebral fractures. The explanation for this finding is uncertain. It has been postulated that impaired bone quality is responsible. However, a vertebral fracture alters the load distribution on neighboring vertebral bodies, which might explain the clustering of fractures in the midthoracic and lower thoracic/upper lumbar spine.

The HOS also reported that prevalent nonvertebral fractures also increased the risk of vertebral fractures [2] (Fig. 5). It has also been reported that wrist fractures increase the risk of hip fractures [6] and that hip fractures increase the risk of contralateral hip fractures [7,8].

Clearly the patient with both a nonviolent fracture and a low bone density represents a more serious, and less treatable, problem than the patient with low bone density alone. It has therefore been proposed that the goal of fracture risk management should be prevention of the *first* fracture [9]. In the patient with hypertension,

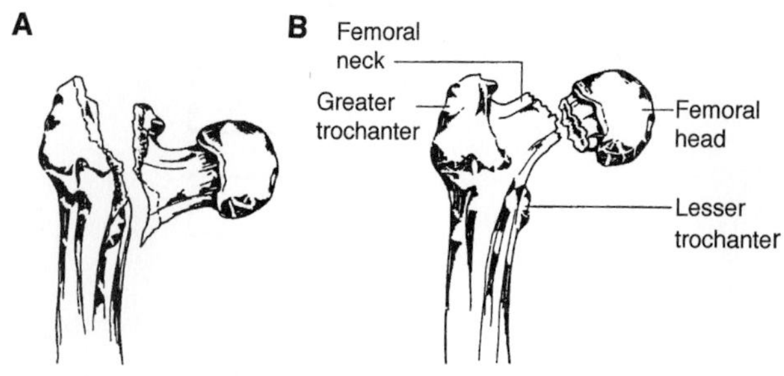

FIGURE 4 Intertrochanteric fracture (A) and femoral neck fracture (B).

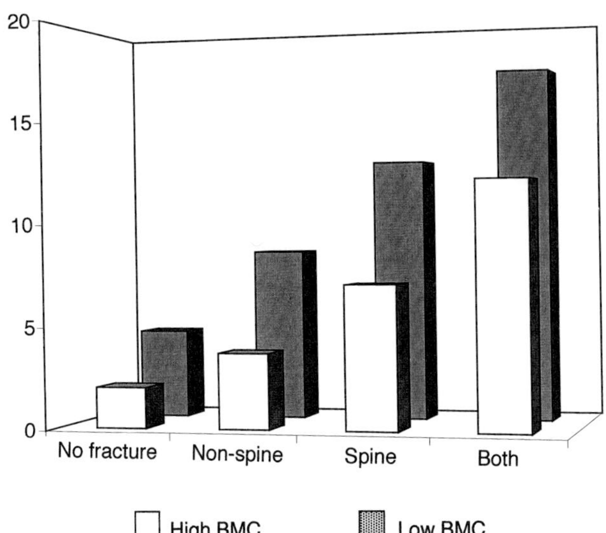

FIGURE 5 Age-adjusted rate ratios for new spine fractures for women with low heel bone density (≤50th percentile) compared with women with high bone density, and further categorized according to the presence or absence of prevalent fractures.

it is considered good practice to prevent the onset of complications, such as stroke or renal failure. Likewise, early identification of a high fracture risk offers greater opportunity to prevent future fractures.

Although the prevention of hip fractures is certainly desirable, that should not be the sole goal of management. A reduction in the incidence of all osteoporotic fractures is a more prudent policy than a narrow focus on hip fractures alone.

References

1. Ross, P. D., Davis, J. W., Epstein, R. S., Wasnich, R. D. Pre-existing fractures and bone mass predict vertebral fracture incidence in women. *Ann. Intern. Med.* **114,** 919–923 (1991).
2. Wasnich, R. D., Davis, J. W., and Ross, P. D. Spine fracture risk is predicted by non-spine fractures. *Osteoporosis Int.* **4,** 1–5 (1994).
3. Ross, P. D., Kim, S., Wasnich, R. D. Bone density predicts vertebral fracture risk in both men and women. *J. Bone Min. Res.* **11,** 1275 (1996).
4. Seeley, D. G., Browner, W. S., Nevitt, M. C., *et al.* Which fractures are associated with low appendicular bone mass in elderly women? *Ann. Intern. Med.* **115,** 837–842 (1991).
5. Gardsell, P., Johnell, O., Nilsson, B. E., Nilsson, J. A. The predictive value of fracture, disease and falling tendency due to fragility fractures in women. *Calcif. Tissue Res.* **45,** 327–330 (1989).
6. Owen, R. A., Melton, L. J. III, Ilstrup, D. M., Johnson, K. A., Riggs, B. L. Colles' fracture and subsequent hip fracture risk. *Clin. Orthop.* **152,** 35–43 (1980).
7. Melton, L. J. III, Ilstrup, D. M., Beckenbaugh, R. D., Riggs, B. L. Hip fracture recurrence: A population-based study. *Clin. Orthop.* **167,** 131–138 (1982).
8. Stewart, T. M. Fracture of neck of femur: Survival and contralateral fracture. *BMJ* **2,** 922–924 (1957).

CHAPTER 29

Epidemiology and Consequences of Osteoporotic Fractures

PHILIP D. ROSS, ARTHUR SANTORA, AND A. JOHN YATES
Merck & Co., Inc., Rahway, New Jersey

HEALTH CARE COSTS OF OSTEOPOROTIC FRACTURES

Hip and other fractures related to osteoporosis result in a greater number of hospital bed days than many other conditions among women, including myocardial infarction, diabetes, and breast cancer (Fig. 1) [1]. Although hip fractures represent only about 9% of all osteoporotic fractures and outpatient services related to osteoporotic fractures [2,3], almost all hip fracture cases require hospitalization, and about half are discharged to nursing homes or other chronic care institutions in the United States [4,5]. As a result, hip fractures account for approximately 63% of fracture-related health care costs, 3.4 million hospital bed days, 60,000 admissions to nursing homes, and more than 7 million days of restricted activity each year in the United States [3,6–8]. In the United States, the average cost of hip fracture was $33,000 [8]; in Sweden, it was $26,000 [9]. Worldwide, the average cost is approximately $21,000 per hip fracture [10]. The annual incidence of hip fracture in the United States is approximately 250,000. Thus, based on these figures, annual health care costs attributable to hip fractures in the United States are approximately $8.3 billion, and total costs for all fractures are approximately $13 billion. Similar estimates ($6–20 billion for all fractures combined) have been derived using health care records [7,11–13]. Although hip fractures account for a major share of economic costs, other fractures contribute substantially to health care costs. Furthermore, fractures other than hip generally occur earlier in life, and there is mounting evidence that they may rival or even surpass hip fractures in terms of aggregate morbidity and debilitation.

HOW COMMON IS OSTEOPOROSIS?

Low bone mineral density (BMD) is an important risk factor for osteoporotic fractures—it can identify people at risk before fractures have occurred. People with low bone density will not always develop fractures, but the probability of fracture is increased (just as most smokers are not currently diagnosed with lung cancer or cardiovascular disease, but are at increased risk). There is a continuous relationship, i.e., fracture probability increases progressively as bone density declines. However, fracture probability is also influenced by age and other risk factors. For example, a history of a previous nonviolent (due to moderate trauma or less, such as a fall at floor level) fracture(s) is an independent predictor of future fracture risk. Therefore, both BMD and fracture history have been used to categorize the severity of osteoporosis and fracture risk. The World Health Organization has proposed that individuals with BMD values higher than 2.5 (others have proposed 2.0) standard deviations (SD) below the mean for young adults be classified as having osteoporosis and that people with BMD in this range together with a history of nonviolent fracture be classified as having severe osteoporosis [14,110]. Low bone mass (osteopenia) has been defined as BMD values between 1.0 and 2.5 (or 2.0) SD below the mean for young, healthy adults. The choice of different BMD cutoffs for defining osteoporo-

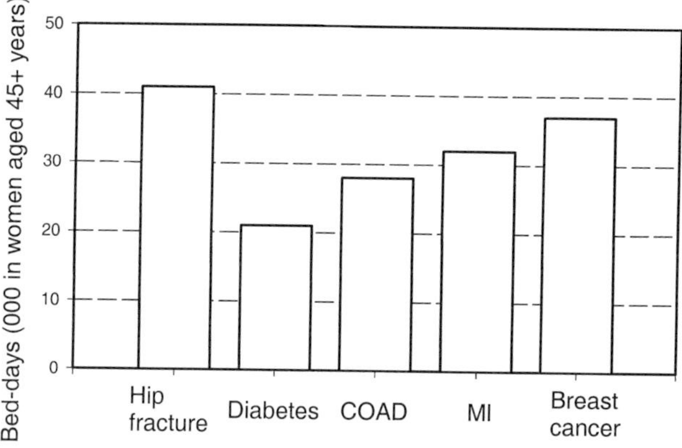

FIGURE 1 Hospital bed occupancy in women aged 45 years or more according to diagnostic category in the Trent region of England (9% of the U.K. population). COAD, chronic obstructive airways disease; MI, myocardial infarction. From Kanis *et al.* [1], with permission.

sis reflects the continuous nature of the relationship between BMD and fracture risk—risk increases progressively with decreasing BMD, and there is no objective reason for choosing a single cutoff, except for the fact that definitives are necessary.

Given that most women will eventually sustain at least one osteoporotic fracture during their lifetime if left untreated, it is essential that preventive treatment be initiated as early as possible. Patients with low bone mass and no prior nonviolent fracture currently have a moderate risk of fracture. Prevention of further bone loss will help ensure that their fracture risk remains moderate, whereas treatments that increase BMD will reduce their risk of fractures. Patients with osteoporosis who have not yet had fractures are already at high risk. Treatment should be initiated to increase BMD and to reduce the risk of fractures (as well as to prevent further progression of bone loss). Although treatment can increase BMD and reduce fracture risk, it is not possible to completely reverse the loss of bone mass and impairment of bone microarchitecture that have already occurred, and fracture risk may therefore remain moderately elevated. Patients who have already had fractures are most likely to experience additional fractures if left untreated [15,16] and require the most aggressive therapy. Although effective treatments can reduce this risk substantially, the risk of additional fractures cannot be eliminated entirely. Effective treatments can increase BMD and reduce the risk of additional fractures by approximately half within 1–3 years and will also prevent subsequent BMD declines that would otherwise increase fracture risk further [1].

Over the average life span, women lose approximately half of their bone mass; men experience declines of approximately 30% [18]. Each reduction of 10–15% doubles fracture risk. There may be considerable differences between individuals in the cumulative amount of bone loss, and the ages over which this bone loss occurs. Among women, some evidence shows that bone density may begin to decline prior to menopause. Around the time of menopause, however, the rate of bone loss increases dramatically, averaging approximately 2 to 3% per year, with some individuals losing as much as 20 to 30% over a period of 5 years or less [18–21]. Thereafter, bone loss continues throughout life at a slower rate, approximately 0.5 to 1% per year, on average [19,22–24]. For men, the rate of bone loss after age 60 is approximately half that of women. After age 70, the rate of loss may increase for both men and women, perhaps due to declines in health and activity [22,25,26]. There are enormous differences in fracture risk between individuals who are identified by BMD measurement. These differences result not only from variations in the amount of peak bone density accrued during development, but also from differences in the rate of bone loss later in life [22,23,27,28], as well as to the quality of the bone.

Among the elderly, low bone density increases the risk of almost all types of fractures [2]. Most fractures among the elderly result from mild to moderate trauma, such as a fall from standing height or less [29]. As a result of the large lifetime declines in BMD and accompanying declines in bone strength, the incidence of most fractures increases progressively and exponentially with age (Fig. 2) [30]. Currently, most postmenopausal women will live at least to the age of 80. Approximately 70% of women over 80 have osteoporosis as defined by BMD values more than 2.5 SD below the mean for young healthy women [14,31,32].

The spine is the most common site of osteoporotic fractures [2,33]. As many as half of all women have radiographic evidence of vertebral fractures after age 80, and half of those with fractures have more than one affected vertebra [15,16,34–36]. However, only about one-third of all vertebral fractures are currently identified in clinical settings [34,37,38]. The incidence of hip and vertebral fractures is negligible prior to menopause, but increases with age, reaching 3% per year, or more, after age 80 [30,36,39,40].

The lifetime risk of having at least one fracture is greater than 50% for white women; this includes lifetime risks of approximately 32% for vertebral fracture, 16% for hip fracture, 15% for wrist fracture, and 8% for humerus fractures [41–44]. Because of the rapid increase in risk with age, the risk of hip fracture is twice as high (compared to the usual life span) for people who live to age 90: 32% for women and 17% for men [11]. Furthermore, as more than half of women will experience osteoporotic fractures, people with above average risk are more likely than not to have a fracture, and many people will have more than one. For comparison, the lifetime risks of breast and endometrial cancers

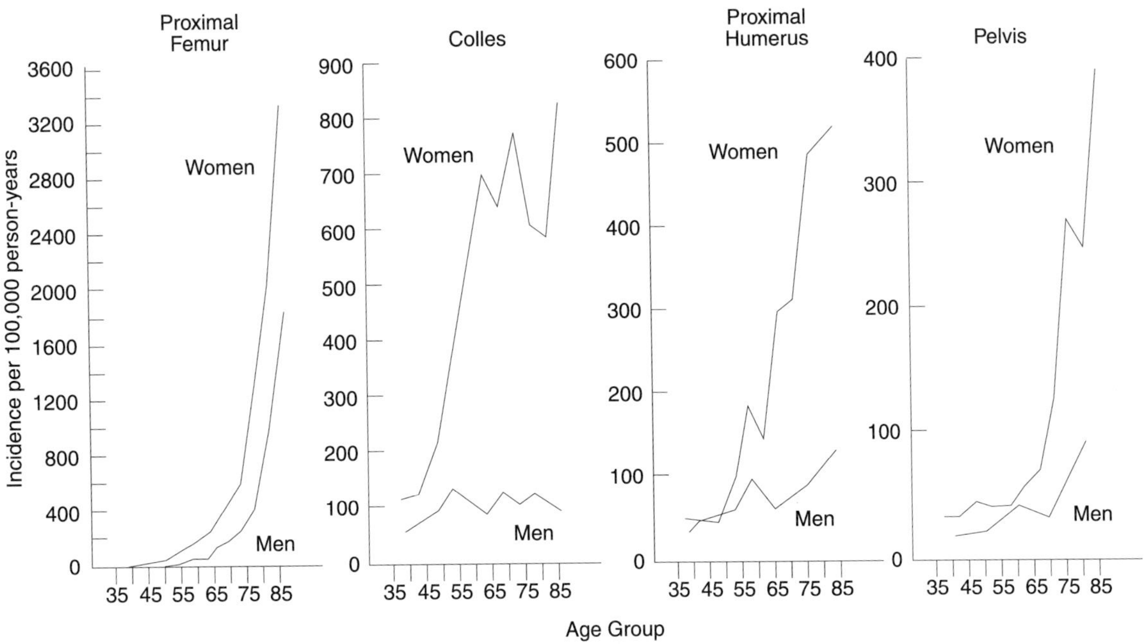

FIGURE 2 Age- and sex-specific incidence rates among residents of Rochester, Minnesota, for four age-related fracture sites. Note that the vertical scale varies for each fracture site. From Melton [30], with permission.

are only approximately 9 and 3%, respectively [41]. Considering that hip fractures represent approximately 9% of all fractures among the elderly and that only one-third of all vertebral fractures are diagnosed clinically, the total number of fractures per year in the United States is likely to be approximately 3.2 million [2,34,37,38].

MORTALITY AND MORBIDITY

The risk of death is two to five times higher during the first 6 to 12 months after a hip fracture compared to other people of similar age [4,5,39,45]. White women in the United States have almost a 3% lifetime chance of dying from the consequences of a hip fracture, compared to 31% for coronary heart disease, 2.8% for breast cancer, and 0.7% for endometrial cancer. As with fracture probability, these averages do not reflect individual differences—some people have a lower than average risk of heart disease, but a higher risk of fractures. A higher death rate has also been reported for women with vertebral fractures and for men and women with low bone density [45–49].

Although the risk of death is increased somewhat among people with osteoporosis, pain, disability, and reduced quality of life are more common outcomes that are often profound and may persist for many years. Serious declines in physical performance due to fractures can lead to loss of independence. For example, one prospective study of hip fracture showed that among those who were able to walk and climb stairs at baseline, 50% were unable to walk independently and 87% were unable to climb stairs without assistance a year later [50]. Another study reported that 31% of surviving hip fracture cases were bedridden 6 years later, and only 9% could walk outdoors by themselves, whereas only 1.5% of the control group was bedridden and 55% of the controls could walk outdoors [51]. Surveys of hip fracture cases after 6 to 12 months have found that 20 to 60% are unable to perform numerous other types of routine activities that they had been able to do prior to the fracture [50,52,53].

Half of all women with radiographic evidence of vertebral fractures do not recall having had typical back pain reflecting the acute event. While symptoms generally resolve within a few months, symptoms among the remaining women with vertebral fractures range from mild to intolerable, and chronic pain sometimes persists for years [38,54–62]. The majority of women (60–87%) with chronic pain from vertebral fractures reported problems with routine activities such as walking, carrying, lifting, shopping, and housework [63]. Furthermore, many women rate changes in appearance such as height loss and kyphosis as important contributors to decreased quality of life as a result of vertebral fractures. The risk of pain and physical impairment increases progressively with the number and severity of vertebral fractures (Table I) [54,60,62–68].

Fractures other than those of the hip and spine also impair physical function and quality of life. Compared to women without prior fracture, women with fractures

TABLE I Proportion (%) of Women (n = 2992) with the Indicated Outcome by Number of Vertebral Fractures[a]

Proportion (%) of women with outcome of	Number of severe[b] fractures			
	0	1	2	>2
Disability score[c] greater than 6	4	7	14	27
Height loss more than 4 cm	23	43	67	81
Moderate/severe back pain	42	56	55	77

[a] Data from Ettinger *et al.* [62].
[b] Vertebral height more than 4 SD below mean.
[c] On a scale of 0 to 18.

that had occurred an average of 7 years prior to interview were two to six times more likely to report difficulty with activities such as walking, getting in or out of a car, climbing or descending stairs, reaching above the head, bending and lifting, cooking, shopping, and other routine activities [66]. These physical impairments, plus fears of additional fractures and falls, often cause people to restrict their activities, which reduces their independence. Reduced physical activity also accelerates declines in bone density, muscle mass, and physical performance, thereby increasing the risk of falls, fractures, and institutionalization. Some people with osteoporotic fractures suffer declines in quality of life that are more important than measurable physical impairments [63,64,69].

RISK FACTORS FOR BONE LOSS AND FRACTURES

Low bone strength (a consequence of low peak bone mass or bone loss) and falls both contribute to fracture risk. Recognizing risk factors for bone loss and risk factors for falls can help reduce the impact of factors contributing to fracture risk. Such risk factors can also identify those who could benefit most from preventive therapy *before* fractures occur.

Low BMD (whether due to low peak BMD, bone loss, or both) is a major risk factor for fractures. The range of BMD values among older adults represents differences in fracture risk of at least 10–15 times. Many factors influence the attainment of peak BMD and the rate of subsequent loss. Current BMD represents the cumulative, combined influence of all such factors, known and unknown. As a result, it is not possible to accurately estimate BMD from an assessment of risk factors, and BMD must be measured directly [70–72]. However, it is still useful to recognize risk factors for bone loss to determine which patients are more likely to need treatment to prevent bone loss and because some (such as smoking, excess alcohol, dietary deficiencies, sedentary life-style) are amenable to intervention (Table II) [73].

Important risk factors for accelerated bone loss include corticosteroid use (losses increase with dose and duration), hypogonadism (including menopause), and immobilization (bedridden, casted fractures, wheelchair-bound, etc.) [74–78]. Low body weight is a risk factor for bone loss and for hip fractures [79,80]. Ensuring adequate calcium and vitamin D intake can reduce the rate of bone loss, particularly in the elderly or those with nutritional deficiencies, but is not sufficient to prevent bone loss completely, especially during the early postmenopausal period [81,82]. Poor nutrition can also lead to loss of muscle mass and other health declines, increasing the risk of falls and fractures. Other factors reported to contribute to bone loss are smoking, a sedentary life-style, endocrine disorders (such as hyperthyroidism, hypercortisolism, or hyperparathyroidism) or other health problems, and caffeine [71,73,83–86]. However, the skeletal benefits of life-style interventions alone are often small in comparison to the magnitude of lifetime declines in BMD, and many women require more effective (i.e., pharmacological) therapy to prevent fractures.

Treatment of postmenopausal women with estrogen increases BMD initially and reduces the long-term rate of bone loss by an average of 40%. After 6 or more years of treatment, fracture risk is reduced by half compared to women who do not use estrogen [87–89]. However, rapid bone loss occurs upon discontinuation of estrogen, and the benefits of previous HRT therapy disappear within a few years [90,91]. Treatment with bisphosphonates such as alendronate increases BMD, reduces bone turnover (as measured by biochemical markers), and reduces osteoporotic fracture risk by about half within 1–3 years [92,93]. Progressive increases in BMD occur during alendronate use, at least over the first 3–5 years. Discontinuation does not appear to be associated with accelerated bone loss, but the effects of cessation on fracture risk are currently not known [94].

Bone turnover (as measured by biochemical markers and by histomorphometry) increases after menopause. In the adult, increases in bone turnover lead to loss of bone because of the inefficiency in the processes associated with bone remodelling. An excess of resorption over formation leads to a reduction in the amount of bone mass. When bone turnover is high, the decline in bone loss is greater. Strong data indicate that patients with high turnover are at increased risk of fracture relative to those with lower rates of turnover and that this risk is independent of current BMD (Fig. 3) [95,96].

TABLE II Common Risk Factors for Fractures, Bone Loss, and Falls[a,b]

Attribute	Risk factor for fractures?	Risk factor for bone loss?[c]	Risk factor for falls?[c]	Modifiable?
Low bone density	↑ ↑	NA	—	Yes
Age	↑	↑	↑	No
History of fragility fractures	↑ ↑	?	?	No
History of frequent falls	↑	—	↑ ↑	No
Hypogonadism (including postmenopausal estrogen deficiency)	↑	↑ ↑	?	Yes
Female gender	↑	↑	↑	No
Caucasian race	↑	—	↑	No
Low body mass	↑	↑	↑	Yes
Immobility/inactivity	↑	↑ ↑	↑	Yes
Biochemical markers of bone turnover	↑ ↑	↑ ↑	—	Yes
Bone geometry (longer hip axis length)	↑	—	—	No
Alcohol abuse	↑	↑	↑ ↑	Yes
Cigarette smoking	↑	↑	↑	Yes
Caffeine excess	↑	↑	—	Yes
Calcium deficiency	↑	↑	—	Yes
Vitamin D deficiency	↑	↑	?	Yes
Poor physical function (muscle weakness, etc.)	↑	?	↑ ↑	Yes
Chronic health problems	↑	↑	↑	Some
Poor vision	↑	—	↑	Yes
Long life expectancy (duration of exposure to risk)	↑	↑	↑	No
Genetics (family history)	↑	?	?	No
Thyroid hormone excess	↑	↑	—	Yes
Anticonvulsants	↑	?	?	Yes
Long-acting benzodiazepines	↑	—	↑	Yes
Corticosteroid use	↑	↑ ↑	?	Yes
Estrogen replacement therapy (women)	↓	↓	?	Yes

[a] ↑, risk increases as the attribute increases; ↑ ↑, risk increases strongly as the attribute increases; ↓, risk decreases as the attribute increases; NA, not applicable; ?, association possible, but not confirmed; and —, no association.
[b] From Ross [73], reprinted with permission.
[c] Falls and bone loss are risk factors for fractures. It can be inferred that attributes that magnify these two factors will also increase the risk of fractures, even if direct associations with fracture risk have not yet been demonstrated.

Thus, while further studies to characterize this relationship are needed, the finding of high bone turnover in conjunction with other factors that increase fracture risk may be of value in determining the need for treatment.

Fracture risk factors that are partly independent of BMD include increasing age and the number of previous nonviolent fractures. The risk of future fractures is doubled or tripled by each preexisting fracture [15–17,97,98]. A family history of hip or wrist fractures also doubles fracture risk [17]. Spine radiographs should be obtained to identify vertebral fractures among people with osteoporosis because the probability of existing vertebral fractures is high, but only one-third are diagnosed in most clinical settings.

The higher fracture risk among women compared to men appears to be accounted for primarily by bone loss after menopause. Differences in BMD between races are small in comparison to the magnitude of lifetime bone loss [99–101]. However, mean BMD in blacks is, on average, about 10 to 25% higher than that in whites or Asians, which probably accounts for the reduced hip fracture incidence in blacks, which is approximately half that of other races [40,100,111]. Nonetheless, osteoporosis is a significant problem in women and men of all races, and measuring BMD is much more informative than race.

Falls are the main source of trauma resulting in osteoporotic fractures. Older people fall more often and have

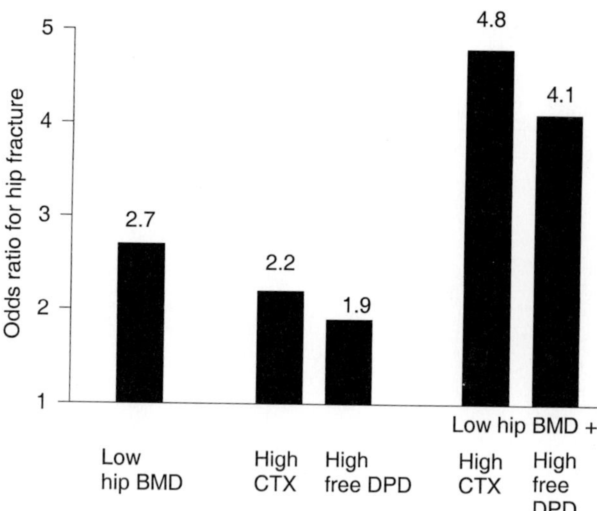

FIGURE 3 Separate and combined value of hip BMD and two resorption markers, urinary collagen cross-links (CTX) and deoxypyridinoline (DPD), for predicting hip fracture. A low hip BMD is defined as >2.5 SD below the young mean; high markers are >2 SD above the young mean. All odds ratios are statistically significant ($P < 0.05$). From Garnero *et al.* [96], with permission.

reduced protective mechanisms, both of which increase fracture risk. Approximately 20–30% of older women fall each year, and half of these fall more than once [102–104]. Risk factors for falls include low muscle strength, poor balance, poor vision, poor general health, use of multiple medications (especially psychoactive agents), and a history of past falls (Table II) [80,98,103–108]. Multiple risk factors indicate an especially high risk of falls [80,109].

In summary, fracture risk increases with the number of risk factors [15,16,80] (Fig. 4). Current BMD is one of the most important because it can quantify a much larger range of risk than other characteristics such as race, gender, body size, diet, or physical activity. BMD represents the combined effects of all prior and current influences on the skeleton and must be measured directly because it cannot be predicted accurately from life-style or health history. Biochemical markers provide an indication of the current rate of bone turnover and the rate of future bone loss and complement BMD for predicting fracture risk. Other risk factors, such as history of nonviolent fractures, family history of osteoporosis, and use of certain medications, can also complement BMD and markers to quantify the risk of rapid bone loss and fractures.

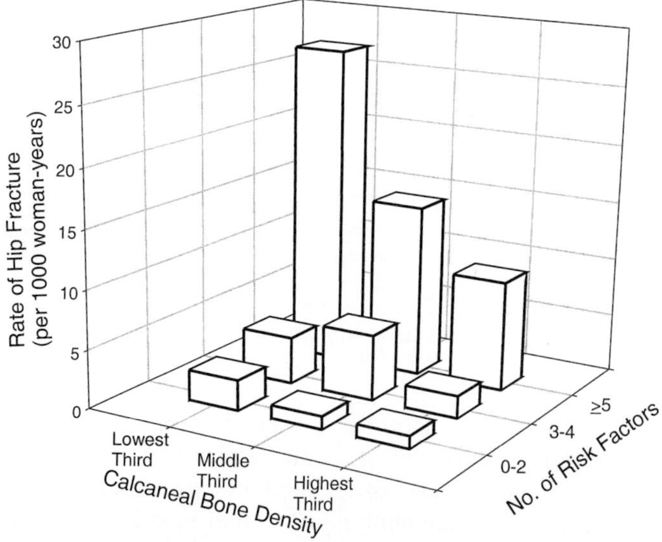

FIGURE 4 Annual risk of hip fracture according to the number of risk factors and age-specific calcaneal bone density. Risk factors include age ≥80; maternal history of hip fracture; any fracture (except hip) since the age of 50; fair, poor, or very poor health; previous hyperthyroidism; current long-acting benzodiazepine therapy; current weight less than at age 25; height at the age of 25 ≥168 cm; caffeine intake more than the equivalent of two cups of coffee per day; on feet ≤4 hr/day; no walking for exercise; inability to rise from chair without using arms; lowest quartile (standard deviation >2.44) of depth perception; lowest quartile (≤0.70 unit) of vision contrast sensitivity; and pulse rate >80/min. From Cummings *et al.* [17], with permission.

References

1. Kanis, J. A., Delmas, P., Burckhardt, P., *et al.* Guidelines for diagnosis and management of osteoporosis. *Osteoporos. Int.* **7,** 390–406 (1997).
2. Seeley, D. G., Browner, W. S., Nevitt, M. C., Genant, H. K., Scott, J. C., and Cummings, S. R. Which fractures are associated with low appendicular bone mass in elderly women? *Ann. Intern. Med.* **115,** 837–842 (1991).
3. Phillips, S., Fox, N., Jacobs, J., and Wright, W. E. The direct medical costs of osteoporosis for American women aged 45 and older, 1986. *Bone* **9,** 271–279 (1988).
4. Magaziner, J., Simonsick, E. M., Kashner, T. M., *et al.* Survival experience of aged hip fracture patients. *Am. J. Public Health* **79,** 274–278 (1989).
5. U.S. Congress, Office of Technology Assessment, "Hip Fracture Outcomes in People Age Fifty and Over." Background paper, OTA-BP-H-120, US Government Printing Office, Washington, DC, 1994.
6. Melton, L. J., III. Hip fractures: A worldwide problem today and tomorrow. *Bone* **14**(Suppl), S1–S8 (1993).
7. Holbrook, T. L., Grazier, K., Kelsey, J. L., and Stauffer, R. N., "The Frequency of Occurrence, Impact, and Cost of Selected Musculoskeletal Conditions in the United States." American Academy of Orthopaedic Surgeons, Chicago, 1984.
8. Melton, L. J., III, Thamer, M., Ray, N. F., *et al.* Fractures attributable to osteoporosis: Report from the National Osteoporosis Foundation. *J. Bone Miner. Res.* **12**(1), 16–23 (1997).
9. Sernbo, I., and Johnell, O. Consequences of a hip fracture: A prospective study over 1 year. *Osteoporos. Int.* **3,** 148–153 (1993).
10. Johnell, O. The socioeconomic burden of fractures: Today and in the 21st century. *Am. J. Med.* **103,** 20S–26S (1997).
11. Grisso, J. A., Chiu, G. Y., Maislin, G., *et al.* Risk factors for hip fractures in men: A preliminary study. *J. Bone Miner. Res.* **6,** 865–868 (1991).
12. Peck, W. A., Riggs, B. L., Bell, N. H., *et al.* Research directions in osteoporosis. *Am. J. Med.* **84,** 275–282 (1988).
13. Praemer, A., Furner, S., and Rice, D. P., "Musculoskeletal Conditions in the United States." American Academy of Orthopaedic Surgeons, Park Ridge, IL, 1992.
14. Kanis, J. A., Melton, L. J., III, Christiansen, C., *et al.* The diagnosis of osteoporosis. *J. Bone Miner. Res.* **9,** 1137–1141 (1994).
15. Ross, P. D., Davis, J. W., and Epstein, R. S. Pre-existing fractures and bone mass predict vertebral fracture in women. *Ann. Intern. Med.* **114,** 919–923 (1991).
16. Ross, P. D., Genant, H. K., Davis, J. W., *et al.* Predicting vertebral fracture incidence from prevalent fractures and bone density among non-black, osteoporotic women. *Osteoporos. Int.* **3,** 120–127 (1993).
17. Cummings, S. R., Nevitt, M. C., Browner, W. S., *et al.* Risk factors for hip fracture in white women. *N. Engl. J. Med.* **332,** 767–773 (1995).
18. Riggs, B. L., Wahner, H. W., Seeman, E., *et al.* Changes in bone mineral density of the proximal femur and spine with aging: Differences between the postmenopausal and senile osteoporosis syndromes. *J. Clin. Invest.* **70,** 716–723 (1982).
19. Sowers, M. R., Clark, M. K., Hollis, B., *et al.* Radial bone mineral density in pre- and postmenopausal women: A prospective study of rates and risk factors for loss. *J. Bone Miner. Res.* **7,** 647–657 (1992).
20. Hagino, H., Yamamoto, K., Teshima, R., *et al.* Radial bone mineral changes in pre- and postmenopausal healthy Japanese women: Cross-sectional and longitudinal studies. *J. Bone Miner. Res.* **7,** 147–152 (1992).
21. Nilas, L., and Christiansen, C. Rates of bone loss in normal women: Evidence of accelerated trabecular bone loss after the menopause. *Eur. J. Clin. Invest.* **18,** 529–534 (1988).
22. Davis, J. W., Ross, P. D., Wasnich, R. D., *et al.* Comparison of cross-sectional and longitudinal measurements of age-related changes in bone mass. *J. Bone Miner. Res.* **4,** 351–357 (1989).
23. Harris, S., and Dawson-Hughes, B. Rates of change in bone mineral density of the spine, heel, femoral neck and radius in healthy postmenopausal women. *Bone Miner.* **17,** 87–95 (1992).
24. Hansen, M. A., Overgaard, K., and Christiansen, C. Spontaneous postmenopausal bone loss in different skeletal areas—followed up for 15 years. *J. Bone Miner. Res.* **10,** 205–210 (1995).
25. Davis, J. W., Ross, P. D., and Vogel, J. M. Age-related changes in bone mass among Japanese-American men. *Bone Miner.* **15,** 227–236 (1991).
26. Nguyen, T. V., Sambrook, P. N., and Eisman, J. A. Bone loss, physical activity, and weight change in elderly women: The Dubbo Osteoporosis Epidemiology Study. *J. Bone Miner. Res.* **13**(9), 1458 (1998).
27. Ross, P. D. Risk factors for fracture. *In* "Spine: State of the Art Reviews: Vertebral Osteoporosis" (C. Cooper and J. Reeve, eds.), Vol. 8, pp. 91–110. Hanley and Belfus, Philadelphia, 1994.
28. Riis, B. J., Hansen, M. A., Jensen, A. M., *et al.* Low bone mass and fast rate of bone loss at menopause: Equal risk factors for future fracture: A 15-year follow-up study. *Bone* **19**(1), 9–12 (1996).
29. Melton, L. J., III, Ilstrup, D. M., Riggs, B. L., and Beckenbaugh, R. D. Fifty-year trend in hip fracture incidence. *Clin. Orthop.* **162,** 144–149 (1982).
30. Melton, L. J., III. Epidemiology of age-related fractures. *In* "The Osteoporotic Syndrome: Detection, Prevention, and Treatment" (Avioli, ed.), 3rd Ed., pp. 17–38. Wiley-Liss, New York, 1993.
31. Looker, A. C., Wahner, H. W., Dunn, W. L., Calvo, M. S., Harris, T. B., Heyse, S. P., Johnston, C. C., and Lindsay R. Updated data on proximal femur bone mineral levels of US adults. *Osteoporos. Int.* **8,** 469–489 (1998).
32. Melton, L. J., III. How many women have osteoporosis now? *J. Bone Miner. Res.* **10,** 175–177 (1995).
33. Melton, L. J., III, and Cummings, S. R. Heterogeneity of age-related fractures: Implications for epidemiology. *Bone Miner.* **2,** 321–331 (1987).
34. Cooper, C. Epidemiology of vertebral fractures in western populations. *In* "Spine: State of the Art Reviews: Vertebral Osteoporosis" (C. Cooper and J. Reeve, eds.), Vol. 8, pp. 1–21. Hanley and Belfus, Philadelphia, 1994.
35. Ross, P. D., Fujiwara, S., Huang, C., *et al.* Japanese women in Hiroshima have greater vertebral fracture prevalence than Caucasians or Japanese-Americans in the U.S. *Int. J. Epidemiol.* **24**(6), 1171–1177 (1995).
36. Ross, P. D., Wasnich, R. D., and Vogel, J. M. Detection of pre-fracture spinal osteoporosis using bone mineral absorptiometry. *J. Bone Miner. Res.* **3,** 1–11 (1988).
37. Cooper, C., Atkinson, E. J., O'Fallon, W. M., Melton, and L. J., III. Incidence of clinically diagnosed vertebral fractures: A population-based study in Rochester, Minnesota, 1985–1989. *J. Bone Miner. Res.* **7,** 221–227 (1992).
38. Ross, P. D., Davis, J. W., Epstein, R. S., and Wasnich, R. D. Pain and disability associated with new vertebral fractures and other spinal conditions. *J. Clin. Epidemiol.* **47,** 231–239 (1994).
39. Fisher, E. S., Baron, J. A., Malenka, D. J., *et al.* Hip fracture incidence and mortality in New England. *Epidemiology* **2,** 116–122 (1991).
40. Farmer, M. E., White, L. R., Brody, J. A., and Bailey, K. R. Race and sex differences in hip fracture incidence. *Am. J. Public Health* **74,** 1374–1380 (1984).

41. Cummings, S. R., Black, D. M., and Rubin, S. M. Lifetime risks of hip, Colles', or vertebral fracture and coronary heart disease among white postmenopausal women. *Arch. Intern. Med.* **149,** 2445–2448 (1989).
42. Lauritzen, J. B., Schwarz, P., Lund, B., *et al.* Changing incidence and residual lifetime risk of common osteoporosis-related fractures. *Osteopor. Int.* **3,** 127–132 (1993).
43. Cooper, C. The crippling consequences of fractures and their impact on quality of life. *Am. J. Med.* **103**(2A), 12S–19S (1997).
44. Melton, L. J., III. Socio-economic impact. *In* "Osteoporosis in Clinical Practice: A Practical Guide for Diagnosis and Treatment" (P. Geusens, ed.). Springer-Verlag, London, 1998.
45. Cooper, C., Atkinson, E. J., Jacobsen, S. J., *et al.* Population-based study of survival after osteoporotic fractures. *Am. J. Epidemiol.* **137,** 1001–1005 (1993).
46. Weiss, N. S., Liff, J. M., Ure, C. L., *et al.* Mortality in women following hip fracture. *J. Chron. Dis.* **36,** 879–882 (1983).
47. Browner, W. S., Seeley, D. G., Vogt, T. M., and Cummings, S. R. Non-trauma mortality in elderly women with low bone mineral density. *Lancet* **338,** 355–358 (1991).
48. Browner, W. S., Pressman, A. R., Nevitt, M. C., *et al.* Association between low bone density and stroke in elderly women. The study of osteoporotic fractures. *Stroke* **24,** 940–946(1993).
49. Gärdsell, P., and Johnell, O. Bone mass—a marker of biologic age? *Clin. Orthop.* **287,** 90–93 (1993).
50. Magaziner, J., Simonsick, E. M., Kashner, T. M., *et al.* Predictors of functional recovery one year following hospital discharge for hip fracture: A prospective study. *J. Gerontol. Med. Sci.* **45,** M101–M107 (1990).
51. Jalovaara, P., and Virkkunen, H. Quality of life after hemiarthroplasty for femoral neck fracture. *Acta Orthop. Scand.* **62,** 208–217 (1991).
52. Marotolli, R. A., Berkman, L. F., and Cooney, L. M. Decline in physical function following hip fracture. *J. Am. Geriatr. Soc.* **40,** 861–866 (1992).
53. Cummings, S. R., Phillips, S. L., Wheat, M. E., *et al.* Recovery of function after hip fracture. *J. Am. Geriatr. Soc.* **36,** 801–806 (1988).
54. Huang, C., Ross, P. D., and Wasnich, R. D. Vertebral fractures and other predictors of back pain among older women. *J. Bone Miner. Res.* **11**(7), 1025–1031 (1996).
55. Lyritis, G. P., Mayasis, B., Tsakalakos, N., *et al.* The natural history of the osteoporotic vertebral fracture. *Clin. Rheumatol.* **8**(Suppl. 2), 66–69 (1989).
56. Gold, D. T. The clinical impact of vertebral fractures: Quality of life in women with osteoporosis. *Bone* **18**(Suppl), 185S–189S (1996).
57. Patel, U., Skingle, S., Campbell, G. A., *et al.* Clinical profile of acute vertebral compression fractures in osteoporosis. *Br. J. Rheum.* **30,** 418–421 (1991).
58. Ryan, P. J., Evans, P., Gibson, T., and Fogelman, I. Osteoporosis and chronic back pain: A study with single-photon emission computed tomography bone scintigraphy. *J. Bone Miner. Res.* **7**(12), 1455–1460 (1992).
59. Ryan, P. J., Blake, G., Herd, R., and Fogelman, I. A clinical profile of back pain and disability in patients with spinal osteoporosis. *Bone* **15,** 27–30 (1994).
60. Nevitt, M. C., Ettinger, B., Black, D. M., Stone, K., Jamal, S., Ensrud, K., Segal, M., Genant, H. K., and Cummings, S. R. The association of radiographically detected vertebral fractures with back pain and function: A prospective study. *Ann. Intern. Med.* **128**(10), 793 (1998).
61. Ross, P. D., Davis, J. W., and Epstein, R. S. Pain and disability associated with new vertebral fractures and other spinal conditions. *J. Clin. Epidemiol.* **47,** 231–239 (1994).
62. Ettinger, B., Black, D. M., Palermo, L., *et al.* Contribution of vertebral deformities to chronic back pain and disability. *J. Bone Miner. Res.* **7**(4), 449–456 (1992).
63. Cook, D. J., Guyatt, G. H., Adachi, J. D., *et al.* Quality of life issues in women with vertebral fractures due to osteoporosis. *Arthritis Rheum.* **36,** 750–756 (1993).
64. Ross, P. D., Ettinger, B., Davis, J. W., *et al.* Evaluation of adverse health outcomes associated with vertebral deformities. *Osteoporos. Int.* **1**(3), 134–140 (1991).
65. Huang, C., Ross, P. D., and Davis, J. W. Contributions of vertebral fractures to stature loss among elderly Japanese-American women in Hawaii. *J. Bone Miner. Res.* **11**(3), 408–411 (1996).
66. Greendale, G. A., Barrett-Connor, E., Ingles, S., and Haile, R. Late physical and functional effects of osteoporotic fracture in women: The Rancho Bernardo Study. *J. Am. Geriatr. Soc.* **43,** 955–961 (1995).
67. Huang, C., Ross, P. D., and Wasnich, R. D. Vertebral fracture and other predictors of physical impairment and health care utilization. *Arch. Intern. Med.* **156,** 2469–2475 (1996).
68. Ross, P. D. Clinical consequences of vertebral fractures. *Am. J. Med.* **103**(2A), 30S–43S (1997).
69. Greendale, G. A., and Barrett-Connor, E. Outcomes of osteoporotic fractures. *In* "Osteoporosis" (R. Marcus, D. Feldman, and J. Kelsey, eds.), pp. 635–643. Academic Press, San Diego, 1996.
70. Ribot, C., Tremollieres, F., and Pouilles, J.-M. Can we detect women with low bone mass using clinical risk factors? *Am. J. Med.* **98**(Suppl 2A), 52S–55S (1995).
71. Bauer, D. C., Browner, W. S., Cauley, J. A., *et al.* Factors associated with appendicular bone mass in older women. *Ann. Intern. Med.* **118,** 657–665 (1993).
72. Slemenda, C. W., Hui, S. L., Longcope, C., *et al.* Predictors of bone mass in perimenopausal women. *Ann. Intern. Med.* **112,** 96–101 (1990).
73. Ross, P. D. Prediction of fracture risk, II: Other risk factors. *Am. J. Med. Sci.* **312**(6), 260–269 (1996).
74. Reid, I. R. Steroid osteoporosis. *In* "Spine: State of the Art Reviews: Vertebral Osteoporosis" (C. Cooper and J. Reeve, eds.), Vol. 8, pp. 111–131. Hanley and Belfus, Philadelphia, 1994.
75. Minaire, P. Immobilization osteoporosis: A review. *Clin. Rheumatol.* **852,** 95–103 (1989).
76. Andersson, S. M., and Nilsson, B. E. Changes in bone mineral content following tibia shaft fractures. *Clin. Orthop. Rel. Res.* **144,** 226–229 (1979).
77. Kannus, P., Leppala, J., Lehto, M., *et al.* A rotator cuff injury produces permanent osteoporosis in the affected extremity, but not in those with whom the shoulder function has returned to normal. *J. Bone Miner. Res.* **10,** 1263–1271 (1995).
78. Prince, R. L., Price, R. I., and Ho, S. Forearm bone loss in hemiplegia: A model for the study of immobilization osteoporosis. *J. Bone Miner. Res.* **3,** 305–310 (1988).
79. Grisso, J. A., Kelsey, J. L., and Strom, B. L. Risk factors for falls as a cause of hip fracture in women. *N. Engl. J. Med.* **324**(19), 1326–1331 (1991).
80. Cummings, S. R., Nevitt, M. C., Browner, W. S., *et al.* Risk factors for hip fracture in white women. *N. Engl. J. Med.* **332,** 767–773 (1995).
81. Dawson-Hughes, B., Dallal, G. E., Krall, E. A., *et al.* Effect of vitamin D supplementation on wintertime and overall bone loss in healthy postmenopausal women. *Ann. Intern. Med.* **115,** 505–512 (1991).
82. Heaney, R. P. Thinking straight about calcium. *N. Engl. J. Med.* **328,** 503–505 (1993).
83. Sowers, M. R., Clark, M. K., Hollis, B., *et al.* Radial bone mineral density in pre- and postmenopausal women: A prospective study

of rates and risk factors for loss. *J. Bone Miner. Res.* **7,** 647–657 (1992).

84. Nilas, L., and Christiansen, C. Rates of bone loss in normal women: Evidence of accelerated trabecular bone loss after the menopause. *Eur. J. Clin. Invest.* **18,** 529–534 (1988).
85. Prior, J. C., Vigna, Y. M., Schechter, M. T., and Burgess, A. E. Spinal bone loss and ovulatory disturbances. *N. Engl. J. Med.* **323,** 1221–1227 (1990).
86. Rigotti, N. A., Nussbaum, S. R., Herzog, D. B., and Neer, R. M. Osteoporosis in women with anorexia nervosa. *N. Engl. J. Med.* **311,** 1601–1606 (1984).
87. Ettinger, B., Genant, H. K., and Cann, C. E. Long-term estrogen replacement therapy prevents bone loss and fractures. *Ann. Intern. Med.* **102,** 319–324 (1985).
88. Krieger, N., Kelsey, J. L., Holford, T. R., and O'Connor, T. An epidemiologic study of hip fracture in postmenopausal women. *Am. J. Epidemiol.* **116,** 141–148 (1982).
89. Cauley, J. A., Seeley, D. G., Ensrud, K., *et al.* Estrogen replacement therapy and fractures in older women. Study of Osteoporotic Fractures Research Group. *Ann. Intern. Med.* **122,** 9–16 (1995).
90. Horsman, A., Nordin, B. E., and Crilly, R. G. Effect on bone of withdrawal of oestrogen therapy. *Lancet* **2,** 33 (1979).
91. Lindsay, R., Hart, D. M., MacLean, A., *et al.* Bone response to termination of oestrogen treatment. *Lancet.* **1,** 1325–1327 (1978).
92. Cummings, S. R., Black, D. M., Thompson, D. E., *et al.* Effect of alendronate on risk of fracture in women with low bone density but without vertebral fractures. *JAMA.* Dec 23/30, **280**(24), 2077–2082 (1998).
93. Black, D. M., Cummings, S. R., Karpf, D., *et al.* Randomized trial of effect of alendronate on risk of fracture in women with existing vertebral fractures. *Lancet* **348,** 1535–1541 (1996).
94. Chesnut, C. H., III., McClung, M. R., Ensrud, K. E., *et al.* Alendronate treatment of the postmenopausal osteoporotic woman: effect of multiple dosages on bone mass and bone remodeling. *Am. J. Med.* **99,** 144–152 (1995).
95. Ross, P. D. Using bone turnover markers to assess bone loss and fracture risk. *Female Patient* (OB/GYN edition) **23**(9), 59.
96. Garnero, P., Hausherr, E., Chapuy, M.-C., *et al.* Markers of bone resorption predict hip fracture in elderly women: The EPIDOS prospective study. *J. Bone Miner. Res.* **11,** 1531–1538 (1996).
97. Lauritzen, J. B., Schwarz, P., McNair, P., *et al.* Radial and humeral fractures as predictors of subsequent hip, radial or humeral fractures in women, and their seasonal variation. *Osteoporos. Int.* **3,** 133–137 (1993).
98. Gärdsell, P., Johnell, O., Nilsson, B. E., and Nilsson, J. A. The predictive value of fracture, disease, and falling tendency for fragility fractures in women. *Calcif. Tissue Int.* **45,** 327–330 (1989).
99. Ross, P. D., He, Y.-F., Yates, A. J., *et al.,* for the EPIC Study Group. Body size accounts for most differences in bone density between Asian and Caucasian women. *Calcif. Tissue Int.* **59,** 339–343 (1996).
100. Cummings, S. R., Cauley, J., Palermo, L., *et al.* Racial differences in hip axis length might explain racial differences in rates of hip fracture. *Osteoporos. Int.* **4,** 226–229 (1994).
101. Cundy, T., Cornish, J., Evans, M. C., *et al.* Sources of interracial variation in bone mineral density. *J. Bone Miner. Res.* **10**(3), 368–373 (1995).
102. Davis, J. W., Ross, P. D., Nevitt, M. C., and Wasnich, R. D. Incidence rates of falls among Japanese men and women living in Hawaii. *J. Clin. Epidemiol.* **50**(5), 589–594 (1997).
103. O'Loughlin, J. L., Robitaille, Y., Boivin, J. F., and Suissa, S. Incidence of and risk factors for falls and injurious falls among the community-swelling elderly. *Am. J. Epidemiol.* **137,** 342–354 (1993).
104. Campbell, A. J., Borrie, M. J., and Spears, F. Risk factors for falls in a community-based prospective study of people 70 years and older. *Gerontol.* **44,** M112–M117 (1989).
105. Lord, S. R., Sambrook, P. N., Gilbert, C., *et al.* Postural stability, falls, and fractures in the elderly: Results from the Dubbo Osteoporosis Epidemiology Study. *Med. J. Aust.* **160**(11), 684–685 (1994).
106. Lord, S. R., Clark, R. D., and Webster, A. W. Physiological factors associated with falls in an elderly population. *J. Am. Geriatr. Soc.* **39,** 1194–2000 (1991).
107. Nevitt, M. C., Cummings, S. R., Kidd, S., and Black, D. Risk factors for recurrent nonsyncopal falls. A prospective study. *JAMA* **261,** 2663–2668 (1989).
108. Tinetti, M. E., Speechley, M., and Ginter, S. F. Risk factors for falls among elderly persons living in the community. *N. Engl. J. Med.* **319,** 1701–1707 (1988).
109. Tinetti, M. E., Baker, D. I., McAvay, G., *et al.* A multifactorial intervention to reduce the risk of falling among elderly people living in the community. *N. Engl. J. Med.* **331,** 821–827 (1994).
110. Nordin, B. E. C. The definition and diagnosis of osteoporosis. *Calcif. Tissue Int.* **40,** 57–58 (1987).
111. Daniels, E. D., Pettifor, J. M., Schnitzler, C. M., Moodley, G. P., and Zachen, D. Differences in mineral homeostasis, volumetric bone mass and femoral neck axis length in black and white South African women. *Osteopor. Int.* **7,** 105–112 (1997).

CHAPTER 30

Osteoporosis and Fragility Fractures in the Elderly

MICHAEL C. NEVITT Department of Epidemiology and Biostatistics, University of California, San Francisco, San Francisco, California 94105

INTRODUCTION

Osteoporosis and fractures affect a substantial proportion of the older population in the United States and other Western nations. Older Caucasian women are at greatest risk, but older Caucasian men and Asian, Hispanic, and African American older women are also frequently affected. Fractures in the elderly occur at many diverse skeletal sites in addition to those traditionally considered "osteoporotic" (Fig. 1), which adds substantially to the overall burden of the disease. A better understanding of the factors contributing to the risk of these many diverse fractures in the elderly is needed to guide the search for their causes and new approaches to prevention.

FREQUENCY OF OSTEOPOROSIS AND LOW BONE MASS

Because bone mineral is strongly correlated with the strength of the skeleton [1] and is established as a strong determinant of the risk of fractures in older white women [2,3] and men [4], the prevalence of osteoporosis can be assessed in terms of the proportion of the population with low bone mass. An expert panel of the World Health Organization has defined low bone mass (osteopenia) in women as a bone density between 1.0 and 2.5 SD below the mean for young adult women and osteoporosis as a bone density more than 2.5 SD below the young adult mean. Women in the latter group who have already experienced one or more fractures are considered to have "established" osteoporosis [5]. Because the risk of fracture in individuals is a function of both bone density and other age-related risk factors [6,7], these definitions are useful for defining the prevalence of the condition but are limited as treatment thresholds. Moreover, the relationship between bone density and fracture risk is continuous [2] and there is little evidence for a biomechanical threshold at which fractures occur [1].

Bone density measurements at the hip, spine, and radius in a random sample of women from Rochester, Minnesota, have been used to estimate the prevalence of low bone mass or osteoporosis at one or more of these measurement sites for the 1990 population of U.S. white women age 50 and over [8]. According to this study, 30% (9.4 million) of postmenopausal white women have osteoporosis and another 54% (16.8 million) have low bone mass. The prevalence of osteoporosis was similar using each of the individual bone density measurement sites (16–17%). About half of the women with osteoporosis and 16% of all postmenopausal white women (4.8 million) meet the criteria for established osteoporosis. The prevalence of osteoporosis at any site increased dramatically with age, from about 15% in women aged 50–59 to 70% in those aged 80 and older. These estimates are valuable because they are based on bone density measurements at multiple sites, but are derived from a limited racial and geographic sample.

An estimate of the broader scope of the disease in the older U.S. population for 1990 to 1993, although based on bone density of the hip only, is provided by national probability sample data from the third National

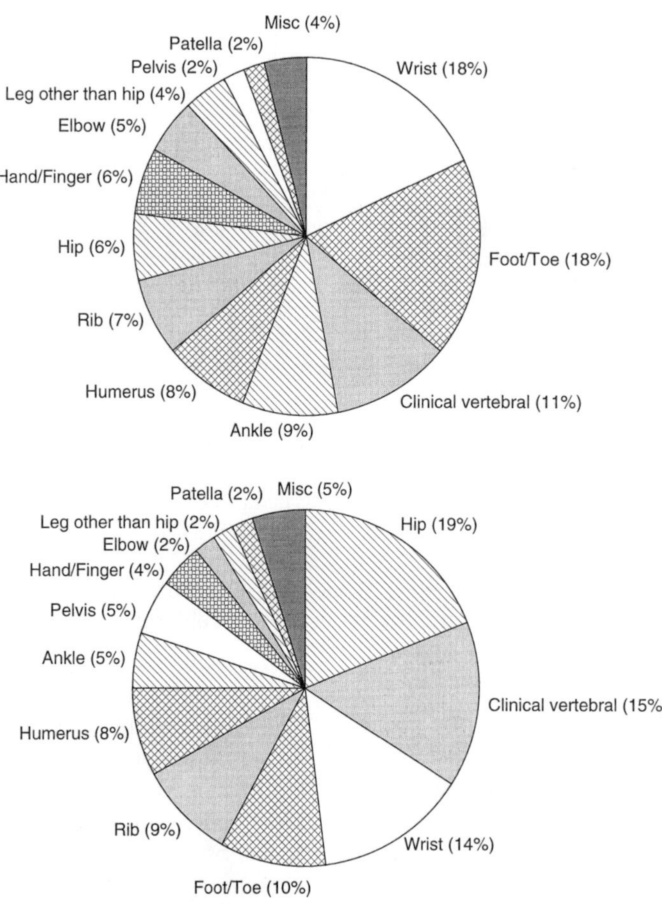

FIGURE 1 Types of fractures occurring in women ages 65–74 (top) and ages 80 and over (bottom). From Seeley *et al.* [35].

Health and Nutrition Examination Survey (NHANES) [9]. Reference ranges for young normals were obtained from 409 non-Hispanic white women and 382 non-Hispanic white men aged 20–29. Using total femur bone density, 17% (5 million) of U.S. white women age 50 and over have osteoporosis and another 42% (12 million) have low bone mass. Prevalence estimates varied by region of interest in the hip and were about 20% higher when based on bone density of the femoral neck. As expected, NHANES data indicate a decreased prevalence of femoral osteoporosis and low bone mass in white women compared to the estimates based on multiple bone density sites. However, the estimated prevalence of femoral osteoporosis was similar in the two studies.

Based on the total femur bone density cutoff values for white women, NHANES data suggest that 8% (0.3 million) of non-Hispanic black women and 12% (0.1 million) Mexican American women have osteoporosis and another 28% (0.9 million) and 37% (0.3 million), respectively, have low bone mass. For men aged 50 and over, a sufficient sample was available to estimate the prevalence of low bone mass for all races combined. Based on bone density cutoff values for the total femur derived from young males, 4% of all men have osteoporosis and another 33% have low bone mass. Similar to the finding for women, prevalence estimates varied by region of interest in the hip and were about 40–50% higher when based on bone density of the femoral neck. Using total femur bone density cutoff values derived from young white women reduced the estimated prevalence of osteoporosis and low bone mass by about one-half. Given uncertainty about whether cutoff values for defining osteoporosis should be gender specific, there is a large range in estimates of the number of U.S. men affected (0.25–2.0 million). However, a study from The Netherlands [10] suggests that the relationship between absolute bone density and hip fracture incidence is similar in men and women of the same age, which lends support to using cutoff values derived from young women and thus for the lower estimates of prevalence in men

By any yardstick, the numbers of older women in the United States with an increased risk of fracture because of osteoporosis or low bone mass are substantial (Table I) and approach or exceed the number with other common conditions of aging, including hypertension, diabetes, and high blood cholesterol [8]. NHANES data provide the first look at the substantial magnitude of the problem of osteoporosis among several racial and ethnic subgroups of older U.S. women. Although the validity of applying bone density cutoffs derived from white women to define osteoporosis in other race and ethnic groups is uncertain, the age-adjusted prevalence ratios for white compared to non-white women obtained from NHANES are consistent with known differences in the incidence of fracture between these groups [11–14]. Nevertheless, studies of the relationship between bone density and fracture risk in racial and ethnic subgroups in the United States are needed to validate the NHANES prevalence estimates for these groups. Prevalence estimates for other nations using the World Health Organization definitions are not yet available. One preliminary estimate for the United Kingdom suggests that the prevalence of femoral osteoporosis in older women (23%) is very similar to the NHANES estimates for the United States [15].

FREQUENCY AND ECONOMIC COST OF OSTEOPOROTIC FRACTURES

Fractures associated with osteoporosis are extremely common in the older population (Table I). One study done in the mid-1980s estimated that 1.3 million fractures per year in the United States could be attributed to osteoporosis [16]. This estimate assumed that 70% of all fractures in the elderly are due, at least in part, to low bone mass. A report relying on expert group judgement concluded that for white women aged 65–84, osteoporosis is responsible for about 90% of hip and spine fractures, 70% of wrist fractures, and 50% of all other fractures [17]. In contrast, estimates of the population attributable risk for hip fracture based on actual data on the relationship between bone mass and fracture risk in women suggest that a much lower proportion of hip fractures (21–25%) is attributable to low bone mass [3]. The latter may underestimate the true contribution of osteoporosis if aspects of bone quality affected adversely by the disease contribute to fracture risk independently of bone density.

Table I Frequency and Impact of Osteoporosis in the United States[a]

Persons with femoral osteoporosis or osteopenia	
White women	17–21 million
Non-white women	1.5–1.8 million
Men	4–15 million
Lifetime risk of hip, wrist, or vertebral fracture	
50-year-old white women	40%
50-year-old white man	13%
Fractures per year due to osteoporosis	1.3 million
Hip fractures per year	250,000–300,000
Hospitalization per year for osteoporotic fractures	432,000
Outpatient visits per year for osteoporotic fractures	3.4 million
Medical expenditures for osteoporotic fractures in 1995	$13.8 billion

[a] See text for sources of data.

In 1995 there were an estimated 432,000 hospital discharges for osteoporotic fractures in the United States involving persons age 45 and older; 57% (246,600) of these were hip fractures, 3% (13,400) were forearm fractures, 7% (29,400) were spine fractures, and 33% (142,700) were other fractures [18]. Another report suggests that the actual number of hip fractures may be as high as 300,000 per year [19]. Women accounted for 80% of all hospitalizations for fracture and 77% of those for hip fracture. The corresponding proportions for white women were 74 and 72%, respectively. With the exception of hip fractures, however, the vast majority of fractures were treated on an outpatient basis. This same study estimated that osteoporotic fractures were responsible for a total of 3.4 million outpatient physician, hospital, and emergency room visits, of which nearly two-thirds were for fractures at sites other than hip, spine, and forearm, and 179,222 nursing home stays, of which 77% were for hip fractures.

The economic burden resulting from osteoporotic fractures is substantial and rising. Total direct medical expenditures for osteoporotic fractures in the mid-1980s in the United States were estimated to be about $5–6 billion [20,21]. Direct U.S. medical expenditures in 1995 for osteoporotic fractures were estimated at $13.8 billion [18]. In a more recent study, 75% of expenditures were for the treatment of white women, 18% for white men, and 7% for the treatment of non-whites. Nearly 30% of expenditures were for fractures other than hip, spine, or wrist. As the number of elderly in the population increases, these costs are expected to rise rapidly. According to one projection, the number of hip fractures and their associated costs could triple by the year 2040 due to demographic changes alone [22].

Globally, Cooper and colleagues [23] have estimated that 1.66 million hip fractures occurred in 1990, with 71% of these involving women and about 45% occurring in countries outside Europe and North America. They project that by 2050, aging of the global population will nearly quadruple the annual number of hip fractures worldwide in both men and women. Because aging of the population will be relatively more rapid in Asia, Latin America, and Africa, 70% of hip fractures will occur in these regions.

Hip fracture rates vary substantially by geographic area and race [24,25]. Age-adjusted hip fracture incidence rates are highest (>6 per 1000 per year) in largely Caucasian populations of Scandinavia and North America. Intermediate age-adjusted rates of 4–6 per 1000 per year have been observed in Great Britain, New Zealand, and Finland, whereas rates of 2–4 per 1000 per year have been found in Hong Kong and Japan and in Asian, black, and Hispanic populations in the United States. Even lower rates have been reported for some Asian countries and blacks in South Africa. In the higher incidence rate populations, the ratio of female to male incidence is around 2 to 1, but this ratio tends to decline as the overall incidence rate declines. These geographic variations in hip fracture incidence are only partly explained by intercountry differences in the way hip fractures are defined, treated, and ascertained [25]. Variations in bone mass, bone size and geometry, physical activity, diet, and other life-style factors may also contribute to geographic and racial differences in fracture risk [26].

LIFETIME RISK OF FRACTURE

The risk of fracture in the remaining life of an individual is influenced by the life expectancy of that person and the risk of fracture at any given age. These competing factors have been modeled in several studies [27–29] that have produced consistent estimates of the lifetime risk of fracture for an average risk 50-year-old white woman and white man (Table II). Lifetime risks of hip fracture for blacks have been reported from one study [29], but there are insufficient data for other fractures or racial groups. The three- to fivefold greater lifetime risks for 50-year-old white women compared to white men and blacks (hip fracture only) are consistent with the relative prevalence of low bone mass and osteoporosis in each group (see earlier discussion), coupled with the longer life expectancy of white women. The lifetime risk at age 50 of having a hip, wrist, or clinical vertebral fracture is about 40% in white women and 13% in white men [27]. A 50-year-old white woman has a 30% lifetime risk of having a fracture other than hip, wrist, or spine and a 70% risk of a fracture at any site (unpublished data from the Study of Osteoporotic Fractures).

TABLE II Lifetime Risk of Fracture at Age 50 Years in Persons with Average Risk

	Hip fracture (%)	Distal forearm (%)	Vertebral fracture: Clinical (%)	Vertebral fracture: Radiographic (%)
White women	16–17[a,b,c]	15–16[a,b,c]	16[c]	35[a]
White men	5–6[a,b,c]	2–3[a,b,c]	5[c]	?
Black women	6[b]	?	?	?
Black men	3[b]	?	?	?

[a] From Chrischilles *et al.* [28].
[b] From Cummings *et al.* [29]
[c] From Melton *et al.* [27]

A lifetime risk of fracture at age 50 is useful for weighing the public health burden of osteoporosis and comparing the long-term risk of various conditions. Estimates of lifetime risk at a variety of different ages must take into account the shorter life expectancy of older persons with high short-term risk as well as the age-related increase in fracture risk likely to occur in younger persons with low short-term risk [30]. For example, the lifetime risk of hip fracture for an 80-year-old white woman (14%) or man (7%) is very similar to that of a 50-year-old woman or man because both hip fracture risk and mortality increase exponentially with age [29]. In contrast, the lifetime risk of wrist fractures, the incidence of which does not increase much with age, is much lower at age 80 in white women (4%) and men (0.5%) than at age 50 [29]. Because people may place greater importance on events likely to occur in the near future, estimates of the intermediate term risk (e.g., next 5 years) faced by people who have already reached a given age will be useful when weighing the benefits and risks of treatment.

Because fracture risk and mortality [31] are both strongly related to a person's bone density at a given age, attempts have been made to incorporate these relationships into estimates of lifetime fracture risk [30,32]. For example, Black *et al.* [32] estimated that a 50-year-old white woman has a 19% lifetime risk of hip fracture if her radial bone mass is at the 10th percentile for her age and an 11% lifetime risk if her bone mass is at the 90th percentile. The difference in lifetime risk of hip fracture between women with high and low bone density will be even greater for estimates based on hip bone density, which is more strongly related to hip fracture risk than bone density at other sites [33], but these estimates are not yet available. Paradoxically, a 50-year-old woman with average radial bone density for her age has a 16% lifetime risk of hip fracture, but an 80-year-old woman with the same absolute bone density has only about a 6% risk in her remaining life [32]. Only a very small fraction of white women, however, have a bone density this "high" by the time they are 80 years old [8].

HETEROGENEITY IN THE RELATIONSHIP OF DIFFERENT TYPES OF FRACTURES TO GENDER, AGE, AND BONE DENSITY

The hallmark epidemiological characteristic of osteoporotic fractures are incidence rates that are higher among women than men and that increase sharply with age [34]. Hip, vertebral, distal forearm, proximal humerus, and pelvis fractures have traditionally been considered to share these broad characteristics, and although they represent only a small fraction of all the skeletal sites affected by fracture in old age, they account for about one-half of clinical fractures in white women aged 65 and over (Fig. 1) [35] and about one-third of fractures in men [4]. Direct assessment of the association between bone density and fracture risk, however, shows that most types of fractures in white women are related to low bone mass and are therefore, at least in part, due to osteoporosis [35,36]. There is considerable heterogeneity in the relationship of different types of fracture with these epidemiological markers of "osteoporotic" fracture (Table III), which may provide clues about differences in their pathogenesis [37].

A higher incidence of fractures in older women compared to men may reflect a lower peak bone mass and greater bone loss with age among women. The female-to-male ratio for age-adjusted incidence rates in Rochester, Minnesota, for clinical vertebral, hip, pelvis, proximal humerus, and distal forearm fractures ranges from about 2 to 1 to 5 to 1. The ratio for all other limb fractures combined is 1 to 1 (Fig. 2) [37,38]. In a population-based European study of radiographically detected vertebral deformities, no difference in the age-adjusted prevalence between men and women aged 50 to 79 was found [38]. The female-to-male ratio of prevalent deformities increased with age, however, suggesting that traumatic fractures at younger ages in men may contribute to an overall gender similarity in prevalence [39]. A detailed breakdown for a variety of less well-studied fracture sites using an elderly Tennessee Medicaid population found that ankle, femoral shaft, tibia/fibula, and patellar fractures each had an age-adjusted relative risk of 2 or more for female gender. In contrast, the risks of rib, hand, foot, clavicle/scapula, and skull fractures were weakly, or not at all, related to gender (Table III) [14].

An increasing risk of fracture with age may reflect a continuation of bone loss into advanced age at most skeletal sites [40,41]. However, the relationship of incidence to increasing age among older women also varies considerably by type of fracture (Fig. 3). Hip fracture incidence is observed to climb exponentially with age

Table III Types of Fracture in the Elderly Associated with Gender, Age, Bone Density, and Falls[a]

Type of fracture	Fracture rates/risk associated with: Female gender	Increased age	BMD[b]	% of fractures associated with a fall[c]
Hip	+	+	++	>90
Wrist	+	–	++	>90
Vertebral	+[d]	+[d]	++[e]	<50[d]
Proximal humerus	+	+	++	>90
Pelvis	+	+	++	80–90
Rib	–	+	++	50–79
Clavicle	–	–	++	<50
Femur shaft	+	+	++	50–79
Patella	+	–	++	80–90
Tibia/fibula	+	–	++	50–79
Ankle	+	–	+	80–90
Heel	NA	–	++	NA
Foot	–	–	+	<50
Toe	NA	–	+	<50
Elbow	NA	–	+	>90
Hand	–	–	++	50–79
Finger	NA	–	+	50–79
Face	–	–	–	50–79

[a] From Griffin *et al.* [14], Seeley *et al.* [35,36], Melton and Cummings [37], and Nevitt *et al.* [92].

[b] +, relative risk ≥1.2–1.7 per SD decrease in BMD at one or more peripheral and axial measurement sites; ++, relative risk ≥1.8 per SD decrease in BMD at one site.

[c] Fall from standing height or less.

[d] Clinical vertebral fractures.

[e] Radiographically detected vertebral deformities.

in both women and men [26]. The incidence of clinical vertebral fractures in both genders [4,38] and in radiographically detected vertebral deformities in women [42] also increases sharply with age. Of the remaining skeletal sites, only the incidence of proximal humerus, pelvis, rib, and femoral shaft fractures has shown a strong relationship to age in older women and, to a lesser extent, in older men [4,14,35–7,43]. Incidences of most other types of fracture appear to be weakly, or not at all, related to increasing age (Table III) [14,35].

Heterogeneity in the relationship of different fractures to age is reflected in changes with age in the mix of fractures that occur in an older population (Fig. 1). In the Study of Osteoporotic Fractures, composed of a large community-based cohort of elderly white women, distal extremity fractures predominate among women aged 65–74. Among women age 80 and over, distal

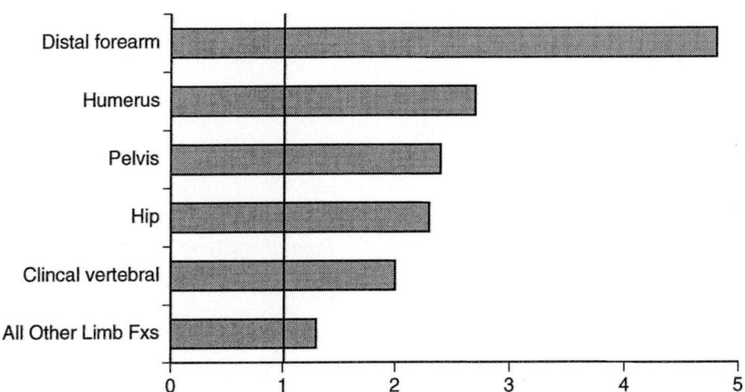

FIGURE 2 Ratio of female to male age-adjusted fracture incidence rates: Rochester, Minnesota, residents age ≥35. From Melton and Cummings [37] and Cooper *et al.* [39].

extremity fractures are still important, but hip, vertebral, rib, and pelvis fractures make up a much larger proportion of the total in these women. In both age groups, however, fractures occur at many diverse sites.

The risk of nearly all types of fracture increases with decreasing bone density [3,35,36,44], including several types that are not associated with gender or age (Table III). Bone density at any commonly measured site in the peripheral or axial skeleton has a similar predictive ability for the risk of a given type of fracture and for all fractures combined. [2,3]. Only hip bone density and hip fracture have demonstrated a uniquely strong site-specific association [3,33]. However, the strength of the association between fracture risk and bone density varies substantially by the site of fracture. In a comprehensive evaluation of diverse types of fracture [35,36], Seeley and colleagues report that only face fractures were not associated with either peripheral or axial bone density. Finger, elbow, ankle, foot, and toe fractures were moderately related to bone density, with relative risks ranging from 1.2 to 1.7 per standard deviation (SD) decrease in bone density. All other fractures sites were strongly related to bone density, with a relative risk of 1.8 or greater per SD decrease at one or more peripheral or axial bone density sites.

POSSIBLE CAUSES OF HETEROGENEITY IN AGE-RELATED FRACTURES

Site-specific differences in bone loss with age may contribute to heterogeneity among fractures in their broad demographic patterns and relationship to bone density. Bone loss at the hip and calcaneus appears to accelerate in the very old [40,41], but this pattern is less clear for other sites. One study suggests that cortical bone loss in the forearm may slow after age 60 in women [45]. These differences are consistent with the plateau in the incidence of wrist fractures around age 60, in

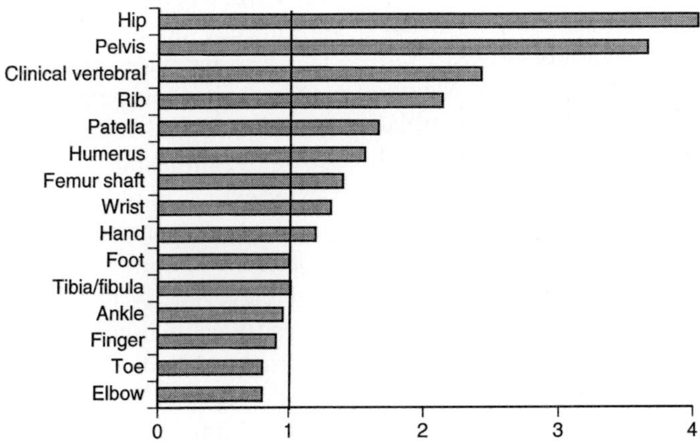

FIGURE 3 Ratio of fracture incidence rates in women age ≥75 versus women aged 65–74. From Nevitt [54].

contrast with the continued sharp increase in hip fractures with age.

It is likely, however, that other age-related factors also play a role in site-specific fracture risk, including the frequency and type of falls and other trauma, neuromuscular changes, and the effects of bone quality on bone strength. Falls are the most common source of trauma in the elderly. The risk of falling doubles between the ages of 60 and 80 and is greater in women than men at most ages [47], consistent with the age and gender incidence patterns for some types of fracture. Over 80% of nonspine fractures in older white women are the result of a fall from a standing height or less (generally considered to represent mild to moderate trauma) [45,46], but the proportion attributable to falls varies widely by type of fracture (Table III). Several types of fracture that are nearly always associated with falls, such as hip, wrist, proximal humerus, and pelvis, tend also to be strongly associated with female gender and age (Table III). Foot, toe, hand, finger, and face fractures, however, are much less likely to be due to falls and also have inconsistent or weak relationships to gender and age. Sources of trauma in the elderly not due to falls are poorly understood. Types of fracture that are nearly always due to falls also tend to have a stronger relationship to bone density than those frequently associated with other types of trauma, although there are notable exceptions (e.g., vertebral fractures) (Table III). Several studies have found that bone density is related more strongly to fractures that are the result of falls compared to its association with the same types of fracture when these are due to more severe forms of trauma [35,45].

Fewer than 5% of falls result in fracture and less than 1% in a hip fracture [46]. Biomechanical factors such as the orientation, height, and potential energy of a fall, the effectiveness of protective arm and leg responses, and energy absorbed by soft tissues affect the location and force of impact of a fall and therefore determine which bone is at risk and whether a fracture will occur [1]. Variations in these biomechanical factors by gender and age may help explain, for example, the failure of wrist fracture incidence to increase with age in contrast to the sharp rise in hip fracture incidence, despite a strong association of both types of fracture with bone density and falls. Age-related slowing of gait and loss of neuromuscular coordination may make it less likely that an older faller will land on the wrist and more likely that they will land on another bone, especially the hip [48,49]. Several studies have found that falls directly onto the hip, and especially falls to the side, carry an extremely high risk of hip fracture [48,50]. An increased frequency of these unprotected falls with age may contribute to the exponential rise in hip fracture incidence with age. Age-related loss of soft tissue padding would be more likely to affect the risk of some fractures (e.g., hip, humerus) than others (wrist, lower leg).

About 30% of clinically diagnosed vertebral fractures are associated with a fall from a standing height or less. Women are more than three times as likely as men to have a vertebral fracture due to moderate or minimal trauma, including falls, whereas men have a twofold higher risk of fracture due to severe trauma [39]. Common activities such as standing while holding an object in outstretched arms, holding an object with trunk flexed, and arms extended or lifting a moderate weight object from the floor can generate forces in the spine sufficient to fracture the lumbar vertebrae of an older osteoporotic woman [1]. Gender- and age-related characteristics such as vertebral body size, degree of kyphosis, the distribution of body weight, weakness of spinal musculature, and the presence of degenerative disc disease may affect the strength of the vertebrae or alter the magnitude of forces in the spine during common activities. The effect of these factors on the risk of vertebral fractures is not known, but should be a high priority for future study.

Age-related decrements in bone quality, including loss of trabecular continuity, increased cortical porosity, abnormalities of mineralization, and the accumulation of microfractures, are thought to contribute to increased bone fragility in the elderly [51] and may have varying effects on different types of fractures. The extent to which the possible effects of bone quality on fracture risk are independent of bone density is not known. However, an independent effect of age and prior fractures on subsequent fracture risk, after adjusting for bone density, is sometimes interpreted as a marker for an independent effect of bone quality on fracture risk. After adjustment for bone density and other risk factors, age and previous fractures remain significantly associated with the risk of hip [6] and vertebral fractures [52]. In contrast, age and previous fracture do not affect risk of proximal humerus fractures, another fracture whose incidence increases sharply with age, after adjusting for bone density [53]. Methods for the direct assessment of bone quality are needed for a better understanding of its contribution to the risk of various age-related fractures.

SUMMARY

A variety of pathophysiological mechanisms lead to reduced bone strength and an increased risk of fracture in the elderly. White women are most frequently and severely affected, but the risk of osteoporosis in men and non-whites is also substantial and is only beginning to be fully appreciated. Fractures occur at many diverse skeletal sites in the elderly. Although the classical osteoporotic fracture sites of hip, spine, wrist, and proximal humerus account for about one-half of fractures and more than two-thirds of the medical costs of osteoporosis in the elderly, fractures at other skeletal sites make a substantial contribution to the overall burden of the disease. The lifetime risk of having any type of fracture for a 50-year-old white woman is about 70%. The many different types of fracture that occur in the elderly have a diverse and heterogeneous relationship to key risk factors such as gender, age, and bone density. These broad patterns point to potential heterogeneity in the underlying pathophysiological mechanisms that contribute to the risk of different fractures. An examination of these differences may lead to a better appreciation of the complex and diverse causes of fragility fractures in the elderly and guide the search for new approaches to prevention in this fast-growing segment of the population.

References

1. Bouxsein, M. L., Myers, E. R., and Hayes, W. C. Biomechanics of age-related fractures. *In* "Osteoporosis" (R. Marcus, D. Feldman, and J. Kelsey, eds.), pp. 373–393. Academic Press, San Diego, 1996.
2. Black, D., Cummings, S., Genant, H., Nevitt, M., Palermo, L., and Browner, W. Axial and appendicular bone density predict fractures in older women. *J. Bone Miner. Res.* **7**(6), 633–638 (1992).
3. Marshall, D., Johnell, O., and Wedel, H. Meta-analysis of how well measures of bone mineral density predict occurrence of osteoporotic fractures. *Br. Med. J.* **312,** 1254–1259 (1996).
4. Nguyen, T. V., Eisman, J. A., Kelly, P. J., and Sambrook, P. N. Risk factors for osteoporotic fractures in elderly men. *Am. J. Epidemiol.* **144**(3), 255–263 (1996).
5. World Health Organization. "Assessment of Fracture Risk and Its Application to Screening for Postmenopausal Osteoporosis," WHO Technical Report Series, WHO, Geneva, 1994.
6. Cummings, S. R., Nevitt, M. C., Browner, W. S., *et al.* Risk factors for hip fracture in white women. *N. Engl. J. Med.* **332,** 767–773 (1995).
7. Nguyen, T., Sambrook, P., Kelly, P., *et al.* Prediction of osteoporotic fractures by postural instability and bone density. *Br. Med. J.* **307,** 1111–1115 (1993).
8. Melton, L. J. How many women have osteoporosis now? *J. Bone Miner. Res.* **10,** 175–177 (1995).
9. Looker, A. C., Orwoll, E. S., Johnston, C. C., Jr., Lindsay, R. L., Wahner, H. W., Dunn, W. L., Calvo, M. S., Harris, T. B., and Heyse, S. P. Prevalence of low femoral bone density in older U.S. adults from NHANES III. *J. Bone Miner. Res.* **12**(11), 1761–1768 (1997).
10. De Laet, C. E. D. H., van Hout, B. A., Burger, H., Hofman, A., and Pols, H. A. P. Bone density and risk of hip fracture in men and women: Cross sectional analysis. *Br. Med. J.* **315,** 221–225 (1997).
11. Kellie, S. E., and Brody, J. A. Sex-specific and race-specific hip fracture rates. *Am. J. Public Health* **80,** 326–328 (1990).
12. Silverman, S. L., and Madison, R. E. Decreased incidence of hip fracture in Hispanics, Asians, and Blacks: California hospital discharge data. *Am. J. Public Health* **78**(11), 1482–1483 (1988).
13. Farmer, M. E., White, L. R., Brody, J. A., and Bailey, K. R. Race and sex differences in hip fracture incidence. *Am. J. Public Health* **74,** 1374–1380 (1984).
14. Griffin, M. R., Ray, W. A., Fought, R. L., and Melton, L. J., III. Black–white differences in fracture rates. *Am. J. Epidemiol.* **136,** 1378–1385 (1992).
15. Cooper, C., and Melton, L. J., III. Magnitude and impact of osteoporosis and fractures. *In* "Osteoporosis" (R. Marcus, D. Feldman, and J. Kelsey, eds.), pp. 419–434. Academic Press, San Diego, 1996.
16. Kelsey, J. L. Osteoporosis: Prevalence and incidence. *In* "Osteoporosis, Proceedings of the NIH Consensus Development Conference;" pp. 25–28. Held April 2 through April 4, 1984.
17. Melton, L. J., III, Thamer, M., Ray, N. F., Chan, J. K., Chesnut, C. H., III, Einhorn, T. A., Johnston, C. C., Raisz, L. G., Silverman, S. L., and Siris, E. S. Fractures attributable to osteoporosis: Report from the National Osteoporosis Foundation. *J. Bone Miner. Res.* **12**(1), 16–23 (1997).
18. Ray, N. F., Chan, J. K., Thaemer, M., and Melton, L. J., III. Medical expenditures for the treatment of osteoporotic fractures in the United States in 1994. *J. Bone Miner. Res.* **12,** 24–35 (1997).
19. U. S. Congress Office of Technology Assessment, "Hip Fracture Outcomes in People Age 50 and Over—Background Paper." OTA-BP-H-120, U. S. Government Printing Office, Washington, DC, 1994.
20. Philips, S., Fox, N., Jacobs, J., and Wright, W. E. The direct medical costs of osteoporosis for American women aged 45 and older, 1986. *Bone* **9,** 271–279 (1988).
21. Holbrook, T. L., Grazier, K., Kelsey, J. L., and Stauffer, R. N., "The Frequency of Occurrence, Impact and Cost of Selected Musculoskeletal Conditions in the United States." American Academy of Orthopedic Surgeons, Chicago, 1984.
22. Schneider, E. L., and Guralnik, J. M. The aging of America: Impact on health care costs. *JAMA* **263,** 2335–2350 (1990).
23. Cooper, C., Campion, G., and Melton, L. J., III. Hip fractures in the elderly: A world-wide projection. *Osteopor. Int.* **2,** 285–289 (1992).
24. Maggi, S., Kelsey, J. L., Litvak, J., *et al.* Incidence of hip fractures in the elderly: A cross-national analysis. *Osteopor. Int.* **1,** 232–241 (1991).
25. Villa, M. L., and Nelson, L. Race, ethnicity, and osteoporosis. *In* "Osteoporosis" (R. Marcus, D. Feldman, and J. L., Kelsey, eds.), pp. 435–437. Academic Press, San Diego, 1996.
26. Cumming, R. G., Nevitt, M. C., and Cummings, S. R. Epidemiology of hip fractures. *Epidemiol. Rev.* **19**(2), 244–257 (1997).
27. Melton, L., Chrischilles, E., Cooper, C., Lane, A., and Riggs, B. How many women have osteoporosis? *J. Bone Miner. Res.* **7**(9), 1005–1010 (1992).
28. Chrischilles, E. A., Butler, C. D., Davis, C. S., and Wallace, R. B. A model of lifetime osteoporosis impact. *Arch. Intern. Med.* **151,** 2026–2032 (1991).
29. Cummings, S. R., Black, D. M., and Rubin, S. M. Lifetime risks of hip, Colles' or vertebral fracture and coronary heart disease among white postmenopausal women. *Arch. Intern. Med.* **149,** 2445–2448 (1989).
30. Suman, V. J., Atkinson, E. J., O'Fallon, W. M., Black, D. M., and Melton, L. J., III. A nomogram for predicting lifetime hip fracture risk from radius bone mineral density and age. *Bone* **14,** 843–846 (1993).
31. Browner, W. S., Seeley, D. G., Vogt, T. M., Cummings, S. R., and the Study of Osteoporotic Fractures Research Group. Non-trauma mortality in elderly women with low bone density. *Lancet* **338,** 355–358 (1991).

32. Black, D. M., Cummings, S. R., and Melton, L. J., III. Appendicular bone mineral and a woman's lifetime risk of hip fracture. *J. Bone Miner. Res.* **7**(6), 639–646 (1992).
33. Cummings, S. R., Black, D. M., Nevitt, M. C., *et al.* Bone density at various sites for prediction of hip fractures. *Lancet* **341,** 72–75 (1993).
34. Melton, L. J., III. Epidemiology of fractures. *In* "Osteoporosis: Etiology, Diagnosis, and Management" (B. L. Riggs and L. J. Melton, eds.), pp. 133–154. Raven Press, New York, 1988.
35. Seeley, D. G., Browner, W. S., Nevitt, M. C., Genant, H. K., Scott, J. C., and Cummings, S. R., for the Study of Osteoporotic Fractures Research Group. Which fractures are associated with low appendicular bone mass in elderly women? *Ann. Intern. Med.* **115,** 837–842 (1991).
36. Seeley, D. G., Browner, W. S., Nevitt, M. C., Genant, H. K., and Cummings, S. R. Almost all fractures are osteoporotic. *J. Bone Miner. Res.* **10**(S1), 468 (1995).
37. Melton, L. J., III, and Cummings, S. R. Heterogenity of age-related fractures: Implications for epidemiology. *Bone Miner* **2,** 321–331 (1987).
38. O'Neill, T. W., Felsenberg, D., Varlow, J., Cooper, C., Kanis, J. A., Silman, A. J., and the European Vertebral Osteoporosis Study Group. The prevalence of vertebral deformity in European men and women: The European Vertebral Osteoporosis study. *J. Bone Miner. Res.* **11**(7), 1010–1018 (1996).
39. Cooper, C., Atkinson, E. J., O'Fallon, W. M., Melton, L. J., III. Incidence of clinically diagnosed verterbral fractures: A population-based study in Rochester, Minnesota, 1985–1989. *J. Bone Miner. Res.* **7,** 221–227 (1992).
40. Ensrud, K. E., Palermo, L., Black, D. M., *et al.* Hip and calcaneal bone loss increase with advancing age: Longitudinal results from the study of osteoporotic fractures. *J. Bone Miner. Res.* **10**(11), 1778–1787 (1995).
41. Jones, G., Nguyen, T., Sambrook, P., Kelly, P. J., and Eisman, J. A. Progressive loss of bone in the femoral neck in elderly people: Longitudinal findings of the Dubbo osteoporosis epidemiology study. *Br. Med. J.* **309,** 691–695 (1994).
42. Melton, L. J., III, Lane, A. W., Cooper, C., Eastell, R., O'Fallon, W. M., and Riggs, B. L. Prevalence and incidence of vertebral deformities. *Osteopor. Int.* **3,** 113–119 (1993).
43. Arneson, T. J., Melton, L. J., III, Lewallen, D. G., and O'Fallon, W. M. Epidemiology of diaphyseal and distal femoral fractures in Rochester, Minnesota, 1965–1984. *Clin. Orthop.* **234,** 188–194 (1988).
44. Melton, L. J., III, Atkinson, E. J., O'Fallon, M., Wahner, H. W., and Riggs, B. L. Long-term fracture prediction by bone mineral assessed at different skeletal sites. *J. Bone Miner. Res.* **8,** 1227–1233 (1993).
45. Hui, S. L., Wiske, P. S., Norton, J. A., and Johnston, C. C. A prospective study of change in bone mass with age in postmenopausal women. *J. Chronic Dis.* **35,** 715–725 (1982).
46. Nevitt, M., and Cummings, S. R. Falls and fractures in older women. *In* "Falls, Balance and Gait Disorders in the Elderly" (B. Vellas, M. Toupet, L. Rubenstein, J. Albarede, and Y. Christen, eds.), pp. 69–80. Elsevier, Paris, 1992.
47. Nevitt, M. Falls in older persons: Risk factors and prevention. *In* "The Second Fifty Years: Promoting Health and Preventing Disability" (R. Berg, ed.), pp. 263–289. National Academy Press, Washington, 1990.
48. Nevitt, M. C., and Cummings, S. R. Type of fall and risk of hip and wrist fractures: The study of osteoporotic fractures. *J. Am. Geriatr. Soc.* **41**(11) (1993).
49. Cummings, S. R., and Nevitt, M. C. A hypothesis: The causes of hip fractures. *J. Gerontol. Med. Sci.* **44,** M107–M111 (1989).
50. Greenspan, S. L., Myers, E. R., Maitland, L. A., Resnick, N. M., and Hayes, W. C. Fall severity and bone mineral density as risk factor for hip fracture in ambulatory elderly. *JAMA* **217,** 128–133 (1994).
51. Melton, L. J., III, Chao, E. Y. S., and Lane, J. Biomechanical aspects of fracture. *In* "Osteoporosis: Etiology, Diagnosis, and Management" (B. L. Riggs and L. J. Melton III, eds.), pp. 133–154. Raven Press, New York, 1988.
52. Nevitt, M. C., Cummings, S. R., Black, D. M., Genant, H. K., Fox, K., and Stone, K. Risk factors for first and recurrent vertebral fractures. *J. Bone Miner. Res.* **10**(S1), 468 (1995).
53. Kelsey, J., Browner, W., Seeley, D., Nevitt, M., Cummings, S., and Group, S. R. Risk factors for fractures of the distal forearm and proximal humerus. *Am. J. Epidemiol.* **135**(5), 477–489 (1992).
54. Nevitt, M. C. *Rheum. Dis. Clin. N. Am.* **20,** 535–559 (1994).

CHAPTER 31

The Aging Maxillofacial Skeleton

MEREDITH AUGUST AND LEONARD B. KABAN
Department of Oral and Maxillofacial Surgery, Massachusetts General Hospital, Boston, Massachusetts 02114

INTRODUCTION

Aging of the maxillofacial complex produces important functional and aesthetic changes. The jaws may reflect the aging process and metabolic changes taking place throughout the skeleton, but they also show unique patterns of resorption and remodeling. Alterations in dentition, supporting alveolar bone and attachments of the muscles of mastication, account for the significant morphologic consequences of aging and alterations in masticatory efficiency. Structural and functional changes in the temporomandibular joint can also affect mastication. Osteopenia and osteoporosis of the maxilla and mandible are less well understood. The capacity of osteopenic jaws to heal normally and to integrate dental implants are important issues for dental practitioners. This chapter reviews skeletal changes in the maxilla and mandible from birth to maturity. Changes in the morphology of the bones and the relationship to tooth loss, the secondary effect of decreased muscle mass, and the effects of systemic physiologic alterations and osteoporosis are discussed.

SKELETAL CHANGES FROM BIRTH TO MATURITY

To better understand the changes that take place in the facial skeleton as a consequence of aging, the basic principles of facial growth should be understood. Enlow and Hans [1] describe two basic types of movement in the developing jaws, namely *remodeling* and *displacement.* Remodeling is the term Enlow has chosen to describe the phenomenon of bony deposition and resorption that creates changes in size. Bone biologists more commonly refer to this movement as "modeling" and, for consistency, it will be so called in the remainder of this discussion. With modeling, each component of the bone sequentially relocates to allow for enlargement and changes in shape. These changes accommodate different functions. In contrast, displacement is defined as a physical movement of the entire bone away from other bones in direct articulation to it. Both modeling and displacement occur simultaneously as the facial skeleton grows.

The Mandible

With growth, the mandible is displaced away from its articulation in the glenoid fossa. The condyle and ramus then grow upward and backward into the space created by the displacement process. With modeling, the ramus becomes progressively longer and wider to accommodate the functional demands of mastication and the widening pharyngeal space. The condyle itself is no longer considered as a pace-setting "master" growth center for the lower jaw. It is, however, a major field of growth. Injury to this area at a young age can have significant consequences on function and symmetry of the jaws [1].

The development of the inferior alveolar nerve (IAN) and its final position in the adult mandible should be well understood to avoid injury during mandibular procedures such as the removal of third molar teeth and jaw osteotomies. Examination of human embryos and fetal specimens has shed light on the development of this nerve and its relation to the growing mandible. The appearance of nerve tissue precedes ossification, and early bone formation is found in close relation to the developing nerve. Three separate canals appear to develop from the lingual aspect of the mandibular ramus and, with them, three distinct nerve branches to different tooth groups. Rapid prenatal growth and modeling in the ramus region result in eventual coalescence of these to form the single mandibular foramen that is evident at birth [2]. In adults, this foramen lies, on average, 4 mm above the plane of the teeth and 2 cm below the sigmoid notch (Fig. 1). Distal to its insertion into the intrabony canal through which the nerve courses, an alveolar branch is given off that supplies the posterior teeth. Before exiting the bone at the mental foramen, other fibers leave the nerve and form an intricate plexus apical to the roots of the incisor teeth. The mental nerve is the large terminal branch of the IAN. It exits the bone at the mental foramen and innervates the skin of the lower lip and chin as well as the mucosa and gingiva of the incisor region [3].

The Maxilla

Both types of growth are also observed in the maxilla. Lengthening in the sagittal plane is produced by modeling in the region of the maxillary tuberosity. It is here that backward-facing periosteal surfaces expand the bony volume. The alveolar arch widens as deposition takes place on the lateral surfaces, and growth along the midpalatal suture results in progressive widening of the bone. The entire maxilla also undergoes a simultaneous process of primary displacement in an anterior and inferior direction (Fig. 2). As this displacement occurs, the osteogenic sutural regions form new bone that enlarges the entire maxilla [1].

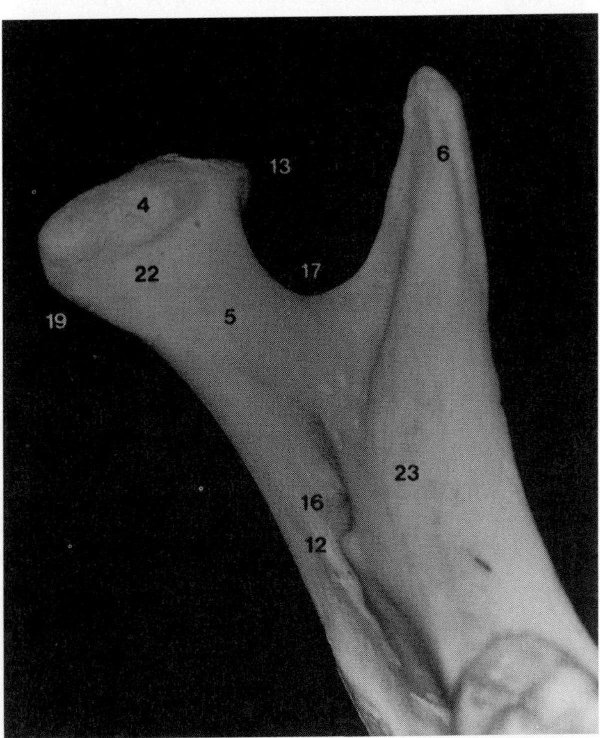

FIGURE 1 Inner aspect of the left hemimandible demonstrating the position of the lingula (12) and its relationship to the entry into the bone of the inferior alveolar nerve (16) and the inferior aspect of the sigmoid notch (17). The articular surface of the condyle is indicated by 4. The last molar tooth is visible at the bottom right. Reproduced with permission from McMinn *et al.* [52].

Dentition

The formation and eruption of teeth takes place in both jaws during the process of growth. As tooth buds develop, the roots gradually enlarge and eruption takes place. After eruption, a process described as "drift" allows the teeth to move as the maxilla and mandible grow. Dentition thus changes position and keeps pace with the rapidly enlarging mandible and maxilla. The teeth and their enveloping bone sockets move as a unit. This process of drift is distinct from the simple extrusion of teeth, which is sometimes observed with loss of opposing occlusal contact.

The maxillofacial complex has a timetable of growth and development related to the changing airway, masticatory muscle function, influence of the fifth and seventh cranial nerves, and eruption of the teeth. Once skeletal maturity is reached, it is the physiologic and functional consequences of aging that produce subsequent alterations in the jaws [1].

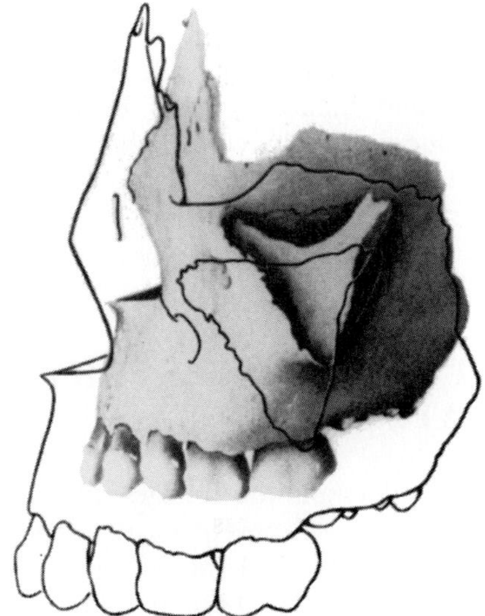

FIGURE 2 The entire maxilla undergoes displacement in an anterior and inferior direction with growth. The immature maxillary skeleton is depicted by the stipled drawing and the adult maxilla by the outline. Reproduced with permission from Moyers and Enlow [53].

SKELETAL CHANGES AFTER MATURITY ASSOCIATED WITH TOOTH LOSS

Major alterations in the morphology of the jaw bones with aging are usually secondary to tooth loss and progressive atrophy. Fortunately, with the advent of widely available dental care and preventive measures, the incidence of edentulism has decreased. Large cohort studies in Sweden have shown a decrease in the edentulous population over the decade of 1972 to 1982 from 52 to 34% [4]. Similar trends have been observed in the United States [5]. However, the progressive effects of periodontal disease, loss of tooth-supporting bone, and deleterious habits such as tobacco use on bone mineral content remain leading causes of tooth loss and consequent jaw atrophy.

Factors associated with ridge resorption are categorized as either local or systemic. Local factors, in addition to loss of teeth, include previous bone loss secondary to periodontal disease, the duration of edentulism, and occlusal forces transmitted to the ridge from denture prostheses. Denture forces may accelerate alveolar atrophy in some cases. Systemic factors that have an adverse effect on bone mineralization include age, female gender, low calcium intake, osteoporosis, other metabolic bone disorders, and the use of medications such as corticosteroids.

The Mandible

The changes in morphology of the mandible after tooth loss have been studied extensively. In addition, long-term reduction of the residual ridge and its effect on jaw occlusal relationships have been investigated. Atwood [6] studied the observable patterns of mandibular atrophy and classified residual ridge form into six orders that have gained wide acceptance (Fig. 3). These range from the dentate alveolus through the early changes with tooth loss and finally loss of basal mandibular bone.

Ulm *et al.* [7] evaluated the position of the mandibular canal and its alteration with progressive atrophy. Edentulous lower jaw halves ($n = 43$) were sectioned between the mental foramina and third molar regions. Mandibles were classified according to residual ridge order as described earlier. The distance between the mandibular canal and the lingual (medial) and buccal (lateral) cortical plates was not found to be affected by the atrophic process. However, the distance between the mandibular canal and the superior and inferior borders changed in a statistically significant fashion. The decrease in distance

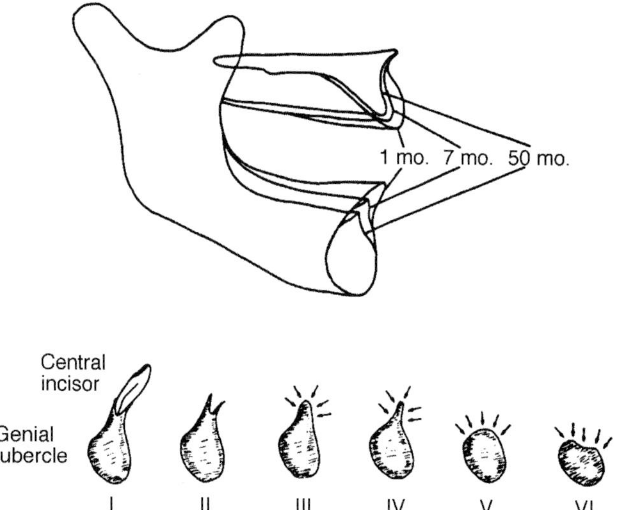

FIGURE 3 Six orders of residual ridge form of the mandible from the preextraction stage (I) to severe resorption of basal bone (V and VI). The tracings represent changes in the maxilla and mandible at 1, 7, and 50 months postextraction. Reproduced with permission from Atwood [54].

from the canal to the superior border of the atrophic ridge was most striking. These changes were most evident in the edentulous first molar region. This often complicates dental implant placement into the posterior mandible. If the height above the inferior alveolar nerve canal is less than the requisite amount required for even the shortest dental implants, placement may not be possible. Impingement on the inferior alveolar nerve and nerve injury has been reported under these circumstances (Fig. 4). In addition, resorption of bone overlying the mental foramen and mental nerve can result in impingement and pain from an overlying denture.

There appear to be gender-related differences in the bone mineral density of atrophic mandibles. Solar *et*

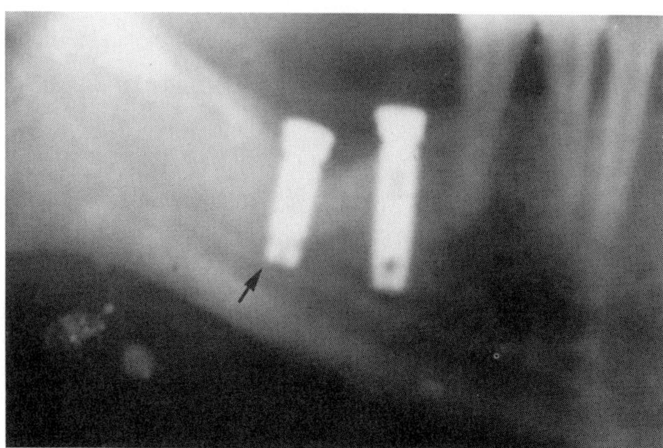

FIGURE 4 Dental radiograph demonstrating the proximity of a root-form endosseous implant to the inferior alveolar nerve canal (noted by arrow) of the mandible.

al. [8] measured the mineral content in 25 edentulous mandibles with dual-photon absorptiometry. With advancing age, mineral density in the mandibles of men was found to increase slightly whereas those in women tended to decrease. It was also found that the inner cortical bone in male atrophic mandibles increased in width. This was determined to be an adaptive response to stabilize the severely thinned bone. However, it was not observed in women and the role of osteoporosis in limiting this adaptation should be explored.

The Maxilla

The maxilla demonstrates more rapid and severe resorption than the mandible after tooth loss, presumably because of its thin medullary and cortical architecture. The pattern of bone loss commonly observed is described as centripetal (tending to narrow the bone) on three-dimensional analysis. This is distinct from the centrifugal resorption noted in the mandible, which results in an overall widening as basal bone is resorbed. A frequently encountered width discrepancy between the two bones in long-term edentulous patients is seen [9]. This problem complicates prosthetic rehabilitation in that the two dental arches are no longer compatible.

Without teeth, there is little functional stimulation or load on the jaws. This is compounded in denture wearers when focal pressure from an overlying prosthesis accelerates bone loss. The maxillary alveolus initially thins in a labiopalatal direction with retention of alveolar height. This results in what is commonly described as a "knife-edged" ridge (Fig. 5). Use of dental implants in such sites frequently results in perforation of the labial bone. Similarly, this ridge form is less than ideal for comfortable denture use and retention. As bone loss continues, alveolar height is lost and buccinator and other muscle attachments obliterate labial vestibular depth, further compromising denture retention. The pneumatized maxillary sinuses are prominent in edentulous individuals and progressive loss of bone height is occasionally seen to the level of the antral floor (Fig. 6).

Resorption of the anterior maxilla can lead to prominence of the anterior nasal spine and yet another impediment to comfortable denture use. Placement of dental implants in the maxilla is also complicated by the anatomy. Insufficient bone below both the antra and nasal cavities necessitates bone grafting procedures if implants are to placed. In addition, this progressive bone loss results in soft tissue changes to the upper lip and face and resultant esthetic problems. In both men and women, there is progressive thinning of soft tissue in the region of the anterior nasal spine with age [10]. The maxilla moves progressively superiorly and posteriorly in space, resulting in decreased lower face height.

SKELETAL CHANGES AFTER MATURITY WITHOUT TOOTH LOSS

Mandibular Changes

If the teeth are maintained, very little morphologic change is noted in the anatomical landmarks of the

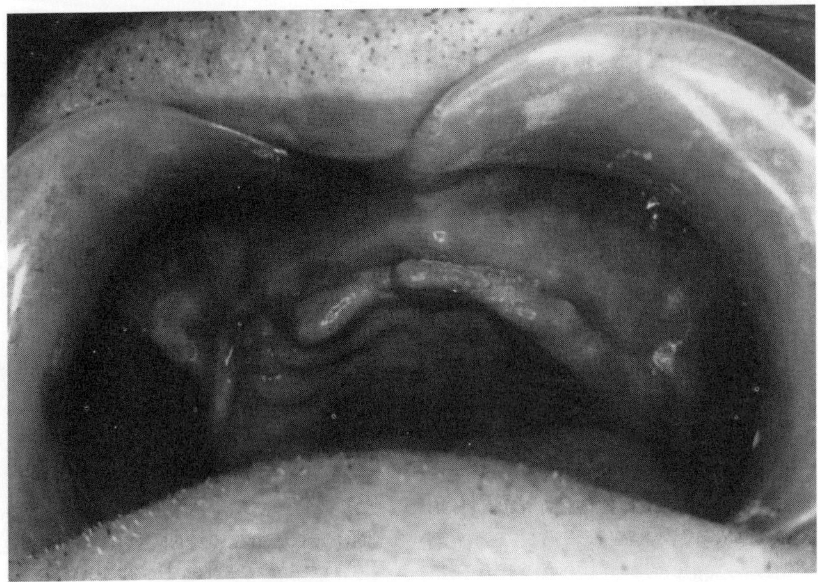

FIGURE 5 Clinical photograph of maxillary resorption in the labiopalatal direction resulting in a knife-edge configuration.

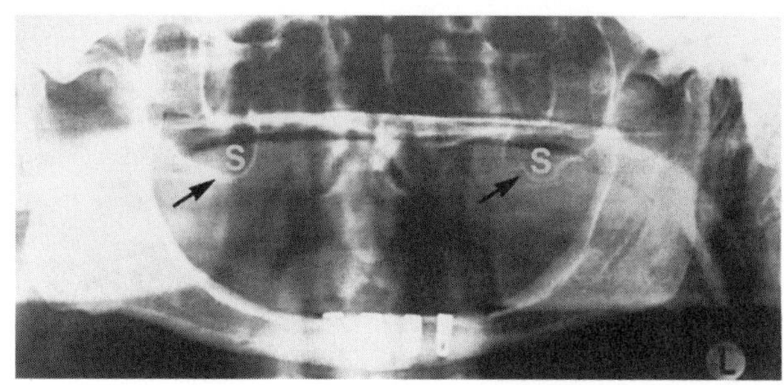

FIGURE 6 Panoramic radiograph demonstrating pneumatization of the maxillary sinuses (S) to the level of the resorbed alveolar bone (arrows).

mandible with age [11]. The distance from the lingula (the foramen through which the inferior alveolar nerve and vessels enter the mandible) to the anterior edge of the ramus does not change over time. Similarly, the ramus dimensions, coronoid process, and lingula–mental foramen distance are all stable throughout life. Only in the area of the mandibular symphysis are bony changes noted with age. In females, there is appositional bone growth in the region of the chin (pogonion), making it appear more prominent. The loss of vertical dimension associated with tooth loss, attrition of teeth, and jaw overclosure further add to the prominence of the chin point (Fig. 7). In addition, progressive thickening of the mentalis muscles and overlying soft tissue occurs with aging.

Maxillary Changes

If the teeth are not lost, the maxilla remains relatively stable with aging. Doual *et al.* [12] evaluated changes in maxillary anatomic structures with age and found stability in the size of the sinuses as well as the position of the premaxilla. That group noted a subtle but progressive increase in posterior maxillary height as well as a downward and forward pivoting of the palatine processes over time. It is not known whether this is associated with functional changes in bite force and occlusion.

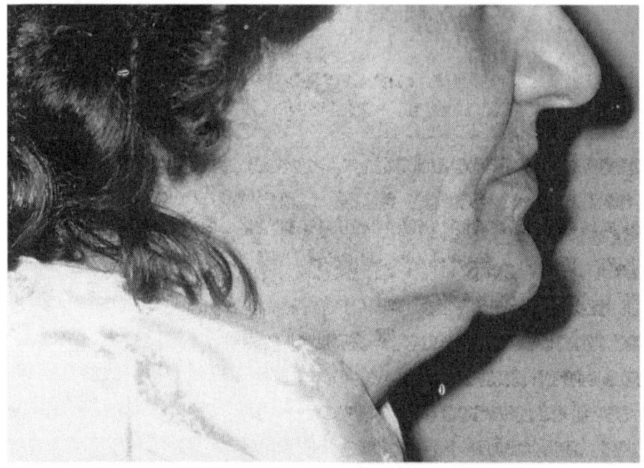

FIGURE 7 Lateral photograph demonstrating the loss of vertical dimension and jaw overclosure frequently observed with tooth loss and aging. Note the resultant prominence of the chin point and deepened nasolabial fold, also described in the "aging face."

CHANGES IN THE TEMPOROMANDIBULAR JOINT ASSOCIATED WITH AGING

The temporomandibular joint comprises the mandibular condyle, its articulation with the glenoid fossa of the temporal bone, the interposing meniscus, and associated muscle and ligamentous attachments. Although not a weight-bearing joint, it is the recipient of significant loading forces secondary to both normal masticatory function and the effects of parafunctional habits such as bruxism. Manifestations of osteoarthrosis and bony degeneration as well as rheumatologic abnormalities in this joint have been described [13,14].

Strattman *et al.* [15] evaluated the effect of aging on the temporomandibular joint (TMJ) and its associated cartilaginous meniscus. That group evaluated 100 postmortem TMJ specimens in patients 65–85 years of age. Measurements were made of meniscal thickness at five discrete points. Of note is that 27% of specimens showed lateral and laterocentral perforations of the meniscus and 8% showed thinning of the lateral surface of the disk so as to render it translucent. These changes in the disk had been reported previously [16]. Some authors believe this to be secondary to overloading of the lateral portion of the meniscus during excursive movements and bruxism. Because the meniscus is composed of fibrocartilage and possesses no regenerative capacity, perforation is an end stage abnormality [17,18]. Discal thinning and perforation may be part of the normal aging process and not pathologic. It is estimated that such perforations may be anticipated in more than 80% of patients over the age of 80 years. Despite the large number of meniscal abnormalities, gross degenerative changes in the condyle itself were noted in only 3% of the specimens in this study. Milder degenerative changes have been reported more frequently with increasing age [13].

Radiologic evaluation of the condyle in the fifth and sixth decades of life showed that less than 40% of condyles had a smooth, regular, and convex form. Deterioration and notching of the cortical plate were seen routinely after the seventh decade. These changes were characterized by a polygonal or flattened shape with sclerosis of the bone on radiograph (Fig. 8) [19].

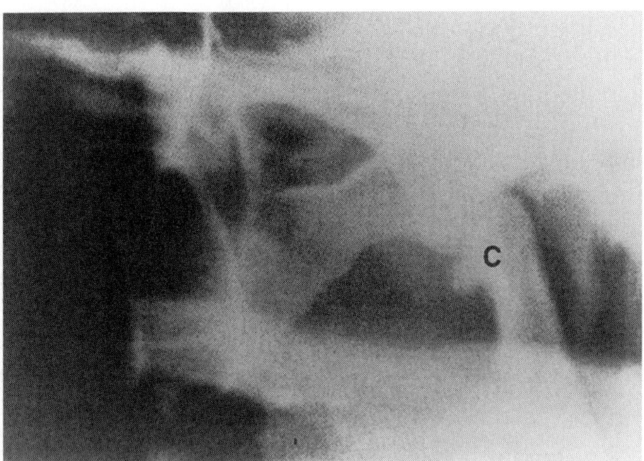

FIGURE 8 Tomogram of the condyle (C) of the mandible demonstrating severe flattening, sclerosis, and osteophyte formation associated with degenerative disease. Reproduced with permission from Norman and Bramley [55].

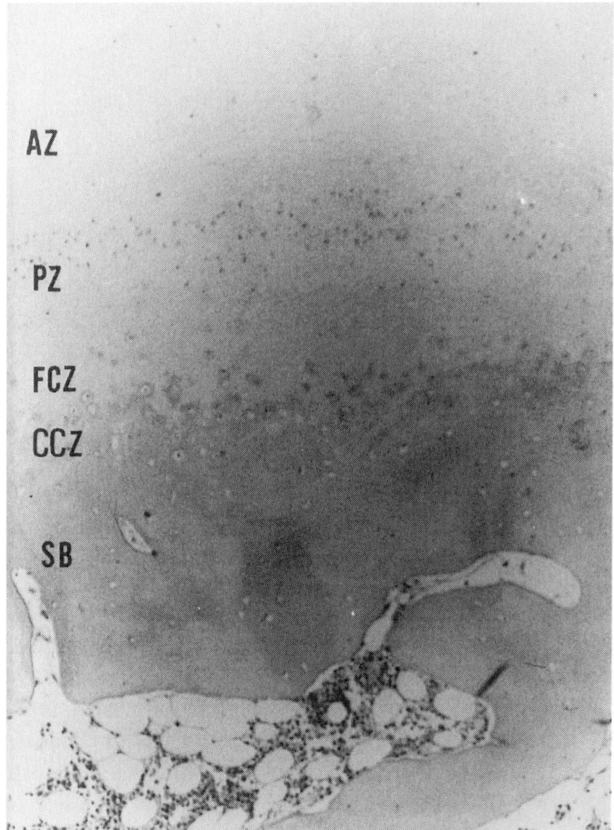

FIGURE 9 The four histologic zones of the articular cartilage of the condyle are noted: articular zone (AZ), proliferative zone (PZ), fibrocartilaginous zone (FCZ), and calcified cartilaginous zone (CCZ). SB represents the subchondral bone of the condyle. Reproduced with permission from Ishibashi *et al.* [13].

Histologic studies of the cartilaginous zones of the condyle at different ages similarly show reproducible patterns of change [13]. In the fifth and sixth decades, the articular zone was found to be thickened with a compact arrangement of the collagen fibers. In the seventh decade, the number of undifferentiated mesenchymal cells and chondrocytes was decreased with less production of extracellular matrix. In more than 50% of specimens, there was a horizontal split between fibrocartilaginous and calcified cartilaginous zones. These zones are illustrated in Fig. 9. Because undifferentiated mesenchymal cells and chondrocytes are related to the ability of the articular surface to remodel and regenerate, the depression noted with aging may play a role in the development of osteoarthritis.

One of the more commonly described symptoms associated with temporomandibular joint dysfunction is the presence of joint noise (clicking and/or crepitation) that is secondary to meniscal movement and to degenerative changes. If these sounds are not associated with symptoms of pain or limitation of movement, further diagnostic efforts are not warranted. Most studies indicate that the presence of joint sounds increases with age and tooth loss and is more frequently observed in women. Mandibular dysfunction as well as crepitation are most common in edentulous individuals [20].

Maximal interincisal opening is measured as the vertical distance between maxillary and mandibular central incisors. This measurement is usually greater in men than women and ranges from 40 to 55 mm [21]. Studies on large elderly populations have shown significant decreases with age for both sexes. The percentage of individuals over age 65 unable to open to 40 mm was 15.8% in one large study [22]. The functional consequences of the progressive decrease in jaw motion in the elderly is not understood.

CHANGES IN BITE FORCE AND CHEWING EFFICIENCY WITH AGE

Investigators have documented changes in bite force associated with aging [23–25]. The number of remaining teeth have a strong impact on variation in measured forces. Direct measurements of the capacity to reduce a test-food bolus to small particles showed that chewing efficiency decreases as the natural occlusion deteriorates. Full-denture wearers have substantially lower bite force than dentate subjects as measured by electromyography [26]. Tallgren *et al.* [27] suggested that changes in jaw and occlusal relationships due to resorptive processes mentioned earlier and settling of denture protheses also affect jaw muscle activity. These local factors appear to be more important variables than age. In general, bite force is stronger in men than in women.

In women, it is found to increase until 25 years of age and then shows a slow but progressive decrease with age. In men, this decrease is not observed until age 45 [28].

Newton *et al.* [29] evaluated changes in cross-sectional area and density of the muscles of mastication using computed tomography. Both masseter and medial pterygoid muscles demonstrated significant reduction in cross-sectional area throughout the age range studied (20–90 years). These values were lower in women and both muscles showed a greater decrease in density in edentulous versus dentate patients of all ages. The authors concluded that changes in density and cross-sectional area of the muscles of mastication were consistent with general age-related changes in other muscles of the body and may account for the diminution of masticatory forces observed in elderly individuals. The clinical implication of this reduction in bite force and masticatory ability is that partially and completely edentulous patients may self-impose dietary restrictions that can compromise overall nutritional status. This may be compounded by other age-associated economic, social, and physical limitations and collectively pose a considerable health maintenance problem for these patients.

OSTEOPOROSIS AND METABOLIC BONE DISEASE: EFFECTS ON THE MAXILLA AND MANDIBLE

The role of osteopenia and osteoporosis in oral bone loss and periodontal disease is not well understood. Although the craniofacial area is often noted to be "spared" from bone loss in osteoporosis, this conclusion is likely based on the limitations of dental and panoramic radiographs to adequately reflect changes in bone density [30]. It has been estimated that more than a 40% reduction of bone density is required before osteopenia is appreciated on these X rays. In addition, sustained negative calcium balance in adults thins cortical bone from the inner surface to the outer surface. Because the outer dimensions of the jaw bones are therefore maintained, low bone mass may not be appreciated on plain radiographs.

Bone Density

Henrickson *et al.* [31] compared the density of long bones with that of edentulous mandibles using dual photon absorptiometry. That study showed a statistically significant correlation between mineral density of the mandible and that of the radius. The authors concluded that osteoporotic changes similarly affect the two parts of the skeleton in much the same way. It has also been reported that during skeletal depletion secondary to stimulation of the parathyroid gland, alveolar bone may be affected before other parts of the skeleton such as ribs, vertebrae, and long bones [32]. Kribbs and colleagues [33] reviewed 85 post-menopausal women with a diagnosis of osteoporosis and found that mandibular alveolar ridge height correlated significantly with total body calcium and mandibular bone mass. Von Wowern *et al.* [34] compared the pattern of alveolar atrophy in osteoporotic postmenopausal women and nonosteoporotic age-matched controls. Bone mineral content was measured *in vivo* by dual photon absorptiometry. The densities of the mandibles and forearm bones of the osteoporotic group were significantly lower than controls [34]. Of note, sagittal X rays were found to be identical in the two groups, again demonstrating the limitations of plain radiography in the assessment of bone density.

Histomorphometric evaluation of mandibular bone in osteoporotic patients demonstrated an increased volume of osteoid seam and active osteoclastic resorption [35]. Disturbances in calcium homeostasis and resultant hyperfunction of the parathyroid glands are likely to play roles in severe atrophy. Thus, as more sensitive techniques are used to measure bone density in the maxillofacial complex, "sparing" is not observed.

Periodontal Disease

The bacterial etiology of periodontal disease is well established. Osteoporosis, immune dysfunction, nutritional deficiencies, medications, cigarette smoking, diabetes, pregnancy, and other hormonal alterations are secondary risk factors [36,37]. Inflammation of the supporting tissue of the teeth is usually progressive and destructive and leads to loss of bone and periodontal ligament attachment. It is estimated that some form of periodontal disease affects 75% of the general population. In its severe form (Fig. 10), it is found to affect 14% of adults and up to 30% of older adults and remains a common cause of tooth loss in the elderly [38].

The association between skeletal density and tooth loss has been investigated by numerous authors. Krall and co-workers [39] found that bone mineral density of both the spine and the distal radius correlated statistically with the number of remaining teeth. This group sought to determine, in prospective fashion, whether estrogen replacement therapy (ERT) in a population at risk would improve tooth retention. Four hundred and eighty-seven women were included as part of the Framingham Osteoporosis Study. The duration of estrogen replacement therapy was found to be an indepen-

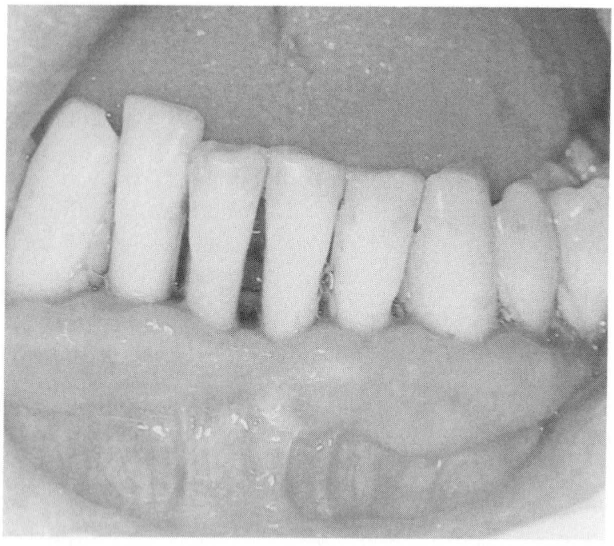

FIGURE 10 Typical pattern in moderate to severe periodontal bone loss. Note loss of interdental papillae and the long clinical crowns of the teeth that have lost crestal bone support.

dent predictor of tooth retention. Long-term ERT users (defined as 10 years or greater) had an average of three more teeth than nonusers. The association between ERT and tooth retention was most striking for anterior teeth. In addition, case-control studies have demonstrated a significantly greater periodontal attachment loss in osteoporotic women than in normal women.

In a prospective study of 70 postmenopausal women in Buffalo, New York, the association between bone mineral density and periodontal measurements was evaluated. The variables in this group included age, years since menopause, estrogen use, body mass index, and smoking. A positive correlation was found between bone mineral density of the spine and alveolar crestal height, and the authors concluded that alveolar crestal height and tooth loss are related to osteopenia in this patient population [38].

Radiographic Evaluation

Assessing bone mineral density of the jaw by plain radiography is difficult. Benson *et al.* [40] described the use of panoramic radiographs and defined the panoramic mandibular index. The number of teeth present, mandibular cortical width at the mental region, the degree of mandibular alveolar bone resorption, and the morphologic classification of the mandibular inferior cortex are components of this index and suggested indicators of osteopenia. Some authors have generated an index of mandibular alveolar resorption by dividing the total mandibular height by the height from the center of the mental foramen to the inferior border of the mandible. The mandibular inferior cortex has been classified into three grades: grade 1, the endosteal margin of the cortex is even and sharp on both sides; grade 2, the endosteal margin shows semilunar defects (lacunar resorption); and grade 3, the cortical layer is thin and clearly porous. These patterns are illustrated in Fig. 11. However, attempts to correlate these grades with generalized osteopenia have proved disappointing.

Klemetti *et al.* [41] evaluated three panoramic-based indices and compared these to the bone mineral density by dual photon absorptimetry. That study concluded that panoramic radiographs were not useful for measuring bone density. Hildebolt *et al.* [42] used small dental films (bitewing radiographs) and were able to detect 5%

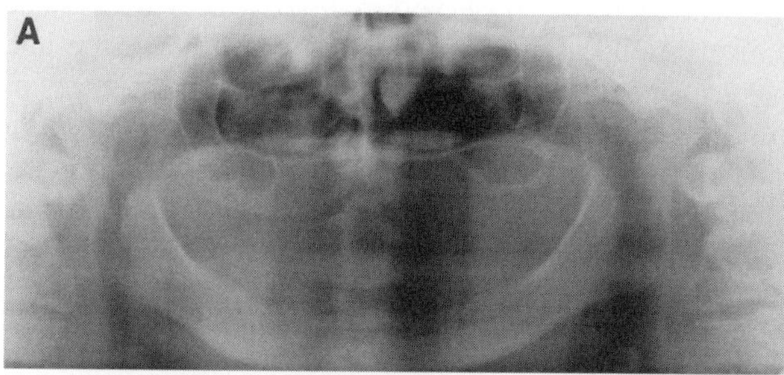

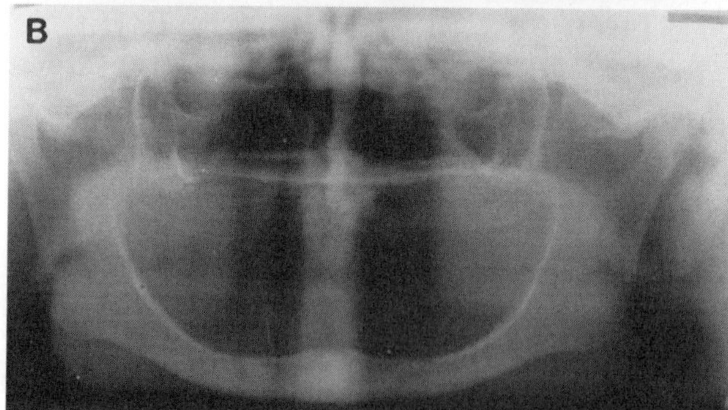

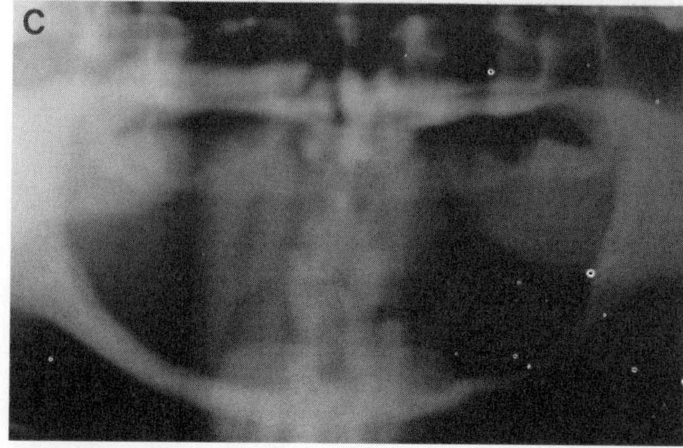

FIGURE 11 (A) Panoramic radiograph demonstrating an even and well-preserved endosteal margin at the inferior border of the mandible (grade 1). (B) Loss of the discreet cortical margin noted at the inferior mandibular border (grade 2). (C) A thinned and porous inferior border is seen with semilunar defects at the inferior border (grade 3).

or greater change in the alveolar bone mineral content. These routine dental films appear to be more sensitive indicators of alveolar bone loss than panoramic films.

Endosseous Implants and Osteopenia

The role of decreased bone mineral density in the healing of endosseous implants in the jaws is currently under investigation. Endosseous dental implants are inserted into the jaw bone and can be used to support single crown, bridges, or overdenturea prostheses. They have become a mainstay in the oral rehabilitation of patients who have lost some or all of their natural dentition. Because the recipient population is largely elderly, assessing bone mineral status and understanding its effect on the healing of implants are important. In a rabbit osteopenic model, Mori *et al.* [43] found that new bone formation adjacent to implants was both delayed and inadequate. Several authors have advocated medical treatment of osteoporosis before the placement of endosseous implants to improve their prognosis, but little convincing data are available to support this assumption [44,45]. The authors demonstrated a statistically lower rate of osseointegration of maxillary and mandibular implants in postmenopausal women compared to the general population [46].

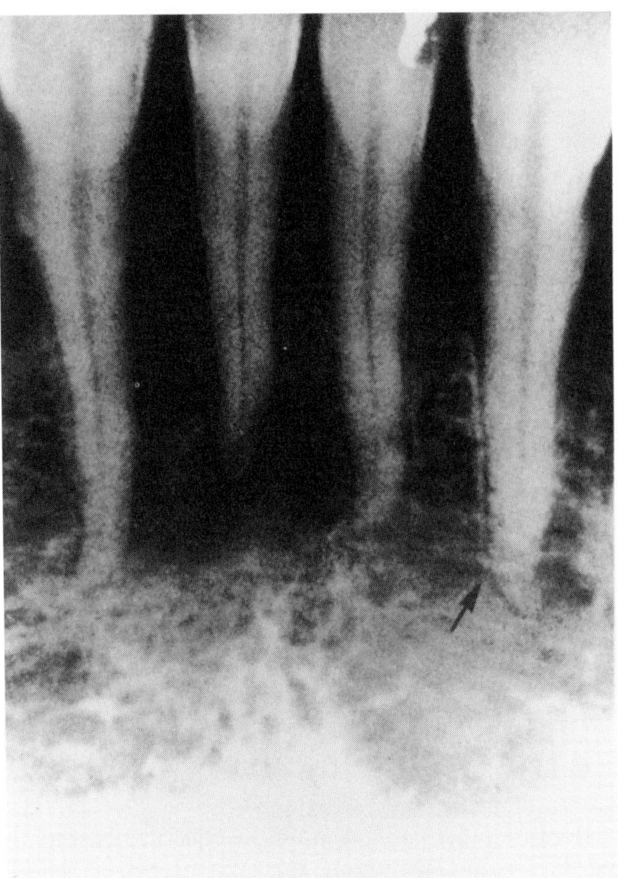

FIGURE 12 Periapical dental radiograph demonstrating changes of hyperparathyroidism, including, loss of the lamina dura surrounding the teeth in contrast to the intact lamina dura noted on the right (arrow). Note the ground glass appearance to the alveolar bone with evident loss of density.

Hyperparathyroidism

In patients with primary hyperparathyroidism, the loss of calcium and phosphorus from the bone results in a generalized osteoporosis with impaired bony healing if pathologic fracture occurs. Tooth drifting, spacing, and resultant malocclusion have been described. Jaw radiographs in hyperparathyroidism have been described as having a ground glass appearance. In addition, a commonly noted finding on dental radiographs is a partial loss of lamina dura structure around teeth and abnormal appearing alveolar bone (Fig. 12). Secondary hyperparathyroidism, most commonly associated with end-stage renal disease, may show the same manifestations in the jaws [47].

Paget's Disease of Bone

Osteitis deformans (Paget's disease of bone) occurs primarily in patients over the age of 40. Its incidence increases proportionately with increasing age. Paget's disease results in well-recognized alterations in bone quality and has multiple orofacial manifestations. The onset and progression of disease can be insidious. Facial pain, deafness, and visual loss secondary to the compression of cranial nerves is reported. Progressive enlargement of the skull is seen commonly. Involvement of the jaws is reported in up to 20% of cases with the maxilla affected more frequently than the mandible. The entire bone may enlarge with resultant widening of the alveolar ridge and loosening, migration, and spacing of teeth (Fig. 13). Jaw enlargement may progress to the point where patients are unable to seal their lips over the teeth and gingiva. Difficulty with the fit of dentures and partial dentures is also a problem. The bone-forming or osteoblastic phase of the disease is most commonly recognized on radiographs. Affected areas may be patchy in distribution, resulting in the so-called "cotton wool" appearance of the bone. The teeth themselves may manifest hypercementosis with bulbous distortion of the root morphology as well as loss of the lamina dura surrounding the teeth (Fig. 14). This problem often complicates exodontia in affected individuals [47,48].

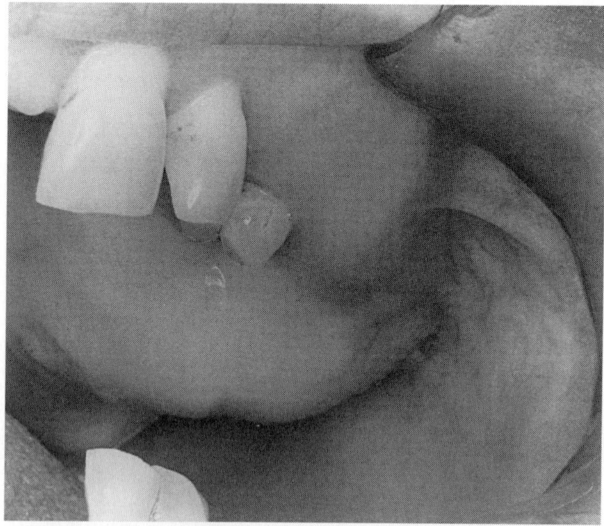

FIGURE 13 Clinical photograph demonstrating widening of the maxillary alveolar process and tooth spacing observed in a patient with Paget's disease of bone. Reproduced with permission from Cawson and Eveson [56].

CHANGES IN DENTITION WITH AGING

Because older patients are more consistently retaining their natural dentition, specific patterns of dental alteration and special dental needs are encountered. The increased incidence of periodontal bone loss and its association with age has been mentioned. In addition, periodontal disease is more rapidly progressive in diabetic patients and this is a disease seen more commonly in the elderly. The severity of periodontal disease in diabetics is secondary to the altered immune response and small vessel damage to the periodontal tissues. Along with apical migration of the epithelial attachment, root surfaces of the teeth become exposed to the oral environment and susceptible to a specific pattern of decay known as root surface caries (Fig. 15). This is exacerbated by decreased salivary production in elderly patients secondary to loss of functional acinar tissue, fibrofatty replacement of major salivary glands, and the xerostomic effects commonly associated with many medications. These teeth, undermined in this neck of tooth location, are more vulnerable to coronal fracture. Evidence shows that the cementum itself becomes more susceptible to decay because of structural changes in cementocytes as the tooth ages [49]. These cells show a rapid decrease in number as well as size, with pyknosis of the nuclei and loss of cytoplasmic volume. An increase in number of both vacuoles and lysosomes is indicative of impending cell death.

The internal structure of teeth also changes with age. Standard endodontic therapy may be difficult in the elderly because of calcification of the pupal tissue. Studies on the morphology of the wall of the root canal by scanning electron microscopy have demonstrated calcospherite formation in the upper root and irregular calcifications noted at the midroot level. This is seen histologically in Fig. 16. In addition, irregular formation of secondary dentin within the pulp is an expected part of normal aging of the root. Animal studies show changes in the pupal nerve fibers of teeth as they age. Both the internodal length and the fiber diameter are found to decrease with age. Myelin changes, such as

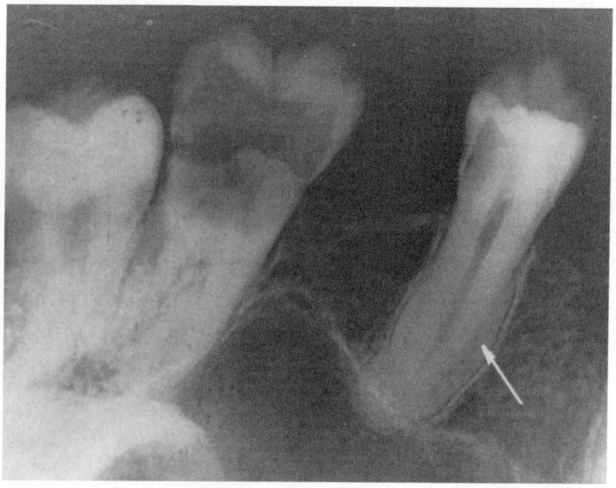

FIGURE 14 Periapical dental radiograph demonstrating hypercementosis of the root in a patient with Paget's disease of bone. The area of root enlargement is designated by the white arrow. Reproduced with permission from Shafer *et al.* [47].

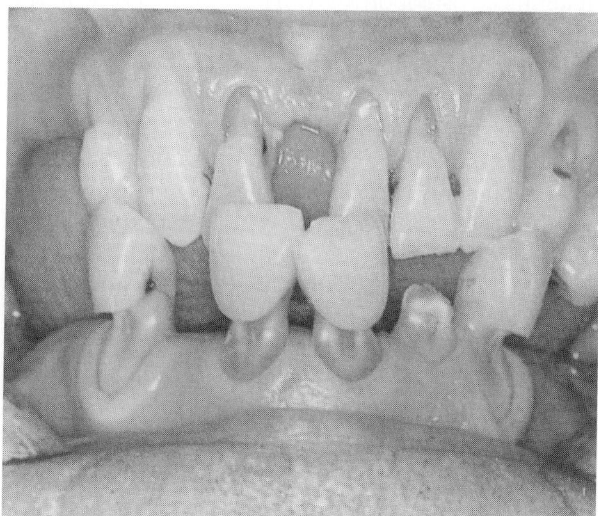

FIGURE 15 Clinical photograph in which both carious and abrasive involvement of the root surfaces of the necks of the teeth are seen. If progressive, this undermining will result in tooth fracture as seen here. Reproduced with permission from Cawson and Eveson [56].

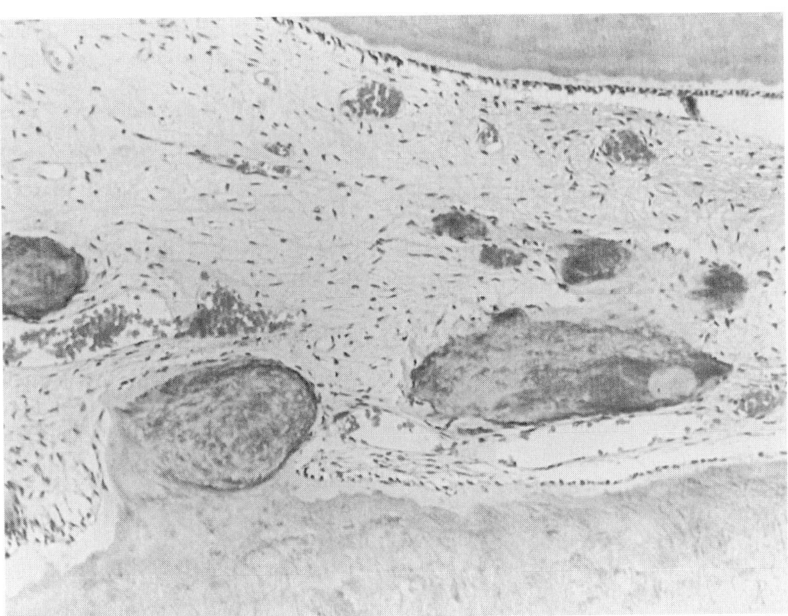

FIGURE 16 Histologic section demonstrating calcified pulp stones within the pulp chamber of an aging tooth. Reproduced with permission from Cawson and Eveson [56].

shortening of intercalated internodes, wrinkling, nodal lengthening, and the formation of myelin ovoids, have all been described. The relationship of these changes and altered dental sensitivity and proprioception remains to be studied in the aging population [50].

Tooth wear and dental attrition can reach significant proportions in the elderly population (Fig. 17). Both normal function and the long-term effect of parafunctional habits such as clenching and nocturnal bruxing account for the cumulative loss of enamel structure. Various indices have been described to assess tooth wear and are utilized for age evaluation in both anthropology and forensics. Not surprisingly, the highest mean wear scores in the elderly are observed on the occlusal and incisal surfaces of the teeth. With the exception of the palatal aspect of the maxillary anterior teeth, no significant attrition is found on the buccal and lingual surfaces of the dentition of the elderly. Attrition is more severe in elderly men than women, most likely due to the increased forces generated during parafunctional movements of the jaws and the overall increased bite forces generated [51].

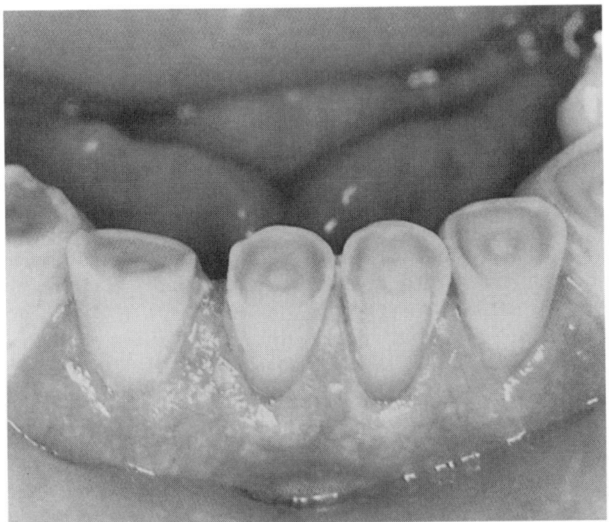

FIGURE 17 Clinical photograph demonstrating advanced attrition of the teeth secondary to longstanding parafunctional habits such as nocturnal bruxism. Exposed dentin is noted on the occlusal surfaces of these teeth.

SUMMARY

The changes observed in the maxillofacial skeleton with aging have significant functional consequences. With progressive loss of teeth, subsequent alveolar atrophy complicates prosthetic rehabilitation and challenges dental practitioners and reconstructive surgeons. If teeth are maintained throughout life, alveolar atrophy is generally not encountered, However, associated periodontal disease, root surface exposure, and decay make ongoing care of these patients essential to maintain dental and general health. Changes in the masticatory muscles with age alter bite forces, and a patient's ability to maintain a normal diet may be compromised, especially if compounded by tooth loss. The development of osteoarthrosis in the temporomandibular joint can lead to limited motion and occasionally pain with jaw function. The profound effect that metabolic bone disease has on the skeleton is certainly observed in the maxillofacial region. Problems with bone healing, more advanced periodontal disease, a decreased capacity to integrate endosseous implants, and more advanced and rapid alveolar atrophy have been described in patients with osteoporosis. Even the internal and external structures of teeth alter with age and may further complicate efforts to maintain optimal health in the elderly. Understanding the particular changes seen in the maxillofacial complex in elderly patients is essential if proper care and guidance are to be provided.

References

1. Enlow, D. H., and Hans, M. G., "Essential of Facial Growth," pp. 18–98. Saunders, Philadelphia, 1996.
2. Chavez-Lomeli, M. E., Mansilla, L. J., Pompa, J. A., *et al.* The human mandibular canal arises from three separate canals innervating different tooth groups. *J. Dent. Res.* **75**(8), 1540–1544 (1996).
3. Hollingshead, W. H., "Anatomy for Surgeons," 2nd Ed., Vol. I, pp. 403–406. Harper and Row, Hagerstown, MD, 1968.
4. Osterberg, T., and Mellstrom, D. Tobacco smoking: a major risk factor for loss of teeth in three 70-year-old cohorts. *Community Dent. Oral Epidemiol.* **14,** 367–370 (1986).
5. Kapur, K. K. Management of the edentulous elderly population. *Gerodontics* **3**(1), 51–54 (1987).
6. Atwood, D. A. Reduction of residual ridges: a major oral disease entity. *J. Prosthet. Dent.* **26**(3), 266–278 (1971).
7. Ulm, C. W., Solar, P., Blahout, R., *et al.* Location of the mandibular canal within the atrophic mandible. *Br. J. Oral Maxillofac. Surg.* **31,** 370–375 (1993).
8. Solar, P., Ulm, C., Lill, W., *et al.* Precision of three-dimensional CT-assisted model production in the maxillofacial area. *Eur. Radiol.* **2,** 473–477 (1992).
9. Eufinger, H., Gellrich, N. C., Sandmann, D., *et al.* Descriptive and metric classification of jaw atrophy. *Int. J. Oral Maxillofac. Surg.* **26,** 23–28 (1997).
10. Doual, J. M., Doual-Bisser, A., Crocquet M., *et al.* Facial aging. The evolution of the soft tissues. *Bull Group Rech. Sci. Stomatol Odontol.* **34**(1), 11–15 (1991).
11. Ulm, C. W., Pechmann, U., Ertl, L., *et al.* Anatomy of the atrophic mandible. *Z. Stomatol.* **86**(8), 491–503 (1989).
12. Doual, J. M., Ferri, J., and Laude, M. The influence of senescence on craniofacial and cervical morphology in humans. *Surg. Radiol. Anat.* **19**(3), 175–183 (1997).
13. Ishibashi, H., Takenoshita, Y., Ishibashi, K., *et al.* Age-related changes in the human mandibular condyle: a morphologic, radiologic and histologic study. *J. Oral Maxillofac. Surg.* **53**(9), 1016–1023 (1995).
14. Dibbets, J. M., and van der Weele, L. T. Signs and symptoms of temporomandibular disorder (TMD) and craniofacial form. *Am. J. Orthod. Dentofac. Orthop.* **110**(1), 73–78 (1996).
15. Stratmann, U., Schaarschmidt, K., and Santamaria, P. Morphologic investigation of condylar cartilage and disc thickness in the human temporomandibular joint: significance for the definition of osteoartrotic changes. *J. Oral Pathol. Med.* **25**(5), 200 (1996).
16. Hansson, T., and Nordstrom, B. Thickness of the soft tissue layers and articular disc in the temperomandibular joint with deviations in form. *Acta. Odontol. Scand.* **35,** 281–288 (1977).
17. Toller, P. A. Osteoarthrosis of the mandibular condyle. *Br. Dent. J.* **134,** 223–231 (1973).
18. Wilkes, C. H. Internal derangements of the temporomandibular joint. Pathological variation. *Arch. Otolaryngol. Head Neck Surg.* **115,** 469–477 (1989).
19. de Leeuw, R., Boering, G., Stegenga, R., *et al.* Radiographic signs of temporomandibular joint osteoarthrosis and internal derangement 30 years after nonsurgical treatment. *Oral Surg. Oral Med. Oral Pathol. Oral Radiol. Endod.* **79**(3), 382–392 (1995).
20. Morse, D. E., Katz, R. V., Nikoukari, H., *et al.* Temporomandibular joint sounds in an edentulous elderly population. *J. Craniomand. Disord. Facial Oral Pain* **6,** 47–55 (1992).
21. Agerberg, G. Maximal mandibular movements in young men and women. *Swed. Dent. J.* **67,** 81–100 (1974).
22. Agerberg, G., and Bergenholtz, A. Craniomandibular disorders in adult populations of West Bothnia, Sweden. *Acta. Odontol. Scand.* **47,** 129–140 (1989).
23. Yukstas, A. A. The effect of missing teeth on masticatory performance and efficiency. *J. Pros. Dent.* **4**(1), 120–123 (1954).
24. Carlsson, G. E. Masticatory efficiency: the effect of age, the loss of teeth and prosthetic rehabilitation. *Int. Dent. J.* **34**(2), 93–97 (1984).
25. Bakke, M., Holm, B., Jensen, B. L., *et al.* Unilateral, isometric bite force in eight 68-year-old women and men related to occlusal factors. *Scand. J. Dent. Res.* **98,** 149–158 (1990).
26. Wayler, A. H., Muench, M. E., Kapur, K. K., *et al.* Masticatory performance and food acceptability in persons with removable partial dentures, full dentures and intact natural dentition. *J. Gerontol.* **39**(3), 284–289 (1984).
27. Tallgren, A., Holden, S., Lang, B. R., *et al.* Correlations between EMG jaw muscle activity and facial morphology in compete denture wearers. *J. Oral Rehabil.* **10,** 105 (1983).
28. Carlsson, G. E. Bite force and chewing efficiency. *Front. Oral Physiol.* **1,** 265 (1974).
29. Newton, J. P., Yemm, R., Abel, R. W., *et al.* Changes in human jaw muscles with age and dental state. *Gerodontology* **10**(1), 16–22 (1993).
30. Jeffcoat, M. K., and Chesnut, C. H. Systemic osteoporosis and oral bone loss: evidence shows increased risk factors. *JADA* **124,** 49–56 (1993).
31. Henrickson, P. A., Wallenluis, K., and Astrand, K. The mandible and osteoporosis. Method for determining mineral content of the mandible and radius. *J. Oral Rehabil.* **1,** 75–84 (1974).
32. Lufwak, L., Singer, F. R., and Urisi, M. R. Current concepts of bone metabolism. *Ann. Intern. Med.* **80,** 630–644 (1974).
33. Kribbs, P. J., Smith, D., and Chesnut, C. H. Oral findings in osteoporosis: relationship between residual ridge and alveolar bone resorption and generalized skeletal osteopenia. *J. Prosthet. Dent.* **507,** 719–724 (1983).
34. von Wowern, N., Klausen, B., Kollerup G. Osteoporosis: a risk factor in peridontal disease. *J. Periodent.* **65,** 1134–1138 (1994).
35. Wical, J., and Swoope, C. Studies of residual ridge resorption. *J. Prosthet. Dent.* **32,** 13–17 (1974).
36. Norderyd, O. M., Grossi, S. G., Macheci, E. E., *et al.* Peridontal status of women taking postmenopausal estrogen supplementation. *J. Periodontol.* **64**(10), 957–962 (1993).
37. Ciancio, S. G. Medications as risk factors for peridontal disease. *J. Periodontal.* **67**(10 Suppl.), 1055–1059 (1996).
38. Wacrawski-Wende, J., Grossi, S. G., Trevisan, M., *et al.* The role of osteopenia in oral bone loss and peridontal disease. *J. Periodontol.* **67**(10 Suppl.), 1076–1084 (1996).

39. Krall, E. A., Garcia, R. I., and Dawson-Hughes, B. Increased risk of tooth loss is related to bone loss at the body, hip and spine. *Calcif. Tissue Int.* **59,** 433–437 (1996).
40. Benson, B. W., Prihoda, T. J., and Glass, B. J. Variations in adult cortical bone mass as measured by a panoramic mandibular index. *Oral Surg. Oral Med. Oral Pathol.* **71,** 349–359 (1991).
41. Klemetti, E., Collin, H. L., Forss, H., *et al.* Mineral status of skeleton and advanced peridontal disease. *J. Clin. Periodontol.* **21**(3), 184–188 (1994).
42. Hildebolt, C. F., Rupich, R. C., Vannier, M. W., *et al.* Interrelationships between bone mineral content measures, Dual energy radiography (DER) and bitewing radiographs (BWX). *J. Clin. Periodontol.* **20,** 739–745 (1993).
43. Mori, H., Manabe, M., Horiguchi, J. L., *et al.* Effect of bone density on the dental implant. *J. Dent. Res.* **74,** IADR (1995). [Abstract 278]
44. Baxter, J. C., and Fattore, L. Osteoporosis and osseointegration of implants. *J. Prosthod.* **2,** 120–125 (1993).
45. Shapiro, S., Romberg, T. J., Benson, B. W., *et al.* Postmenopausal osteoporosis: dental patients at risk. *Gerodontics* **1,** 220–225 (1985).
46. August, M., Mita, A. J., Stephens, W. L., *et al.* Evaluation of implants in postmenopausal women: a pilot study. *J. Oral Maxillofac. Surg.* **56**(8), Supplement 4, 32 (1998).
47. Shafer, W. G., Hine, M. K., and Levy, B. M. Oral aspects of metabolic disease. *In* "A Textbook of Oral Pathology," pp. 658–661. Saunders, Philadelphia, 1983.
48. Stevenson, J. C. Pagets disease of bone. *in* "Metabolic Bone Disease," pp. 266–273. Butterworth and Co., United Kingdom, 1990.
49. Ohno, Y. Fine structural observations of age changes in cementocytes of human permanent teeth. *Shika Kiso Igakkar Zasshi* **31**(6), 656–670 (1989).
50. Fried, K., and Erdelyi, G. Changes with age in canine tooth pulp-nerve fibres of the cat. *Arch. Oral Biol.* **29**(8), 581–585 (1984).
51. Donachie, M. A., and Walls, A. W. Assessment of tooth wear in an aging population. *J. Dent.* **23**(3), 157–164 (1995).
52. McMinn, R., Hutchings, R., and Logan, B., "Color Atlas of Head and Neck Anatomy," p. 35. Year Book, Chicago, 1981.
53. Enlow, D., and Hans, M. "Essentials of Facial Growth," p. 82. Saunders, Philadelphia, 1996.
54. Atwood, D. A. *J. Prosthet. Dent.* **13,** 817 (1963).
55. Norman, J., and Bromby, P. "Textbook and Color Atlas of the Temporomandibular Joint," p. 4. Wolfe, London, 1990.
56. Cawson, R., and Eveson, J. "Oral Pathology and Diagnosis." Saunders, Philadelphia, 1987.

CHAPTER 32

Fractures: Effects on Quality of Life

DEBORAH T. GOLD[*,‡,†] AND KENNETH W. LYLES[‡,f,§,||]

*Department of Psychiatry and Behavioral Sciences; ‡Center for the Study of Aging and Human Development; fDepartment of Medicine; §Sarah W. Stedman Nutrition Center; Duke University Medical Center, Durham, North Carolina 27710; †Department of Sociology, Duke University, Durham, North Carolina 27708; ||GRECC, Veterans Administration Medical Center, Durham, North Carolina 27705

INTRODUCTION

Improvements in sanitation, medical care, health promotion, and disease prevention have lead to substantial increases in life expectancy in the United States during the 20th century. This has translated into older adults increasing in both number and proportion, with the fastest growing population group being those age 85 and older. However, although years have been added to the end of life, the tenor of life during those years has diminished substantially for many individuals. As a result, issues of quality of life have become central to research on aging, in part because many have come to believe that living long and experiencing good life quality are mutually exclusive. Although compression of morbidity suggested by Fries [1,2] is most desirable, many doubt that it is viable. These same issues are also central to research on chronic illness because most chronic conditions of late life contribute to poor quality of life.

The conjunction of aging and chronic illness at quality of life raises some critical research questions. First, does aging itself reduce quality of life or is the real cause of diminished life quality in old age the chronic illnesses often experienced by the elderly? If both these conditions (i.e., aging and chronic illness) contribute to diminished life quality, is one or the other a more formidable cause? Thus far, there have been no good answers to these questions as they relate to osteoporosis.

This chapter examines osteoporosis as a specific chronic condition of elderly women and assesses the influence of its most common outcome—fractures—on life quality. To do this, we first define *quality of life* two ways: as a global construct and as a complex set of specific dimensions. We then examine the differential impact of osteoporotic fractures by age. Finally, we suggest ways in which the future impact of fractures on life quality can be diminished.

OSTEOPOROTIC FRACTURES

Although we frequently speak as if osteoporosis itself is the cause of diminished quality of life, that is not in fact true. Many older women live with low bone mass for substantial lengths of time yet never realize that they have osteoporosis. In fact, osteoporosis is "the silent disease" because it can develop significantly without noticeable symptoms [3].

However, untreated low bone density leads to microarchitectural deterioration and atraumatic fractures. Some women experience vertebral compression fractures with minimal or no pain and remain unaware of their osteoporosis. In fact, the pain that may result from "silent fractures" is usually attributed to arthritis or disk problems. In a study that screened 185 older women (mean age of 82) by x-ray for the presence of at least one 20% or greater compression fracture, nearly 30% of these women were unaware of their fracture [4]. This experience is the same as that described by Black *et al.* [5] in the Fracture Intervention Trial. These investigators found that only one-third of subjects with vertebral fractures were recognized clinically.

Nonetheless, fractures do not remain asymptomatic indefinitely, especially when several occur. The accumulated deficits resulting from a hip fracture or from multiple vertebral fractures lead to outcomes that include pain [6], deformity [7], functional limitations [8], and psychosocial impairments [9]. These secondary effects of fractures are direct causes of diminished quality of life, and it is these issues that are focused on in this chapter.

QUALITY OF LIFE: A DEFINITION

Before we describe specific ways in which osteoporotic fractures in combination with age diminish quality of life, it seems critical to define quality of life. There are probably as many different definitions of quality of life as there are scholars who study it, yet each of those definitions contains similar core elements. It is not enough to say that life quality is the absence of problems. Instead, as used here, quality of life is a generalized sense of psychosocial and physical well-being. Although we still lack consensus on the precise parameters to be examined in a quality of life study, most individuals understand what is meant when asked the question, "How would you rate your overall quality of life?" Therefore, a global approach to quality of life can be useful.

However, we would be remiss if we examined only the overall construct of life quality in relation to osteoporotic fractures and aging. Therefore, for the purposes of this chapter, the construct of quality of life will be divided into four dimensions. Those dimensions include physical health, financial resources, social relations, and psychological well-being. We will briefly review how osteoporotic fractures affect each of these dimensions; then we will discuss how these effects are likely to differ between younger and older people.

Let us also note that several investigators have now developed survey instruments to measure quality of life in women with osteoporosis. Virtually all of these are for use with women who have vertebral compression fractures. In general, the scales differ by purpose. For example, the instrument designed by Cook and colleagues [10] was designed specifically to measure the quality of life in women with vertebral compression fractures and pain. Lydick and colleagues [11] took a different approach in designing their scale (OPTQoL) for use in the general population. Lips and colleagues [12] devised a quality of life scale (Qualeffo) to be used with Europeans who had osteoporosis. Thus, investigators must select carefully when choosing an instrument. (See Table I for a list of osteoporosis-specific quality of life instruments and references.)

Measuring the impact of osteoporotic fractures on quality of life is a challenge, but living with that impact

TABLE I Instruments for the Measurement of Quality of Life in Patients with Osteoporosis

Instrument name	Reference
Osteoporosis Health-Related Quality of Life Scale	Cook *et al.* [10]
Osteoporosis Functional Disability Questionnaire (OFDQ)	Helmes *et al.* [43]
Qualeffo (Quality of Life from the European Foundation for Osteoporosis)	Lips *et al.* [12]
Osteoporosis-Targeted Quality of Life (OPTQoL)	Lydick *et al.* [11]
Osteoporosis Assessment Questionnaire (OPAQ)	Silverman *et al.* [56]

can be devastating for anyone who experiences them. Older adults in particular face greater difficulties with osteoporotic fractures and have fewer resources with which to manage these difficulties. It has not been shown empirically that the quality of life of older women is more compromised by fractures than that of younger women, but it would be easy to assume so. There might be two potential explanations for these age differences. First, it could be that the actual impact of the fracture is greater on older than younger people (e.g., older people have more severe fractures; older people take longer to heal). According to Mccalden and colleagues [13], the compressive strength of bone decreases 8.5% with each decade. Second, however, it is possible that older and younger people have similar fracture impact but cope differently with it. Whether this is an actual difference in coping capacity or is related to the amount of stress with which older adults need to cope is not yet clear.

DIMENSIONS OF QUALITY OF LIFE

For the purposes of this chapter, four specific dimensions of quality of life are discussed: physical well-being, financial resources, social relations, and psychological well-being. We define these below and discuss the impact of osteoporotic fractures on each.

Physical Well-Being

Of all aspects of life quality, physical well-being is perhaps the most influenced by osteoporosis and fractures. Fractures result in three specific negative outcomes for physical well-being: deformity, functional limitation, and pain.

PHYSICAL WELL-BEING AND DEFORMITY

The deformity caused by osteoporosis typically centers on pathological changes in the spine [7]. Multiple vertebral compression fractures led to kyphosis, a convex curvature of the thoracic spine. This change in configuration affects multiple parts of the body. The lumbar lordosis flattens (decreases) in response to kyphosis as the rib cage nears the iliac crest. The head is bent forward uncomfortably, and the lungs and stomach are constricted by loss of space in the thoracic and abdominal cavities. The abdomen protrudes, and the waistline disappears. Kyphotic severity is dictated by the number and position of vertebral fractures as well as overall musculoskeletal health. Indeed, the entire body shifts to accommodate the results of these fractures. Kyphosis also has a substantial negative impact on day-to-day functioning [14].

Deformity and Age Needless to say, kyphosis is undesirable and affects the health and mood of all those who develop it. Do older women who have spinal fractures experience more difficulty from kyphosis than younger women? The answer to this question is unclear. Of course, aging itself causes height loss independent of vertebral fractures; therefore, age-related height loss might exacerbate the severity of kyphosis. Second, other age-related changes in appearance—from changes in muscle strength to loss of intervertebral disk height—might exaggerate the kyphosis or make it more prominent. However, this is speculation as no empirical findings in this area exist.

Younger women may have factors protecting them against deformity from fractures. If women experience fractures early in life, they may prevent future fractures with some success. Second, younger musculoskeletal systems are, as a whole, more resilient. Third, younger women exercise more frequently and may therefore keep the paraspinal and other back muscles stronger.

PHYSICAL WELL-BEING AND FUNCTIONAL LIMITATIONS

Functional limitations are caused or exacerbated by osteoporotic fractures. Perhaps the most powerful example of osteoporotic fracture-related disability results from hip fractures. Once women have hip fractures, the residual morbidity and mortality are profound [15]. According to the Office of Technology Assessment in the Congress of the United States [16], women who experienced a hip fracture had the following limitations 1 year later: 40% could not ambulate independently, 60% required at least some assistance with activities of daily living (ADL), and nearly 80% required help with at least one instrumental activity of daily living (IADL).

Similar functional limitations occur after vertebral compression fractures [17]. Although a single compression fracture usually has little impact on function, the cumulated effect of multiple fractures is substantial [6]. As noted earlier, the kyphotic changes resulting from multiple spinal fractures make the challenge of even the simplest movements formidable. When reaching, twisting, or bending are difficult, many daily activities (e.g., cleaning, laundry, and vacuuming) are no longer manageable. When those movements become impossible, the completion of fundamental self-care activities can necessitate full-time assistance or institutionalization.

In a study designed to identify the relative impact of osteoporosis and osteoarthritis on functional impairment, Lyles *et al.* [8] compared two groups of women on measures of physical performance and functional status. The control group (mean age = 80 years) was fracture free but had substantial degenerative changes in the spine. The osteoporotic group (mean age = 82) had similar arthritic changes in their spines but also had at least two 30% or greater anterior wedge deformities. Both groups were tested on six functional performance measures including maximal trunk extension torque using the B-200 Isostation, (Isotechnologist, Inc. Hillsborough NC), thoracic and lumbar spine motion [18], functional reach [19], mobility skills [20], and 6-min walk [21]. On five of the six, women with fractures performed significantly less well than did those without fractures. On the Functional Status Index [22], a self-report measure of current functional capability, women with fractures again scored significantly worse than the control group. Thus, although both groups may have experienced limitations imposed by osteoarthritis, those women with osteoporotic fractures were substantially more impaired than those without.

Functional Limitations and Age As noted earlier, functional limitations can result from multiple chronic health conditions, and it is difficult to identify the pathology that causes a specific limitation. For that reason alone, osteoporotic fractures have a greater likelihood of negative outcomes for older women than for younger ones. Chronic disease typically starts in late middle age and is often well established by age 65 or 70. Comorbid conditions in older women certainly can cause osteoporotic fractures or can combine with them to create severe functional limitations [23]. In the osteoarthritis and osteoporosis study cited earlier [8], the presence of osteoarthritis alone caused functional limitations; the scores of the arthritis-only group were worse than would have been expected from a group without functional limitation. The fact that over 50% of women over age 65 report having osteoarthritis [24] provides but one example of the likely impact of comorbidity on the quality of life of older women.

Osteoporotic fractures add to the challenge of comorbidity that older adults face. Several geriatric conditions including orthostatic hypotension, syncope, vision problems, and inner ear disorders, increase the likelihood of falls, and 5 to 10% of falls in the elderly result in significant injuries [25]. Falls are clearly linked not only to the occurrence of fractures but also to their severity [26].

A final issue on age differences in the impact of osteoporotic fractures on functional limitations relates to something called health resilience. One of the major differences in how well women respond to osteoporotic fractures depends on their physical reserve. A fracture in a young woman resolves more quickly than one in an older woman. In part, this may result from better overall health status, but it is also a result of the younger woman's reservoir of health-related physical resources. One obvious example of these reserves at work can be seen in hip fracture recovery. Extended bed rest following hip fracture is debilitating. For the younger woman, however, recovery from that debilitation can occur more quickly and with less intense effort because her initial physical condition is superior and her reserve deeper than those of the older woman. Thus, for the younger woman, the odds of developing other pathological conditions (such as pneumonia) during recovery are reduced, and a less complicated period of recuperation inevitably leads to a more complete and uncomplicated recovery.

PHYSICAL WELL-BEING AND PAIN

A third result of osteoporotic fractures that compromises physical well-being is pain. Acute fracture pain (i.e., bone pain) typically takes 6 to 8 weeks to resolve and may respond to analgesics (including calcitonin [27]); physical therapy modalities (ice, heat, massage, TENS) are also useful for short-term pain management. But the intolerable pain associated with fractures is chronic and usually muscular in nature. When multiple vertebral fractures result in changed spinal configuration, the position of soft tissue near the spine is also compromised. The paraspinal muscles take additional responsibility for erect posture, something that requires additional muscle strength and bulk. When those muscles are untrained, this extra pressure causes substantial muscular pain. Unfortunately, this pain is frequently nonresponsive to analgesia and may be severe regardless of location. Physical therapy modalities bring temporary relief, but women with osteoporotic fractures who cope with chronic pain rarely know relief [6,17].

It is important to note that Ettinger and colleagues [28,29] report results that suggest a deformity–pain relationship. In their large sample, only those women with the most extreme vertebral deformity had symptoms that were predictable. This sample appears to underrepresent the group of women with the most serious pain complications from vertebral fractures. Cook and colleagues [10] also report results apparently at odds with Ettinger's findings until the sample source is examined. Given that Cook's sample was clinic based as was the authors [9,30], it may be this difference that accounts for the discrepancies in reported level of pain. However, it is important to remember that some fractures result in little or no pain at all.

The authors believe that the key to managing chronic fracture pain is regular exercise [6,9,26]. Women with severe kyphoses are especially in need of back extensor muscle-strengthening exercises. If nothing is done over time to strengthen these muscles, daily activities will exacerbate the pain.

Pain and Age For most young women, the experience of chronic pain is virtually unknown, and for many older women, pain is not a constant companion. However, for the woman of any age with multiple osteoporotic fractures, successful coping with chronic pain is essential. If chronic pain is uncontrolled, damage can occur to many aspects of life. Social relations and psychological well-being suffer as much as physical well-being [6]. For those who try to find a cure for chronic pain, financial resources can be depleted rapidly. Visits to pain clinics, acupuncturists, physical therapists, psychiatrists, and other alternative health care providers are costly and only rarely have positive, long-lasting effects. A discussion of the scope of chronic pain and its quality of life impact is beyond this chapter, but a great deal of research has been done on the impact of chronic pain on quality of life (see, for example, [10] or [31]). (For an excellent review on issues of older women and chronic pain, see Roberto [32].)

Of all the dimensions that relate to overall quality of life, physical well-being is the most important as it relates to osteoporotic fractures. Indeed, the changes that occur to physical well-being when multiple fractures occur have impacts on all three of the other dimensions as well. The following section discusses the issue of financial resources and the ways in which they are critical for the woman with osteoporotic fractures.

Financial Resources

In terms of health care, financial resources help women purchase the best physicians, the newest medications and other therapies, and the best overall care. When a woman experiences fractures related to osteoporosis, her financial status can be important in terms of purchasing immediately needed care; however, it is also important in terms of resource availability in the future. As with any chronic disease, costs with osteoporotic fractures are ongoing. Because fractures are the "acute" phases of osteoporosis, women with this disease should expect to have periodically higher costs resulting from the need for acute care.

Two distinct aspects combine into the phrase "financial resources." The first relates to income and assets. It is no surprise to find that those with the best income also have the best assets. The second aspect of financial resources related to health care is the type and presence of health insurance. Good benefit packages tend to accompany good salaries. Thus, in general, we have polarized groups of the "haves" and "have nots," with the polarization getting stronger. In order to best understand how we meet current costs of osteoporotic fractures and how changes can be made in the health care delivery system to improve access to care, we need to identify the real costs of this disease.

What are the costs associated with osteoporotic fractures? Health problems have some universal costs, regardless of their specific nature. For fractures, these include physician's fees (and surgeon's fees for hip setting or replacement), hospital charges (for all hip fractures and some vertebral fractures), medications (many of which are not available in generic forms), and physical therapy. Depending on the location and severity of the fracture, costs can extend beyond the period of hospital care to include paid service providers to complete routine tasks at home. This list of costs is by no means exhaustive, but it does serve to identify the common financial burdens caused by fractures.

National Costs

Fracture costs occur at two distinct levels. On the national level, the annual direct medical costs of osteoporosis are staggering. National health care expenditures attributable to osteoporotic fractures exceeded $13 billion in 1995 [33]. Costs for rehabilitation after hip fracture are among the highest, regardless of the place in which that fracture occurs [33,34]. Although we are currently unable to estimate total overall costs of vertebral and other nonhip fractures because many do not require hospitalization, others have estimated costs in the range of $5 billion annually [33]. The dollar price on this disease is overwhelming.

Individual Costs

While national costs are borne by all of us, osteoporotic fractures also take a major fiscal toll out of patients. When fractures lead to major ADL and IADL limitations, hiring others to clean, cook, and provide personal care on a part- or full-time basis can be expensive. Many women are fortunate to have family and friends to help during a crisis, but this kind of assistance cannot be routinely given without some cost, and when savings or current salary is spent on current medical costs, that leaves individuals concerned about ongoing financial resources.

Financial Resources and Aging

Direct costs for standard procedures (x-rays, hip replacement, spinal fusion) do not differ in this country by age. Ideally, then, costs of health care provided to fracture victims should also be unaffected by age. Realistically, however, the escalating chronic health problems of the elderly result in higher overall costs for them. Increased comorbidity appears to be the culprit that complicates all aspects of health care for older women with fractures. For example, a younger woman with overall good health who suffers a hip fracture has standard costs and a straightforward recuperation. For an older woman, however, multiple problems may result. The general deterioration of her skeleton may make surgery or hip replacement more complicated. Chronic COPD may put her at increased risk of pneumonia while recuperating. Osteoarthritis in her knees may limit her physical therapy rehabilitation program. In this scenario, costs increase insidiously because of other age-related frailty. The differences in cost for these women result from differential reimbursement by the older woman's insurance company.

If we stop to consider, however, what insurance coverage that older woman has, it is obvious that this problem extends beyond the individual. Over 95% of adults over age 65 have Medicare coverage for their health insurance needs [35]. For costs incurred during hospitalization, Medicare coverage may be adequate; however, subsequent rehabilitation, outpatient care, and institutional costs may not be included in Medicare coverage [36]. Because charges for outpatient physical therapy, ambulatory devices, extensive home health care, and prescription medicines are not covered in most cases, most chronic illnesses result in substantial out-of-pocket payments by older women.

For those older women with Colles or vertebral fractures, the coverage of outpatient costs is poor. However, these costs are minimal when compared to the skilled nursing care necessary for recuperation from hip fracture. Again, the disparity in out-of-pocket costs between older and younger women results not only from different insurance coverage but also from differences in living situations. Over 40% of women over age 65 live alone [37], necessitating either paid live-in help or institutionalization as their only alternatives for postfracture care. Both options drain extant financial resources rapidly. Thus, a second dimension of quality of life that is diminished more for older women by osteoporotic fractures is identified. A third dimension, social relations, is discussed next.

Social Relations

The chronic illness literature is replete with studies showing that women with strong social relations have better illness outcomes than those who face their diseases alone [38,39]. Further, for many women, seeking social support is, in itself, an effective coping strategy. Social relations enhance feelings of adaptation and commitment as well as the sense of being cared for. However, in the face of chronic illness, the absence of positive social relations can have serious negative effects on quality of life.

The impact of osteoporotic fractures on social relations can be profound. Although there is excess morbidity and mortality associated with hip fracture [40,41], low bone density itself is not terminal. In fact, the woman with one spinal fracture or Colles' fracture may not see her social relations influenced at all. However, the woman with a hip fracture or multiple spinal fractures has little control; these fractures will recast nearly every social relationship she has. How family and nonkin relations are changed by fractures and how women with osteoporosis can lose their social roles are discussed next.

Social Relations: The Family

Family relations are most likely to change after fracture but are also most likely to survive this stress. Reciprocity, i.e., mutual sharing and assistance is in effect in families most of the time. However, family members, especially women, contribute routinely to the family support bank without immediate recompense [42]. Therefore, down the road when women experience fractures and need help, they can draw on that account. If fractures always resulted in acute needs, no problem would exist, but when a hip fracture terminates independent living, it also eliminates future deposits in support accounts.

Reciprocal relationships, especially with a spouse or an adult child, can rapidly transform into dependent caregiving when osteoporotic fractures are serious. Unfortunately, independence lost to a hip or multiple vertebral fractures may never return. Both partners in this dependent relationship come to resent it. The care recipient perceives herself as overbenefitted while the caregiver senses that she or he is underbenefitted. Unless the imbalance of benefits can be corrected to some degree, it can ultimately lead to destruction of the relationship.

Social Relationships: Nonkin Bonds

Although family bonds in this country have the highest value, nonfamily relations are influenced by osteoporotic fractures as well. Comfortable patterns of social interaction are essential for most adults and may include widely varying activities such as church or synagogue attendance, card or game playing, group exercise, movie going, or travel. Osteoporotic fractures minimize or terminate participation in these social activities. Especially when fractures result in chronic pain, routine exertions can require superhuman efforts. The most common shared behaviors become difficult and painful. Riding in a car can be agonizing, sitting in a hard pew can be uncomfortable, and standing or walking even short distances can be excruciating. It does not take long for women to realize that refusing certain social invitations will protect them from unwanted pain and that leisure activities, as well as social interaction, will need substantial modification.

In addition to the relationship problems just described, women with osteoporotic fractures also experience social role loss. Each time a woman becomes unable to do something, she is at jeopardy of losing the role in which she would do that activity. For example, if a woman plants annuals every spring and is then told not to do so by her physician, she loses the social role of "gardener." If she can no longer prepare meals or clean, she is no longer a housekeeper or a cook. What is perhaps most unfortunate about this process is that there are not large numbers of roles with which women can replace lost ones. A substantial void in social location can develop over time.

Social Relations and Aging

Once again, the impact of fractures on social relations appears to be more substantial for older women. Several reasons for this exist. First, as women age, they experience continuing losses of social network members to death or infirmity. This rarely happens on a large scale for women under 60. Thus, fractures increase or expand the network losses for them while, for the younger woman, fractures may cause most of the network departures they experience. Thus, the number of such losses is likely to be higher in old age.

This same general pattern is true for social role losses as well. Older women expect to lose some roles and, in fact, surrender them gladly. For example, after 40 years of raising children, a woman is ready to give up the "active mother" role and have her children leave home. Most older women comment that they are ready to retire when that time comes. However, the readiness or willingness to abandon one role is often predicated on having another to step into. When "mother" becomes "grandmother" and "worker" becomes "traveler," the adjustment to role changes is easier, but in those instances where new role adaptation is difficult, the loss of an important existing role can be painful.

Some of the other role losses associated with aging are also undesirable. Widowhood is the most obvious example of these changes and perhaps the most problematic for the woman with fractures. Not only are personal interactions destroyed by a husband's death, but social channels are cut off as well. Many adult activities are predicated on being a part of a couple. While some older women remarry, the lack of available age-appropriate men makes remarriage difficult. For the older woman who participates only in minimal social activities, the act of finding potential mates is exacerbated by fractures. Although younger women with fractures may experience the same barriers in terms of social activities, age-appropriate men are more available to women in their 30s and 40s than in their 70s and 80s.

In this way, osteoporotic fractures can make an active social life stagnant. If demographic and other health factors are included into this equation, we again find that the older woman has further-reaching effects of an osteoporotic fracture than the younger. The absence of an active social life and strong social relations leads to a discussion of our final dimension of quality of life: psychological well-being.

Psychological Well-Being

Just as physical well-being is central to outstanding quality of life, so too is the issue of mental health or psychological well-being. Just as osteoporotic fractures have negative consequences for physical well-being and quality of life, similar phenomena occur in the psychological realm as well. There are three areas of psychological well-being typically affected by osteoporotic fractures: anxiety/depression, self-esteem, and mastery/autonomy. We will concentrate on these three constructs as they relate to quality of life and osteoporotic fractures.

Psychological Well-Being and Anxiety

When in the disease course of osteoporosis does anxiety first appear? Typically, a woman responds with anxiety when she receives the diagnosis of osteoporosis or when she has her first fracture [43]. In order to prevent another fracture from occurring, women sometimes adapt a confined life-style. They avoid going out in public (especially to crowded places such as malls) because they fear being pushed or falling. They stop shopping because lifting and carrying can be difficult. They stop attending church or synagogue because of the pain it causes. Symbolically they make their lives into padded cells in the hope that, if only they are careful enough, a fracture cannot occur.

Psychological Well-Being and Depression

Of course, there is no guarantee that future fractures will not occur. When they do, despite the best efforts of these women, the anxiety transforms into depression. Depression is most likely to develop when functional limitations or pain result from osteoporotic fractures. Further, although no research has specifically addressed this question, the financial and social consequences of these fractures may also result in overwhelming despair.

Depression is a common outcome of chronic illness in general. Although only 6% of adults suffer from depression, the prevalence soars to over 50% when the sample is limited to those with chronic illness [44]. Unfortunately, depression often remains undiagnosed and untreated, especially among older adults, and untreated depression has profoundly negative effects on quality of life.

If the prevalence of depression in persons with chronic illness is so high, why do only a few studies of osteoporosis patients evaluate depression as a potential outcome? The answer is unclear. Many studies of osteoporosis and its fractures are run by specialists (either endocrinologists or rheumatologists) who do not have extensive experience in identifying or treating depression. Several studies have, however, considered the role of depression in the management of osteoporosis. The authors' own studies of patients indicate that women with vertebral fractures report depressive symptoms, although often there are insufficient symptoms for a diagnosis of clinical depression [30]. In addition Leidig-Bruckner and colleagues [45] measured depression in their clinic sample of 63 women with at least one vertebral compression fracture. Forty percent of these women (mean age 65 $\pm$ 7.9 years) reported at least 16 symptoms on the CES-D (Center for Epidemiological) [46], indicating surprisingly high levels of clinically relevant depression.

Is the comorbid depression in women with osteoporotic fractures entirely a psychological or a psychosocial phenomenon? A recent preliminary study suggests a possible physiological link between depression and low bone density, the precursor of osteoporosis. Michelson and colleagues [47] compared 24 premenopausal women with histories of major depression with 24 nondepressed women. Individuals in both groups were matched on several categories (including exercise habits, calcium intake, family history, childbearing history). Bone density measurements were then done at five sites (two spinal and three hip sites). Remarkably, results showed statistically significantly lower bone density in the depressed women than in the nondepressed women in all five sites. Without a prospective study, the association between depression and bone density is merely hypothetical. However, if there is a physiological association between depression and low bone mass, timely treatment of that depression would become essential in osteoporosis management.

Psychological Well-Being and Self-Esteem

A second psychological outcome of osteoporotic fractures in women is diminished self-esteem. In the United States today, women's self-esteem has two cornerstones: her competence (what she does) and her presentation of self (how she looks). Osteoporosis robs women of their self-esteem by deforming them, debilitating them, and disabling them. In a society that has treated women as second-class citizens for a long time, it should perhaps not be surprising to hear that this illness outcome minimizes both appearance and efficacy, two essential components of today's working woman.

In order to be competent, women must be productive. Whether that productivity occurs in the home, the office, or the volunteer organization does not seem important. However, we tolerate a lack of productivity poorly, and individual worth is measured by how much a woman can do and how good her work is. We also set youth and its concomitant physical attractions as a aspiration throughout adulthood. Women employ a variety of products (e.g., hair dye, makeup) and strategies (e.g., face lift, exercise) to achieve this. Under normal circumstances, women have difficulty in maintaining their dreams for youth and productivity [48]. Osteoporotic fractures can make achieving that goal futile.

Self-Esteem and Age

Self-esteem is an area in which age differences frequently occur. Because the United States values productivity and judges people on their appearance and conduct, older women fare poorly in comparison to younger women. In general, this society does not view the elderly as important to our society's health and well-being. As a matter of fact, we do extraordinarily poorly at providing support for self-worth to "old people." If we have a goal for them at all, it is to keep them from being dependent.

Psychological Well-Being and Autonomy or Mastery

The gerontological literature is replete with research on physical dependence and disability that stretches from needing minimal IADL assistance to institutionalization caused by chronic illness [49,50,51], but little has been written about either physical or emotional dependence, especially in osteoporosis. In the Leidig-Bruckner *et al.* [45] article mentioned earlier, the authors note the relationship between spinal deformity and functional limitation and examine the impact of functional loss on depression and general well-being. Unfortunately, we lack reliable and valid ways to measure emotional dependence, especially as it relates to osteoporotic fractures.

Most women with multiple vertebral fractures or with hip fracture lack autonomy or mastery in their lives. If they are limited in terms of physical health, financial situation, and social relations, that leaves them without the means by which they can make their own decisions. If physical condition is severely compromised and they have been permanently institutionalized, autonomy may be lost forever. The nursing home is, perhaps, the perfect example of nonautonomous living. Residents cannot decide when they want meals, what they want for meals (except within certain parameters), when to go to sleep, and when to bathe. From what, then, can the dependent nursing home patient get a sense of competence or success?

Autonomy and Aging

Without question, physical and emotional dependence occur most frequently among older women. Whether caused by poor physical health, social problems, financial losses, or psychological pain, dependence is found most frequently among those at the ends of their lives. How do fractures enter into the equation of dependence? Hip fracture devastates the individual by destroying her capabilities in nearly every quality of life dimension. Although some older women recover well from hip fracture, many do not. A substantial proportion of nursing home residents have suffered hip fractures, either as the precipitating incident or while in the institutional facility. In the case of older adults, the hip fracture may be only one part of a long chain leading to institutional placement. Because younger women are likely to have overall better health, stronger social support systems, income replacement, and more effective coping strategies, they may be better able to achieve good physical and mental health outcomes than older women. However, younger women tend not to have religious faith that is as strong as that of older women [52]. But while spirituality can improve older women's emotional status [53], it does not usually improve the woman's physical condition [54]. Thus, older women need substantially more than religion as a means by which to keep going through health crises that plague them.

FUTURE DIRECTIONS

Living longer, although desirable in many ways, also has disadvantages. One of these is a greater vulnerability to chronic illness. As life expectancy continues to increase into the new century, osteoporosis will increase in prevalence. Currently, postmenopausal and age-associated osteoporosis are now responsible for nearly 300,000 new hip fractures and 700,000 new vertebral fractures annually in the United States. Further, one of every two women over 50 years of age will suffer an osteoporosis-related fracture in her lifetime, and one in four will experience a vertebral fracture [55]. If these statistics are projected into the 21st century, the numbers continue to increase.

There are, however, bright spots on the horizon. First, the increasing availability of antiresorptive medication allows physicians to treat the physical aspects of osteoporosis in ways that simply were not available 30 or 40 years ago. Further, our knowledge of diet, exercise, support groups, and coping strategies has become sophisticated enough to contribute in meaningful ways to improving many disease outcomes. Finally, prevention strategies, if implemented with adolescents and young adults, should reduce the risk of lifetime osteoporotic fractures in today's younger cohorts.

However, in light of prevention efforts, we must not lose sight of the 28 million Americans with or at risk of the devastating effects of osteoporotic fractures. For these women (and men), the management of fractures and tertiary prevention efforts need to be accelerated. Although we may not yet have a cure for the osteoporosis itself, we can affect positive changes in physical health, financial status, social relations, and psychological well-being in ways that improve quality of life for women with osteoporotic fractures.

Acknowledgments

This work was supported by NIH Grants AG42110 and HD30442 (Gold and Lyles) as well as by research grants from the AARP/Andrus Foundation (Gold) and the Veterans Affairs Medical Research Service (Lyles).

References

1. Fries, J. F. The compression of morbidity. *Ann. Acad. Med. (Singapore)* **12,** 358–367 (1983).
2. Fries, J. F. Physical activity, the compression of morbidity, and the health of the elderly. *J. Royal Soc. Med.* **89,** 64–68 (1996).
3. Holmes, S. Osteoporosis: the hidden illness. *Nurs. Times* **94,** 20–23 (1998).
4. Gold, D. T., Shipp, K. M., Pieper, C. F., and Lyles, K. W. "Osteoporosis and Disability in Life-Care Community Women." Randomized clinical trial funded by the National Institute of Child Health and Human Development, 1998.
5. Black, D. M., Cummings, S. R., Karpf, D. B., Cauley, J. A., Thompson, D. E., Nevitt, M. C., Bauer, D. C., Genant, H. K., Haskell, W. L., Marcus, R., Ott, S. M., Torner, J. C., Quandt, S. A., Reiss, T. F., and Ensrud, K. E. Randomised trial of effect of alendronate on risk of fracture in women with existing vertebral fractures. *Lancet* **348,** 1535–1541 (1996).
6. Gold, D. T. Chronic musculoskeletal pain: Older women and their coping strategies. *J. Women Aging* **6,** 43–58 (1994).
7. Shipp, K. M., Pieper, C. F., Gold, D. T., Purser, J. L., and Lyles, K. W. Is spinal deformity related to function and disability? Submitted for publication.
8. Lyles, K. W., Gold, D. T., Shipp, K. M., Pieper, C. F., Martinez, S., and Mulhausen, P. L. Association of osteoporotic vertebral compression fractures with impaired functional status. *Am. J. Med.* **94,** 595–601 (1993).
9. Gold, D. T., Stegmaier, K., Bales, C. W., Lyles, K. W., Westlund, R. E., and Drezner, M. K. Psychosocial functioning and osteoporosis in late life: Results of a multidisciplinary intervention. *J. Women's Health* **2,** 149–155 (1993).
10. Cook, D. J., Guyatt, G. H., Adachi, J. D., Clifton, J., Griffith, L. E., Epstein, R. S., and Juniper, E. F. Quality of life issues in women with vertebral fractures due to osteoporosis. *Arthritis Rheum.* **36,** 750–756 (1993).
11. Lydick, E., Zimmerman, S. I., Yawn, B., Love, B., Kleerekoper, M., Ross, P., Martin, A., and Holmes, R. Development and validation of a discriminative quality of life questionnaire for osteoporosis (OPTQOL). *J. Bone Miner. Res.* **12,** 456–463 (1997).
12. Lips, P., Agnusdei, D., Caulin, F., Cooper, C., Johnell, O., Kanis, J., Liberman, U., Minne, H., Reeve, J., Reginster, J. Y., de Vernejoul, M. C., and Wiklund, I. The development of a European questionnaire for quality of life in patients with vertebral osteoporosis. *Scand. J. Rheum.* **103,** 84–85 (1996).
13. McCalden, R. W., McGeough, J. A., and Courtbrown, C. M. Age-related changes in the compressive strength of cancellous bone: the relative importance of changes in density and trabecular architecture. *J. Bone Joint Surg.* **79A,** 421–427 (1997).
14. Ryan, S. D., and Fried, L. P. The impact of kyphosis on daily functioning. *J. Am. Geriatr. Soc.* **45,** 1479–1486 (1997).
15. Magaziner, J., Lydick, E., Hawkes, W., Fox, K. M., Zimmerman, S. I., Epstein, R. S., and Hebel, J. R. Excess mortality attributable to hip fracture in white women aged 70 years and older. *Am. J. Public Health* **87,** 1630–1636 (1997).
16. U.S. Congress, Office of Technology Assessment. "Hip Fracture Outcomes in People Age 50 and Over." Report No. OTA-BP-H-120. Government Printing Office, Washington, DC, 1994.
17. Tamayo-Orozco, J., Arzac-Palumbo, P., Peon-Vidales, H., Mota-Bolfeta, R., and Fuentes, F. Vertebral fractures associated with osteoporosis: patient management. *Am. J. Med.* **103,** 44S–48S (1997).
18. Ohien, G., Spangfort, E., and Tirgvall, C. Measurement of spinal sagittal configuration and mobility with Debrunner's Kyphometer. *Spine* **14,** 580–583 (1988).
19. Duncan, P., Weiner, D., Chandler, J., and Studenski, S. Functional reach: a new clinical measure of balance. *J. Gerontol.* **46,** M192–197 (1990).
20. Hogue, C. C., Studenski, S., and Duncan, P. Assessing mobility: the first step in falls prevention. *In* "Key Aspects of Recovery: Improving Nutrition, Rest and Mobility" (E. M. Tornquist, S. G., Funk, M. T. Champagne, L. A., Capp, and R. A. Wiese, eds.), pp. 275–280. Springer, New York, 1990.
21. Guyatt, G. H., Sullivan, M. J., Thompson, P. J., Fallen, E. L., Pugsley, S. O., Taylor, D. W., and Berman, L. B. The 6 minute walk: a new measure of exercise capacity in patients with chronic heart failure. *Can. Med. Assoc. J.* **132,** 818–822 (1985).
22. Jette, A. M. Functional Status Index: reliability of a chronic disease evaluation instrument. *Arch. Phys. Med. Rehabil.* **61,** 395–401 (1980).

23. Johnell, O., and Obrant, K. J. What is the impact of osteoporosis? *Baillieres Clin. Rheum.* **11,** 459–477 (1997).
24. National Center for Health Statistics, "Health, United States, 1995." Public Health Service, Hyattsville, MD, 1996.
25. Tinetti, M. E., Speechley, M., and Ginter, S. P. Risk factors for falls among elderly persons living in the community. *N. Engl. J. Med.* **319,** 1701–1707 (1988).
26. Prior, J. C., Barr, S. I., Chow, R., and Faulkner, R. A. Physical activity as therapy for osteoporosis. *Can. Med. Assoc. J.* **155,** 940–944 (1996).
27. Lyritis, G. P., Tsakalakos, N., Magiasis, B., Karachalios, T., Yiatzides, A., and Tsekoura, M. Analgesic effect of salmon calcitonin in osteoporotic vertebral fractures: a double blind placebo-controlled clinical study. *Calcif. Tissue Int.* **49,** 369–372 (1991).
28. Ettinger, B., Black, D. M., Nevitt, M. C., Rundle, A. C., Cauley, J. A., Cummings, S. R., and Genant, H. K. Contribution of vertebral deformities to chronic back pain and disability. *J. Bone Miner. Res.* **7,** 449–456 (1992).
29. Ettinger, B., Block, J. E., Smith, R., Cummings, S. R., Harris, S. T., and Genant, H. K. An examination of the association between vertebral deformities, physical disabilities, and psychosocial problems. *Maturitas* **10,** 283–296 (1988).
30. Gold, D. T., Smith, S. D., Bales, C. W., Lyles, K. W., Westlund, R. E., and Drezner, M. K. Osteoporosis in late life: Does health locus of control affect psychosocial adaptation? *J. Am. Geriatr. Soc.* **39,** 670–675 (1991).
31. Leidig, G., Minne, H. W., Sauer, P., Wuster, C., Wuster, J., Lojen, M., Raue, F., and Ziegler, R. A study of complaints and their relation to vertebral destruction in patients with osteoporosis. *Bone Miner.* **8,** 217–229 (1990).
32. Roberto, K. A., ed., Older Women with Chronic Pain. Haworth Press, New York, 1994.
33. Ray, N. F., Chan, J. K., Thamer, M., and Melton, L. J., III. Medical expenditures for the treatment of osteoporotic fractures in the United States in 1995: report from the National Osteoporosis Foundation. *J. Bone Miner. Res.* **12,** 24–33, (1997).
34. Randell, A., Sambrook, P. N., Nguyen, T. V., Lapsley, H., Jones, G., Kelly, P. J., and Eisman, J. A. Direct clinical and welfare costs of osteoporotic fractures in elderly men and women. *Osteopor. Int.* **5,** 427–432 (1995).
35. Palmer, R. M., Saywell, R. M., Jr., Zollinger, T. W., Erner, B. K., LaBov, A. D., Freund, D. A., Garber, J. E., Misamore, G. W., and Throop, F. B. The impact of the prospective payment system on the treatment of hip fractures in the elderly. *Arch. Intern. Med.* **149,** 2237–2241 (1989).
36. Komisar, H. L., Hunt-McCool, J., and Feder, J. Medicare spending for elderly beneficiaries who need long-term care. *Inquiry* **34,** 302–310 (1997–1998).
37. Barer, B. M. Men and women aging differently. *J. Aging Hum. Dev.* **38,** 29–40 (1994).
38. Von Korff, M., Gruman, J., Schaefer, J., Curry, S. J., and Wagner, E. H. Collaborative management of chronic illness. *Ann. Intern. Med.* **127,** 1097–1102 (1997).
39. Hatchett, L., Friend, R., Symister, P., and Wadhwa, N. Interpersonal expectations, social support, and adjustment to chronic illness. *J. Personal. Soc. Psychol.* **73,** 560–573 (1997).
40. Magaziner, J., Simonsick, E. M., Kashner, T. M., Hebel, J. R., and Kenzora, J. E. Predictors of functional recovery one year following hospital discharge for hip fracture: a prospective study. *J. Gerontol.* **45,** M101–M107 (1990).
41. Keene, G. S., Parker, M. J., and Pryor, G. A. Mortality and morbidity after hip fractures. *Br. Med. J.* **307,** 1248–1250 (1993).
42. Hogan, D. P., Eggebeen, D. J., and Clogg, C. C. The structure of intergenerational exchanges in American families. *Am. J. Soc.* **98,** 1428–1458 (1993).
43. Helmes, E., Hodsman, A., Lazowski, D., Bhardwaj, A., Crilly, R., Nichol, P., Drost, D., Vanderburgh, L., and Pederson, L. A questionnaire to evaluate disability in osteoporotic patients with vertebral compression fractures. *J. Gerontol.* **50A,** M91–98 (1995).
44. Lamberg, L. Treating depression in medical conditions may improve quality of life. *JAMA* **276,** 857–858 (1996).
45. Leidig-Bruckner, G., Minne, H. W., Schlaich, C., Wagner, G., Scheidt-Nave, C., Bruckner, T., Gebest, H. J., and Ziegler, R. Clinical grading of spinal osteoporosis: quality of life components and spinal deformity in women with chronic low back pain and women with vertebral osteoporosis. *J. Bone Miner. Res.* **12,** 663–675 (1997).
46. Radloff, L. S. The CES-D scale: a self-report depression scale for research in the general population. *Appl. Psychol. Meas.* **1,** 385–401 (1977).
47. Michelson, D., Stratakis, C., Hill, L., Reynolds, J., Galliven, E., Chrousos, G., and Gold, P. Bone mineral density in women with depression. *N. Engl. J. Med.* **335,** 1176–1181 (1996).
48. Rijken, M., Komproe, I. H., Ros, W. J., Winnubst, J. A., and van Heesch, N. C. Subjective well-being of elderly women: conceptual differences between cancer patients, women suffering from chronic ailments and healthy women. *Br. J. Clin. Psychol.* **34,** 289–300 (1995).
49. Rozzini, R., Frisoni, G. B., Ferrucci, L., Barbisoni, P., Bertozzi, B., and Trabucchi, M. The effect of chronic diseases on physical function. Comparison between activities of daily living scales and the Physical Performance Test. *Age Aging* **26,** 281–287 (1997).
50. Rudberg, M. A., Parzen, M. I., Leonard, L. A., and Cassel, C. K. Functional limitation pathways and transitions in community-dwelling older persons. *Gerontologist* **36,** 430–440 (1996).
51. Van de Water, H. P. Health expectancy and the problem of substitute morbidity. *Phil. Trans. Roy. Soc. Lond. Seri. B. Biol. Sci.* **352,** 1819–1827 (1997).
52. Levin, J. S., and Taylor, R. J. Age differences in patterns and correlates of the frequency of prayer. *Gerontologist* **37,** 75–88 (1997).
53. Koenig, H. G., George, L. K., and Peterson, B. L. Religiosity and remission of depression in medically ill older patients. *Am. J. Psychiat.* **155,** 536–542 (1998).
54. Lindsey, E. Health within illness: experiences of chronically ill/disabled people. *J. Adv. Nurs.* **24,** 465–472 (1996).
55. Melton, L. J., III. Epidemiology of spinal osteoporosis. *Spine* **22,** S2–S11 (1997).
56. Silverman, S., Go, K., and Herson, J. What is the relative impact of osteoporotic vertebral fractures as compared to aging on quality of life? *J. Bone Miner. Res.* **12,** S363 (1997).

CHAPTER 33

General Orthopedic Principles

JEFFREY D. MOFFETT AND THOMAS A. EINHORN
Department of Orthopedic Surgery, Boston University School of Medicine, Boston, Massachusetts 02118

INTRODUCTION

It will come as no surprise that the aging skeleton is at greater risk for fracture than its counterpart in young, healthy individuals. In the majority of cases, osteoporosis is the underlying pathology. The clinical significance of osteoporosis-related fractures is emphasized by the sheer number of fractures seen in the elderly. As many as 40% of white women and 13% of white men will have at least one fragility fracture after the age of 50 [1]. Most will have osteoporosis as a comorbidity, and 90% of all hip and spine fractures in elderly white women can be attributed to osteoporosis [2]. In 1990 hip fractures alone accounted for 250,000 fractures in the United States (1.7 million worldwide) and the incidence of hip fractures is expected to reach 750,000 (6.3 million worldwide) per year by 2050. Presently, the total cost incurred per patient in the first year following a hip fracture is as high as $34,000, resulting in annual health care expenditures of 8.7 billion dollars [3]. The scope of the problem demands the attention of not only orthopedic surgeons, but all physicians.

The spine, hip, and wrist are the most common locations for osteoporosis-related fractures, but other sites, including the bones around the shoulder, elbow, and knee, are clinically important as well. Approximately 35% of women will sustain a vertebral fracture, 18% a hip fracture, and 17% a wrist fracture in their lifetime [1]. This chapter attempts to address some of the unique problems encountered in treating fractures in the aging skeleton as well as general principles in the management of specific fractures.

FRACTURES IN THE AGING SKELETON

Fractures in the elderly are unique entities for several reasons. First, they are intimately associated with osteoporosis, which complicates fracture management, and second, they occur in a patient population that has a high incidence of comorbid medical conditions that have the potential to alter fracture healing. Polypharmacy is also present in the elderly and the effect of these drugs on fracture healing is largely unknown. The effects of increasing age on fracture healing is also poorly understood. Studies in rats have demonstrated that there are fewer bone progenitor cells in elderly rats, which is associated with a decreased bone repair capacity [4]. It is also known that there are age-related deficits in the fracture-healing process in elderly rats [5]. Comorbid conditions such as diabetes and osteoporosis may also have an effect on fracture healing. Streptozotocin-induced diabetic rats were found to have decreased tensile strength, collagen synthesis, and cellularity of callus in healing fractures compared to those in nondiabetic rats [6]. Another study using ovarectomized rats as a model for osteoporosis showed that short-term ovariectomy impaired fracture healing of closed femoral fractures [7].

The effect of antiosteoporosis drugs on fracture healing is also being examined. Of the bisphosphonates, alendronate has been shown to have no untoward effects on fracture healing in dogs [8], but etidronate may adversely affect fracture healing at high doses such as 20 mg/kg/day. Calcitonin, estrogen, and vitamin D do not interfere with fracture healing and may be helpful.

Nonsteroidal anti-inflammatory drugs are also commonly used in the elderly population and have been shown to have an inhibitory effect on fracture healing that may be reversible upon cessation of the medicine, depending of the particular drug in question [9]. When interpreting these data, it is important to keep the information in context. All the mentioned studies utilize animal models and exactly how the data should be extrapolated to humans is not known.

When fractures occur in osteoporotic bone there is an increased likelihood of complex fracture patterns with high degrees of comminution. Low energy mechanisms may produce the same degree of comminution seen only in high energy fractures in strong healthy bone. Furthermore, when high energy mechanisms are applied to weak, osteoporotic bone, extensive comminution may occur, making reconstruction very difficult. Both high and low energy fractures in the osteoporotic skeleton pose challenging problems for the orthopedist. Specifically, osteoporotic bone does not support internal fixation nearly as well as healthy bone and these fractures are associated with more comminution, making reduction and fixation difficult. In fact, some fractures meeting operative criteria in a younger population may be treated without surgery in specific groups of elderly patients due to problems with fixation and, in some cases, poor preinjury functional status.

In general, however, the goals of treatment are rapid mobilization and a return to normal activities. Conservative fracture management with prolonged periods of immobilization place the patient at risk for pulmonary decompensation, thromboembolic disease, decubitus formation, and further skeletal deterioration from disuse osteopenia [10].

GUIDELINES FOR THE MANAGEMENT OF OSTEOPOROTIC FRACTURES

The goal of operative intervention is to achieve stable fracture fixation and permit early return of function. For the lower extremity, this is dictated by the ability of the patient to return to a weight-bearing status early in the treatment period. Although anatomic restoration is important for intraarticular fractures, metaphyseal and diaphyseal fractures require early stabilization with perfect anatomic reduction being less important.

The inability of osteoporotic bone to support internal fixation devices makes subsequent hardware failure more common than in healthy bone. Because the strength of bone is directly related to the square of its mineral density [11], osteoporotic bone may lack the strength to support rigid fixation devices such as plates and screws. Moreover, comminution of osteoporotic bone often dictates fixation devices that allow for compaction and settling of fracture fragments into stable patterns that minimize stress at the bone–implant interface. Finally, implants should be chosen that minimize stress shielding in order to avoid further regional bone loss. For these reasons, sliding nail-plate devices, intramedullary systems, and tension band wiring constructs that allow load sharing and compaction are generally preferred over static plates with screws or other rigid systems.

Although the events of fracture healing proceed normally in almost all osteoporotic patients, an inadequate calcium intake may result in deficits in callus mineralization or remodeling [12]. Because many elderly patients are malnourished, including orthopedic patients specifically, fracture healing may be enhanced when nutritional deficiencies are corrected [12,13]. Therefore, for optimal results, nutritional assessment should be included in patient evaluation. Several parameters may help identify at-risk groups for nutritional depletion. Arm-muscle circumference, total lymphocyte count, serum albumin level, serum transferrin concentration, and skin antigen testing represent some objective parameters that may be measured. Abnormalities in those tests are associated with increased susceptibility to postoperative complications [13]. A prospective assessment of the nutritional status and complications in patients with hip fractures revealed a 70% mortality within 11 months of fracture in patients with a serum albumin of less than 3.0, compared with a mortality rate of 18% in patients with an albumin greater than or equal to 3.0 [14]. A multidisciplinary approach including nutritional assessment and support programs staffed by physicians, dietitians, and nurses provides optimal patient care [13]. In patients with osteoporosis, discharge from the hospital on a multivitamin or vitamin D supplementation may be beneficial [15].

LOWER EXTREMITY FRACTURES

Hip Fractures

It is well known that hip fractures are a significant source of morbidity and mortality in the elderly population and as such the topic has been examined extensively throughout the years. While percentages vary, a recent prospective, multifactorial study quotes posthip fracture mortality as 6 to 22% depending on the health of the patient. Unhealthy patients included those with poor cardiac status, pneumonia, cancer history, bowel obstruction, malnutrition, dehydration, stroke history, renal failure, or cirrhosis. Twenty-two percent of this group died within 1 year of the hip fracture compared to 6% of the healthy group. Age was also examined as an independent variable after factoring out health status and was found to be associated with higher death rates only in patients greater than 85 years old [16]. In accordance with its profound clinical importance, the topic of hip fractures is given major emphasis in this chapter.

Hip fractures can be divided into three major types according to location of the fracture: femoral neck, intertrochanteric, and subtrochanteric fractures (Fig. 1). Although guidelines exist for the treatment of hip fractures, clinical decision making can be quite difficult. An understanding of hip fracture pathoanatomy is important for basic treatment principles. Subdivision of hip fractures into intracapsular and extracapsular fractures is based on one such pathoanatomic distinction related to the blood supply of the femoral head. Extracapsular, intertrochanteric, and subtrochanteric fractures are at much less risk for avascular necrosis (AVN) of the femoral head than intracapsular, femoral neck fractures.

The blood supply to the femoral head is derived primarily from the medial circumflex femoral artery, which forms an extracapsular arterial ring at the base of the femoral neck (Fig. 2). Extending from the ring proximally up the neck are small ascending cervical arteries that form another subsynovial intracapsular arterial ring providing the majority of the femoral head blood supply. Displaced intracapsular fractures of the femoral neck frequently disrupt this blood supply, resulting in a 16% incidence of AVN and a 33% incidence of nonunion [17]. Another factor contributing to nonunion of intracapsular hip fractures is that the synovial fluid that bathes the fracture contains angiogenic inhibitors that may interfere with the healing process [18]. Extracapsular fractures are rarely associated with AVN.

Femoral neck (intracapsular) fractures are described as subcapital (just below the head), transcervical (through the middle of the neck), and basicervical (at

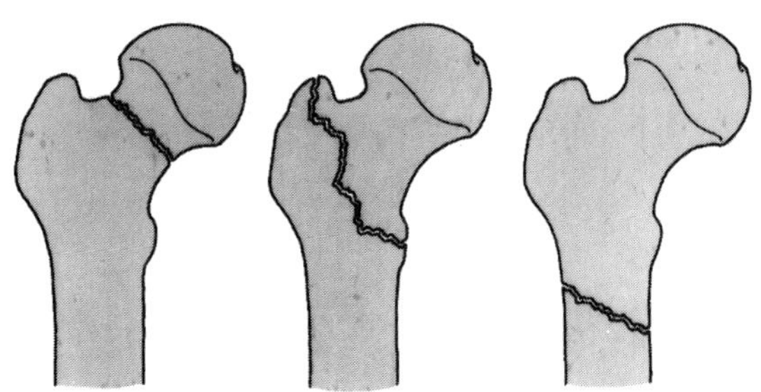

FIGURE 1 Common types of hip fractures: intracapsular (femoral neck), intertrochanteric, and subtrochanteric. Reprinted with permission from Einhorn [49].

the base of the neck). Basicervical fractures are generally grouped as extracapsular as their rate of AVN and type of fixation they require are the same as intertrochanteric fractures. The Garden classification, although subject to intra- and interobserver discrepancies, is the most commonly used system for classifying femoral neck fractures as it can help to direct treatment (Fig. 3). A more simple way to group femoral neck fractures is to divide them into two categories: nondisplaced (Garden I and II) and displaced (Garden III and IV) as treatment is generally dictated by displacement. Garden I and II fractures are essentially nondisplaced fractures and as such are associated with low rates of AVN warranting attempts at preserving the femoral head. These are generally treated by hip pinning with three 7.3-mm cannulated screws placed in a triangular configuration (Fig. 4). This fixation allows the bone to heal, usually by 3 months, and results in patients retaining their own femoral head and articular cartilage. Severely osteoporotic bone, however, may be prone to having the implants dislodge and cut through the soft bone of the femoral head upon weight bearing.

Garden III and IV fractures are displaced fractures that potentially disrupt the blood supply to the femoral head, greatly increasing the chance of AVN. Although reports vary, an 11–19% incidence of AVN can be expected [17]. Hence, treatment involves sacrifice of the femoral head and replacement with a prosthesis (Fig. 5). This may be accomplished by unipolar or bipolar hemiarthroplasty or total hip arthroplasty. A unipolar prosthesis is composed of a single unit femoral stem and head, whereas a bipolar prosthesis is composed of a femoral stem and small head that internally articulates with a larger femoral head. With a bipolar prosthesis, a significant amount of motion occurs between the small head and the large head, which decreases motion at the large head–acetabular interface. This theoretically decreases acetabular wear, prolonging the development of acetabular osteoarthritis. Total hip arthroplasty overcomes the problem of acetabular arthritis by replacing the acetabulum with a prosthetic cup in addition to the femoral head. Unipolar arthroplasties are used commonly in nonambulators and household ambulators; bipolar prostheses are used in community ambulators; and total hip arthroplasty (acetabular and femoral replacement) is generally indicated in those with preexisting osteoarthritis of the hip. As a matter of practice, however, unipolar and bipolar prostheses are used interchangeably and total hip arthroplasty is performed less frequently for hip fractures.

Prosthetic replacement is also indicated in nondisplaced fractures in patients who exhibit any of the "three P's"—Parkinson's disease, Paget's disease, or 'Porosis (osteoporosis) [19]. Parkinson's disease is associated

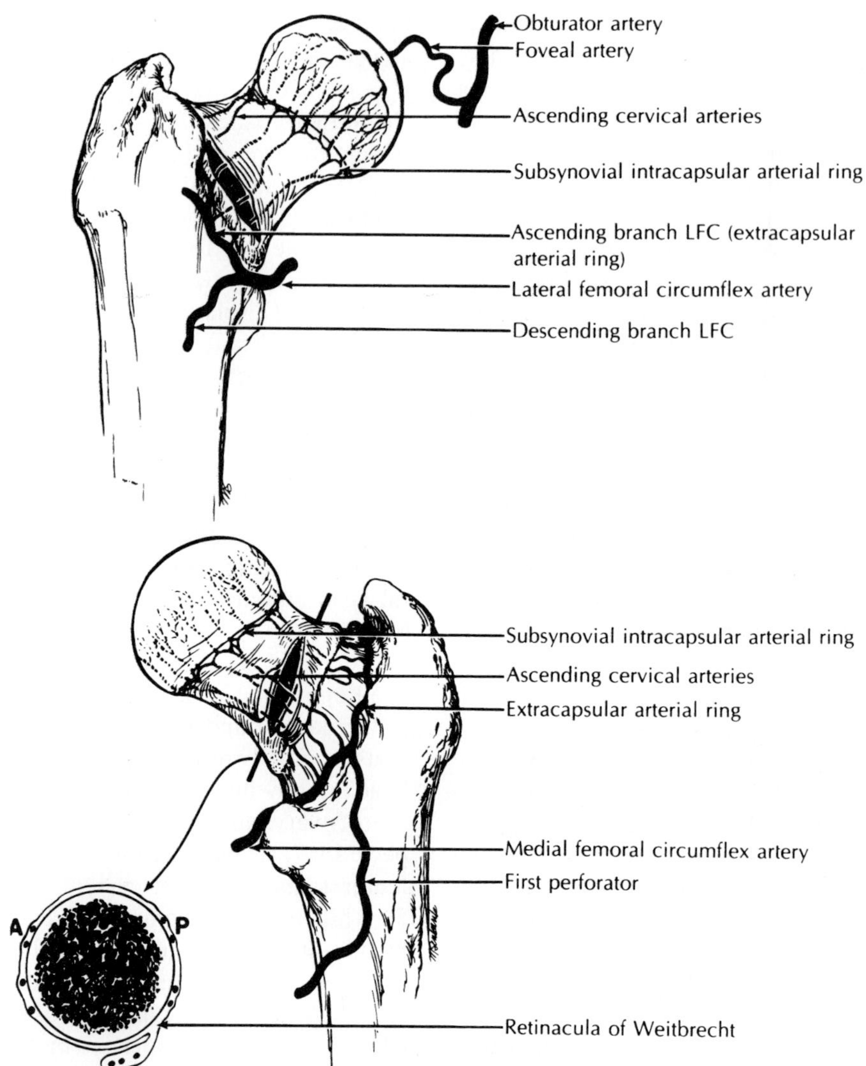

FIGURE 2 Arterial anatomy of the proximal femur. The medial circumflex femoral artery provides the majority of blood flow to the femoral head through the ascending cervical arteries. Reprinted with permission from DeLee [19].

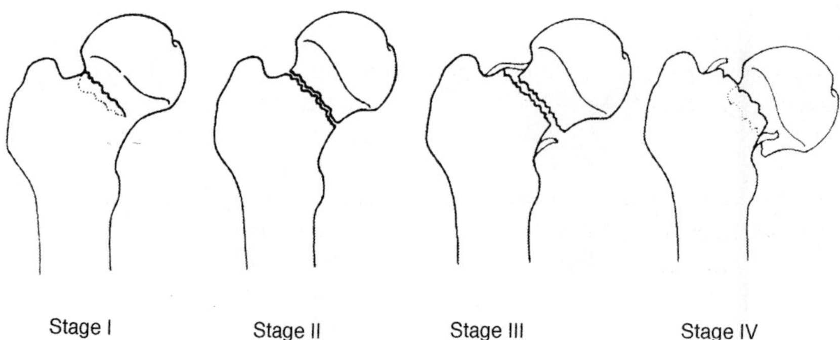

FIGURE 3 Garden Classification of femoral neck fractures. Stage I: Incomplete, valgus-impacted fracture. Stage II: Complete, nondisplaced fracture. Stage III: Complete, partially displaced fracture. Stage IV: Complete, fully displaced fracture. Reprinted with permission from Einhorn [10].

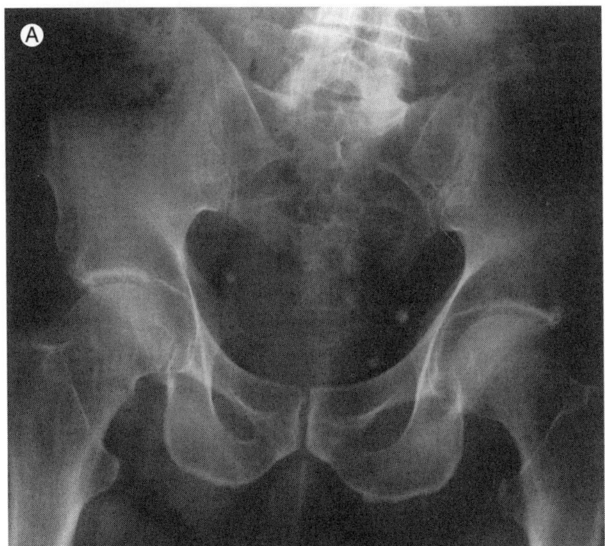

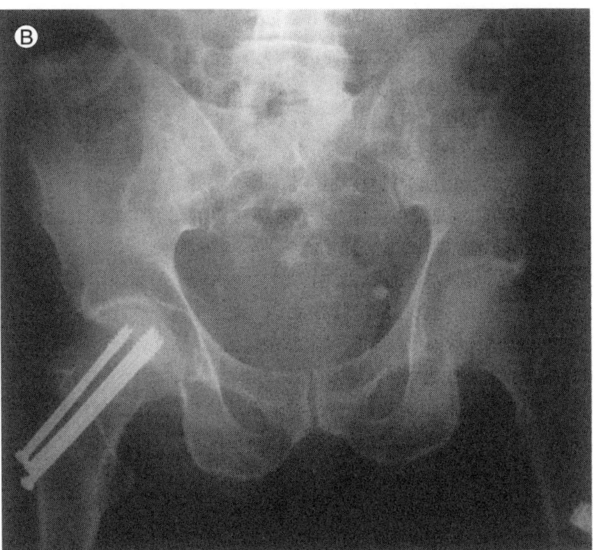

FIGURE 4 (A) AP pelvis radiograph demonstrating a right valgus-impacted (Garden I) femoral neck fracture. (B) Postoperative radiograph demonstrating fixation with three 7.3-mm cannulated screws placed in a triangular configuration.

with increased muscle tone, which can lead to implant failure prior to fracture healing, and Pagetoid bone does not heal as well as normal bone. In addition, severely osteoporotic bone may not support internal fixation devices. Some form of cemented arthroplasty is indicated in all three situations. With current cement techniques, arthroplasty (hemi or total) offers immediate and full weight bearing postoperatively without risk of implant failure. The surgery, however, is more complex than hip pinning and is associated with increased blood loss and operative time. In addition, there is a small risk of intraoperative hypotension during cementing of the femoral prosthesis as the cement (methyl methacrylate) monomer is a direct acting vasodilator.

Though these guidelines exist, relatively younger aged and active patients may sway the orthopedist toward performing closed reduction and pinning of displaced fractures in order to preserve the patient's own femoral head and articular surface. If AVN, nonunion, or implant failure occurs conversion to arthroplasty is possible. This conservative strategy offers the advantage of performing a relatively quick and simple procedure

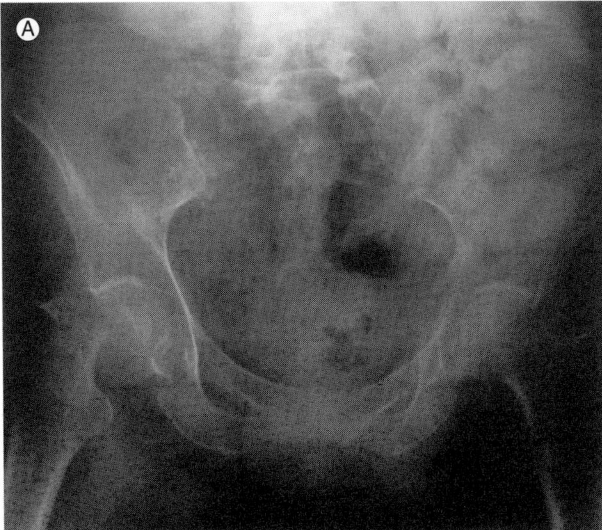

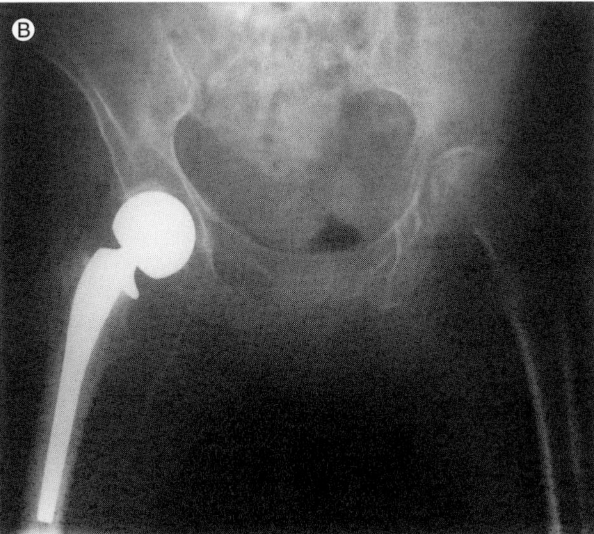

FIGURE 5 (A) AP pelvis radiograph demonstrating a completely displaced (Garden IV) femoral neck fracture. (B) Postoperative radiograph after treatment with a unipolar hemiarthroplasty. Note the patients acetabulum is unaltered.

when the patient is in the least stable condition and a more involved elective operation when the patient is medically optimized.

Intertrochanteric fractures occur between the greater and the lesser trochanters of the femur. They are subdivided into two-, three-, or four-part fractures depending on the number of fragments produced (Fig. 6). A single fracture line produces two-part fractures composed of the femoral head and neck and the femoral metaphysis and shaft. Three-part fractures have a separate lesser trochanteric or greater trochanteric fragment, and four-part fractures are composed of the femoral head and neck, greater trochanter, lesser trochanter, and femoral metaphysis and shaft. In general, fracture instability is directly proportional to the number of fragments. Other complicating factors include comminution, especially of the medial calcar, and reverse obliquity fractures where the fracture line is perpendicular to a line connecting the greater and lesser trochanters. Both factors make the fractures highly unstable.

Most intertrochanteric fractures, however, can be treated with open reduction and internal fixation (ORIF) using some variation of the dynamic hip screw (DHS). This screw and side plate configuration is especially important in osteoporotic bone as it is dynamic in nature and allows controlled settling of the femoral head and neck into a stable configuration (Fig. 7). Some unstable fractures require special fixed-angle (nondynamic) devices or screw and intramedullary nail combinations to provide adequate stability. Although AVN is not a significant factor in intertrochanteric fractures, resultant morbidity from nonunion, mal-union, and implant failure is important.

Subtrochanteric fractures, which occur just below the lesser trochanter, are less common than femoral neck or intertrochanteric fractures. They can be very difficult fractures to treat and require special types of fixation, including reconstruction intramedullary nails, blade plates, or other similar devices. The DHS and side plate used for intertrochanteric fractures do not

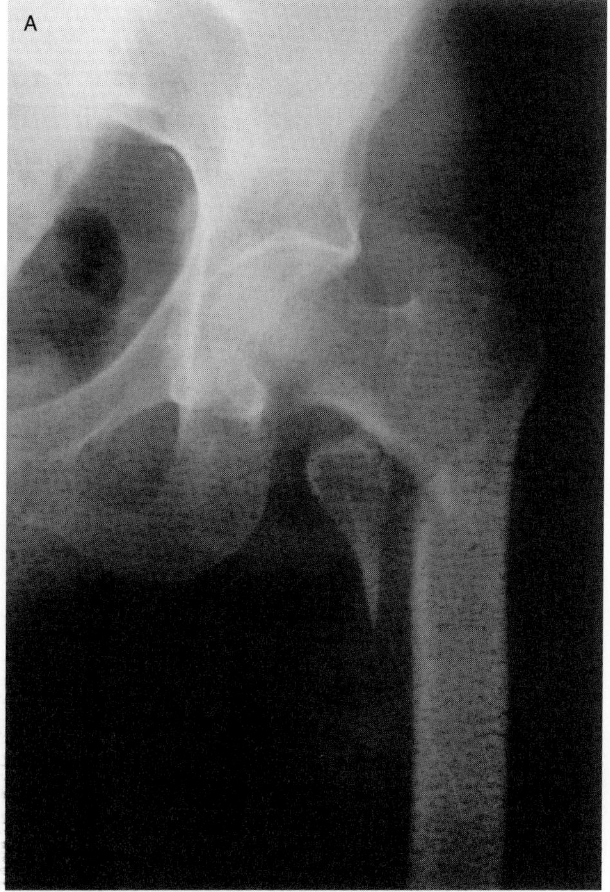

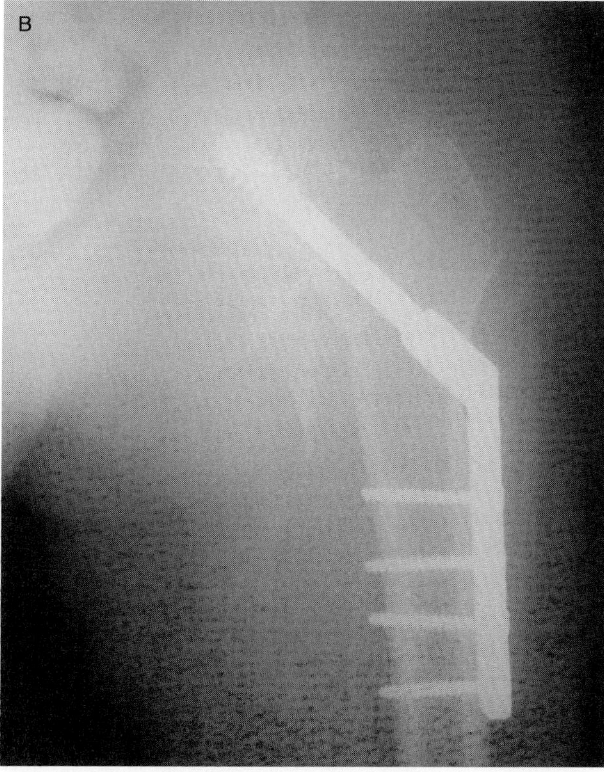

FIGURE 6 (A) Typical four-part intertrochanteric hip fracture with a head and neck fragment, lesser trochanter fragment, greater trochanter fragment, and metaphysis and shaft fragment. (B) Postoperative radiograph showing fixation with a dynamic hip screw and side plate. Note the lesser trochanter does not have to be included in the fixation for healing to occur.

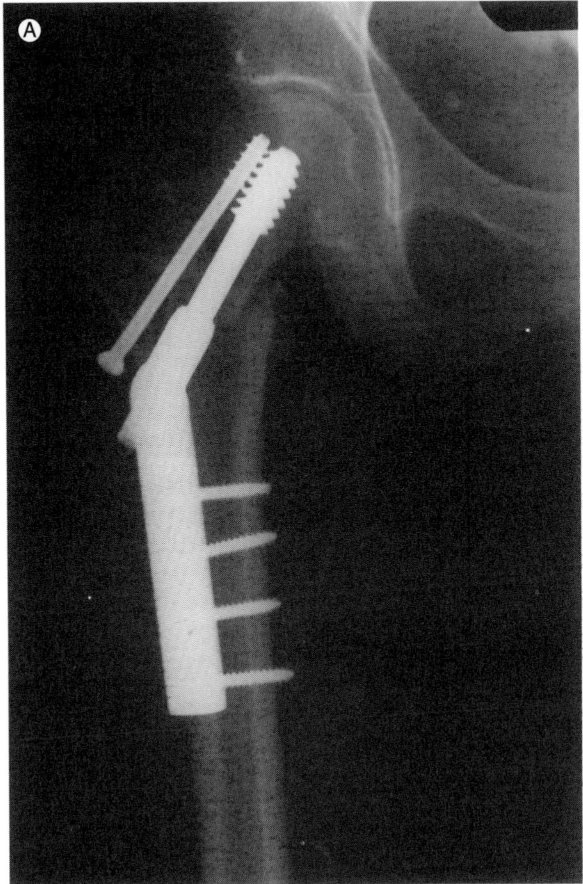

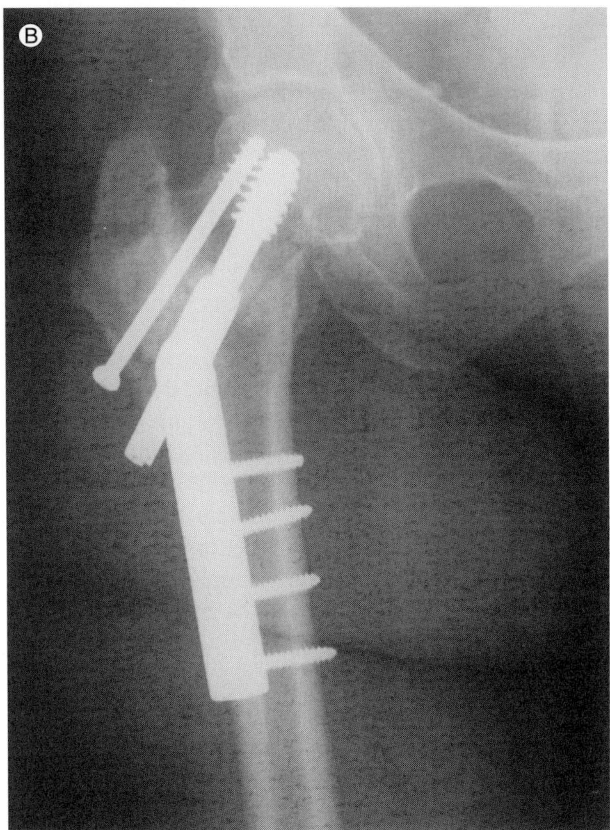

FIGURE 7 (A) This radiograph shows a high intertrochanteric (basi-cervical femoral neck) fracture treated with a dynamic hip screw (DHS) and side-plate combination. Note that the large screw extending from the plate into the femoral head is free to slide within the barrel of the plate fixed to the lateral femur. The smaller screw is present to help provide rotational stability. (B) This radiograph taken several months after initial fixation shows how the DHS system has allowed the large dynamic screw to collapse into the barrel of the plate. This allows the femoral neck to settle into a stable configuration where solid healing can occur. Note how much more of the DHS screw is protruding laterally from the plate in Fig. 6B vs 6A as a result of fracture settling.

provide adequate fixation for subtrochanteric fractures. Nonunion and hardware failure is problematic with these fractures.

Clinical decision making with regard to hip fractures extends not only to the appropriate type of fixation for a given fracture, but also to the timing of the operation. Despite many attempts at studying the morbidity and mortality associated with immediate (less than 12 hr after arrival) versus early (within 2 days of arrival) versus delayed (2 days after arrival) surgery, there is no conclusive evidence to support an optimum time for surgery. A recent study prospectively examined outcomes of hip fractures (femoral neck and intertrochanteric) in cognitively intact, ambulatory patients living at home prior to injury. It concluded that an operative delay of more than 2 calendar days is an important predictor of mortality within 1 year of the time of the fracture [20]. General recommendations include surgery as early as possible, provided that other comorbid conditions are controlled and that the patient is medically stable [21].

One final consideration is whether a particular patient benefits from operative intervention at all. It is well accepted that operative fixation of proximal femoral fractures provides decreased morbidity and mortality and improved outcomes. However, nonoperative management of hip fractures is appropriate for a select group of patients consisting of truly senile, demented, nonambulatory, nursing home patients. Proponents believe that nonoperative therapy is safer, more cost effective, and more humane than hospitalization [22,23]. Notwithstanding, this treatment algorithm can be associated with problems centering around the difficulty of knowing a patient's preinjury status and rehabilitation potential. Primary care providers and geriatricians must play an important role in this decision making [24].

Once the hip fracture has been fixed, attention turns to the postoperative management and rehabilitation of the patient. This is best accomplished with a multidisciplinary team approach to patient care, including orthopedic surgeons, geriatricians, clinical nurse specialists, physical therapists, and case managers who meet on a regular basis to discuss patient care. Proponents of this type of system have shown that a geriatric hip fracture program decreases postoperative complications and transfers to other facilities for acute medical problems, shortens hospital stay, and increases independent ambulation and the chance of returning home rather than discharge to a nursing home [25,26].

Supracondylar Femur Fractures

Supracondylar femur fractures are less common than hip, spine, and wrist fractures, but the exceptionally large mechanical forces placed on this region of the femur make these very difficult fractures to treat and lead to increased morbidity and complications. While these fractures exist as the result of high energy trauma in younger patients, osteoporosis predisposes the elderly to fractures about the knee with relatively low energy injuries. Complications, regardless of treatment type, approach 40% in the elderly population and mortality after 1 year is as high as 22% [27].

Supracondylar femur fractures are defined as metaphyseal fractures of the distal femur with or without intraarticular extension (Fig. 8A). A minor slip or fall on a flexed knee with a valgus or varus stress is usually responsible for these fractures. Extensive comminution is common in osteoporotic bone. As these fractures involve a major weight-bearing joint, disability secondary to malalignment and stiffness is common. Treatment has evolved from closed reduction with casting or traction, which is associated with high rates of stiffness and knee pain, to aggressive operative internal fixation with early motion. Primary above the knee amputation is reserved for the most severe of injuries.

Nondisplaced or incomplete fractures as well as impacted metaphyseal fractures are amenable to cast immobilization. Conversion to a cast brace as soon as pos-

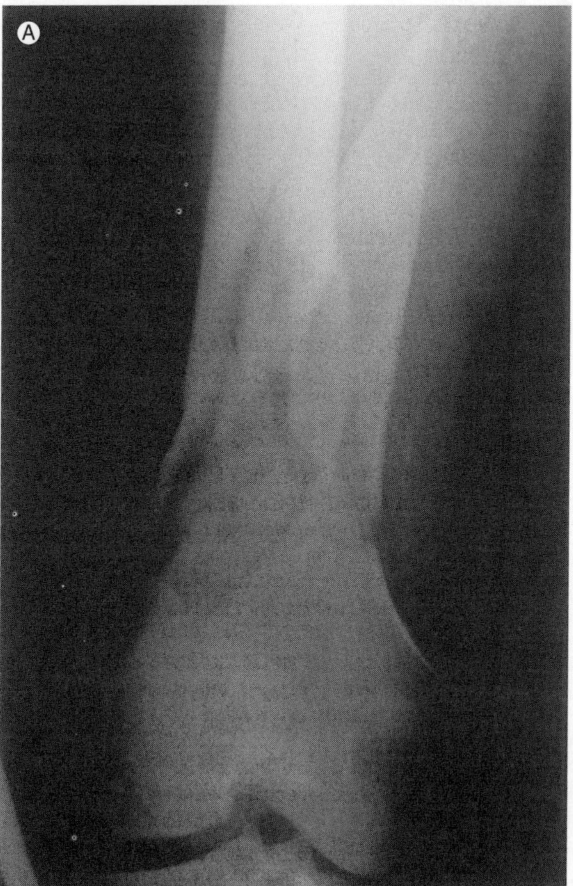

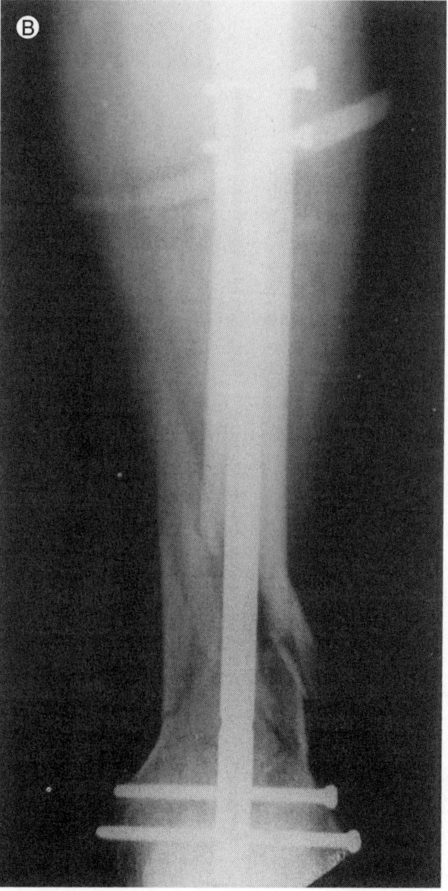

FIGURE 8 (A) AP radiograph of a distal femur with a comminuted, metaphyseal supracondylar femur fracture. (B) Postoperative radiograph demonstrating the use of a retrograde intramedullary nail for fixation. Note the reduction is not anatomic, but stable fixation is achieved.

sible is preferred to allow early knee range of motion [28]. When operative intervention is required, stable internal fixation can be difficult to achieve because of osteoporosis and extensive comminution. Consequently, various devices have been developed to treat supracondylar fractures.

Restoration of length and axial alignment with stable fixation and early functional rehabilitation are goals in the younger patient. Elderly osteoporotic patients may be treated best with impaction of metaphyseal fragments, accepting a small amount of shortening and malalignment as a trade-off for rapid fracture union [28]. Two major types of internal fixation devices are commonly used to treat supracondylar femur fractures: condylar plates and screws and intramedullary nails. Condylar plates provide rigid fixation with some variation of a buttress plate combined with different forms of distal femoral fixation, including standard AO screws, a compression screw (similar to a DHS), or a blade plate (Fig. 9). Intramedullary nails placed in a retrograde fashion through the knee offer the advantage of being load-sharing devices and having the potential to stabilize complex fractures with minimal soft tissue dissection [28] (Fig. 8B). Anterograde nails placed through the proximal femur have a more limited use and are appropriate for high metaphyseal fractures without intraarticular involvement.

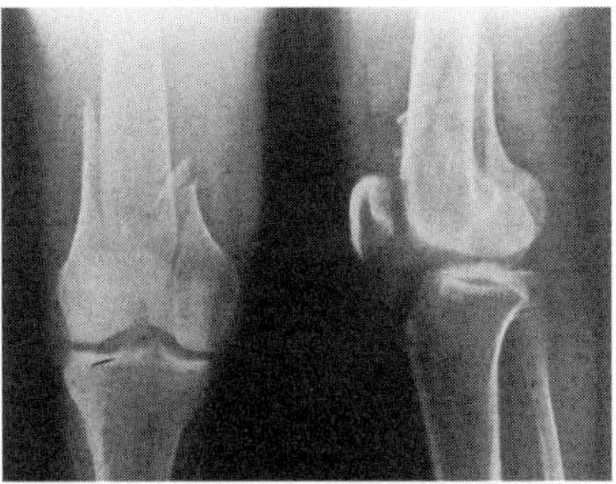

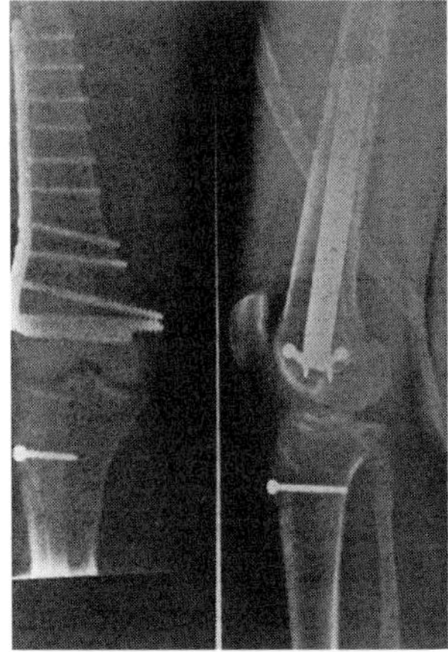

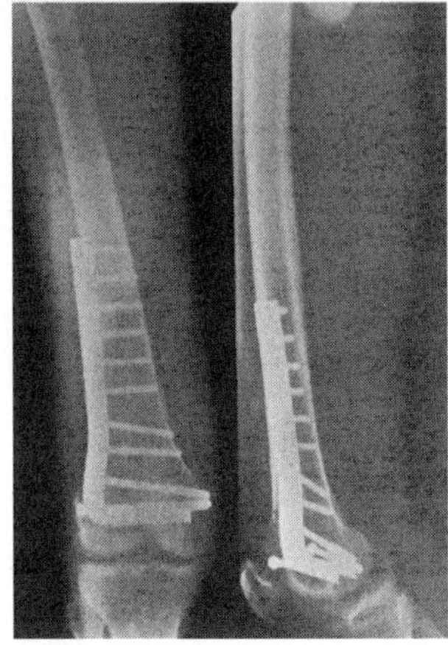

FIGURE 9 Pre- and postoperative radiographs of a comminuted intraarticular supracondylar femur fracture stabilized with an AO blade plate. In this case, near-anatomic reduction of the joint surface, as well as restoration of the normal length of the femur, was obtained. Reprinted with permission from Wiss *et al.* [28].

Rehabilitation with emphasis on knee range of motion is imperative for good functional outcome regardless of treatment method. Continuous passive motion (CPM) machines have offered advances in postoperative management of these injuries. These machines continuously cycle the knee through a range of motion, thus providing constant physical therapy. They are best at helping patients reclaim flexion and are less effective at restoring extension. Therefore, several hours per day are spent off the machine, allowing patients to work on regaining extension. No CPM machine is a substitute for physical therapy and these machines should be used in conjunction with a well-defined physical therapy program. When used in such a fashion, CPM machines have allowed patients to more quickly restore a greater range of motion of their injured knees.

Tibial Plateau Fractures

Like supracondylar femur fractures, fractures of the tibial plateau involve a major weight-bearing joint and can have a significant impact on the ambulatory status of an individual. By definition they are intraarticular fractures and, like intraarticular supracondylar femur fractures, require extensive rehabilitation to regain motion and function of the knee.

Their mechanism of injury parallels that of supracondylar femur fractures and is most commonly axial loading with a varus or valgus stress. The femoral condyle is driven into the tibia with resultant fracture of the medial or lateral tibial plateau, depending on whether the stress is from a varus or valgus force, respectively. The Schatzker classification is the most frequently used system for describing these fractures (Fig. 10).

Axial loading with a valgus moment produces lateral plateau fractures, which are most commonly of the Schatzker II type in the elderly [29]. Depression of the tibial plateau (Schatzker II and III) is common in the osteoporotic patient as the metaphyseal cancellous bone is the first to fail when significant force is applied to the plateau. Type I fractures (isolated split fractures) are seen almost exclusively in young patients with strong, compact cancellous bone [28]. Axial loading and a varus moment may produce medial plateau fractures (Schatzker IV) and are associated with higher energy mechanisms and concomitant knee dislocations. Vascular injury is more common in this group and careful evaluation, including arteriography, may be indicated if vascular embarrassment is present. Schatzker V and VI fractures result from high energy injuries in some

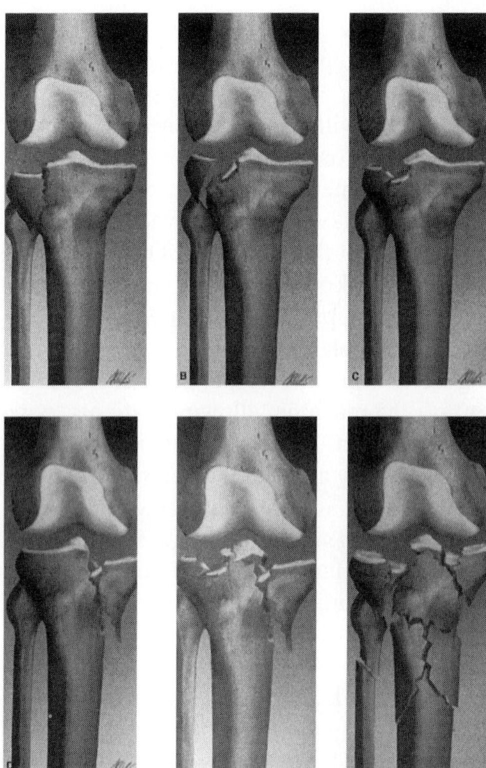

FIGURE 10 Schatzker classification of tibial plateau fractures. (A) Schatzker I: Isolated split of the lateral tibial plateau. (B) Schatzker II: Combined split and depression of lateral tibial plateau. (C) Schatzker III: Isolated depression of lateral tibial plateau. (D) Schatzker IV: Medial plateau fracture. (E) Schatzker V: Combined medial and lateral tibial plateau fractures. (F) Schatzker VI: Combined medial and lateral tibial plateau fractures with associated metaphyseal fracture. Reprinted with permission from Wiss *et al.* [28].

patients, but in the elderly, severe osteoporosis may sufficiently weaken bone, causing these fractures to occur with less energy. These can be very challenging fractures to manage, regardless of the age of the patient.

Radiographic evaluation includes plain radiographs in multiple projections, CT scan, or magnetic resonance imaging (MRI). MRI has played a more important role in the evaluation of these injuries as the literature suggests MRI is equivalent or superior to two-dimensional CT reconstruction for the depiction of fracture configuration and provides the added benefit of soft tissue evaluation of the menisci, collateral ligaments, and cruciate ligaments [30].

Optimal functional outcome depends on joint congruity, stability, and correct load distribution of the injured knee. Restoration of the joint surface is the goal; open reduction and stable internal fixation enabling early rehabilitation is recommended in all displaced articular fractures of the tibial plateau [31]. Operative stabilization takes many forms, depending on the particular fracture configuration, but the reduction of displaced intraarticular fragments and internal fixation with a buttress plate and screws is the mainstay. Any depressed articular fragments are elevated and supported with bone graft and internal fixation. Arthroscopy may be used in conjunction with bone grafting and limited internal fixation, especially in isolated depression fractures (Schatzker III). This approach limits soft tissue dissection and provides excellent visualization of the joint surface during the reduction. External fixation is another option for stabilizing tibial plateau fractures, especially when there are major soft tissue concerns or wounds. As mentioned previously, early motion with physical therapy as well as continuous passive motion machines has been shown to improve functional outcomes [29].

UPPER EXTREMITY FRACTURES

Distal Radius Fractures

Although not life threatening, distal radius fractures are common in the elderly and can carry significant morbidity if treatment fails. The Colles' fracture is the most common type of wrist fracture and represents a metaphyseal fracture with dorsal displacement and angulation. It may extend into the radiocarpal or the distal radioulnar joint. Clinically, the fracture presentation ranges from mild swelling at the distal radius to the so-called silver-fork deformity associated with significant dorsal displacement of the distal radius (Fig. 11). The mechanism for such a fracture is a fall on an outstretched hand with transmission of force as a bending moment to the distal radius. Shear and compression forces are common causes of intraarticular fractures.

Classification of these fractures can be cumbersome, but interpreting three basic radiographic parameters can help direct treatment: dorsal angulation, radial shortening, and intraarticular displacement. While anatomic reduction is preferred, it is not necessary for a good outcome. Exact numbers vary in the literature, but residual dorsal angulation greater than 20°, radial shortening greater than 5 mm, and intraarticular displacement greater than 2 mm is associated with decreased motion, grip strength, and wrist stability [32].

Closed reduction and plaster immobilization remains the mainstay of treatment. Loss of reduction or "slippage" of the fracture, however, is common after manipulation, especially with the severe dorsal comminution seen in osteoporotic bone. Dorsal angulation deteriorates by an average of 11° after reduction [33]. In elderly patients, there is some support for accepting as much as 30° of dorsal angulation and 5 mm of radial shortening without attempting a reduction. Functional outcomes

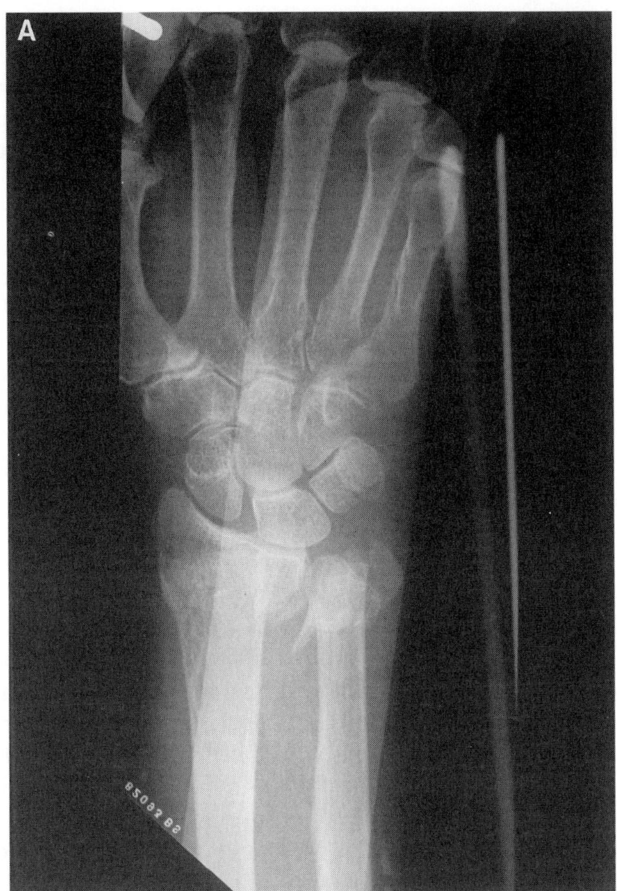

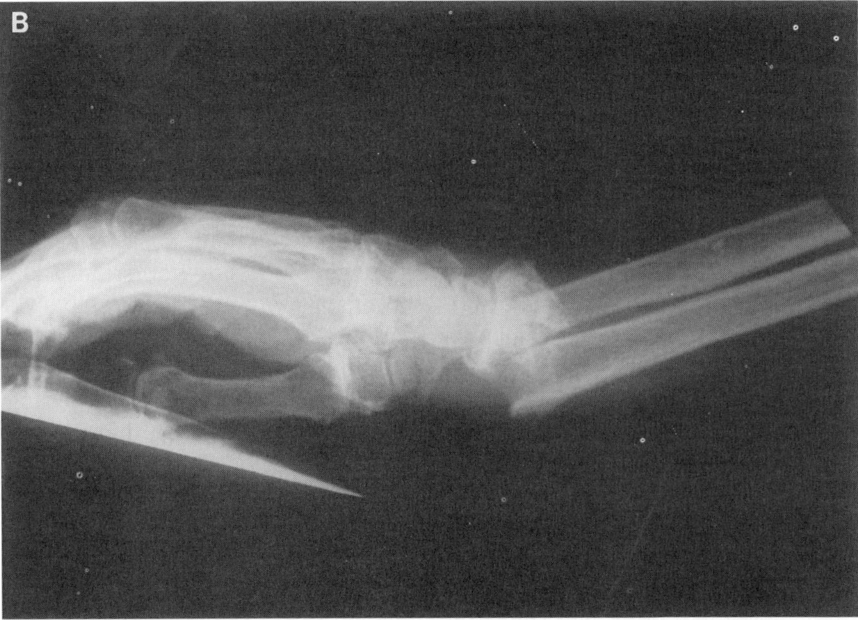

FIGURE 11 AP and lateral radiograph of the wrist demonstrating a dorsally displaced and angulated distal radius and ulna fracture. The lateral radiograph is the X-ray depiction of the clinical silver-fork deformity.

were shown to be the same in this group compared with patients who underwent attempted closed reduction [33]. Casting is continued for approximately 6 weeks at which time occupational therapy for range of motion is instituted. When these criteria are not met, surgical intervention is warranted. The options range from closed reduction with percutaneous pinning to external fixation with percutaneous pinning to ORIF. ORIF is required most frequently for the restoration of displaced intraarticular fractures to prevent posttraumatic degenerative changes at the wrist joint.

Proximal Humerus Fractures

Proximal humerus fractures represent 76% of humerus fractures in elderly patients. The fracture usually results from a fall on an outstretched hand from a standing height or less. A direct blow to the shoulder may also produce the fracture, but a twisting mechanism with the humeral head becoming locked against the acromion with subsequent failure at the surgical neck has been described in osteoporotic individuals [34]. Severe trauma rarely plays a significant role in the development of these fractures in the elderly. Proximal humerus fractures almost always occur at the surgical neck of the humerus, dividing the proximal humerus into as few as two or as many as four parts. The head, greater tuberosity, lesser tuberosity, and shaft make up the four possible fragments as described by Neer [35]. Technically, to qualify as a separate part the fragment must be displaced 1 cm or angulated 45°. Correct radiographic evaluation is extremely important in delineating fracture configuration. Internal and external rotation views of the humerus are inadequate to evaluate the position of the humeral shaft relative to the humeral head. A complete shoulder trauma series consisting of a true AP view of the shoulder (in the plane of the scapula), scapular Y view (perpendicular to the plane of the scapula), and an axillary view is mandatory. Unrecognized displacement of fracture fragments and missed humeral head dislocations may result from inadequate radiographic evaluation. A CT scan may be helpful in the evaluation of three- and four-part fractures to determine the true number of fragments and their suitability for ORIF.

Two-part fractures dividing the shaft and proximal humerus at the surgical neck are the most common configuration and are usually nondisplaced. Sling and swathe immobilization is instituted until pain subsides followed by pendulum exercises at 1 to 2 weeks provided the two fragments move as a unit. Full passive motion is started by 3 weeks and active motion by 5 to 6 weeks. Displaced two-part fractures can usually be managed by closed reduction and impaction followed by the previously mentioned protocol. If closed reduction results in a reduced but unstable fracture, percutaneous pin fixation may be employed.

Three-part fractures (head, a tuberosity fragment, and shaft) are usually unstable and require ORIF. However, osteoporotic bone frequently does not support fixation and hemiarthroplasty is an effective alternative. When ORIF is chosen, various methods may be used, including pin fixation, tension band wiring with or without intramedullary flexible rods, clover plate and screws, or a cannulated blade plate. Impingement against the acromion is a common complication with these types of fixation.

Four-part fractures place the humeral head at risk for AVN (13–34%) and hemiarthroplasty is the treatment of choice, especially in elderly individuals [34]. Two further fracture patterns should be mentioned. The head-splitting fracture that divides the head itself into two separate pieces almost always requires hemiarthroplasty as the rate of AVN is the highest with this fracture pattern. It can be easily overlooked if an axillary view or CT scan is not obtained. Finally, displaced fractures at the anatomic neck of the humerus are also associated with a significant rate of AVN and frequently require hemiarthroplasty.

Humeral Shaft and Distal Humerus Fractures

Humeral shaft and distal humerus fractures are much less common than proximal humerus fractures. Most fractures of the humeral shaft can be treated nonoperatively with a coaptation splint, hanging arm cast, cuff and collar, or fracture brace. Only occasionally is intramedullary fixation or ORIF with plates and screws required. Significant angular deformities and shortening are tolerated as much of upper extremity positioning can be compensated by motion at the elbow and shoulder.

Distal humerus fractures involving the elbow include supracondylar and intracondylar fractures and are serious injuries with frequent morbidity. Intraarticular fractures are associated with significant stiffness and loss of motion at the elbow, despite aggressive ORIF and early motion. Like other intraarticular fractures elsewhere in the body, anatomic reduction is the goal, but even when this is obtained, range of motion may be limited, although functional outcomes are acceptable [36]. Alternatives to ORIF include the "bag of bones" technique where no attempt at reduction or fixation is made and emphasis is placed on early motion. This method is rarely used today, but may be indicated in the very aged with poor preinjury function. Primary total elbow arthroplasty represents the opposite end of the treatment spectrum. It is a viable alternative for severely comminuted fractures in elderly patients [37]. However, this approach is taken only at a limited number of specialized institutions where total elbow arthroplasty is performed in nonfracture patients on a regular basis.

SPINE AND PELVIS FRACTURES

Vertebral Fractures

The spine is the most common site for osteoporotic fractures. Thirty to 50% of women and 20 to 30% of men will develop vertebral fractures during their lifetime. Clinically, these fractures can range from asymptomatic to chronically disabling [38]. Approximately two-thirds of all vertebral fractures are subclinical [39]. Symptomatic complaints include pain, limitations in mobility, and loss of independence. Radiographically, vertebral fractures can be described as biconcave, wedge, or crush (Fig. 12). Acute crush fractures tend to be the most likely to cause pain.

Treatment is centered around a multidisciplinary approach to improve mobility, flexibility, speed of movement, and independence. Goals in treating asymptomatic patients include the prevention of new fractures, physical rehabilitation, restoration of independence, and conservation of bone mass. Fractures associated with acute pain are initially treated with bed rest and analgesics. This pain is usually self-limited and resolves within 4 to 6 weeks. Mobilization and rehabilitation are started after 1 week of rest. Support devices such as braces can be used thereafter to help decrease pain with mobilization. Most agree it is best to discontinue bracing as soon as possible because immobilization of the spine leads to weakening of the paraspinal muscles, which function to stabilize the spine by sharing the mechanical load transmitted through the vertebral column [39].

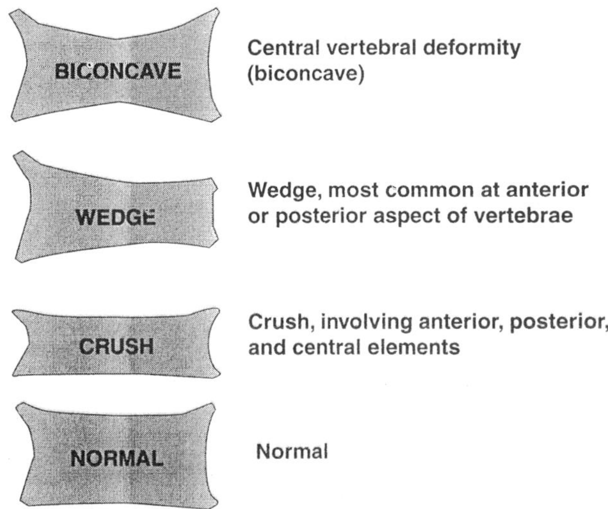

FIGURE 12 Classification of vertebral compression fractures. Reprinted from *American Journal of Medicine,* **103,** Tamayo-Orozco, J., Arza-Palumbo, P., Peon-Vidales, H., Mota-Bolfeta, R., Fuentes, F. Vertebral fractures associated with osteoporosis: Patient management, 448–508 (1997), with permission from Elsevier Science.

For those patients who have not responded to appropriate medical therapy and continue to have intolerable pain, another therapeutic alternative exists. Percutaneous vertebroplasty is a technique by which polymethylmethacrylate (bone cement) is injected percutaneously by a transpedicular or posterolateral approach under flouroscopic or CT guidance into a collapsed vertebral body. Several studies have shown excellent pain relief in 90% of patients immediately following injection [40–42]. Few long-term studies exist but short-term outcomes are promising. Complications from the procedure are uncommon (0–10%) but include extravasation of cement into the spinal canal, neural foramina, paravertebral veins, and adjacent disks. Neurologic compromise requiring operative intervention is exceedingly rare (1 in 258) and most neurologic symptoms are transitory and felt to be due to local inflammation, which resolves over time [42].

Fractures confined to the thoracic spine are more easily rehabilitated than those of the thoracolumbar or lumbar spine. Fractures above the sixth thoracic vertebrae should lead one to suspect malignancy or causes other than osteoporosis because this portion of the spine is well stabilized and less commonly fractured. For those with chronic pain, steroid injections are sometimes used, but detailed study to detect neurologic, myofascial, or other orthopedic conditions should be undertaken. In actuality, neurologic compromise secondary to osteoporotic vertebral fractures is exceedingly rare. Operative stabilization of the spine is also rarely indicated but can be required in fractures of the lumbar vertebrae [39].

Pelvic Insufficiency Fractures

Insufficiency fractures are a subset of stress fractures that occur when normal or physiologic stresses are applied to bone with deficient elastic resistance or mineral content [43,44]. Osteoporosis is the main underlying cause of these fractures, placing the elderly at increased risk. The sacrum and pubic rami are common sites for insufficiency fractures and usually occur in elderly, postmenopausal women. Prolonged immobilization, recent increased physical activity, or minor trauma may predate the fracture. Unfortunately, insufficiency fractures of the pubic rami subsequent to hip and knee surgery are well documented. Fractures may occur a few weeks to several months or years following surgery and may be more frequent after the second operation in patients with bilateral total hip arthroplasty. The fractures are in part due to the patient's ability to enjoy pain-free activity postarthroplasty with resultant increased physical demands on bones that are weakened from previous inactivity [44]. Cautioning patients to slowly increase their activity over months, as well as treating any underlying osteoporosis in conjunction with informing the patients of the signs and symptoms of stress fractures, may reduce this problem. No studies, however, provide any definitive suggestions to decrease the incidence of postarthroplasty stress fractures.

Presentation includes inguinal pain related to activity and is relieved by rest, limping, a waddling gait, or an inability to walk. Low back pain may represent sacral fractures. The diagnosis is often delayed and plain radiographs may overlook the fractures. Bone scintigraphy is extremely useful and is the most sensitive modality for demonstrating these fractures. H-shaped sacral uptake, parasymphyseal uptake, or both are representative of sacral or pubic rami fractures. A CT scan may also be useful, although less sensitive than a bone scan [45].

Bed rest and reduced weight bearing are usually prescribed followed by a gradual progression of weight bearing. These fractures usually heal within a few weeks if diagnosed in a timely fashion. Occasionally, slow healing and osteolysis result from delayed diagnosis and treatment. Treatment for the underlying osteoporosis should also be implemented [44].

FUTURE DIRECTIONS IN THE TREATMENT OF OSTEOPOROTIC FRACTURES

One new treatment option for fractures in osteoporotic bone is a new calcium phosphate-based cement that may be used to augment fracture fixation. This paste-like material (Norian SRS, Norian Corp., Cupertino, CA) can be injected into a fracture site where it hardens into carbonated hydroxyapatite, providing structural support. Currently this substance is being evaluated clinically in the treatment of distal radius fractures. Preliminary studies suggest use of this bone cement following the manipulation of fractures may allow fracture healing without loss of reduction as well as decrease the need for external fixation and shorten immobilization time [46,47]. It may also play a role in augmenting fracture fixation of femoral neck fractures [48]. If successful, this innovative treatment modality may change fracture management throughout the body in both the young and the aged patient.

SUMMARY

Fractures of the aging skeleton have a significant impact on the health care system because of their frequent occurrence and oftentimes costly treatment. Their substantial morbidity and mortality make them important clinical entities. Fractures of the spine, hip, and wrist are the most common and generally are associated with underlying osteoporosis. The fragility of the elderly skeleton, which makes these fractures so common, also complicates the management of fractures in this population. The treating physician must keep this in mind when choosing nonoperative versus operative treatment, as well as the particular type of fixation used if operative intervention is chosen. The basic tenets of anatomic reduction, rigid internal fixation, and early motion may be modified slightly to allow modest degrees of displacement with stable but dynamic fixation. Early motion and an emphasis on rehabilitation remain key to obtaining good functional outcomes. Sound clinical judgment with an understanding of the unique problems posed by the osteoporotic skeleton will become increasingly important as the elderly population grows in the coming decade.

References

1. Cooper, C. The crippling consequences of fractures and their impact on quality of life. *Am. J. Med.* **103**(2A), 12S–17S (1997).
2. Melton, L. J., III, Thamer, M., Ray, N. F., Chan, J. K., Chestnut, C. H., III, Einhorn, T. A., Johnston, C. C., Raisz, L. G., Silverman, S. L., and Siris, E. S. Fractures attributable to osteoporosis: report from the National Osteoporosis Foundation. *J. Bone Miner. Res.* **12**(1), 16–23 (1997).
3. Johnell, O. The socioeconomic burden of fractures: today and in the 21st century. *Am. J. Med.* **103**(2A), 20S–25S (1997).
4. Quarto, R., Thomas, D., and Liang, C. T. Bone progenitor cell deficits and the age-associated decline in bone repair capacity. *Calcif. Tissue Int.* **56**(2), 123–129 (1995).
5. Bak, B., and Andreassen, T. T. The effect of aging on fracture healing in the rat. *Calcif. Tissue Int.* **45**(5), 292–297 (1989).
6. Macey, L. R., Kana, S. M., Jingushi, S., Terek, R. M., Borretos, J., and Bolander, M. E. Defects of early fracture-healing in experimental diabetes. *J. Bone Joint Surg.* **71**(5), 722–733 (1989).
7. Walsh, W. R., Sherman, P., Howlett, C. R., Sonnabend, D. H., and Ehrick, M. G. Fracture healing in a rat osteopenia model. *Clin. Orthop. Rel. Res.* **342,** 218–227 (1997).
8. Peter, C. P., Cook, W. O., Nunamaker, D. M., Provost, M. T., Seedor, J. G., and Rodan, G. A. Effect of alendronate on fracture healing and bone remodeling in dogs. *J. Orthop. Res.* **14**(1), 7–9 (1996).
9. Altman, R. D., Latta, L. L., Keer, R., Renfree, K., Hornicek, F. J., and Banovac, K. Effect of nonsteroidal antiinflammatory drugs on fracture healing: a laboratory study in rats. *J. Orthop. Trauma* **9**(5), 392–400 (1995).
10. Einhorn, T. A. Orthopaedic complications of osteoporosis. *In* "Primer on Metabolic Bone Diseases and Disorders of Mineral Metabolism" (M. J. Fravus, ed.), 3rd Ed., pp. 293–299. Lippincott-Raven, Philadelphia, 1996.
11. Carter, D. R., and Hayes, W. C. The compressive behavior of bone as a two-phase porous structure. *J. Bone Joint Surg.* **59,** 954–962 (1977).
12. Einhorn, T. A., Bonnarens, F., and Burstein, A. H. The contributions of dietary protein and mineral to the healing of experimental

fractures: A biomechanical study. *J. Bone Joint Surg.* **68A,** 1389–1395 (1986).

13. Jensen, J. E., Jensen, T. G., Smith, T. K., Johnston, D. A., and Dudrick, S. J. Nutrition in orthopaedic surgery. *J. Bone Joint Surg.* **64**(9), 1263–1272 (1982).
14. Foster, M. R., Heppenstall, R. B., Friedenberg, Z. B., and Hozak, W. J. A prospective assessment of nutritional status and complications in patients with fractures of the hip. *J. Orthop. Trauma* **4**(1), 49–57 (1990).
15. LeBoff, M. S., Kohlmeier, L., Franklin, J., Haden, S., Hurwitz, S., Wright, J., and Glowacki, J. Compared with osteoporotic controls acute hip fracture patients show high PTH and low Vitamin D levels. Abstract. *J. Amer. Med. Assoc.* (1999). In press.
16. Mullen, J. O., and Mullen, N. L. Hip fracture mortality. A prospective, multifactorial study to predict and minimize death risk. *Clin. Orthop. Rel. Res.* **280,** 214–222 (1992).
17. Lu-Yao, G. L., Keller, R. B., Littenberg, B., and Wennberg, J. E. Outcomes after displaced fractures of the femoral neck. A meta-analysis of one hundred and six published reports. *J. Bone Joint Surg.* **76**(1), 15–25 (1994).
18. Guyton, J. L. Fracture of hip, acetabulum, and pelvis. *In* "Campbell's Operative Orthopaedics" (S. T. Canale, ed.), 9th Ed., Vol. III, pp. 2181–280. Mosby-Year Book, St. Louis, 1998.
19. DeLee, J. C. Fractures and dislocations of the hip. *In* "Rockwood and Green's Fractures in Adults" (C. A. Rockwood, D. P. Green, R. W. Bucholz, and J. D. Heckman, eds.), 4th Ed., Vol. II, pp. 1659–1825. Lippincott-Raven, Philadelphia, 1996.
20. Zuckerman, J. D., Skovron, M. L., Koval, K. J., Aharonoff, G., and Frankel, V. H. Postoperative complications and mortality associated with operative delay in older patients who have a fracture of the hip. *J. Bone Joint Surg.* **77**(10), 1551–1556 (1995).
21. Lyons, A. R. Clinical outcomes and treatment of hip fractures. *Am. J. Med.* **103**(2A), 51S–63S (1997).
22. Lyon, L. J., and Nevins, M. A. Nontreatment of hip fractures in senile patients. *J. Am. Med. Assoc.* **238,** 1175 (1977).
23. Lyon, L. J., and Nevins, M. A. Management of hip fractures in nursing home patients: To treat or not to treat. *J. Am. Geriatr. Soc.* **32,** 391 (1984).
24. Winter, W. G. Nonoperative treatment of proximal femoral fractures in the demented, nonambulatory patient. *Clin. Orthop. Rel. Res.* **218,** 97–103 (1987).
25. Zuckerman, J. D., Fabian, D. R., Aharanoff, G., Koval, K. J., and Fran, V. H. Enhancing independence in the old fracture patient. *Geriatrics* **48**(5), 76–79 (1993).
26. Kennie, D. C., Reid, J., Richardson, I. R., Kiamari, A. A., and Kelt, C. Effectiveness of geriatric rehabilitative care after fractures of the proximal femur in elderly women: a randomized clinical trial. *Br. Med. J.* **297**(6656), 1083–1086 (1988).
27. Karpman, R. R., and Del Mar, N. B. Supracondylar femoral fractures in the frail elderly. Fractures in need of treatment. *Clin. Orthop. Rel. Res.* **316,** 21–24 (1995).
28. Wiss, D. A., Watson, T., and Johnson, E. E. Fractures of the knee. *In* "Rockwood and Green's Fractures in Adults" (C. A. Rockwood, D. P. Green, R. W. Bucholz, and J. D. Heckman, eds.), 4th Ed., Vol. II, pp. 1919–1999. Lippincott-Raven, Philadelphia, 1996.
29. Biyani, A., Reddy, N. S., Chaudhury, J., Simison, A. J., and Klenerman, L. The results of surgical management of displaced tibial plateau fractures in the elderly. *Injury* **26**(5), 291–297 (1995).
30. Kode, L., Lieberman, J. M., Motta, A. O., Wilber, J. H., Vasen, A., and Yagan, R. Evaluation of tibial plateau fractures: efficacy of MR imaging compared with CT. *Am. J. Roentgenol.* **163**(1), 141–147 (1994).
31. Tscherne, H., and Lobenhoffer, P. Tibial plateau fractures. Management and expected results. *Clin. Orthop. Rel. Res.* **292,** 87–100 (1993).
32. Cooney, W. P., III, Linsheid, R. L., and Dobyns, J. H. Fractures and dislocations of the wrist. *In* "Rockwood and Green's Fractures in Adults" (C. A. Rockwood, D. P. Green, R. W. Bucholz, and J. D. Heckman, eds.), 4th Ed., Vol. I, pp. 745–867. Lippincott-Raven, Philadelphia, 1996.
33. Kelly, A. J., Warwick, D., Crichlow, T. P., and Bannister, G. C. Is manipulation of moderately displaced Colles' fractures worthwhile? *Injury* **28**(4), 283–287 (1997).
34. Bigliani, L. U., Flatow, E. L., and Pollock, R. G. Fractures of the proximal humerus. *In* "Rockwood and Green's Fractures in Adults" (C. A. Rockwood, D. P. Green, R. W. Bucholz, and J. D. Heckman, Eds.), 4th Ed., Vol. I, pp. 1055–1107. Lippincott-Raven, Philadelphia, 1996.
35. Neer, C. S. Displaced proximal humeral fractures: I. Classification and evaluation. *J. Bone Joint Surg.* **52A,** 1077–1089 (1970).
36. Pereles, T. R., Koval, K. J., Gallagher, M., and Rosen, H. Open reduction and internal fixation of the distal humerus: functional outcome in the elderly. *J. Trauma* **43**(4), 578–584 (1997).
37. Cobb, T. K., and Morrey, B. F. Total elbow arthroplasty as primary treatment for distal humeral fractures in elderly patients. *J. Bone Joint Surg.* **79**(6), 826–832 (1997).
38. Ross, P. D. Clinical consequences of vertebral fractures. *Am. J. Med.* **103**(2A), 30S–42S (1997).
39. Tamayo-Orozco, J., Arzac-Palumbo, P., Peon-Vidales, H., Mota-Bolfeta, R., and Fuentes, F. Vertebral fractures associated with osteoporosis: Patient management. *Am. J. Med.* **103**(2A), 44S–50S (1997).
40. Jensen, M. E., Evans, A. J., Mathis, J. M., Kallmes, D. F., Cloft, H. J., and Dion, J. E. Percutaneous polymethylmethacrylate vertebroplasty in the treatment of osteoporotic vertebral body compression fractures: Technical aspects. *Am. J. Neuroradiol.* **18,** 1897–1904 (1997).
41. Ganji, A., Kastler, B. A., and Dietemann, J. Percutaneous vertebroplasty guided by a combination of CT and fluoroscopy. *Am. J. Med.* **15,** 83–86 (1994).
42. Connen, A., Boutry, N., Cortet, B., Assaker, R., Demondion, X., Leblond, K., Chastanet, P., Duquesnoy, B., and Deramond, H. Percutaneous vertebroplasty: state of the art. *RadioGraphics* **18,** 311–320 (1998).
43. Peh, W. C., and Evans, N. S. Pelvic insufficiency fractures in the elderly. *Ann. Acad. Med. Singapore* **22**(5), 818–822 (1993).
44. Schapira, D., Militeanu, D., Israel, O., and Scharf, Y. Insufficiency fractures of the pubic ramus. *Sem. Arthritis Rheumatol.* **25**(6), 373–382 (1996).
45. Gotis-Graham, I., McGuigan, L. Diamond, T., Portek, I., Quinn, R., Sturgess, A., and Tulloch, R. Sacral insufficiency fractures in the elderly. *J. Am. Bone Joint Surg.* **76**(6), 882–886 (1994).
46. Jupiter, J. B., Winters, S., Sigman, S., Lowe, C., Pappas, C., Ladd, A. L., Van Wagoner, M., and Smith, S. T. Repair of five distal radius fractures with an investigational cancellous bone cement: a preliminary report. *J. Orthop. Trauma* **11**(2), 110–116 (1997).
47. Kopylov, P., Jonsson, K., Thorngren, K. G., and Aspenberg, P. Injectable calcium phosphate in the treatment of distal radial fractures. *J. Hand Surg.* **21**(6), 768–771 (1996).
48. Stankewich, C. J., Swiontkowski, M. F., Tencer, A. F., Yetkinler, K. N., and Poser, R. D. Augmentation of femoral neck fracture fixation with an injectable calcium-phosphate bone mineral cement. *J. Orthop. Res.* **14**(5), 786–793 (1996).
49. Einhorn, T. A. *Resident Staff Phys.* **34,** 97–113 (1988).

CHAPTER 34

Nutritional Approaches to Healing Fractures in the Elderly

RENÉ RIZZOLI AND JEAN-PHILIPPE BONJOUR
Department of Internal Medicine, Division of Bone Diseases, World Health Organization Collaborating Center for Osteoporosis and Bone Diseases, University Hospital, 1211 Geneva 14, Switzerland

INTRODUCTION

Osteoporosis is widely recognized as a major public health problem in the elderly. Fracture of the proximal femur, which represents the most dramatic expression of the disease, increases as the population ages [1–5]. A variety of different factors determine the risk of osteoporosis, including genetics, sex hormone deficiency, reduced physical exercise, and various environmental risk factors. Among the determinants of osteoporosis in the elderly, nutritional deficiencies certainly play a significant role. Indeed, undernutrition is often observed in the elderly; it appears to be more severe in patients with hip fracture than in the general aging population [6–13]. Thus, deficiency in nutritional elements could play an important role in the pathogenesis of osteoporotic fracture. Not only can undernutrition accelerate age-dependent bone loss, but it also increases the propensity to fall. Although calcium supplementation reduces bone loss and fracture incidence in vitamin D-replete elderly subjects [14–17], the level of protein intake could also influence calcium–phosphate metabolism, bone mass, or the risk of osteoporotic fracture [18,19]. However, two different views argue that either a deficient or an excessive protein intake could each negatively affect calcium balance and mineral homeostasis [18,19]. Uncertainty regarding the benefits of protein supplementation on calcium balance and bone mass is due to several factors. These variables include whether protein supplementation was given to well-nourished or undernourished people and in what form it was provided: natural food products, purified extracts, or mixtures of amino acids. In addition, the source of protein, either animal (e.g., casein) or vegetable (e.g., soya) is a factor that needs to be considered. Some investigations have been short term or long term; some have modified other nutritional factors such as energy and/or calcium. The published literature, therefore, gives a mixed view of the subject at this time. However, there is general agreement on the point that protein intake far below RDA could be particularly detrimental both for the acquisition of bone mass and for the conservation of bone integrity with aging. Within the range generally recommended [20] [i.e., 2 g/kg (children); 1 g/kg (adolescents); 0.75 g/kg (adults)] the prevailing physiological or clinical conditions determine whether an increase or a reduction in protein intake will produce a change in the calcium–phosphate balance and bone mass.

PROTEIN AND BONE MINERAL MASS ACQUISITION

Total bone content at a given age is determined by minerals acquired during growth (leading to the so-called peak bone mass) and by subsequent bone loss [21]. Protein undernutrition during childhood and adolescence results in a reduction of height, weight, and overall lean body tissue [22], thereby affecting peak bone mass.

Studies in experimental animals indicate that isolated protein deficiency leads to reduced bone mass and strength (i.e., to osteoporosis), without histomorphometric evidence of a mineralization defect [18,19,23]. Thus, an inadequate supply of protein appears to play a central role in the pathogenesis of delayed skeletal growth and reduced bone mass observed in undernourished children. The question arises whether variations in the protein intake within the "normal" range can influence skeletal growth and thereby modulate the genetic potential for attainment of peak bone mass in "well-nourished" children and adolescents [24].

In a prospective survey carried out in about 200 female and male adolescents aged 9 to 19 years, food intake was assessed twice, at a 1-year interval, using a 5-day food diary method with the weighing of all consumed foods [24–26]. With respect to macronutrients, results indicated that the total energy intake, which remained within the recommended dietary allowances, was influenced significantly by both pubertal maturation and gender when expressed in absolute terms, but only by pubertal stages when adjusted per kilogram body weight. The intake of protein, two-thirds of which was from animal sources, was above RDA. In this adolescent cohort, the relationship between increments in bone mass and protein intake was analyzed. It was not surprising to find a positive correlation between these two variables in both girls and boys. The correlation was still statistically significant after adjustment for the influence of age and/or pubertal stage. The association between bone mass gain and protein intake was observed in both genders at the level of the lumbar spine, the proximal femur, and the midfemoral shaft. The association appeared to be particularly significant from pubertal stage P_1 to P_4. However, these results should not be interpreted as evidence for a causal relationship between bone mass gain and protein intake. Indeed, it is quite possible that protein intake reflects the overall amount of ingested calories in this cohort and was, to a large extent, determined by growth requirements during childhood and adolescence. In agreement with this interpretation, rats treated with growth hormone spontaneously select a high protein diet [27]. Nevertheless, as is the case for other nutrients such as calcium, only prospective studies can ascertain whether variations in protein intake within the range recorded in our western "well-nourished" population can affect bone mass accrual during growth. Such prospective studies are needed to delineate the crucial years during which modifications in nutrition would be particularly effective for bone mass accumulation in children and in adolescents [21].

PROTEIN MALNUTRITION

Osteoporosis is certainly due to several factors [28]. Bone mass in the elderly in particular is affected by many conditions in which dietary factors are likely to be involved [29–31].

Undernutrition appears to play a key role in the rising incidence of osteoporotic hip fracture among the elderly. Protein undernutrition can favor the occurrence of hip fracture by increasing the propensity to fall as a result of muscle weakness and impaired coordination. Protective mechanisms, such as reaction time and muscle strength, become impaired, reducing the energy required to fracture an osteoporotic bone [11]. Furthermore, any reduction in the protective layer of adipose tissue (padding) decreases the force required to fracture [32–35]. In a survey carried out in hospitalized elderly patients, low protein intake was associated with reduced femoral neck areal bone mineral density (BMD) and poor physical performances [36] (Fig. 1). The study was composed of female and male patients with mean ages of 82 and 80 years, respectively. They were divided into two groups according to their spontaneous dietary protein intake, as determined on 3 nonconsecutive days during the first 28 days in hospital while on a regular diet. The group with the higher protein intake (more than 1.0 g per kg of ideal body weight) also had greater energy, carbohydrate, lipid, and calcium intakes. The remarkable steadiness in the intakes recorded in each subject during the 4 weeks following admission suggested that the inter-individual variation corresponded to long-term nutritional habits rather than to the medical conditions that prompted hospitalization. The group with higher intakes and greater BMD, particularly at the femoral neck, also had a better improvement of

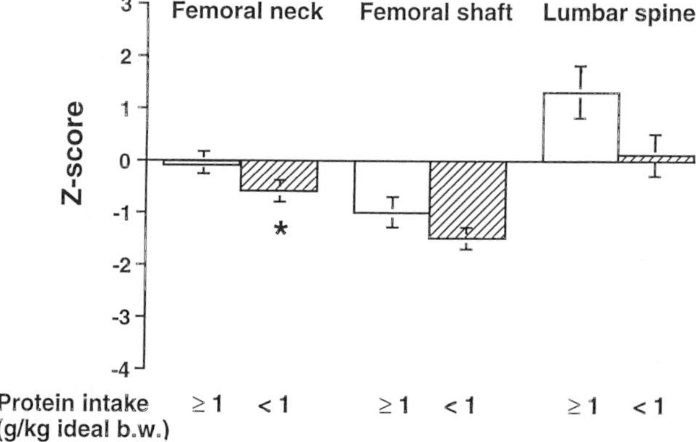

FIGURE 1 Bone mineral density in the elderly with a spontaneous daily protein intake lower or higher than 1 g per kg body weight (*$p < 0.05$). Results are adapted from Geinoz *et al.* [36], with permission.

biceps and quadriceps muscle strength and performance, as indicated by increased capacity to walk and climb stairs, after 4 weeks of hospitalization [36]. Because the mean body weight was not significantly different in this cohort, the lower energy intake may represent a lower degree of energy expenditure, assuming similar metabolic rates. Thus, the difference may also be the reflection of various levels of physical activity, with a possible positive influence of exercising on both bone mass and muscle strength.

Undernutrition could also accelerate age-dependent bone loss [29–31,37,38]. This observation is in keeping with several studies in which a state of undernutrition was documented in elderly patients with hip fracture [6,7,10,11,39]. A low plasma albumin level has been found repeatedly in patients with hip fracture as compared to age-matched healthy subjects or patients with osteoarthritis [7,10,12,40]. In hip fracture patients in whom a lower femoral neck BMD at the level of the proximal femur has been demonstrated [41], a dietary survey based on 50 daily precise measurements of food intake confirmed that nutritional requirements were not met while the patients were in hospital, although adequate quantities of food were offered [12]. The voluntary oral intake energy was about 1100 kcal (RDA: 1800 kcal), protein was 34 g (RDA: 60–70 g), and calcium was 400 mg (RDA: 1000–1500 mg).

Thus, it appears that the integrity of the skeleton in the elderly could be affected, not only by an inadequate supply of bone mineral elements and vitamin D [14–16], but also by an inappropriately low protein intake. Whereas a gradual decline in caloric intake with age can be considered an adequate adjustment to the progressive reduction in energy expenditure, the parallel reduction in protein intake may be detrimental for maintaining the integrity and function of muscle and bone [42–44]. In association with the progressive age-dependent decrease in both protein intakes and bone mass, several reports have documented a decrement in insulin-like growth factor (IGF)-I plasma levels [45,46].

Various studies have found a relationship between the level of protein intake and calcium–phosphate or bone metabolism [18,19,47,48] and reached the conclusion that either a deficient or an excessive protein supply could negatively affect the balance of calcium. The issue of a relationship between fracture incidence and protein intake has been addressed in several epidemiological studies. Hip fracture appeared to be more frequent in countries with a high protein intake of animal origin [49], but, as expected, countries with the highest incidence are those with the longest life expectancy. In contrast, a trend for hip fracture incidence inversely related to protein intake has been reported [50]. Similarly, hip fracture was higher with low energy intake, low serum albumin levels, and low muscle strength in the NHANES I study [51]. In a prospective study carried out on more than 40,000 women in Iowa, a higher protein intake was associated with a reduced risk of hip fracture [52]. Similarly, a reduced relative risk of hip fracture was found with a higher intake of milk [53]. In another survey, although no association between hip fracture and nondairy animal protein intake could be detected, fracture risk was increased when a high protein diet was accompanied by a low calcium intake [54]. There was a negative correlation between bone mass and spontaneous protein intake in premenopausal women [48]. Bone mineral mass was directly proportional to serum albumin in hip fracture patients [55]. In a longitudinal follow-up of the Framingham study, the rate of bone mineral loss was correlated inversely to dietary protein intake [56]. In contrast, in a cross-sectional study, a protein intake close to 2 g/kg body weight was associated with reduced bone mineral density but only at one of two forearm sites in young college women [47]. Despite these uncertainties, most studies strongly suggest that low protein intake per se could be particularly detrimental for both the acquisition of bone mass and the conservation of bone integrity with aging both in experimental animals and in human subjects.

In the elderly, underweight due to inappropriate nutrition is more common as a risk factor for death than overweight resulting from excessive food intake with respect to energy expenditure [43,44]. Low serum albumin, taken as a reflection of nutritional state, is a determinant of hospital length of stay, of mortality, and of rate of readmission [57].

NUTRITIONAL CONTROL OF INSULIN-LIKE GROWTH FACTOR-I AND BONE HOMEOSTASIS

Experimental and clinical studies suggest that dietary proteins could control bone anabolism by influencing both the production and the action of growth factors, particularly the growth hormone (GH) insulin-like growth factor system [58–60]. The hepatic production and plasma level of IGF-I is under the influence of dietary proteins [61,62]. Protein restriction has been shown to reduce IGF-I plasma levels by inducing a resistance to the hepatic actions of GH [63,64] and by an increase of the IGF-I metabolic clearance rate [65]. Resistance to GH depends on a reduction in GH hepatic-binding sites and on postreceptor defects [66,67]. Indeed, liver IGF-I mRNA is reduced by protein restriction through a transcriptional alteration [68] and, in addition, the hepatic IGF-I translational process could also be affected by protein deprivation [66]. The effects of protein restriction could also be mediated by a reduction in the hepatic supply of essential amino acids. Indeed, culture medium deprived in tryptophan or lysine is associated with a selective reduction of the production of IGF-I by cultured rat hepatocytes without affecting cell viability [69]. Decreased levels of IGF-I have been found in states of undernutrition such as marasmus, anorexia nervosa, celiac disease, or HIV-infected patients [63,70–73]. Refeeding these patients led to an increase of IGF-I [70,74]. Furthermore, an elevated protein intake is able to prevent the decrease in IGF-I usually observed in hypocaloric states [61,75].

In addition, protein restriction could render target systems less sensitive to IGF-I. When IGF-I was given to rats maintained on a low protein diet at amounts leading to normal plasma levels, skeletal longitudinal growth was not improved [76]. It has also been shown that IGF-I receptors in bone cells could be increased by treatment with calcitriol [77]. The production of IGF-binding proteins (IGFBP) is also influenced by protein-calorie restriction. IGFBP-1, IGFBP-2, and IGFBP-4, which are possible inhibitors of the action of IGF-I, were increased by protein restriction and in patients with recent hip fracture [68,78,79], whereas IGFBP-3 levels were lowered [80,81].

IGF-I is an essential factor for longitudinal bone growth [82], as it stimulates proliferation and differentiation of chondrocytes in epiphyseal plate [60,83]. IGF-I also plays a role in trabecular and cortical bone formation. This factor can stimulate both proliferation and differentiation of osteoblasts; it increases type I collagen synthesis, alkaline phosphatase activity, and osteocalcin production [83]. IGF-I has also been shown to inhibit the degradation of collagen produced by osteoblastic cells [60,83]. Furthermore, by its renal action on the tubular reabsorption of phosphate and on the synthesis of calcitriol through a direct action on renal cells [84–87], IGF-I can be considered an important controller of the intestinal absorption and of the extracellular concentration of both calcium and phosphate, the main elements of bone mineral. IGF-I can selectively stimulate the transport of inorganic phosphate across the plasma membrane in some osteoblastic cell lines [88]. This effect could be important in the process of bone formation, as phosphate is an essential element for cell growth.

Before puberty, a deficiency in IGF-I or a resistance to its action results in a diminution in skeletal longitudinal growth [89,90] and of the level of peak bone mass [91,92]. Long-term repletion with GH during adolescence can restore peak bone mass to a normal level [92] or increase bone mineral mass in the elderly [93,94]. Finally, similar to peak bone mass values [95], a study in twins has shown that plasma levels of IGF-I are also determined genetically [96]. In adult animals, administration of IGF-I can also affect bone mass positively. Thus, the influence of IGF-I on BMD delivered by subcutaneous osmotic minipumps in adult rats made osteoporotic by ovariectomy was investigated (Fig. 2). BMD was measured by dual-energy X-ray absorptiometry at the lumbar spine and proximal and total tibia. A 6-week infusion of IGF-I induced a dose-dependent increment of BMD at the three skeletal sites [97]. In this animal model, the increase in BMD induced by IGF-I was not due merely to an increase in bone growth. It was associated with an increase in the resistance to mechanical strain and in bone shaft outer dimensions [97–99] (Fig. 2).

Osteogenic cells are equipped with specific IGF-I receptors, and also IGF-I-producing machinery. Several factors, including GH, estradiol, parathyroid hormone, calcitriol, glucocorticoids, and triiodothyronine, have the capacity to modulate *in vitro* the expression of IGF-I mRNA and the accumulation of immunoreactive IGF-I in bone culture systems [60,83]. It has been demonstrated that, following local administration of GH, epiphyseal cartilage can produce IGF-I [100]. This observation suggests the possibility of an autocrine or a paracrine mechanism operating in the epiphyseal chondrocytes [82]. The biological importance of these effects in terms of bone formation needs to take into account possible simultaneous variations in the production of IGF-binding proteins [83,101,102] and in the number or affinity of membrane-associated IGF-I receptors in osteogenic cells. Regarding a possible influence of the local environment in proteins or amino acids

Experimental conditions

	OVX (vehicle)	OVX + Pamidronate	OVX + IGF-I	OVX + Pamidronate +IGF-I
Experimental data				
Ext. Diam.	2.81 ± 0.04	2.82 ± 0.05	2.91 ± 0.03	2.98 ± 0.06 *
Cort. Thick.	0.63 ± 0.01	0.68 ± 0.02 *	0.64 ± 0.02	0.71 ± 0.01 *
Bone Surf.	4.51 ± 0.12	4.55 ± 0.16	4.61 ± 0.11	5.10 ± 0.13 *

Conceptual view

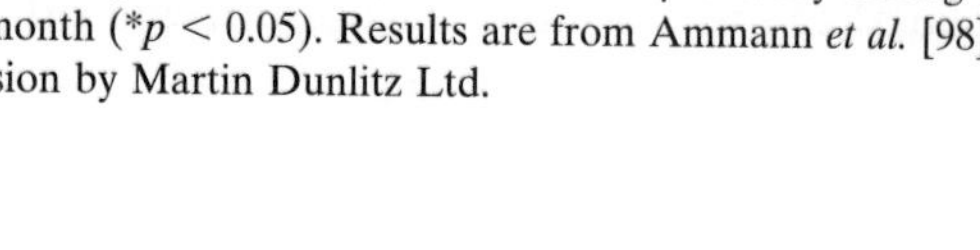

FIGURE 2 Effects of IGF-I and/or of the bisphosphonate pamidronate in aged rats made osteopenic by ovariectomy (OVX). Bone were collected 8 weeks after the beginning of IGF-I treatment delivered by intraperitoneal osmotic minipump at a dose of 2 mg/kg BW · day for 6 weeks or of pamidronate at a dose of 1.6 μmol/day during 5 days every month (*$p < 0.05$). Results are from Ammann *et al.* [98], with permission by Martin Dunlitz Ltd.

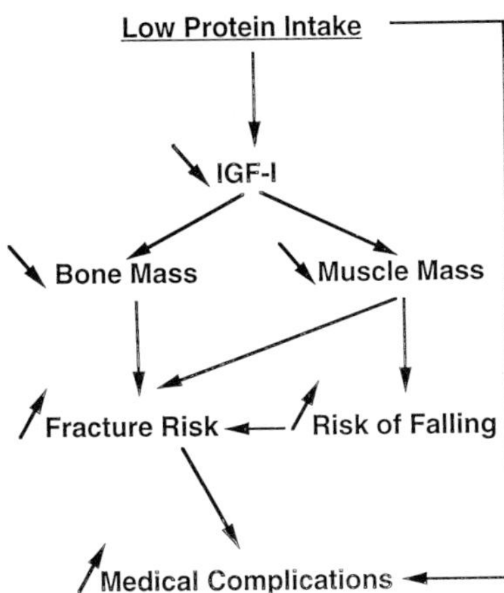

Figure 3 Possible role of IGF-I in the pathogenesis of osteoporotic hip fracture and postfracture medical complications in the elderly.

on IGF-I production by bone cells, it has been found that the amino acids arginine or lysine increased IGF-I production and collagen synthesis by a mouse osteoblastic cell line in a time- and concentration-dependent manner [103]. These results highlight the potential role of locally produced IGF-I and the influence of extracellular amino acid concentration in the regulation of osteoblast function.

Thus, IGF-I can exert anabolic effects on bone mass not only during growth, but also during adulthood. Taking into account the described experimental and clinical observations, the conclusion arises that the axis "protein intake → IGF system → bone mass" plays a significant role in the pathophysiology and prevention of osteoporosis (Fig. 3). Furthermore, restoration of this altered system in the elderly by protein replenishment is likely to favorably influence not only bone mineral density, but also muscle mass and strength [104,105]. Whether the progressive age-dependent decrease in plasma level of IGF-I [45,46] and bone mineral mass, which is thus associated with a decrement in protein intake, could be prevented by maintaining an absolute intake of proteins, remains to be documented.

OUTCOME OF FRACTURE OF THE PROXIMAL FEMUR

In accordance with several studies in which a state of undernutrition has been documented in elderly patients with hip fracture [6,7,9,11,39], low protein intake was associated with reduced femoral neck areal BMD and poor physical performance [36]. Several studies support the notion that a state of malnutrition on admission followed by an inadequate food intake during hospital stay can adversely influence the clinical outcome of elderly patients with hip fracture [11,12,40]. The first evidence was obtained by intervention studies using supplementary feeding by a nasogastric tube or parenteral nutrition [106]. The clinical course of these patients could also be improved by providing a simple oral dietary preparation, as this way of correcting the deficient food intake has obvious practical and psychological advantages over nasogastric tube feeding or parenteral nutrition [12]. In these patients, who displayed very low femoral neck BMD [41] and had a self-selected intake of protein and energy insufficient during their hospitalization [12], the clinical outcome after hip fracture was improved significantly by a daily oral nutritional supplement that normalized protein intake.

This dietary supplementation increased the mean intake of energy by about 25%, protein by 60%, and calcium by 130%. It should be emphasized that a 20-g protein supplement brought the intake from low to a level still below RDA, thus avoiding the risk of an excess of dietary protein. The supplement was given at a time of the day so that it did not interfere with scheduled meals and thus did not probably reduce voluntary oral intakes. Ingestion of the supplement was associated with biochemical evidence of nutritional improvement as assessed by an increase in the plasma albumin level. The clinical outcome was significantly better in supplemented groups compared to controls. Follow-up showed a significant difference in the clinical course, with supplemented patients doing better. Overall, 56% of individuals in the supplemented group had a favorable course as compared to 13% in the controls. Although the mean duration of dietary supplementation did not exceed 30 days, the significantly lower rate of complications (bedsore, severe anemia, intercurrent lung or renal infections, 44% vs 87%) and deaths was still observed at 6 months (40% vs 74%) [12]. The duration of hospital stay of elderly patients with hip fracture is determined not only by the actual medical condition, but also by domestic and social factors [5,11,107]. Nevertheless, in this study, the total length of stay in the orthopedic ward and convalescent hospital was significantly shorter in supplemented patients than in controls (median: 24 days vs 40 days). Differences in the biochemical and clinical course between the two groups suggested that the nutritional status was improved rapidly by oral supplementation, whereas the clinical benefit of supplementation was apparent only after the acute phase (fracture, operation, and early postoperative days).

In a subsequent study, it was shown that the normalization of protein intake, independent of energy, calcium, and vitamin D, was in fact responsible for this more favorable outcome [108]. Indeed, in addition to protein, various minerals and vitamins were also present in the supplement, as in previous reports using parenteral or nasogastric infusion [106]. The question as to whether protein represented the key nutrient responsible for the beneficial effect was addressed by comparing the clinical outcome of elderly patients with hip fracture (mean age 82 years) receiving two different dietary supplements that differed only by their protein contents [108]. The clinical course was significantly better in the group receiving protein, with 79% having a favorable course as compared to 36% in the control group during the stay in the recovery hospital (Fig. 4). The rate of complications and deaths was also significantly lower in the protein-supplemented vs the control group (52% vs 80%) 7 months after hip fracture. The median hospital stay was significantly lower in the protein-supplemented group (69 days vs 102 days). Thus, results of this trial indicated that protein appeared to be the critical nutrient responsible for the clinical benefits. That a better clinical course in the protein-supplemented patients was apparent in the recovery hospital and at 7 months, although the dietary treatment had been discontinued on average after 36 days, could be explained by an increase in the voluntary food intake that would have been initiated by the protein supplement taken during the preceding weeks. Such a process would tend to break the vicious circle mentioned earlier with protein malnutrition increasing the propensity to develop infectious diseases or other clinical complications, which in turn further worsen the state of protein malnutrition. It should be stressed that the oral supplement increased the overall protein intake from a low to a normal level. Although still a matter of controversy, it is possible that a supplementation that would increase the protein intake above RDA should be avoided, as it might lead to a negative calcium balance [30,31].

In the undernourished elderly with a recent hip fracture, an increase in protein intake from low to normal can also be beneficial for bone integrity [81]. Indeed, in a double-blind, placebo-controlled study, the effects of protein repletion were investigated in patients with a recent hip fracture. Within 1 week after an osteoporotic hip fracture, 82 patients (80.7 ± 1.2 years) were randomly allocated to a daily 20-g protein supplement, which nearly corrected protein deficiency, or to an isocaloric placebo for 6 months. All were given 200,000 IU vitamin D once at baseline and 550 mg/day of calcium. BMD, bone remodeling, calciotropic hormones, biochemical nutritional or immunological status, and muscle strength were assessed at 6 and 12 months. As compared with healthy controls, patients with hip fractured had lower proximal femur BMD, lower serum levels of albumin, prealbumin, IGF-I, IGF-binding protein 3, or calcidiol and higher parathyroid hormone, IGF-binding protein 2, and lower upper extremity muscle strength at baseline [72]. In agreement with previous results [12,108], protein repletion after hip fracture was associated with a more favorable outcome, including a shorter rehabilitation hospital stay. In a multiple regression analysis, baseline IGF-I concentrations and biceps muscle strength, together with the presence of protein supplements, accounted for more than 30% of the variance of the length of stay in rehabilitation hopitals ($r^2 = 0.312$, $p < 0.001$). As compared to the placebo group, the protein-supplemented patients had significantly greater gains in serum prealbumin, in IGF-I (Fig. 5), and in IgM (Table I). In protein-supplemented patients, the proximal femur BMD decrease observed at 1 year in the placebo group was attenuated by approximately 50% (Fig. 6). These results are in agreement with the hypothesis that the beneficial effects of protein repletion after hip fracture, with respect to a more favorable outcome and a shorter stay in rehabilitation hospitals, could be associated with a stimulation of the IGF-I system.

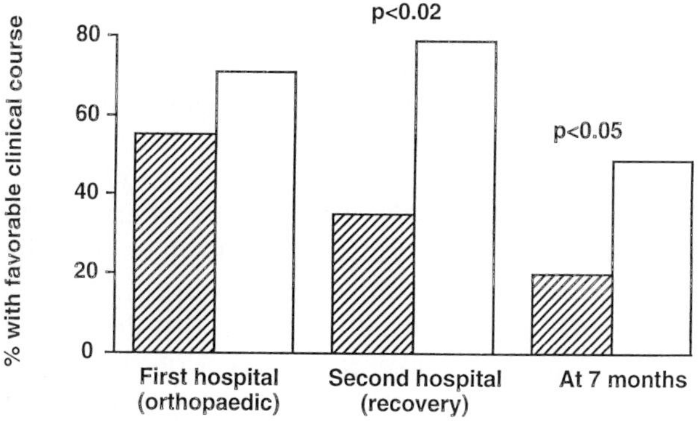

FIGURE 4 Effects on the medical complication rate of a milk protein daily supplement of 20 g in the elderly with a recent hip fracture. Hashed bars, controls; dashed bars, protein-supplemented patients. Results are from Tkatch *et al.* [108], with permission.

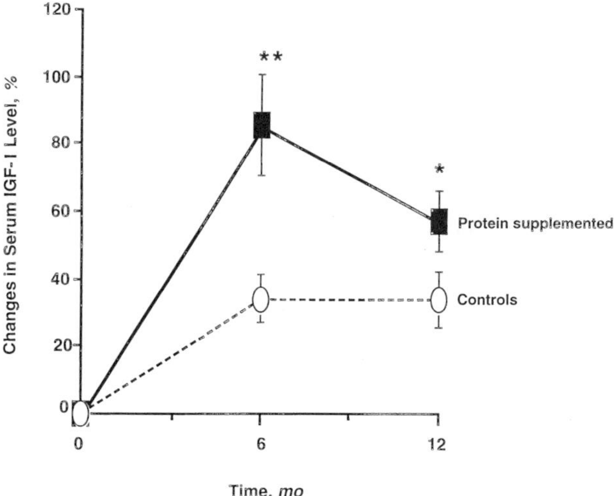

FIGURE 5 Effects on serum IGF-I levels of a milk protein supplement of 20 g in the elderly with a recent hip fracture (*$p < 0.06$; **$p < 0.005$). Results are from Schürch *et al.* [81], with permission.

TABLE I Effects of Protein Supplements in the Elderly with a Recent Fracture of the Proximal Femur[a,b]

Changes from baseline (%)	Placebo	Protein supplemented	p value
Prealbumin[c] (%)	56.1 ± 8.8	86.1 ± 13.9	0.075
IGF-I[c] (%)	34.1 ± 7.2	85.6 ± 14.8	0.003
IgM[c] (%)	40.2 ± 5.8	65.8 ± 8.8	0.016
Femoral neck BMD[d] (%)	−4.7 ± 0.9	−2.0 ± 1.2	0.079
Trochanter BMD[d] (%)	−4.8 ± 0.8	−2.8 ± 0.5	0.048
Proximal femur BMD[d] (%)	−4.7 ± 0.8	−2.3 ± 0.7	0.029
Length of stay in rehabilitation hospital (days)	53.0 ± 4.6 (median: 54)	42.2 ± 6.6 (median: 33)	0.018

[a] Results are adapted from Schürch *et al.* [81], with permission.
[b] Results are mean ± SEM. Biochemical and BMD values are expressed as percentage of baseline.
[c] At 6 months.
[d] At 1 year.

The lower incidence of medical complications observed after such a supplement [12,108] is also compatible with the hypothesis of IGF-I improving the immune status, as this growth factor can stimulate the proliferation of immunocompetent cells and modulate immunoglobulin secretion [109]. These results raise the question whether the protein repletion of frail elderly could prevent the age-dependent decrease in IGF-I levels, thereby helping to prevent falls and to increase bone mass [110,111]. However, the effects of protein repletion in frail elderly at risk of osteoporotic fracture remain to be tested.

SUMMARY

Undernutrition, particularly protein undernutrition, contributes to the occurrence of osteoporotic fracture by lowering bone mass and altering muscle strength. Furthermore, the rate of medical complications after fracture can also be increased by nutritional deficiency. The IGF-I system appears to be involved directly in the pathogenetic mechanisms leading to osteoporotic hip fracture in the elderly and to its complications. In the presence of adequate calcium and vitamin D supplies, protein supplements that increase intakes from low to normal, increase IGF-I levels, improve, the clinical outcome after hip fracture, and attenuate the decrease in proximal femur bone mineral density in the year following the fracture. This nutritional approach was associated with a significant reduction of the stay in a rehabilitation hospital. This underscores the importance of nutritional support to prevent and to heal osteoporotic fractures.

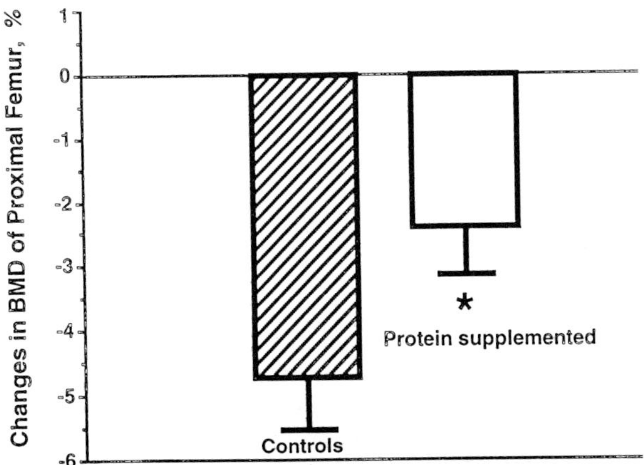

FIGURE 6 Effects on proximal femur bone mineral density of a daily milk protein supplement in the elderly with a recent hip fracture (*$p < 0.05$). Results are adapted from Schürch *et al.* [81], with permission.

Acknowledgments

We thank Mrs. M. Perez for her secretarial assistance. The studies from our group were supported by the Swiss National Research Foundation (Grant No. 32-32415.91 and 32-49957.96).

References

1. Cummings, S. R., Kelsey, J. L., Nevitt, M. C., and O'Dowd, K. J. Epidemiology of osteoporosis and osteoporotic fractures. *Epidemiol. Rev.* **7,** 178–199 (1985).
2. Nydegger, V., Rizzoli, R., Rapin, C. H., Vasey, H., and Bonjour, J. P. Epidemiology of fractures of the proximal femur in Geneva: Incidence, clinical and social aspects. *Osteopor. Int.* **2,** 42–47 (1991).
3. Cooper, C., and Melton, J., III. Epidemiology of osteoporosis. *Trends Endocrinol. Metab.* **3,** 224–229 (1992).
4. Sernbo, I., and Johnell, O. Consequences of a hip fracture: a prospective study over 1 year. *Osteopor. Int.* **3,** 148–153 (1993).
5. Schürch, M. A., Rizzoli, R., Mermillod, B., Vasey, H., Michel, J. P., and Bonjour J. P. A prospective study on socioeconomic

aspects of fracture of the proximal femur. *Bone Miner. Res.* **11,** 1935–1942 (1996).

6. Young, G. A., Chem, C., and Hill, G. L. Assessment of protein-caloric malnutrition in surgical patients from plasma proteins and anthropometric measurements. *Am. J. Clin. Nutr.* **31,** 429–435 (1978).
7. Wootton, R., Brereton, P. J., Clark, M. B., Hesp, R., Hodkinson, H. M., Klenerman, L., Reeve, J., Slavin, G., and Tellez-Yudilevich, M. Fractured neck of the femur in the elderly: an attempt to identify patients at risk. *Clin. Sci.* **57,** 93–101 (1979).
8. Older, M. W. J., Edwards, D., and Dickerson, J. W. T. A nutrient survey in elderly women with femoral neck fractures. *Br. J. Surg.* **67,** 884–886 (1980).
9. Jensen, J. E., Jensen, T. G., Smith, T. K., Johnston, D. A., and Dudrick, S. J. Nutrition in orthopaedic surgery. *J. Bone Joint Surg.* **64,** 1263–1272 (1982).
10. Rapin, C. H., Lagier, R., Boivin, G., Jung, A., and MacGee, W. Biochemical findings in blood of aged patients with femoral neck fractures: a contribution to the detection of occult osteomalacia. *Calcif. Tissue Int.* **34,** 465–469 (1982).
11. Bastow, M. D., Rawlings, J., and Allison, S. P. Undernutrition, hypothermia, and injury in elderly women with fractured femur: an injury response to altered metabolism? *Lancet* **i,** 143–146 (1983).
12. Delmi, M., Rapin, C. H., Bengoa, J. M., Delmas, P. D., Vasey, H., and Bonjour, J. P. Dietary supplementation in elderly patients with fractured neck of the femur. *Lancet* **i,** 1013–1016 (1990).
13. Fiatarone, M. A., O'Neill, E. F., Ryan, N. D., Clements, K. M., Solares, G. R., Nelson, M. E., Roberts, S. B., Kehayias, J. J., Lipsitz, L. A., and Evans, W. J. Exercise training and nutritional supplementation for physical frailty in very elderly people. *N. Engl. J. Med.* **330,** 1769–1775 (1994).
14. Chapuy, M. C., Arlot, M. E., Duboeuf, F., Brun, J., Crouzet, B., Arnaud, S., Delmas, P. D., and Meunier, P. J. Vitamin D3 and calcium to prevent hip fractures in elderly women. *N. Engl. J. Med.* **327,** 1637–1642 (1992).
15. Chevalley, T., Rizzoli, R., Nydegger, V., Slosman, D., Rapin, C. H., Michel, J. P., Vasey, H., and Bonjour, J. P. Effects of calcium supplements on femoral bone mineral density and vertebral fracture rate in vitamin D-replete elderly patients. *Osteopor. Int.* **4,** 245–252 (1994).
16. Dawson-Hughes, B. Calcium supplementation and bone loss: a review of controlled clinical trials. *Am. J. Clin. Nutr.* **54,** 274S–280S (1991).
17. Dawson-Hughes, B., Harris, S. S., Krall, E. A., and Dallal, G. E. Effect of calcium and vitamin D supplementation on bone density in men and women 65 years of age or older. *N. Engl. J. Med.* **337,** 670–676 (1997).
18. Orwoll, E. S. The effects of dietary protein insufficiency and excess on skeletal health. *Bone* **13,** 343–350 (1992).
19. Bonjour, J. P., Schürch, M. A., and Rizzoli, R. Nutritional aspects of hip fractures. *Bone* **18**(Suppl. 3), S139–S144 (1996).
20. Recommended Daily Allowances, "National Research Council (U.S.)," 10th ed. National Academy Press, Washington, 1989.
21. Bonjour, J. P., Theintz, G., Law, F., Slosman, D., and Rizzoli, R. Peak bone mass. *Osteopor. Int.* **4**(Suppl. 1), 7–14 (1994).
22. Pellett, P. L. Food energy requirements in humans. *Am. J. Clin. Nutr.* **51,** 711–722 (1990).
23. Ferretti, J. L., Tessaro, R. D., Delgado, C. J., Bozzini, C. E., Alippi, R. M., and Barcelo, A. C. Biochemical performance of diaphyseal shafts and bone tissue of femur from protein-restricted rats. *Bone Min.* **4,** 329–339 (1988).
24. Clavien, H. H., Theintz, G., Rizzoli, R., and Bonjour, J. P. Does puberty alter dietary habits in adolescents living in a Western society? *J. Adolesc. Health* **19,** 68–75 (1996).
25. Bonjour, J. P., Theintz, G., Buchs, B., Slosman, D., and Rizzoli, R. Critical years and stages of puberty for spinal and femoral bone mass accumulation during adolescence. *J. Clin. Endocrinol. Metab.* **73,** 555–563 (1991).
26. Theintz, G., Buchs, B., Rizzoli, R., Slosman, D., Clavien, H., Sizonenko, P. C., and Bonjour, J. P. Longitudinal monitoring of bone mass accumulation in healthy adolescents: evidence for a marked reduction after 16 years of age at the levels of lumbar spine and femoral neck in female subjects. *J. Clin. Endocrinol. Metab.* **75,** 1060–1065 (1992).
27. Roberts, T. J., Azain, M. J., Douglas White, B., and Martin, R. J. Rats treated with somatotropin select diets higher in protein. *J. Nutr.* **125,** 2669–2678 (1995).
28. WHO Technical Report Series, "Assessment of Fracture Risk and Its Application to Screening for Postmenopausal Osteoporosis." Report of a WHO Study Group, 843, World Health Organization, Geneva, 1994.
29. Seeman, E., and Riggs, B. L. Dietary prevention of bone loss in the elderly. *Geriatrics* **36,** 71–79 (1981).
30. Parfitt, A. M. Dietary risk factors for age-related bone loss and fractures. *Lancet* **ii,** 1181–1184 (1983).
31. Schaafsma, G., Van Beresteyn, E. C. H., Raymakers, J. A., and Duursma, S. A. Nutritional aspects of osteoporosis. *World Rev. Nutr. Diet.* **49,** 121–159 (1987).
32. Grisso, J. A., Kelsey, J. L., Strom, B. L., Chiu, G. Y., Maislin, G., O'Brien, L. A., Hoffman, S., Kaplan, F., and the Northeast Hip Fracture Study Group. Risk factors for falls as a cause of hip fracture in women. *N. Engl. J. Med.* **324,** 1326–1331 (1991).
33. Vellas, B. J., Albarede, J. L., and Garry, P. J. Diseases and aging: patterns of morbidity with age: relationship between aging and age-associated diseases. *Am. J. Clin. Nutr.* **55**(Suppl. 6) 1225S–1230S (1992).
34. Vellas, B., Baumgartner, R. N., Wayne, S. J., Conceicao, J., Lafont, C., Albarede, J. L., and Garry, P. J. Relationship between malnutrition and falls in the elderly. *Nutrition* **8,** 105–108 (1992).
35. Dargent-Molina, P., Favier, F., Grandjean, H., Baudoin, C., Schott, A. M., Hausherr, E., Meunier, P. J., and Breart, G. Fall-related factors and risk of hip fracture: the EPIDOS prospective study. *Lancet* **348,** 145–149 (1996).
36. Geinoz, G., Rapin, C. H., Rizzoli, R., Kraemer, R., Buchs, B., Slosman, D., Michel, J. P., and Bonjour, J. P. Relationship between bone mineral density and dietary intakes in the elderly. *Osteopor. Int.* **3,** 242–248 (1993).
37. Garn, S. M., and Kanzas, J. Protein intake, bone mass, and bone loss. *In* "Osteoporosis: Recent Advances in Pathogenesis and Treatment" (H. F. De Luca, H. Frost, W. Jee, C. Johnston, A. M. Parfitt, eds), pp. 257–263. University Park Press, Baltimore, 1981.
38. Garn, S. M., Guzman, M. A., and Wagner, B. Subperiostal gain and endosteal loss in protein-calorie malnutrition. *Am. J. Phys. Anthropol.* **30,** 153–155 (1969).
39. Tinetti, M. E., Speechley, M., and Ginter, S. F. Risks factors for falls among elderly persons living in the community. *N. Engl. J. Med.* **319,** 1701–1707 (1988).
40. Patterson, B. M., Cornell, C. N., Carbone, B., Levine, B., and Chapman, D. Protein depletion and metabolic stress in elderly patients who have a fracture of the hip. *J. Bone Joint Surg.* **74A,** 251–260 (1992).
41. Chevalley, T., Rizzoli, R., Nydegger, V., Slosman, D., Tkatch, L., Rapin C. H., Vasey, H., and Bonjour, J. P. Preferential low

bone mineral density of the femoral neck in patients with a recent fracture of the proximal femur. *Osteopor. Int.* **1,** 147–154 (1991).
42. Chandra, R. K. Nutritional regulation of immunity and risk of infection in old age. *Immunology* **67,** 141–147 (1989).
43. Morley, J. E., and Miller, D. K. Malnutrition in the elderly. *Hosp. Pract.* **27,** 95–116 (1992).
44. Munro, H., and Schlierf, G., "Nutrition of the Elderly." Nestlé Nutrition Workshop Series, Vol. XIX. Raven Press, New York, 1992.
45. Hammerman, M. R. Insulin-like growth factors and aging. *Endocrinol. Metab. Clin. North Am.* **16,** 995–1011 (1987).
46. Quesada, J. M., Coopmans, W., Ruiz, B., Aljama, P., Jans, I., and Bouillon, R. Influence of vitamin D on parathyroid function in the elderly. *J. Clin. Endocrinol. Metab.* **75,** 494–501 (1992).
47. Anderson, J. J. B., and Metz, J. A. Adverse association of high protein intake to bone density. *Challenges Modern Med.* **7,** 407–412 (1995).
48. Cooper, C., Atkinson, E. J., Hensrud, D. D., Wahner, H. W., O'Fallon W. M., Riggs, B. L., and Melton, L. G., III. Dietary protein intake and bone mass in women. *Calcif. Tissue Int.* **58,** 320–325 (1996).
49. Abelow, B. J., Holford, T. R., and Insogna, K. L. Cross-cultural association between dietary animal protein and hip fracture: a hypothesis. *Calcif. Tissue Int.* **50,** 14–18 (1992).
50. Feskanich, D., Willett, W. C., Stampfer, M. J., and Colditz, G. A. Protein consumption and bone fractures in women. *Am. J. Epidemiol.* **143,** 472–479 (1996).
51. Huang, Z., Himes, J. H., and McGovern, P. G. Nutrition and subsequent hip fracture risk among a national cohort of white women. *Am. J. Epidemiol.* **144,** 124–134 (1996).
52. Munger, R. G., Cerhan, J., Chiu, B., Yang, S., and Allnutt, K. Protein intake and risk of hip fracture in a cohort of older IOWA women. *Am. Soc. Clin. Nutr.* (1995). [Abstract]
53. Johnell, O., Gullberg, B., Kanis, J. A., Allander, E., Elffors, L., Dequeker, J., Dilsen, G., Gennari, C., Vaz, A. L., Lyritis, G., Mazzuoli, G., Miravet, L., Passeri, M., Cano, R. P., Rapado, A., and Ribot, C. Risk factors for hip fracture in European women: the MEDOS study. *J. Bone Miner. Res.* **10,** 1802–1815 (1995).
54. Meyer, H. E., Pedersen, J. I., Løken, E. B., and Tverdal, A. Dietary factors and the incidence of hip fracture in middle-aged Norwegians. A prospective study. *Am. J. Epidemiol.* **145,** 117–123 (1997).
55. Thiébaud, D., Burckhardt, P., Costanza, M., Sloutskis, D., Gilliard, D., Quinodoz, F., Jacquet, A. F., and Burnand, B. Importance of albumin, 25(OH)-vitamin D and IGFBP-3 as risk factors in elderly women and men with hip fracture. *Osteopor. Int.* **7,** 457–462 (1997).
56. Hannan, M. T., Tucker, K., Dawson-Hughes, B., Felson, D. T., and Kiel, D. P. Effect of dietary protein on bone loss in elderly men and women: the Framingham Osteoporosis Study. *J. Bone Miner. Res.* **12**(Suppl. 1), S151 (1997).
57. Herrmann, F. R., Safran, C., Levkoff, S. E., and Minaker, K. L. Serum albumin level on admission as a predictor of death, length of stay, and readmission. *Arch. Intern. Med.* **152,** 125–130 (1992).
58. Rosen, C. Growth hormone, insulin-like growth factors, and the senescent skeleton: Ponce de Leon's fountain revisited? *J. Cell Biochem.* **56,** 348–356 (1994).
59. Rosen, C. J., and Donahue, L. R. Insulin-like growth factors: potential therapeutic options for osteoporosis. *Trends Endocrinol. Metab.* **6,** 235–241 (1995).
60. Canalis, E., McCarthy, T. L., and Centrella, M. Growth factors and cytokines in bone cell metabolism. *Annu. Rev. Med.* **42,** 17–24 (1991).
61. Isley, W. L., Underwood, L. E., and Clemmons, D. R. Dietary components that regulate serum somatomedin-C concentrations in humans. *J. Clin. Invest.* **71,** 175–182 (1983).
62. Thissen, J. P., Ketelslegers, J. M., and Underwood, L. E. Nutritional regulation of the insulin-like growth factors. *Endocr. Rev.* **15,** 80–101 (1994).
63. Thissen, J. P., Triest, S., Maes, M., Underwood, L. E., and Ketelslegers, J. M. The decreased plasma concentrations of insulin-like growth factor-I in protein-restricted rats is not due to decreased number of growth hormone receptors on isolated hepatocytes. *J. Endocrinol.* **124,** 159–165 (1990).
64. VandeHaar, M. J., Moats-Staats, B. M., Davenport, M. L., Walker, J. L., Ketelslegers, J. M., Sharma, B. K., and Underwood, L. E. Reduced serum concentrations of insulin-like growth factor-I (IGF-I) in protein-restricted growing rats are accompanied by reduced IGF-I mRNA levels in liver and skeletal muscle. *J. Endocrinol.* **130,** 305–312 (1991).
65. Thissen, J. P., Davenport, M. L., Pucilowska, J., Miles, M. V., and Underwood, L. E. Increased serum clearance and degradation of (125I)-labeled IGF-I in protein-restricted rats. *Am. J. Physiol.* **262,** E406–E411 (1992).
66. Thissen, J. P., Triest, S., Moats-Statts, B. M., Underwood, L. E., Mauerhoff, T., Maiter, D., and Ketelslegers, J. M. Evidence that pretranslational and translational defects decrease serum IGF-I concentrations during dietary protein restriction. *Endocrinology* **129,** 429–435 (1991).
67. Maiter, D., Fliesen, T., Underwood, L. E., Maes, M., Gerard, G., Davenport, M. L., and Ketelslegers, J. M. Dietary protein restriction decreases insulin-like growth factor I independent of insulin and liver growth hormone binding. *Endocrinology* **124,** 2604–2611 (1989).
68. Straus, D. S., and Takemoto, C. D. Effect of dietary protein deprivation on insulin-like growth factor (IGF)-I and (IGF)-II, IGF binding protein-2, and serum albumin gene expression in rat. *Endocrinology* **127,** 1849–1860 (1990).
69. Harp, J. B., Goldstein, S., and Phillips, L. S. Molecular regulation of IGF-I by amino acid availability in cultured hepatocytes. *Diabetes* **40,** 95–101 (1991).
70. Pucilowska, J. B., Davenport, M. L., Kabir, I., Clemmons, D. R., Thissen, J. P., Butler, T., and Underwood, L. E. The effect of dietary protein supplementation on insulin-like growth factors (IGFs) and IGF-binding proteins in children with shigellosis. *J. Clin. Endocrinol. Metab.* **77,** 1516–1521 (1993).
71. Hill, K. K., Hill, D. B., McClain, M. P., Humphries, L. L., and McClain, C. J. Serum insulin-like growth factor-I concentrations in the recovery of patients with anorexia nervosa. *J. Am. Coll. Nutr.* **4,** 475–478 (1993).
72. Sullivan, D. H., and Carter, W. J. Insulin-like growth factor I as an indicator of protein-energy undernutrition among metabolically stable hospitalized elderly. *J. Am. Coll. Nutr.* **13,** 184–191 (1994).
73. Ketelslegers, J. M., Maiter, D., Maes, M., Underwood, L. D., and Thissen, J. P. Nutritional regulation of insulin-like growth factor-I. *Metabolism* **44,** 50–57 (1995).
74. Clemmons, D. R., Underwood, L. E., Dickerson, R. N., Brown, R. O., Hak, L. J., MacPhee, R. D., and Heizer, W. D. Use of plasma somatomedin-C/insulin-like growth factor-I measurements to monitor the response to nutritional repletion in malnourished patients. *Am. J. Clin. Nutr.* **41,** 191–198 (1985).
75. Musey, V. C., Goldstein, S., Farmer, P. K., Moore, P. B., and Phillips, L. S. Differential regulation of IGF-I and IGF-binding protein-I by dietary composition in humans. *Am. J. Med. Sci.* **305,** 131–138 (1993).

76. Thissen, J. P., Underwood, L. E., Maiter, D., Maes, M., Clemmons, D. R., and Ketelslegers, J. M. Failure of insulin-like growth factor-I (IGF-I) infusion to promote growth in protein-restricted rats despite normalization of serum IGF-I concentrations. *Endocrinology* **128,** 885–890 (1991).
77. Kurose, H., Yamaoka, K., Okada, S., Nakajima, S., and Seino, Y. 1,25-dihydroxyvitamin-D3 [1,25-(OH)2D3] increases insulin-like growth factor-I (IGF-I) receptors in clonal osteoblastic cells—study on interaction of IGF-I and 1,25-(OH)2D3. *Endocrinology* **126,** 2088–2094 (1990).
78. Rosen, C., Donahue, L. R., Hunter, S., Holick, M., Kavookjian, H., Kirschenbaum, A., Mohan, S., and Baylink, D. J. The 24/25-kDa serum insulin-like growth factor-binding protein is increased in elderly women with hip and spine fractures. *J. Clin. Endocrinol. Metab.* **74,** 24–27 (1992).
79. Straus, D. S., Burke, E. J., and Marten, N. W. Induction of insulin-like growth factor binding protein-1 gene expression in liver of protein-restricted rats and in rat hepatoma cells limited for a single amino acid. *Endocrinology* **132,** 1090–1100 (1993).
80. Smith, W. J., Underwood, L. E., and Clemmons, D. R. Effects of caloric or protein restriction on insulin-like growth factor-I (IGF-I) and IGF-binding proteins in children and adults. *J. Clin. Endocrinol. Metab.* **80,** 443–449 (1995).
81. Schürch, M. A., Rizzoli, R., Slosman, D., Vadas, L., Vergnaud, P., and Bonjour, J. P. Protein supplements increase serum insulin-like growth factor-I levels and attenuate proximal femur bone loss in patients with recent hip fracture. A randomized, double-blind, placebo-controlled trial. *Ann. Intern. Med.* **128,** 801–809 (1998).
82. Froesch, E. R., Schmid, C., Schwander, J., and Zapf, J. Actions of insulin-like growth factors. *Annu. Rev. Physiol.* **47,** 443–467 (1985).
83. Schmid, C., and Ernst, M. Insulin-like growth factors. *In* "Cytokines and Bone Metabolism" (M. Gowen, ed.), pp. 229–265. CRC Press, Boca Raton, FL, 1992.
84. Caverzasio, J., and Bonjour, J. P. Insulin-like growth factor I stimulates Na-dependent Pi transport in cultured kidney cells. *Am. J. Physiol.* **257,** F712–F717 (1989).
85. Menaa, C., Vrtovsnik, F., Friedlander, G., Corvol, M., and Garabedian, M. Insulin-like growth factor I, a unique calcium-dependent stimulator of 1,25-dihydroxyvitamin D-3 production. Studies in cultured mouse kidney cells. *J. Biol. Chem.* **270,** 25461–25467 (1995).
86. Caverzasio, J., Montessuit, C., and Bonjour, J. P. Stimulatory effect of insulin-like growth factor-I on renal Pi transport and plasma 1,25-dihydroxyvitamin D3. *Endocrinology* **127,** 453–459 (1990).
87. Palmer, G., Bonjour, J. P., and Caverzasio, J. Stimulation of inorganic phosphate transport by insulin-like growth factor-I and vanadate in opossum kidney cells is mediated by distinct protein tyrosine phosphorylation processes. *Endocrinology* **137,** 4699–4705 (1996).
88. Palmer, G., Bonjour, J. P., and Caverzasio, J. Expression of a newly identified phosphate transporter/retrovirus receptor in human SaOS-2 osteoblast-like cells and its regulation by insulin-like growth factor I. *Endocrinology* **138,** 5202–5209 (1997).
89. Daughaday, W. H., and Trivedi, B. Absence of serum growth hormone binding protein in patients with growth hormone receptor deficiency (Laron dwarfism). *Proc. Natl Acad. Sci. USA* **84,** 4636–4640 (1987).
90. Merimee, T. J., Zapf, J., Hewlett, B., and Cavalli-Sforza, L. L. Insulin-like growth factors in pygmies. *N. Engl. J. Med.* **316,** 906–911 (1987).
91. Hyer, S. L., Rodin, D. A., Tobias, J. H., Leiper, A., and Nussey, S. S. Growth hormone deficiency during puberty reduces adult bone mineral density. *Arch. Dis. Child* **67,** 1472–1474 (1992).
92. Saggese, G., Baroncelli, G. I., Bertelloni, S., and Barsanti, S. The effect of long-term growth hormone (GH) treatment on bone mineral density in children with GH deficiency. Role of GH in the attainment of peak bone mass. *J. Clin. Endocrinol. Metab.* **81,** 3077–3083 (1996).
93. Rudman, D., Feller, A. G., Nagraj, H. S., Gergans, G. A., Lalitha, P. Y., Goldberg, A. F., Schlenker, R. A., Cohn, L., Rudman, I. W., and Mattson, D. E. Effects of human growth hormone in men over 60 years old. *N. Engl. J. Med.* **323,** 1–6 (1990).
94. Papadakis, M. A., Grady, D., Black, D., Tierney, M. J., Gooding, G. A., Schambelan, M., and Grunfeld, C. Growth hormone replacement in healthy older men improves body composition but not functional ability. *Ann. Intern. Med.* **124,** 708–716 (1996).
95. Pocock, N. A., Eisman, J. A., Hopper, J. L., Yeates, M. G., Sambrook, P. N., and Eberl, S. Genetic determinants of bone mass in adults—a twin study. *J. Clin. Invest.* **80,** 706–710 (1987).
96. Kao, P. C., Matheny, A. P., Jr., and Lang, C. A. Insulin-like growth factor-I comparisons in healthy twin children. *J. Clin. Endocrinol. Metab.* **78,** 310–312 (1994).
97. Ammann, P., Rizzoli, R., Muller, K., Slosman, D., and Bonjour, J. P. IGF-I and pamidronate increase bone mineral density in ovariectomized adult rats. *Am. J. Physiol.* **265,** E770–E776 (1993).
98. Ammann, P., Rizzoli, R., Meyer, J. M., and Bonjour, J. P. Bone density and shape as determinants of bone strength in IGF-I and/or pamidronate-treated ovariectomized rats. *Osteopor. Int.* **6,** 219–227 (1996).
99. Rosen, H. N., Chen, V., Cittadini, A., Greenspan, S. L., Douglas, P. S., Moses, A. C., and Beamer, W. G. Treatment with growth hormone and IGF-I in growing rats increases bone mineral content but not bone mineral density. *J. Bone Miner. Res.* **10,** 1352–1358 (1995).
100. Underwood, L. E., D'Ercole, A. J., Clemmons, D. R., and Van Wyk, J. J. Paracrine functions of somatomedins. *Clin. Endocrinol. Metab.* **15,** 59–77 (1986).
101. Cohick, W. S., and Clemmons, D. R. The insulin-like growth factors. *Annu. Rev. Physiol.* **55,** 131–153 (1993).
102. Jones, J. I., and Clemmons, D. R. Insulin-like growth factors and their binding proteins: biological actions. *Endocr. Rev.* **16,** 3–34 (1995).
103. Chevalley, T., Rizzoli, R., Manen, D., Caverzasio, J., and Bonjour, J. P. Arginine increases insulin-like growth factor-I production and collagen synthesis in osteoblast-like cells. *Bone* **23,** 103–109 (1998).
104. Aniansson, A., Zetterberg, C., Hedberg, M., and Henriksson, K. Impaired muscle function with aging. *Clin. Orthop.* **191,** 193–201 (1984).
105. Castaneda, C., Gordon, P. L., Fielding, R. A., Evans, W. J., and Crim, M. C. Low-protein dietary intake results in reduced plasma IGF-I levels and skeletal muscle fiber atrophy in elderly women. *FASEB J.* **11,** (1997) [Abstract 1374]
106. Bastow, M. D., Rawlings, J., and Allison, S. P. Benefits of supplementary tube feeding after fractured neck of femur: a randomised controlled trial. *Br. Med. J.* **287,** 1589–1592 (1983).
107. Sullivan, D. H., Patch, G. A., Walls, R. C., and Lipschitz, D. A. Impact of nutrition status on morbidity in a select population of geriatric rehabilitation patients. *Am. J. Clin. Nutr.* **51,** 749–758 (1990).
108. Tkatch, L., Rapin, C. H., Rizzoli, R., Slosman, D., Nydegger, V., Vasey, H., and Bonjour, J. P. Benefits of oral protein supple-

ment in elderly patients with fracture of the proximal femur. *J. Am. Coll. Nutr.* **11,** 519–525 (1992).

109. Auernhammer, C. J., and Strasburger, C. J. Effects of growth hormone and insulin-like growth factor I on the immune system. *Eur. J. Endocrinol.* **133,** 635–645 (1995).

110. Uauy, R., Scrimshaw, N. S., and Young, V. R. Human protein requirements: nitrogen balance response to graded levels of egg protein in elderly men and women. *Am. J. Clin. Nutr.* **31,** 779–785 (1978).

111. Gersovitz, M., Motil, K., Munro, H. N., Scrimshaw, N. S., and Young, V. R. Human protein requirements: assessment of the adequacy of the current recommended dietary allowance for dietary protein in elderly men and women. *Am. J. Clin. Nutr.* **35,** 6–14 (1982).

CHAPTER 35

Analgesic Management

PETER LEONG AND KATHLEEN FORTI-GALLANT
Pain Program, Penobscot Pain Management, Bangor, Maine 04402

INTRODUCTION

Pain management is an integral part of the treatment of osteoporosis. People with osteoporosis may suffer with acute and chronic pain from fractures. The most common sites are the hip, spine, and wrist as pain is usually the result of the fracture, not the disease process. This chapter focuses on strategies to relieve pain, not to make the diagnosis of the osteoporotic fracture. Treatment must be individualized to meet each patient's needs with the usual goals of treatment being pain relief, increased function, quality of life, and prevention of future fractures.

FRACTURES AND PAIN ASSESSMENT

Fracture Sites

It is estimated that 25% of females over the age of 50 in the United States will have one or more vertebral fractures due to osteoporosis in their lifetime [1] and 80% of these will experience acute pain [2]. However, not all patients are symptomatic with fractures. The patient's subjective history, physical exam, and radiographs diagnose fractures. There are three types of vertebral fractures: biconcave, anterior wedge (usually T7–L2), and crush deformity (L1–L4). Anterior–posterior radiographs and symptomatology are key. A bone scan can aid in assessing fracture age. Periosteal irritation, cytokine release from bleeding, and muscle spasm can cause acute pain from a fracture.

Chronic pain arises from vertebral deformity that alters joint articulation and accelerates degenerative changes. Loss of height and change of alignment decrease abdominal and thoracic cavities, which can lead to decreased lung volume and early satiety. Spinal extensor muscles may weaken and promote kyphosis. Spinal stenosis may be a late complication characterized by buttock and lower extremity pain with walking. Ileus and urinary retention may also be present [2]. The patient may develop costo-iliac impingement syndrome from the ribs overlapping the iliac crests, which may require surgical resection if postural and more conservative approaches fail. Neurological signs such as radicular pain, paresthesias, weakness, gait disturbance, and incontinence are rare but may be signs of cord compression and warrant investigation.

Proper diagnosis of the etiology of pain dictates treatment. Therefore, it is important to review some differential diagnoses, such as neoplasm, disk herniation, osteoporosis, facet arthropathy, infection, aortic aneurysm, abdominal etiologies, osteomyelitis, and epidural abscess before starting treatment [1,3]. Insufficiency fractures are seen in patients with osteoporosis and may be overlooked in radiographs. Symptoms include low back and buttock pain without neurological deficits or instability [4]. A CT scan is useful for ruling out other etiologies, and if uncertainty about a fracture exists after radiographs, a bone scan may be helpful, as cortical bone is not well defined in MRI. [5] Hip fractures are associated with higher morbidity than the other fractures and may have referred pain patterns. Colles wrist fractures, as well as proximal humerus fractures, are other common painful sites.

Pain Assessment

Patient self-report is the primary assessment tool using a visual analog scale as shown in Fig. 1 [6]. Pain assessment should also include history; location(s); quality; duration; severity; aggravating and relieving factors; effects of pain on activity, appetite, sleep, mood, and relationships; daily functioning; coexisting symptoms; treatments previously utilized; and examination. The assessment of patient expectations, psychiatric or substance abuse history, beliefs, and barriers all are useful for furthering patient education and treatment. [6]

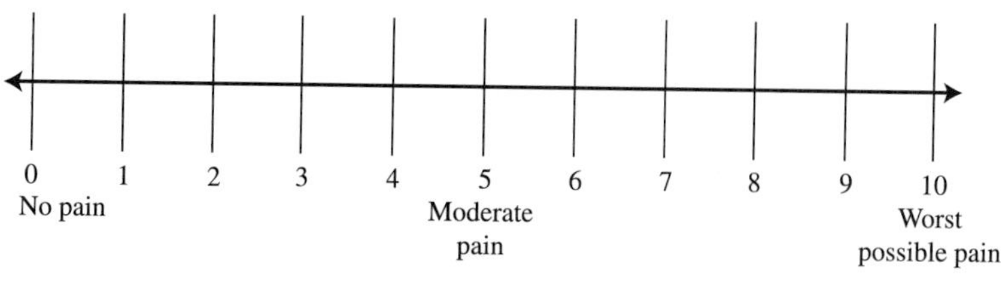

FIGURE 1

TREATMENT MODALITIES

Asymptomatic Fractures

Asymptomatic osteoporotic fractures require no analgesic treatment. The goals are to maintain bone mass, prevent new fractures, and increase function [7].

Acute Pain Management of Vertebral Compression Fractures

ACTIVITY MODIFICATION

Short-term bed rest for a few days to several weeks provides an opportunity for the pain to subside. Prolonged bedrest can cause bone loss, but significant aggravation of bone loss is not likely to occur in 2–3 weeks of bed rest. Modifications in sleeping posture can be instituted by simply placing a thin pillow under the knees to avoid undue strain on the spine. Some patients may have less pain lying on their side rather than supine or prone.

Early, slow, progressive mobilization with rest periods, decreases the hazards of mobility for these elderly patients [3,8].

REGIONAL TREATMENTS

Ice massage provides initial temporary analgesia during the acute phase of a fracture. Ice can be applied every hour if necessary and to the point of numbness and burning. This modality provides an effect similar to a temporary regional nerve block [9]. After several days, moist heat and massage may be applied, especially if significant muscle spasm is involved [1].

PHARMACOLOGIC TREATMENTS

Pharmacologic intervention should be tailored to the severity of the pain and loss in function and should be instituted in a logical and stepwise manner.

Nonsteroidal Anti-inflammatory Drugs (NSAIDs). The numerous NSAIDs available in the United States belong to several chemical classes (Table I). Prostaglandin E (PGE) inhibition accounts for much of the antiinflammatory activity of the NSAIDs [6].

With the exception of Ketorolac (Toradol), these are administered orally up to four times per day. In the elderly, however, the gastrointestinal and renal side effects and cardiovascular toxicity of the NSAIDS may limit utilization. In addition to side effects, there may be a ceiling effect with continued use. Despite the reported role of PGEs in done turnover, there is no evidence to suggest that NSAIDs preserve or enhance bone turnover.

Giving a daily maintenance dose of an NSAID can often reduce the need for additional analgesics.

Muscle Relaxants There are several muscle relaxants utilized for concomitant pain arising from myofascial etiology. In general though, the elderly do not tolerate muscle relaxants well because of their anticholinergic side effects. They may be useful as adjuvants to NSAIDs and may be instituted cautiously as a nighttime dose (Tables II and III) [1,10].

Narcotics When narcotics are used in the acute stage, careful dosing and follow-ups are required in the elderly and narcotic-naive population. These medications have significant side effects, including decreased respiratory drive, decreased bowel motility, urinary retention, nausea, vomiting, and excessive sedation.

For patients reporting a pain score of 4 to 6 on a 0 to 10 scale, a weaker schedule II narcotic medication, such as codeine, hydrocodone, or tramadol, should be added if NSAIDs are insufficient in relieving the pain.

Stronger opioids are sometimes necessary and are suggested for use when pain is reported at ≥6 on a 0 to 10 scale. Commonly used medications in the category are morphine, hydromorphine (Dilaudid), Fentanyl (Duragesic patch), and the synthetic codeine (oxycodone) (see Tables II and III) [6].

Calcitonin Calcitonin is an endogenous polypeptide hormone secreted by the parafollicular cells of the thyroid gland. Exogenously, it can be administered in subcutaneous or intranasal forms. Since the mid-late 1970s, calcitonin has been considered to have analgesic proper-

TABLE I NSAIDs and Adjuvants

General name	Brand name	Daily dose range (oral)	Half-life($t½$)
Commonly used nonsteroidal analgesics			
Asprin		1300–4000 mg	0.5–3 hr
Acetaminophen	Tylenol	Up to 4000 mg	1–3 hr
Oxaprozin	Daypro	Up to 1800 mg	42–50 hr
Ibuprofen	Motrin	Up to 3200 mg	1.8–2.5 hr
Etodolac	Lodine	800–1200 mg	7.3 hr
Naproxen	Naprosyn	500–1000 mg	12–15 hr
Nabumetone	Relafen	1000–2000 mg	22.5–30 hr
Ketoprofen	Oruvail	100–300 mg	2–4 hr
Commonly Used Muscle Relaxants			
Cyclobenzaprine	Flexeril	20–60 mg	1–3 days
Baclofen	Lioresal	15–80 mg	3.5 hr
Carisoprodol	Soma	1000–1400 mg	8 hr
Orphenadrine	Norflex	200 mg	14–16 hr
Commonly Used Anticonvulsants for Neuropathic Pain			
Carbamazepine	Tegretol	200–1200 mg	18–54 hr
Phenytoin	Dilantin	100–300 mg	Dose dependent
Gabapentin	Neurontin	300–1800 mg	5–7 hr
Clonazepam	Klonopin	1.5–20 mg	18–60 hr

ties. Pain relief from osteoporotic vertebral fractures from calcitonin might be due to decreased inflammation by the reduction of prostaglandin synthesis, changes in local nerve transmission, or increased serum levels of β-endorphins. [11,12] Salmon calcitonin is more potent and appears to provide more analgesia than synthetic

TABLE II Opioids and Adjuvants

General name	Brand name	Daily dose range (oral)	Half-life($t½$)
Commonly used opiod analgesics			
Morphine sulfate			
Controlled release	MS Contin	30–90 mg	2–4 hr
Immediate release	MSIR	60–180 mg	1.5–2 hr
Oxycodone			
Controlled release	OxyContin	20 mg	ND
Immediate release	Roxicodone	20 mg	ND
Oxycodone/acetaminophen	Percocet	Up to 4000 mg acetaminophen	ND
Hydrocodone/acetaminophen	Vicodin, Anexsia	Up to 4000 mg acetaminophen	3–8 hr
Acetaminophen/codeine	Tylenol No. 3	120–360 mg (based on codeine)	
Propoxyphene/acetaminophen	Darvocet-N 100	Up to 600 mg propoxyphene napsylate	
Propoxyphene	Darvon HCL	Up to 390 mg	6–12 hr
	Napsylate	Up to 600 mg	
Fentanyl patch	Duragesic	25–300 mcg/hr transdermal	1.5–6 hr
Hydromorphone	Dilaudid	8–24 mg	2–3 hr
Commonly used antidepressant adjuvants			
Tricyclics			
Amitriptyline	Elavil	50–100 mg	31–46 hr
Desipramine	Norpramin	25–300 mg	12–24 hr
Doxepin	Adapin	50–300 mg	8–24 hr
Trazodone	Desyrel	150–600 mg	4–9 hr
Imipramine	Tofranil	75–150 mg	11–25 hr
Antiseratonergics			
Fluoxetine	Prozac	10–40 mg	2–9 days
Sertraline	Zoloft	50–150 mg	1–4 days
Paroxetine	Paxil	20–50 mg	10–24 hr

fractures. Short term use of braces helps relieve fatigue and allow more rapid mobilization and return to function [17]. There are many different commercially available back braces for lumbar and thoracic uses. These include the Taylor brace, the Jewett hyperextension brace, the posture training support, and the lumbar corset. In general, braces must be practical, lightweight, easy to apply, and properly fitted to assure comfort and patient compliance.

Nerve Blocks

The modality of epidural nerve blocks with steroids and local anesthetics in patients with acute vertebral compression fractures is still controversial. Much of the reservation about this modality centers on the systemic effects of steroids administered by this route, even in an acute setting. In the author's experience, the epidural injection of steroids and analgesic agents remains an alternative for the management of pain related to compression fractures in certain clinical situations:

a. Patients who are unresponsive to conservative treatment as mentioned earlier.
b. Patients who are severely debilitated and are at high risk because of concurrent diseases, such as chronic obstructive pulmonary disease and coronary artery disease.

Unlike cancer pain management, the efficacy of various epidural, and intrathecal pumps with home infusion is still unknown. There is a great need for creative approaches to pain relief for patients with severe pain who do not respond to usual conservative treatments.

Chronic Pain Management of Vertebral Compression Fractures

Relief of pain is usually indicative of fracture healing. Those patients in whom pain is persistent for 4–6 weeks require a detailed examination to detect neurologic, myofascial, or orthopedic complications that can lead to long-term problems.

Physical Exercise

After 4 to 6 weeks, a daily aerobic exercise program of mobilization, such as walking, swimming, and stretching exercises, should be instituted. These exercises will reverse some of the muscle deconditioning. If the patient is successful in incorporating these aerobic exercises, the next step is to incorporate back-strengthening exercises under the direction of a physical therapist. The use of extension exercises is currently favored. Flexion exercises are not recommended as these can increase vertebral compression forces on the body of the vertebral bones and increase the possibility of occurrence of compression fractures and further increase the kyphosis.

Pharmacologic

a. Calcitonin. As previously described.

b. Analgesic medications. The principles of pain management of utilizing analgesic medications in the chronic setting are similar to the acute setting, except in the area of the narcotic medications. Currently, there is significant controversy in the area of opioid therapy for chronic nonmalignant pain. There are significant legal, practical, moral, and ethical issues that need to be answered in addition to long-term controlled studies. The author uses a moderate approach and adheres closely to the guidelines proposed by H. L. Fields and J. C. Liebeskind, "Opioid Therapy for Chronic Nonmalignant Pain: Current Status." Generally, these narcotic medications have been used cautiously to increase function and improve quality of life. Patients are immediately detoxified if they exhibit drug-seeking behavior.

Nerve Blocks

There is no evidence to support that epidural injections are indicated in the chronic setting strictly for vertebral compression fracture. However, other indications, such as spinal stenosis or facet arthropathy, may exist as a concomitant condition. In these situations, an epidural injection or facet injection may be diagnostic and/or therapeutic.

Vertebroplasty

Percutaneous vertebroplasty is an alternative that needs further evaluation. The procedure involves injecting the affected vertebrae with polymethyl methacrylate percutaneously under fluoroscopic guidance. The resulting reinforcement of the fractured vertebra is reported to eliminate the pain and need for narcotic analgesics [18]. This technique offers a new therapeutic option for pain relief in appropriately selected cases when conservative or more conventional therapy has failed. It is not a recognized standard treatment and is invasive with significant risks.

Spinal Infusions

Implantable pumps for chronic pain are options for patients with refractory pain from osteoporotic fractures. Because of its invasive nature, risk, expense, and follow-up management needs, implantable pumps are utilized infrequently. More studies are needed for efficacy with chronic pain from osteoporotic fractures. However, several types can be utilized in tertiary cases. Opioids, local anesthetics, Baclofen, and Clonidine have been utilized epidurally and intrathecally for other pain conditions and require a pain management specialist and monitoring.

ALTERNATIVE MODALITIES

Electromagnetic [1], transcutaneous electrical nerve stimulation, and acupuncture may also be beneficial in the acute setting. However, there is a lack of good controlled studies for these modalities. Cognitive therapies such as education, relaxation, imagery, biofeedback, distraction, music [6], and therapeutic touch may provide some pain relief.

EDUCATION

Patient and family education about pain management options can alleviate anxiety, as well as encourage the patient to be an active participant in their care. Patient education regarding osteoporosis, its treatment, lifestyle changes, diet, fall prevention, and medications are part of long-term treatment. [7,8]

SUMMARY

Pain from fractures due to osteoporosis affects millions of people annually. A stepwise approach, sometimes with trial and error, utilizing the patient's report of pain and function as a guide, involving members of a health care team, is the optimal approach.

The mainstay for acute pain management is rest; early mobilization, various oral medications such as NSAIDs, tricyclics, and muscle relaxants, bracing, as needed, noninvasive modalities such as ice or heat, calcitonin, and possibly epidural injections.

Chronic pain management utilizes some oral medications, exercise, education, and noninvasive techniques, including psychological treatment as needed, promotion of function, pain relief, and quality of life.

References

1. Von Feldt, J. M. Managing osteoporotic fractures: Minimizing pain and disability. *Revue Du Rhumatisme (English Ed.),* **64,**(6, suppl), 785–805 (1997, June 30).
2. Lukert, B. P. Vertebral compression fractures: How to manage pain, avoid disability. *Geriatrics,* **496,** 22–26 (1994, February).
3. Portenoy, R. K. Opioid therapy for chronic non-malignant pain: clinicians' perspective. *Journal of Law, Medicine, and Ethics,* **24**(4), 296–309 (1996, Winter).
4. Weber, M., Hasler, P., and Gerber, H. Insufficiency fractures of the sacrum. Twenty cases & review of the literature. *Spine,* **18**(6), 2507–2512 (1993).
5. Leroux, J. L., Denat B., Thomas, E., Blotman, F., and Bonnel, F. *Spine,* **18**(16), 2502–2506 (1993).
6. Acute Pain Management Guideline Panel. Acute Pain Management: Operative or Medical Procedures and Trauma. Clinical Practice Guideline. AHCPR Pub. No. 92-0032. Rockville, MD. Agency for Health Care Policy and Research, Public Health Service, US Dept. of Health and Human Services. Government Printing Office: Washington, DC (1992, Feb).
7. Tamayo-Orozco, J., Arzac-Palumbo, P., Mota-Bolfeta, R., and Fuentes, F. Vertebral fractures associated with osteoporosis, patient management. *American Journal of Medicine,* **103**(2A), 445–485 (1997, August 18).
8. Myers, A. Osteoporosis & low back pain. *Comprehensive Therapy,* **23**(1), 57–59 (1997).
9. Carr, D. B., Paris, P. M., and Turturro, M. A. Treat pain as a medical emergency. *Patient Care,* 60–83 (1995, August 15).
10. Montauk, S. L., and Martin, J. Treating chronic pain. *American Family Physician,* **55**(4), 1151–1161 (1997, March).
11. Gennari, C., Agnusdei, D., and Camporeale, A. Use of calcitonin in the treatment of bone pain associated with osteoporosis. *Calcified Tissue International,* **49**(suppl. 2), 9–13 (1991).
12. Kapuscinski, P., Tatataj, M., Borowicz, J., Marcinowska-Suchowierska, E., and Brzozowski, R. An analgesic effect of synthetic human calcitonin in patients with primary osteoporosis. *Materia Medica Polona,* **28**(3,98), 83–86. 1996, July–September).
13. Pontiroli, A. E., Pajetta, E., Scaglia, L., Rubinacci, A., Resmini, G., Arrigoni, M., and Pozza, G. *Aging Clin. Exp. Res.,* **6**(6), 459–463 (1994, December).
14. Body, J. J. Calcitonin for prevention and treatment of postmenopausal osteoporosis. *Clinical Rheumatology, 14 Suppl.* (3), 18–21 (1995, September).
15. Lyritis, G. P., Paspati, I., Karachalios, T., Ioakimidis, D., Skarantavos G., and Lyritis, P. G. Pain relief from nasal salmon calcitonin in osteoporotic vertebral crush fractures. *Acta Orthop Scand (suppl 275),* **68,** 112–114 (1997).
16. Tolino, A., Romano, L., Ronsini, S., Riccio, S., and Montemagno, U. Treatment of postmenopausal osteoporosis with salmon calcitonin nasal spray: evaluation by bone mineral content and biochemical patterns. *International Journal of Clinical Pharmacology, Therapy, and Toxicology,* **31**(7), 358–360 (1993, July).
17. Kaplan, R. S., and Sinaki, M. Posture training support: Preliminary report on a series of patients with diminished symptomatic complications of osteoporosis. *Mayo Clinic Proceedings,* **68,** 1171–1176 (1993).
18. Mathis, J. M., Petri, M., and Noff, N. Percutaneous vertebroplasty treatment of steroid-induced osteoporotic compression fractures. *Arthritis & Rheumatism* **41**(1), 171–175 (1998).

Part VI

Therapeutics

CHAPTER 36

Complications of Joint Replacement in the Elderly

MITCHELL J. WINEMAKER AND THOMAS S. THORNHILL
Brigham and Women's Hospital, Harvard Medical School, Boston, Massachusetts 02115

INTRODUCTION

As with most diseases, the best treatment of arthritis is prevention. Educating patients regarding a healthy lifestyle, including proper nutrition, weight control, and physical fitness, is beneficial. Nevertheless, there are numerous causes of joint disease that at present cannot be prevented. For many patients, there are treatment alternatives that may preserve function and delay joint replacement, including oral and injectable medications, physical therapy, arthroscopy, and limb realignment procedures. These and other modalities are often used to delay the progression of joint arthrosis and the subsequent need for joint replacement. Despite numerous long-term studies of total joint replacement showing successful relief of pain and improvement in function in greater than 90% of patients, the life span of an artificial joint is limited. In addition, results of revising a failed arthroplasty are inferior to the primary procedure. For these reasons, prosthetic joint replacement is reserved for the aging population except in circumstances where severe joint destruction is compromising activities of daily living and there is no better treatment alternative.

The appropriate selection of patients is key to the avoidance of many complications. Those ideally suited to joint replacement are arthritic elderly, low-demand patients in otherwise good general medical condition who have failed other appropriate treatment options. There are few contraindications to prosthetic arthroplasty in severely disabled patients, however, provided that they are adequately informed and both the patient and surgeon agree that the benefits outweigh the potential complications. The only absolute contraindications to joint replacement are active sepsis and medical conditions that preclude adequate anesthesia. There are other factors that may compromise the result of joint replacement and are often listed as relative contraindications. These include a vital nonfunctioning structure such as the extensor mechanism in knee replacement, neuropathic arthropathy, a well-functioning arthrodesis, previous adjacent osteomyelitis, significant peripheral vascular disease, and a variety of medical illnesses that increase perioperative risk. Appropriate history, physical examination, and radiologic assessment as well as ancillary investigations will help identify those patients who are inappropriate surgical candidates.

The single most important factor determining the success of total joint replacement is the surgeon. Appropriate handling of the soft tissues during surgical exposure will help avoid infection and skin necrosis. Proper restoration of limb alignment, prosthetic component orientation, and balancing of the soft tissues will optimize joint stability, function and longevity. Choosing prosthetic components with a design and material of proven long-term success will help ensure patient satisfaction and prevent early failure of the prosthesis.

RESULTS OF JOINT REPLACEMENT

Consistently successful results have been reported in the literature for total joint replacement in various locations. This chapter focuses primarily on large joint replacement of the hip and knee and to a lesser extent on the shoulder and elbow. Modern hip joint replacement began in the late 1960s and is credited to Sir John Charnley, whose pioneering work remains essentially unchanged today. There have been some changes in surgical technique (e.g., surgical approach, cement technique) and component design (e.g., cementless component fixation, new metal alloys, new bearing surfaces, and increased modularity of components) that have evolved over the years, some leading to improved prosthesis longevity and some leading to catastrophic failure. As high success rates are realized, surgeons are expanding the indications for total joint replacement, performing them increasingly in younger patients.

The success of a total joint replacement is assessed by long-term function and the absence of any need for revision surgery; this requires at least a decade to evaluate. Most surgical techniques and component designs have been altered since these long-term studies were reported. As a result of this constant evolution of joint replacement surgery, outcomes have become difficult to measure and compare. For example, Schulte *et al.* [1] reported a minimum 20-year follow-up on the outcome of the original Charnley total hip arthroplasty by one surgeon. Of the original 262 patients receiving total hips between 1970 and 1972 by that surgeon, 83 patients were still living. Eighty-five percent of these had no pain. Fifteen percent of the hip replacements in patients who were alive at the time of study ultimately required revision surgery; 3% were for infection and loosening, 11% were for aseptic loosening, and 1% was for dislocation. Of the 322 hips in 262 patients for which the outcome was known after a minimum of 20 years, 90% of patients retained the original implant until death or most recent follow-up examination. Most of us would agree that these are impressive results for modern joint replacement that had been performed in its early days. Nonetheless, very few surgeons still perform total hip arthroplasty using the same surgical technique and component design that was used in that study. One would hope that the alterations made by surgeons today will continue to improve the success and longevity of hip replacements. Unfortunately, experience has shown us that what appears to be a step forward can sometimes be two steps backward. Thus, one must use caution when interpreting results of total joint replacement and compare outcomes between similar patient populations, using similar techniques and component design with adequate long-term follow-up.

Excellent results with greater than 10-year follow-up have now been reported using newer "second-generation cementing techniques" and cementless hip replacements with a survivorship of greater than 90% [2,3]. The current trend is toward a cemented femoral component and an uncemented acetabular component, also known as a "hybrid" total hip replacement. Comparable long-term results have also been reported in the knee, shoulder, and elbow [4–6].

PATIENT CONSIDERATIONS

Systemic Illness and the Aged

Comorbid illness is frequent in the aging patient population, requiring total joint replacement. Medical and anesthesia consultations are an essential part of perioperative patient care to identify these comorbid conditions and minimize any adverse events. Most patients are evaluated in a preadmission clinic where appropriate evaluation, investigations, medication alterations, and teaching about joint replacement are performed. Unless preoperative management needs to be monitored in the hospital, such as reversal of anticoagulation, most patients are now admitted on the day of surgery. Joint replacement is an elective procedure and the benefits must outweigh the risks to proceed with surgery.

Most preoperative testing is geared toward assessing risk and optimizing the medical condition of the patient by evaluating each organ system. The Goldman criteria have been used to assess preoperative cardiac risk and those with unstable angina, decompensated congestive heart failure, severe aortic stenosis, or recent myocardial infarction are at greatest risk [7]. Any cardiac condition should be medically or surgically optimized prior to considering prosthetic replacement. Generally, a patient will be required to wait at least 3 months following an acute myocardial infarction before consideration will be given to joint replacement. One possible exception may be following a femoral neck fracture where the risk of postponing joint replacement may exceed the risk of proceeding with surgery in an elderly frail individual.

Pulmonary complications are increased in patients with a history of heavy smoking, asthma, obesity, and chronic obstructive pulmonary disease. These patients should be evaluated with pulmonary function studies and arterial blood gases. Those with hypercapnia and a FEV1 $<$ 1L are at greatest risk [8]. Chronic smokers are at additional risk for wound healing problems. Patients should be encouraged to stop smoking preoperatively and chest physiotherapy is encouraged. Control of cardiopulmonary disease with blood pressure control, antianginal medication, bronchodilators, and corticosteroids are continued perioperatively.

Renal disease can cause hypertension and volume and electrolyte abnormalities, as well as chronic anemia and platelet dysfunction that can increase bleeding and infection. Doses of renally excreted medications may need adjusting and nephrotoxic medications should be avoided [9]. Patients on dialysis usually develop severe renal osteodystrophy and should be advised that this can lead to early aseptic loosening of their joint replacement. This is possibly due to continued bone resorption at the cement–bone interface [10].

Patients with liver disease need to be assessed for coagulopathy, blood pressure, volume, and electrolyte abnormalities [11].

Diabetes mellitus predisposes patients to poor wound healing and infection after joint replacement [12,13]. Antibiotic prophylaxis is essential perioperatively to rule out other potential sources of infection, such as skin ulcers or urinary tract infections. These patients may have coexisting cardiac disease, peripheral vascular disease, neuropathy, and nephropathy, all of which add to the perioperative risk. Many surgeons will avoid the use of a tourniquet in prosthetic knee replacement in the presence of significant peripheral vascular disease. Diabetics require close monitoring of their blood sugar in the perioperative period. Oral hypoglycemics are discontinued the night prior to surgery and short-acting insulin is begun the morning of surgery often intravenously with 5% dextrose solution.

The aged are more susceptible to postoperative confusion, which can lead to further complications and poorer postoperative function. These patients should be evaluated carefully to rule out and treat an underlying cause. These can include structural or metabolic causes, including alcohol withdrawal, narcotic medication, stroke, fat embolism, pulmonary embolism, infection, and electrolyte abnormalities.

Musculoskeletal Disease and the Aged

There are certain musculoskeletal conditions that are prevelant in the aging skeleton that either result in joint destruction and/or pose an increased risk of complications with joint replacement. These include osteoporosis, osteoarthritis, rheumatoid arthritis, neuromuscular disease, Paget's disease, ankylosing spondylitis, and metastatic disease.

Osteoporosis

The aged are at increased risk for osteoporosis, particularly thin, white postmenopausal females who are sedentary and have not taken estrogen replacement. Osteoporosis does not result in arthritis but may coexist in patients with joint disease, particularly in rheumatoid arthritis. Conversely, a negative relationship between osteoarthritis and osteoporosis has been demonstrated in some studies. A cross-sectional study of 4855 women older than 64 years showed that women with grade 3–4 hip osteoarthritis had a higher age-adjusted bone mineral density at all sites [14]. There has also been the suggestion that estrogen replacement may help protect against osteoarthritis of the hip in elderly white females [15]. Osteoporosis increases the risk of periprosthetic fractures during total joint replacement [16]. The relationship between osteoporosis and aseptic loosening of a joint prosthesis has not been studied extensively. Preoperative bone mass was not correlated with mechanical loosening around hip replacements in one study [17]. Although bony ingrowth into uncemented joint replacements has been successful, some surgeons prefer the use of cemented components in osteoporotic bone to avoid the increased risk of fracture during the implantation of press-fit components.

Osteoarthritis

The vast majority of joint replacements are performed in patients with degenerative joint disease or osteoarthritis of primary or secondary cause [18]. Osteoarthritis is more prevalent with advancing age; however, there are other genetic and environmental factors that are associated with the disorder, including female gender, obesity, previous meniscectomy, and trauma to name a few [18]. Biologic factors (e.g., matrix metalloproteinases, cytokines, and growth factors) and mechanical events are both thought to be involved in the pathogenesis of osteoarthritis, resulting in cartilage destruction [19]. This is clinically manifested as pain, swelling, deformity, reduced range of motion, and limited function. Radiographic signs confirming the diagnosis are joint space narrowing, subchondral sclerosis, subchondral cysts, and osteophyte formation. Hip and knee joints are affected most frequently, requiring replacement. The most successful joint replacements are those performed in patients with primary osteoarthritis.

Rheumatoid Arthritis

Rheumatoid arthritis is the most common inflammatory joint disease that requires joint replacement in the aged. Both immunogenetic and environmental factors are involved in the pathogenesis of the disease. Clinically, pain predominates; however, these patients often have significant joint swelling acutely and severe deformity following persistent long-standing disease. Diagnosis is made primarily on clinical grounds as outlined by the American Rheumatism Association [20]. Radiographically, rheumatoid arthritis can be distinguished from classic osteoarthritis by noting the distinctive osteopenia, marginal erosions, lack of osteophytes, joint space narrowing, frequent deformity, and joint subluxation. Rheumatoid arthritis is classically a symmetrical polyarthritis affecting the entire joint, in contrast to osteoarthritis, which is often asymmetric, affecting only part of the joint (e.g., medial compartment osteoarthritis of the knee).

Virtually every organ system can be affected by rheumatoid arthritis, posing additional risk at the time of surgery [21]. Access to the airway may be difficult for the anesthesiologist secondary to temporomandibular, cricoarytenoid, and cervical spine involvement (e.g., atlantoaxial instability). Preoperative assessment of the cervical spine for signs of myelopathy (e.g., clonus, hyperreflexia, Llermitt's sign) should be performed routinely, and lateral flexion–extension radiographs are used to assess the degree of static and dynamic instability. Pleuritis, carditis, and nephritis can impair function in these vital organs, necessitating careful preoperative assessment of cardiopulmonary and renal function. Medications such as nonsteroidal anti-inflammatory drugs (NSAID) increase the risk of perioperative bleeding complications and should be discontinued at least 1 week prior to joint replacement. During that time, pain can be controlled with other analgesic agents. Steroids predispose patients to infection, skin breakdown, and gastrointestinal bleeding ulcers. In fact, rheumatoid patients taking steroids were found to carry a higher risk of infection following total knee arthroplasty in a retrospective review [22]. Nonetheless, perioperative steroids should be used in all patients who have taken oral steroids within a year of their planned surgery to prevent a potential crisis of adrenal insufficiency. The effect of methotrexate on wound healing and infection is controversial, and withholding this medication for 2 weeks during the perioperative period has been recommended [23]. Because of the severe joint deformity and osteopenia found at the time of surgery, joint replacement can be challenging in the elderly patient with rheumatoid arthritis. Even so, the overall long-term results are excellent [24].

Neuropathic Arthropathy

Neuropathic arthropathy (Charcot joint) is often considered a contraindication to joint replacement due to the increased rate of early failure. Nonetheless, moderately successful attempts at total knee replacement have been made with the adequate restoration of limb alignment, stability, and range of motion [25,26]. Total hip replacement is considered contraindicated in Charcot arthropathy due to the increased risk of failure and recurrent dislocation [10].

Neuromuscular Disease

Parkinson's disease patients often present with femoral neck fractures and occasionally arthritic knees. As with other neuromuscular diseases, they are at an increased risk of hip dislocation and generally a lateral approach to the hip and insertion of a bipolar hemiarthroplasty is recommended following femoral neck fracture to minimize the risk of dislocation [27]. Knee replacement has been associated with early failure of the prostheses due to hamstring rigidity [28].

Other neuromuscular disease less commonly seen in the aged, such as cerebral palsy and poliomyelitis, also have an increased risk of loosening and joint instability [29–31].

Paget's Disease

The incidence of Paget's disease in the general population over 40 years old is between 2 and 4% [10]. Up to 50% of these patients develop symptomatic hip arthritis and 10% develop knee arthritis [10]. Nonoperative management includes NSAID, calcitonin, and bisphosphonates, but occasionally joint replacement is needed. Paget's disease can make joint replacement more technically challenging because of acquired bony deformity that can result in component malpositioning. An osteotomy in conjunction with prosthetic replacement is sometimes required to address this problem. An increased incidence of heterotopic ossification has been noted around joint replacements in Paget's patients [32]. Pagetic bone tends to be very vascular and blood loss is a concern. Preoperative calcitonin and/or bisphosphonates have been advocated to control the disease and reduce blood loss. The overall results of joint replacement in Paget's disease are inferior to those for primary osteoarthritis [32–34]. Uncemented components have not been recommended due to the theoretical reduced bone ingrowth potential of Pagetic bone.

Ankylosing Spondylitis

Ankylosing spondylitis leads to an arthritic hip in approximately 30% of patients and is often bilateral. Ambulation may be severely restricted when severe hip flexion contractures are combined with associated thoracolumbar kyphosis. Cardiopulmonary assessment should be carefully assessed preoperatively due to the increased prevalence of restrictive lung disease in these patients. Total hip arthroplasty may improve function; however, a high incidence of significant heterotopic ossification has been noted (23%) that may compromise outcome [35]. Low-dose irradiation or indomethacin has been used successfully to reduce the incidence of heterotopic ossification.

Metastatic Disease

Metastatic disease to bone is most commonly from the lung, breast, prostate, kidney, and thyroid. Occasionally a lesion may be located in a periarticular region and cause pain or impending fracture. As a palliative measure, prosthetic replacement may be performed, provided the patient can medically withstand the surgery and has a reasonable life expectancy.

SURGICAL CONSIDERATIONS

Anesthesia

When undergoing total joint replacement, patients are often more concerned about the risks of the anesthetic than those of the surgery. With current monitoring, including a pulse oximeter, capnograph, blood pressure cuff, cardiac monitor, temperature probe, plus or minus invasive cardiac monitoring (Swan-Ganz, arterial monitoring), and current anaesthetic agents, the risk of a catastrophic event related to the anesthetic is exceedingly low. The type of anesthetic chosen at surgery is made primarily by the anesthesiologist. Significant benefits can be achieved using regional anesthesia, including reduced blood loss, decreased incidence of deep vein thrombosis, and a convenient and effective modality for postoperative pain control [36]. Conversely, regional anesthesia often requires more technical expertise, can be more time-consuming, and occasionally fails, necessitating a general anesthetic. The risk of cardiac complications is similar between general and regional anesthesia [37].

Total joint replacement may often be a prolonged operation, particularly in the revision of a failed arthroplasty, and, as a result, appropriate positioning of the patient is crucial. Both the anesthetist and the surgeon must be vigilant during patient positioning. They must ensure that the skin is well padded to prevent skin breakdown, the eyes are protected to prevent corneal damage or acute glaucoma, the neck is positioned appropriately to avoid injury, especially in the rheumatoid population, and the extremities are well padded to prevent compressive neuropathies.

Early Complications

BLOOD LOSS

Blood loss may be a significant concern during joint replacement due to the long duration of surgery, the wide exposure necessary for prosthetic implantation, and the exposed medullary canal where bleeding is difficult to control. In addition, many of these patients are on nonsteroidal anti-inflammatory medication to control their joint disease, which may compound the bleeding problem. These medications should be discontinued at least a week prior to surgery to restore platelet function. Preoperative hemoglobin, hematocrit, platelet count, prothrombin, and partial thromboplastin time are routine prior to joint replacement, especially in patients with a history of blood dyscrasia, anemia, or coagulopathy. Medical consultation should be sought in patients at risk of bleeding. Patients on chronic anticoagulation should be evaluated for perioperative management of their medications to minimize the risk of bleeding during surgery versus clotting perioperatively [38].

Studies show that blood loss after primary total hip replacement averages between 500 and 1000 ml and that postoperative drain losses are 200 to 600 ml. Blood loss after revision hip arthroplasty can be as high as 2000 ml.

Allogeneic blood transfusion is given judiciously because of the concerns of disease transmission, immunomodulation, and increased perioperative infection and transfusion reactions. Current rigorous screening of donated blood has reduced the risk of hepatitis C at 1 in 3000 to 1 in 5000, hepatitis B to 1 in 200,000 units, and HIV at 1 in 200,000 to 1 in 800,000 [39,40]. Several studies suggest that the risk of disease transmission is no less with directed donation than nondirected homologous transfusion. As a result, surgeons are generally recommending autologous transfusion where indicated and otherwise nondirected homologous transfusion following the National Institute of Health guidelines [39]. Patients must have a sufficient hemoglobin (110 g/dl) and cardiac reserve to predonate blood and must not have an active infection.

Autologous blood donation can be costly, and because a significant number of predonated units may be wasted [41], others have attempted to predict which patients will ultimately require transfusion. Friedman *et al.* [42] showed that patients with a preoperative hemoglobin level less than 10.5 g/dl had greater than a 90% chance of requiring a transfusion. The risk decreased in a linear fashion as the hemoglobin level increased and was negligible over 14 g/dl. Similarly, Hatzidakis *et al.* [43] found that only 3% of donors less than 65 years old undergoing primary total joint arthroplasty with preoperative hemoglobin greater than 13 g/dl needed transfusion. They also found an increased need for blood transfusion in patients undergoing revision total joint replacement. This information allows us to appropriately designate those patients for autologous blood donation while containing costs. For such patients, it is recommended that 1 to 2 units of autologous blood be donated for primary unilateral hip and knee surgery and 3 to 4 units for bilateral or revision surgery.

Other important modalities used to prevent blood loss in joint replacement include a meticulous surgical technique, hypotensive anesthesia, preoperative hemodilution, washed or unwashed perioperative autologous red blood cell salvage, preoperative erythropoietin, and other less proven pharmacological agents, including aprotinin and ε-aminocaproic acid [40,44].

Various surgical techniques can minimize blood loss. The choice of surgical implant fixation can influence blood loss and is often reduced using cemented versus porous-ingrowth components as cement effectively tamponades the intramedullary canal. The use of a tourniquet where appropriate reduces blood loss. Controversy exists whether a tourniquet should be deflated prior to closure of the wound following total knee replacement. The senior author routinely deflates the tourniquet in total knee arthroplasty prior to closure to assure hemostasis of the geniculate vessels, which reveals the occasional patient who may otherwise have persistent postoperative bleeding. Others have found blood loss to increase with intraoperative deflation of the tourniquet in combination with immediate continuous passive motion [45]. There was less blood loss when the tourniquet was released after application of a compressive dressing with delayed continuous passive motion. The use of closed suction drainage postoperatively in both the hip and the knee has been challenged, with authors suggesting no difference in wound drainage, hematoma, or transfusion requirements [46,47]. The senior author still recommends the use of drains because the risk of a hematoma or persistent drainage increases the potential for infection.

Various anesthetic techniques can be used to reduce blood loss. Hypotensive anesthesia is helpful in reducing blood loss but cannot always be used effectively in elderly patients with poor cardiac reserve, labile blood pressure, significant cerebrovascular disease, or low flow states to the liver or kidney. Regional anesthesia has been shown to reduce blood loss after total hip replacement [40].

Pharmacological agents have been used to reduce blood loss. Recombinant human erythropoietin is a stimulator of red blood cell production. It has been shown to reduce the need for allogeneic transfusion perioperatively and can enhance the predonation of autologous blood by maintaining an acceptable hemoglobin level preoperatively [40]. At this time, the U.S. Food and Drug Administration has not approved erythropoietin for use in the predonation of autologous blood and it is not used currently for routine orthopedic procedures. It may be considered for simultaneous bilateral or complex revision joint replacement or in patients with chronic anemia from renal failure, AIDS, nonmyeloid malignant disease, and Jehovah's Witnesses [40].

Preoperative hemodilution involves removing whole blood and replacing it with crystalloid or colloid to maintain intravascular volume while reducing the hematocrit. This can improve blood rheology and cardiac output, which is beneficial, but it can also increase myocardial oxygen demand, which is detrimental in some elderly patients. The whole blood removed can be reinfused as necessary. This technique has not gained popularity for orthopedic procedures due to the additional manpower, time, and risk of using this method [44].

Washed red blood cell salvage has been used during revision joint replacement where blood loss is expected to exceed 1 liter [44]. It retrieves about 60% of the red blood cells lost during the procedure [44]. It is not cost effective for primary joint replacement because it requires additional equipment and qualified personnel such as a perfusionist. It should not be used in the presence of active infection or malignancy. The use of unwashed autologous blood salvage postoperatively from closed suction drains is controversial due to the risk of contamination from fat particles, polymethylmethacrylate, fibrin degradation products, vasoactive mediators, clotting factors, and free hemoglobin [40].

Careful patient assessment and planning will allow the surgeon to select which techniques are appropriate for a given patient to effectively minimize blood loss.

Fat Embolism Syndrome

Fat embolism is a frequent occurrence following hip and knee replacement, but the clinical syndrome of fat emboli is rare [48]. The majority occur following the use of long-stemmed implants or intramedullary instrumentation for limb alignment [49]. Fat embolism syndrome has been seen more commonly in rheumatoid arthritis [50].

Mortality is high following fat embolism syndrome and thus measures must be taken to prevent its occurrence. When using intramedullary instrumentation, it is recommended that gentle insertion, overdrilling of the canal, and slotted alignment stems should be used to reduce intramedullary pressures that may lead to fat emboli. During preparation for cemented stem insertion, canal plugging and removal of loose intramedullary debris may help minimize fat emboli [48].

Fat embolism syndrome often presents as confusion secondary to hypoxemia during the first few days following surgery. Other causes of confusion must be ruled out [51]. The classic axillary and subconjunctival petechiae are often not present on physical examination. Several authors have tried to establish criteria to make the diagnosis of fat embolism syndrome [52,53]. Once established, fat embolism syndrome is treated with hemodynamic and respiratory support. Corticosteroids have been used in some cases.

Wound/Infection

While infrequent, a deep infection around a joint replacement is one of the most dreaded and costly complications for both the patient and the surgeon. The incidence of deep infection is less than 1% in some of the larger series. The incidence of late infection is approximately 0.6%. A variety of factors have been cited as increasing the risk of infection around a total joint replacement [22]. These include rheumatoid arthritis, associated skin breakdown, prior surgery, concomitant urinary tract infection, obesity, and other conditions where a patient may be immunocompromised such as diabetes mellitus, renal failure, and malignant disease. Because the incidence of infection around total joint replacements is so low, it is difficult to definitively implicate some of these factors in the pathogenesis of infection.

In addition to standard operating room procedure, high air exchange rates in the operating room, ultraviolet lights, whole body exhaust-ventilated suits, intraoperative wound towels, and closed suction drainage have all been employed to reduce the periprosthetic infection rate. An important variable in reducing infection is the administration of perioperative antibiotics. A single preoperative dose of antibiotic has been shown to be as effective as a 48-hr regimen [54].

Diagnosis and treatment of infection must be prompt to prevent an adverse outcome. One-third of all deep periprosthetic infections occur within 3 months. Pain is the most frequent symptom; however, the clinical presentation may be variable. Delayed infection implies hematogenous seeding of the prosthetic joint and is often heralded by a history of infection from another site. A history should be obtained in search of other common sources such as dental, genitourinary, gastrointestinal, and skin infections. Persistent warmth and swelling, erythema, wound drainage, and occasionally fever may be present. An elevated white blood count with an increased proportion of polymorphonuclear leukocytes, a persistently elevated erythrocyte sedimentation rate (ESR), or C-reactive protein should alert the physician to the possibility of infection. An elevated ESR in isolation may be difficult to interpret because it may be elevated up to a year following total joint arthroplasty and should be interpreted along with other clinical findings. Plain radiographs are limited in the diagnosis of infection because an effusion, new periosteal bone, and osteolysis may also be seen with aseptic loosening of a prosthesis. Some advocate the use of Technetium bone scans or indium-labeled leukocyte scans to diagnose periprosthetic infection [55]. False-positive scans may occur, particularly within the first year of prosthetic replacement. Preoperative joint aspiration under sterile technique for cell count, gram stain, culture, and antibiotic sensitivity has proven to have up to 95% specificity in the detection of infection. False-negative aspiration may occur in 15% of patients, and false positives may occur rarely with specimen contamination. A white cell count greater than 100,000 is considered an infection until proved otherwise. A white cell count of 20,000 to 40,000 often indicates an inflammatory process, but in the presence of other findings, it may be consistent with infection. Repeat aspiration is recommended in cases where the findings of the aspirate do not correlate with the clinical picture. The current gold standard for the diagnosis of infection is cultures from tissue and fluid obtained intraoperatively. Even in this scenario, a definitive organism is identified in only 80 to 90% of patients. Newer techniques such as polymerase chain reaction may improve the accuracy and speed with which infection can be detected.

Most surgeons agree that prophylactic antibiotics should be administered routinely for invasive dental, genitourinary, and gastrointestinal procedures following joint replacement. Data regarding the use of antibiotic prophylaxis for routine dental cleaning are more controversial. Certainly patients at increased risk for infection should take prophylactic antibiotics for these procedures [56]. The current recommendation is for routine prophylactic antibiotic use for 2 years following joint replacement with 2 g Amoxicillin before dental procedures. One gram of erythromycin before dental cleaning is substituted in the case of penicillin allergy.

The management of periprosthetic infection depends on the timing of presentation, virulence of the organism, and patient comorbidity. Options for treatment include debridement and synovectomy, antibiotic suppression, primary or delayed exchange of the prosthesis, arthrodesis, and resection arthroplasty. The distinction between acute and chronic infection is arbitrary. The senior author designates an acute infection as one that has persisted less than 3 weeks and a chronic infection as one present for longer than that period. If an infection with an antibiotic sensitive organism presents acutely and the components are well fixed, then an open debridement and a 6-week course of intravenous antibiotic therapy may be attempted with approximately a 50% success rate. If the component is loose, as indicated by bone–cement demarcation or the organism is considered virulent, such as a gram-negative organism, then the components should be removed. A primary exchange of the components is considered in the elderly and infirmed patient with an approximately 83% success rate. Synovectomy, delayed exchange, and antibiotic therapy is recommended for the majority of patients and has the highest success rate (90%) at resolving the infection [57]. The delayed exchange protocol includes preoperative aspiration, culture and sensitivity, removal of the prosthesis, wound debridement and synovectomy, insertion of an antibiotic cement-laden spacer, and closed suction drainage for 24–48 hr. Intravenous antibiotics are maintained for 4 to 6 weeks and the joint is subsequently reaspirated prior to reimplantation of a new prosthetic joint. Continued oral antibiotic suppression is recommended if there is a chronic source of infection, such as the skin, urinary tract, or oropharynx. Resection arthroplasty or arthrodesis is considered when a delayed exchange has failed. Finally, amputation is considered when other attempts at irradicating the infection have failed and the existing limb has a higher morbidity than amputation.

Venous Thromboembolic Disease

Venous thromboembolic disease is primarily a concern in lower extremity joint replacement surgery. Total joint replacement predisposes patients to Virchow's classic triad of stasis, hypercoagulability, and endothelial damage. Patients are frequently sedentary prior to and during the perioperative period due to their joint disease, which leads to poor venous return. In addition, many of these patients are obese, which limits their mobility. The actual trauma of surgery releases procoagulants and also causes stretching and kinking of vessels, which can contribute to venous thromboembolic disease. The true incidence of thromboembolic disease following prosthetic replacement is difficult to determine. Patients are quite often asymptomatic and confirmatory tests are not always performed or may be unreliable in certain circumstances. Despite these limitations, the incidence of deep vein thrombosis (DVT) after hip or knee replacement is approximately 50%. Less than half of these are in the proximal deep veins, which are of most clinical significance. Pulmonary emboli occur in approximately 5% of patients, and less than 1 in 5 of these are fatal. Overall, the incidence of significant proximal DVT seems to be slightly higher in the hip than in the knee [58].

The clinical diagnosis of DVT is notoriously unreliable, with a sensitivity of 33% and a specificity of 50% in high-risk patients examined by experienced clinicians [58]. Classically, peak thrombus formation occurs 5 to 7 days following surgery and diminishes once the patient is mobile. Some reports suggest that it can frequently occur weeks after hospital discharge [59,60]. Patients may complain of calf pain or swelling and signs of calf tenderness, edema, or pain with ankle dorsiflexion (Homan's sign). A pulmonary embolus typically presents as chest pain or shortness of breath, although sudden death in the perioperative period may be secondary to a pulmonary embolus.

The gold standard for confirmation of a DVT is venography; however, it is not frequently used because of its invasiveness. Duplex ultrasonography is the most widely used investigation for DVT because it is noninvasive, can be repeated easily, and is relatively inexpensive. Sensitivity of 93% and specificity of 98% have been reported; however, the accuracy is variable and relies heavily on the operator's technical expertise [58]. The gold standard for investigation of pulmonary embolism is angiography and because of its invasiveness, a ventilation–perfusion (V/Q) lung scan is often performed instead. In patients with V/Q mismatch for other reasons such as atelectasis or pneumonia, the test may be indeterminate and angiography may be required for diagnosis.

Treatment of a confirmed DVT is recommended to prevent the risk of fatal pulmonary emboli, postphlebitic syndrome, and recurrent DVT. Generally, either asymptomatic or symptomatic DVT diagnosed following joint replacement is treated with 5–7 days of heparin followed by 3–6 months of warfarin. Treatment of DVT located distal to the knee is more controversial since the rate of propagation beyond the knee ranges from 0 to 40% [58]. The current recommendation is to either follow these patients with serial duplex ultrasound or treat with 3 months of warfarin.

Prophylaxis of DVT is a routine part of joint replacement due to its high incidence and potentially serious consequences. Regional anesthesia at the time of joint replacement has been shown to decrease the frequency of DVT [61]. Postoperative early mobilization and rehabilitation are encouraged to both improve joint function and minimize DVT. External pneumatic compression has been shown to be effective in the reduction of DVT by improving venous flow and stimulating the fibrinolytic system [58,62]. Compliance can sometimes be a problem, but pneumatic compression boots are used commonly as an adjunct in prophylaxis of DVT. Aspirin has been advocated because of its ease of administration and lack of need for monitoring. The effectiveness in reducing DVT in joint replacement is controversial and further prospective randomized trials are needed. It is some experts practice to place patients on 6 weeks to 3 months of aspirin following a negative duplex ultrasound prior to hospital discharge. Warfarin remains the mainstay of prophylactic treatment for DVT in prosthetic replacement. The reported rates of DVT while on warfarin are 10–20% [58]. The rates fall to between 5 and 10% for proximal DVT and there is a reported 1–3% risk of major bleeding [58]. Most patients are kept on warfarin following discharge from the hospital for 6–12 weeks and are most effectively monitored via an outpatient anticoagulant clinic. More recently, low molecular weight heparin has been shown to have similar efficacy and safety as warfarin in the prophylaxis of DVT; however, some experts are concerned about the potential for increased wound drainage and bleeding [63–65]. Despite the potential serious and even life-threatening problems due to DVT, there is no consensus on treatment for this condition and the surgeon must choose one or more of several prophylactic regimens in the perioperative period.

NEUROVASCULAR INJURY

Neurovascular injuries following primary total joint replacement are rare, with an overall incidence of less than 1% [66,67]. They result from excessive traction, compression, or ischemia during joint replacement surgery. As the complexity of the surgery increases, particularly with revision joint replacement or severe periarticular deformity, the risk of neurovascular injury increases. Thorough knowledge of the regional anatomy is essential in minimizing these risks.

Neurologic injury following primary total knee replacement most commonly occurs following correction of severe valgus deformity and concomitant flexion contracture in rheumatoid patients [68,69]. Despite this finding, most surgeons do not expose the peroneal nerve in this setting. Initial management of an acute peroneal nerve palsy includes the removal of compressive dressings and flexion of the knee approximately 30°. The role for surgical decompression remains controversial. It has been advocated by some authors if recovery does not progress after 3 months of nonoperative treatment [66].

Revision total hip replacement has been associated with a 1.4–7.5% incidence of nerve injury related to more extensive, difficult exposure, and altered anatomy [67]. High-riding hip dysplasia poses the greatest risk of neurologic injury due to the altered anatomy and overly aggressive attempts at limb lengthening. Acute limb lengthening more than 6% or roughly 4 cm has been associated with nerve injury in as high as 28% of patients and should be discouraged [70,71]. Other potential sources of neurologic injury include prosthetic dislocation, excessive soft tissue retraction, hematoma secondary to over anticoagulation, wires passed circumferentially around the femur, extruded cement, and screws placed in the anterior quadrants of the acetabulum [72–77]. The vast majority of these complications are preventable by adhering to careful operative technique [67]. Intraoperative neural monitoring is not used commonly in joint replacement surgery as its efficacy in reducing neural injury is not well established.

The treatment of neurologic injury involves careful assessment and documentation of the patient's neurological and vascular status. Acutely, observation is recommended unless there is clear evidence of a compressive hematoma that may be evacuated or when there is reason to believe that a major direct injury, such as surgical transection or encirclement of the nerve, has occurred during wire placement. Further treatment includes a foot drop splint, passive stretching exercises, and electrophysiologic monitoring at 3 weeks and 3 months to document any recovery. Late exploration is rarely performed unless there is no sign of recovery.

Neurologic injury in the upper extremity following joint replacement should be approached in a manner similar to the lower extremity. The most common nerve injury after shoulder replacement is the musculocutaneous nerve, followed by the axillary nerve. The ulnar nerve is most at risk in total elbow replacement; however, the median and radial nerves may also be injured.

Vascular injuries after joint replacement are rare, accounting for less than 0.25% of complications [78]. Mechanisms of vascular injury are similar to those causing neural damage but may manifest as thrombosis, traumatic aneurysm, arteriovenous fistula, or direct transection. Thrombosis is the most common injury and occurs more commonly in patients with preexisting vasculopathy [79]. It may be prompted by manipulation of the extremity or by tourniquet inflation causing arteriosclerotic plaque disruption. The prevention of vascular injury involves a precise surgical technique, avoiding tourniquet use in vasculopathic patients, and appropriate preoperative vascular consultation. Close postoperative monitoring for the recognition of ischemia to an extremity is essential. Treating physicians should have a low threshold for using angiography to confirm the diagnosis of a vascular injury. Treatment must be immediate and includes revascularization using a venous bypass graft and fasciotomy.

PERIPROSTHETIC FRACTURE

Periprosthetic fractures occur in approximately 1% of patients [80,81]. Risk factors for periprosthetic fracture include both patient factors and surgical factors. Patient factors include conditions leading to osteopenic bone (e.g., rheumatoid arthritis, chronic steroid therapy), neurologic conditions causing unsteady gait and joint stiffness, or "arthrofibrosis," especially during joint manipulation [82]. Surgical factors increasing periprosthetic fracture risk are revision joint replacement, often due to compromised bone stock, and insertion of uncemented components, due to the need for a tight press fit for initial implant stability. Inadvertent notching of the anterior femoral cortex likely increases the risk of supracondylar femur fracture after total knee replacement, particularly in osteopenic bone [83,84].

The important issues that guide management of periprosthetic fractures are the location and severity of the fracture, the quality of the bone, and the fixation of the implant [85,86]. Implants that are not well fixed to bone following a periprosthetic fracture will require revision of the implant and stabilization of the fracture with an intramedullary stem approximately two cortical diameters beyond the fracture. A well-fixed implant requires supplemental fracture fixation with conventional devices, including cerclage wires, screws, plates, allograft bone, and intramedullary devices (Fig. 1). In the aged with osteopenic bone, nonoperative management may

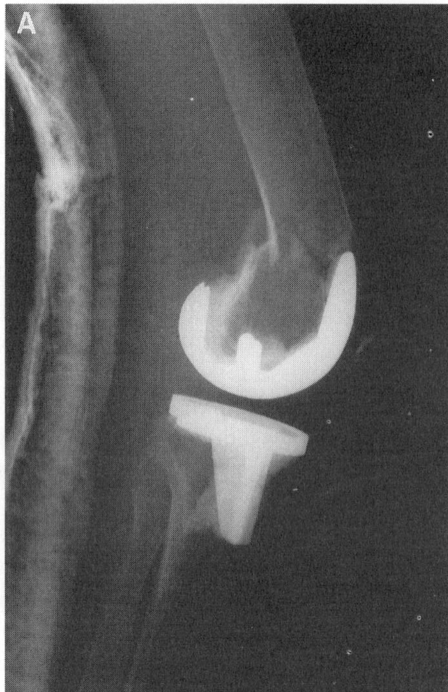

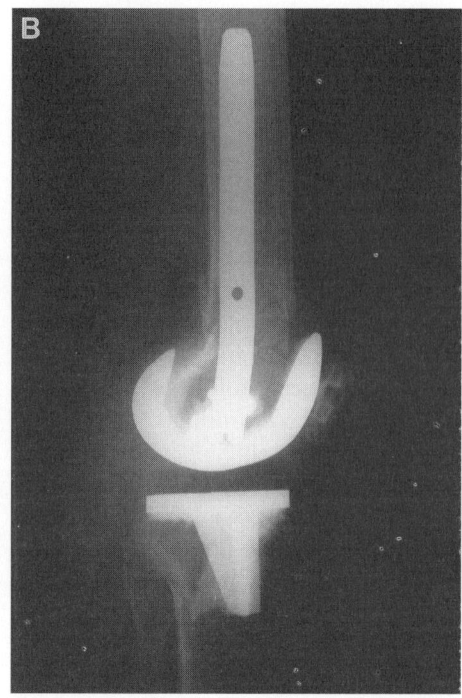

FIGURE 1 Lateral radiographs illustrating (A) a supracondylar femur fracture around a well-fixed prosthesis in a patient with rheumatoid arthritis and (B) intramedullary rod fixation of the fracture maintaining the prosthesis and restoring bony alignment.

be considered, especially in minimally displaced fractures that do not extend beyond the prosthetic implant. The current trend, however, is to operatively fix most periprosthetic fractures in the elderly to facilitate early mobilization and thus prevent the pulmonary and thromboembolic complications associated with prolonged bed rest.

INSTABILITY AND DISLOCATION

Dislocation following total hip arthroplasty occurs in 2–5% of patients. Factors such as neurologic disorders and noncompliance during rehabilitation predispose patients to dislocation. Ekelund *et al.* [87] reported a dislocation rate of 9.2% in a group of patients over 80 years of age undergoing prosthetic hip replacement. Surgical factors that involve appropriate placement of the components, restoration of abductor muscle tension, and removal of impinging bone, soft tissue, or cement are critical in minimizing the chance of dislocation (Fig. 2). As with most surgical complications, greater technical experience can reduce the incidence of dislocation [88]. Exposure of the hip through a posterior approach has been associated with a higher incidence of dislocation compared to the lateral approach. The dislocation rate using the posterior approach has been reduced significantly in recent years with the routine repair of capsule and external rotators. Despite the concerns of dislocation, many surgeons still favor the posterior approach because of the wide and familiar exposure that it offers without risk of compromise to the abductor muscles.

Posterior dislocation of the hip occurs frequently following an attempt to rise from a seated position; the patient's hip will appear flexed and internally rotated. An anterior dislocation often occurs while a patient turns in bed away from the prosthetic hip, forcing it into external rotation. In this case, the limb appears shortened and externally rotated. Once recognized, referral should be made to the orthopedist for prompt reduction of the hip. Provided the limb remains neurovascularly intact, hip reduction is not emergent; however, a long delay may make the reduction more difficult. Occasionally, a closed reduction of the hip is not possible and an open reduction may be necessary with revision of the malpositioned implants. If a closed reduction of the hip is achieved and the implants are positioned appropriately on the radiographs, a brief period of bed rest (1–2 days) and use of a prefabricated abduction orthosis or hip spica may be used until the soft tissues heal enough to prevent recurrent dislocation (6–12 weeks). Morrey [89] reported that dislocations occuring within 3 months of total hip replacement are treated successfully in this manner two-thirds of the time. Hedlundh *et al.* [90] reported in their series of dislocated hips that only 35% did not go onto recurrent dislocation within a year. Operative correction of an unstable hip replacement has been successful if the

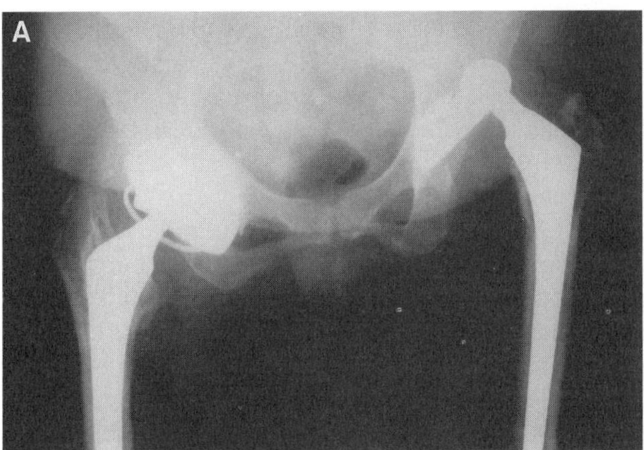

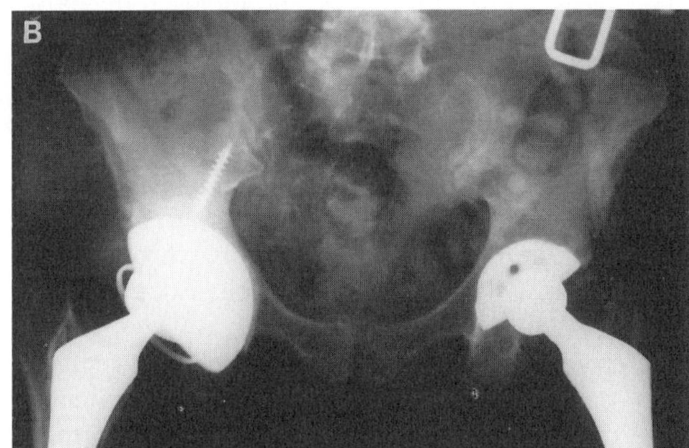

FIGURE 2 Anteroposterior pelvic radiographs of a 66-year-old female with a history of recurrent dislocations on the right hip necessitating a constrained liner who has (A) dislocated her left total hip arthroplasty postoperatively. (B) She underwent a closed reduction of the hip and the radiograph shows the acetabular component malpositioned with inadequate anteversion.

cause has been identified preoperatively and addressed accordingly at the time of surgery [90,91].

Dislocation of the tibiofemoral joint is a very rare complication after total knee replacement; however, patellofemoral dislocation or subluxation is more frequent [92–94]. Strict attention to the surgical technique in restoring anatomic bony alignment and soft tissue tension will minimize the risk of instability (Fig. 3). A tibiofemoral dislocation is most likely to occur in a prosthetic knee with a posterior-stabilized design that is loose in flexion. This knee should be reduced promptly, particularly if there is neurovascular compromise. As with prosthetic hip dislocation, the best results of surgery for knee instability are those in which the cause is identified preoperatively and can be addressed appropriately by realigning the limb, by revising malpositioned components, or by restoring soft tissue balance.

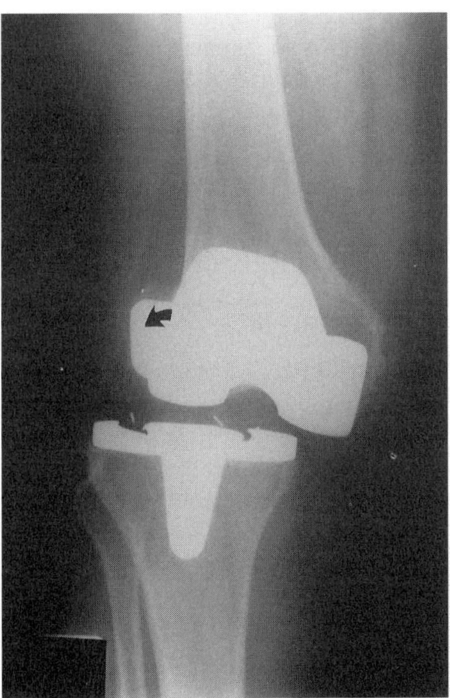

FIGURE 3 Anteroposterior radiograph of a 70-year-old male showing total knee replacement with lateral tibial subluxation and lateral patellar dislocation (arrow) as a result of malpositioning of the components and improper soft tissue balancing.

Instability can occur after shoulder and unconstrained elbow replacement and is caused by soft tissue imbalance, component malposition, muscle deficiency or dysfunction, and bony deficiency [95–97]. The principles of management are similar to the hip and knee and can be successful if the etiology is identified and corrected [98].

Late Complications

STIFFNESS AND HETEROTOPIC OSSIFICATION

Poor joint motion following total knee replacement is a common patient complaint. One of the most important predictors of a stiff joint following prosthetic replacement is a poor preoperative range of motion related to chronic soft tissue contracture [99]. Other etiologic factors include general patient factors such as poor rehabilitation and neurologic disorders (e.g., reflex sympathetic dystrophy, Parkinson's disease) as well as local factors such as mechanical impediments (e.g., osteophytes, cement, heterotopic ossification), soft tissue scarring or arthrofibrosis, component malposition, bony malalignment, soft tissue imbalance, and infection. Appropriate history, physical examination, and radiographs should be evaluated to determine the cause of joint stiffness. If there is mechanical impediment, bony/component malposition, or infection, further surgery will be necessary to address these problems. If the etiology cannot be identified easily, aggressive physical therapy and manipulation under general anesthesia can be performed in the first 6–12 weeks following surgery. Epidural anesthesia and continuous passive motion are effective acutely following manipulation to maintain the range of motion. Persistent stiffness due to soft tissue contracture can be addressed by either arthroscopic or open lysis of adhesions and occasionally revision of the implants.

Heterotopic bone formation around joint replacements occurs commonly, but causes significant pain and limitation of motion in few patients [100]. It occurs most commonly after total hip arthroplasty with an incidence of severe heterotopic ossification causing pain and limited motion in as many as 7% of patients [101] (Fig. 4). Risk factors for heterotopic bone formation include previous heterotopic bone in the ipsilateral or contralateral hip, heterotopic osteoarthritis, and active ankylosing spondylitis. A multitude of other factors have been implicated in the formation of heterotopic ossification and a few of the more common factors cited include males with osteoarthritis, age greater than 60, transtrochanteric and lateral exposures of the hip, revision surgery, and extensive soft tissue stripping. The precise etiology of heterotopic ossification is not well understood, but it is related to the differentiation of primordial mesenchymal cells into osteoprogenitor cells that synthesize bone. The initiation of this process is thought to be related to muscle trauma, subsequently leading to ossification. This process may begin as early as 16 hr postoperatively and peaks at 32 hr [101]. Radiographically, heterotopic bone can be seen at 3–4 weeks and matures up to a year postoperatively.

The prevention of heterotopic ossification, at least in patients with established risk factors, is currently recommended in the form of radiation or nonsteroidal anti-inflammatory medication. Bisphosphonate therapy has not been found to be effective in the prevention or treatment of heterotopic ossification. Irradiation alters the DNA of rapidly dividing cells and presumably prevents the differentiation of pluripotential mesenchymal cells into osteoblasts. Administration of irradiation to the periarticular muscles is currently recommended in one to two fractions totaling 700 to 800 rads between postoperative day 1 and 4 [102,103]. Because irradiation may inhibit bony ingrowth around an uncemented implant, this area should be shielded. NSAID reduce heterotopic ossification presumably through prostaglandin inhibition and dampening of the inflammatory response thought to be associated with this phenomenon. There is some controversy as to the dosage, duration, and choice of NSAID to be administered. Both 650 mg of aspirin administered twice daily for 6 weeks and 25 mg of indomethacin administered three times daily for 2 weeks were effective in the prevention of heterotopic bone formation after hip replacement surgery [104]. Concerns regarding NSAID use include the potential inhibition of bony ingrowth around cementless implants and the added risk of bleeding, especially in those patients taking warfarin for DVT prophylaxis.

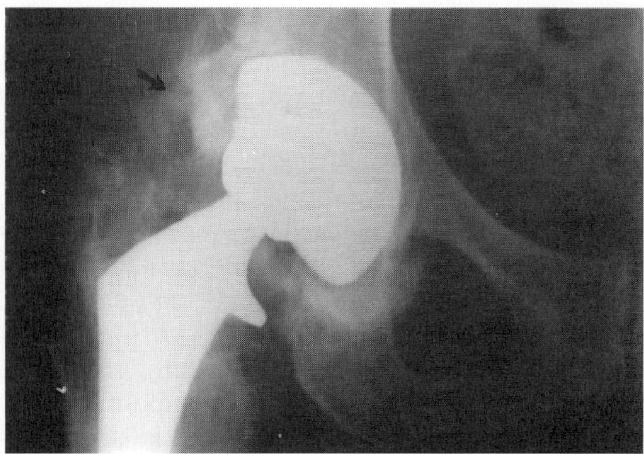

FIGURE 4 An anteroposterior radiograph following routine right total hip replacement illustrating heterotopic ossification in the abductor muscles, causing limitation of hip motion.

Once heterotopic bone is established, surgical excision may be considered in patients having pain and severe restriction of motion. Excision should be delayed until the heterotopic bone is matured and no longer progressing, which is usually beyond 6 months from joint replacement. A cold bone scan and a normal serum alkaline phosphatase have been used to confirm the maturation of heterotopic bone. Surgical excision is technically challenging and vital structures must be protected during the procedure. Successful pain relief and improved range of motion has been reported in a small series of patients following surgical excision and postoperative irradiation [105].

MECHANICAL FAILURE AND OSTEOLYSIS

Mechanical failure following joint replacement can result from implant fatigue or fracture or from loosening of the bone–implant interface. Although more common with earlier designs, fracture of the metallic portion of an implant is rare. When it occurs, it is often at junction points where the implant changes shape or texture or in areas where there is deficient bony support.

Aseptic loosening of the bone–implant interface is the leading cause of late joint replacement failure necessitating revision. A conservative estimate of the aseptic loosening rate of prosthetic replacement necessitating a revision operation is estimated to be less than 10% at 10 years. Osteolysis refers to the resorption of bone that occurs around both cemented and uncemented implants that may be loose. Clinically, it results from both mechanical and biologic factors.

Wear results from implant surface irregularities and materials of different hardness contacting one another and producing debris. Wear-debris generation has been characterized by different modes termed abrasion, adhesion, fatigue, fretting, corrosion, and third-body wear [106,107]. Implant materials such as polyethylene, polymethyl methacrylate, and metal can all produce wear debris that incites a host macrophage response that leads to bone resorption or osteolysis (Fig. 5). The macrophage engulfs particulate debris, resulting in the release of cell mediators and cytokines that resorb bone [108,109]. Retrieval studies from biologically active periprosthetic membranes have implicated polyethylene debris as the major contributor to osteolysis.

A multitude of patient, component, and surgical factors have been shown to contribute to wear and aseptic loosening [110]. Patient factors include increased body weight, activity level, and young age. Component factors include polyethylene thickness $<$6 mm, gamma sterilization of polyethylene in air, long polyethylene shelf-life, type of polyethylene (e.g., Hylamer due to its brittleness), increasing modularity of implants [111], increasing prosthetic constraint, and type of implant used (e.g., metal-backed patella, acetabular shells with screw holes). Surgical factors that increase wear and loosening include malpositioning of the implants (e.g., varus positioning of the hip or knee) and inadequate initial fixation, such as poor or outdated cementing techniques or inadequate fit and fill of an uncemented stem.

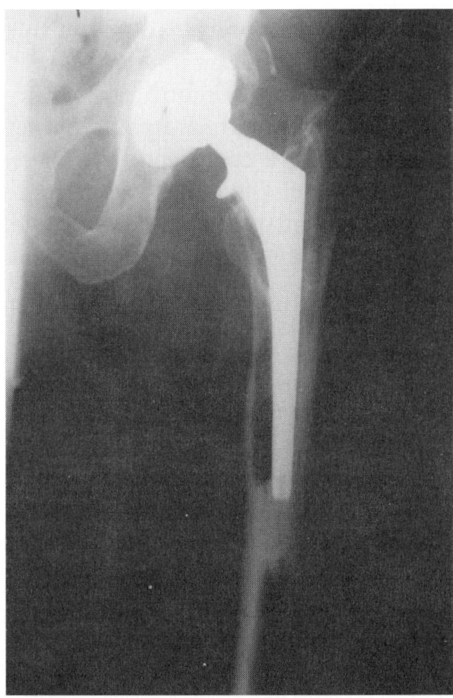

FIGURE 5 An anteroposterior radiograph 7 years following a left total hip replacement showing extensive osteolysis around the femoral component, causing pain and prosthesis loosening.

Diagnosis of a loose implant is confirmed by a history of gradually increasing pain, often exacerbated by activity or with provocation on range-of-motion testing. Radiographs aid in confirming a loose implant as evidenced by subsidence, migration, implant fracture, or progressive radiolucencies at the bone–implant interface. Arthrographic dye tracking in the bone–implant interface is sometimes helpful in diagnosis but has significant false negatives and positives. Nuclear medicine studies can also aid in diagnosis but has the limitation of being nonspecific. Infection should always be considered and ruled out as a cause of implant loosening.

Treatment of a loose implant generally requires surgical revision of the prosthesis to resolve pain and to prevent the increasing chance of catastrophic failure and bone destruction. If a patient is symptomatic and a large osteolytic focus is identified around a well-fixed implant, the current recommendation is to currettage the osteolytic membrane, consider bone grafting the defect, and change the polyethylene liner [112]. Some surgeons find it difficult to achieve adequate exposure of the defect and advocate removal of the component and replacement with a new implant. If the patient is asymptomatic with a large osteolytic defect, management is more controversial. Bisphosphonate therapy has not been approved for use in preventing or delaying the progression of osteolysis, although some effect has been observed in an animal model [113]. Most surgeons will follow the osteolytic defect radiographically every 3 to 6 months and will recommend surgery if the defect progresses, becomes symptomatic, or if wear through to the metal backing is imminent.

LEG LENGTH DISCREPANCY

Leg length inequality is the most common complication of total hip arthroplasty leading to malpractice suits [114]. There is a tendency to lengthen the limb of the prosthetic hip by an average of 1 cm due to the fact that increased length allows greater abductor tension and hip stability [115]. It is estimated that most people can tolerate a leg length discrepancy of 1 to 2 cm without compromising gait and it is estimated that less than 5% of patients would be lengthened enough to require a shoe lift using current surgical techniques [114].

Prevention of limb length inequality involves the careful assessment of gait, true and apparent limb lengths, pelvic obliquity, and femoral length comparison with the knees flexed. Moreover, restoration of the femoral offset is critical in reestablishing abductor tension and in preventing either limb lengthening or instability.

It is also important to compare the clinical length difference with that found on radiographic measurements. Occasionally a scanogram can aid in the investigation of leg length inequality. A discussion regarding patient perception of limb length discrepancy and the possibility of it persisting or requiring a shoe lift postoperatively should be routine. One should account for the effect of adduction and flexion contractures on limb length differences. Most importantly, a preoperative, intraoperative, and postoperative method of assessment of limb lengths should be performed by the surgeon. Preoperative templates from the implant manufacturer are used to estimate the level of femoral neck resection necessary to restore equal leg lengths, which can be measured from the lesser or greater trochanter. Intraoperative methods of assessment include matching up the operative and nonoperative leg, assessing tension or "shuck" in the reduced prosthetic hip, and using markers or Steinmann pins above the acetabulum and distal to the femoral neck with the leg in a standard position prior to femoral neck resection. This last method requires that the measurement be reproduced by the replaced hip in the case of equal preoperative leg lengths.

Most persistent leg length discrepancies may be treated with a shoe lift. Very rarely, a more severe leg length discrepancy requires surgical correction in the form of implant modification with trochanteric advancement or a constrained cup to maintain hip stability or a subtrochanteric osteotomy.

UNDIAGNOSED PAIN

Rarely, there is a patient with persistent pain following total joint replacement for which an etiology is not identified easily. In this situation, a very careful history must be performed to characterize the severity, location, quality, timing, and precipitating and relieving factors surrounding the pain. The patient's expectations following joint replacement should be discussed. Previous surgery, complications, and rehabilitation as well as comorbid illness and infection should be investigated. The level of disability with activities of daily living, social, psychiatric, and medication history should be obtained. Original radiographs prior to surgery should be reviewed and suspicion should be raised if the arthritic change was mild in proportion to the patient's pain preoperatively. Occult infection, instability, wear and loosening, arthrofibrosis, stress fracture, and vascular, muscle, or neurologic disorders should all be entertained in the etiology of undiagnosed pain.

A careful physical examination should be performed on the joint that has been replaced, as well as the surrounding joints, spine, and other organ systems as pain occasionally may be referred. For example, a fourth lumbar radiculopathy can easily mimic pain around a total knee replacement. Systematic assessment of gait, limb alignment, skin status, temperature, tenderness, swelling, range of motion, stability, muscle strength, and neurovascular status should be performed.

Radiographs should initially be performed to verify component position and to rule out malalignment, osteolysis, loosening, and fracture. Occasionally, a dynamic problem such as instability can be verified under fluoroscopy or with stress view radiographs. Nuclear medicine scans can be helpful in identifying occult loosening, stress fracture, and infection, remembering that they are frequently hot in a normal joint replacement up to a year postoperatively [116]. Arthrography has been used to identify dye tracking at the bone–prosthesis interface following loosening of a joint replacement, but the accuracy of this test is poor. Magnetic resonance imaging (MRI) has not been used with much frequency in the investigation of undiagnosed pain because of the metal artifact that obscures interpretation. Newer MRI techniques enable excellent visualization around metal implants, which may expand its indications for the diagnosis of unidentified pain. Vascular studies and consultation should be considered in patients with poor peripheral circulation and symptoms of vascular claudication.

Reflex sympathetic dystrophy is an uncommon cause of undiagnosed pain and usually presents as pain out of proportion to other findings [117]. Quite often, these patients have poor pain control postoperatively and are slow to rehabilitate and regain joint motion. Cutaneous hypersensitivity and temperature changes consistent with sympathetic stimulation are noted in the affected limb. Diagnosis may be confirmed by pain relief with sympathetic blockade. The key to successful treatment is early recognition and institution of aggressive physical therapy combined with sympathetic blockade.

Arthroscopic surgery has been used for both diagnostic and therapeutic purposes following undiagnosed pain and total knee replacement [118–120]. Retained foreign material or soft tissue, traumatic hemarthrosis, arthrofibrosis, patellar clunk syndrome, and patellar maltracking are some of the unidentified causes of pain that may be addressed at the time of arthroscopic surgery. Arthroscopy can also be useful in diagnosing polyethylene wear [118,121].

Embarking on surgery for undiagnosed pain often results in failed surgery and persistent pain [122]. A systematic approach must be used to aid in diagnosis. Failing this, a second physician for consultation is advised. A specific diagnosis must be obtained prior to considering surgical intervention.

Special Problems

PATELLOFEMORAL COMPLICATIONS AND KNEE ARTHROPLASTY

Patellofemoral problems, including instability, patella fracture, component loosening and failure, patellar clunk syndrome, and rupture of the extensor mechanism after total knee replacement, comprise up to 50% of the surgical complications [80,123]. The issue of whether to resurface the patella following routine total knee arthroplasty is controversial [124–126]. One approach is to reserve nonresurfacing for patients with noninflammatory arthritis, minimal chondromalacia, normal patellar tracking, patellar thickness greater than 15 mm, minimal osteophytes, and young age.

As mentioned previously, patellofemoral instability is very dependent on the surgical technique and often represents poor restoration of bony alignment or soft tissue balance. Results of isolated patellar component revision have been poor, and treatment must adequately address the underlying cause [127].

Patella fracture is an uncommon complication following total knee arthroplasty, but common risk factors include osteopenia, avascular necrosis of the patella, trauma, excessive patellar resection, patellar malalignment, and component design [80]. As with periprosthetic fractures elsewhere, management depends on quality of the bone, location of the fracture, and whether the component is loose. Loose components should be revised if bone stock permits and other fractures may be managed nonoperatively if displaced minimally or by conventional means of open reduction and internal fixation.

Patellar failure has primarily been noted following the use of metal-backed designs, which are no longer used by most surgeons [128]. Risk factors for failure of the patellar component include obesity, increased postoperative knee flexion beyond 115°, increased activity, male gender, component oversizing, and malpositioning [128–130]. Clinical presentation includes pain, swelling, and crepitus aggravated particularly by stair climbing, squatting, or rising from a chair. Once a loose prosthesis has been confirmed, revision surgery is recommended.

Patellar clunk syndrome results from a nodule of fibrous scar tissue that develops at the superior pole of the patella and inferior quadriceps junction (Fig. 6). As the knee moves from flexion to extension at 30–45°, the nodule gets caught in the intercondylar notch of the femoral prosthesis and produces a painful "clunk" as it exits the notch. This phenomenon occurs primarily but not exclusively following posterior-stabilized total knee designs [131]. It is prudent to remove any redundant tissue in this area prior to closure of the knee replacement. Once a painful, persistent "clunk" is established, the nodule can be treated successfully by arthroscopic or open debridement and occasionally requires patellar component revision [131].

Extensor mechanism disruption is a rare but disabling complication following total knee replacement because of the difficulty with reconstruction. Reported incidence is 0.17% in one series of 8288 procedures [132]. It often occurs during exposure of a stiff or scarred knee, following excessive patellar resection, and secondary to devascularization of the patellar ligament or component impingement. When it occurs postoperatively, a large extensor lag will be noted on physical examination. Treatment includes primary repair, which often leads to failure versus reconstruction with tendon augmentation (e.g., semitendonosis) or extensor mechanism allograft [133].

LIGAMENT OR MUSCLE DEFICIENCY

The results of prosthetic replacement are compromised severely in the presence of ligament or muscle deficiency. In total shoulder arthroplasty, severe rotator cuff arthropathy is treated with a large hemiarthroplasty; however, the results are disappointing. Deltoid paresis is a relative contraindication to shoulder arthroplasty. Similarly, triceps dysfunction compromises total elbow arthroplasty severely. Abductor dysfunction in total hip arthroplasty leaves patients with a severe Trendelenburg lurch compromising function. This is not infrequently seen in the take down of a previously arthrodesed hip. Extensor mechanism incompetence is a relative contraindication to total knee replacement; however, allograft reconstruction has been performed with some success, provided that the quadriceps muscles are functioning. Ligament deficiency primarily leads to instability of the prosthetic joint replacement but some of this may be addressed by more constrained implants or by allograft reconstruction in some rare cases.

COMPLICATIONS AND REVISION PROSTHETIC REPLACEMENT

Virtually every complication occurs with higher frequency following repeat joint replacement. Quite often, patients are older and more medically ill. The soft tissues around the replaced joint are often scarred and more poorly vascularized and the bone is often more deficient (Fig. 7). Surgical reconstruction is often more technically difficult with increased surgical time and blood loss than primary joint replacement. With an increased aging population and with the expanding indications for pros-

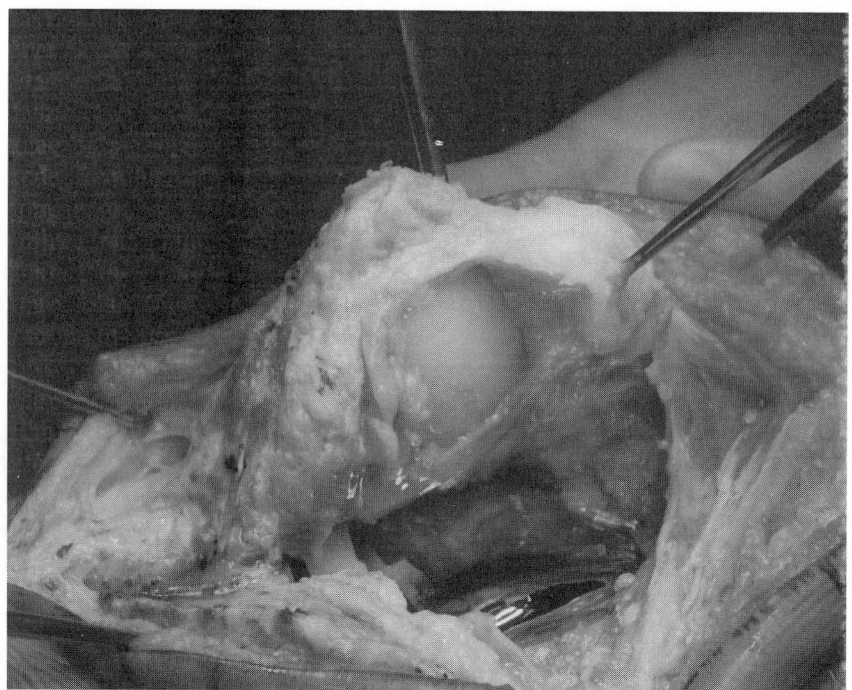

FIGURE 6 An intraoperative view of scar tissue above the superior pole of the patella responsible for patellar "clunk" following a posterior stabilized total knee arthroplasty.

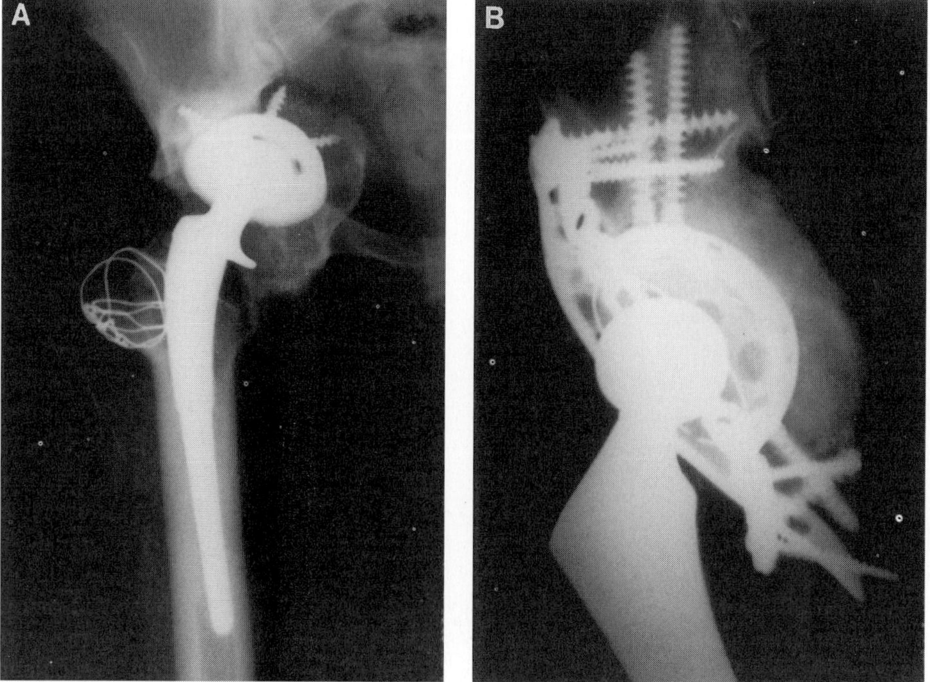

FIGURE 7 (A) An anteroposterior radiograph of a hip showing acetabular protrusio of a hip prosthesis due to a progressive loss of bony support. (B) An anteroposterior radiograph showing revision of acetabular bony deficiency with bone graft, a reconstruction ring, and plates and screws.

thetic joint replacement in younger patients, there will be an increasing need for revision surgery.

SUMMARY

Improved implant designs, patient selection, preoperative investigation, and surgical technique have all played a major role in the current success of total joint replacement. Nevertheless, complications continue to occur both early and late following surgery. Age-related systemic disease and specific musculoskeletal disease add to the perioperative surgical risk and technical demands of surgery as well as the postoperative rehabilitation. Long-term, well-designed clinical studies are necessary to determine the success rates, risk factors, complications, and adjunctive treatments that will optimize the management of joint disease in the aged. Unfortunately, joint replacement technology is evolving prior to long-term testing of new designs and techniques, making it difficult to draw conclusions about the status of some joint replacements being performed today.

Currently, little is known about the effects of physiological factors in the aging population such as nutrition, osteoporosis, and estrogen replacement therapy, for example, on the long-term success of joint replacement. Development of relevant experimental models and increased collaborations among orthopedists, physicians, and basic scientists are needed to resolve these issues that affect the aging skeleton.

Acknowledgment

Karen Aneshansley is gratefully appreciated for her skillful assistance in the preparation of this chapter.

References

1. Schulte, K. R., Callaghan, J. J., Kelley, S. S., and Johnston, R. C. The outcome of Charnley total hip arthroplasty with cement after a minimum twenty-year follow-up: The results of one surgeon. *J. Bone Joint Surg.* **75A,** 961–975 (1993).
2. Mulroy, R. D., Jr., and Harris, W. H. The effect of improved cementing techniques on component loosening in total hip replacement. *J. Bone Joint Surg.* **72B,** 757 (1990).
3. Engh, C. A., Jr., Culpepper, W. J., and Engh, C. A. Long-term results of use of the anatomic medullary locking prosthesis in total hip arthroplasty. *J. Bone Joint Surg.* **79A,** 177–184 (1997).
4. Rand, J. A., and Ilstrup, D. M. Survivorship analysis of total knee arthroplasty. *J. Bone Joint Surg.* **73A,** 397–409 (1991).
5. Wirth, M. A., and Rockwood, C. A., Jr. Complications of shoulder arthroplasty. *Clin Orthop.* **307,** 47–69 (1994).
6. Morrey, B. F., and Adams, R. A. Semiconstrained arthroplasty for the treatment of rheumatoid arthritis of the elbow. *J. Bone Joint Surg.* **74A,** 479–490 (1992).
7. Goldman, L. Cardiac risks and complications of noncardiac surgery. *Ann. Intern. Med.* **98,** 504–513 (1983).
8. Jackson, M. C. V. Preoperative pulmonary evaluation. *Arch. Intern. Med.* **148,** 2120–2127 (1988).
9. Burke, J. F., Jr., and Francos, G. C. Surgery in the patient with acute or chronic renal failure. *Med. Clin. North Am.* **71,** 489–497 (1987).
10. Lachiewicz, P. F. Total joint replacement in special medical conditions. *In* "Orthopaedic Knowledge Update: Hip and Knee Reconstruction" (J. J. Callaghan *et al.,* ed.), pp. 79–86. American Academy of Orthopaedic Surgeons, Rosemont, IL, 1995.
11. Friedman, L. S., and Maddrey, W. C. Surgery in the patient with liver disease. *Med. Clin. North Am.* **71,** 453–476 (1987).
12. England, S. P., Stern, S. H., Insall, J. N., and Windsor, R. E. Total knee arthroplasty in diabetes mellitus. *Clin. Orthop.* **260,** 130–134 (1990).
13. Moeckel, B., Huo, M. H., Salvati, E. A., and Pellicci, P. M. Total hip arthroplasty in patients with diabetes mellitus. *J. Arthroplasty.* **8,** 279–284 (1993).
14. Nevitt, M. C., Lane, N. E., Scott, J. C., Hochberg, M. C., Pressman, A. R., Genant, H. K., and Cummings, S. R. Radiographic osteoarthritis of the hip and bone mineral density. The study of osteoporotic fractures research group. *Arthritis Rheum.* **38,** 907–916 (1995).
15. Nevitt, M. C., Cummings, S. R., Lane, N. E., Hochberg, M. C., Scott, J. C., Pressman, A. R., Genant, H. K., and Cauley, J. A. Association of estrogen replacement therapy with the risk of osteoarthritis of the hip in elderly white women. Study of Osteoporotic Fractures Research Group. *Arch. Intern. Med.* **156,** 2073–2080 (1996).
16. Taylor, M. M., Meyers, M. H., and Harvey, J. P., Jr. Intraoperative femur fractures during total hip replacement. *Clin Orthop.* **137,** 96–103 (1978).
17. Carlsson, A. S., and Nilsson, B. E. The relationship of bone mass and loosening of the femoral component in total hip replacement. *Acta Orthop. Scand.* **51,** 285–288 (1980).
18. Creamer, P., and Hochberg, M. C. Osteoarthritis. *Lancet* **350,** 503–508 (1997).
19. Ling, S. M., and Bathon, J. M. Osteoarthritis in older adults. *J. Am. Geriatr. Soc.* **46,** 216–225 (1998).
20. Arnett, F. C., and Committee. The 1987 revised ARA criteria for classification of rheumatoid arthritis. *Arthritis Rheum.* **31,** 315 (1988).
21. MacKenzie, C. R., and Sharrock, N. E. Perioperative medical considerations in patients with rheumatoid arthritis. *Rheum. Dis. Clin. North. Am.* **24,** 1–17 (1998).
22. Wilson, M. G., Kelley, K., and Thornhill, T. S. Infection as a complication of total knee-replacement arthroplasty: Risk factors and treatment in sixty-seven cases. *J. Bone Joint Surg.* **72A,** 878–883 (1990).
23. Bridges, S. L., Jr., and Moreland, L. W. Perioperative use of methotrexate in patients with rheumatoid arthritis undergoing orthopedic surgery. *Rheum. Dis. Clin. North Am.* **23,** 981–993 (1998).
24. Sledge, C. B., Ruddy, S., Harris, E. D., Jr., and Kelley, W. N., "Arthritis Surgery," Chaps. 43 and 44, pp. 780–817. Saunders, Philadelphia, 1994.
25. Soudry, M., Binazzi, R., Johanson, N. A., Bullough, P. G., and Insall, J. N. Total knee arthroplasty in Charcot and Charcot-like joints. *Clin. Orthop.* **208,** 199–204 (1986).
26. Yoshino, S., Fujimori, J., Kajino, A., Kiowa, M., and Uchida, S. Total knee arthroplasty in Charcot's joint. *J. Arthroplasty.* **8,** 335–340 (1993).

27. Staeheli, J. W., Frassica, F. J., and Sim, F. H. Prosthetic replacement of the femoral head for fracture of the femoral neck in patients who have Parkinson disease. *J. Bone Joint Surg.* **70A,** 565–568 (1988).
28. Oni, O. O., and MacKenney, R. P. Total knee replacement in patients with Parkinson's disease. *J. Bone Joint Surg.* **67A,** 424–425 (1985).
29. Buly, R. L., Huo, M., Root, L., Binzer, T., and Wilson, P. D., Jr. Total hip arthroplasty in cerebral palsy. *Clin. Orthop.* **296,** 148–153 (1993).
30. Root, L., Goss, J. R., and Mendes, J. The treatment of the painful hip in cerebral palsy by total hip replacement or hip arthrodesis. *J. Bone Joint Surg.* **68A,** 590–598 (1986).
31. Patterson, B. M., and Insall, J. N. Surgical management of gonarthrosis in patients with poliomyelitis. *J. Arthroplasty* **7(Suppl.),** 419–426 (1992).
32. McDonald, D. J., and Sim, F. H. Total hip arthroplasty in Paget's disease. *J. Bone Joint Surg.* **69A,** 766–772 (1987).
33. Merkow, R. L., Pellicci, P. M., Hely, D. P., and Salvati, E. A. Total hip replacement for Paget's disease of the hip. *J. Bone Joint Surg.* **66A,** 752–758 (1984).
34. Gabel, G. T., Rand, J. A., and Sim, F. H. Total knee arthroplasty for osteoarthritis in patients who have Paget's disease of bone at the knee. *J. Bone Joint Surg.* **73A,** 739–744 (1991).
35. Walker, L. G., and Sledge, C. B. Total hip arthroplasty in ankylosing spondylitis. *Clin. Orthop.* **262,** 198–204 (1991).
36. Hyderally, H. Anesthetic problems in joint replacement surgery. *Mt. Sinai J. Med.* **65,** 313–316 (1987).
37. Manolio, T. A., Beattie, C., Christopherson, R., and Pearson, T. A. Regional versus general anesthesia in high-risk surgical patients: the need for a clinical trial. *J. Clin. Anesth.* **1,** 414–421 (1989).
38. Kearon, C., and Hirsh, J. Management of anticoagulation before and after elective surgery. *N. Engl. J. Med.* **336,** 1506–1511 (1997).
39. Consensus conference. Perioperative red blood cell transfusion. *JAMA* **260,** 2700–2703 (1988).
40. Lemos, M. J., and Healy, W. L. Current concepts review: Blood transfusion in Orthopaedic operations. *J. Bone Joint Surg.* **78A,** 1260–1270 (1996).
41. Bierbaum, B. E., Galante, J. O., Rubash, H. E., Tooms, R. E., and Welch, R. B., "Prediction of Red Cell Transfusion in Orthopaedic Surgery," p. 251 Presented AAOS 65th annual meeting, 1998.
42. Friedman, R. J., Zimlich, R. H., Butler, J., and Schutte, H. D., Jr., "Preoperative Hemoglobin as a Predictor of Transfusion Risk in Total Hip and Knee Arthroplasty," p. 252 Presented AAOS 65th annual meeting, 1998.
43. Hatzidakis, A. M., Mendlick, R. M., McKillop, T., Reddy, R. R., and Garvin, K. L., "The Effect of Preoperative Autologous Donation and Other Factors on the Frequency of Transfusion after Total Joint Arthroplasty," p. 252. Presented AAOS 65th annual meeting, 1998.
44. Sculco, T. P. Blood management in Orthopaedic surgery. *Am. J. Surg.* **170,** 60S–63S (1995).
45. Lotke, P. A., Faralli, V. J., Orenstein, E. M., and Ecker, M. L. Blood loss after total knee replacement. Effects of tourniquet release and continuous passive motion. *J. Bone Joint Surg.* **73A,** 1037–1040 (1991).
46. Beer, K. J., Lombardi, A. B., Mallory, T. H., and Vaughn, B. K. The efficacy of suction drains after routine total joint arthroplasty. *J. Bone Joint Surg.* **73A,** 584–587 (1991).
47. Ritter, M. A., Keating, E. M., and Faris, P. M. Closed wound drainage in total hip or total knee replacement. *J. Bone Joint Surg.* **76A,** 35–38 (1994).
48. Lewallen, D. G., and Ereth, M. H. Intraoperative mortality. *In* "Reconstructive Surgery of the Joints" (B. F., Morrey, ed.), 2nd Ed., Vol. 1, pp. 197–205. Churchill Livingstone, New York.
49. Levy, D. The fat embolism syndrome: A review. *Clin. Orthop.* **26,** 281–286 (1990).
50. Monto, R. R., Garcia, J., and Callaghan, J. J. Fatal fat embolism following total condylar knee arthroplasty. *J. Arthroplasty* **5,** 291–299 (1990).
51. Gurd, A. R. Fat embolism: an aid to diagnosis. *J. Bone Joint Surg.* **52B,** 732–737 (1970).
52. Schonfeld, S. A., Ploysongsang, Y., Dilisio, R., Crissman, J. D., Miller, E., Hammerschmidt, D. E., and Jacob, H. S. Fat embolism prophylaxis with corticosteroids. A prospective study in high-risk patients. *Ann. Intern. Med.* **99,** 438–443 (1983).
53. Lindeque, B. G. P., Schoeman, H. S., Dommisse, G. F., Boeyens, M. C., and Vlok, A. L. Fat embolism and the fat embolism syndrome: A double-blind therapeutic study. *J. Bone Joint Surg.* **69B,** 128–131 (1987).
54. Mauerhan, D. R., Nelson, C. L., Smith, D. L., Fitzgerald, R. H., Jr., Slama, T. G., Petty, R. W., Jones, R. E., and Evans, R. P. Prophylaxis against infection in total joint arthroplasty. *J. Bone Joint Surg.* **76A,** 39–45 (1994).
55. Johnson, J. A., Christie, M. J., Sandler, M. P., Parks, P. F., Homra, L., and Kaye, J. J. Detection of occult infection following total joint arthroplasty using sequential technetium-99m HDP bone scintigraphy and indium-111 WBC imaging. *J. Nuclear Med.* **29,** 1347–1353 (1988).
56. Thornhill, T. S. Total knee infection. *In* "Orthopaedic Knowledge Update: Hip and Knee Reconstruction" (J. J. Callaghan *et al.,* eds.), pp. 297–300. American Academy of Orthopaedic Surgeons, Rosemont, IL, 1995.
57. Windsor, R. E., Insall, J. N., Urs, W. K., Miller, D. V., and Brause, B. D. Two-stage reimplantation for the salvage of total knee arthroplasty complicated by infection. *J. Bone Joint Surg.* **72A,** 272–278 (1990).
58. Paiement, G. D., and Green, H. Thromboembolic disease in hip and knee replacement patients. *In* "Orthopaedic Knowledge Update: Hip and Knee Reconstruction" (J. J. Callaghan *et al.,* eds.), pp. 1–7. American Academy of Orthopaedic Surgeons, Rosemont, IL, 1995.
59. Oishi, C. S., Grady-Benson, J. C., Otis, S. M., Colwell, C. W., Jr., and Walker, R. H. The clinical course of distal deep venous thrombosis after total hip and total knee arthroplasty, as determined with duplex ultrasonography. *J. Bone Joint Surg.* **76A,** 1658–1663 (1994).
60. Pellegrini, V. D., Jr., Clement, D., Lush-Ehmann, C., Keller, G. S., and Evarts, C. M. The John Charnley Award. Natural history of thromboembolic disease after total hip arthroplasty. *Clin. Orthop.* **333,** 27–40 (1996).
61. Dalldorf, P. G., Perkins, F. M., Totterman, S., and Pellegrini, V. D., Jr. Deep venous thrombosis following total hip arthroplasty. *J. Arthroplasty* **9,** 611–616 (1994).
62. Fahmy, N. R., and Patel, D. G. Hemostatic changes and postoperative deep-vein thrombosis associated with use of a pneumatic tourniquet. *J. Bone Joint Surg.* **63A,** 461–465 (1981).
63. Colwell, C. W., Jr., Spiro, T. E., Trowbridge, A. A., Morris, B. A., Kwaan, H. C., Blaha, J. D., Comerota, A. J., and Skoutakis, V. A. Use of Enoxaparin, a low-molecular-weight heparin, and unfractionated heparin for the prevention of deep venous thrombosis after elective hip replacement. *J. Bone Joint Surg.* **76A,** 3–14 (1994).
64. Leclerc, J. R., Geerts, W. H., Desjardins, L., Jobin, F., Laroche, F., Delorme, F., Haviernick, S., Atkinson, S., and Bourgouin, J. Prevention of deep vein thrombosis after major knee surgery—A

randomized, double-blind trial comparing a low molecular weight heparin fragment (Enoxaparin) to placebo. *Thromb. Haemost.* **67,** 417–423 (1992).
65. RD Heparin Arthroplasty Group. RD heparin compared with warfarin for prevention of venous thromboembolic disease following total hip or knee arthroplasty. *J. Bone Joint Surg.* **76A,** 1174–1185 (1994).
66. Mont, M. A., Dellon, A. L., Chen, F., Hungerford, M. W., Krackow, K. A., and Hungerford, D. S. The operative treatment of peroneal nerve palsy. *J. Bone Joint Surg.* **78A,** 863–869 (1996).
67. Lewallen, D. G. Neurovascular injury associated with hip arthroplasty. *J. Bone Joint Surg.* **79A,** 1870–1880 (1997).
68. Knutson, K., Leden, I., Sturfelt, G., Rosen, I., and Lidgren, L. Nerve palsy after knee arthroplasty in patients with rheumatoid arthritis. *Scand. J. Rheumatol.* **12,** 201–205 (1983).
69. Rose, H. A., Hood, R. W., Otis, J. C., Ranawat, C. S., and Insall, J. N. Peroneal-nerve palsy following total knee arthroplasty. *J. Bone Joint Surg.* **64A,** 347–351 (1982).
70. Johanson, N. A., Pellicci, P. M., Tsairis, P., and Salvati, E. A. Nerve injury in total hip arthroplasty. *Clin. Orthop.* **179,** 214–222 (1983).
71. Edwards, B. N., Tullos, H. S., and Noble, P. C. Contributory factors and etiology of sciatic nerve palsy in total hip arthroplasty. *Clin. Orthop.* **218,** 136–141 (1987).
72. Simmons, C., Jr., Izant, T. H., Rothman, R. H., Booth, R. E., Jr., and Balderston, R. A. Femoral neuropathy following total hip arthroplasty. Anatomic study, case reports, and literature review. *J. Arthroplasty* **6(Suppl.)** S57–S66 (1991).
73. Fleming, R. E., Jr., Michelsen, C. B., and Stinchfield, F. E. Sciatic paralysis. *J. Bone Joint Surg.* **61A,** 37–39 (1979).
74. Mallory, T. H. Sciatic nerve entrapment secondary to trochanteric wiring following total hip arthroplasty. A case report. *Clin. Orthop.* **180,** 198–200 (1983).
75. Oleksak, M., and Edge, A. J. Compression of the sciatic nerve by methylmethacrylate cement after total hip replacement. *J. Bone Joint Surg.* **74B,** 729–730 (1992).
76. Siliski, J. M., and Scott, R. D. Obturator-nerve palsy resulting from intrapelvic extrusion of cement during total hip replacement. *J. Bone Joint Surg.* **67A,** 1225–1228 (1985).
77. Wasielewski, R. C., Cooperstein, L. A., Kruger, M. P., and Rubash, H. E. Acetabular anatomy and the transacetabular fixation of screws in total hip arthroplasty. *J. Bone Joint Surg.* **72A,** 501–508 (1990).
78. Nachbur, B., Meyer, R. P., Verkkala, K., and Zürcher, R. The mechanisms of severe arterial injury in surgery of the hip joint. *Clin. Orthop.* **141,** 122–133 (1979).
79. Calligaro, K. D., DeLaurentis, D. A., Booth, R. E., Rothman, R. H., Savarese, R. P., and Dougherty, M. J. Acute arterial thrombosis associated with total knee arthroplasty. *J. Vasc. Surg.* **20,** 927–932 (1994).
80. Ayers, D. C., Dennis, D. A., Johanson, N. A., and Pellegrini, V. D., Jr. Common complications of total knee arthroplasty. *J. Bone Joint Surg.* **79A,** 278–311 (1997).
81. Lewallen, D. G., and Berry, D. J. Periprosthetic fracture of the femur after total hip arthroplasty. *J. Bone Joint Surg.* **79A,** 1881–1890 (1997).
82. Culp, R. W., Schmidt, R. G., Hanks, G., Mak, A., Esterhai, J. L., Jr., and Heppenstall, R. B. Supracondylar fracture of the femur following prosthetic knee arthroplasty. *Clin Orthop.* **222,** 212–222 (1987).
83. Aaron, R. K., and Scott, R. D. Supracondylar fracture of the femur after total knee arthroplasty. *Clin. Orthop.* **219,** 136–139 (1987).
84. Ritter, M. A., Faris, P. M., and Keating, E. M. Anterior femoral notching and ipsilateral supracondylar femur fracture in total knee arthroplasty. *J. Arthroplasty* **3,** 185–187 (1988).
85. Duncan, C. P., and Masri, B. A. Fractures of the femur after hip replacement. *Instr. Course Lect.* **44,** 293–304 (1995).
86. DiGioia, A. M., III, and Rubash, H. E. Periprosthetic fractures of the femur after total knee arthroplasty. A literature review and treatment algorithm. *Clin. Orthop.* **271,** 135–142 (1991).
87. Ekelund, A., Rydell, N., and Nilsson, O. S. Total hip arthroplasty in patients 80 years of age and older. *Clin. Orthop.* **281,** 101–106 (1992).
88. Hedlundh, U., Ahnfelt, L., Hybbinette, C. H., Weckstrom, J., and Fredin, H. Surgical experience related to dislocations after total hip arthroplasty. *J. Bone Joint Surg.* **78,** 206–209 (1996).
89. Morrey, B. F. Difficult complications after hip joint replacement. *Clin Orthop.* **344,** 179–187 (1997).
90. Hedlundh, U., Sanzen, L., and Fredin, H. The prognosis and treatment of dislocated total hip arthroplasties with a 22 mm head. *J. Bone Joint Surg.* **79B,** 374–378 (1997).
91. Daly, P. J., and Morrey, B. F. Operative correction of an unstable total hip arthroplasty. *Bone Joint Surg.* **74A,** 1334–1342 (1992).
92. Sharkey, P. F., Hozack, W. J., Booth, R. E., Balderston, R. A., and Rothman, R. H. Posterior dislocation of total knee arthroplasty. *Clin. Orthop.* **278,** 128–133 (1992).
93. Cameron, H. U., and Fedorkow, D. M. The patella in total knee arthroplasty. *Clin. Orthop.* **165,** 197–199 (1982).
94. Kirk, P., Rorabeck, C. H., Bourne, R. B., Burkart, B., and Nott, L. Management of recurrent dislocation of the patella following total knee arthroplasty. *J. Arthroplasty* **7,** 229–233 (1992).
95. Connor, P. M., and D'Alessandro, D. F. Inflammatory arthritis of the shoulder. *In* "Orthopaedic Knowledge Update: Shoulder and Elbow" (T. R. Norris, ed.), pp. 215–240. American Academy of Orthopaedic Surgeons, Rosemont, IL, 1997.
96. Morrey, B. F. Complications of elbow replacement surgery. *In* "The Elbow and Its Disorders" (B. F. Morrey, ed.), 2nd Ed., pp. 665–675. Saunders, Philadelphia, 1993.
97. Ewald, F. C., Simmons, E. D., Jr., Sullivan, J. A., Thomas, W. H., Scott, R. D., Poss, R., Thornhill, T. S., and Sledge, C. B. Capitellocondylar total elbow replacement in rheumatoid arthritis. Long-term results. *J. Bone Joint Surg.* **75A,** 498–507 (1993).
98. Moeckel, B. H., Altchek, D. W., Warren, R. F., Wickiewicz, T. L., and Dines, D. M. Instability of the shoulder after arthroplasty. *J. Bone Joint Surg.* **75A,** 492–497 (1993).
99. Anouchi, Y. S., McShane, M., Kelly, F., Jr., Elting, J., and Stiehl, J. Range of motion in total knee replacement. *Clin. Orthop.* **331,** 87–92 (1996).
100. Thomas, B. J. Heterotopic bone formation after total hip arthroplasty. *Orthop. Clin. North Am.* **23,** 347–358 (1992).
101. Vaughn, B. K. Other complications of total hip arthroplasty. *In* "Orthopaedic Knowledge Update: Hip and Knee Reconstruction" (J. J. Callaghan *et al.,* Eds.), pp. 163–170. American Academy of Orthopaedic Surgeons, Rosemont, IL, 1995.
102. Pellegrini, V. D., Konski, A. A., Gastel, J. A., Rubin, P., and Evarts, C. M. Prevention of heterotopic ossification with irradiation after total hip arthroplasty. *J. Bone Joint Surg.* **74A,** 186–200 (1992).
103. Maloney, W. J., Jasty, M., Willett, C., Mulroy, R. D., Jr., and Harris, W. H. Prophylaxis for heterotopic bone formation after total hip arthroplasty using low-dose radiation in high-risk patients. *Clin. Orthop.* **280,** 230–234 (1992).
104. Kjaersgaard-Anderson, P., and Ritter, M. A. Short-term treatment with nonsteroidal anti-inflammatory medications to prevent heterotopic bone formation after total hip arthroplasty. *Clin. Orthop.* **279,** 157–162 (1992).

105. Warren, S. B., and Brooker, A. F. Excision of heterotopic bone followed by irradiation after total hip arthroplasty. *J. Bone Joint Surg.* **74A,** 201–210 (1992).
106. Litsky, A. S., and Spector, M. Biomaterials. *In* "Orthopaedic Basic Science" (S. R. Simon, ed.), pp. 447–486. American Academy of Orthopaedic Surgeons, IL, 1994.
107. Friedman, R. J., Black, J., Galante, J. O., Jacobs, J. J., and Skinner, H. B. Current concepts in orthopaedic biomaterials and implant fixation. *Instr. Course Lect.* **43,** 233–255 (1994).
108. Chiba, J., Rubash, J. E., Kim, K. J., and Iwaki, Y. The characterization of cytokines in the interface tissue obtained from failed cementless total hip arthroplasty with and without femoral osteolysis. *Clin. Orthop.* **300,** 304–312 (1994).
109. Thornhill, T. S., Ozuna, R. M., Shortkroff, S., Keller, K., Sledge, C. B., and Spector, M. Biochemical and histological evaluation of the synovial-like tissue around failed (loose) total joint replacement prostheses in human subjects and a canine model. *Biomaterials* **11,** 69–72 (1990).
110. Jacobs, J. J., Shanbhag, A., Glant, T. T., Black, J., and Galante, J. O. Wear debris in total joint replacements. *J. Am. Acad. Orthop. Surg.* **4(2),** 212–220 (1994).
111. Barrack, R. L. Modularity of prosthetic implants. *J. Am. Acad. Orthop. Surg.* **2(1),** 16–25 (1994).
112. Maloney, W. J., Herzwurm, P., Paprosky, W., Rubash, H. E., and Engh, C. A. Treatment of pelvic osteolysis associated with a stable acetabular component inserted without cement as part of a total hip replacement. *J. Bone Joint Surg.* **79A,** 1628–1634 (1997).
113. Shanbhag, A. S., Hasselman, C. T., and Rubash, H. E. The John Charnley Award. Inhibition of wear debris mediated osteolysis in a canine total hip arthroplasty model. *Clin. Orthop.* **344,** 33–43 (1997).
114. Trousdale, R. T., and Morrey, B. F. Leg length inequality. *in* "Reconstructive Surgery of the Joints" (B. F. Morrey, ed.), 2nd Ed., Vol. 2, pp. 1297–1306. Churchill Livingstone, New York, 1996.
115. Abraham, W. D., and Dimon, J. H., III. Leg length discrepancy in total hip arthroplasty. *Orthop. Clin. North Am.* **23,** 201–209 (1992).
116. Hunter, J. C., Hattner, R. S., Murray, W. R., and Genant, H. K. Loosening of the total knee arthroplasty: Detection by radionuclide bone scanning. *Am. J. Roentgenol.* **135,** 131–136 (1980).
117. Katz, M. M., Hungerford, D. S., Krackow K. A., and Lennox, D. W. Reflex sympathetic dystrophy as a cause of poor results after total knee arthroplasty. *J. Arthroplasty.* **1,** 117–124 (1986).
118. Diduch, D. R., Scuderi, G. R., Scott, W. N., Insall, J. N., and Kelly, M. A. The efficacy of arthroscopy following total knee replacement. *Arthroscopy* **13,** 166–171 (1997).
119. Bocell, J. R., Thorpe, C. D., and Tullos, H. S. Arthroscopic treatment of symptomatic total knee arthroplasty. *Clin. Orthop.* **271,** 125–134 (1991).
120. Jerosch, J., Schroder, M., Steinbeck, J., and Halm, H. Arthroscopy in patients with knee endoprostheses. *Knee Surg. Sports Traumatol. Arthrosc.* **1,** 218–222 (1993).
121. Mintz, L., Tsao, A. K., McCrae, C. R., Stulberg, S. D., and Wright, T. The arthroscopic evaluation and characteristics of severe polyethylene wear in total knee arthroplasty. *Clin Orthop.* **273,** 215–222 (1991).
122. Jacobs, M. A., Hungerford, D. S., Krackow, K. A., and Lennox D. W. Revision total knee arthroplasty for aseptic failure. *Clin. Orthop.* **226,** 78–85 (1988).
123. Brick, G. W., and Scott, R. D. The patellofemoral component of total knee arthroplasty. *Clin. Orthop.* **231,** 163–178 (1988).
124. Barrack, R. L., Wolfe, M. W., Waldman, D. A., Milicic, M., Bertot, A. J., and Myers, L. Resurfacing of the patella in total knee arthroplasty. A prospective, randomized, double-blind study. *J. Bone Joint Surg.* **79A,** 1121–1131 (1997).
125. Feller, J. A., Bartlett, R. J., and Lang, D. M. Patellar resurfacing versus retention in total knee arthroplasty. *J Bone Joint Surg.* **78B,** 226–228 (1996).
126. Boyd, A. D., Jr., Ewald, F. C., Thomas, W. H., Poss, R., and Sledge, C. B. Long-term complications after total knee arthroplasty with or without resurfacing of the patella. *J. Bone Joint Surg.* **75A,** 674–681 (1993).
127. Berry, D. J., and Rand, J. A. Isolated patellar component revision of total knee arthroplasty. *Clin. Orthop.* **286,** 110–115 (1993).
128. Rosenberg, A. G., Andriacchi, T. P., Barden, R., and Galante, J. O. Patellar component failure in cementless total knee arthroplasty. *Clin. Orthop.* **236,** 106–114 (1988).
129. Bayley, J. C., Scott, R. D., Ewald, F. C., and Holmes, G. B. Failure of the metal-backed patellar component after total knee replacement. *J. Bone Joint Surg.* **70A,** 668–674 (1988).
130. Stulberg, D. S., Stulberg, B. N., Hamati, Y., and Tsao, A. Failure mechanisms of metal-backed patellar components. *Clin. Orthop.* **236,** 88–105 (1988).
131. Beight, J. L., Yao, B., Hozack, W. J., Hearn, S. L., and Booth, R. E., Jr. The patellar 'clunk' syndrome after posterior stabilized total knee arthroplasty. *Clin. Orthop.* **299,** 139–142 (1994).
132. Rand, J. A., Morrey, B. F., and Bryan, R. S. Patellar tendon rupture after total knee arthroplasty. *Clin. Orthop.* **244,** 233–238 (1989).
133. Emerson, R. H., Head, W. C., and Malinin, T. I. Reconstruction of patellar tendon rupture after total knee arthroplasty with an extensor mechanism allograft. *Clin. Orthop.* **260,** 154–161 (1990).

Shape and Size of an Osteoporotic Woman

MEHRSHEED SINAKI Department of Physical Medicine and Rehabilitation, Mayo Clinic and Mayo Foundation, and Mayo Medical School, Rochester, Minnesota 55905

INTRODUCTION

Osteoporosis silently drains bones of their calcium. One cannot separate the effects of nutrition, exercise, hormones, and life-style; they indeed intertwine. The statement "your life-style can make or break your bones" (read by the author at the IX Congresso Nazionale S.I.O.P., Parma, Italy, 1997) explains it well. Reduction in the biomechanical competence of the axial skeleton can result in challenging complications. In men and women, the combination of aging and reduction of physical activity can affect musculoskeletal health and contribute to the development of bone fragility.

In general, women's muscle strength and bone mineral density at any time in life are significantly lower than those of men. The level of bone mass in adults depends on the peak bone mass acquired during skeletal maturity and on the rate of bone loss thereafter. That the bone mineral density of the spine decreases with age is a well-accepted fact. This reduction has been shown to be significantly correlated with the reduction of back extensor strength [1,2] (Fig. 1). The rate of bone loss varies in different skeletal areas. There is a higher loss of trabecular bone from the axial skeleton with age. This loss is almost 47% throughout life in women and about 30% in men. In women, age-related bone loss becomes rapid and exponential after the start of ovarian failure. This loss of 2–3% per year continues for about 5–7 years. Therefore, postural changes due to loss of bone, muscle mass, and back strength are more significant in women with increasing age and decreased physical activity, as are skeletal deformities. A study of a relatively homogeneous ethnic group of healthy women aged 30 to 79 years demonstrated that height decreased significantly with increasing age [3].

Peak muscle strength is achieved at about age 20 to 30 years [4]. After age 35 to 40 years in nonathletic individuals, the reduction in muscle mass starts. Muscle mass and strength decrease with aging in men and women [5] (Fig. 2). Aging is not the only factor that contributes to sarcopenia; reduction of physical activity also plays a significant role (Fig. 3). Muscle loss may contribute to osteoporosis because muscle mass is directly related to bone mass [6]. During physical activity, muscle contractions apply direct force and strain to the attached bones. Women who have osteoporosis also perform strenuous daily physical activities. A study of normal versus osteoporotic women [7] found that the level of physical activity in osteoporotic women was comparable to that in age-matched controls without evidence of osteoporosis. Therefore, it is not surprising that small-framed osteoporotic individuals experience compression fractures during their activities of daily living.

MUSCULOSKELETAL CONSEQUENCES OF OSTEOPOROSIS

Osteoporosis can affect women and men of all shapes and sizes. However, individuals of small frame and lower muscle and bone mass can be affected even more. The reduction of muscle strength and bone mass is not without consequences. The major loss of muscle mass is from the axial skeleton [5]. If not well supported, the fragile skeleton, especially in the axial area, can go through significant disfiguration [8]. These musculoskeletal changes may result in kyphoscoliosis and subse-

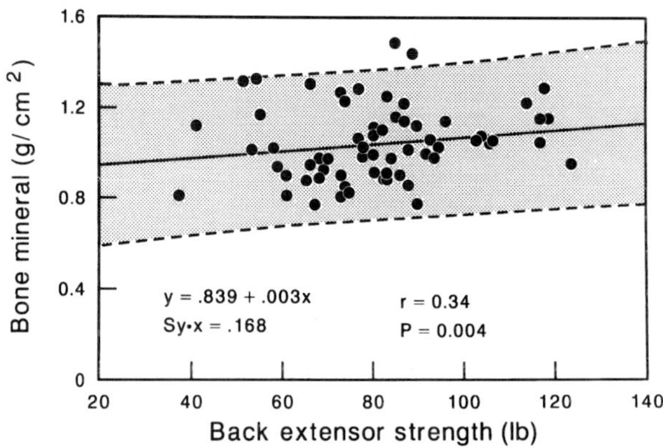

FIGURE 1 Relationship between bone mineral density of second to fourth lumbar vertebrae and strength of back extensors. Linear regression and 95% confidence intervals for individual predicted values are shown. From Sinaki *et al.* [1], with permission of Mayo Foundation.

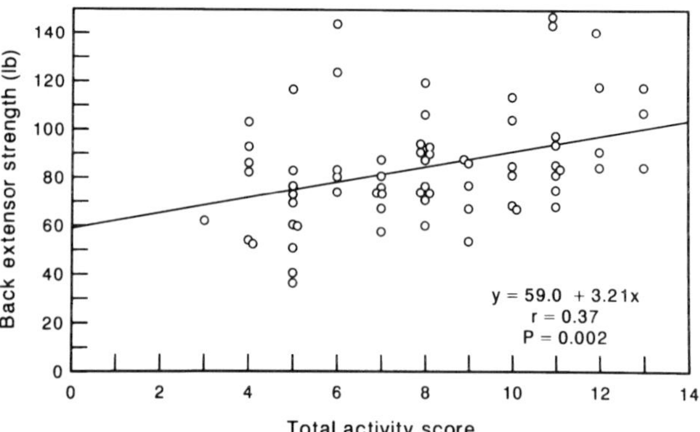

FIGURE 3 Relationship between physical activity score and back extensor strength. From Sinaki and Offord [2], with permission of the American Congress of Rehabilitation Medicine and American Academy of Physical Medicine and Rehabilitation.

quently kyphotic posture (Fig. 4). Kyphotic posture not only is psychologically taxing but also creates chronic pain associated with iliocostal friction (Fig. 5).

Fractures associated with the reduction of bone mass and osteoporosis are not uncommon, particularly in elderly white women. Spinal disfiguration can contribute to an increment in vertebral fractures and the risk of falling [9,10]. An increase in the number of vertebral fractures is associated with kyphosis (Fig. 6), loss of height, back pain, chronic pain syndrome, fear of falling, and, most importantly, negative self-image and increased mortality. Twenty percent of hip fractures in women result in death. This percentage is even higher for men because hip fractures usually occur at an older age in men. Axial skeletal fractures, such as fracture of the sacral alae and pubic rami, may not be found until radiographic changes are detected (Fig. 7).

Imposing a significant mechanical load on a spine depleted of bone and poorly supported by muscles can result in kyphosis or kyphoscoliosis (or both) according to the direction of the force.

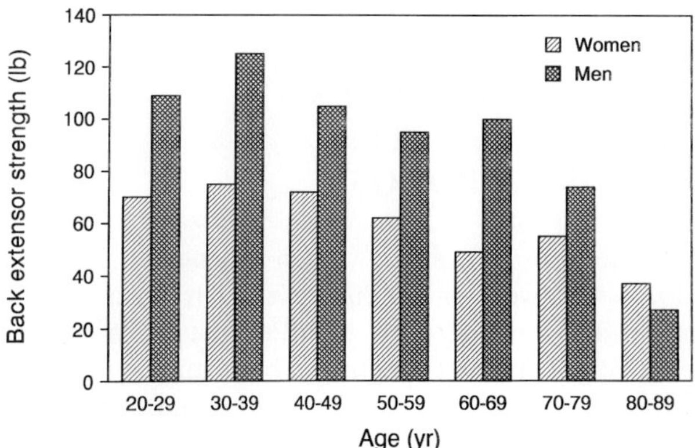

FIGURE 2 Both men and women lose muscle strength with aging. In general, women's muscle strength is lower than that of men at any time in adulthood. (Phillips, B., and Sinaki, M., unpublished data.)

Scoliosis develops in 58% of patients with idiopathic osteoporosis, and osteoporosis develops in 76% of patients with idiopathic kyphoscoliosis [11]. Scoliosis adds to the complications related to changes in shape. Obviously, the main objective of rehabilitative measures is to prevent fractures and disfiguration rather than to treat the consequences. Therefore, preventive methods such as orthotics that distribute the weight evenly over the vertebral end plates are desirable and can be helpful for decreasing the incidence of vertebral disfiguration.

Axial disfiguration results in back pain, which is usually the patient's main complaint [12,13]. Vertebral compression fractures often occur in the midthoracic and upper lumbar vertebral bones, followed in order of frequency by low thoracic and lower lumbar vertebral bones [14] (Fig. 8). The outcome of compression fractures and wedging is loss of height, kyphosis, or both. The cervical and upper thoracic vertebrae are rarely, if ever, involved. Compression fractures are manifested by the occurrence of pain in the involved level of the spine. The pain related to compression fractures may come on gradually or occur suddenly after a heavy object has been lifted or after strenuous physical activity.

Acute pain that occurs in the absence of a previous fracture is usually due to compression fractures in the vertebrae. Sometimes a minor fall or even an affectionate hug may lead to a compression fracture. The compressed vertebra may not be apparent on radiographs for up to 4 weeks after the injury [15]. Compression fracture usually results in acute pain that later resolves, but the spinal deformity as a result of the fracture can produce chronic pain [16].

Kyphotic postural change is the most physically disfiguring and psychologically damaging effect of osteopo-

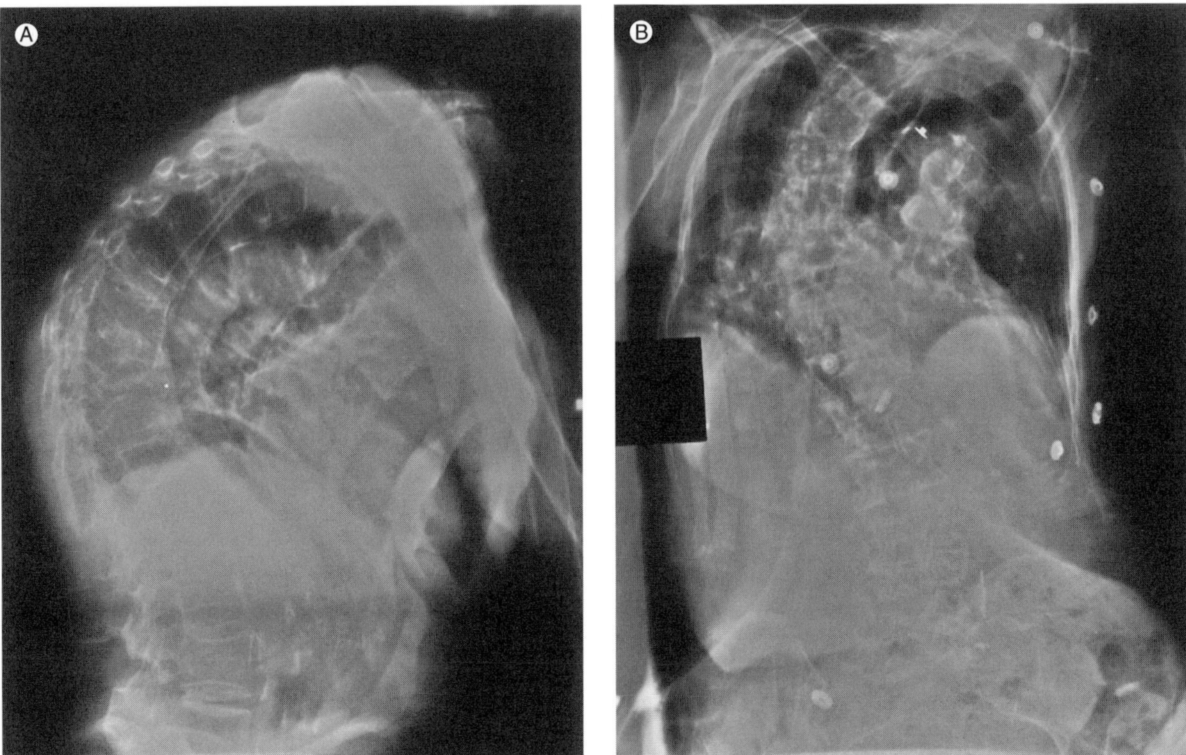

FIGURE 4 Radiographic findings in an 86-year-old woman with severe osteoporosis, kyphosis, and scoliosis. (*A*) Lateral view. (*B*) Anterior view showing severe scoliosis.

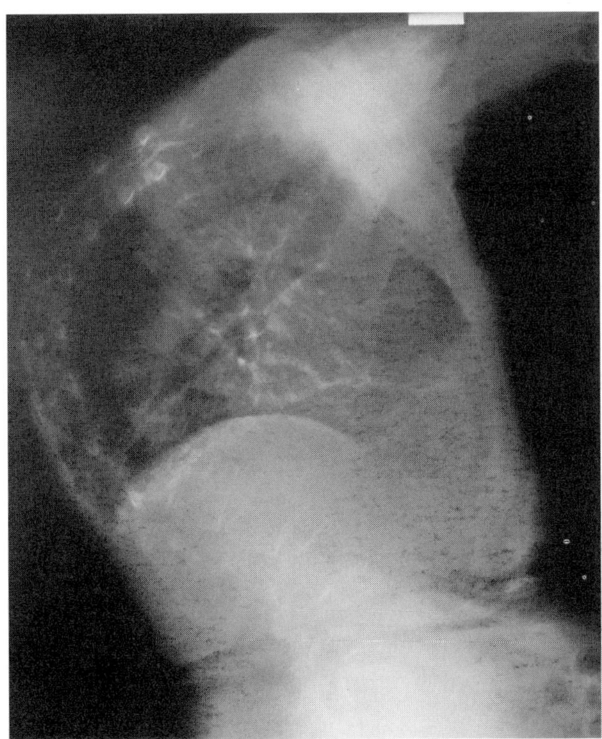

FIGURE 5 Radiographic findings in an 81-year-old woman with severe kyphotic posturing and iliocostal friction syndrome.

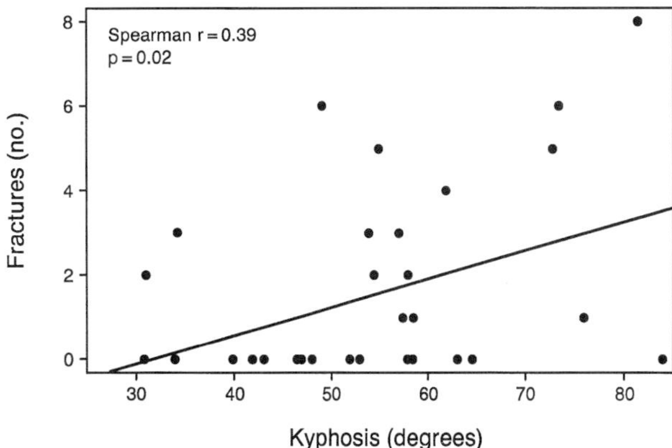

FIGURE 6 Correlation of number of vertebral fractures with degree of kyphosis in women with osteoporosis. From Sinaki *et al.* [9], with permission of Mayo Foundation.

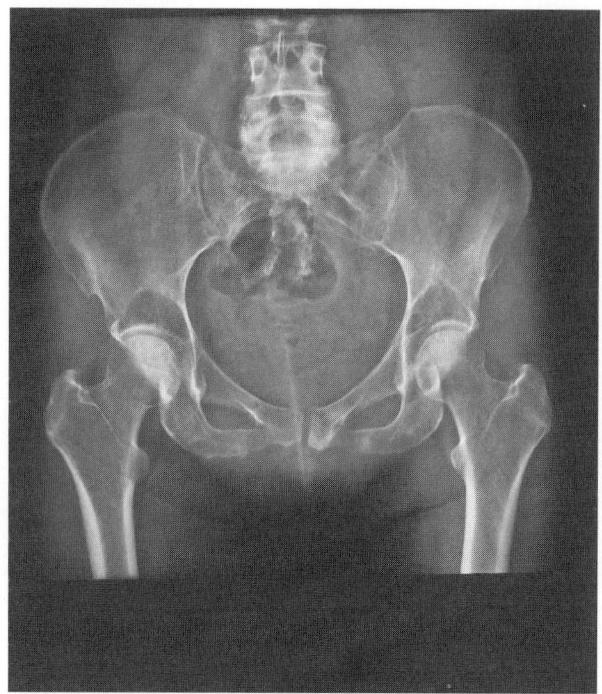

FIGURE 7 A 55-year-old woman with osteopenia, healing fractures of the left pubis and right inferior pubic ramus. Areas of sclerosis in the right superior pubic ramus, left inferior pubic ramus, and both sacral ala are consistent with the insufficiency-type fracture.

rosis [17] (Fig. 9). Kyphotic posture creates a problem for proper application and fitting of a back brace to support the spine and to decrease pain related to the compression fracture. The incidence of osteoporosis-related fractures and deformities can be decreased substantially in the high-risk patient population by early detection and subsequent intervention. A disproportionate weakness in back extensor musculature relative to body weight or trunkal flexor strength contributes significantly to compression of the vertebrae in the fragile osteoporotic spine. Improvement of trunkal muscle strength will enhance the ability to maintain proper vertical alignment [18]. Protective measures to decrease compressive forces on the spine during strenuous activities can also decrease the risk of spinal fractures. The geriatric population has an increased risk for debilitating postural changes as a result of several factors, including a greater prevalence of osteoporosis with age, involutional loss of functional muscle motor units, and reduction in resilience of the intervertebral disks [19,20].

Because postmenopausal osteoporosis principally affects the trabecular bone of the thoracic and lumbar spine, the back extensor strength of women who had osteoporosis was compared with that of normal women [7]. The study showed that back extensor strength in osteoporotic women was significantly lower (controlled for age) than that in normal women (Fig. 10).

Acute compression fracture requires bracing. If conventional thoracolumbar braces (Figs. 11A–11C) are not tolerated because of deformity, a weighted kyphoorthosis (posture training support, PTS) is an alternative option (Fig. 11D). The PTS works on the basis of two principles: It counteracts the mechanical load that contributes to kyphotic posture and it induces awareness of kyphotic posturing through proprioception. One of three types of PTS can be prescribed according to the

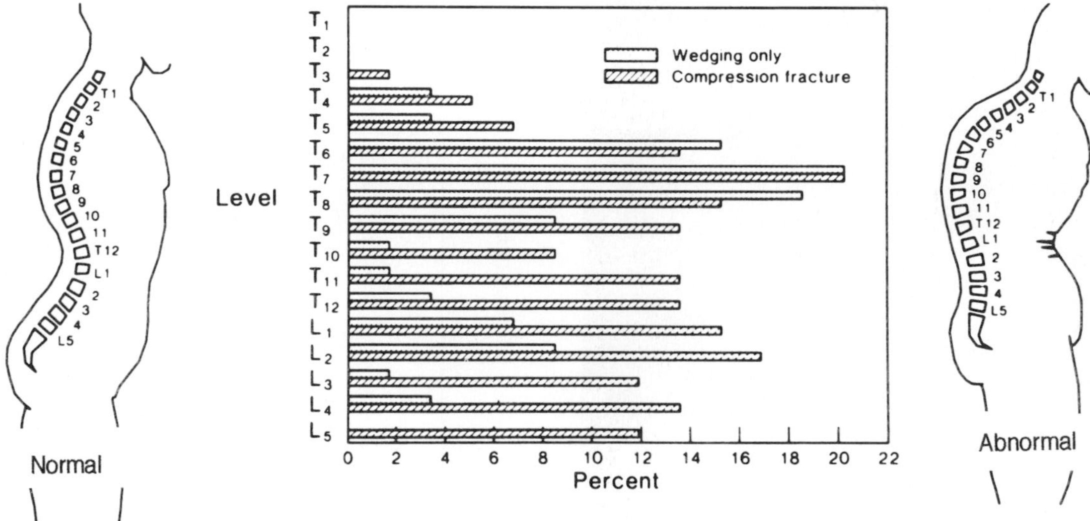

FIGURE 8 Osteoporosis-related incidence of wedging and compression fractures at various levels of the spine on radiographic evaluation. From Sinaki and Mikkelsen [14], with permission of the American Congress of Rehabilitation Medicine and the American Academy of Physical Medicine and Rehabilitation.

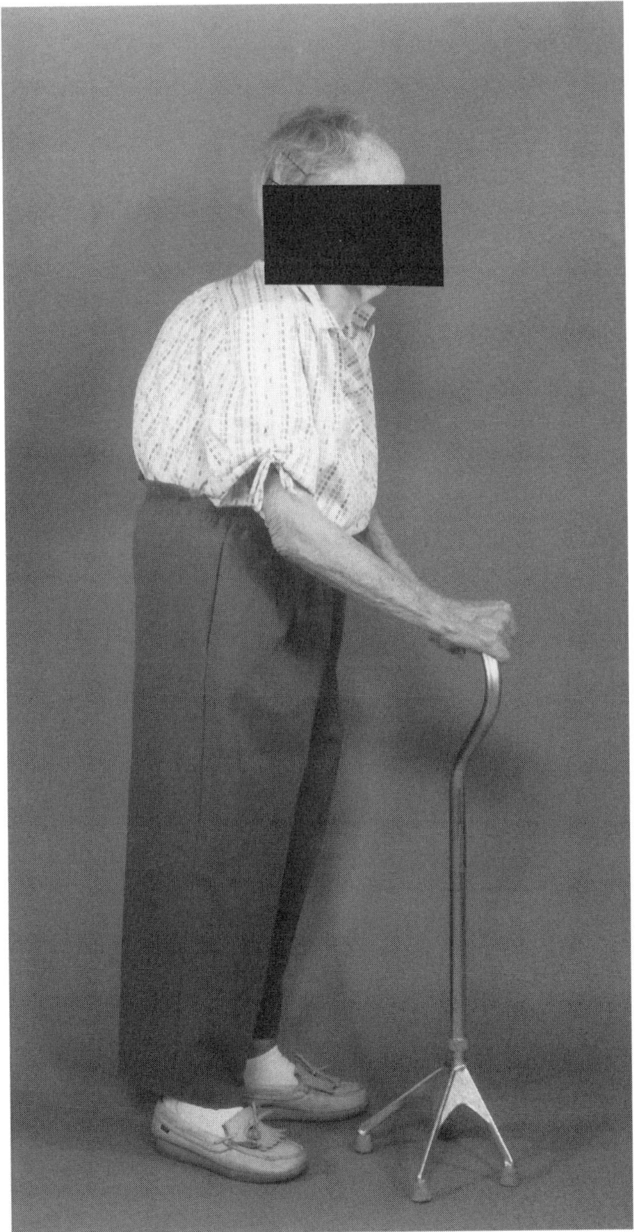

FIGURE 9 An 80-year-old woman with postural disfiguration and loss of height due to compression of multiple vertebral bodies and narrowing of L4 and lumbosacral interspaces.

patient's needs. The PTS should be fitted in such a way that the weight is positioned below the inferior angles of the scapulae. This program requires postural exercises, which need to be prescribed to encourage use of paraspinal muscles (Figs. 12A–12C). Sedative physical therapy such as application of cold and, later, heat is also important. Acute pain should be well managed during the early stages to discourage chronic pain behavior, thereby significantly reducing pain-related postural disfiguration.

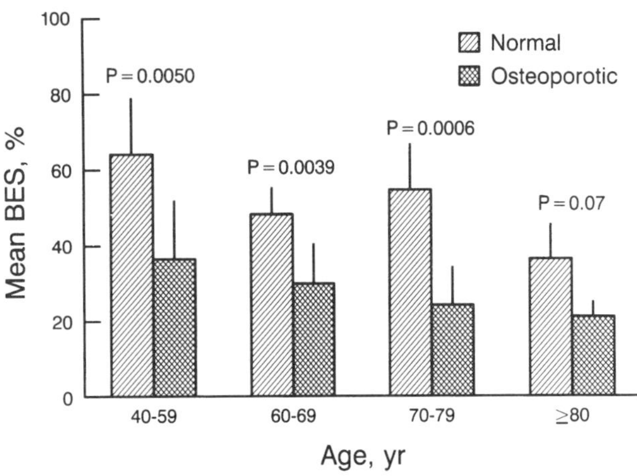

FIGURE 10 Relationship of back extensor strength (BES) in pounds to age for normal and osteoporotic subjects. *P* values at levels of 0.05 or less were considered statistically significant. Data from Sinaki *et al.* [7].

Chronic pain may be due to the development of deformity resulting from vertebral wedging and compression. The intervertebral disks undergo the most dramatic age-related changes of all connective tissues [21]. With aging, the number and diameter of the collagen fibril portion of the disk increase. This change is accompanied by a progressive decrease in disk compliance. Eventually, loss of distinction between the nucleus pulposus and the annulus fibrosus occurs.

Chronic back pain is related to postural changes caused by vertebral fractures and ligamentous stretch [22,23]. Pain is not the only problem that can be created with multiple compression fractures. The negative self-image associated with a disfigured spine is more psychologically damaging. Strong back muscles contribute to good posture and skeletal support [9]. It is hard to differentiate the loss of muscle strength before spinal compression fractures with that of muscle loss due to pain and the related immobility after fracture. The pain and skeletal deformity associated with osteoporosis may reduce muscle strength secondarily. The reduction in muscle strength could, potentially, further exacerbate the postural abnormalities associated with this condition. Management of chronic pain should include measures to sedate the pain and the use of spinal supports along with back-strengthening exercises [24] (Figs. 12D–12G).

HYPERKYPHOSIS AND FALLS

The prevention of falls and fractures in patients with osteoporosis is as important as attempts to improve the bone mineral density of the skeleton. Because aging and osteoporosis are associated with a reduction of

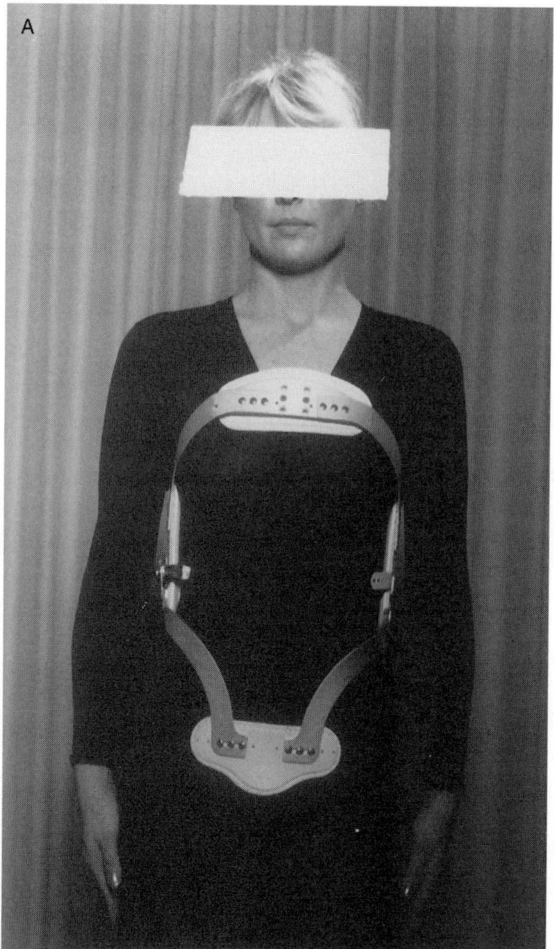

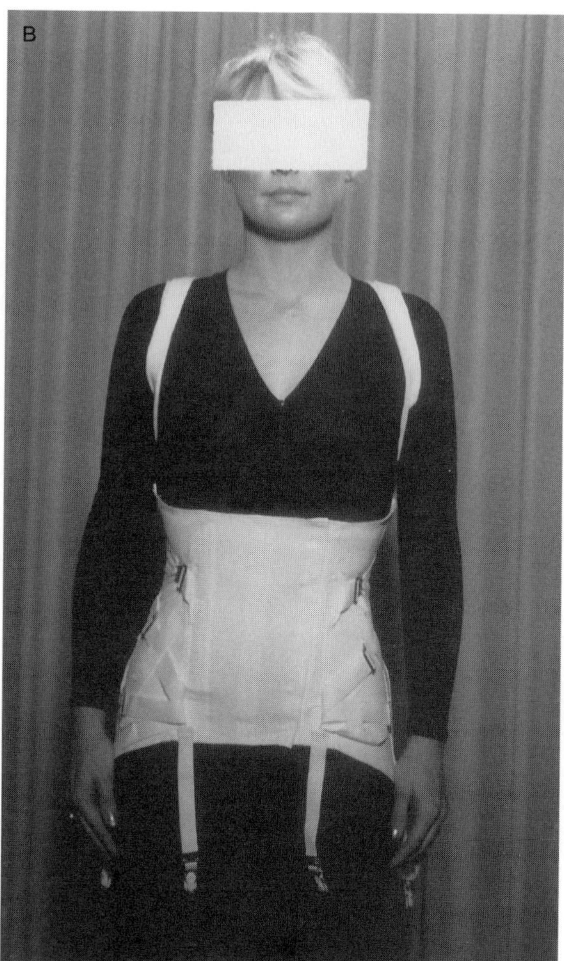

FIGURE 11 (*A*) A Jewett brace is used to prevent lumbar and thoracic flexion when the patient has acute pain due to recent compression fracture of the spine. Proper fitting requires proper contact at the base of sternum and over the pubic bone. (*B*) Thoracolumbar support with rigid or semirigid stays. The addition of shoulder straps further decreases kyphotic posture or reminds patient to avoid severe stooping. Padding can be added to shoulder straps to decrease pressure over bony prominences. From Sinaki [24], with permission of Mayo Foundation. (*C*) Rigid back support, or bivalved body jacket. The brace is made of polypropylene and is custom-fitted. From Sinaki [31], with permission. (*D*) Weighted kyphoorthosis, PTS universal (top) and PTS vest (bottom). Biomechanical approach appropriately positions weights below inferior angles of the scapulae to counteract the tendency to bend forward. With permission of Mayo Foundation.

axial muscle strength, strengthening exercises are highly recommended. One study showed that back extensor strength had a significant negative correlation with thoracic kyphosis and a positive correlation with lumbar lordosis and sacral inclination [25]. Results indicated that the stronger the back extensors, the less the thoracic kyphosis and the more the lumbar lordosis and sacral inclination. The study concluded that back extensor strength is an important determinant of posture in healthy women but that back extensor strengthening exercises alone may also increase lumbar lordosis, which is not desirable. Therefore, one should prescribe back extensor strengthening exercises in combination with lumbar flexor strengthening exercises.

The change in the normal orientation of the line of gravity to the spine results in disturbed balance and unsteadiness of gait. A reduction in the size of the thoracic vertebral column and increased forward flexion create problems such as orthopnea and decreased endurance. Development of kyphotic posture not only can predispose the individual to postural back pain but also can increase the risk of falls. Individuals with more kyphosis (Cobb angle of more than 54°) have more postural sway and greater use of hip strategies than ankle strategies to maintain balance than individuals with less kyphosis [10]. Some patients have disturbance of their dynamic and static posturing because of either reduction of their muscle strength or neurogenic reduction of the lower extremity sensory system with aging or age-

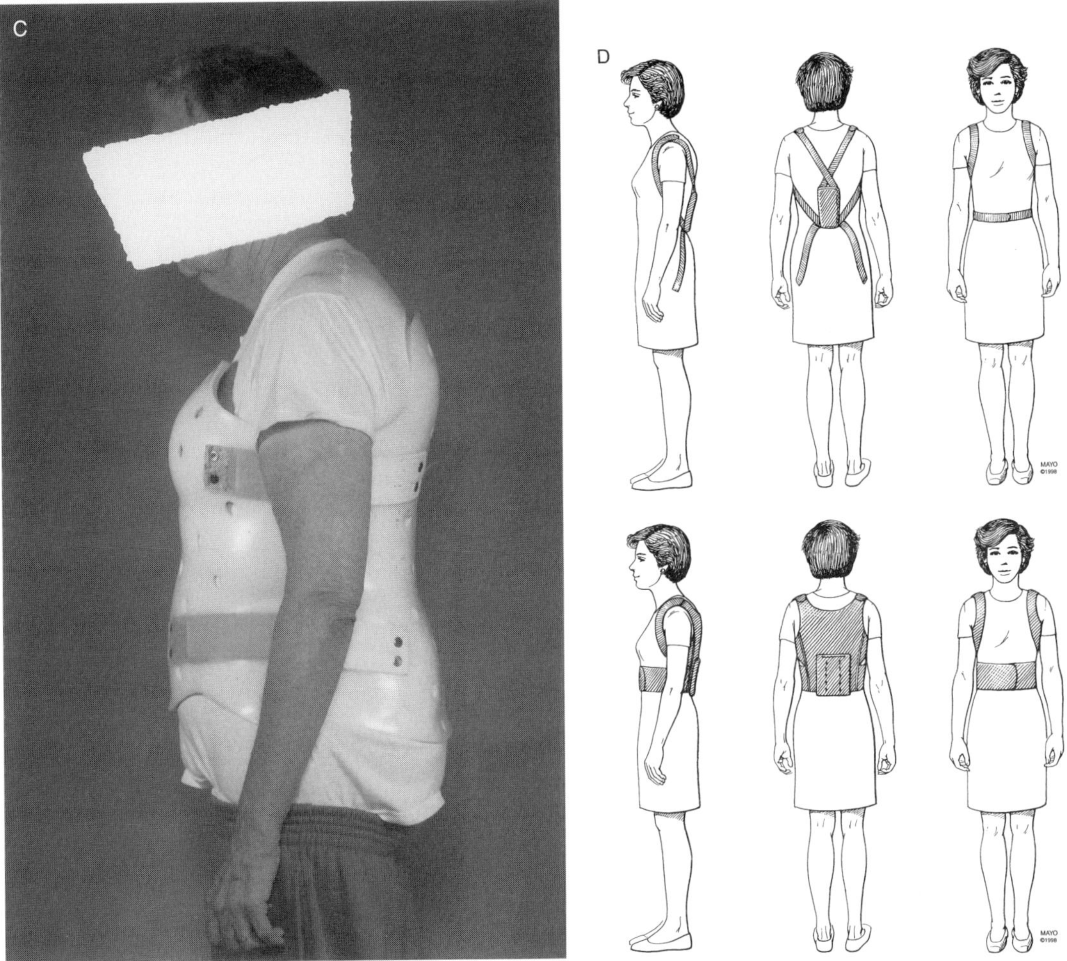

FIGURE 11 *(continued)*

related rigidity. Coordination exercises for the lower extremities (Frenkel's exercises) can be of help.

Several complications can result from hyperkyphosis and changes in the axial skeletal shape that can affect an individual's quality of life. Loss of height and hyperkyphosis can decrease vital capacity. Hyperkyphosis can also decrease the iliocostal space, which can lead to iliocostal friction syndrome (Fig. 5) and pain [26]. The proper fitting of a brace becomes difficult with these changes in shape (Fig. 9). Application of a weighted kyphoorthosis along with a posture training exercise program can reduce this pain [27] (Fig. 13).

CAMOUFLAGING POSTURAL DISFIGURATION

Development of a negative self-image is another problem that is related concomitantly to postural disfiguration. Pain and deformities related to axial musculoskeletal changes create problems with fitting of clothes and finding the proper clothes. A hemline of a favorite dress that seems much longer than it was a few years ago might be a woman's first indication of postural changes. Needless to say, because of such a difficulty, most women lose interest in shopping for clothes. Some women admit that they prefer to avoid this formerly pleasurable task because seeing their own disfigured spine makes them even more depressed. Through the proper selection of clothing, however, men and women with osteoporosis can improve their physical image and put their best, most attractive, self forward. After analyzing the postural changes due to osteoporosis, suggestions can be offered to encourage the patient to select clothing that deemphasizes postural change. For example, a woman with severe kyphosis may consider adding shoulder pads to her loose-fitting jacket to camouflage or reduce the visual detection of the "dowager's hump." Fitted clothes accentuate the waistline and kyphotic posturing, whereas loose-fitting clothes can camouflage postural changes. A beautiful scarf around the neck can focus attention away from the deformed posture. A

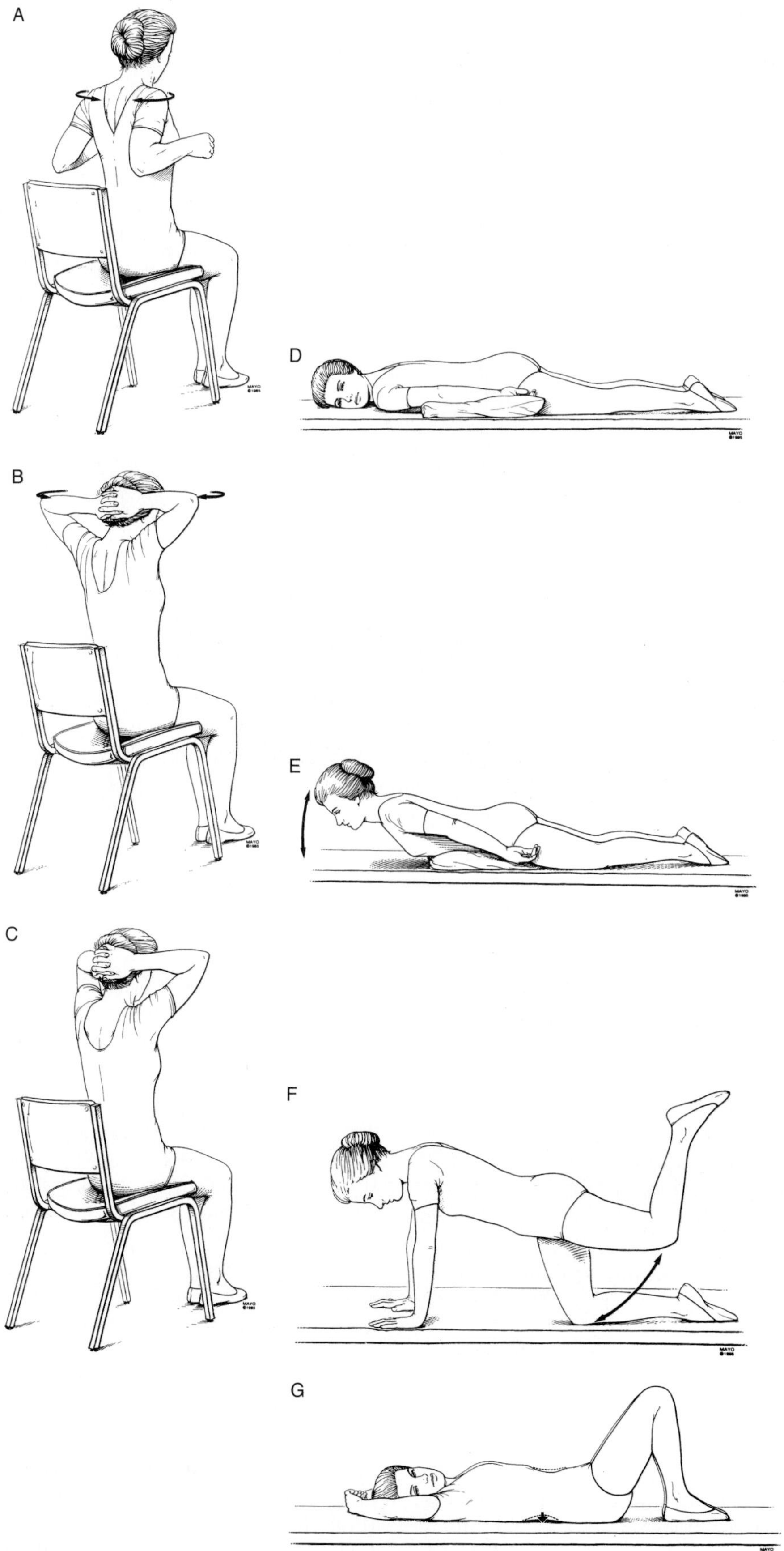

Figure 12

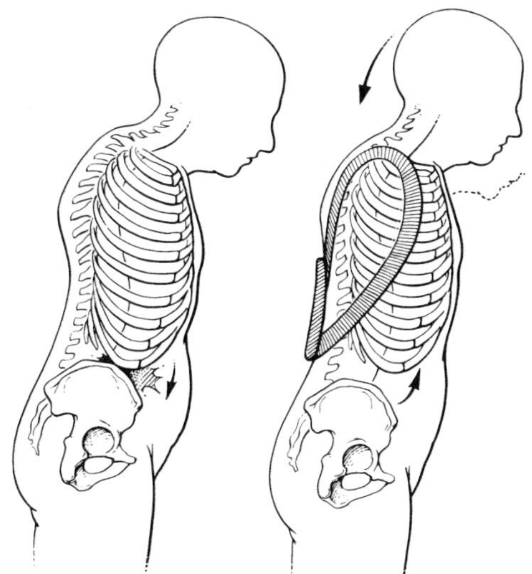

FIGURE 13 Severe thoracic kyphosis can result in iliocostal contact or iliocostal friction syndrome (left). Application of a weighted kyphoorthosis (Posture Training Support) provides counteracting forces that enable users to contract their erector spinae muscles better and decrease kyphotic posturing (right). From Sinaki [27], with permission.

reduction of kyphotic posturing through the application of a weighted kyphoorthosis can be of some help. A posture training exercise program can also be helpful. With application of a weighted postural support, one can camouflage the kyphosis while improving posture (Fig. 14).

EXERCISE AND THE OSTEOPOROTIC SPINE

Proper weight-bearing and resistive exercise [28] (including recreational exercises) in combination with good nutrition [29] and the proper hormone level [30] can contribute significantly to an individual's well-being. Small-framed, extremely thin women lack proper protection for absorbing the contact energy of a fall. Building gluteal muscles through resistive exercises can improve natural hip protection. Not all types of exercises are safe for the osteoporotic spine [14]. Before an exercise program is initiated in persons age 50 years or older, the beneficial effects of exercise on bone should be evaluated for both the healthy, nonosteoporotic skeleton and the osteoporotic skeleton. In men and women, there is an age-related decrease in cardiorespiratory fitness. Exercises that are beneficial for fitness and cardiovascular conditioning are not necessarily weight-bearing and effective for the improvement of bone mineral density. With increasing age, cardiovascular fitness

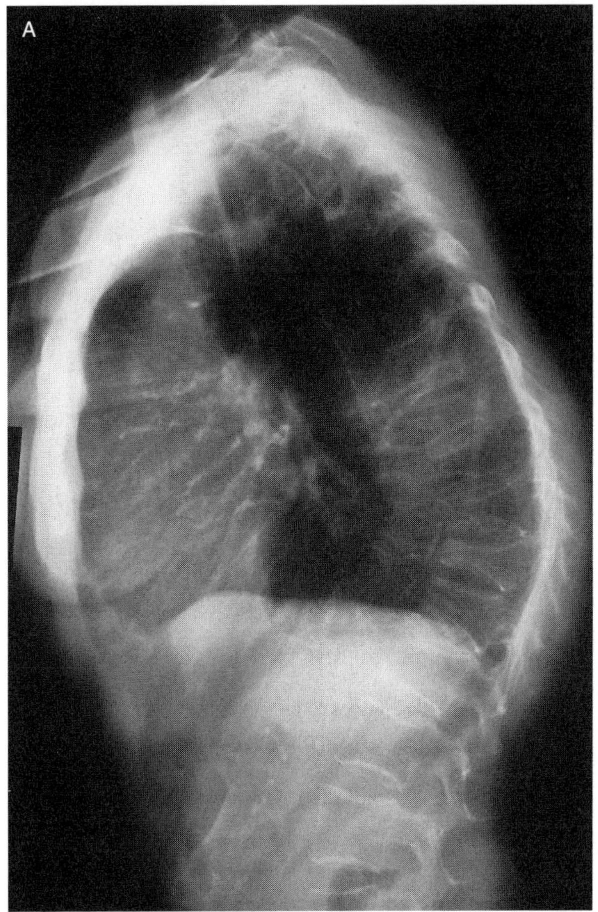

FIGURE 14 A 72-year-old woman with osteoporosis. (*A*) Radiograph shows thoracic kyphosis and compression fractures of multiple lower thoracic and upper lumbar vertebral bodies. (*B*) Lateral view of patient's posture without support. (*C*) Patient wearing Posture Training Support-thoracolumbar. (*D*) Same patient demonstrating improvement of posture with application of support. (*E*) Proper clothing can camouflage the kyphosis and the spinal support.

FIGURE 12 (*A*) Back extension exercise in the sitting position. This position avoids or minimizes pain in patients with severe osteoporosis. From Sinaki [24], with permission of Mayo Foundation. (*B* and *C*) Deep-breathing exercise combined with pectoral stretching and back extension exercise. Patient sits on a chair, locks hands behind head, inhales deeply while gently extending elbows backward, and, while exhaling, returns to starting position. This exercise is repeated 10 to 15 times. (*B*, redrawn from Sinaki [12]. *C*, from Sinaki [24]. With permission of Mayo Foundation.) (*D* and *E*). Back extension exercise in prone position. (*F*) Back extension exercise for improving strength in lumbar extensors and gluteus maximus muscles. (*G*) Exercise to decrease lumbar lordosis with isometric contraction of lumbar flexors. From Sinaki [24], with permission of Mayo Foundation.

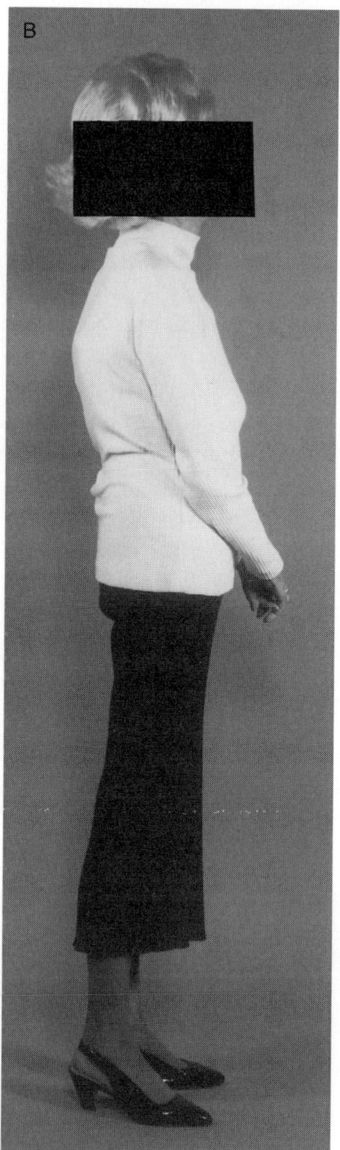

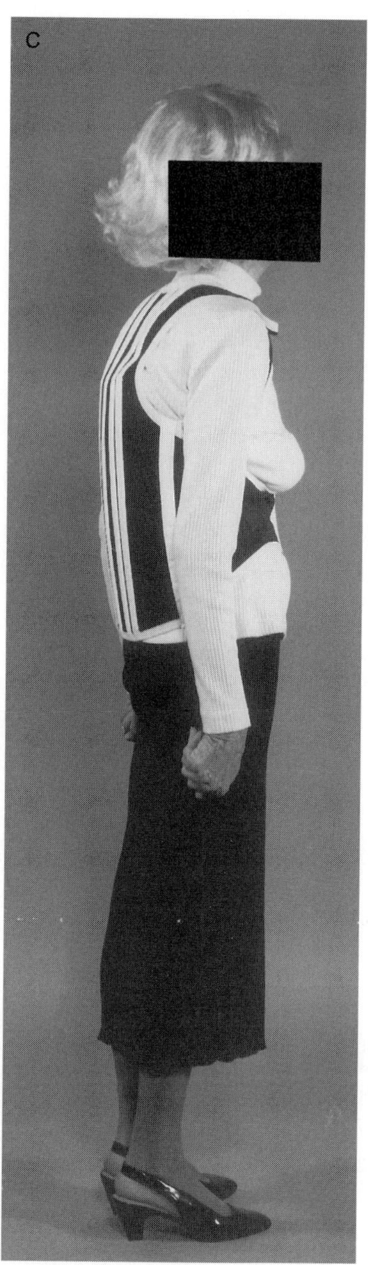

FIGURE 14 *(continued)*

decreases by about 1% per year. After age 50 years, an exercise program needs to be weight-bearing to be osteogenic and resistive to increase muscle mass. For maintenance of flexibility, range-of-motion exercises are recommended to improve coordination. Frenkel's exercises are important. When prescribing an exercise program for an osteoporotic patient, consideration should be given to (1) the objective of the exercise program, (2) the biomechanical competence of the spine and musculoskeletal health in general, (3) the status of neuromuscular health, (4) cardiovascular fitness, (5) past history of sports activity and interests, and (6) a patient's environment.

As women and men age, their body shape changes. Maintenance of muscle mass and strength can reduce the risk of fracture and secondary axial disfiguration. Prevention of changes in shape can contribute to a more positive self-image with aging. Proper nutrition and an active life-style can slow down and minimize these changes to some extent. The osteoporotic woman should be encouraged to focus on a positive self-image and good self-esteem, both of which can greatly enhance the

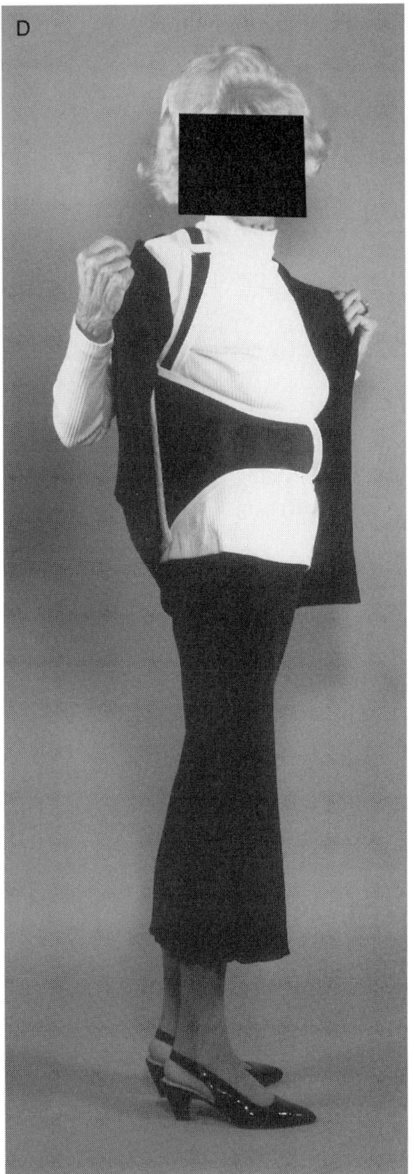

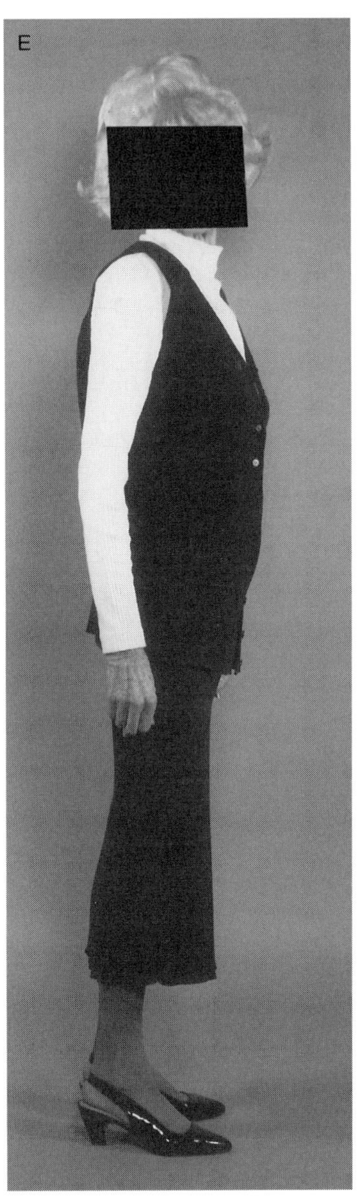

FIGURE 14 *(continued)*

quality of life and enthusiasm for facing the challenges of daily life.

References

1. Sinaki, M., McPhee, M. C., Hodgson, S. F., Merritt, J. M., and Offord, K. P. Relationship between bone mineral density of spine and strength of back extensors in healthy postmenopausal women. *Mayo Clin. Proc.* **61,** 116–122 (1986).
2. Sinaki, M., and Offord, K. P. Physical activity in postmenopausal women: Effect on back muscle strength and bone mineral density of the spine. *Arch. Phys. Med. Rehabil.* **69,** 277–280 (1988).
3. Limburg, P. J., Sinaki, M., Rogers, J. W., Caskey, P. E., and Pierskalla, B. K. A useful technique for measurement of back strength in osteoporotic and elderly patients. *Mayo Clin. Proc.* **66,** 39–44 (1991).
4. Hettinger, T., "Physiology of Strength." Charles C Thomas, Springfield, IL, 1961.
5. Sinaki, M., Opitz, J. L., and Wahner, H. W. Bone mineral content: Relationship to muscle strength in normal subjects. *Arch. Phys. Med. Rehabil.* **55,** 508–512 (1974).
6. Doyle, F., Brown, J., and Lachance, C. Relation between bone mass and muscle weight. *Lancet* **1,** 391–393 (1970).
7. Sinaki, M., Khosla, S., Limburg, P. J., Rogers, J. W., and Murtaugh, P. A. Muscle strength in osteoporotic versus normal women. *Osteopor. Int.* **3,** 8–12 (1993).
8. Sinaki, M. Rehabilitation of osteoporotic fractures of the spine. *In* "Physical Medicine and Rehabilitation: State of the Art Reviews" (A. J. Mehta, ed.), Vol. 9, pp. 105–123. Hanley & Belfus, Philadelphia, 1995.

9. Sinaki, M., Wollan, P. C., Scott, R. W., and Gelczer, R. K. Can strong back extensors prevent vertebral fractures in women with osteoporosis? *Mayo Clin. Proc.* **71,** 951–956 (1996).
10. Lynn, S. G., Sinaki, M., and Westerlind, K. C. Balance characteristics of persons with osteoporosis. *Arch. Phys. Med. Rehabil.* **78,** 273–277 (1997).
11. Healey, J. H., and Lane, J. M. Structural scoliosis in osteoporotic women. *Clin. Orthop.* **195,** 216–223 (1985).
12. Sinaki, M. Postmenopausal spinal osteoporosis: Physical therapy and rehabilitation principles. *Mayo Clin. Proc.* **57,** 699–703 (1982).
13. Urist, M. R. Orthopaedic management of osteoporosis in postmenopausal women. *Clin. Endocrinol. Metab.* **2,** 159–176 (1973).
14. Sinaki, M., and Mikkelsen, B. A. Postmenopausal spinal osteoporosis: Flexion versus extension exercises. *Arch. Phys. Med. Rehabil.* **65,** 593–596 (1984).
15. Nordin, B. E., Horsman, A., Crilly, R. G., Marshall, D. H., and Simpson, M. Treatment of spinal osteoporosis in postmenopausal women. *Br. Med. J.* **280,** 451–455 (1980).
16. Sinaki, M. Musculoskeletal rehabilitation. *In* "Osteoporosis: Etiology, Diagnosis, and Management" (B. L. Riggs and L. J. Melton III, eds.), 2nd Ed., pp. 435–473. Lippincott-Raven, Philadelphia, 1995.
17. Sinaki, M., and Grubbs, N. C. Back strengthening exercises: Quantitative evaluation of their efficacy for women aged 40 to 65 years. *Arch. Phys. Med. Rehabil.* **70,** 16–20 (1989).
18. Sinaki, M. Beneficial musculoskeletal effects of physical activity in the older woman. *Geriatr. Med. Today* **8,** 53–72 (1989).
19. Gutmann, E. Age changes in the neuromuscular system and aspects of rehabilitation medicine. *In* "Neurophysiologic Aspects of Rehabilitation Medicine: Proceedings of the International Conference on Neurophysiologic Aspects of Rehabilitation Medicine, January, 1974, University of California, Irvine, California" (A. A. Buerger and J. S. Tobis, eds.), pp. 42–61. Charles C Thomas, Springfield, IL, 1976.
20. McComas, A. J., Fawcett, P. R., Campbell, M. J., and Sica, R. E. Electrophysiological estimation of the number of motor units within a human muscle. *J. Neurol. Neurosurg. Psychiat.* **34,** 121–131 (1971).
21. Adams, P., Eyre, D. R., and Muir, H. Biochemical aspects of development and ageing of human lumbar intervertebral discs. *Rheumatol. Rehabil.* **16,** 22–29 (1977).
22. Itoi, E., and Sinaki, M. Effect of back-strengthening exercise on posture in healthy women 49 to 65 years of age. *Mayo Clin. Proc.* **69,** 1054–1059 (1994).
23. Sinaki, M., Wahner, H. W., Offord, K. P., and Hodgson, S. F. Efficacy of nonloading exercises in prevention of vertebral bone loss in postmenopausal women: A controlled trial. *Mayo Clin. Proc.* **64,** 762–769 (1989).
24. Sinaki, M. Exercise and physical therapy. *In* "Osteoporosis: Etiology, Diagnosis, and Management" (B. L. Riggs, Jr., and L. J. Melton III, eds.), pp. 457–479. Raven Press, New York, 1988.
25. Sinaki, M., Itoi, E., Rogers, J. W., Bergstralh, E. J., and Wahner, H. W. Correlation of back extensor strength with thoracic kyphosis and lumbar lordosis in estrogen-deficient women. *Am. J. Phys. Med. Rehabil.* **75,** 370–374 (1996).
26. Hirschberg, G. G., Williams, K. A., and Byrd, J. G. Medical management of iliocostal pain. *Geriatrics* **47,** 62–63 (1992).
27. Sinaki, M. The influence of exercise on bone and the rehabilitation of osteoporosis patients. *In* "The Opinion of the Orthopedist and Physiatrist" (M. Passeri, ed.). EDIMES Publishing, Pavia, Italy, 1995.
28. Sinaki, M. Metabolic bone disease. *In* "Basic Clinical Rehabilitation Medicine" (M. Sinaki, ed.), 2nd Ed., pp. 209–236. Mosby Year Book, Chicago, 1993.
29. Heaney, R. P. Nutritional factors in bone health. *In* "Osteoporosis: Etiology, Diagnosis, and Management" (B. L. Riggs and L. J. Melton III, eds.), pp. 359–372. Raven Press, New York, 1988.
30. Lindsay, R. Osteoporosis and its relationship to estrogen. *Contemp. Obstet. Gynecol.* **63,** 201–224 (1984).
31. Sinaki, M. *In* "Osteoporotic Fractures in the Elderly: Clinical Management and Prevention" (J. D. Ringe and P. J. Meunier, eds.), pp. 99–115. Georg Thieme Verlag, Stuttgart, 1996.
32. PTS, Posture Training Support Brochure Y3255. Camp International, Jackson, MI, 1993.

CHAPTER 38

Prevention of Falls

DOUGLAS P. KIEL Harvard Medical School Division on Aging and Hebrew Rehabilitation Center for Aged Research and Training Institute, Boston, Massachusetts 02131

INTRODUCTION

A textbook devoted to the aging skeleton would be noticeably incomplete without a thorough recognition of trauma from falls as a major contributing factor to the occurrence of osteoporotic fractures. Falls are not only one of the most common problems that threaten the independence of older persons, but they are also of significant enough force to exceed the breaking strength of most aged bones. Falls are sometimes viewed as an inevitable consequence of aging by medical providers because of their common occurrence. As is the case for many geriatric syndromes, falls usually result when impairments in multiple domains compromise the compensatory ability of the individual [1]. The prevention of falls requires an understanding of etiology and an appreciation that research in the field has made significant gains over the past decade.

EPIDEMIOLOGY OF FALLS

Incidence

The incidence of falls increases with age and varies according to living status. Results from multiple cohort studies reveal that between 30 and 40% of community-dwelling elderly over the age of 65 years will fall each year [2–4]. Among those with a history of a fall in the previous year, the annual incidence of falls is close to 60% [5]. In the long-term care setting, about half of all persons fall each year [6,7].

Fall Outcomes

Most falls result in an injury of some type, usually minor soft tissue injuries, such as bruises and scrapes; however, 10–15% result in fracture [5]. The majority of fractures, especially hip fractures, occur because of a fall. It may be surprising that at least one-third of clinically diagnosed vertebral fractures also are associated with falls [8]. In fact, results from case-control studies [9,10] have shown that characteristics of the fall are clearly related to fracture risk independent of the underlying bone density. Falls to the side or straight down are associated with hip fracture, whereas falls forward and landing on a hand are associated with wrist fractures. In general, falls are associated with subsequent declines in functional status, a greater likelihood of nursing home placement, and an increased use of medical services [11,12]. Fallers are also more likely to develop fear of falling, which itself is associated with lower self-efficacy than nonfallers [13]. Of those elderly persons who fall, only half are able to get up without help, resulting in the so-called "long lie." The significance of this group of fallers is that long lies are associated with lasting declines in functional status [14].

Death following a fall occurs far less frequently than do injuries; however, complications resulting from falls are the leading cause of death from injury in men and women older than age 65 [15]. The death rate attributable to falls increases with age, with white men aged 85 years and older having the highest death rate (greater than 180 deaths per 100,000 population) [15]. In a large epidemiologic study of elderly persons seeking emergency care after a fall, 2.2% of injurious falls resulted in death [16].

Economic Costs

The true costs of falls in terms of health care dollars are difficult to ascertain. It has been estimated that the lifetime costs of fall-related injuries for persons older than age 65 is $12.6 billion [17]. Because many falls result in injury, there is a significant increase in the use of emergency room facilities among fallers. Based on studies from the early 1990s, almost 8% of persons older than age 70 go to emergency rooms each year because of a fall-related injury [16], and close to a third of these individuals are admitted to the hospital [15,18] for a median length of stay of 8 days. A population-based study conducted in Washington state using a state abstract reporting system identified 149,504 patients aged 65 years of age and older discharged from Washington state hospitals in 1989. Of these, 7873 (5.3%) were hospitalized for injuries from falls. Of the $995,499,233 in hospital charges in 1989 for persons in Washington state aged 65 and older, $53,346,191 (5.3%) were attributable to hospitalization of patients with fall-related trauma [19]. In terms of health care expenditures attributable to osteoporotic fractures, 1995 estimates were $13.8 billion for the entire U.S. population [20].

ETIOLOGY OF FALLS

Conceptual Model of Falls

Falls in older people are rarely due to a single cause, which is a common theme throughout the literature on geriatric syndromes [1]. Falls usually occur when a threat to the normal homeostatic mechanisms that maintain postural stability is superimposed on underlying age-related declines in balance, ambulation, and cardiovascular function. In some cases this may involve an acute illness such as infection, fever, dehydration, and arrhythmia or an environmental stress such as a newly initiated drug or an unsafe walking surface. Whether it is an intrinsic stress or an extrinsic, environmental stress, the elderly person is unable to compensate because of either age-related declines in function or chronic disease-related declines. It is unlikely for an extrinsic stress to completely explain the circumstances of a fall [21]. The interactions among these factors were characterized nicely in a review by King and Tinnetti [17] and are shown in Fig. 1. This conceptual model highlights that older persons, by virtue of their age alone, experience declines in physiologic function, have greater numbers of chronic diseases, acute illnesses, and hospitalizations, and use multiple medications. Superimposed on these age-related characteristics, challenges to postural control may have a greater impact in aged persons according to their risk-taking behavior and opportunity to fall. Thus, those individuals who are completely immobile may not be at risk of falling despite multiple predisposing factors. However, persons who are either vigorous or somewhat frail may be at increased risk compared to individuals in between these extremes [22]. Vigorous elderly persons may take more risks, whereas frail elderly individuals may not be able to compensate for threats to postural stability.

Why Falls Cause Fractures

An important concept for the understanding of osteoporosis and related fractures in elderly individuals is that decreased bone strength, as reflected by bone mineral density, is probably not the most important contributor to fracture risk. Other factors that contribute to the occurrence of hip fracture include a propensity to fall, an inability to correct a postural imbalance, orientation of the fall, adequacy of local tissue shock absorbers, and underlying skeletal strength. For its part, the resistance

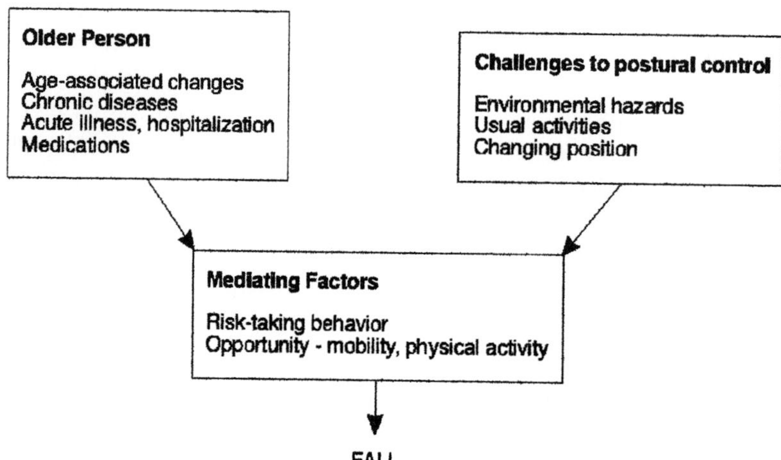

FIGURE 1 Conceptual model of the etiology of falls in elderly persons. After King and Tinnetti [17].

of a skeletal structure to failure (i.e., fracture) depends on the geometry of the bone, the mechanical properties of the calcified tissue, and the location and direction of the loads to which the bone is subjected (i.e., during a fall). Estimations of the forces generated within the bone in response to a given load can be estimated using basic engineering principles. The forces can then be compared with the strengths of the tissue. The ratio of the impact force expected during a fall to the force required to cause the bone to fail may be thought of as the structure's "factor of risk." When the factor of risk is high (close to or more than 1), the structure is at great risk of fracture.

In the elderly, simple stance and normal ambulation involve a factor of risk at the femoral neck of about 0.3. For stair climbing, it is about 0.6. In falls, the factor of risk probably ranges from 1 to greater than 7 [23]. The calculations are complicated by considerable uncertainty about the loads to which hips are actually subjected during falls. For one thing, skeletal structures at high risk for age-related fracture, such as the hip, change their geometry with aging and bone remodeling. These changes make it difficult to ascertain the force of failure *in vivo*.

Despite the difficulties of determining the force of failure *in vivo*, *in vitro* testing of femurs can provide data on the work required to fracture a bone. Studies in young persons have estimated the potential energies liberated by a fall from standing height to be close to 600 J. By the time the hip strikes the floor, 70% of the potential energy has been dissipated during the descent phase, leaving about 170 J of energy just before impact [24]. It is not known whether elderly fallers are also able to dissipate the same amount of energy during a fall or whether they, in effect, "fall harder" than young adults. Nevertheless, this amount of energy is two orders of magnitude greater than the energy required to fracture elderly femurs during *in vitro* studies. These findings confirm that a simple fall is easily capable of fracturing the proximal femur.

Falls themselves are not simple events. In particular, the total energy of a fall is not entirely delivered to the trochanter. Potentially important factors that can influence the amount of force imposed include the presence of energy-absorbing soft tissues over the greater trochanter and the state of leg muscle contraction at the time of the fall. Threefold increases in the thickness of soft tissue overlying skeletal structures reduce the predicted peak impact force of a fall by 20% and may explain the observation that heavier persons have a reduced risk of hip fracture [25]. It has been proposed that padding the trochanter may be an option for preventing hip fracture [26]. Falling in a muscle-relaxed state reduces the peak force by more than 50% [25].

Risk Factors for Falls

Prospective Studies of Risk Factors

Multiple community-based prospective cohort studies of risk factors for falls have been published over the past decade. As shown in Table I, the risk factors for falls that were found in at least two of the five studies reviewed included age, female gender, past history of a fall, cognitive impairment, lower extremity weakness, balance problems, psychotropic drug use, and arthritis. The five studies differed significantly in the types of risk factors evaluated, the types of population studied (e.g., past fall history was sometimes an entry criteria), and the outcome (one fall, two or more falls, injurious falls). The fact that different risk factors were found across studies highlights the multifactorial nature of falls and suggests there may be other circumstances surrounding falls that are not accounted for in studies of this type. In general, the risk of falling increases with the number of risk factors [2,4,5], although some falls occur in individuals with no risk factors.

Age-Related Changes and Falls

The clinical approach to fall prevention in the elderly population requires a knowledge of age-related changes that increase the risk of falls. The ability to maintain an upright posture is dependent on sensory input from several systems, including vision, proprioception, and vestibular. With aging there are declines in all three systems. For example, the visual system demonstrates reductions in acuity, depth perception, contrast sensitivity, and dark adaptation. With aging, the vestibular system demonstrates a loss of labyrinthine hair cells, vestibular ganglion cells, and nerve fibers. The proprioceptive system also loses sensitivity in the lower extremities.

Even with knowledge of these age-related changes in sensory systems, it has been difficult to quantify the age-related changes in postural control that are independent of disease. In general, when postural stability is tested in young and old subjects with no apparent musculoskeletal or neurological impairment, age-related differences in measured sway are most pronounced when moderately severe pertubations of stance are administered, such as changing the support surface, changing body position, altering the visual input, or moving the support surface horizontally or rotationally [27]. This occurs because these perturbations stress the redundancy of the sensory systems in their ability to maintain postural stability. In addition, other age-related

TABLE I Independent Risk Factors for One or More Falls or Injurious Falls in Six Prospective Community-Based Studies

	Tinetti *et al.* [2]	Campbell *et al.* [4]	Nevitt *et al.* [42]	Nevitt *et al.* [5][a]	O'Loughlin [78]	Tinetti [79][a]
Age		↑	↑	↑		
Female				↑		↑
White race			↑			
Past fall			↑	↑		
Cognitive impairment	↑			↑		↑
Lower extremity weakness	↑	↑				
Balance/gait problems	↑					↑
Very active					↑	
Inactive					↑	
Dizziness					↑	
Problem walking					↑	
Multiple medications		↑				
Psychotropic/sedative medications	↑	↑				
Arthritis		↑	↑			
Stroke		↑				
Chronic lung disease			↑			
Body sway		↑				
Alcohol consumption					↓	
Low body habitus						↑
Multiple chronic conditions						↑
Slow reaction time				↑		
Visual problems				↑		
Parkinson's disease			↑			
Foot problems	↑					

[a] Injurious falls.

changes in the central nervous system may also affect postural control, including loss of neurons and dendrites, and depletion of neurotransmitters, such as dopamine, within the basal ganglia [28].

Because it is difficult to find elderly subjects without at least subtle neurologic findings, some of the young–old differences may be due to these factors. During formal testing of postural control, some of the most striking differences between young and old relate to the order or grouping of muscle activation patterns. Thus, in response to perturbations of the support surface, older persons tend to activate the proximal muscles such as the quadriceps before the more distal muscles such as the tibialis anterior [29]. This contrasts with the distal-to-proximal responses observed in younger persons and may not be an efficient way to maintain postural stability. Similarly, in the elderly, there may be greater cocontraction of antagonistic muscles, and the onset of the muscle activation and associated joint torque may be delayed [30]. Finally, the ability to recover balance upon a postural disturbance may be compromised by an age-related decline in the ability to rapidly develop joint torque using muscles of the lower extremity [31]. All of these strategies potentially undermine upright posture.

Another important physiologic contributor to the successful maintenance of upright posture is the regulation of systemic blood pressure. The failure to perfuse the brain, which accompanies hypotension, increases the risk of a fall, usually in association with syncope. In addition to the age-related declines in baroreflex sensitivity to hypotensive stimuli, manifested as a failure to cardioaccelerate, everyday stresses such as posture change, eating a meal, or an acute illness may result in hypotension [32]. Because many elderly persons have a resting cerebral perfusion that is compromised by vascular disease, even slight reductions in blood pressure may produce cerebral ischemic symptoms, resulting in falls. Finally, with aging, there is a reduction in total body water, which places older individuals at increased risk of dehydration with acute illness, diuretic use, or hot weather conditions. Because there is a progressive decrease in basal and stimulated renin levels and a decrease in aldosterone production with aging, dehydrating stresses may lead to orthostatic hypotension and a fall.

CHRONIC CONDITIONS AND FALLS

In addition to the just-mentioned age-related physiologic changes that threaten postural control, a number of age-related chronic conditions deserve special mention because of their association with fall risk. Parkinson's disease, in particular, increases the risk of falls through several mechanisms, including the rigidity of lower extremity musculature, the inability to correct sway trajectory due to the slowness in initiating movement, hypotensive drug effects, and, in some cases, cognitive impairment. Another common disease contributing to falls is osteoarthritis. When present in the knee, osteoarthritis may affect mobility, the ability to step over objects and maneuver, and the tendency to avoid complete weight bearing on a painful joint.

MEDICATION USE AND FALLS

One of the most modifiable risk factors for falls that has been demonstrated repeatedly in observational studies is medication use. Thus, individual classes of medications, such as benzodiazepines, tricyclic antidepressants, the newer class of antidepressants (SSRIs) [32a,32b] and neuroleptics, have been associated with an increased risk of hip fracture [33–35]. In addition to these specific drug classes, recent changes in the dose of a medication, and the total number of prescriptions have been associated with an increased risk of falling [36,37].

ENVIRONMENTAL FACTORS

The relative importance of environmental factors to the risk of falling has not been well quantified because they interact so frequently with risk factors intrinsic to the individual. Well-designed intervention studies have focused on improving the risk factor profile of the individual [38] or have combined individual interventions with environmental manipulation [39], making it difficult to partition out the contributions of the environmental factors. Nevertheless, attention to safety hazards in the home environment would appear to be worthwhile. A home assessment by a physical therapist is one approach to addressing this need.

CLINICAL APPROACH

Many falls never come to clinical attention for a variety of reasons, including the following: the patient never mentions the event to a health care provider, there is no injury at the time of the fall, the provider fails to query the patient about a history of falls, or the invalid assumption that falls are an inevitable part of the aging process. It is not uncommon that treatment of injuries resulting from falls rarely includes an investigation of the etiology of the fall that led to the injury. It is common in emergency rooms and on orthopedic services to suture the laceration, immobilize the sprain, or repair the fracture without any further evaluation of the etiology of the fall.

Clinical Evaluation

HISTORY

In the clinical evaluation of the geriatric patient who is not specifically being seen for a problem with falling, it is still important that an assessment of fall risk be integrated into the history and physical examination. The most important point in the history is the previous history of a fall as this is a strong risk factor for future falls [40–42]. In the case of a patient presenting with a fall, important components of the history include the activity of the faller at the time of the incident, prodromal symptoms (lightheadedness, imbalance, dizziness), where the fall occurred, and when the fall occurred. Loss of consciousness is associated with injurious falls and should raise important considerations, such as orthostatic hypotension, cardiac, or neurologic disease. Information on previous falls should be collected to identify patterns that may help target risk factor modification strategies. A complete medication history should focus specifically on vasodilators, diuretics, and sedative hypnotic drug use because these agents have been associated with an increased risk of falls. In addition to inquiring about the circumstances surrounding the fall, the history should attempt to identify environmental factors that may have contributed. Thus, information on lighting, floor covering, door thresholds, railings, and furniture may add important clues.

STANDARD PHYSICAL EXAMINATION

The physical examination of the individual who has fallen should focus on those aspects related to the just-mentioned risk factors. Thus the examination should begin with an assessment of postural vital signs to rule out orthostatic hypotension [43]. Blood pressure and heart rate should be taken supine, then after 1 and 3 min of standing. If the patient is unable to stand, some information may be derived from sitting vital signs. An assessment of visual acuity should be performed as it was at the time of the fall, as this factor has been linked to the risk of hip fracture in several studies [44,45]. If the patient was not wearing corrective lenses, then the visual acuity should be checked with and without glasses. Hearing may be assessed using the whisper test or a hand-held audiometer [46], as eighth cranial nerve deficits may be associated with vestibular dysfunction. Examination of the extremities may uncover deformities of the feet that may contribute to the risk of falling, such as bunions, callouses, and arthritic deformities. Sensory neuropathies also increase the risk of falls [47]. Footwear may also be an important factor to consider. In one small study of older men tested for balance wearing a variety of shoe types, shoes with thin, hard soles produced the best results in terms of balance testing, although these shoes were perceived as less comfortable than thick, soft midsoled shoes such as running shoes [48].

EXAMINATION OF GAIT AND BALANCE

Probably the most important part of the physical examination is to include an assessment of integrated musculoskeletal function by performing one or more tests of postural stability. One of the best known tests is commonly referred to as the "get up and go test [49], which was originally described using a graded 1–5 scale. Later versions employed a timed performance [50] approach. The "get up and go" consists of a subject rising from a standard arm chair, walking a fixed distance across the room, turning around, walking back to the chair, and sitting back down. Observation of the different components of this test may help in identifying deficits in leg strength, balance, vestibular dysfunction, and gait.

Duncan and colleagues have also developed a simple maneuver called the "functional reach" test, which is a practical approach to testing the integrated neuromuscular base of support (51) and which has predictive validity for falls in elderly males [52]. This test is performed using a leveled yardstick secured to a wall at the height of the acromion. The person being tested assumes a comfortable stance without shoes or socks and stands so that his or her shoulders are perpendicular to the yardstick. The individual makes a fist and extends the arm forward as far as possible without taking a step or losing balance. The total reach is measured along the yardstick and recorded (Fig. 2). In its initial description, the functional reach correlated with other physical performance measures such as walking speed ($r = 0.71$), tandem walk using an ordinal scale ($r = 0.67$), and standing on one foot measured as number of seconds that a one-footed stance could be maintained ($r = 0.64$).

A more comprehensive performance-oriented assessment of balance has been used by Tinetti; it includes measures of sitting and standing balance, ability to withstand a nudge on the sternum, and ability to reach up, bend down, and extend the back and neck [53]. Each of these performance measures attempts to identify components of postural stability that complement the standard physical examination.

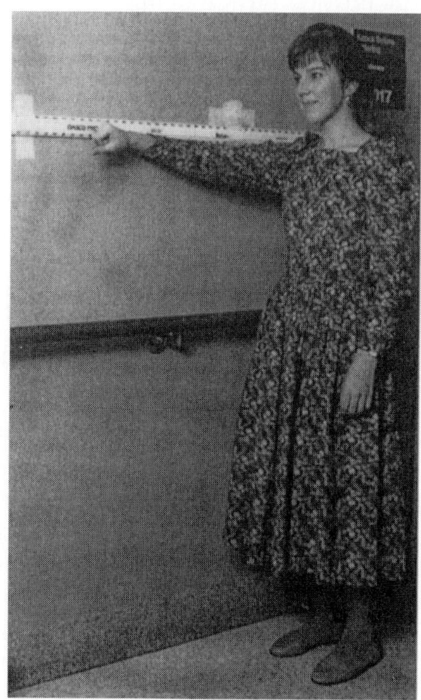

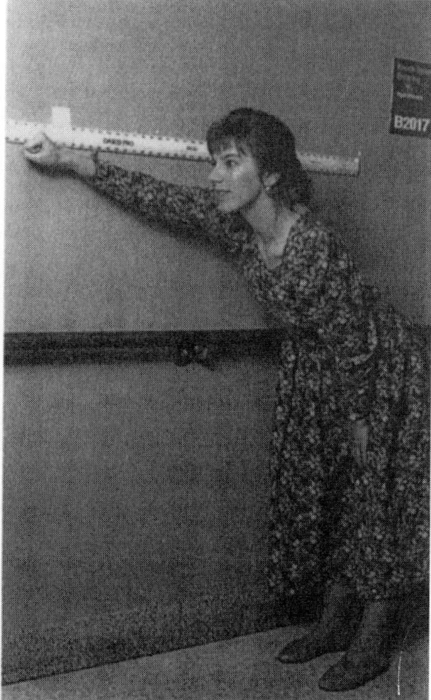

FIGURE 2 The functional reach measure. After Weiner *et al.* [51].

LABORATORY AND OTHER DIAGNOSTIC TESTING

Based on the history and physical examination, including the evaluation of postural stability, gait, and mobility, further diagnostic testing may be indicated. There is no "standard" diagnostic evaluation of an individual with falls or with a high risk of falls. Obviously laboratory tests such as hemoglobin, serum urea nitrogen, creatinine, or glucose can help to rule out causes of falling such as anemia, dehydration, and hyperglycemia with hyperosmolar dehydration. There is no proven value of routinely performing Holter monitoring of individuals who have fallen [54]. Similarly, the decision to perform echocardiography, brain imaging, or radiographic studies of the spine should be driven by the findings of the history and physical examination. Thus echocardiograms should be reserved for those with heart murmurs believed to contribute to the maintenance of blood flow to the brain. Spine radiographs or magnetic resonance imaging may be useful in patients with gait disorders, abnormalities on neurologic examination, lower extremity spasticity, or hyperreflexia to rule out cervical spondylosis or lumbar stenosis.

TREATMENT AND PREVENTION

Preventing Falls

As described earlier, data on risk factors for falling in community-dwelling older people are derived from multiple observational studies. Not all studies have identified the same intrinsic and environmental risk factors. Nevertheless, based on these reported risk factors, multiple preventive intervention studies have been conducted over the past decade, including programs to improve strength or balance, educational programs, optimization of medications, and environmental modifications in homes or institutions. Some interventions have targeted single-risk factor modification, whereas others have attempted to address multiple interventions.

In a systematic review of interventions to reduce the incidence of falling in the elderly, only studies that included elderly individuals randomized to an intervention versus control, or into one of two interventions, were considered. As of May 1997, 18 individual study reports meeting the inclusion criteria and one preplanned meta-analysis were identified. Of the 18 studies, 14 reported the effect of interventions in subjects living in the community [39,55–67], 2 were set in long-term care institutions [68,69], and 2 were hospital based, either in a rehabilitation hospital [70] or in an acute geriatric assessment and treatment unit [71]. Five of the studies compared a physical exercise intervention with an attention control visit, education only, or no intervention [61,62,64,67,69]. Reinsch *et al.* [64] also included a cognitive intervention, whereas Means *et al.* [63] compared a more intense exercise program with a lower intensity program. In nine of the studies, the intervention was targeted to risk factors identified on an initial assessment, including intrinsic risk factors and environmental factors. The other studies employed a variety of interventions, including physician referrals with or without a formal recommendation; health visitor assessments of nutrition, medical conditions, environmental hazards, and physical fitness; multifactorial interventions based on geriatric assessment; targeted risk factor intervention; counseling; and even hormone replacement therapy [55]. The hospital-based studies evaluated the effectiveness of a bed alarm system [71] and the use of blue identification bracelets [70] for the prevention of falls in high-risk elderly inpatients.

Results of this systematic review revealed that neither an untargeted exercise intervention alone versus usual care nor an untargeted exercise and health education or health education alone versus usual care significantly reduced the risk of falls. There was a suggestion that untargeted behavioral interventions targeting risk factors might reduce the risk of falls. The most favorable results were observed in studies in which health screening was followed by targeted interventions. Pooling of data from five studies suggested that an intervention in which older people are assessed by a health professional trained to identify intrinsic and environmental risk factors is likely to reduce the fall rate (odds ratio = 0.79; 95% CI 0.65–0.96) [72]. These results are summarized graphically in Figs. 3–8. The costs of implementing such a program with a multidimensional health assessment followed by targeted interventions have been explored in one of the five studies to investigate such an approach. Based on the results of that study, targeted intervention appears cost effective [73].

Since the time of this review of clinical trials to reduce the incidence of falling in the elderly, an additional randomized controlled trial was published by Buchner and colleagues [74]. This study tested the effect of strength and endurance training on gait, balance, physical health status, fall risk, and health services use in older adults. This single-blinded, randomized controlled trial enrolled 105 elderly subjects from a health maintenance organization with at least mild deficits in strength and balance. There were three exercise groups (strength training using weight machines, endurance training using bicycles, and strength and endurance training) and a control. After 6 months of intervention, with all exercise groups combined versus the control group, there was a significant beneficial effect of exercise on time to the first fall (relative hazard = 0.53, 95% CI 0.30–0.91), despite the fact that there was virtually no effect on

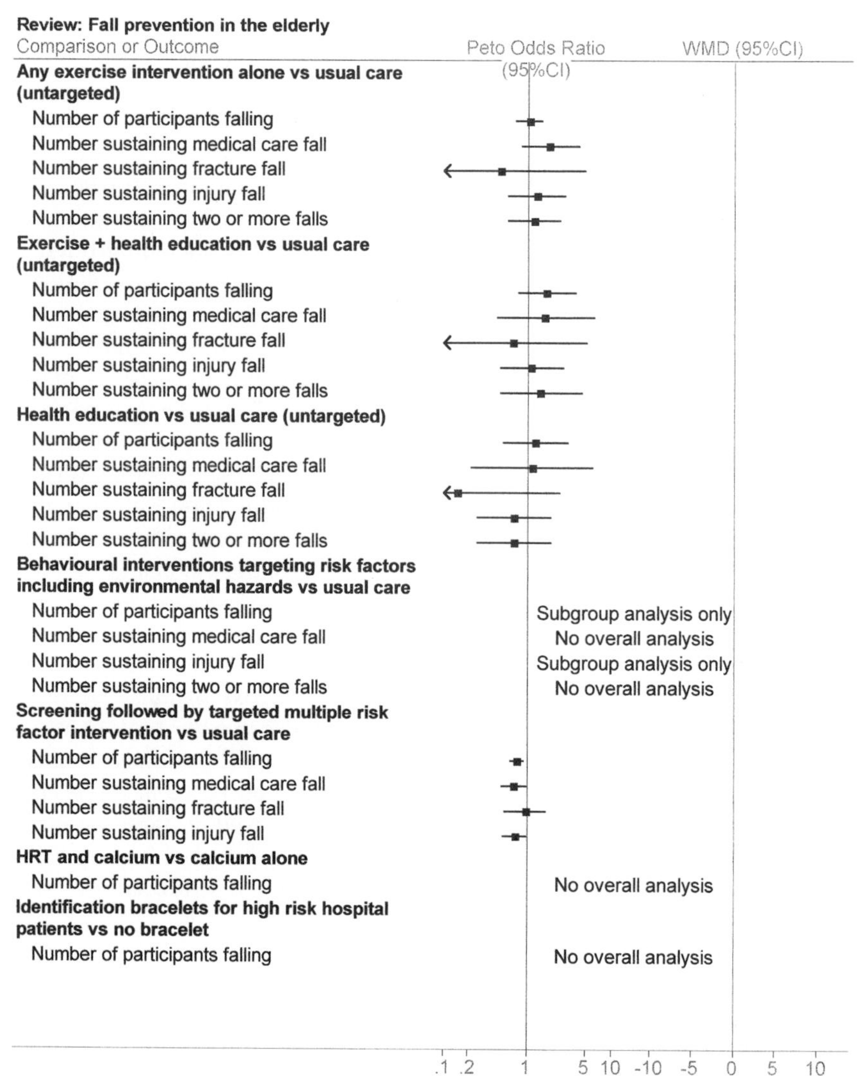

FIGURE 3 Results of meta-analysis of studies using various interventions to prevent falls in the elderly. From Gillespie *et al.* [72].

intermediate outcomes such as gait and balance. Similar results emerged when a person–time analysis was done to address whether exercise subjects had fewer total falls during follow-up. The fall rate in controls (0.81 falls/year) was significantly higher than the rate in exercise subjects (0.49 falls/year) (relative risk = 0.61, 95% CI 0.39–0.93). These findings differed from the meta-analysis of the related intervention studies called the FICSIT studies, even though this study was included in the meta-analysis [38]. This meta-analysis suggested that strength and endurance training may not affect fall risk, which is similar to the conclusions of the systematic review. Of course it is possible that only some endurance and strength training protocols are effective and possibly only effective in certain subgroups. All of these studies highlight the need for clarification of the effect of exercise on groups of elderly persons with different functional status.

Preventing Fractures Using Passive Protective Systems

Because falls to the side that impact on the hip are the primary determinant of hip fracture [9,10], there is considerable interest in the design and evaluation of protective trochanteric padding devices. In early trials, padding devices were found to reduce hip fracture risk, but subject compliance was relatively low [26]. Newer padding systems are designed to lower femoral impact force by shunting energy away from the femur and into the surrounding soft tissues. Laboratory methods of im-

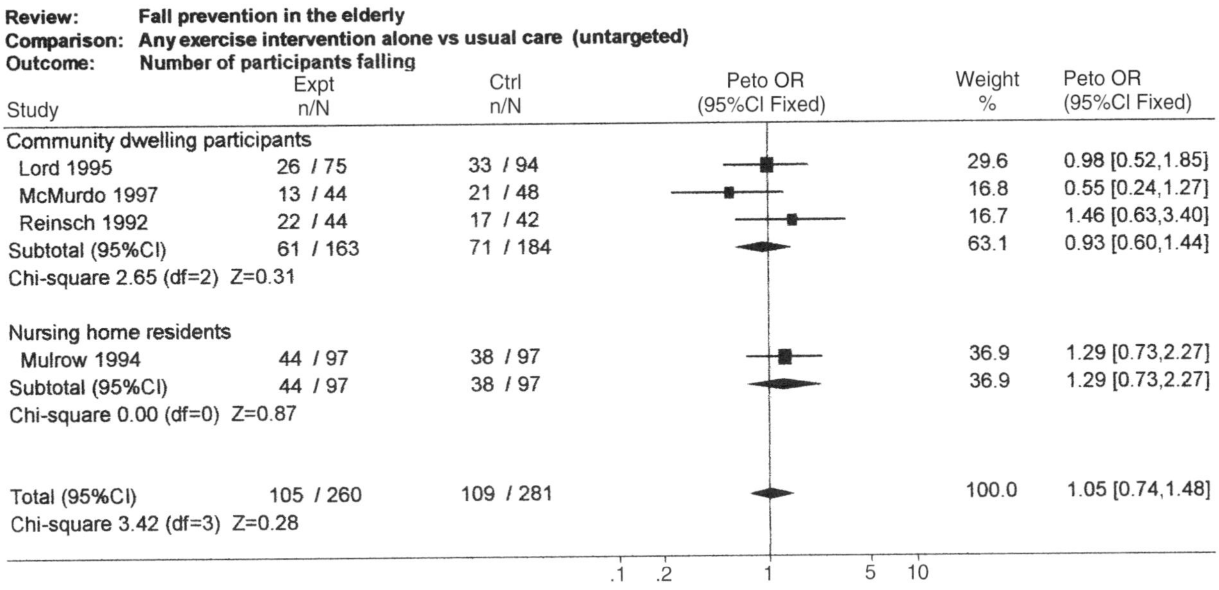

Review: **Fall prevention in the elderly**
Comparison: **Any exercise intervention alone vs usual care (untargeted)**
Outcome: **Number of participants falling**

Study	Expt n/N	Ctrl n/N	Peto OR (95%CI Fixed)	Weight %	Peto OR (95%CI Fixed)
Community dwelling participants					
Lord 1995	26 / 75	33 / 94		29.6	0.98 [0.52,1.85]
McMurdo 1997	13 / 44	21 / 48		16.8	0.55 [0.24,1.27]
Reinsch 1992	22 / 44	17 / 42		16.7	1.46 [0.63,3.40]
Subtotal (95%CI)	61 / 163	71 / 184		63.1	0.93 [0.60,1.44]
Chi-square 2.65 (df=2) Z=0.31					
Nursing home residents					
Mulrow 1994	44 / 97	38 / 97		36.9	1.29 [0.73,2.27]
Subtotal (95%CI)	44 / 97	38 / 97		36.9	1.29 [0.73,2.27]
Chi-square 0.00 (df=0) Z=0.87					
Total (95%CI)	105 / 260	109 / 281		100.0	1.05 [0.74,1.48]
Chi-square 3.42 (df=3) Z=0.28					

.1 .2 1 5 10

FIGURE 4 Results of meta-analysis of studies examining fall prevention in the elderly (studies of community-dwelling older persons and nursing home residents) in which the intervention was exercise alone versus usual care. From Gillespie *et al.* [72].

Review: **Fall prevention in the elderly**
Comparison: **Exercise + health education vs usual care (untargeted)**
Outcome: **Number of participants falling**

Study	Expt n/N	Ctrl n/N	Peto OR (95%CI Fixed)	Weight %	Peto OR (95%CI Fixed)
Reinsch 1992	33 / 61	17 / 42		100.0	1.72 [0.78,3.75]
Total (95%CI)	33 / 61	17 / 42		100.0	1.72 [0.78,3.75]
Chi-square 0.00 (df=0) Z=1.35					

.1 .2 1 5 10

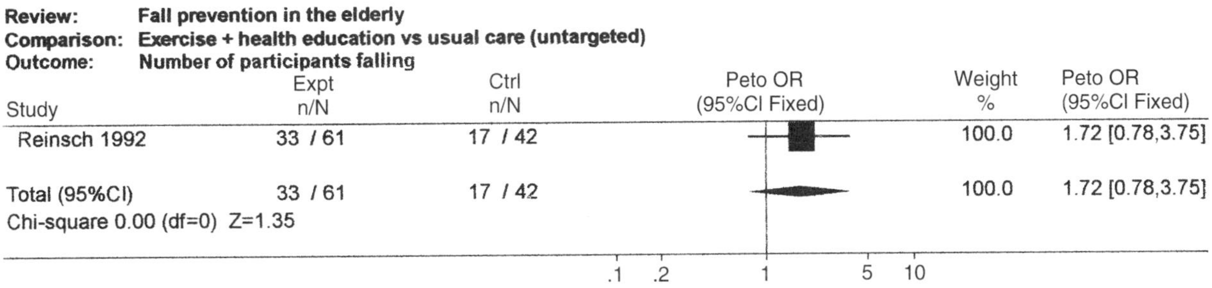

FIGURE 5 Results of meta-analysis of studies examining fall prevention in the elderly in which the intervention was exercise plus health education versus usual care. From Gillespie *et al.* [72].

Review: **Fall prevention in the elderly**
Comparison: **Health education vs usual care (untargeted)**
Outcome: **Number of participants falling**

Study	Expt n/N	Ctrl n/N	Peto OR (95%CI Fixed)	Weight %	Peto OR (95%CI Fixed)
Reinsch 1992	17 / 37	17 / 42		100.0	1.25 [0.51,3.03]
Total (95%CI)	17 / 37	17 / 42		100.0	1.25 [0.51,3.03]
Chi-square 0.00 (df=0) Z=0.49					

.1 .2 1 5 10

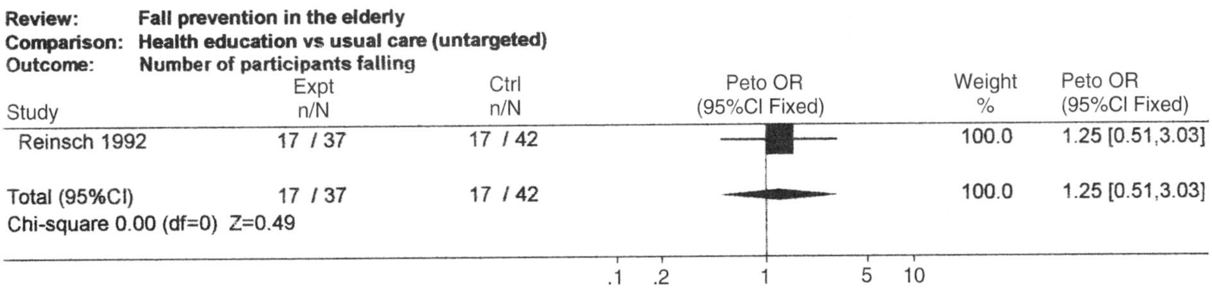

FIGURE 6 Results of meta-analysis of studies examining fall prevention in the elderly in which the intervention was health education versus usual care. From Gillespie *et al.* [72].

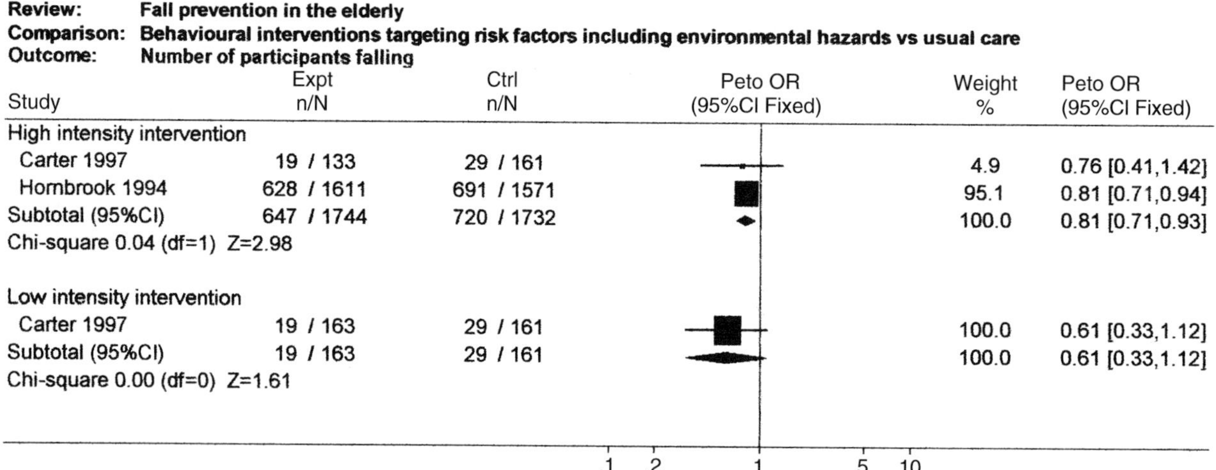

Review: **Fall prevention in the elderly**
Comparison: **Behavioural interventions targeting risk factors including environmental hazards vs usual care**
Outcome: **Number of participants falling**

Study	Expt n/N	Ctrl n/N	Weight %	Peto OR (95%CI Fixed)
High intensity intervention				
Carter 1997	19 / 133	29 / 161	4.9	0.76 [0.41,1.42]
Hornbrook 1994	628 / 1611	691 / 1571	95.1	0.81 [0.71,0.94]
Subtotal (95%CI)	647 / 1744	720 / 1732	100.0	0.81 [0.71,0.93]
Chi-square 0.04 (df=1) Z=2.98				
Low intensity intervention				
Carter 1997	19 / 163	29 / 161	100.0	0.61 [0.33,1.12]
Subtotal (95%CI)	19 / 163	29 / 161	100.0	0.61 [0.33,1.12]
Chi-square 0.00 (df=0) Z=1.61				

FIGURE 7 Results of meta-analysis of studies examining fall prevention in the elderly in which the intervention was behavioral, targeting risk factors including environmental hazards, versus usual care. From Gillespie *et al.* [72].

Review: **Fall prevention in the elderly**
Comparison: **Screening followed by targeted multiple risk factor intervention vs usual care**
Outcome: **Number of participants falling**

Study	Expt n/N	Ctrl n/N	Peto OR (95%CI Fixed)	Weight %	Peto OR (95%CI Fixed)
Fabacher 1994	14 / 100	22 / 95		5.9	0.55 [0.27,1.12]
Rubenstein 1990	64 / 79	68 / 81		4.7	0.82 [0.36,1.84]
Tinetti 1994	52 / 147	68 / 144		14.2	0.61 [0.39,0.98]
Vetter 1992	95 / 240	65 / 210		20.7	1.46 [0.99,2.14]
Wagner 1994	175 / 635	223 / 607		54.4	0.66 [0.52,0.83]
Total (95%CI)	400 / 1201	446 / 1137		100.0	0.77 [0.64,0.91]
Chi-square 13.96 (df=4) Z=2.97					

.1 .2 1 5 10

FIGURE 8 Results of meta-analysis of studies examining fall prevention in the elderly in which the intervention was screening followed by targeted mutliple risk factor intervention versus usual care. From Gillespie *et al.* [72].

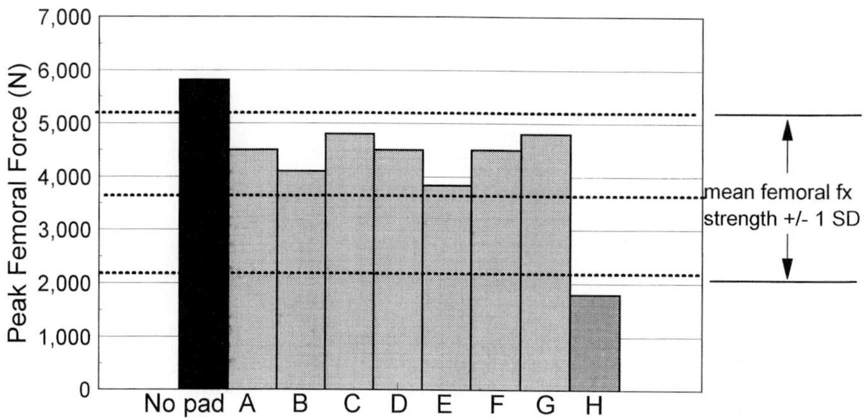

FIGURE 9 Impact tests with a laboratory apparatus measuring force attenuation of eight energy-shunting pads compared with no pad. Bars show mean peak femoral force from five repeated measures, with error bars displaying 1 standard deviation. Pad H is the pad currently being tested by the author in collaboration with Dr. Wilson C. Hayes. After Robinovitch *et al.* [75].

pact testing are available for comparing the ability of such devices to attenuate the forces of a fall on the trochanter. Using such laboratory tests, there are wide ranges of energy reducing potential of the pads currently available [75]. Not all pads attenuate the forces of a fall on the trochanter to levels that would be expected to reduce the risk of hip fracture. As optimal pad design evolves, it is expected that these devices may enjoy widespread use by elderly individuals who are at the highest risk of fall-related fractures, such as nursing home residents. As with any therapeutic intervention, the hip pad would be expected to have the greatest protection among persons who are prone to fall to the side and who have very little soft tissue overlying the trochanter (Fig. 9).

Related to protective trochanteric padding devices, another way to reduce the energy delivered to the hip during a fall is to design flooring materials that will absorb energy rather than deliver the energy of a fall directly to the trochanter. Toward this goal, such flooring materials are being tested with the goal of using them in high-risk environments such as nursing homes.

CLINICAL GUIDELINES

For patients who have sustained a fall, the following approach has been suggested by one expert in the field [76]. This guideline synthesizes much of the data from the previous discussions of risk factors and multidimen-

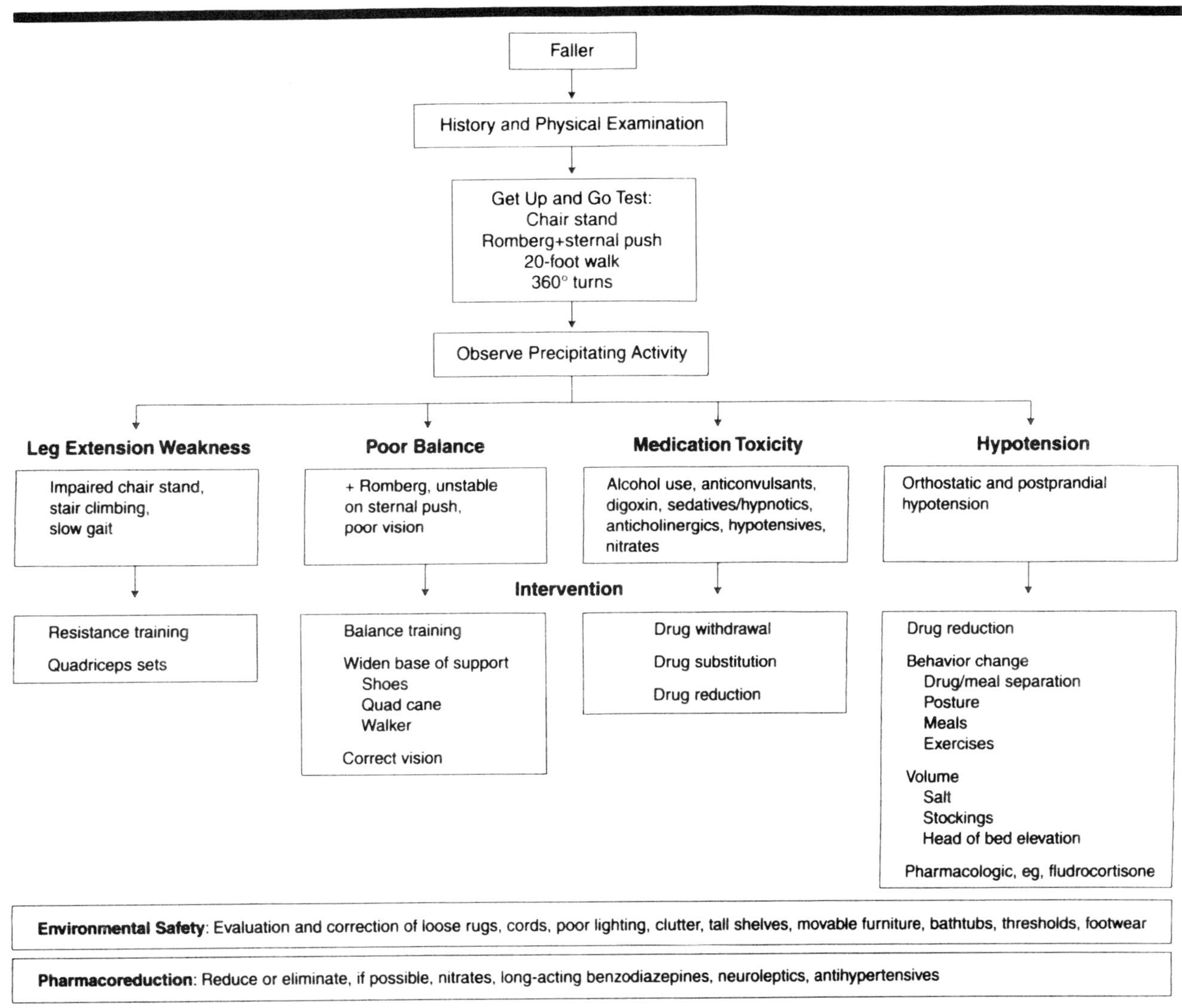

FIGURE 10 A therapeutic approach to a patient with falls. The interventions entitled Environmental Safety and Pharmacoreduction are appropriate for all patients with falls. After Lipsitz [76].

TABLE II Approach to Fall Risk Assessment and Targeted Interventions to Reduce Falls

Risk Factors	Interventions
Postural hypotension	Behavioral recommendation such as ankle pumps or hand clenching; elevate head of bed
Use of any benzodiazepines or other sedative-hypnotics	Education about appropriate use of these medications; nonpharmacologic treatment of sleep problems; medication taper and discontinuation
At least four prescription drugs	Medication review with patient
Unsafe tub and toilet transfers	Transfer training; environmental manipulations such as grab bars and raised toilet seats
Environmental fall or tripping hazards	Appropriate manipulations such as hazard removal, safer furniture, and structures such as grab bars or stair handrails
Any gait impairment	Gait training, appropriate assistive device, balance or strengthening exercises if indicated
Any transfer or balance impairment	Balance exercises, transfer training if indicated, environmental manipulations (walking devices, reachers, adaptive furniture such as higher chairs)
Impairment of lower and upper extremity muscle strength or joint range of motion	Resistive exercises

sional assessment and targeted intervention. For elderly persons who have no history of falling, it would seem reasonable to approach the patient through the use of the traditional multidimensional geriatric assessment with targeted interventions as risk factors are identified. (Fig. 10 and Table II). This is adapted from the findings of Tinetti and colleagues [39,77].

SUMMARY

It is clear from this review that an integrated approach to the reduction of osteoporotic fractures requires attention to the falling risk. The contribution of falling to the etiology of fractures is considerable and probably more important in the aged individual who often has underlying low bone mass. Based on recent prospective cohort studies, multiple risk factors for falls have been identified. The best approach to reducing falls and thereby lowering fracture risk is to comprehensively assess the older person and to intervene in multiple domains as identified from the assessment. This approach can be cost effective and will potentially lead to a better quality of life for the aging population.

References

1. Tinetti, M. E., Inouye, S. K., Gill, T. M., and Doucette, J. T. Shared risk factors for falls, incontinence, and functional dependence. *JAMA* **273,** 1348–1353 (1995).
2. Tinetti, M. E., Speechley, M., and Ginter, S. F. Risk factors for falls among elderly persons living in the community. *N. Engl. J. Med.* **319,** 1701–1707 (1988).
3. Graafmans, W. C., Ooms, M. E., Hofstee, H. M. A., Bezemer, P. D., Bouter, L. M., and Lips, P. Falls in the elderly: A prospective study of risk factors and risk profiles. *Am. J. Epidemiol.* **143,** 1129–1136 (1996).
4. Campbell, A. J., Borrie, M. J., and Spears, G. F. Risk factors for falls in a community-based prospective study of people 70 years and older. *J. Gerontol.* **44,** 112–117 (1989).
5. Nevitt, M. C., Cummings, S. R., and Hudes, E. S. Risk factors for injurious falls: A prospective study. *J. Gerontol.* **46,** M164-M170 (1991).
6. Purushottam, B. T., Brockman, K. G., Gideon, P., Fought, R. L., and Ray, W. A. Injurious falls in nonambulatory nursing home residents: A comparative study of circumstances, incidence, and risk factors. *J. Am. Geriatr. Soc.* **44,** 273–278 (1996).
7. Tinetti, M. E., Liu, W., and Ginter, S. F. Mechanical restraint use and fall-related injuries among residents of skilled nursing facilities. *Ann. Intern. Med.* **116,** 369–374 (1992).
8. Cooper, C., Atkinson, E. J., O'Fallon, M., and Melton, L. J. Incidence of clinically diagnosed vertebral fractures: A population-based study in Rochester, Minnesota, 1985–1989. *J. Bone Miner. Res.* **7,** 221–227 (1992).
9. Nevitt, M. C., Cummings, S. R., and Group, and The Study Of Osteoporotic Fractures Research Group. Type of fall and risk of hip and wrist fractures: The study of osteoporotic fractures. *J. Am. Geriatr. Soc.* **41,** 1226–1234 (1993).
10. Greenspan, S. L., Myers, E. R., Maitland, L. A., Resnick, N. M., and Hayes, W. C. Fall severity and bone mineral density as risk factors for hip fracture in ambulatory elderly. *JAMA* **271,** 128–133 (1994).
11. Kiel, D. P., O'Sullivan, P., Teno, J. M., and Mor, V. Health care utilization and functional status in the aged following a fall. *Med. Care* **29,** 221–228 (1991).
12. Tinetti, M. E., and Williams, C. S. Falls, injuries due to falls, and the risk of admission to a nursing home. *N. Engl. J. Med.* **337,** 1279–1284 (1997).
13. Tinetti, M. E., Mendes de Leon, C. F., Doucette, J. T., and Baker, D. I. Fear of falling and fall-related efficacy in relationship to functioning among community-living elders. *J. Gerontol.* **49,** M140–M147 (1994).
14. Tinetti, M. E., Liu, W. L., and Claus, E. B. Predictors and prognosis of inability to get up after falls among elderly persons. *JAMA* **269,** 65–70 (1993).
15. Sattin, R. W. Falls among older persons: A public health perspective. *Annu. Rev. Public Health* **13,** 489–508 (1992).
16. Sattin, R. W., Huber, D. A. L., DeVito, C. A., Rodriauez, J. G., Ros, A., Bacchelli, S., Stevens, J. A., and Waxweiler, R. J. The incidence of fall injury events among the elderly in a defined population. *Am. J. Epidemiol.* **131,** 1028–1037 (1990).

17. King, M. B., and Tinnetti, M. E. Falls in community-dwelling older persons. *J. Am. Geriatr. Soc.* **43,** 1146–1154 (1995).
18. Grisso, J. A., Schwartz, D. F., Wolfson, V., Polansky, M., and LaPann, K. The impact of falls in an inner-city elderly African-American population. *J. Am. Geriatr. Soc.* **40,** 673–678 (1992).
19. Alexander, B. H., Rivara, F. P., and Wolf, M. E. The cost and frequency of hospitalization for fall related injuries in older adults. *Am. J. Public Health* **82,** 1020–1023 (1992).
20. Ray, N. F., Chan, J. K., Thamer, M., and Melton, L. J. Medical expenditures for the treatment of osteoporotic fractures in the United States in 1995: Report from the National Osteoporosis Foundation. *J. Bone Miner. Res.* **12,** 24–35 (1997).
21. Nickens, H. Intrinsic factors in falling among the elderly. *Arch. Intern. Med.* **145,** 1089–1093 (1985).
22. Speechley, M., and Tinetti, M. Falls and injuries in frail and vigorous community elderly persons. *J. Am. Geriatr. Soc.* **39,** 46–52 (1991).
23. Hayes, W. C., "Biomechanics of Cortical and Trabecular Bone: Implications for Assessment of Fracture Risk." Raven Press, New York, 1991.
24. van den Kroonenberg, A. J., Hayes, W. C., and McMahon, T. A. Hip impact velocities and body configurations for voluntary falls from standing height. *J. Biomech.* **29,** 807–811 (1996).
25. Hayes, W. C., Myers, E. R., Robinovitch, S. N., Kroonenberg, A. V. D., Courtney, A. C., and McMahon, T. A. Etiology and prevention of age-related hip fractures. *Bone* **18,** 77S–86S (1996).
26. Lauritzen, J. B., Petersen, M. M., and Lund, B. Effect of external hip protectors on hip fractures. *Lancet* **341,** 11–13 (1993).
27. Alexander, N. B. Postural control in older adults. *J. Am. Geriatr. Soc.* **42,** 93–108 (1994).
28. Scheibel, A. B. Falls, motor dysfunction, and correlative neurohistologic changes in the elderly. *Clin. Geriatr. Med.* **1,** 671–677 (1985).
29. Woollacott, M. H., Shumway-Cook, A., and Nashner, L. M. Aging and posture control: Changes in sensory organization and muscular coordination. *Int'l. J. Aging Hum. Dev.* **23,** 97–114 (1986).
30. Maki, B. E., and McIlroy, W. E. Postural control in the older adult. *Clin. Geriatr. Med.* **12,** 635–658 (1996).
31. Thelen, D. G., Schultz, A. B., Alexander, N. B., and Ashton-Miller, J. A. Effect of age on rapid ankle torque development. *J. Gerontol. Med. Sci.* **51A,** M226–M232 (1996).
32. Jonsson, P. V., Lipsitz, L. A., Kelley, M. M., and Koestner, J. S. Hypotensive responses to common daily activities in institutionalized elderly: A potential risk for recurrent falls. *Arch. Intern. Med.* **150,** 1518–1524 (1990).
32a. Liu, B., Anderson, G., Mittman, N., *et al.* Use of selective serotonin-reuptake inhibitors or tricyclic antidepressants and risk of hip fractures in elderly people. *Lancet* **351,** 1303–1307 (1998).
32b. Thapa, P. B., Gideon, P., Cost, T. W., *et al.* Antidepressants and the risk of falls among nursing home residents. *N. Engl. J. Med.* **339,** 875–882 (1998).
33. Ray, W. A., Griffin, M. R., and Schaffner, W. Psychotropic drug use and the risk of hip fracture. *N. Engl. J. Med.* **316,** 363–369 (1987).
34. Ray, W. A., Griffin, M. R., and Malcolm, E. Cyclic antidepressants and the risk of hip fracture. *Arch. Intern. Med.* **151,** 754–756 (1991).
35. Ray, W. A., Griffin, M. R., and Downey, W. Benzodiazepines of long and short elimination half-life and the risk of hip fracture. *JAMA* **262,** 3303–3307 (1989).
36. Cumming, R. G., Miller, J. P., Kelsey, J. L., *et al.* Medications and multiple falls in elderly people: The St. Louis OASIS study. *Age Ageing* **20,** 455–461 (1991).
37. Buchner, D. M., and Larson, E. B. Falls and fractures in patients with alzheimer-type dementia. *JAMA* **257,** 1492–1495 (1987).
38. Province, M. A., Hadley, E. C., Hornbrook, M. C., Lipsitz, L. A., Miller, J. P., Mulrow, C. D., Ory, M. G., Sattin, R. W., Tinetti, M. E., and Wolf, S. L. The effects of exercise on falls in elderly patients: A preplanned meta-analysis of the FICSIT trials. *JAMA* **273,** 1341–1347 (1995).
39. Tinetti, M. E., Baker, D. I., and McAvay, G. A multifactorial intervention to reduce the risk of falling among elderly people living in the community. *N. Engl. J. Med.* **331,** 821–827 (1994).
40. Teno, J., Kiel, D. P., and Mor, V. Multiple stumbles: A risk factor for falls in community-dwelling elderly. *J. Am. Geriatr. Soc.* **38,** 1321–1325 (1990).
41. Myers, A. H., Baker, S. P., Van Natta, M. L., Abbey, H., and Robinson, E. G. Risk factors associated with falls and injuries among elderly institutionalized persons. *Am. J. Epidemiol.* **133,** 1179–1190 (1991).
42. Nevitt, M. C., Cummings, S. R., Kidd, S., and Black, D. Risk factors for recurrent nonsyncopal falls: A prospective study. *JAMA* **261,** 2663–2668 (1989).
43. Lipsitz, L. A. Orthostatic hypotension in the elderly. *N. Engl. J. Med.* **321,** 952–957 (1989).
44. Felson, D. T., Anderson, J. J., Hannan, M. T., Milton, R., Wilson, P. W. F., and Kiel, D. P. Impaired vision and hip fracture: The Framingham Study. *J. Am. Geriatr. Soc.* **37,** 495–500 (1989).
45. Cummings, S. R., Nevitt, M. C., Browner, W. S., Stone, K., Fox, K. M., Ensrud, K. E., Cauley, J., Black, D., and Vogt, T. M. Risk factors for hip fracture in white women. *N. Engl. J. Med.* **332,** 767–773 (1995).
46. Lichtenstein, M. J., Bess, F. H., and Logan, S. A. Validation of screening tools for identifying hearing impaired elderly in primary care. *JAMA* **259,** 2875–2878 (1988).
47. Richardson, J. K., and Hurvitz, E. A. Peripheral neuropathy: A true risk factor for falls. *J. Gernotol.* **50A,** M211–M215 (1995).
48. Robbins, S., Gouw, G. J., and McClaran, J. Shoe sole thickness and hardness influence balance in older men. *J. Am. Geriatr. Soc.* **40,** 1089–1094 (1992).
49. Mathias, A., Nayak, U. S. L., and Isaacs, B. Balance in elderly patients: The "get up and go" test. *Arch. Phys. Med. Rehab.* **67,** 387–389 (1986).
50. Posiadlo, D., and Richardson, S. The timed "Up & Go": A test of basic functional mobility for frail elderly persons. *J. Am. Geriatr. Soc.* **39,** 142–148 (1991).
51. Weiner, D. K., Duncan, P. W., Chandler, J., and Studenski, S. A. Functional reach: A marker of physical frailty. *J. Am. Geriatr. Soc.* **40,** 203–207 (1992).
52. Duncan, P. W., Studenski, S., Chandler, J., and Prescott, B., Functional reach: Predictive validity in a sample of elderly male veterans. *J. Gerontol.* **47,** M93–M98 (1992).
53. Tinetti, M. E. Performance-oriented assessment of mobility problems in elderly patients. *J. Am. Geriatr. Soc.* **34,** 119–126 (1986).
54. Rosado, J. A., Rubenstein, L. Z., Robbins, A. S., Heng, M. K., Schulman, B. L., and Josephson, K. R. The value of holter monitoring in evaluating the elderly patient who falls. *J. Am. Geriatr. Soc.* **37,** 430–434 (1989).
55. Armstrong, A. L., Osborne, J., Coupland, C. A. C., Macpherson, M. B., Bassey, E. J., and Wallace, W. A. Effect of hormone replacement therapy on muscle performance and balance in post-menopausal women. *Clin. Sci.* **91,** 685–690 (1996).
56. Carpenter, G. I., and Demopoulos, G. R. Screening the elderly in the community: Controlled trial of dependency surveillance using a questionnaire administered by volunteers. *Br. Med. J.* **300,** 1253–1256 (1990).
57. Carter, S., Campbell, E., and Sanson-Fisher, R. A trial of two strategies aimed at reducing falls and other unintentional events

through home modification and medication review. submitted for publication.

58. Fabacher, D., Josephson, K., Pietruszka, F., Linderborn, K., Morley, J. E., and Rubenstein, L. Z. An in-home preventive assessment programme for independent older adults. *J. Am. Geriatr. Soc.* **42,** 630–638 (1994).
59. Gallagher, E. M., and Brunt, H. Head over heels: Impact of a health promotion program to reduce falls in the elderly. *Can. J. Aging* **15,** 84–96 (1996).
60. Hornbrook, M. C., Stevens, V. J., Wingfield, D. J., Hollis, J. F., Greenlick, M. R., and Ory, M. G. Preventing falls among community-dwelling older persons: Results from a randomized trial. *Gerontologist* **34,** 16–23 (1994).
61. Lord, S. R., Ward, J. A., Williams, P., and Sturdwick, M. The effect of a 12-month exercise trial on balance, strength, and falls in older women: A randomized controlled trial. *J. Am. Geriatr. Soc.* **43,** 1198–1206 (1995).
62. McMurdo, M. E. T., Mole, P. A., and Paterson, C. R. Controlled trial of weight bearing exercise in older women in relation to bone density and falls. *Br. Med. J.* **314,** 596 (1997).
63. Means, K. M., Rodell, D. E., O'Sullivan, P. S., and Cranford, L. A. Rehabilitation of elderly fallers: Pilot study of a low to moderate intensity exercise programme. *Arch. Phys. Med. Rehab.* **77,** 1030–1036 (1996).
64. Reinsch, S., MacRae, P., Lachenbruch, P. A., and Tobis, J. S. Attempts to prevent falls and injury: A prospective community study. *Gerontologist* **32,** 450–456 (1992).
65. Vetter, N. J., Lewis, P. A., and Ford, D. Can health visitors prevent fractures in elderly people? *Br. Med. J.* **304,** 888–890 (1992).
66. Wagner, E. H., LaCroix, A. Z., Grothaus, L., Leveille, S. G., Hecht, J. A., Artz, K., Odle, K., and Buchner, D. M. Preventing disability and falls in older adults: A population-based randomized trial. *Am. J. Public Health* **84,** 1800–1806 (1994).
67. Wolf, S. L., Barnhart, H. X., Kutner, N. G., McNeely, E., Coogler, C., and Xu, T. Reducing frailty and falls in older persons: An investigation of Tai Chi and computerized balance training. *J. Am. Geriatr. Soc.* **44,** 489–497 (1996).
68. Rubenstein, L. Z., Robbins, A. S., Josephson, K. R., Schulman, B. L., and Osterweil, D. The value of assessing falls in an elderly population. A randomized clinical trial. *Ann. Intern. Med.* **113,** 308–316 (1990).
69. Mulrow, C. D., Gerety, M. B., Kanten, D., Cornell, J. E., DeNino, L. A., Chiodo, L., Aguilar, C., O'Neil, M. B., Rosenberg, J., and Solis, R. M. A randomized trial of physical rehabilitation of very frail nursing home residents. *JAMA* **271,** 519–524 (1994).
70. Mayo, N. E., Gloutney, L., and Levy, A. R., *Arch. Phys. Med. Rehab.* **75,** 1302–1308 (1994).
71. Tideiksaar, R., Feiner, C. F., and Maby, J. Falls prevention: The efficacy of a bed alarm system in an acute-care setting. *Mt. Sinai J. Med.* **60,** 522–527 (1993).
72. Gillespie, L. D., Gillespie, W. J., Cumming, R., Lamb, S. E., and Rowe, B. H. Interventions to reduce the incidence of falling in the elderly. *Cochrane Database of Systematic Reviews* (1998).
73. Rizzo, J. A., Baker, K. I., McAvay, G., and Tinetti, M. E. The cost-effectiveness of a multifactorial targeted intervention program for falls among community elderly persons. *Med Care* **34,** 954–969 (1996).
74. Buchner, D. M., Cress, M. E., de Lateur, B. J., Esselman, P. C., Margherita, A. J., Price, R., and Wagner, E. H. The effect of strength and endurance training on gait, balance, fall risk, and health services use in community-living older adults. *J. Gerontol.* **52A,** M218–M224 (1997).
75. Robinovitch, S. N., Hayes, W. C., and McMahon, T. A. Energy-shunting hip padding system attenuates femoral impact force in a simulated fall. *J. Biomech. Eng.* **117,** 409–413 (1995).
76. Lipsitz, L. A. An 85-year old woman with a history of falls. *JAMA* **276,** 59–66 (1996).
77. Tinetti, M. E., Baker, K. I., Garrett, P. A., Gottschalk, M., Koch, M. L., and Horwitz, R. I. Yale FICSIT: risk factor abatement strategy for fall prevention. *J. Am. Geriatr. Soc.* **41,** 315–320 (1993).
78. O'Loughlin, J. L., Robitaille, Y., Boivin, J. F., Suissa, S. Incidence of and risk factors for falls and injurious falls among the community-dwelling elderly. *Am. J. Epidemiol.* **137,** 342–354 (1993).
79. Tinetti, M. E., Doucette, J., Claus, E., Marottoli, R. Risk factors for serious injury during falls by older persons in the community. *J. Am. Geriatr. Soc.* **43,** 1214–1221 (1995).

Impact of Physical Activity on Age-Related Bone Loss

BELINDA BECK AND ROBERT MARCUS

Geriatrics Research, Education and Clinical Center, Veterans Affairs Medical Center, Palo Alto, and Department of Medicine, Stanford University Stanford, California 94304

INTRODUCTION

Exercise is frequently promoted as a natural panacea for the age-related deterioration of body functions. As with most generalizations, there may be substance to this concept, but the degree to which it can be embraced is limited by exceptions to the rule. The aim of this chapter is to examine the evidence that physical activity can attenuate age-related bone loss.

Peak bone mass, the amount of bone present at skeletal maturity, is attained during the third decade of life, after which time the skeleton undergoes a gradual loss of mass. As the consequence of this loss is bone fragility and increased risk of fracture, substantial effort has been directed toward identifying behaviors that may reduce it. This chapter describes the nature of age-related changes to the skeleton, the typical response of normal bone tissue to controlled mechanical loading, and the effect of exercise intervention on the skeleton during aging. It also considers the modulating influence of factors such as muscle strength, calcium supplementation, and hormone replacement therapy on this effect.

Previous examinations of the role of physical activity in osteoporosis prevention have concluded that regular weight bearing and resistance exercise may increase bone mass or at least retard bone loss [1–15]. However, the evidence underlying these conclusions must be interpreted with caution due to common limitations in study design such as the subject selection bias inherent in cross-sectional studies. In addition, methodological shortcomings, including unreliable measurement technique and inappropriate skeletal site evaluation, often confound definitive generalizations. Consequently, this chapter emphasizes as much as possible, those reports that utilized a rigorous methodological technique (randomized, controlled intervention trials, unless otherwise stated), measured bone regions specifically loaded in the course of the intervention, and utilized instruments of bone mass measurement with the smallest degree of precision error. The authors acknowledge that this approach substantially reduces the large offering of published studies and may exclude a number of traditionally cited works. The authors consider the increased reliability of data adequate justification for such omissions.

THE NATURE OF AGE-RELATED BONE LOSS

Mechanisms of Bone Loss

Normal bone tissue exists in a state of ongoing remodeling, a coupled process of osteoclastic bone removal followed by osteoblastic bone replacement. It is thought that the fundamental role of bone remodeling is to minimize the accumulation of fatigue damage that occurs with repetitive loading. The generalized loss of bone subsequent to the acquisition of peak skeletal mass reflects an inherent inefficiency in the remodeling process, i.e., the amount of bone formed does not fully match that which has been resorbed so that small deficits in bone mass accumulate with each successive remodeling cycle. The degree of remodeling inefficiency increases with age, infirmity, and some medications. Thus, although remodeling provides a buffer against tissue fatigue, its long-term consequence is progressive bone loss. Therefore, anything that promotes an increase in whole body bone remodeling, such as nutrient or hormonal deficiency, will accelerate the loss of bone, whereas successful efforts to lower remodeling activity will conserve it.

Age-Related Adaptations in Bone Geometry

Bone strength is influenced not only by its material properties, such as mineral density, but also by its macro- and microscopic geometry. Macroscopic geometry refers to the shape and dimension of a bone as a whole, whereas microscopic geometry pertains to the orientation of osteons and microporosity within the bone tissue. To illustrate, the ability of a vertebral body to withstand a compressive force is equal to its mineral density squared times its cross-sectional area.

Until recently, very little attention has been given to age-related changes in bone geometry or the effect of exercise on it. In fact, some of the losses in long bone strength that might be expected to occur as age-related bone loss progresses appear to be ameliorated by compensatory modifications in bone geometry. For example, age-related bone loss from endosteal surfaces of the femoral diaphysis (shaft) is attended by a concurrent increase in diaphyseal width [16]. Diaphyseal expansion creates an increased *cross-sectional moment of inertia* (CSMI), an expression of the resistance of an object to bending. CSMI is related to an object's cross-sectional area and the *distribution* of structural material in relation to the axis about which the bone bends. The greater the distance bone tissue is distributed from the bending axis, the more resistance to bending (strength) the bone as a whole will have.

Preindustrial skeletal remains indicate no gender-specific differences in age-related geometric adaptation [17], but in modern times, men appear to have maintained the ability to expand diaphyseal widths to a greater extent than women [16,18,19]. Although the forearm bones of older women do exhibit greater cross-sectional moments of inertia than those of younger women, the magnitude of diaphyseal expansion may not fully compensate for excessive endosteal bone loss [20]. Changes in physical activity patterns from pre- to post-industrial society likely account for the gender differences that exist today in age-related geometric adaptation.

SKELETAL EFFECTS OF MECHANICAL LOADING

Skeletal Adaptation

Among its several roles, providing a rigid structure that enables an organism to withstand the effects of gravity is the raison d'etre for the skeleton. Normal bone tissue exhibits a remarkable ability to adapt to changes in patterns of habitual loading in a manner that minimizes the long-term risk of structural failure (fracture). Loads applied to the skeleton are generally described in terms of stress and strain. *Stress* is the force applied per unit area to an object. *Strain* is a measure of bone deformation in response to the application of stress and can be calculated by dividing the change in bone length by its original value. One strain unit equals a 0.1% deformation.

The ability of bone to modify its size and form to accommodate new patterns of loading is commonly referred to as Wolff's law. It is achieved in a site-specific manner by temporary alterations in bone resorption and formation activity. These alterations persist until bone mass and trabecular orientation approach an optimized functional state. The functional parameter, which is optimized, is not known with certainty, but seems likely to be the amount of strain experienced per unit of bone. Support for this concept comes from measurements of strains from the bones of different species during habitual forms of loading. Regardless of species or activity type, typical forms of loading produce bone surface strains between 2000 and 3000 microstrain, or 0.2–0.3% deformation [21].

One of the most concrete descriptions of the adaptative response of bone to loading is the mechanostat theory of Harold Frost [22]. Therein, Frost suggested that skeletal responses differ selectively according to the magnitude of engendered bone strain. He introduced the concept of bone modeling, which, when associated with load-related adaptation, refers to bone formation, which is uncoupled from resorption. According to the mechanostat theory, when bone is loaded above 2500 microstrain, modeling occurs via increased bone formation, effecting periosteal expansion and reduced endosteal resorption. This adaptive combination ultimately produces a bone that is more resistant to deformation. However, when applied loads engender only 200 microstrain or less, modeling is inhibited and intracortical and endosteal remodeling is stimulated. Substantial reductions in chronic loading are thus associated with increased cortical porosity, expansion of the marrow cavity, thinning of the bone cortex, and, ultimately, bone that is less resistant to bending. Frost referred to the level of strain, which, when habitually applied to bone, will prevent bone loss, as the "minimum effective strain" (MES). Findings of animal studies support the concept of bone as a mechanostat [23–26], although the control of bone adaptation is clearly related to more complex load signals than simple peak strains, since even very low loads can induce bone formation if applied at sufficiently high frequencies [27].

The Curvilinear Nature of Skeletal Response

Complete skeletal immobilization leads rapidly to marked bone loss. In contrast, imposition of even substantial training regimens on normally ambulatory humans or animals appears to increase bone mass by only a few percent. This phenomenon is illustrated in Fig. 1, where the effect of walking on bone mass is schematized. As an individual goes from immobility to full ambulation, the duration of time spent walking becomes a progressively less efficient stimulus for increasing bone mass. A person who habitually walks 6 hr each day might require another 4–6 hr of walking just to add a few more percent bone mineral density. However, adding a more rigorous stimulus, such as high impact loading, for even a few cycles would increase the bone response slope.

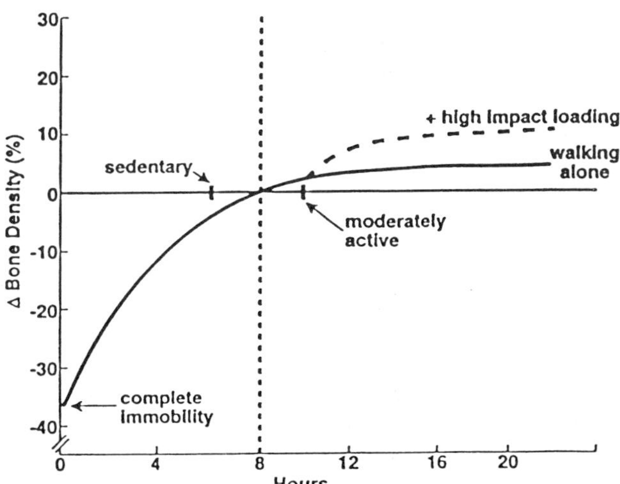

FIGURE 1 The curvilinear nature of the skeletal response to exercise. From Marcus [124].

EFFECTS OF PHYSICAL ACTIVITY ON AGING BONE

Bone Measurement Terminology

It is essential to recognize a number of terms commonly employed to quantify bone mass. *Bone mineral content* (BMC) is a measure (in grams) of the total amount of mineral within a defined region of bone. To adjust for differences in bone size among individuals, the amount of mineral must be divided by the volume of bone measured. Computed tomography (CT) permits true volumetric estimates of *bone mineral density* (BMD), but other measurement techniques that expose patients to substantially less ionizing radiation than CT are used more commonly. Two-dimensional projection techniques such as dual energy X-ray absorptiometry (DXA) provide estimates of *areal bone mineral density* wherein BMC is divided by the area of bone measured and is expressed as grams per centimeters squared. Although areal BMD has great clinical utility, it is confounded to some degree when extreme differences in bone size exist. To adjust for those differences, calculation of a pseudo-volumetric quantity, *bone mineral apparent density* (BMAD), provides an approximation of volumetric bone density [28,29]. BMAD is calculated from densitometry-derived bone area and other skeletal length dimensions and is expressed in grams per centimeters cubed.

The Role of Progressive Sloth: Skeletal Unloading

It has been argued frequently that a reduction in bone mass with age reflects the reduced mechanical loading of an increasingly sedentary life-style rather than aging per se [30,31]. It is certainly well known that chronic reductions in mechanical loading such as immobilization, bed rest, spinal cord injury, and exposure to microgravity precipitate generalized skeletal loss, particularly in bones that bear weight under normal conditions [32,33–35]. Other factors undoubtedly contribute to age-related bone loss and fragility, however. The ability of bone to adapt to mechanical loading appears to be greater during the growing years, particularly during adolescence, than after maturity [36,37]. Number and vigor of cell populations, concentrations of circulating growth factors, and production of bone matrix proteins all decline with age [38,39] and may all contribute to an age-related attenuation of the adaptive response.

Exercise Intervention

Animal Trials

Studies of animals have produced inconsistent results with respect to the durability of the adaptive response with age. Three-, 8-, 11-, 17-, 25-month-old rats are considered young, mature, middle age, early stage aging, and senescent, respectively [40]. Imposition of a running program on 8-month old (mature) rats produced a 52% increase in vertebral trabecular bone volume (TBV) compared to sedentary animals, while cortical bone maintained compactness and increased calcium content by about 25%. In contrast, rats initiating training at 11 or 17 months (i.e., middle age and older) did not increase either TBV or calcium content when compared to age-matched controls. Others concur that training efficacy diminishes with age [36,40–43]. Evidence also suggests that the *nature* of the skeletal response may change with age. In studies of treadmill exercise, young female rats increased cortical mineralization in a site-specific manner whereas older animals responded with a more generalized skeletal effect [44].

Other reports, however, have shown no age differences in exercise effect. Raab and associates [45] found that training effects were not limited by age in female rats; relatively old male rats restored BMC to young adult values after initiation of a running program [46] and 1 h/week of running for 1 year prevented continued high bone turnover in adult rats with NH_4Cl-induced osteoporosis [47].

Human Trials

A plethora of cross-sectional investigations have pronounced that individuals who engage in regular weight-bearing physical activity, particularly those participating during childhood, have skeletons of greater mass than sedentary people. Talmage and colleagues [48] observed a reduced rate of age-related bone loss in athletic versus nonathletic women aged 18–98 years. A comparison of the relationship of distal radius BMD to age in athletic versus nonathletic women is illustrated in Fig. 2. These pronouncements fit conveniently within the edict of exercise as a natural panacea and, given current understanding of the effects of mechanical loading on bone, appear intuitive. The inherent subject selection bias of cross-sectional studies, however, necessitates confirmation of such assertions with evidence from controlled, randomized intervention trials that utilize subjects of all ages and both sexes.

As osteoporosis currently affects a greater proportion of the female population than male, exercise intervention trials have historically focused on women to a greater extent than men. Consequently, reviews of the topic, including this chapter, appear to contain a disproportionate emphasis toward women. For a comprehensive review of male exercise studies, see Beck and Marcus [49]. For this discussion, studies will be stratified according to sex, subject age, and type of exercise intervention.

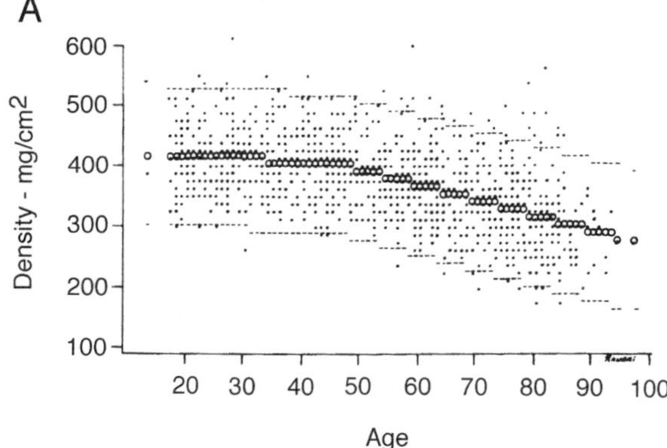

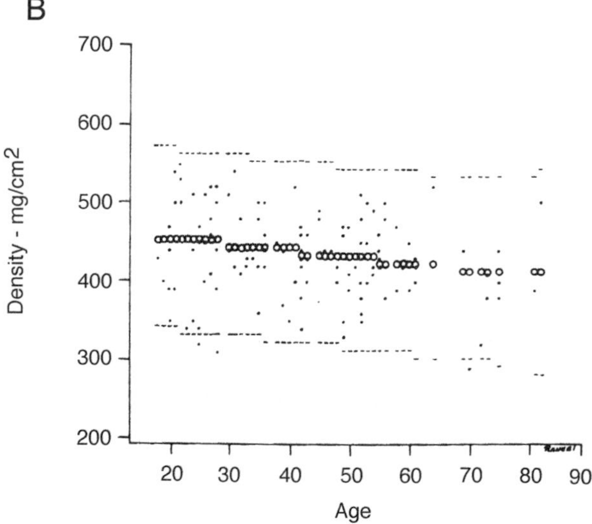

FIGURE 2 (Top) Individual BMD values of the distal radius in nonathletic women plotted as a function of age with mean and 95% confidence limits superimposed. (Bottom) Individual BMD values of the distal radius in athletic women. From Talmage *et al.* [48].

Young Adult Women Exercise training programs have been observed to enhance the bone density of young women in a site-specific manner. Both resistance and endurance exercise programs effectively increased lumbar spine BMD in women with a mean age of 20 years [50]. A 2-year combined program of aerobic and weight training similarly increased spine, femoral, and calcaneal BMD of women aged 20–35 [51]. Resistance training effected a small increase in the lumbar spine BMD, but no change in the bones of the whole body, arm, or leg of 28- to 39-year-old women [52]. High-impact exercises increased femoral neck but not radius BMD in 35- to 45-year-old women [53].

Young Adult Men Although many fewer intervention trials with male cohorts have been reported, exercise likely exerts a similar effect on the skeletons of young men. Following 9 months of marathon training, the amount of change in calcaneal BMC of consistent runners significantly exceeded that of nonexercising controls [54]. The correlation between average distance run and percentage change in BMC also indicated a strong positive relationship.

Perimenopausal Women Only a few studies have addressed the skeletal response to loading in the years just prior to menopause. Heinonen and colleagues [55] found that previously sedentary women aged 52–53 who engaged in 18 months of endurance exercise maintained femoral neck BMD to a greater extent than controls and women who participated in a program of calisthenics. Interestingly, the distal radius of the endurance exercisers showed a significant negative linear trend in comparison to the other groups. No significant differences were found between groups at the spine and calcaneus. Others have found that 40- to 50-year-old premenopausal women maintained spine BMD following 6 months of resistance exercise designed to primarily load the spine and hip compared to controls [56]. Both controls and exercisers appeared to gain femoral BMD, an effect which, in the former group, may be attributed to calcium supplementation during the course of the trial.

Early Menopausal Women One of the strongest confounding factors affecting the study of exercise in older women is the impact of menopause. As it is known that bone loss is particularly rapid in the years immediately subsequent to menopause, exercise intervention studies that combine both early and late postmenopausal women may fail to distinguish the factor exerting the greatest influence on bone. Thus, whether the rapid menopause-related bone loss can be curbed by exercise intervention remains unclear. The lone existing investigation of early postmenopausal women suggests that resistance exercise may benefit the lumbar spine but provide insufficient stimulus to prevent hormone-related bone loss at other skeletal sites [57].

Postmenopausal Women: Long-Term Resistance Exercise Controlled, randomized intervention trials of 9 to 24 months duration with postmenopausal women engaged in resistance/weight training programs generally (although not uniformly [58–60]) report an increase or maintenance of BMD (compared to losses in controls) at the whole body [61], lumbar spine [57,61–64], proximal femur [62,64,65], and radius [65].

Older Men: Long-Term Resistance Exercise Results from exercise intervention trials with older men are similarly conflicting. McCartney and associates [66] reported that 42 weeks of weight training in 60- to 80-year-old men increased muscle strength and functional ability but did not improve whole body or spine BMD. Conversely, Welsh and Rutherford [67] found that trochanteric BMD increased significantly in 50- to 73-year-old men performing step and jumping exercises. It is possible that the discrepancy of results is attributable to methodological shortcomings in McCartney's trial, such as limitations of ^{153}Gd-based dichromatic densitometry and inadequate consideration of subject anthropometric characteristics.

Postmenopausal Women: Long-Term Endurance Exercise Controlled, weight-bearing impact/endurance exercise interventions of 7 to 18 months duration with postmenopausal women also generally report exercise benefits (increases or maintenance of BMD compared to losses in control subjects) at the whole body [61,67], lumbar spine [67–71], proximal femur [61,67], radius [71], and calcaneus [54,72]. Nonweight-bearing endurance exercise may also improve BMD in postmenopausal women. Bloomfield and colleagues [73] reported that 8 months of moderate intensity cycle ergometry increased lumbar spine (but not femoral) BMD compared to controls who lost bone.

In contrast, Cavanaugh and Cann [74] found that walking did not prevent loss of spinal trabecular bone mineral in postmenopausal women. In a finding illustrative of the site specificity of exercise on bone mass, Kohrt and others [61] found that weight-bearing exercise did not increase forearm BMD.

Older Men: Long-Term Endurance Exercise No randomized, controlled intervention trials of this nature have been reported.

Postmenopausal Women: Short-Term Exercise The time required for bone to undergo a full modeling or remodeling cycle in response to altered patterns of loading is approximately 4 and 6 months, respectively. As such, bone mass evaluations before and after exercise interventions less than 6 months in duration may not accurately reflect either the effectiveness of the exercise stimulus or the relative responsiveness of bone to loading. With this precautionary remark in mind, the following studies are included for consideration.

Five months of diverse, dynamic, high strain, and high rate of strain forearm exercises significantly increased forearm bone density in osteoporotic, postmenopausal women [75,76]. Six months of a combined walking and resistance exercise program also increased vertebral trabecular BMC in osteoporotic, postmenopausal women compared to controls who continued to lose bone [77]. Again illustrating the curvilinear response of bone to loading, the magnitude of skeletal response to exercise likely depends on an individual's initial bone mass [6,8], i.e., individuals with very low initial bone mass stand to gain the greatest amount of bone following exercise intervention. The positive findings of these short duration trials may thus arise from the very low starting bone mass of the study participants.

Men: Short-Term Exercise Not surprisingly, 3 months of walking and running training were insufficient to increase BMC in 25- to 52-year-old men [78]. However, young Army recruits completing 14 weeks of intensive physical training were observed to increase right and left leg BMC by 8.3 and 12.4%, respectively [79]. In a similar trial, a 7.5% increase in tibial bone density was observed in Army recruits after 14 weeks of basic training [80]. Again, recruits who began the training period with the lowest bone density gained the greatest amount. It is notable that 10% of recruits actually lost bone density, an effect likely due to resorption-related porosity that had not yet been matched by replacement formation due to the short time frame of the study. The discrepancy in results across recruits highlights the substantial individual variation that characterizes bone adaptation.

Fujimura and associates [81] found that 4 months of high-intensity resistance training of 23- to 31-year-old Asian males increased the serum concentrations of biochemical markers of bone formation (osteocalcin and bone-specific alkaline phosphatase) within 1 month of initiating training, and that values were persistently elevated throughout the training period. Markers of bone resorption (plasma procollagen type I and urinary deoxypyridinoline) did not increase. Although these findings led the authors to conclude that resistance training stimulates bone formation but not bone resorption, no significant changes in BMD were evident following training to confirm the assertion.

Sex Comparison in Exercise Response Only a modicum of data exists comparing male and female responses to exercise, and information regarding any interaction of age with a sex-specific exercise response is essentially nonexistent. Welsh and Rutherford [67] observed the effect of 12 months of high-impact aerobics two to three times a week on hip, spine, and total body BMD of elderly men and women. They found that both groups increased BMD a similar amount (men: approximately 1.2%, women: approximately 1.3%) at all sites, whereas controls lost BMD.

Relationship between Skeletal and Muscular Aging Although the primary focus of this chapter is bone, the relationship of age-associated reductions in muscle strength to skeletal disability is of more than tangential relevance. In keeping with his mechanostat theory, Frost [22] stated that declining muscle strength in aging individuals decreases loads on bone that has previously adapted to strains generated by stronger, young adult muscle contraction. The resultant reduction in muscle-imposed bone strain to levels below the MES constitutes a form of bone unloading so that disuse-osteopenia ensues. According to this reasoning, as long as muscle strength continues to decrease, bone will lose mass.

Indeed, muscle force appears to be an essential component of the bone-loading milieu. Some authors state that muscles place substantially greater loads on bones than those imposed by gravitational forces [82] and that they may account for more than 70% of bone-bending moments [83]. Consequently, demonstrations of a relationship between muscle strength and bone mass should not be unexpected [84–86]. Loss of muscle strength precedes the loss of bone and the recovery of muscle strength precedes the recovery of bone mass, albeit with a substantial delay, reflecting the different rates of adaptation for these two tissues [87]. Something of a conundrum remains, however, as muscle strength gains following resistance training programs are not always accompanied by gains in BMD [58,88].

With age, characteristic changes occur in muscle fiber morphology and function. These changes include atrophy of type II (fast-twitch) fibers, with an increasing predominance of type I (slow-twitch) muscle fibers, and degenerative changes in peripheral nerve and neuromuscular junctions [89–95]. The extent to which these changes reflect fundamental effects of age per se, as opposed to diminished activity or altered hormonal milieu, remains uncertain. However, their significance may be profound as muscle weakness consistently emerges as a risk factor for falls and hence for fracture [96].

The muscle strength of older men and women responds dramatically to the imposition of resistance exercise [97,98]. Strength gains vary from 30% to more than 100% in various muscle groups and, as indicated by histomorphometric analysis of muscle fiber areas from percutaneous muscle biopsies, are associated with true muscle fiber hypertrophy [98,99]. The relatively poor correlation of changes in muscle fiber area to changes in strength in these studies suggests that simultaneous improvement in the efficiency of motor unit recruitment or synchrony may underlie some of the strength gains [100]. Training-induced strength gains are initially rapid but tend to plateau after 12–14 weeks, even with progressive increases in loads [99].

In healthy young men and women, strength gains due to resistance training are characteristically greatest when the training regimen emphasizes load magnitude rather than frequency. This does not seem to be the case for older individuals, in whom a year-long clinical trial comparing low-intensity, high-repetition training and high-intensity, low-repetition training resulted in comparable strength gains [58]. Thus, to achieve and maintain improved muscle strength, it does not appear to be necessary to subject older people to high-intensity, potentially high-risk training regimens.

Some have stated that age-related bone loss cannot be primarily a consequence of decreased muscle strength because significant declines do not become evident until the fifth decade or beyond, i.e., long after age-related bone loss can be documented [91,101–103]. A number of authors, however, state that the onset of loss in muscle strength occurs shortly after age 30 [104,105]. Discrepant findings of this sort reflect the substantial interindividual variation in muscle strength and highlight the necessity for rigorous, population-based studies of muscle strength from which conclusions may be drawn most reliably. It seems most likely that age-related bone loss is truly a multifactorial phenomenon and that loss of mechanical stimulation as a consequence of declining muscular function will prove to be one of several important contributors.

Interaction between Calcium and Exercise Intervention The effect of exercise on BMD may be greatest when combined with calcium supplementation [106,107]. From a review of 17 trials, Specker [106] reported that physical activity affects BMD only when mean calcium intake surpasses 1000 mg/day and that the effect is more pronounced in the lumbar spine than at the radius. Indeed, Prince and colleagues [108] found that calcium supplementation and exercise combined were more effective at reducing bone loss in postmenopausal women than calcium supplementation alone.

There is some dissent on this issue. A cross-sectional study of 422 women indicated that while both high levels of physical activity and high calcium intake were associated with a higher total body BMC than low-activity levels and low calcium intake, no significant interaction between the two variables was found [109]. More pointedly, in a 2-year program of combined aerobics and weight training that increased the BMD of young women, calcium supplementation neither enhanced the exercise benefit nor improved BMD in the absence of exercise [51]. Similarly, 9 months of walking, jogging, and stair climbing, plus 1500 mg of daily supplemental calcium, increased lumbar BMC in postmenopausal women compared to no change in a control group who also received the calcium supplement [68]. Nelsen and associates [110] also found that a nonrandomized 1-year walking and weights program maintained lumbar spine BMD in postmenopausal women compared to BMD loss in the control group, but no interactive effect of calcium supplementation was observed. At the femur, BMD was maintained in women consuming high dietary levels of calcium compared to BMD loss in those who consumed only moderate amounts. In this case, there was no effect of exercise. Clearly, the skeletal interactions of exercise and calcium require further scrutiny.

Interaction between Hormone Replacement and Exercise Intervention: Women In young bone, the mechanical environment is thought to be the predominant modulator of the balance between bone resorption and formation. Disruption of the normal hormonal mileu, such as occurs at menopause and other estrogen-deficient states, precipitates bone loss due to increased osteoclast activation frequency and bone resorption.

Human studies in this area are limited and somewhat inconclusive due in part to ethical limitations surrounding the manipulation of hormone status in this population. However, the recent focus on hormone replacement therapy (HRT) of menopausal women has sparked research concerning its efficacy in comparison to, and in combination with, exercise. Some findings suggest that exercise enhances the bone-conserving effect of HRT. For example, 1 year of resistance exercise significantly increased spine, total body, and radial midshaft BMD in estrogen-replaced, surgically menopausal women compared to estrogen-replaced, nonexercising controls who merely maintained BMD [111]. Similarly, whereas 9 months of weight-bearing training (walking, jogging, stairs) and HRT increased total body and lumbar spine BMD in 60- to 72-year-old postmenopausal women supplemented to 1500 mg calcium/day, the combination of HRT plus exercise was more effective than exercise or HRT alone [112]. Prince and associates [113] found that exercise with estrogen supplementation increased forearm bone density in postmenopausal women. Exercise and calcium supplementation merely prevented bone loss compared to an exercise-alone control group and a nonexercising control group.

Other studies, however, have found otherwise. One hour of resistance exercise plus 2 hr per week of walking or running for 1 year did not enhance the positive effect of estrogen supplementation on lumbar vertebral or femoral neck BMD in postmenopausal women [114]. Similarly, BMD loss at the lumbar spine and proximal femur was prevented by two different regimens of HRT in early postmenopausal women, but 3 hr of exercise loading had no additional skeletal effect despite a positive effect of exercise on BMD in a hormone placebo group [88].

Interaction between Hormone Replacement and Exercise Intervention: Men Equivalent studies of reproductive hormone (testosterone) interactions with exercise have not been studied effectively in men. However, other forms of hormone supplementation have been investigated. Four months of progressive resistance exercise training 4 days/week, with or without growth hormone supplementation, did not increase whole body, spine, or proximal femur BMD in elderly men (mean age 67) with normal BMD [115]. Similarly, 6 months of resistance exercise training, with and without recombinant human growth hormone, increased muscle strength to an equivalent degree, but effected no change in BMD of older men [116,117] (D. R. Taaffe, personal communication).

IMPACT OF PHYSICAL ACTIVITY ON FALLING AND FRACTURE

There is general agreement that exercise occupies a central role in the maintenance of muscle strength, flexibility, and balance and in the prevention of falls, thereby reducing osteoporosis-related fractures and promoting functional independence [2,7]. However, as exercise itself transiently exposes the participant to an increased risk for falls and trauma, it is not certain that the skeletal and muscular benefits achieved from physical activity will necessarily be attended by a reduction in fractures. In one report, participants in a 2-year program of brisk walking conserved femoral BMD, but the effect was tempered by an increased cumulative incidence of falls [118]. As Nelsen and associates [110] reported that walking itself did not improve muscle strength, optimal exercise prescription for decreasing the incidence of fracture may require specific attention to improving muscle strength, as well as to loading bone in a weight-bearing manner.

With regard to an association between exercise and an increased incidence of fracture, a report from a yearlong Canadian osteoporosis prevention program in postmenopausal women offered more encouraging results. Exercise was found to improve bone mass, VO_{2max} and well-being, stamina, mobility, and pain tolerance, no fractures occurred in the course of the study [119]. More recently, other studies have described a beneficial relationship between exercise and fracture risk. The Study of Osteoporotic Fractures, a large, prospective, community-based, observational study of healthy older Caucasian women, found that moderately to vigorously active women had significant reductions in hip and vertebral fracture incidence compared to inactive women [120]. Similarly, a Norwegian survey of 12,270 men and women found that of individuals aged 45 years and older, the most physically active experienced fewer fractures in weight-bearing bones than the most sedentary. No difference in fracture incidence was found in the nonweight-bearing skeleton [121].

THERAPEUTIC RECOMMENDATIONS

Primarily reflecting a lack of consistency in the research, no consensus exists as to the precise intensity, frequency, duration, and type of activity that most benefits bone. Although one meta-analysis concluded that exercise intensity and rate do not influence the effect of intervention [3], other writers on this subject maintain that only vigorous aerobic and resistance training regimens enhance bone density and that walking is a relatively ineffective means to prevent osteoporosis [9,13,74]. In fact, Krall and Dawson-Hughes [122] reported that women who walked more than 7.5 miles/week had higher whole body, leg, and trunk BMD than women who walked less than 1 mile/week. The implication of these results is tempered by the cross-sectional nature of the study design, but supplemental longitudinal observations from the same study showed that walking was related to a retardation of bone loss in the legs. More convincingly, Hatori and colleagues [70] reported that 7 months of thrice-weekly walking above the anaerobic threshold increased lumbar spine BMD.

The most osteogenic forms of loading are those that include unusual strain distributions, high strains, and high strain rates. Few loading cycles are necessary to obtain an effect if such exercises are employed [123]. An aggressive approach to bone mass maintenance then would be an exercise regimen, not necessarily prolonged, but inclusive of novel forms of rapid loading with relatively high resistance. Examples of such activities are aerobics, jump rope, stair climbing and descending, zig-zag running, and arm wrestling. The recommendation to exercise in this manner must be applied with an understanding of the attendant risks, which include cardiovascular stress and/or falls. Screening physical examinations should avert the former, and good design and supervision of exercise programs should prevent the latter. Individuals with advanced osteoporosis with or without a history of vertebral compression fractures should not engage in high-impact activities or deep forward flexion exercises such as rowing.

Emphasis on exercise as a means to influence bone mass, however, misses several important points. First, it is a fact that the adult populations of most Western industrialized societies are relatively sedentary. Indeed, according to the President's Council on Fitness, less than 25% of adult Americans participate in *any* recreational physical activity as often as once each week. Therefore, the most effective recommendation is one that will increase the overall level of activity of an inactive person to any degree and that will also achieve the greatest degree of long-term compliance. In this respect, walking remains a very attractive option, given the associated cardiovascular and neuromuscular benefits in addition to those relating strictly to the skeleton.

Second, the most important skeletal issue to be addressed by exercise is fracture reduction, not BMD conservation per se. The fracture that most devastates quality of life, carries the greatest repercussions for survival, and confers the largest societal cost occurs at the hip. Hip fracture is a morbid event that in 95% of instances is the immediate and direct consequence of a fall. Falls also underlie a nontrivial proportion of vertebral fractures (M. L. Bouxsein, personal communication). Thus, the major skeletally relevant goal to be accomplished with exercise is a reduction in falls. Muscle weakness consistently emerges as an important antecedent factor for falls and an independent risk factor for hip fracture [96]. Therefore, the recommendation to incorporate leg-strengthening exercises into conditioning programs has a rational basis.

Older men and women may prove a uniquely refractory group for instituting an exercise program. Limitations of mobility and overall deconditioning stemming from a lifetime of sedentary habits may overwhelm an intellectual understanding that exercise would be a good thing to do. It is even more difficult to conceive that sedentary elders would undertake more than one type of exercise program. It would certainly prove futile to recommend an aerobics program for cardiovascular conditioning, a stretching program for flexibility, and resistance exercise for leg strength. An important research challenge remains to consolidate these diverse goals into a single exercise prescription that could be undertaken long term, simply and safely at home or in the local community, with minimal imposition on time and resources. Clearly, walking will remain an important component of such a prescription, perhaps accompanied by some form of leg-strengthening activity.

SUMMARY

Many factors contribute to age-related bone loss. In designing effective interventions to minimize such loss, one must consider as many of these factors as possible and the degree to which they can be modified. Important factors contributing to bone loss during adult life include bone remodeling inefficiency, sedentary life-style with associated reduced habitual bone loading, inadequate nutrient intake and assimilation (particularly calcium), reduced muscle strength, and age-related attenuation of the adaptive capacity of bone. Of these, reduced skeletal loading and muscle weakness constitute obvious targets for exercise intervention.

The weight of evidence supports a conclusion that exercise is an effective strategy for the maintenance of skeletal health. Intervention trials in humans suggest that certain forms of exercise may, at a minimum, halt or slow age-related bone loss and, in some instances, actually improve bone mass in a site-specific manner. Increments in bone mass with exercise are most evident in individuals with low baseline values of bone density and in those whose baseline level of activity is the least, i.e., healthy, moderately active men and women may achieve fewer bone mass gains than sedentary osteopenic cohorts who are otherwise comparable.

The basis for substantial interindividual variations in the response of bone to exercise is unexplained. Better understanding of the mechanism by which mechanical load signals are transduced to bone cells may help clarify this issue and remains the key to the successful application of skeletal adaptation theory to the practical world of exercise prescription.

Finally, the concept of exercise as a panacea requires additional consideration. Many exercise enthusiasts currently choose to rely solely on physical activity for skeletal protection at times when other forms of protection may also be indicated. For example, some menopausal women may abstain from estrogen replacement therapy because of their belief that exercise, alone or with calcium, will suffice. The available evidence provides little support for this belief. Professor Robert Heaney has invoked the model of a three-legged stool to represent skeletal health. One can diligently lavish attention on any two legs, but if neglected, the third leg will give way when the stool is sat upon. Extending this metaphor to bone, the three legs correspond to mechanical loading, nutrient intake, and reproductive hormone status. Although these elements are not completely independent of one another, proper attention to all three is required for optimal skeletal health, and overzealous attention to any one or two elements will not make up for negligence to the others.

References

1. Aisenbrey, J. A. Exercise in the prevention and management of osteoporosis. *Phys. Ther.* **67,** 1100–1104 (1987).
2. Allen, S. H. Exercise considerations for postmenopausal women with osteoporosis. *Arthritis Care Res.* **7,** 205–214 (1994).

3. Berard, A., Bravo, G., and Gauthier, P. Meta-analysis of the effectiveness of physical activity for the prevention of bone loss in postmenopausal women. *Osteopor. Int.* **7,** 331–337 (1997).
4. Birge, S. J., and Dalsky, G. The role of exercise in preventing osteoporosis. *Public Health Rep.* **104**(Suppl.) 54–58 (1989).
5. Block, J. E., Smith, R., Friedlander, A., and Genant, H. K. Preventing osteoporosis with exercise: a review with emphasis on methodology. *Med. Hypoth.* **30,** 9–19 (1989).
6. Dalsky, G. P. The role of exercise in the prevention of osteoporosis. *Compr. Ther.* **15,** 30–37 (1989).
7. Drinkwater, B. L. Exercise in the prevention of osteoporosis. *Osteopor. Int.* **3,** 169–171 (1993).
8. Forwood, M. R., and Burr, D. B. Physical activity and bone mass: exercises in futility? *Bone Miner* **21,** 89–112 (1993).
9. Gutin, B., and Kasper, M. J. Can vigorous exercise play a role in osteoporosis prevention. A review. *Osteopor. Intl.* **2,** 55–69 (1992).
10. Prior, J. C., Barr, S. I., Chow, R., and Faulkner, R. A. Prevention and management of osteoporosis: consensus statements from the Scientific Advisory Board of the Osteoporosis Society of Canada. 5. Physical activity as therapy for osteoporosis. *CMAJ* **155,** 940–944 (1996).
11. Smith, E. L., and Raab, D. M. Osteoporosis and physical activity. *Acta Med. Scand. Suppl.* **711,** 149–156 (1986).
12. Stacey, T. A. Osteoporosis: exercise therapy, pre- and post-diagnosis. *J. Manipulative Physiol. Ther.* **12,** 211–219 (1989).
13. Swezey, R. L. Exercise for osteoporosis—is walking enough? The case for site specificity and resistive exercise. *Spine* **21,** 2809–2813 (1996).
14. Thomas, W. C., Jr. Exercise, age, and bones. *South Med. J.* **87,** S23–S25 (1994).
15. Yeater, R. A., and Martin, R. B. Senile osteoporosis. The effects of exercise. *Postgrad. Med.* **75,** 147–159, 163 (1984).
16. Martin, R. B., and Atkinson, P. J. Age and sex-related changes in the structure and strength of the human femoral shaft. *J. Biomech.* **20,** 223–231 (1977).
17. Ruff, C. B., and Hayes, W. C. Cross-sectional geometry of Pecos pueblo femora and tibiae—a biomechanical investigation: II. Sex, age, and side differences. *Am. J. Phys. Anthropol.* **60,** 383–400 (1983).
18. Ruff, C. B., and Hayes, W. C. Sex differences in age-related remodeling of the femur and tibia. *J. Orthopaed. Res.* **6,** 886–896 (1988).
19. Burr, D. B., and Martin, R. B. The effects of composition, structure and age on the torsional properties of the human radius. *J. Biomech.* **16,** 603–608 (1983).
20. Bouxsein, M. L., Myburgh, K. H., van der Meulen, M. C. H., Lindenberger, E., and Marcus, R. Age-related differences in cross-sectional geometry of the forearm bones in healthy women. *Calcif. Tissue Intl.* **54,** 113–118 (1994).
21. Rubin, C. T., and Lanyon, L. E. Dynamic strain similarity in vertebrates: An alternative to allometric limb bone sealing. *J. Theor. Biol.* **107,** 321–327 (1984).
22. Frost, H. M. Bone "mass" and the "mechanostat". *Anat. Rec.* **219,** 1–9 (1987).
23. Hillam, R. A., and Skerry, T. M. Inhibition of bone resorption and stimulation of formation by mechanical loading of the modeling rat ulna in vivo. *J. Bone Miner. Res.* **10,** 683 (1995).
24. Newhall, K. M., Rodnick, K. J., Van Der Meulen, M. C., Carter, D. R., and Marcus, R. Effects of voluntary exercise on bone mineral content in rats. *J. Bone Min. Res.* **6,** 289–296 (1991).
25. Raab, D. M., Crenshaw, T. D., Kimmel, D. B., and Smith, E. L. A histomorphometric study of cortical bone activity during increased weight-bearing exercise. *J. Bone Miner. Res.* **6,** 741–749 (1991).
26. Rubin, C. T., and Lanyon, L. E. Regulation of bone mass by mechanical strain magnitude. *Calcif. Tissue Intl.* **37,** 411–417 (1985).
27. Rubin, C. T., and McLeod, K. J. *In* "Osteoporosis" (R. Marcus, D. Feldman, and J Kelsey, eds.), pp. 351–371. Academic Press, San Diego, 1996.
28. Katzman, D. K., Bachrach, L. K., Carter, D. R., and Marcus, R. Clinical and anthropometric correlates of bone mineral acquisition in healthy adolescent girls. *J. Clin. Endocrinol. Metab.* **73,** 1332–1339 (1991).
29. Carter, D. R., Bouxsein, M. L., and Marcus, R. New approaches for interpreting projected bone density. *J. Bone Miner. Res.* **7,** 137–145 (1992).
30. Dishman, R. K., and Steinhardt, M. Health locus of control predicts free-living, but not supervised, physical activity: a test of exercise-specific control and outcome-expectancy hypotheses. *Res. Q. Exerc. Sport* **61,** 383–394 (1990).
31. Rowe, J. W., and Kahn, R. L. Human aging: usual and successful. *Science* **237,** 143–149 (1987).
32. Krolner, B., and Toft, B. Vertebral bone loss: an unheeded side effect of therapeutic bed rest. *Clin. Sci.* **64,** 537–540 (1983).
33. Donaldson, C. L., *et al.* Effect of prolonged bed rest on bone mineral. *Metabolism* **19,** 1071–1084 (1970).
34. Tilton, F. E., Degioanni, J. J., and Schneider, V. S. Long-term follow-up of Skylab bone demineralization. *Aviat. Space Environ. Med.* **51,** 1209–1213 (1980).
35. Leblanc, A. D., Schneider, V. S., Evans, H. J., Engelbretson, D. A., and Krebs, J. M. Bone mineral loss and recovery after 17 weeks of bed rest. *J. Bone Miner. Res.* **5,** 843–850 (1990).
36. Rubin, C. T., Bain, S. D., and McLeod, K. J. Suppression of the osteogenic response in the aging skeleton. *Calcif. Tissue Intl.* **50,** 306–313 (1992).
37. Parfitt, A. M. The two faces of growth: benefits and risks to bone integrity. *Osteopor. Int.* **4,** 382–398 (1994).
38. Termine, J. D. Cellular activity, matrix proteins, and aging bone. *Exp. Gerontol.* **25,** 217–221 (1990).
39. Benedict, M. R., *et al.* Dissociation of bone mineral density from age-related decreases in insulin-like growth factor-1 and its binding proteins in the male rat. *J. Gerontol.* **49,** B224–B230 (1994).
40. Silbermann, M., *et al.* Long-term physical exercise retards trabecular bone loss in lumbar vertebrae of aging female mice. *Calcif. Tissue Int.* **46,** 80–93 (1990).
41. Turner, C. H., Takano, Y., and Owan, I. Aging changes mechanical loading thresholds for bone formation in rats. *J. Bone Miner. Res.* **10,** 1544–1549 (1995).
42. Steinhagen-Thiessen, E., Reznik, A., and Hilz, H. Negative adaptation to physical training in senile mice. *Mech. Ageing Dev.* **12,** 231–236 (1980).
43. Reznick, A. Z., Steinhagen-Thiessen, E., Gellersen, B., and Gershon, D. The effect of short- and long-term exercise on aldolase activity in muscles of CW-1 and C57/BL mice of various ages. *Mech. Ageing Dev.* **23,** 253–258 (1983).
44. McDonald, R., Hegenauer, J., and Saltman, P. Age-related differences in the bone mineralization pattern of rats following exercise. *J. Gerontol.* **41,** 445–452 (1986).
45. Raab, D. M., Smith, E. L., Crenshaw, T. D., and Thomas, D. P. Bone mechanical properties after exercise training in young and old rats. *J. Appl. Physiol.* **68,** 130–134 (1990).
46. Beyer, R. E., Huang, J. C., and Wilshire, G. B. The effect of endurance exercise on bone dimensions, collagen, and calcium in the aged male rat. *Exp. Gerontol.* **20,** 315–323 (1985).

47. Myburgh, K. H., Noakes, T. D., Roodt, M., and Hough, F. S. Effect of exercise on the development of osteoporosis in adult rats. *J. Appl. Physiol.* **66,** 14–19 (1989).
48. Talmage, R. V., Stinnett, S. S., Landwehr, J. T., Vincent, L. M., and McCartney, W. H. Age-related loss of bone mineral density in non-athletic and athletic women. *Bone Miner.* **1,** 115–125 (1986).
49. Beck, B. R., and Marcus, R. *In* "Male Osteoporosis" (E. Orwoll, ed.). Academic Press, San Diego, 1999, in press.
50. Snow-Harter, C., Bouxsein, M., Lewis, B. T., Carter, D. R., and Marcus, R. Effects of resistance and endurance exercise on bone mineral status of young women: A randomized exercise intervention trial. *J. Bone Miner. Res.* **7,** 761–769 (1992).
51. Friedlander, A. L., Genant, H. K., Sadowsky, S., Byl, N. N., and Gluer, C. C. A two-year program of aerobics and weight-training enhances BMD of young women. *J. Bone Miner. Res.* **10,** 574 (1995).
52. Lohman, T., *et al.* Effects of resistance training on regional and total bone mineral density in premenopausal women: a randomized prospective study. *J. Bone Miner. Res.* **10,** 1015 (1995).
53. Heinonen, A., *et al.* Randomised controlled trial of effect of high-impact exercise on selected risk factors for osteoporotic fractures [see comments]. *Lancet* **348,** 1343–1347 (1996).
54. Williams, J. A., Wagner, J., Wasnich, R., and Heilbrun, L. The effect of long-distance running upon appendicular bone mineral content. *Med. Sci. Sports Exer.* **16,** 223–227 (1984).
55. Heinonen, A., Oja, P., Sievanen, H., Pasanen, M., and Vuori, I. Effect of two training regimens on bone mineral density in healthy perimenopausal women: A randomized controlled trial. *J. Bone Miner. Res.* **13,** 483–490 (1998).
56. Dornemann, T. M., McMurray, R. G., Renner, J. B., and Anderson, J. J. B. Effects of high intensity resistance exercise on bone mineral density and muscle strength of 40-50 year old women. *J. Sports Med. Phys. Fitness* **37,** 246–251 (1997).
57. Pruitt, L. A., Jackson, R. D., Bartells, R. L., and Lehnhard, H. J. Weight-training effects on bone mineral density in early postmenopausal women. *J. Bone Miner. Res.* **7,** 179–185 (1992).
58. Pruitt, L. A., Taaffe, D. R., and Marcus, R. Effects of a one-year high-intensity versus low-intensity resistance training program on bone mineral density in older women. *J. Bone Miner. Res.* **10,** 1788–1795 (1995).
59. Sinaki, M., Wahner, H. W., Offord, K. P., and Hodgson, S. F. Efficacy of nonloading exercises in prevention of vertebral bone loss in postmenopausal women: a controlled trial. *Mayo Clin. Proc.* **64,** 762–769 (1989).
60. Bassey, E. J., and Ramsdale, S. J. Weight-bearing exercise and ground reaction forces: A 12-month randomized controlled trial of effects on bone mineral density in healthy postmenopausal women. *Bone* **16,** 469–476 (1995).
61. Kohrt, W. M., Ehsani, A. A., and Birge, S. J., Jr. Effects of exercise involving predominantly either joint-reaction or ground-reaction forces on bone mineral density in older women. *J. Bone Miner. Res.* **12,** 1253–1261 (1997).
62. Nelson, M. E., *et al.* Effects of high-intensity strength training on multiple risk factors for osteoporotic fractures. A randomized controlled trial. *JAMA* **272,** 1909–1914 (1994).
63. Revel, M., Mayoux-Benhamou, M. A., Rabourdin, J. P., Bagheri, F., and Roux, C. One-year psoas training can prevent lumbar bone loss in postmenopausal women: a randomized controlled trial. *Calcif. Tissue Int.* **53,** 307–311 (1993).
64. Smidt, G. L., Lin, S. Y., O'Dwyer, K. D., and Blanpied, P. R. The effect of high-intensity trunk exercise on bone mineral density of postmenopausal women. *Spine* **17,** 280–285 (1992).
65. Kerr, D., Morton, A., Dick, I., and Prince, R. Exercise effects on bone mass in postmenopausal women are site-specific and load-dependent. *J. Bone Miner. Res.* **11,** 218–225 (1996).
66. McCartney, N., Hicks, A. L., Martin, J., and Webber, C. E. A longitudinal trial of weight training in the elderly: continued improvements in year 2. *J. Gerontol.* **51**(Ser. A), B425–B433 (1996).
67. Welsh, L., and Rutherford, O. M. Hip bone mineral density is improved by high-impact aerobic exercise in postmenopausal women and men over 50 years. *Eur. J. Appl. Physiol. Occup. Physiol.* **74,** 511–517 (1996).
68. Dalsky, G. P., *et al.* Weight-bearing exercise training and lumbar bone mineral content in postmenopausal women. *Ann. Intern. Med.* **108,** 824–828 (1988).
69. Grove, K. A., and Londeree, B. R. Bone density in postmenopausal women: high impact vs low impact exercise. *Med. Sci. Sports Exerc.* **24,** 1190–1194 (1992).
70. Hatori, M., *et al.* The effects of walking at the anaerobic threshold level on vertebral bone loss in postmenopausal women. *Calcif. Tissue Int.* **52,** 411–414 (1993).
71. Krolner, B., Toft, B., Nielsen, S. P., and Tondevold, E. Physical exercise as prophylaxis against involutional vertebral bone loss: a controlled trial. *Clin. Sci.* **64,** 544–546 (1983).
72. Rundgren, A., Aniansson, A., Ljungberg, P., and Wetterqvist, H. Effects of a training programme for elderly people on mineral content of the heel bone. *Arch. Gerontol. Geriatr.* **3,** 243–248 (1984).
73. Bloomfield, S. A., Williams, N. I., Lamb, D. R., and Jackson, R. D. Non-weightbearing exercise may increase lumbar spine bone mineral density in healthy postmenopausal women. *Am. J. Phys. Med. Rehabil.* **72,** 204–209 (1993).
74. Cavanaugh, D. J., and Cann, C. E. Brisk walking does not stop bone loss in postmenopausal women. *Bone* **9,** 201–204 (1988).
75. Ayalon, J., Simkin, A., Leichter, I., and Raifmann, S. Dynamic bone loading exercises for postmenopausal women: effect on the density of the distal radius. *Arch. Phys. Med. Rehabil.* **68,** 280–283 (1987).
76. Simkin, A., Ayalon, J., and Leichter, I. Increased trabecular bone density due to bone-loading exercises in postmenopausal osteoporotic women. *Calcif. Tissue Int.* **40,** 59–63 (1987).
77. Dilsen, G., Berker, C., Oral, A., and Varan, G. The role of physical exercise in prevention and management of osteoporosis. *Clin. Rheumatol.* **8**(Suppl. 2) 70–75 (1989).
78. Dalen, N., and Olsson, K. E. Bone mineral content and physical activity. *Acta Orthop. Scand.* **45,** 170–174 (1974).
79. Margulies, J. Y., *et al.* Effect of intense physical activity on the bone-mineral content in the lower limbs of young adults. *J. Bone Joint Surg.* **68,** 1090–1093 (1986).
80. Leichter, I., *et al.* Gain in mass density of bone following strenuous physical activity. *Orthop. Res.* **7,** 86–90 (1989).
81. Fujimura, R., *et al.* Effect of resistance exercise training on bone formation and resorption in young male subjects assessed by biomarkers of bone metabolism. *J. Bone Miner. Res.* **12,** 656–662 (1997).
82. Pauwels, F., "Gesammelte Abhandlungen zur Funktionellen Anatomie des Bewegungsapparates." Springer, Berlin, 1965.
83. Lu, T. W., Taylor, S. J., O'Connor, J. J., and Walker, P. S. Influence of muscle activity on the forces in the femur: an in vivo study. *J. Biomech.* **30,** 1101–1106 (1997).
84. Slemenda, C. W., *et al.* Influences on skeletal mineralization in children and adolescents: evidence for varying effects of sexual maturation and physical activity. *J. Pediatr.* **125,** 201–207 (1994).
85. Villa, M. L., Marcus, R., Ramirez Delay, R., and Kelsey, J. L. Factors contributing to skeletal health of postmenopausal

Mexican-American women. *J. Bone Miner. Res.* **10,** 1233–1242 (1995).

86. Bauer, D. C., *et al.* Factors associated with appendicular bone mass in older women. The Study of Osteoporotic Fractures Research Group [see comments]. *Ann. Intern. Med.* **118,** 657–665 (1993).
87. Sievanen, H., Heinonen, A., and Kannus, P. Adaptation of bone to altered loading environment: a biomechanical approach using X-ray absorptiometric data from the patella of a young woman. *Bone* **19,** 55–59 (1996).
88. Heikkinen, J., *et al.* HRT and exercise: effects on bone density, muscle strength and lipid metabolism. A placebo controlled 2-year prospective trial on two estrogen-progestin regimens in healthy postmenopausal women. *Maturitas* **26,** 139–149 (1997).
89. Clarkson, P. M., Kroll, W., and Melchionda, A. M. Age, isometric strength, rate of tension development and fiber type composition. *J. Gerontol.* **36,** 648–653 (1981).
90. Gutmann, E., and Hanzlikova, V. Fast and slow motor units in ageing. *Gerontology* **22,** 280–300 (1976).
91. Larsson, L., and Karlsson, J. Isometric and dynamic endurance as a function of age and skeletal muscle characteristics. *Acta Physiol. Scand.* **104,** 129–136 (1978).
92. Larsson, L., Sjodin, B., and Karlsson, J. Histochemical and biochemical changes in human skeletal muscle with age in sedentary males, age 22–65 years. *Acta Physiol. Scand.* **103,** 31–39 (1978).
93. Larsson, L. Physical training effects on muscle morphology in sedentary males at different ages. *Med. Sci. Sports Exerc.* **14,** 203–206 (1982).
94. Oertel, G. Changes in human skeletal muscles due to ageing. Histological and histochemical observations on autopsy material. *Acta Neuropathol.* **69,** 309–313 (1986).
95. Scelsi, R., Marchetti, C., and Poggi, P. Histochemical and ultrastructural aspects of m. vastus lateralis in sedentary old people (age 65–89 years). *Acta Neuropathol.* **51,** 99–105 (1980).
96. Whipple, R. H., Wolfson, L. I., and Amerman, P. M. The relationship of knee and ankle weakness to falls in nursing home residents: an isokinetic study. *J. Am. Geriatr. Soc.* **35,** 13–20 (1987).
97. Frontera, W. R., Meredith, C. N., O'Reilly, K. P., Knuttgen, H. G., and Evans, W. J. Strength conditioning in older men: skeletal muscle hypertrophy and improved function. *Appl. Physiol.* **64,** 1038–1044 (1988).
98. Charette, S. L., *et al.* Muscle hypertrophy response to resistance training in older women. *Appl. Physiol.* **70,** 1912–1916 (1991).
99. Pyka, G., Lindenberger, E., Charette, S., and Marcus, R. Muscle strength and fiber adaptations to a year-long resistance training program in elderly men and women. *J. Gerontol.* **49,** M22–M27 (1994).
100. Milner-Brown, H. S., Stein, R. B., and Lee, R. G. Synchronization of human motor units: possible roles of exercise and supraspinal reflexes. *Electroencephalogr. Clin. Neurophysiol.* **38,** 245–254 (1975).
101. Hurley, B. F. Age, gender, and muscular strength. *J. Gerontol. A Biol. Sci. Med. Sci.* **50,** 41–44 (1995).
102. Marcus, R. Relationship of age-related decreases in muscle mass and strength to skeletal status. *J. Gerontol. A Biol. Sci. Med. Sci.* **50,** 86–87 (1995).
103. Vandervoort, A. A., and McComas, A. J. Contractile changes in opposing muscles of the human ankle joint with aging. *J. Appl. Physiol.* **61,** 361–367 (1986).
104. Aloia, J. F., McGowan, D. M., Vaswani, A. N., Ross, P., and Cohn, S. H. Relationship of menopause to skeletal and muscle mass. *Am. J. Clin. Nutr.* **53,** 1378–1383 (1991).
105. Kallman, D. A., Plato, C. C., and Tobin, J. D. The role of muscle loss in the age-related decline of grip strength: cross-sectional and longitudinal perspectives. *J. Gerontol.* **45,** M82–M88 (1990).
106. Specker, B. L. Evidence for an interaction between calcium intake and physical activity on changes in bone mineral density. *J. Bone Miner. Res.* **11,** 1539–1544 (1996).
107. Kanders, B., Dempster, D. W., and Lindsay, R. Interaction of calcium nutrition and physical activity on bone mass in young women. *J. Bone Miner. Res.* **3,** 145–149 (1988).
108. Prince, R., *et al.* The effects of calcium supplementation (milk powder or tablets) and exercise on bone density in postmenopausal women. *J. Bone Miner. Res.* **10,** 1068–1075 (1995).
109. Uusi-Rasi, K., *et al.* Associations of physical activity and calcium intake with bone mass and size in healthy women at different ages. *J. Bone Miner. Res.* **13,** 133–142 (1998).
110. Nelson, M. E., Fisher, E. C., Dilmanian, F. A., Dallal, G. E., and Evans, W. J. A 1-y walking program and increased dietary calcium in postmenopausal women: effects on bone. *Am. J. Clin. Nutr.* **53,** 1304–1311 (1991).
111. Notelovitz, M., *et al.* Estrogen therapy and variable-resistance weight training increase bone mineral in surgically menopausal women [see comments]. *J. Bone Miner. Res.* **6,** 583–590 (1991).
112. Kohrt, W. M., Ehsani, A. A., and Birge, S. J., Jr. HRT preserves increases in bone mineral density and reductions in body fat after a supervised exercise program. *J. Appl. Physiol.* **84,** 1506–1512 (1998).
113. Prince, R. L., *et al.* Prevention of postmenopausal osteoporosis. A comparative study of exercise, calcium supplementation, and hormone-replacement therapy. *N. Engl. J. Med.* **325,** 1189–1195 (1991).
114. Heikkinen, J., *et al.* Moderate exercise does not enhance the positive effect of estrogen on bone mineral density in postmenopausal women. *Calcif, Tissue Int.* **49,** S83–S84 (1991).
115. Yarasheski, K. E., Campbell, J. A., and Kohrt, W. M. Effect of resistance exercise and growth hormone on bone density in older men. *Clin. Endocrinol.* **47,** 223–229 (1997).
116. Taaffe, D. R., *et al.* Effect of recombinant human growth hormone on the muscle strength response to resistance exercise in elderly men. *J. Clin. Endocrinol. Metab.* **79,** 1361–1366 (1994).
117. Taaffe, D. R., Jin, I. H., Vu, T. H., Hoffman, A. R., and Marcus, R. Lack of effect of recombinant growth hormone (GH) on muscle morphology and GH-insulin-like growth factor expression in resistance-trained elderly men. *J. Clin. Endocrinol. Metab.* **81,** 421–425 (1996).
118. Ebrahim, S., Thompson, P. W., Baskaran, V., and Evans, K. Randomized placebo-controlled trial of brisk walking in the prevention of postmenopausal osteoporosis. *Age Ageing* **26,** 253–260 (1997).
119. Chow, R., Harrison, J., and Dornan, J. Prevention and rehabilitation of osteoporosis program: exercise and osteoporosis. *Int. J. Rehabil. Res.* **12,** 49–56 (1989).
120. Gregg, E. W., Cauley, J. A., Seeley, D. G., Ensrud, K. E., and Bauer, D. C. Physical activity and osteoporotic fracture risk in older women. Study of Osteoporotic Fractures Research Group [see comments]. *Ann. Intern. Med.* **129,** 81–88 (1998).
121. Joakimsen, R. M., *et al.* The Tromso Study: Physical activity and the incidence of fractures in a middle-aged population. *J. Bone Miner. Res.* **13,** 1149–1157 (1998).
122. Krall, E. A., and Dawson-Hughes, B. Walking is related to bone density and rates of bone loss. *Am. J. Med.* **96,** 20–26 (1994).
123. Lanyon, L. E. Using functional loading to influence bone mass and architecture: objectives, mechanisms, and relationship with estrogen of the mechanically adaptive process in bone. *Bone* **18,** 37S–43S (1996).
124. Marcus, R. *In* "Principles of Bone Biology" (J. P. Bilezikian, L. G. Raisz, and G. Rodan, eds.), pp. 1135–1146. Academic Press, San Diego, 1996.

CHAPTER 40

The Rationale for Calcium Supplementation in the Therapeutics of Age-Related Osteoporosis

R. L. PRINCE University Department of Medicine, University of Western Australia
and Department of Endocrinology & Diabetes, Sir Charles Gairdner Hospital,
Nedlands, Western Australia 6009

CALCIUM AND THE AGING SKELETON: RATIONALE FOR INCREASING DIETARY CALCIUM INTAKE

The concept that diets in general and Western-style diets in particular are deficient in calcium has been controversial. In large part this is because there has been little differentiation between the importance of calcium intakes in different age groups. The biological mechanisms involved in skeletal development in childhood and adolescence are completely different from those involved in skeletal maintenance in adult life. In childhood, the principal mechanisms for skeletal development are growth at the physeal growth plate and modeling on bone surfaces, although remodeling is also important in determining the shape of the skeleton. Although it is intuitively obvious that a supply of dietary calcium is required to allow deposition of hydroxyapatite on the collagen framework, it is not clear that under normal Western dietary patterns in childhood and adolescence of around 800 mg of calcium per day that calcium intake is rate limiting in allowing optimal skeletal development at peak bone mass [1]. In early adult life, data that dietary calcium intake is deficient have also been controversial [2]. However, in elderly people there is general agreement that calcium intake may be deficient in many [3]. More recent bone density and fracture end point studies utilizing randomized controlled trial methodology have shown a clear clinical benefit from calcium supplementation. It is, however, important to realize that data on the efficacy of calcium for fracture prevention have been developed in Westernized countries, as to date data have not been fully replicated in other cultures.

CALCIUM BALANCE: EXTRACELLULAR SPACE VERSUS WHOLE BODY

The mechanism of action of any therapeutic intervention must be clearly understood if it is to be used to maximum effect. This is particularly true of dietary calcium supplementation because of several interacting processes that influence its effectiveness in skeletal maintenance. Because the skeleton is the major reservoir of total body calcium, containing over 98% of the

1–2 kg of calcium in the body, it is often thought that total body calcium balance is the same as bone calcium balance. Over the long term this is correct but in the short term it is extracellular calcium balance that is much more important to the survival of the individual. This is because of the vital role calcium pays in all cell signaling. In addition to the central role of calcium as a second messenger in the regulation of all cell activity, it also has a specific role in conduction of the action potential along nerves and in excitation contraction coupling in striated and cardiac muscle.

Often the requirements of maintenance of extracellular calcium homeostasis are in conflict with the maintenance of skeletal hydroxyapatite and thereby the skeletal structure. It is this tension between the requirements of separate body compartments that sets the scene for the importance of calcium nutrition in the prevention and treatment of age-related osteoporosis. The mechanisms that defend the internal milieu from fluctuations in calcium concentration have to contend with the variable intake of dietary calcium. The bone reservoir of calcium is used to smooth out these fluctuations. This occurs by increasing osteoclastic bone resorption, which then entrains osteoblastic bone reformation at the same site to regenerate the calcium supply when the dietary intake of calcium increases. In aging the ability of the kidney and bowel to maintain extracellular calcium homeostasis declines. The reasons for this are complex and will be discussed in detail. The consequence of these defects is that the skeletal bone resorption rises. As a result of a defect in osteoblast activity associated with aging, the regeneration of bone is deficient, resulting in osteoporosis.

Mechanisms of Maintenance of Extracellular Calcium Homeostasis

At an organ level the principal players in extracellular calcium homeostasis are the bone, the gut, and the kidney, as it is these structures that regulate the principal flow of calcium into or out of the extracellular space. The interrelations between these factors are illustrated in Fig. 1. It is critically important to realize that calcium is continually cycling in and out of the bloodstream, bathing these organs in what might be considered a futile cycle. In the kidney, 99% of the calcium filtered at the glomerulus is reabsorbed, i.e., approximately 150 mmol/day. In the bone it can be calculated that 0.05% of the hydroxyapatite in the skeleton is reabsorbed per day, amounting to 5–10 mmol/day. If the individual is in calcium balance this must be replaced in newly formed bone. In the bowel, intestinal calcium excretion is approximately 5 mmol/day; at 50% reabsorption efficiency, approximately 2.5 mmol would be reabsorbed [3]. Thus calcium is continually fluxing in and out of these principal organs of extracellular calcium homeostasis. Similarly, it is continually moving in and out of all the cells of the body. The skin is a further small source of calcium transport loss from the body in perspiration [4].

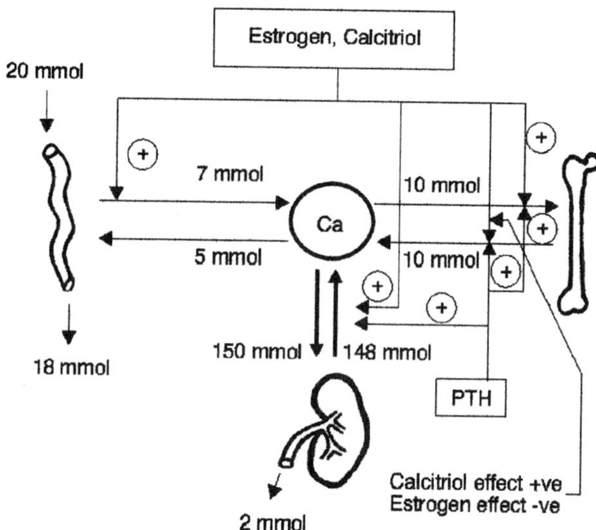

Figure 1 Regulation of organs involved in calcium transport.

Regulation of Mechanisms of Extracellular Calcium Homeostasis

The maintenance of the concentration of plasma calcium and total calcium balance, which is an important consideration for the growth and maintenance of the skeleton, are closely regulated by a number of hormonal and physiological mechanisms. The flow of calcium into and out of the bone, gut, and kidney is regulated by a variety of mechanisms, which are only partly understood but involve the principal hormonal regulator of calcium homeostasis, namely the vitamin D–parathyroid hormone (PTH) system (Fig. 2). In addition, other steroid hormones, such as estrogen and progesterone, are thought to influence calcium transport in the gut, kidney, and possibly the bone [5].

The teleologic question of the purpose of this futile cycling arises as it involves considerable "unnecessary" energy expenditure. It may be that it is easier to precisely control a system in which rapid large fluxes are occurring. This is because it is easier to regulate precisely the amount of calcium entering or being removed from a high-flow rate system than from a low-flow rate system. Thus the critical issue in the control of this sytem is to regulate the relative activity of the various organs and

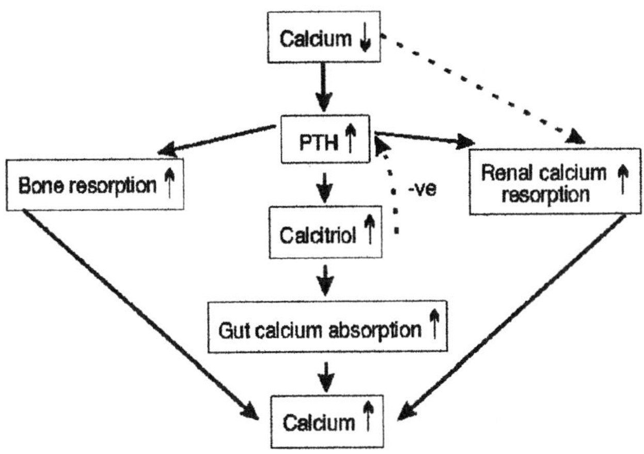

FIGURE 2 PTH and calcitriol regulation of calcium homeostasis.

cells to optimize constancy of the internal milieu. A common stress that the system has to cope with is episodes of low dietary calcium. Under these circumstances, calcium cycles into the bowel and kidney faster relative to the rate in which it cycles out. In the bone compartment, calcium cycles out faster relative to the rate at which it enters the bone compartment.

Epithelial Calcium Transport

The consequences of calcium deficiency are in the end associated with variation in the transport of calcium from one body compartment to another. Thus the mechanisms of calcium transport across membranes will now be reviewed. Transcellular calcium flux in epithelial cells is the result of the specialized structure of these cells resulting in a functional polarity between apical and basolateral membranes due to the different requirements of calcium transport between these two membranes. In the epithelial cell, the apical membrane may be exposed to a relatively high concentration of calcium compared to the low intracellular calcium concentration, so calcium passes across this membrane along a calcium gradient, utilizing specific transport systems. At the basolateral membrane, calcium must move against a calcium gradient, requiring specific transport mechanisms [6,7]. Two distinct transport mechanisms are known to exist in the plasma membranes of renal and intestinal epithelium that remove calcium from the cell, the plasma membrane calcium pump (PMCP), and the Na^+–Ca^{2+} exchanger (NCE). Evidence shows that the activity of PMCP in the bowel is regulated by calcitriol [8] and that the activity of the NCE in kidney is regulated by PTH [9]. Two important calcium-binding proteins also play a role in moving calcium from the apical to basolateral membranes, calbindin D28K, present in distal tubular cells in the kidney, and calbindin D9K, present in intestinal cells. The calbindins have been shown to increase the diffusion rates of physiological levels of calcium [10].

PLASMA MEMBRANE CALCIUM PUMP

The PMCP is a Ca^{2+}–Mg^{2+}–dependent ATPase with a molecular weight of 135,000 [11]. The pump consists of 10 putative transmembrane helices with a high degree of homology in the catalytic domains of the rat and human sequences. The PMCP is coded by four separate genes in both the human and the rat and alternate splicing results in potentially more than 30 isoforms 2 [11]. Calmodulin increases both the affinity and the V_{max} of this system [11] in both kidney and intestine.

SODIUM CALCIUM EXCHANGER

The NCE is a secondary active transport system, using the electrochemical gradient produced by sodium ATPase activity [12]. Three different isoforms have been discovered that are coded from a single gene, with almost identical homology between species. It is a 970 amino acid protein with a primary structure that contains 11 transmembrane-spanning regions and a large cytoplasmic loop between transmembrane segments 6 and 7. The NCE is particularly abundant in cells that handle large fluxes of calcium across their membranes, such as contractile and neuronal cells. The orientation of the NCE is determined by the predominance of two inwardly directed electrochemical gradients generated by plasma membrane sodium and calcium pumps. This electrochemical gradient is determined by the net activity of the PMCP, the sodium pump, cell organelle calcium sequestering, and the membrane potential difference. Depending on these factors it can operate in a calcium influx or calcium efflux mode or, if the gradient is neutral, Na^+–Ca^{2+} exchange ceases [12].

Evidence also shows that both NCE and PMCP calcium transporters exist in bone cells [6,13]. Further, transcellular calcium transport has been shown to be important in dentine mineralization by the odontoblast [14].

Disordered Mechanisms of Calcium Homeostasis and the Etiology of Age-Related Osteoporosis

Critical abnormalities in calcium homeostasis resulting in age-related osteoporosis involve all three main organs of calcium homeostasis (Fig. 3). On the supply side there is a reduction in gut calcium absorption [15–18] that compounds the low dietary intake of many elderly people. The causation of the reduction in absorp-

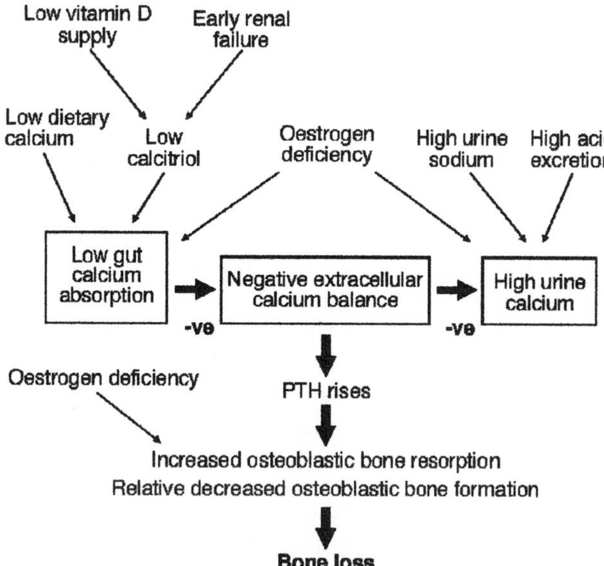

FIGURE 3 Age-related bone loss.

tion is complex, involving intrinsic gut wall defects and abnormalities in vitamin D and estrogen status. On the demand side there is an increase in renal calcium excretion that, in women, occurs at menopause and persists into old age [19]. This increase is, in women, due to an estrogen deficiency and other determinants of renal calcium excretion such as salt and acid base balance. Within the bone the abnormality is in the regeneration of the calcified skeleton for future episodes of calcium deficiency. The causation of this osteoblast defect is uncertain but may, on certain surfaces, be due to a reduction in stress strain effects due to the reduction in physical activity associated with aging.

If there is insufficient gut calcium absorption to compensate for renal and skin loss of calcium, stimulation of bone resorption occurs that involves the stimulation of PTH secretion [20] and the suppression of calcitonin secretion by relative hypocalcemia [21]. The calcium deficiency of age-related bone loss is associated with raised levels of PTH [19,22]. This can be corrected by dietary calcium supplements [23–25]. The effect of the rise in PTH is to stimulate bone resorption from trabecular and cortical bone to maintain extracellular calcium homeostasis.

The rise in PTH in response to relative calcium deprivation is exacerbated by three factors: (1) the relative 1,25-dihydroxyvitamin D deficiency that is noted more than 10 years past menopause [15,19] associated with the early renal failure of aging [26,27], (2) increases in PTH [28,29] as a result of vitamin D deficiency due to reduced sunlight exposure [30], and (3) estrogen deficiency in women [31,32]. These factors will be discussed in relation to the function of principal organs of calcium homeostasis in the bowel and kidney. The principal effect of the rise in PTH on the skeleton is to induce excessive bone resorption, which is not compensated for by an associated adequate increase in bone formation, and thus results in bone loss.

DETERMINANTS OF GUT CALCIUM ABSORPTION

Gut calcium absorption is a critical determinant of extracellular and bone calcium balance in the aging individual. The principal determinants relate to the dietary calcium intake and the fraction absorbed. In the adult human, of the calcium consumed each day, 10 to 60% is absorbed by the intestine, some of which is the reabsorption of calcium secreted into the bowel. Under conditions of low calcium intake it is possible for the unresorbed intestinal secretion of calcium in the feces, the endogenous fecal calcium, to exceed that eaten in the diet. Under these circumstances the individual will have a negative calcium balance in the bowel compartment [33]. Therefore, net calcium absorption is the difference between the net amount of calcium absorbed and the amount lost as fecal calcium excretion.

Gut calcium absorption is determined (1) by the intraluminal concentration of calcium achieved at various points in the bowel and (2) by gut wall factors determining absorption efficiency, including the vitamin D status. The actual site of calcium absorption in the bowel varies, depending on the magnitude of the calcium load in the food and on its rate of transit through the bowel [34]. In general, 95% of calcium absorption occurs in the small bowel [35]. Although having the highest rate of active absorption, duodenal absorption is not the most important site for calcium absorption on a quantitative basis, except at very low calcium intakes [36]. This is because the time that calcium resides within the duodenum is relatively short.

As discussed later, the rate of calcium consumption is critically important in the presence of a defect in active calcium absorption as occurs with aging. This is because passive calcium absorption can effectively compensate for these defects if a high enough intraluminal calcium concentration can be achieved by the rapid ingestion of calcium, as occurs with the use of calcium tablets. The minimum fractional absorption to preserve a positive calcium balance on an intake of 1500 mg of calcium per day in postmenopausal women can be calculated to be about 20% [17,33]. Thus, provided the calcium intake is high enough, a gut calcium absorption efficiency of 20% is sufficient to maintain bone calcium balance.

Dietary Calcium Intake

Intraluminal factors affecting the magnitude of gut calcium absorption are related to the intraluminal concentration of calcium, which is determined by the frequency and magnitude of calcium intake and the nature of the foods that it is consumed with. These factors are important when considering the clinical prescription of the calcium intake for the individual. Before considering methods of improving calcium balance by dietary means it would be desirable to know what the calcium intake of the individual patient actually is. Unfortunately, it is difficult to accurately evaluate dietary calcium intakes even in research studies in which weighed food records are used. This is because intakes vary quite considerably from day to day and over the seasons. Thus for research and clinical practice purposes it is difficult to define an individual's intake accurately, although mean calcium intakes in large groups of individuals can be measured reasonably accurately [37].

In terms of practical patient management it is reasonable to try to detect those with calcium intakes below 400 mg per day as they may respond best to calcium supplementation [38]. To this end the average calcium contents of various foods are listed in Table I. It should be pointed out that calcium fortification of food is practiced in some countries. It is clear from Table I that the major source of calcium is dairy foods, which are not available freely in many countries in the world.

Epidemiological Data on Calcium Intake

Mean data show wide variations in intake among age groups, genders, and countries. These data have been compared with fracture rates in these groups by correla-

TABLE I Foods High in Calcium

Food	mg calcium	Food	mg calcium
Milk, 1 glass, 250 ml	295	1 egg	27
Milk, skim, 250 ml	300	Fish, 150-g fillet	50
Milk, low fat enriched, 250 ml	390	Salmon, canned, 100 g	185
Buttermilk, 250 ml	295	Sardines, canned, 100 g	350
Cheese, cheddar, 30 g	260	Oysters, 12	230
Cheese, Swiss, 30 g	290	Scallops, 6	120
Processed cheese, 1 slice, 21 g	150	Beans, haricot, 1 cup cooked	110
Cream cheese, 50 g	60	Canned baked beans, 1/2 cup	55
Cottage cheese, 1/2 cup	115	Tofu, 100 g	130
Yogurt, natural, 200 g	380	Almonds, 50 g	125
Yogurt, flavored, 200 g	315	Brazil or hazel nuts, 50 g	90
Ice cream, 150 ml	70	Peanuts, 50 g	30
Baked custard, average serving	250	Pistachio nuts, 50 g	65
Cream, 2 tablespoons	35	Walnuts, 50 g	40
Coconut milk, 200 ml	60	Sesame seeds, 20 g	230
Soybean milk, 250 ml	55	Sunflower seeds, 20 g	25
Beans, green, average serving	30	Blackberries, 1/2 punnet	80
Broccoli, average serving	75	Lemon, 1	110
Brussels sprouts, average serving	25	Orange, average	55
Carrots, 1 medium	50	Orange juice, 250 ml	30
Molasses, black, 1 tablespoon	120	Raspberries, 1/2 punnet	50
Molasses, light, 1 tablespoon	35	Rhubarb, 1/2 cup cooked	105
Silverbeet, average serving	75	Strawberries, 1/2 punnet	35
Watercress, 1/2 cup	45	Cabbage, average serving	45
Spinach, average serving	360	Parsley, 1/4 cup	30
Pumpkin, average piece	40	Milk chocolate, 50 g	145
Peas, 1/2 cup	30		

tion analysis. These cross-cultural comparisons show that countries with low calcium intakes have low hip fracture rates [39]. Surprisingly, these data have been taken to mean that an increasing calcium intake increases fracture rates. This conclusion ignores the enormous number of genetic and environmental differences between different cultures. The pitfalls of drawing conclusions from simple correlation of two measures are often covered in basic statistics courses in which it is stated that "correlation does not necessarily imply causation."

Nevertheless, it has to be acknowledged from epidemiological data that high calcium intakes prevent fracture is extremely weak. These data show that there is no or only a very weak effect of high dietary calcium intake on fracture prevention. In contrast, long-term randomized controlled data show that calcium supplementation prevents bone loss and fracture. Although this could be because the methods of measuring regular calcium intake are weak, it also raises the possibility that the intake of calcium in the diet under real conditions is relatively ineffective. This may be because passive calcium absorption is important in the aging bowel. Under these circumstances, high calcium concentrations are required, which may be best achieved with calcium tablets. Nevertheless, provided similar high calcium concentrations can be achieved by other calcium sources, a similar effect on bone density will occur [25].

Effects of Lactose on Calcium Absorption

Lactose intolerance has been associated with the development of osteoporosis [40] and, more recently, has been shown to be a predictor of fracture [41]. The connection between lactose intolerance and osteoporosis would appear to be due to a reduced calcium intake associated with an avoidance of milk products [41]. It is therefore appropriate to determine whether milk products cause abdominal symptoms as this may be an indicator of lactose intolerance. Another aspect is that in subjects with lactose intolerance, lactose will itself induce calcium malabsorption from about 25 to 20% [42]. This effect may be due to the osmotic effects of the lactose reducing the effective concentration of calcium within the bowel [36]. Interestingly, in normal subjects, lactose may increase calcium absorption from 22 to 36% [42]. Unfortunately, lactose was not compared to other carbohydrates so it is uncertain as to whether this effect is specific to lactose.

Effects of Phytates and Fiber on Calcium Absorption

High-fiber diets have been recommended for various benefits on the bowel and cardiovascular system. Studies that have examined the effects of these diets on calcium consumption have not found any significant deleterious effects, at least at moderate consumption of these foods [43]. However, at high-fiber intakes, calcium retention is reduced from 25 to 19% [44]. Although fiber in the form of wheat bran binds calcium within the gut and reduces the fractional absorption of calcium, the actual absorption is independent of carrier load. Thus at high calcium concentrations the fractional absorption in the presence of wheat bran is still 23% so the actual absorption of a 600-mg calcium tablet may still be adequate to preserve bone calcium balance.

Effects of the Chemical Form of Calcium on Absorption

Several studies have examined absorption in relation to the anion that accompanies the calcium [44,45]. In general, this does not make much difference provided that the calcium tablet, if calcium is given in this form, dissolves in the bowel lumen [46,47]. It has been shown in achlorhydric individuals that the absorption of calcium, when administered as calcium carbonate, is less than when administered as calcium citrate. This differential absorption is abolished if the calcium is taken with food [48]. Certainly in terms of bioactivity in preventing bone loss, calcium lactate gluconate was identical to milk powder containing the same amount of calcium [25,49]. After a calcium-restricted diet the absorption of calcium citrate in the fasting state is slightly higher than calcium carbonate [44]. The dietary calcium absorption from various foods has been examined. Spinach calcium is particularly poorly absorbed, whereas milk, bone meal, and kale calcium are absorbed about equally at a fractional absorption of 0.3 to 0.4 [50].

Effects of Calcium on Other Nutrient Intakes

Increasing calcium intake as part of an overall diet message has been shown to be beneficial if combined with advice on fat intake [51]. In view of the combination of dietary deficiencies and excesses in this age group, such a diet may have broad health benefits [52]. In this regard the zinc content of milk powder may confer some benefit [53]. However, there is some concern that calcium supplementation interferes with iron and zinc absorption [34,35,54].

Calcium Transport across the Intestine

The absorption of calcium occurs by transcellular and paracellular mechanisms (Fig. 4). In general the

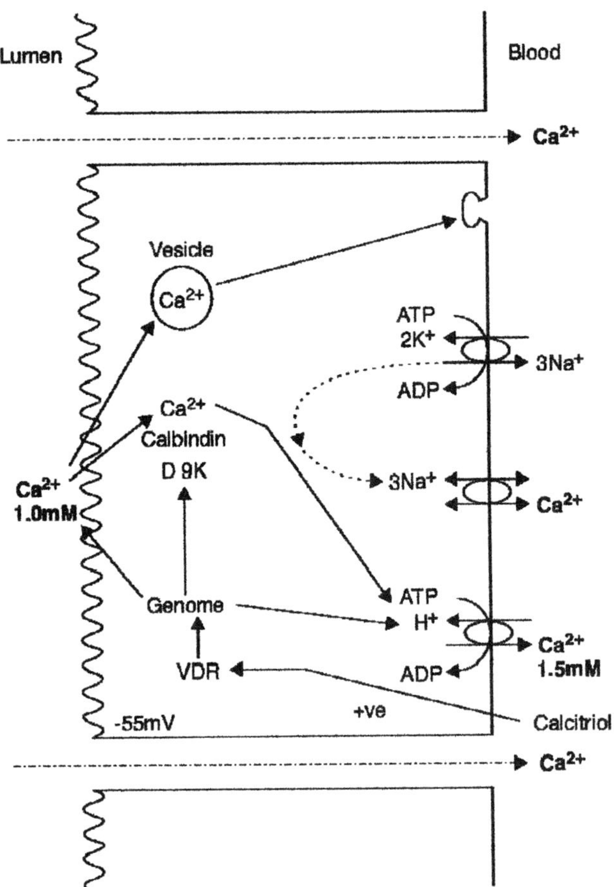

FIGURE 4 Enterocyte calcium transport.

paracellular route is considered to be unregulated, although there is some evidence that vitamin D can stimulate the nonsaturable phase of calcium transport [55]. The driving force behind the paracellular route is thought to be concentration gradient and solvent drag driven. The paracellular movement of calcium takes place throughout the length of the intestine and may account for two-thirds of calcium flux in the rat intestine. In humans, passive paracellular absorption appears to have an absorption efficiency of about 15%. Thus at high dietary intakes it would be possible to supply the calcium requirement to maintain extra cellular homeostasis from this source. Paracellular movement favors absorption in the duodenum only, with paracellular calcium secretion occurring in the jejunum and ileum, indicating that net calcium absorption is determined by transcellular mechanisms as well as the net difference between paracellular absorption and secretion [56].

There are two mechanisms of transcellular transport: active transport and transcellular vesicular transport termed transcaltachia. Transcellular calcium transport in the enterocyte is summarized in Fig. 4. NCE activity has been shown in the intestine in both rats [57] and humans [58] and it appears to have approximately 20% of the calcium-translocating activity of the PMCP in basolateral membrane preparations [57]. This suggests that PMCP is the more important mechanism for the translocation of calcium in the intestine. In support of this is the observation that the activity of the PMCP in the rat declines with age [8] and its activity and mRNA expression appear to be stimulated by calcitriol [8]. The bowel PMCP has a calbindin D9K-binding domain; however, the interaction of calbindin D9K does not appear to result in an increase in PMCP activity [59].

In addition to the just-described mechanism of active transcellular transport, there is evidence of an endocytotic, exocytotic vesicular transport mechanism. The opening of apical membrane calcium channels may increase calcium transport into the cell as the result of rapid, nongenomic stimulation by calcitriol, a process referred to as transcaltachia [60]. In this mechanism, calcitriol stimulates calcium uptake into lysosomes at the apical membrane, with subsequent delivery to the basolateral membrane with a time course in the order of 30 min [61].

Regulation of Intestinal Calcium Transport by Vitamin D

The physiological source of vitamin D is from the action of sunlight on 6-dehydrocholesterol in the skin. There is no doubt that sunlight-deprived individuals, no matter where they live, readily become deficient in cholecalciferol, which may be reflected in reduced 25-hydroxyvitamin D levels. This is particularly prevalent in northern countries in the elderly where skin formation of cholecalciferol may not occur between October and April [62]. That severe vitamin D deficiency can lead to calcium malabsorption is not in dispute. The question that arises is the relative importance of vitamin D status in relation to the other physiological variables affecting calcium absorption in aging.

If gut calcium absorption is measured using a radioactive calcium method with a low calcium dose it has been shown that total 1,25-dihydroxyvitamin D is a strong determinant of calcium absorption [15,16]. However, studies using high calcium intakes in patients with adequate vitamin D stores have not shown a dependence of gut calcium absorption on 1,25-dihydroxyvitamin D levels [18,63]. Clearly the differences in the findings indicate that vitamin D-based mechanisms are less important at high calcium loads.

The role of vitamin D as the active principle in calcium absorption goes back to Nicholyasen, who coined the term "endogenous factor" to specify a regulator of calcium absorption. With the advent of modern biochemical techniques, it became clear that cholecalciferol was metabolized to 25-hydroxyvitamin D.

Eventually, 1,25-dihydroxyvitamin D was isolated [64] and, in the chick bowel receptor assay, was shown to have an affinity for the vitamin D receptor at least 1000 times higher than 25-hydroxyvitamin D [65]. Furthermore, 25-dihydroxyvitamin D was inactive in transport studies in rat bowel as compared to 1,25-dihydroxyvitamin D [55]. Despite the clear physiological role of 1,25-dihydroxyvitamin D compared to 25-hydroxyvitamin D in *in vitro* and animal systems, the physiological importance of either 1,25-dihydroxyvitamin D or 25-hydroxyvitamin D in the physiology of calcium absorption in aging humans has been more controversial.

Renal dysfunction is very common in the aging population, especially in subjects over the age of 70 [19]. The author and others have shown that early renal dysfunction (GFR less than 60 ml/min) is associated with a slight fall in 1,25-dihydroxyvitamin D and a rise in PTH [26,27,66]. Furthermore, there may be a specific defect in the production of 1,25-dihydroxyvitamin D in subjects with osteoporosis compared to age-matched normal subjects, which is more important at low calcium intakes [67]. A further complexity is that there is evidence for a reduction in the end organ activity of 1,25-dihydroxyvitamin D on the bowel in later life [68].

Vitamin D-Binding Proteins

Consideration of binding protein concentrations in the circulation, which can affect the physiologically relevant, free fraction of vitamin D, is important. The vitamin D-binding protein has an affinity for 25-hydroxyvitamin D 10- to 20-fold that for 1,25-dihydroxyvitamin D [69]. Albumin has a much lower affinity for vitamin D metabolites. The free biologically active level of 1,25-dihydroxyvitamin D is about 300 fmol/1 and the free concentration of 25-hydroxyvitamin D is about 60-fold higher [69]. When the 1000-fold higher affinity of 1,25-dihydroxyvitamin D for its receptor and for calcium transport in the everted gut sac is considered it is likely that 1,25-dihydroxyvitamin D is the active entity.

Evaluation of Vitamin D Status

In the presence of deficiency of its precursor 25-hydroxyvitamin D, the 1-hydroxylase enzyme making the active compound is up-regulated to maintain supply. Under these circumstances, the blood level of the active compound may be within the normal reference range. However, it is important to recognize that normal reference ranges do not apply in the presence of substrate deficiency because the physiological requirement is much higher. That this is so is shown by studies of the effects of replacing vitamin D with sun exposure in vitamin D-deficient individuals [30]. When this is done, the plasma levels of 1,25-dihydroxyvitamin D rise much more rapidly than 25-hydroxyvitamin D levels. Thus, to evaluate vitamin D status, it is more useful to measure 25-hydroxyvitamin D than 1,25-dihydroxyvitamin D levels. Furthermore, because the total concentration of 25-hydroxyvitamin D is 1000-fold higher than for 1,25-dihydroxyvitamin D, the assay for 25-hydroxyvitamin D is easier and more precise than for 1,25-dihydroxyvitamin D. A comparison with the evaluation of the thyroid status is apt. Although tri-iodothyronine is the active hormone when compared to thyroxine, its site of action is intracellular. In general, it is more useful to measure thyroxine than tri-iodothyronine when assessing the thyroid status because the concentration of the active hormone, triodothyronine, is maintained.

Data in young healthy subjects with normal baseline vitamin D status consuming a 300-mg calcium meal have confirmed that high doses of 25-hydroxyvitamin D can increase gut calcium absorption [70]. Doses of 50 μg/day, which produced circulating 25-hydroxyvitamin D levels of over 500 nmol/liter, achieved a 25% increase in the fractional absorption of calcium. Extrapolation to more physiological levels suggests that up to 7% of gut calcium absorption of a 300-mg calcium meal may be accounted for by circulating 25-hydroxyvitamin D. Circulating 1,25-dihydroxyvitamin D accounted for approximately 40% of calcium absorption. The remainder was considered to be passive. The relevance of these data to elderly subjects with a marginal vitamin D status remains to be determined.

Elderly subjects with a mean level of 25-hydroxyvitamin D of 35 nmol/liter and a mean calcium intake of 876 mg/day responded to increasing cholecalciferol intake by mouth with a rise in 1,25-dihydroxyvitamin D and a fall in PTH [71]. Unfortunately, such a regiment did not reduce fractures in a similar population [72]. Thus the optimal vitamin D status, as measured by 25-hydroxyvitamin D levels, to prevent fracture is uncertain and is dependent on the calcium intake of the individual.

Relative Importance of Calcium Dose and Vitamin D Status in Calcium Absorption

Dosing studies in young subjects that used bowel washout techniques clearly show the dependence of gut calcium absorption on 1,25-dihydroxyvitamin D concentrations and calcium intakes across the physiological range bowel [73]. Sheikh *et al.* [73] were able to calculate that the vitamin D-independent fraction of calcium absorption in their subjects was about 30% across the range of calcium intakes. 1,25-Dihydroxyvitamin D regulated calcium absorption across the physiological range and was able to stimulate fractional calcium absorption from close to zero at low 1,25-dihydroxyvitamin D concentrations to over 60% at very high concentrations. Thus, in a normal individual with a 1,25-dihydroxyvitamin D concentration of 120 pmol/liter consuming a meal containing 300 mg of calcium, approximately 75 mg of calcium would be absorbed by vitamin D-dependent processes whereas approximately 25 mg would be absorbed by passive processes. However, by extrapolation, if a high calcium intake were consumed, e.g., a 600-mg calcium tablet, it could be calculated that 180 mg of calcium would be absorbed by passive means with no increment in active absorption. These fractional absorption data have been supported by other studies carried out at high calcium doses [74,75]. Thus, assuming that there is no deterioration in the passive absorption of calcium with age if high calcium meals are ingested, the vitamin D status of the individual would have little impact on calcium absorption. If, however, low calcium meals are consumed, as is common in elderly subjects, then the vitamin D status becomes critical. Under these circumstances if there is deficiency of 1,25-dihydroxyvitamin D, there may well be net calcium loss from the bowel [73].

Estrogen Effects on Gut Calcium Absorption

In view of evidence for a reduction in calcium absorption at menopause [17], it has been suggested that there may be a direct effect of estrogen on gut calcium absorption. Other data have suggested that estrogen may potentiate the effect of 1,25-dihydroxyvitamin D on the stimulation of calcium absorption [76]. However, direct evidence for an effect of estrogen on calcium absorption in aging humans remains controversial [5].

ROLE OF THE KIDNEY IN EXTRACELLULAR CALCIUM BALANCE

The kidneys filter approximately 100–200 mmol per 24 hr, of which about 98% is reabsorbed. Because of the high rate at which calcium is cycling across the renal tubular membrane, it is possible for subtle variations in the rate of reabsorption to have profound effects on the extracellular calcium balance. Factors that increase calcium reabsorption are numerous and may include volume depletion, PTH, 1,25-dihydroxyvitamin D, and estrogen. This section outlines the ways in which this may occur. At menopause there is a significant increase in renal calcium excretion that persists indefinitely [19]. This suggests that estrogen deficiency is a major cause of increased renal calcium excretion, which is likely due to a primary effect on the kidney [24].

Calcium Transport in the Kidney

Approximately 70% of calcium reabsorption occurs in the proximal tubule [77] and is largely passive and voltage dependent. It is associated with the active reabsorption of sodium, glucose, and other solutes. In the kidney, paracellular calcium transport is regulated by the extracellular ionized calcium concentration that acts on the calcium-sensing receptor that has been cloned in human [78] and rat [79] kidney. The interaction of calcium with the calcium-sensing receptor results in a decrease in hormone-dependent sodium chloride reabsorption. This is the result of the inhibition of hormone-dependent cyclic AMP production and a decrease in the $Na^{+}K\ 2Cl^{-}$ cotransporter and K^{+} channel activity as a result of phospholipase A activation and the subsequent stimulation of arachadonic acid and 20-HETE. This in turn decreases both the lumen-positive potential that drives paracellular calcium transport and the countercurrent multiplier that concentrates urine, resulting in increased urine calcium excretion [80].

In the distal tubule, sodium and calcium reabsorption can be uncoupled, e.g., with thiazide diuretics [81]. It is in this segment that regulation by PTH and cAMP occurs [81]. This suggests that the fine regulation of calcium excretion by hormonal control of the NCE and the PMCP occurs in the distal tubule. Mechanisms involved in calcium transport and their regulation are outlined in Fig. 5. In the kidney the NCE is located only in the distal tubule and has been shown to be the primary mechanism by which PTH modulates renal calcium reabsorption [9]. The PMCP is present in both proximal and distal tubules, with a higher affinity in the distal tubule, indicating that its role in the proximal tubule may be the maintenance of intracellular calcium levels rather than the translocation of large amounts of calcium [82]. Localization studies in the human kidney using monoclonal antibodies to the human red blood cell calcium pump could only detect the calcium pump in the distal tubule [83], indicating that the lower affinity plasma pump activity observed in proximal tubules is of a different type. A second major factor in transcellular calcium transport in the kidney is calbindin D28K. This calcium-binding protein is colocated with the PMCP in the distal nephron in both human [84] and rat [7] kidney.

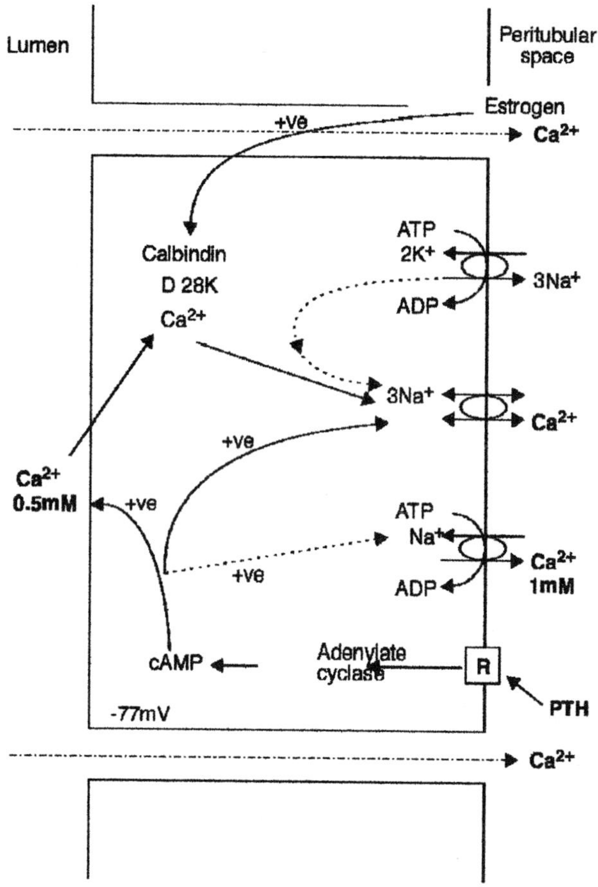

FIGURE 5 Distal tubule calcium transport.

Of particular interest is the evidence for a calbindin D28K stimulatory effect on basolateral membrane PMCP activity [85], suggesting a coordinated role of calbindin D28K and the PMCP in regulating transcellular calcium transport.

Regulation of Renal Calcium Reabsorption by PTH and Estrogen

One of the critical factors regulating renal calcium transport is estrogen [31]. Several studies have supported a role for estrogen in directly reducing renal calcium excretion [24,86]. These data have been supported [87]. Indeed the estrogen effect may be a prominent cause of the rise in PTH with aging [32]. It is of course quite clear that the first effect of estrogen replacement in postmenopausal women is to reduce bone resorption, which may result in secondary hyperparathyroidism if the bone resorption space is large enough. This will result in an increase in renal calcium reabsorption via increasing PTH in addition to the direct effect of estrogen deficiency on renal calcium reabsorption.

Effects of Salt on Calcium Balance

As described earlier, it is clear that sodium can compete with calcium for reabsorption in the proximal and distal tubules. The net result is that there is a strong association between sodium excretion and calcium excretion [88]. However, clinical investigations have revealed that only sodium chloride is associated with increased renal calcium excretion; the other sodium salts, bicarbonate or citrate, do not increase on renal calcium excretion [89,90]. In view of the fact that most sodium intake is associated with chloride, it is likely that the observed relationship between sodium and calcium excretion is in fact an effect of the combination of sodium and chloride.

In a 2-year prospective epidemiological study of the effects of sodium intake measured by 24-hr sodium excretion on bone mass in elderly postmenopausal women, the author was able to show a deleterious effect of sodium on the bone loss. In this study, a high sodium intake was associated with a greater degree of bone loss [91]. In these same patients a high calcium intake prevented bone loss and the interaction of the two factors predicted the change in bone mass better than either alone. The effects of salt on bone mass are probably mediated via effects on extracellular calcium homeostasis, whereby an increased salt intake induces calciuresis. If this reduction in extracellular calcium balance cannot be compensated adequately by increased gut calcium absorption stimulated by an increase in 1,25-dihydroxyvitamin D, then increased PTH-mediated bone resorption appears to take place [92]. In younger subjects, increases in 1,25-dihydroxyvitamin D [93] and therefore gut calcium absorption occur so that the effects on bone are likely to be much less.

Effects of Protein Intake and Acid Base Status on Renal Calcium Excretion

It is generally agreed that dietary protein intake increases renal calcium excretion [94,95]. The effect appears to be related to the excretion of fixed organic acid as a result of protein metabolism, with sulfur-containing amino acids in particular. Certainly the effect can be reversed by increasing alkali intake at the same time [95]. In addition the protein effect may increase the glomerular filtration rate. Whether the calcuretic effect of protein results in bone loss would depend on whether there was a compensatory increase in gut calcium absorption. Although an increase in protein from 44 to 102 g per day induced a negative calcium balance in younger subjects, the effect was not statistically significant. Furthermore, in this study the subject did not have time to adapt to the high protein intake.

These data should not be taken to indicate that an adequate protein intake of around 70 g per day is deleterious to the skeleton in aging. In the author's study of 65-year-old women consuming 78 g of protein per day, the milk powder supplement containing 1000 mg calcium and 30 g protein was as effective as a calcium supplement of 1000 mg [25]. Thus the extra protein was not deleterious. In population studies of the effects of dietary intake in renal calculi, there was no excess risk of intakes over 76 g per day compared to intakes under 42 g per day [96]. In old age there is evidence that a protein supplement will improve bone density and clinical outcomes after hip fracture [97]. Certainly there is a positive association between protein intake and IGF1 levels in postmenopausal women [53].

The effect of alkali in reducing renal calcium excretion is well described and has been attributed to effects on bone resorption [98,99] and renal calcium excretion [100]. The primary effect is uncertain and indeed both may be linked as a method of buffering excess food acid. It is certainly possible that part of the effectiveness of alkaline calcium supplements relates to the fact that they assist in buffering food acid, thereby reducing skeletal resorption.

CLINICAL DATA ON THE EFFECTIVENESS OF CALCIUM SUPPLEMENTATION

Data on the effectiveness of calcium are derived from a variety of sources. The most persuasive are the randomized controlled clinical trials of calcium supplementation with or without vitamin D, all of which show a reduction in fractures. Equally persuasive are the long-term calcium supplementation studies with bone density end points that show prevention or reduction in bone loss. There are also a large number of observational studies using both a case control and a cohort design. In general, these are usually negative. Indeed, a large cohort study showed that calcium supplement use was associated with an increase in fracture rate, not a decrease. Thus there is a significant discrepancy between clinical trial data and observational studies. Before exploring the reasons for this, the data will be reviewed.

Epidemiological Studies of Calcium Intake and Supplementation

A large number of case control and prospective cohort studies have examined the effect of dietary calcium and calcium supplements on fracture rates in women, with some data from men. Three case control studies out of 16 have shown a reduction in hip fracture rates with a high dietary calcium intake [101–103]. In the first, the effect was present only in the men [101]. In the second the effect was found at extremely low calcium intakes typical of eastern cultures and is consistent with the concept that extremely low calcium intakes are deleterious [102]. The most convincing study was undertaken in six southern European countries [104]. In this study, calcium intake was quantitated by asking about the number of glasses of milk consumed at various times of life. These data were combined into a score in which it was apparent that those scoring three or less, corresponding to a milk intake of less than 250 mg of calcium per day, throughout their life were at higher risk than the rest of the population [104]. Balanced against these three studies are 13 others in which there are no convincing data [105]. It may of course be that the estimation of calcium intake is too difficult to allow an evaluation of the effect on fracture risk. However, data on cohort studies are equally weak in showing an antifracture effect [105–111]. In these studies the calcium intake was measured using food frequency or recall methods. In only one was a reduction in fracture rate noted with a high calcium intake [106]. In two studies, calcium intake was estimated from tablet intake. In one [112], calcium tablets were associated with an increased risk of fracture. As indicated by the authors, it could be that patients at high risk of fracture took calcium tablets, thus confounding the analysis. It must also be recognized that the treatment was ineffective under the conditions of the study.

Clinical Trials of Calcium

Clinical trials of calcium supplementation are uniformly positive in showing a fracture effect. There are now four bone density studies lasting 3 to 4 years [49,113–115]. At the hip site there was no evidence of bone loss in calcium-supplemented subjects compared to controls who lost bone at this site [49,113–115]. At the spine there was no loss in the control group in any study, presumably due to degenerative changes. In the three studies that measured total body bone density, there was no loss in calcium-supplemented subjects in two. In all studies, calcium induced a significant reduction in bone loss at all sites [49,113–115]. These data strongly support the previously reported shorter-term studies showing a reduction in bone loss with calcium supplements [33]. Thus the effect of calcium supplementation is not merely a manifestation of a temporary remodeling transient effect but rather a fundamental modification of the bone loss of aging, indicating that in large part the bone loss of aging is due to a negative calcium balance. In these trials the calcium supplement was given once or twice a day in doses of 500 to 600 mg of calcium, usually as a calcium tablet.

Randomized, controlled trials of calcium supplementation with a fracture end point support this conclusion [113,114,116–118]. These show that calcium supplementation with or without vitamin D reduce fracture rates. It must be accepted that several of these studies are rather small with wide confidence intervals on the size of the treatment effect. Nevertheless, data are very suggestive of a beneficial effect of increased calcium intake.

The question of why there is a big discrepancy between epidemiologic data and randomized, controlled data is interesting. It raises the possibility that the population studies made type two errors because the method of measuring the calcium intake was inaccurate. As indicated earlier, in the presence of a reduction in the efficiency of gut calcium absorption, coupled with the increase in renal calcium excretion, it is important to consume calcium supplements that induce a transient high concentration of calcium within the gut. This allows passive calcium absorption to occur most effectively with a reduced dependence on gut wall factors.

Nonskeletal Effects of Calcium Supplementation

In general, very few side effects have been recognized with calcium supplementation. The principal problem with calcium tablets is that they may induce constipation in some subjects, although the size of the problem has not been documented carefully. Another possible problem is that of renal calculi. The risk of renal calculi in postmenopausal women is around 1 case in a 1000 women, which is similar to premenopausal rates. However, epidemiologic studies have suggested a reduction in risk of renal stone in women with increasing calcium intake from dietary sources, principally milk. Under these circumstances, the relative risk of calcium intakes over 1098 mg per day compared to less than 488 mg per day was 0.65 (0.50–0.83) [96]. However, calcium tablet consumption was associated with an increased relative risk of 1.2 (1.02–1.41), although this may be ameliorated if the supplement is taken with food. Clearly the low actual rate of renal stones and the small increase in relative risk do not suggest that the majority of women should avoid using calcium tablets to prevent osteoporotic fracture. The risks of renal calculi are also reduced in men who consume more than 605 mg calcium per day, principally as dairy products, as compared to those who consumed less than 605 mg per day [119]. Calcium tablets did not increase the risk in men.

Other potential deleterious effects of calcium supplementation relate to inhibitory effects of high calcium intakes on iron and zinc absorption [34,35,54]. Thus it may be important to evaluate iron and zinc status in calcium-supplemented individuals. In general, iron deficiency is not a major problem in men or in women after menopause.

In terms of impact on other diseases, an increased calcium intake appears to be beneficial. There is some evidence that a high calcium intake may reduce blood pressure [120–122] and may protect against bowel cancer [123–125].

Calcium as a Therapeutic Agent for Osteoporosis

From the information provided in this chapter it should be clear that a negative calcium balance is clearly the cause of age-related osteoporosis rather than a consequence of a specific bone disorder. This is not to say that there is no abnormality within the bone but that the primary abnormality is a reduction in gut calcium absorption and an increase in renal calcium excretion, which together result in increased bone resorption during episodes of dietary calcium deprivation. Because of the osteoblast defect that occurs with aging, the bone lost during calcium deprivation is not replaced adequately during episodes of high calcium intake. In young individuals there is no osteoblast defect, and bone lost during low calcium intake episodes is replaced during episodes of high calcium intake.

Thus it is in elderly individuals that calcium supplementation is most critical. Discrepancies between clinical trial data and observational data, coupled with evidence that the aging bowel has a specific defect in active calcium transport, suggest that effective treatment is critically dependent on achieving high intraluminal calcium concentrations to allow high levels of passive calcium absorption to occur. This is best achieved with calcium tablets, although milk is probably equally effective, provided it is consumed in large amounts. It is also important to undertake calcium supplementation on a regular basis as the duration of action of calcium to suppress PTH levels is limited.

On the basis of clinical trials and the theoretical considerations discussed earlier, the dose of calcium required to achieve bone balance is around 1000 mg of calcium per day in addition to the normal dietary calcium intake, which may be as low as 500 mg. The precise formulation of the calcium supplement is relatively unimportant, providing the absorbed fraction of the dose is over 20%. This requirement is met by most calcium supplements. As a result of these considerations, dietary calcium supplementation with tablets should be the first step in the therapy of age-related osteoporosis.

References

1. Johnston, C. C., Miller, J. Z., Slemenda, C. W., Reister, T. K., Hui, S., Christian, J. C., and Peacock, M. Calcium supplementation and increases in bone mineral density in children. *N. Engl. J. Med.* **327,** 82–87 (1992).
2. Kanders, B., Dempster, D. W., and Lindsay, R. Interaction of calcium nutrition and physical activity on bone mass in young women. *J. Bone Miner. Res.* **3,** 145–149 (1988).
3. Hannan, M. T., Tucker, K., Dawson-Hughes, B., Felson, D. T., and Kiel, D. P. Effect of dietary protein on bone loss in elderly men and women: the Framingham Osteoporosis Study. *J. Bone Miner. Res.* 12S1–S194 (1997).
4. Charles, P., Eriksen, E. F., Hasling, C., Sendergard, K., and Mosekilde, L. Dermal, intestinal, and renal obligatory losses of calcium: relation to skeletal calcium loss. *Am. J. Clin. Nutr.* **54,** 266S–273S (1991).
5. Prince, R. L. Counterpoint: Estrogen effects on calcitropic hormones and calcium homeostasis. *Endocr. Rev.* **15,** 301–309 (1994).
6. Borke, J. L., Eriksen, E. F., Minami, J., Keeting, P., Mann, K. G., Penniston, J. T., Riggs, B., and Kumar, R. Epitopes of the human erythrocyte Ca2+ -Mg2+ ATPase pump in human osteoblast-like cell plasma membranes. *J. Clin. Endocrinol. Metab.* **67,** 1299–1304 (1988).
7. Borke, J. L., Caride, A., Verma, A. K., Penniston, J. T., and Kumar, R. Plasma membrane calcium pump and 28-kDa calcium binding protein in cells of rat kidney distal tubules. *Am. J. Physiol.* **257,** F842–F849 (1989).
8. Armbrecht, H. J., Boltz, M. A., and Wongsurawat, N. Expression of plasma membrane calcium pump mRNA in rat intestine effect of age and 1,25-dihydroxyvitamin D. *Biochim. Biophys. Acta* **1195,** 110–114 (1994).
9. Bouhtiauy, I., LaJeunesse, D., and Brunette, M. G. The mechanism of parathyroid hormone action on calcium reabsorption by the distal tube. *Endocrinology* **128,** 251–258 (1991).
10. Feher, J. J. Facilitated calcium diffusion by intestinal calcium-binding protein. *Am. J. Physiol.* **244,** C303–C307 (1983).
11. Carafoli, E. The calcium pumping ATPase of the plasma membrane. *Annu. Rev. Physiol.* **53,** 531–547 (1991).
12. Dominguez, J. H., Juhaszovam, M., and Feister, H. A. The renal sodium-calcium exchanger. *J. Lab. Clin. Med.* **119,** 640–649 (1992).
13. White, K. E., Gesek, F. A., and Friedman, P. A. Na+/Ca2+ exchange in rat osteoblast-like UMR 106 cells. *J. Bone Miner. Res.* **11,** 1666–1675 (1996).
14. Lundgren, T., and Linde, A. Calcium ion transport kinetics during dentinogenesis: effects of disrupting odontoblast cellular transport systems. *Bone Miner.* **19,** 31–44 (1992).
15. Gallagher, J. C., Riggs, B. L., Eisman, J., Hamstra, A., Arnaud, S. B., and DeLuca, H. F. Intestinal calcium absorption and serum vitamin D metabolites in normal subjects and osteoporotic patients. *J. Clin. Invest.* **64,** 729–736 (1979).
16. Morris, H. A., Need, A. G., Horowitz, M., O'Loughlin, P. D., and Nordin, B. E. C. Calcium absorption in normal and osteoporotic postmenopausal women. *Calcif. Tissue Int.* **49,** 240–243 (1991).
17. Heaney, R. P., Recker, R. R., Stegman, M. R., and Moy, A. J. Calcium absorption in women: Relationships to calcium intake, estrogen status, and age. *J. Bone Miner. Res.* **4,** 469–475 (1989).
18. Devine, A., Prince, R. L., Kerr, D. A., Dick, I. M., Kent, G. N., Price, R. I., and Garcia Webb, P. Determinants of intestinal calcium absorption in women ten years past the menopause. *Calcif. Tissue Int.* **52,** 358–360 (1993).
19. Prince, R. L., Dick, I. M., Devine, A., Price, R. I., Gutteridge, D. H., Kerr, D., Criddle, A., Garcia-Webb, P., and St. John, A. The effects of menopause and age on calcitropic hormones: a cross sectional study of 655 healthy women aged 35 to 90. *J. Bone Miner. Res.* **10,** 835–842 (1995).
20. Prince, R. L., Dick, I., Garcia-Webb, P., and Retallack, R. W. The effects of the menopause on calcitriol and parathyroid hormone: Responses to a low dietary calcium stress test. *J. Clin. Endocrinol. Metab.* **70,** 1119–1123 (1990).
21. Dick, I. M., and Prince, R. L. Transdermal estrogen replacement does not increase calcitonin secretory reserve in postmenopausal women. *Acta Endocrinol. (Copenh)* **125,** 241–245 (1991).
22. Prince, R. L., Dick, I., Devine, A., Kerr, D., Criddle, R. A., Price, R., and Garcia Webb, P. Importance of bone resorption in the determination of bone density in women more than 10 years past the menopause. *J. Bone Miner. Res.* **8,**(11), 1273–1279 (1993).
23. Horowitz, M., Need, A. G., Philcox, J. C., and Nordin, B. E. C. Effect of calcium supplementation on urinary hydroxyproline in osteoporotic postmenopausal women. *Am. J. Clin. Nutr.* **3a,** 857–859 (1984).
24. Prince, R. L., Smith, M., Dick, I. M., Price, R. I., Garcia Webb, P., Henderson, N. K., and Harris, M. M. Prevention of postmenopausal osteoporosis: A comparative study of exercise, calcium supplementation, and hormone-replacement therapy. *N. Engl. J. Med.* **325,** 1189–1195 (1991).
25. Prince, R. L., Devine, A., Dick, I., Criddle, R. A., Kerr, D., Kent, N., Price, R., and Randell, A. The effects of calcium supplementation (milk powder or tablets) and exercise on bone density in postmenopausal women. *J. Bone Miner. Res.* **10,** 1068–1075 (1995).
26. St. John, A., Thomas, M. B., Davies, C. P., Mullan, B., Dick, I., Hutchison, B., van der Schaff, A., and Prince, R. L. Determinants of intact parathyroid hormone and free 1,25-dihydroxyvitamin D levels in mild and moderate renal failure. *Nephron* **61,** 422–427 (1992).
27. Prince, R. L., Hutchison, B. G., Kent, J. C., Kent, G. N., and Retallack, R. W. Calcitriol deficiency with retained synthetic reserve in chronic renal failure. *Kidney Int.* **33,** 1–7 (1988).
28. Krall, E. A., Sahyoun, N., Tannenbaum, S., Dallal, G. E., and Dawson-Hughes, B. Effect of vitamin D intake on seasonal variations in parathyroid hormone secretion in postmenopausal women. *N. Engl. J. Med.* **321,** 1777–1783 (1989).
29. Dawson-Hughes, B., Dallal, G. E., Krall, E. A., Harris, S., Sokoll, L. J., and Falconer, G. Effect of vitamin D supplementation on wintertime and overall bone loss in healthy postmenopausal women. *Ann. Intern. Med.* **115,** 505–512 (1991).
30. Adams, J. S., Clemens, T. L., Parrish, J. A., and Holick, M. F. Vitamin-D synthesis and metabolism after ultra violet irradiation of normal and vitamin-D-deficient subjects. *N. Engl. J. Med.* **306,** 722–725 (1982).
31. Prince, R. L. Counterpoint: Estrogen effects on calcitropic hormones and calcium homeostasis. *Endocr. Rev.* **15**(3), 301–309 (1994).
32. McKane, W. R., Khosla, S., Risteli, J., Robins, S. P., Muhs, J. M., and Riggs, B. L. Role of estrogen deficiency in pathogenesis of secondary hyperparathyroidism and increased bone resorption in elderly women. *Proc. Assoc. Am. Phys.* **109,** 174–180 (1997).
33. Nordin, B. E. C. Calcium and osteoporosis. *Nutrition* **13,** 664–686 (1997).
34. Wood, R. J., and Zheng, J. J. High dietary calcium intakes reduce zinc absorption and balance in humans. *Am. J. Clin. Nutr.* **65,** 1803–1809 (1997).

35. Reddy, M. B., and Cook, J. D. Effect of calcium intake on nonheme-iron absorption from a complete diet. *Am. J. Clin. Nutr.* **65,** 1820–1825 (1997).
36. Sheikh, M. S., Schiller, L. R., and Fordtran, J. S. In vivo intestinal absorption of calcium in humans. *Miner. Electrolyte Metab.* **16,** 130–146 (1990).
37. Heaney, R. P. Nutrient effects: Discrepancy between data from controlled trials and observational studies. *Bone* **21**(6), 469–471 (1997).
38. Dawson-Hughes, B., Dallal, G. E., Krall, E. A., Sadowski, L., Sahyoun, N., and Tannenbaum, S. A controlled trial of the effect of calcium supplementation on bone density in postmenopausal women. *N. Engl. J. Med.* **323,** 878–883 (1990).
39. Kanis, J. A., and Passmore, R. Calcium supplementation of the diet-2. *Br. Med. J* **298,** 205–208 (1989).
40. Finkenstedt, G., Skrabal, F., Gasser, R. W., and Braunsteiner, H. Lactose absorption, milk consumption, and fasting blood glucose concentrations in women with idiopathic osteoporosis. *Br. Med. J.* **292,** 161–162 (1986).
41. Honkanen, R., Koger, H., Alhava, E., Tuppurainen, M., and Saarikoski, S. Lactose Intolerance Associated with Fractures of Weight-Bearing Bones in Finnish Women Aged 38–57 Years. *Bone* **21**(6), 473–477 (1997).
42. Cochet, B., Jung, A., Griessen, M., Bartholdi, P., Schaller, P., and Donath, A. Effects of lactose on intestinal calcium absorption in normal and lactase-deficient subjects. *Gastroenterology* **84,** 935–940 (1983).
43. Wisker, E., Nagel, R., Tanudjaja, T. K., and Feldheim, W. Calcium, magnesium, zinc, and iron balances in young women: effects of a low-phytate barley-fiber concentrate. *Am. J. Clin. Nutr.* **54,** 553–559 (1991).
44. Harvey, J. A., Zobitz, M. M., and Pak, C. Y. C. Dose dependency of calcium absorption: a comparison of calcium carbonate and calcium citrate. *J. Bone Miner. Res.* **3,** 253–258 (1988).
45. Sheikh, M. S., Santa Ana, C. A., Nicar, M. J., Schiller, L. R., and Fordtran, J. S. Gastrointestinal absorption of calcium from milk and calcium salts. *N. Engl. J. Med.* **317,** 532–536 (1987).
46. Sheikh, M. S., and Fordtran, J. S. Calcium Bioavailability from two calcium carbonate preparations. *N. Engl. J. Med.* **323,** 921 (1991).
47. Whiting, S. J., and Pluhator, M. M. Comparison of in vitro and in vivo tests for determination of availability of calcium from calcium carbonate tablets. *J. Am. Coll. Nutr.* **11,** 553–560 (1992).
48. Recker, R. R. Calcium absorption and achlorhydria. *N. Engl. J. Med.* **313,** 70–73 (1985).
49. Devine, A., Dick, I. M., Heal, S. J., Criddle, R. A., and Prince, R. L. A 4-year follow up study of calcium supplementation on bone density in elderly postmenopausal women. *Osteopor. Int.* **7,** 23–28 (1997).
50. Heaney, R. P., Recker, R., and Weaver, C. M. Absorbability of calcium sources: The limited role of solubility. *Calcif. Tissue Int.* **46,** 300–304 (1990).
51. Devine, A., Prince, R. L., and Bell, R. Nutritional effect of calcium supplementation by skim milk powder or calcium tablets on total nutrient intake in postmenopausal women. *Am. J. Clin. Nutr.* **64,** 731–737 (1996).
52. Devine, A., Prince, R. L., and Bell, R. R. Nutrient intake of postmenopausal women in relation to skeletal and cardiovascular disease. *Aust. J. Nutr. Diet.* **53,** 144–150 (1996).
53. Devine, A., Rosen, C., Mohan, S., Baylink, D., and Prince, R. Effects of zinc and other nutritional factors on IFG1 and IGF1 binding proteins in postmenopausal women. *Am. J. Clin. Nutr.* in press.
54. Preziosi, P., Hercberg, S., Galan, P., Devanlay, M., Cherouvier, F., and Dupin, H. Iron Status of a Healthy French Population: Factors Determining Biochemical Markers. *Ann. Nutr. Metab.* **38,** 192–202 (1994).
55. Boyle, I. T., Omdahl, J. L., Gray, R. W., and DeLuca, H. F. The response of intestinal calcium transport to 25-hydroxy and 1,25-dihydroxyvitamin D in nephrectomized rats. *Endocrinology* **90,** 605–608 (1972).
56. Karbach, U. Paracellular calcium transport across the small intestine. *J. Nutr.* **122,** 641–643 (1992).
57. Hildmann, B., Schmidt, A., and Murer, H. Ca++ transport across basal-lateral membranes from rat small intestinal epithelial cells. *J. Membr. Biol.* **65,** 55–62 (1982).
58. Kikuchi, K., Kikuchi, T., and Ghisan, F. K. Characterization of calcium transport by basolateral membrane vesicles of human small intestine. *Am. J. Physiol.* **255,** G482–G489 (1988).
59. James, P., Vorherr, T., Thulin, E., Forsen, S., and Carafoli, E. Identification and primary structure of a calbindin 9K binding domain in the plasma membrane Ca2+ pump. *FEBS Lett.* **278,** 155–159 (1991).
60. Nemere, I., and Norman, A. W. Transcaltachia, vesicular calcium transport and microtubule-associated calbindin D28k: Emerging views of 1,25-dihydroxyvitamin D3-mediated intestinal calcium absorption. *Minerl. Electrolyte MEtab. Miner. Electrolyte Metab.* **16,** 109–114 (1990).
61. Nemere, I. Vesicular calcium transport in chick intestine. *J. Nutr.* **122,** 657–661 (1992).
62. Webb, A. R., Kline, L., and Holick, M. F. Influence of season and latitude on the cutaneous synthesis of Vitamin D3: Exposure to winter sunlight in Boston and Edmonton will not promote Vitamin D3 synthesis in human skin. *J. Clin. Endocrinol. Metab.* **67,** 373 (1988).
63. Eastell, R., Yergey, A. L., Vieira, N. E., Cedel, S. L., Kumar, R., and Riggs, B. L. Interrelationship among Vitamin D metabolism, true calcium absorption, parathyroid function, and age in women: Evidence of an age-related intestinal resistance to 1,25-dihydroxyvitamin D action. *J. Bone Miner. Res.* **6,** 125–132 (1991).
64. Fraser, D. R., and Kodicek, E. Unique biosynthesis by kidney of a biologically active vitamin D metabolite. *Nature* **228,** 764–766 (1970).
65. Eisman, J. A., and DeLuca, H. F. Intestinal 1,25-dihydroxyvitamin D3 binding protein:specificity of binding. *Steroids* **30,** 245–257 (1977).
66. Prince, R. L., Hutchison, B. G., and Dick, I. The regulation of calcitriol by parathyroid hormone and absorbed dietary phosphorus in subjects with moderate chronic renal failure. *Metabolism* **42,** 834–838 (1993).
67. Prince, R. L., Dick, I. M., Lemmon, J., and Randell, D. The pathogenesis of age-related osteoporotic fracture: effects of dietary calcium deprivation. *J. Clin. Endocrinol. Metab.* **82,** 260–264 (1997).
68. Ebeling, P. R., Sandgren, M. E., DiMagno, E. P., Lane, A. W., DeLuca, H. F., and Riggs, B. L. Evidence of an age-related decrease in intestinal responsiveness to vitamin D: Relationship between serum 1,25-Dihydroxyvitamin D3 and intestinal vitamin D receptor concentrations in normal women. *J. Clin. Endocrinol. Metab.* **75,** 176–182 (1992).
69. Bikle, D. D., Gee, E., Halloran, B., Kowalski, M. A., Ryzen, E., and Haddad, J. G. Assessment of the free fraction of 25-hydroxyvitamin D in serum and its regulation by albumin and the vitamin D-binding protein. *J. Clin. Endocrinol. Metab.* **63,** 954–959 (1986).
70. Heaney, R. P., Barger-Lux, J., Dowell, M. S., Chen, T. C., and Holick, M. F. Calcium absorptive effects of vitamin D and its

major metabolites. *J. Clin. Endocrinol. Metab.* **82,** 4111–4116 (1997).

71. Ooms, M. E., Roos, J. C., Bezemer, P. D., Vijgh, W. J. F. V. D., Bouter, L. M., and Lips, P. Prevention of bone loss by vitamin D supplementation in elderly women: a randomized double-blind trial. *J. Clin. Endocrinol. Metab.* **80,** 1052–1058 (1995).
72. Lips, P., Graafmans, W. C., Ooms, M. E., Bezemer, P. D., and Bouter, L. M. Vitamin D supplementation and fracture incidence in elderly persons. *Ann. Intern. Med.* **124,** 400–406 (1996).
73. Sheikh, M. S., Ramirez, A., and Emmett, M. Role of vitamin D-dependent and vitamin D-independent mechanisms in absorption of food calcium. *J. Clin. Invest.* **81,** 126–132 (1988).
74. Tellez, M., Reeve, J., Royston, J. P., Veall, N., and Wootton, R. The reproducibility of double-isotope deconvolution measurements of intestinal calcium absorption. *Clin. Sci.* **59,** 169–172 (1980).
75. DeGrazia, J. A., Ivanovich, P., Fellows, H., and Rich, C. A double isotope method for measurement of intestinal absorption of calcium in man. *J. Lab. Clin. Med.* **66,** 822–829 (1965).
76. Gennari, C., Agnusdei, D., Nardi, P., and Civitelli, R. Estrogen preserves a normal intestinal responsiveness to 1,25-dihydroxyvitamin D3 in oophorectomized women. *J. Clin. Endocrinol. Metab.* **71,** 1288–1293 (1990).
77. Suki, W. N. Calcium transport in the nephron. *Am. J. Physiol.* **237,** F1–F6 (1979).
78. Aida, K., Koishi, S., Tawata, M., and Onaya, T. Molecular cloning of a putative Ca2+ sensing receptor cDNA from human kidney. *Biochem. Biophys. Res. Commun.* **214,** 524–529 (1995).
79. Riccardi, D., Park, J., Lee, W. S., Gamba, G., Brown, E. M., and Hebert, S. C. Cloning and functional expression of a rat kidney extracellular calcium/polyvalent cation-sensing receptor. *Proc. Natl. Acad. Sci. USA* **92,** 131–135 (1995).
80. Hebert, S. C., Brown, E. M., and Harris, H. W. Role of the Ca2+ sensing receptor in divalent mineral ion homeostasis. *J. Exp. Biol.* **200,** 295–302 (1997).
81. Costanzo, L., and Windhager, E. Calcium and sodium transport by the distal convoluted tubule in the rat. *Am. J. Physiol.* **235,** F492–F506 (1978).
82. Tsukamoto, Y., Saka, S., and Saitoh, M. Parathyroid hormone stimulates ATP-dependent calcium pump activity by a different mode in proximal and distal tubules of the rat. *Biochim. Biophys. Acta* **1103,** 163–171 (1991).
83. Borke, J. L., Minami, J., Verma, A., Penniston, J. T., and Kumar, R. Monoclonal antibodies to human erythrocyte membrane Ca2+-Mg2+ adenosine triphosphate pump recognize an epitope in the basolateral membrane of human kidney distal tubule cells. *J. Clin. Invest.* **80,** 1225–1231 (1987).
84. Borke, J. L., Minami, J., Verma, A. K., Penniston, J., and Kumar, R. Co-localization of erythrocyte Ca++-Mg++ ATPase and vitamin D-dependent 28-kDa-calcium binding protein. *Kidney Int.* **34,** 262–267 (1988).
85. Wasserman, R. H., Chandler, J. S., Meyer, S. A., Smith, C. A., Brindak, M. E., Fullmer, S. A., Penniston, J. T., and Kumar, R. Intestinal calcium transport and calcium extrusion processes at the basolateral membrane. *J. Nutr.* **122,** 662–671 (1992).
86. Nordin, B. E. C., Need, A. G., Morris, H. A., Horowitz, M., and Robertson, W. G. Evidence for a renal calcium leak in postmenopausal women. *J. Clin. Endocrinol. Metab.* **72,** 401–407 (1991).
87. McKane, W. R., Khosla, S., Burritt, M. F., Kao, P. C., Wilson, D. M., Ory, S. J., and Riggs, B. L. Mechanism of renal calcium conservation with estrogen replacement therapy in women in early menopause—a clinical research centre study. *J. Clin. Endocrinol. Metab.* **80,** 3458–3464 (1995).
88. Massey, L. K., and Whiting, S. J. Dietary salt, urinary calcium, and bone loss. *J. Bone Miner. Res.* **11,** 731–736 (1996).
89. Sakhaee, K., Nicar, M., Hill, K., and Pak, Y. C. Contrasting effects of potassium citrate and sodium citrate therapies on urinary chemistries and crystallization of stone-forming salts. *Kidney Int.* **24,** 348–352 (1983).
90. Lemann, J., Gray, R. W., and Pleuss, J. A. Potassium bicarbonate, but not sodium bicarbonate, reduces urinary calcium excretion and improves calcium balance in healthy men. *Kidney Int.* **35,** 688–695 (1989).
91. Devine, A., Criddle, R. A., Dick, I. M., Kerr, D. A., and Prince, R. L. A longitudinal study of the effect of sodium and calcium intakes on regional bone density in postmenopausal women. *Am. J. Clin. Nutr.* **62,** 740–745 (1995).
92. McParland, B. E., Goulding, A., and Campbell, A. J. Dietary salt affects biochemical markers of resorption and formation of bone in elderly women. *Br. Med. J.* **299,** 834–835 (1989).
93. Breslau, N. A., McGuire, J. L., Zerwekh, J. E., and Pak, C. Y. C. The role of dietary sodium on renal excretion and intestinal absorption of calcium and on Vitamin D metabolism. *J. Clin. Endocrinol. Metab.* **55,** 369–373 (1982).
94. Hegsted, M. S., Schuette, S. A., Zemel, M. B., and Linkswiler, H. M. Urinary calcium and calcium balance in young men as affected by level of protein and phosphorus intake. *J. Nutr.* **111,** 553–562 (1981).
95. Lutz, J. Calcium balance and acid-base status of women as affected by increased protein intake and by sodium bicarbonate ingestion. *Am. J. Clin. Nutr.* **39,** 281–288 (1984).
96. Curhan, G. C., Willett, W. C., Speizer, F. E., Spiegelman, D., and Stampfer, M. J. Comparison of dietary calcium with supplemental calcium and other nutrients as factors affecting the risk for kidney stones in women. *Ann. Intern. Med.* **126,** 497–504 (1997).
97. Schurch, M. A., Rizzoli, R., Slosman, D., Vadas, L., Vergnaud, P., and Bonjour, J. P. Protein supplements increase serum insulin-like growth factor-1 levels and attenuate femur bone loss in patients with recent hip fracture. *Ann. Intern. Med.* **128,** 801–809 (1998).
98. Lemann, J., Jr., Litzow, J. R., and Lennon, E. J. The effects of chronic acid loads in normal man: further evidence for the participation of bone mineral in the defence against chronic metabolic acidosis. *J. Clin. Invest.* **45,** 1608–1614 (1966).
99. Barzel, U. S. The skeleton as an ion exchange system: implications for the role of acid-base inbalance in the genesis of osteoporosis. *J. Bone Miner. Res.* **10**(10), 1431–1436 (1995).
100. Sutton, R., Wong, N., and Dirks, J. Effects of metabolic acidosis and alkalosis on sodium and calcium transport in the dog kidney. *Kidney Int.* **15,** 520–533 (1979).
101. Cooper, C., Barker, D. J. P., and Wickham, C. Physical activity, muscle strength, and calcium intake in fracture of the proximal femur in Britain. *Br. Med. J.* **297,** 1443–1446 (1988).
102. Lau, E., Donnan, S., Barker, D. J. P., and Cooper, C. Physical activity and calcium intake in fracture of the proximal femur in Hong Kong. *Br. Med. J.* **297,** 1441–1443 (1988).
103. Meyer, H. E., Henriksen, C., Falch, J. A., Pedersen, J. I., and Tverdal, A. Risk factors for hip fracture in a high incidence area: a case-control study from Oslo, Norway. *Osteopor. Int.* **5,** 239–246 (1995).
104. Johnell, O., Gullberg, B., Kanis, J. A., Allander, E., Elffors, L., Dequeker, J., Dilsen, G., Gennari, C., Vaz, A., Lyritis, G., Mazzuoli, G., Miravet, L., Passeri, M., Cano, R. P., Rapado, A., and Ribot, C. Risk factors of hip fracture in european women: the MEDOS study. *J. Bone Miner. Res.* **10,** 1802–1815 (1995).
105. Cumming, R. G., and Nevitt, M. C. Calcium for the prevention of osteoporotic fractures in postmenopausal women. *J. Bone Miner. Res.* **12,** 1321–1329 (1997).

106. Holbrook, T. L., Barrett-Connor, E., and Wingard, D. L. Dietary calcium and risk of hip fracture: 14 year prospective population study. *Lancet* **2,** 1046–1049 (1988).
107. Wickham, C. A. C., Walsh, K., Cooper, C., Barker, D. J. P., Margetts, B. M., Morris, J., and Bruce, S. A. Dietary calcium, physical activity, and risk of hip fracture: a prospective study. *Br. Med. J.* **299,** 889–892 (1989).
108. Kelsey, J. L., Browner, W. S., Seeley, D. G., Nevitt, M. C., and Cummings, S. R. Risk factors for fractures of the distal forearm and proximal humerus. *Am. J. Epidemiol.* **135,** 477–489 (1992).
109. Cummings, S. R., Nevitt, M. C., Browner, W. S., Stone, K., Fox, K. M., Ensrud, K. E., Cauley, J., Black, D., and Vogt, T. M. Risk factors for hip fracture in white women. *N. Engl. J. Med.* **332,** 767–773 (1995).
110. Looker, A. C., Harris, T. B., Madans, J. H., and Sempos, C. T. Dietary calcium and hip fracture risk: the NHANES I epidemiologic follow-up study. *Osteopor. Int.* **3,** 177–184 (1993).
111. Meyer, H. E., Pedersen, J. I., Loken, E. B., and Tverdal, A. Dietary factors and the incidence of hip fractures in middle-aged Norwegians. *Am. J. Epidemiol.* **145,** 117–123 (1997).
112. Cumming, R. G., Cummings, S. R., Nevitt, M. C., Scott, J., Ensrud, K. E., Vogt, T. M., and Fox, K. Calcium intake and fracture risk: results from the study of osteoporotic fractures. *Am. J. Epidemiol.* **145,** 926–934 (1997).
113. Reid, I. R., Ames, R. W., Evans, M. C., Gamble, G. D., and Sharpe, S. J. Long-term effects of calcium supplementation on bone loss and fractures in postmenopausal women: a randomized controlled trial. *Am. J. Med.* **98,** 331–335 (1995).
114. Dawson-Hughes, B., Harris, S. S., Khall, E. A., and Dallal, G. E. Effect of calcium and vitamin D supplementation on bone density in men and women 65 years of age or older. *N. Engl. J. Med.* **337,** 670–676 (1997).
115. Riggs, B. L., O'Fallon, W. M., Muhs, J., O'Connor, M. K., Kumar, R., and Melton, L. J. Long-term effects of calcium supplementation on serum parathyroid hormone level, bone turnover, and bone loss in elderly women. *J. Bone Miner. Res.* **13,** 168–174 (1998).
116. Chevalley, T., Rizzoli, R., Nydegger, V., Slosman, D., Rapin, C. H., Michel, J. P., Vasey, H., and Bonjour, J.-P. Effects of calcium supplements on femoral bone mineral density and vertebral fracture rate in Vitamin-D-replete elderly patients. *Osteopor. Int.* **4,** 245–252 (1994).
117. Recker, R. R., Hinders, S., Davies, K. M., Heaney, R. P., Stegman, M. R., Lappe, J. M., and Kimmel, D. B. Correcting calcium nutritional deficiency prevents spine fractures in elderly women. *J. Bone Miner. Res.* **11,** 1961–1966 (1996).
118. Chapuy, M. C., Arlot, M. E., Delmas, P. D., and Meunier, P. J. Effect of calcium and cholecalciferol treatment for three years on hip fractures in elderly women. *Br. Med. J.* **308,** 1081–1082 (1994).
119. Curhan, G. C., Willett, W. C., Rimm, E. B., and Stampfer, M. J. A prospective study of dietary calcium and other nutrients and the risk of symptomatic kidney stones. *N. Engl. J. Med.* **328**(12), 833–838 (1993).
120. McCarron, D. A., Morris, C. D., Young, E., Roullet, C., and Drueke, T. Dietary calcium and blood pressure: modifying factors in specific populations. *Am. J. Clin. Nutr.* **54,** 215S–219S (1991).
121. St John, A., Dick, I., Hoad, K., Retallack, R., Welborn, T., and Prince, R. Relationship between calcitrophic hormones and blood pressure in elderly subjects. *Eur. J. Endocrinol.* **130,** 446–450 (1994).
122. Allender, P. S., Cutler, J. A., Follmann, D., Cappuccio, F. P., Pryer, J., and Elliott, P. Dietary calcium and blood pressure: a meta-analysis of randomized clinical trials. *Ann. Intern. Med.* **124,** 825–831 (1996).
123. Slattery, M. L., Sorenson, A. W., and Ford, M. H. Dietary calcium intake as a mitigating factor in colon cancer. *Am. J. Epidemiol.* **128,** 504–514 (1988).
124. Garland, C. F., Garland, F. C., and Gorham, E. D. Can colon cancer incidence and death rates be reduced with calcium and vitamin D? *Am. J. Clin. Nutr.* **54,** 193S–201S (1991).
125. Wargovich, M. J., Lynch, P. M., and Levin, B. Modulating effects of calcium in animal models of colon carcinogenesis and short-term studies in subjects at increased risk for colon cancer. *Am. J. Clin. Nutr.* **54,** 202S–205S (1991).

CHAPTER 41

Estrogen

ROBERT LINDSAY AND FELICIA COSMAN
Clinical Research Center, Helen Hayes Hospital, West Haverstraw, New York 10993

INTRODUCTION

It has been recognized for a long time that estrogens are important in the maintenance of skeletal homeostasis. In the early 1940s, Fuller Albright demonstrated that premenopausal ovariectomy was more common in the patients who presented with vertebral crush fracture syndrome [1]. In 1947 he demonstrated further the importance of estrogen intervention in correcting the abnormality in calcium balance seen in patients with osteoporosis [2]. Since then, the literature has substantiated the importance of estrogen status in regulating skeletal homeostasis throughout life, not only in women but possibly also in men. Estrogen intervention, either as estrogen replacement therapy or hormone replacement therapy (in combination with a progestin), has become the gold standard for prevention and treatment of osteoporosis in many countries.

The exact mechanism of action of estrogens on the skeleton is still not clear. Although it is known that osteoblasts and perhaps also osteoclasts have receptors for estrogen, other cells such as macrophages, fibroblasts, and other constituents of the bone marrow may also be targets in mediating the effects of estrogen on the skeleton [3]. Further, the signals that produce estrogen's effect in reducing the activation of remodeling and perhaps also in restoring the balance between formation and resorption within each remodeling cycle are not clear. A variety of local factors have been implicated, including insulin-like growth factors (IGFs), transforming growth factor β, and interleukins, particularly IL-1, IL-6, and IL-11, as well as prostaglandins [4]. The discovery of a second estrogen receptor, ERβ, has further complicated the issue [5]. Estrogens have also been shown to affect the skeleton indirectly by regulating parathyroid hormone (PTH) secretion and skeletal responsivity to PTH [6]. In addition, the realization that the effects of estrogen on bone can be separated from the effects of estrogen on the uterus with pharmacological agents (selective estrogen receptor modulators) adds to the complexity [7]. This chapter reviews our current understanding of the effects of estrogen on the skeleton throughout life.

ESTROGEN AND GROWTH

Before puberty, bone growth and skeletal mass are essentially identical in both sexes, except in the vertebrae [8]. One study has suggested that even prior to puberty, boys may have a greater vertebral cross-sectional area than girls [9]. The gender-associated difference in bone size is exaggerated during the prepubertal bone growth spurt [10]. The suggestion that the risk of vertebral fracture may be related to the cross-sectional area of the vertebral bodies provides an explanation, at least in part, for the difference in fracture incidence between men and women [11]. It is, however, around the time of puberty, particularly during the prepubertal growth spurt, when this sexual dimorphism becomes more evident [10]. The adolescent growth spurt results from the concerted action of a variety of factors, including growth hormone, IGFs, thyroid hormone, adrenal steroids, and sex steroids [12]. The growth spurt begins approximately 2 years earlier in girls than it does in boys, at around the age of 11, and is characterized by an 80% increase in the rate of linear growth. In boys, the rate of linear growth is slightly more but it does not begin until the age of 13. Eventually, linear growth ceases as the endocrine changes that occur initiate closure of the endochondral growth plates, with growth terminating about 2 years earlier in girls (average age, 15) than it does in boys (average age, 17). It is generally assumed that the growth spurt in boys is more intense than in girls. The growth spurt can account for most of the differences in body size superimposed on an average of 2 more years at the slower growth rate in males.

Changes in body size are accompanied by the development of a larger skeleton in boys than in girls [9,10].

During this adolescent phase, there is a gradual increase in the size of the skeleton, both by linear growth and also in long bone diameter [10]. There is a continued process of acquisition of cortical bone, often called skeletal consolidation, that continues into the third decade, whereas cancellous bone mass peaks during the teens [13].

The transient acceleration of growth during the growth spurt is accompanied by a transient increase in the risk of traumatic fracture in both girls and boys [14,15]. The most common site of occurrence is the distal forearm. Transient fragility may be related to the shifting of calcium within the skeleton as acquisition of new bone for linear growth exceeds the capacity to maintain a positive calcium balance [16].

The fact that estrogens are important for linear bone growth is suggested by the phenotypic expression of Turner syndrome (gonadal dysgenesis) with deletion of one X chromosome [17]. These adults have short stature with low bone mass [18]. In women without adequate gonadal activity or who lose their ovaries prior to the onset of puberty, a eunuchoid stature results with somewhat greater height but with low bone mass. The determinant of final skeletal mass and density is probably closely related to the genes that control body size, but there are significant influences of both nutrition and physical activity [19]. Estrogens also appear to be important in the control of body size and bone mass in men.

Of interest in this regard is a description of a male totally resistant to estrogen because of a mutation in the estrogen receptor gene in both alleles [20]. This individual had normal pubertal development and masculinization, but was tall and continued to grow after puberty with failure to close the epiphyses and low bone density and increased bone turnover. Studies in an osteoporotic young man (age 24) born with aromatase deficiency and an inability to convert androgens to estrogens also demonstrate the importance of estrogen in the developing male skeleton. Thus, even in males, estrogen action is important for bone maturation and mineralization.

PREMENOPAUSAL WOMEN

During adult premenopausal life, the process of bone remodeling, modulated by estrogen, maintains the youthful skeleton. There is some suggestion of variance in the rate of bone turnover across the menstrual cycle [21,21a], although not all data agree. Clearly, when estrogen is removed in the premenopausal population, there is evidence for increased bone turnover and bone loss [22]. Thus, in this setting of amenorrhea, bone mass is lost [23,24]. The same is true when GnRH agonists are used in the treatment of endometriosis [25]. In anorexia nervosa, estrogen deficiency is compounded by malnutrition [26–28]. In amenorrhea due to excessive exercise, the reduction in bone mass is somewhat lessened but not reversed by the beneficial effects of the exercise [29–37] (see Chapter 11).

Conflicting evidence suggests that increasing estrogen supply may provide a small positive benefit in terms of the skeleton in premenopausal women [38–41]. These data come mostly from cross-sectional studies of oral contraceptive use in premenopausal women, which suggest that ethinyl estradiol (25–35 mcg/day), in doses somewhat greater than the equivalent dose of 17β-estradiol, produced on a daily basis by the premenopausal ovary, is associated with a small but significant increase in bone mass. No controlled clinical trials of oral contraception have been performed, however, and not all studies have reported positive effects [42].

A good example of a premenopausal hyperestrogen state is pregnancy. Early data suggested that pregnancy was a protective factor for osteoporotic fractures [43,44]. Bone mass is certainly maintained during pregnancy, despite the demands of the fetus, probably due to changes in calcium homeostasis associated with pregnancy [45]. However, during lactation there are even greater demands for calcium and bone is lost, particularly in adolescent women and those with low calcium intake. In many situations, this a reversible phenomenon, especially if lactation is continued for less than an entire remodeling cycle (average 6–9 months) [46–50].

Some studies show that there is a gradual decline in bone mass in normal healthy premenopausal women, particularly in the hip during the 30s and 40s. It is more apparent, however, that bone loss begins at all skeletal sites prior to the overt appearance of menopause. This may be in part related to declining ovarian function. A study of Johnston *et al* [51] demonstrated that in perimenopausal women, endogenous estrogen supply was an important determinant of the rate of bone loss.

POSTMENOPAUSAL WOMEN

Loss of estrogen supplied by the ovary or its significant reduction as it occurs across the menopause is associated with an increase in the rate of bone remodeling and an absolute decrement in bone mass [51,52]. The change of remodeling that occurs is accounted for primarily by an increase in the activation of remodeling sites [52]. However, the increased remodeling rate per se would result only in a transient decline in bone mass, which should be completely reversible once the insult was removed. Therefore, an ongoing imbalance between the extent of bone resorption and formation is also required to explain persistent bone loss after menopause.

Support for an imbalance between bone resorption and formation was derived originally from studies of the kinetics of calcium transfer into and out of the skeleton [53,54]. These studies clearly demonstrate a negative calcium balance in postmenopausal women, as was noted originally by Fuller Albright, who also suggested that the negative calcium balance was more severe in patients who presented with osteoporotic fractures [1]. This imbalance could result from increased activity of the osteoclast population, resulting in greater bone resorption within each remodeling cycle, or, alternatively, a decline in the recruitment or activity of osteoblasts, resulting in incomplete replacement of the resorbed bone by osteoid and its subsequent mineralization. Although it has never been absolutely determined which mechanism contributes more, data are more suggestive of an increase in osteoclast activity. The more recent evaluation of biochemical markers of bone turnover across menopause and in postmenopausal women suggests that the net increments in total resorption are greater than those seen in formation [55,56]. While this is clearly only indirect evidence, it is certainly suggestive of increased resorptive activity. In addition to imbalance within each remodeling unit, the fact that there is an increased likelihood, within cancellous bone, of complete penetration of trabeculae by remodeling units active on each side of the trabeculae would lead to a stochastically greater chance of loss of the template on which to lay down new bone [57]. This would result in bone formation being unable to follow bone resorption as is the case under normal situations of remodeling. The consequence would be accelerated loss of bone.

As noted earlier, the mechanisms by which estrogen acts on the skeleton are inadequately understood. Consequently, the mechanisms by which estrogen deficiency results in increased bone remodeling and absolute loss of bone mass are also poorly understood. In rodent models, increased IL-6 appears to be a mediator of the effects of estrogen deficiency [58]. In the human model, it has been suggested that increased production of interleukin-1 is the major mediator [59,60]. Prostaglandin E_2 (PGE_2) has also been implicated in rodent models of bone loss [61]. Not all of these agents have been implicated in bone loss in humans. In addition, the mechanisms involved in mediating the changes in resorption and formation clearly occur at the individual cellular level and are also inadequately understood [62]. Possibilities include an increase in the recruitment or activity of osteoclasts or an increase in the longevity of the osteoclast population. In addition, a decline in bone formation may be related to either reductions in osteoblast recruitment or an increase in programmed cell death (apoptosis). These changes could all be mediated directly by effects of estradiol on osteoblasts or, alternatively, by the effects of estradiol on other cell populations, such as the monocyte precursors of osteoclasts, or even more indirectly by effects on the lymphocyte population or other marrow constituents [63].

The consequence of estrogen deficiency, whatever the mechanisms turn out to be, is bone loss. With continued bone loss in the postmenopausal population, the risk of fracture increases [64]. There is a direct relationship between increased fracture risk and decline in bone mass. This is due, at least in part, to architectural changes that accompany the alterations in cancellous bone. When trabecular plates of bone are eroded gradually, complete trabecular units can be lost or replaced by thin-looking flat fibrils or rods of bone [57]. At the same time, endocortical erosion results in what is sometimes called trabecularization of the cortex with resultant thinning of the cortex. Enhanced periosteal bone formation only partially offsets this erosive effect. A relatively modest change in bone mass or a density of approximately 10–12% over the first 5 postmenopausal years may produce a doubling in the risk of osteoporotic fracture.

While a reduction in secretion of estradiol by the ovary is the major endocrine change that occurs at menopause, it is by no means the only change [65,66]. Reductions in progesterone and androgens also occur. Androgens, particularly testosterone, are produced not only by the premenopausal ovary but also, in some individuals, by the postmenopausal ovary. Circulating testosterone levels fall by 25–50% across menopause. Additionally, the adrenal steroid androstenedione, which then becomes the prevalent postmenopausal androgen, is converted to estrone, a process that appears to occur principally in adipose tissue. Thus estrone becomes the principal estrogen in postmenopausal women [67,68], while the principal circulating estrogen in premenopausal women is estradiol. It is likely that the early changes in postmenopausal skeletal remodeling are influenced by these changes in estrogen status [69–73]. Other factors clearly modulate the change in estrogen amount and form on skeletal remodeling, such as the remaining hormonal milieu, [69]. Although the first 5 to 10 years following menopause, appear to reflect most dynamically the state of estrogen deficiency on skeletal remodeling, newer data indicate an influence of estrogen deficiency through-out the postmenopausal years. Superimposed on these changes in sex steroid production are the effects of nutrition and life-style, all of which modulate the effects of the remaining estradiol supply on skeletal remodeling [74].

The site of greatest bone loss in the early postmenopausal years is cancellous bone [75]. This is probably related to the greater surface area available at cancellous sites. With advancing years and loss of more cancellous bone, the continuing effects of estrogen deficiency become more evident at cortical sites [76]. In addition, as individuals age, other factors that are detrimental to bone health become more important, such as declining renal function, declining intestinal efficiency for calcium absorption, reductions in the dermal substrate of Vitamin D, 7-dehydrocholesterol, declining calcium intake, and reduced physical activity [77]. Finally, changes in the sex hormone-binding globulin level, with age can influence effects of the sex steroids on skeletal turnover [79,80].

ESTROGEN REPLACEMENT

Intervention with either estrogen replacement therapy or combined hormone replacement therapy reduces bone turnover and prevents bone loss after menopause [81–108]. Early studies involved evaluation of bone density measured in peripheral bone using single energy X-ray absorptiometry or radiographic changes in radius or metacarpals. More recent studies have evaluated changes in the spine and hip, as well as in total body bone mass. The majority of the studies conducted have been 1 or 2 years in duration and only very few long-term studies have been performed.

In short-term studies, it is clear that estrogens reduce bone turnover, as evidenced by the reduction of biochemical markers of bone remodeling, within 3–6 months from elevated levels more compatible with the premenopausal or estrogen-replete status. These changes, which are assumed to be the converse of the changes that occur across menopause, are indications that bone remodeling has been reduced and perhaps also that the balance between formation and resorption within each remodeling cycle has also been restored. In the majority of studies, especially those in which measurements of the spine are made, there is a transient increase in bone density that varies from 4 to 8% over the course of the first 1–2 years with no major changes in bone density thereafter. A similar pattern of change occurs in the hip, although the increment is quantitatively less, usually being on the order of 2–3%. It has been assumed that the differences in the increase in bone mass between those sites is related to the representation of cancellous bone at each site. The greater the amount of cancellous bone that is present, the greater the increment in bone mass that is seen. This is presumed to be related to the greater surface area of cancellous bone and therefore the greater the magnitude of the effect in terms of reduction of activation frequency that would be seen when this is modified with antiresorptive therapy, such as estrogens.

Measurements of peripheral bone show even smaller effects, with many studies demonstrating the stability of bone mass but no substantial increases. In an early study of the effects of estrogen on bone performed by our group, we demonstrated stability of bone density in the third metacarpal of the right hand measured by single photon absorptiometry. In this case, administration of the three methyl ether of ethinyl estradiol (mestranol) at an average dose of about 24 mcg/day produced long-term maintenance of bone mass at the metacarpal skeletal site. This investigation also demonstrated that, at least in terms of bone density, the earlier that intervention occurred, the better the outcome. It also showed that estrogens could prevent further bone loss even when started well after menopause. Cross-sectional evaluation of the data 10 years after initiation of the study revealed similar protective effects of this estrogen at this dose on bone mass in the spine and the hip [101]. After 10 years of estrogen therapy, bone mass in the spine was 18% higher in the mestranol group than in the placebo population and bone mass in the hip was 13% higher. In another long-term study conducted in the United States, conjugated equine estrogens given at the high dose of 2.5 mg/day prevented bone loss in the radius over a 10-year period [90]. Thus, it is clear that long-term estrogens prevent bone loss, at least in the radius or metacarpal and probably also in the spine and in the hip.

Controlled clinical trials in which vertebral bone mass was formally measured using either dual photon absorptiometry or computed tomography have demonstrated the prevention of vertebral bone loss. Almost all of those studies are of no more than 1–2 years in duration. In all of those studies, the estrogen group performed significantly better than the placebo control group, although the outcome in terms of either gain or stability of bone mass was somewhat variable. The same is true with bone mass measurement on the hip where dual photon absorptiometry or, more recently, dual x-ray absorptiometry are the only available techniques. The largest controlled clinical trial of estrogen intervention in early postmenopause, the progestin/estrogen prevention intervention study, confirmed an increase of 5% over 3 years in the spine and an increase of 3% in the femoral neck over the same time period [105].

The long-term effects of estrogen and bone mass in the spine and hip, i.e., effects over 10 years of therapy, have to be gleaned from either cross-sectional data, as noted earlier, or from observational data [109]. No controlled clinical trials have evaluated bone density over this period of time with hormone replacement therapy intervention. It has been suggested from some studies that after long-term therapy with standard doses of hormone replacement therapy (HRT) or estrogen replacement therapy (ERT), bone loss may begin again in the femoral neck. It is not clear whether the bone loss that is occurring is slower than would be expected or is compatible with a similar rate in untreated individuals. In the control arm of a study of parathyroid hormone treatment performed by our group in which bone density was measured in the spine and the hip, patients on hormone replacement therapy alone showed only very modest insignificant bone loss over a 4-year period in the hip and no evidence of bone loss in the spine (femoral bone mass fell by approximately 1% over the 4-year period) [110].

Comparatively few studies have evaluated the minimum effective dose of estrogen in the prevention of bone loss either in the spine or in the hip. In the early studies, measurements were again mostly made on peripheral bone. In the one study conducted with several doses of conjugated equine estrogens, a modest effect was seen at 0.3 mg/day and a maximum effect at 0.625 mg/day with no additive effects seen by increasing the dose to 1.25 mg/day [89]. In a study performed at approximately the same time, similar results on the radius were found, but measurements of the spine by computed tomography suggested that there was no effect until 0.625 mg and that the maximum effect was also seen at that dose [111]. It is notable that in one of those studies, calcium supplementation was not used and the average intake of calcium was close to the current known average intake in the United States of 500–600 mg/day.

Controlled clinical trials to evaluate the minimum effective dose of esterified estrogen recently completed in the United States suggest that the 0.3-mg/day dose may be somewhat more effective than previous reports and that the average change, while still less than that seen with higher doses, is compatible with the preservation of bone mass in most individuals [107]. Again, it is worth nothing that in that study, calcium supplementation was given along with estrogen and may have had a significant impact on the outcome.

As far as can be ascertained from data available, the route of administration for estrogens appears not to influence its effect on the skeleton. Data are available using percutaneous estrogen, transcutaneous estrogen, transdermal estrogen, and estrogens delivered by vaginal ring [94,106,112–114]. In all situations, if adequate amounts of estrogen are given, reductions in bone turnover are seen and preservation of bone mass occurs. With transdermal estrogen, it is easier to determine the circulating levels of estrogen that might be effective. Estradiol levels of between 40 and 80 pg/ml appear to be needed to preserve bone mass. Because it is impossible to measure all estrogen components in oral estrogen delivery, it is not known whether similar circulating levels of estradiol or equivalent would be required when oral therapy is used.

The addition of a progestin, at least the progestins normally used in the United States, has little influence on the dominant effect of estrogen on the skeleton [105]. Medroxyprogesterone acetate added as 5 mg cyclically or 2.5 mg continuously had no effect on the skeletal outcome in the progestin estrogen prevention intervention study. Micronized progesterone at a dose of 200 mg/day given cyclically also had no effect. It has been suggested that the 19 nortestosterone derivatives, particularly norethindrone acetate (1 mg), may enhance the estradiol effect, at least in terms of bone density outcome.

When estrogens are discontinued, bone loss begins again [91,102,116–118]. There is considerable argument about the rate of bone loss that occurs after discontinuing estrogen, with some data suggesting that the bone loss is rapid with an accelerated return of bone mass to the rate compatible with untreated controls, whereas other data suggest that the rate of bone loss may be parallel to the rate that occurs after ovariectomy in premenopausal women. One cross-sectional study from the United States suggested that within 8 years of stopping estrogen, bone density in the spine appeared to be similar to those who had been untreated [119], implying an accelerated period of bone loss was experienced after estrogen therapy was discontinued.

FRACTURE OUTCOMES

Several epidemiological studies have evaluated the effects of estrogen in reducing the risk of fracture in the aging population [120–127]. Most studies show a lower incidence of the risk of osteoporotic fractures with a reduction in the risk of hip fracture of anywhere between 20 and 75%. In the majority of those studies, "ever use," usually defined as the period of estrogen use of 1 year or more, classified those women who had used estrogen at any time in their postmenopausal life. More recently, however, when evaluating in excess of 9000 women over the age of 65 in the United States, the Study of Osteoporotic Fracture suggested that current use was an important determinant of fracture risk [127]. In addition, fracture data from the cohort supported the conclusion from bone density data that the earlier the intervention was initiated, the greater the effect would be. For those women who had been on estrogen for more than 10 years and were still currently on hormone replacement therapy, reductions on the order of 75% in the risk of both hip and wrist fractures were seen. In contrast, those women who had previously been on estrogen but discontinued it essentially lost most of the protective effect. No controlled clinical trials have been completed to show whether estrogens do reduce hip fracture and/or by what magnitude. One recent randomized clinical trial of continuous combined HRT in patients with established heart disease showed no overall effect of this HRT regimen on heart disease, but also no effect against hip fracture or any symptomatic fracture [128]. This study did not include spinal x-rays, so no conclusions can be drawn regarding effects on spinal deformity.

One controlled primary intervention trial with estrogen showed that a relatively small cohort followed for a long period of time (10 years) experienced a similar reduction in the risk of spine fractures, perhaps by as much as 75–80% [83]. One other short-term clinical trial in osteoporosis patients showed a reduction in vertebral fracture with 1 year of transdermal estradiol administration [112]. Other observational data confirmed the reductions in vertebral fracture, although again, the effects of observational data appear to be somewhat less than that seen in one controlled clinical trial [87].

There is considerable discussion as to the mechanism of estrogen's effects in reducing fracture risk in the spine. Maintaining cancellous structure in the spine may be critically important, but in the hip, the situation may be considerably more complicated. Other covariates, such as body mass, physical activity, and calcium intake, may also be important. The Study of Osteoporotic Fracture also showed that smoking contributed to the risk of hip fracture [129]. It is well known that the use of cigarettes may interfere with the effects of exogenous estrogen on bone turnover and mass and may be another variable important in the epidemiological database, as cigarette consumption appears to be lower among those who use estrogen therapy.

Perhaps the best data have been accrued in studies in which standing height has been measured, substantiating an effect of estrogen on vertebral fracture. Over the lifespan, the average individual can expect height to decline between 1 and 2 inches, primarily because of narrowing of the intervertebral disc spaces but also because of some natural degree of progressive kyphosis, the consequence of the erect posture. Excess height loss, however, is most commonly due to loss of vertebral height. A number of years ago, Henneman and Wallach demonstrated that those women treated by Fuller Albright with estrogen stopped losing height in comparison to untreated women who continued to lose height as vertebrae continued to collapse [130]. Similar data have been shown in a controlled clinical trial of a bisphosphonate, alendronate, supporting the idea that if one could prevent bone loss and vertebral fracture, one could also reduce height loss with age and presumably the resulting excessive kyphosis that results from multiple vertebral fractures [131].

When estrogens are used in a preventive mode, the mean change in bone density is perhaps less important than the proportion of individuals in whom bone loss is completely prevented. Such data are more difficult to obtain. From the progestin estrogen prevention intervention study (PEPI), a dose of 0.625 mg of conjugate equine estrogens prevented significant bone loss in the spine in 97% of individuals [132]. The corresponding value for the femoral neck was 93%. It might be expected that the proportion of individuals who lose bone at lower doses of estrogen would be greater but such data have not been reported.

Estrogen intervention and prevention of osteoporosis addresses only that component of bone loss which relates to estrogen deficiency following menopause or ovariectomy. Bone loss in the aging population has other causes, notably declines in physical activity and in calcium supply or absorption. A consequence of these two latter changes is an element of secondary hyperparathyroidism, which is presumed to be the mechanism by which undernutrition of calcium is associated with bone loss [133]. Consequently, estrogens will not prevent those changes except in a modest way by stimulating 1-hydroxylase in the kidney to produce higher amounts of 1,25-dihydroxyvitamin D and improving calcium absorption across the intestine [134]. Estrogens may also improve calcium homeostasis by reducing the renal loss of calcium, although whether this is a direct or indirect effect is still not clear [135]. Estrogens also increase the resistance of the skeleton to the bone-resorbing effects of parathyroid hormone, a mechanism postulated by Heaney for estrogen effects many years ago [6,136]. Nonetheless, estrogen cannot completely make up for the effects of calcium insufficiency. Recognizing that calcium intake in the United States is on average less than 600 mg/day and considerably less than either the RDA or the new recommended intake of 1200 mg/day led us to the hypothesis that those studies with estrogen in which calcium supplementation was added should have a better outcome than those in which estrogens were given by themselves. We performed an analysis of all the controlled clinical trials that we could find in the published literature in which estrogens had been used and bone density had been the measured outcome. Division of those studies into those in which calcium had been given and those in which calcium had not gives a clear indication that the addition of calcium enhanced the estrogen effect significantly at all skeletal sites at least in terms of bone density [137]. It has been shown in controlled clinical trials that calcium supplementation, particularly in combination with vitamin D supplementation, may reduce the risk of fracture [138,139]. Consequently, it seems reasonable to ensure that when antiresorptive therapy such as estrogen is used, an intake adequate in calcium through diet or calcium supplements be used to ensure that the total calcium intake per day reaches levels of 1200–1500 mg.

ESTROGENS IN OLDER AGE

Data in the early postmenopausal years suggest that there is no real relationship between the estrogen effect and the duration of years that have passed since menopause. However, comparatively few studies have focused on estrogens in older individuals. In part, this is because of the well-known difficulty clinically in initiating estrogen therapy in women over the age of 70. In controlled clinical trials of patients with osteoporosis, this is less of a problem. In those controlled clinical trials, it is clear that estrogens prevent bone loss and indeed increase bone mass in a transient fashion, much as they do in postmenopausal women [140]. Again, the effects of estrogen are seen when given both orally or transdermally. It is not entirely clear whether differences in dose would be required in those patients who have significant osteoporosis in comparison to healthy postmenopausal women. One relatively short-term controlled clinical trial demonstrated a significant reduction in fractures as a consequence of estrogen intervention in patients with osteoporosis [141]. However, no large-scale studies have been done in a controlled fashion to demonstrate whether fracture risk other than vertebral fractures might be reduced by estrogen intervention in either the very elderly or patients with established osteoporosis. Such studies are currently underway.

References

1. Albright, F., Smith, P. H., and Richardson, A. M. Postmenopausal osteoporosis. *JAMA* **116,** 2465–2474 (1941).
2. Albright, F. The effect of hormones on osteogenesis in man. *Recent Prog. Horm. Res.* **1,** 293–353 (1947).
3. Oursler, M. J., Kassem, M., Turner, R., Riggs, B. L., and Spelsberg, T. C. Regulation of bone cell function by gonadal steroids. *In* "Osteoporosis" (R. Marcus, D. Feldman, and J. Kelsey, eds.), pp. 237–260. Academic Press, San Diego, 1996.
4. Kibble, R. B. Alcohol, cytokines, and estrogen in the control of bone remodeling. *Alcohol Clin. Exp. Res.* **21**(3), 385–391 (1997).
5. Kuiper, G. G. J. M., Enmark, E., Pelto-Huikko, M., Nilsson, S., and Gustafsson, J. A. Cloning of a novel estrogen receptor expressed in rat prostate and ovary. *Proc. Natl. Acad. Sci. USA* **93,** 5925–5930 (1996).
6. Cosman, F., Shen, V., Xie, F., Seibel, M., Ratcliffe, A., and Lindsay, R. Estrogen protection against the resorbing effects of (1-34)hPTH infusion. Assessment by use of biochemical markers. *Ann. Intern. Med.* **118**(5), 337–343 (1993).
7. Mitlak, B. H., and Cohen, F. J. In search of optimal long-term female hormone replacement: The potential of selective estrogen receptor modulators. *Horm. Res.* **48,** 155–163 (1997).
8. Glastre, C., Braillon, P., David, L., Cochat, P., Meunier, P., and Delmas, P. Measurement of bone mineral content of the lumbar spine by dual energy x-ray absorptiometry in normal children: Correlations with growth parameter. *J. Clin. Endocrinol.* **70,** 1330–1333 (1990).
9. Gilsanz, V., Boechat, I., Roe, T. F., Loro, M. L., Sayre, J. W., and Goodman, W. G. Gender differences in vertebral body sizes in children and adolescents. *Radiology* **190,** 673–677 (1994).
10. Bonjour, J. P., and Rizzoli, R. Bone acquisition in adolescence. *In* "Osteoporosis" (R. Marcus, D. Feldman, and J. Kelsey, eds.), pp. 465–476. Academic Press, San Diego, 1996.
11. Gilsanz, V., Loro, M. L., Roe, T. F., Sayre, J., Gilsanz, R., and Schulz, E. E. Vertebral size in elderly women with osteoporosis. *J. Clin. Invest.* **95,** 2332–2337 (1995).
12. Juul, A., Beng, P., Hertel, N. T., *et al.* Serum insulin-like growth factor I in 1030 healthy adolescents and adults: Relation to age, sex, stage of puberty, testicular size, and body mass index. *J. Clin. Endocrinol.* **78,** 744 (1994).
13. Recker, R. R., Davies, M., Hinders, S. M., Heaney, R. P., Stegman, M. R., and Kimmel, D. B. Bone gain in young adult women. *JAMA* **268,** 2403–2408 (1992).
14. Landin, L. A. Fracture patterns in children. *Acta. Orthop. Scand.* **54**(Suppl.), 1–109 (1983).
15. Bailey, D. A., Wedge, J. H., McCullogh, R. G., Martin, A. D., and Bernhardson, S. C. Epidemiology of fractures of the distal end of the radius in children as associated with growth. *J. Bone Joint Surg.* **71A,** 1225–1230 (1989).
16. Blimkie, C., Jr., Lefevre, J., Beunen, G. P., Renson, R., Dequeker, J., and Van Damme, P. Fractures, physical activity, and growth velocity in adolescent Belgian boys. *Med. Sci. Sports Exerc.* **25,** 801–808 (1993).
17. Lippe, B. M. Physical and anatomical abnormalities in Turner Syndrome. *In* "Turner Syndrome" (R. G. Rosenfeld, and M. M. Grumbach, eds.), pp. 183–196. Deker, New York, 1990.
18. Beals, R. K. Orthopedic aspects of the XO (Turner's) syndrome. *Clin. Orthop.* **97,** 19–30 (1973).
19. Kelly, P. J., Sambrook, P. N., and Eisman, J. A. The interaction of genetic and environmental influences on peak bone density. *Osteopor. Int.* **1,** 56–60 (1990).
20. Federman, D. Life without estrogen. *N. Engl. J. Med.* **331,** 1088–1089 (1994).
21. Gorai, I., Taguchi, Y., Chaki, O., Kikuchi, R., Nakayama, M., Yang, B. C., Yokota, S., and Minaguchi, H. Serum soluble interleukin-6 receptor and biochemical markers of bone metabolism show significant variations during the menstrual cycle. *J. Clin. Endocrinol. Metab.* **83,** 326–332 (1998).

21a. Lindsay, R. Estrogen deficiency. *In* "Osteoporosis" (B. L. Riggs and L. J. Melton III, eds.), pp. 133–160. Lippincott-Raven, Philadelphia, 1995.

22. Schlechte, J. A., Sherman, B., and Martin, R. Bone density in amenorrheic women with and without hyperprolactinemia. *J. Clin. Endocrinol. Metab.* **56,** 1120–1123 (1983).
23. Klibanski, A., Neer, R. M., and Beitins, I. Z. Decreased bone density in hyperprolactinemic women. *N. Engl. J. Med.* **303,** 1511–1514 (1980).
24. Riis, B. J., Christiansen, C., Johansen, J. S., and Jacobson, J. Is it possible to prevent bone loss in young women treated with luteinizing hormone-releasing hormone agonists? *J. Clin. Endocrinol. Metab.* **70,** 920–924 (1990).

25. Ayers, J. W. T., Gidwani, G. P., and Schmidt, I. M. V. Osteoporosis in hypoestrogenic young women with anorexia nervosa. *Fertil. Steril.* **41,** 224–228 (1984).
26. Biller, B. M. K., Saxe, V., and Herzog, D. B. Mechanisms of osteoporosis in adult and adolescent women with anorexia nervosa. *J. Clin. Endocrinol. Metab.* **68,** 548–554 (1989).
27. Rigotti, N. A., Nussbaum, S. R., and Herzog, D. B. Osteoporosis in women with anorexia nervosa. *J. Engl. J. Med.* **311,** 1601–1606 (1984).
28. Baker, E., and Demers, L. Menstrual status in female athletes: Correlation with reproductive hormones and bone density. *Obstet. Gynecol.* **72,** 683–687 (1988).
29. Cann, C. E., Martin, M. C., and Genant, H. K. Decreased spinal mineral content in amenorrheic women. *J. Am. Med. Assoc.* **251,** 626–629 (1984).
30. Drinkwater, B. L., Nilson, K., and Chesnut. Bone mineral content of amenorrheic and eumenorrheic athletes. *N. Engl. J. Med.* **311,** 277–281 (1984).
31. Drinkwater, B. L., Nilson, K., and Ott, S. Bone mineral density after resumption of menses in amenorrheic athletes. *J. Am. Med. Assoc.* **245,** 380–382 (1986).
32. Feicht, C. B., Johnson, T. S., and Martin, B. J. Secondary amenorrhea in athletes. *Lancet* **1,** 1145–1146 (1978).
33. Lindberg, J. S., Fears, W. B., and Hunt, M. M. Exercise-induced amenorrhea and bone density. *Ann. Int. Med.* **101,** 647–648 (1984).
34. Linnell, S. L., Stager, J. M., and Blue, P. W. Bone mineral content and menstrual regularity in female runners. *Med. Sci. Sports. Exer.* **16,** 343–348 (1984).
35. Marcus, R., Cann, C., and Madvig, P. Menstrual function and bone mass in elite women distance runners. *Ann. Int. Med.* **102,** 158–163 (1985).
36. Warren, M. P., Brooks-Gunn, J., and Hamilton, L. H. Scoliosis and fractures in young ballet dancers. *N. Engl. J. Med.* **314,** 1348–1353 (1986).
37. Goldsmith, N. F., and Johnston, J. O. Bone mineral: Effects of oral contraceptives, pregnancy and lactation. *J. Bone Joint Surg.* **57,** 657–668 (1975).
38. Lindsay, R., Tohme, J., and Kanders, B. The effect of oral contraceptive use on vertebral bone mass in pre- and post-menopausal women. *Contraception* **34,** 333–340 (1986).
39. Seeman, E., Szmukler, G. I., Formica, C., Tsalamandris, C., and Mestrovic, R. Osteoporosis in anorexia nervosa: The influence of peak bone density, bone loss, oral contraceptive use, and exercise. *J. Bone Miner.* **17,** 1467–1474 (1992).
40. Kleerekoper, M., Brienza, R. S., Schultz, L. R., and Johnson, C. C. Oral contraceptive use may protect against low bone mass. *Arch. Intern. Med.* **151,** 1971–1976 (1991).
41. Mazess, R. B., and Barden, H. S. Bone density in premenopausal women: Effects of age, dietary intake, physical activity, smoking and birth-control pills. *Am. J. Clin. Nutr* **53,** 132–142 (1991).
42. Murphy, S., Khaw, K. T., and Compston, J. E. Lack of relationship between hip and spine bone mineral density and oral contraceptive use. *Eur. J. Clin. Invest.* **23,** 108–111 (1993).
43. Paganini-Hill, A., Chao, A., and Ross, R. K. Exercise and other factors in the prevention of hip fracture: The Leisure World Study. *Epidemiology* **2,** 16–25 (1991).
44. Hoffman, S., Grisso, J. A., and Kelsey, J. L. Parity, lactation and hip fracture. *Osteopor. Int.* **3,** 84–89 (1993).
45. Sowers, M. F., Crutchfield, M., Jannausch. A prospective evaluation of bone mineral change in pregnancy. *Obstet. Gynecol.* **77,** 841–845 (1991).
46. Atkinson, P. J., and West, R. R. Loss of skeletal calcium in lactating women. *J. Obstet. Gynaecol. Br.* **77,** 555–560 (1970).
47. Lamke, B., Brundin, J., and Moberg, P. Changes of bone mineral content during pregnancy and lactation. *Acta Obstet. Gynecol. Scand.* **56,** 217–219 (1977).
48. Chan, G. M., McMurry, M., and Westover, K. Effects of increased dietary calcium intake upon the calcium and bone mineral status of lactating adolescent and adult women. *Am. J. Clin. Nutr.* **46,** 319–323 (1987).
49. Kent, G. N., Price, R. I., and Gutterridge, D. H. Human lactation: Forearm trabecular bone loss, increased bone turnover, and renal conservation of calcium and inorganic phosphate with recovery of bone mass following weaning. *J. Bone Miner.* **5,** 361–369 (1990).
50. Sowers, M. F., Corton, G., and Shapiro, B. Changes on bone density with lactation. *JAMA* **269,** 3130–3135 (1993).
51. Johnston, C. C., Jr., Hui, S. L., Witt, R. M., Appledorn, R., Baker, R. S., and Longcope, C. Early menopausal changes in bone mass and sex steroids. *J. Clin. Endocrinol.* **61,** 905–911 (1985).
52. Erikson, E. F. Normal and pathological remodeling of human trabecular bone: Three dimensional reconstruction of the remodeling sequence in normals and in metabolic bone disease. *Endocr. Rev.* **7,** 379–408 (1986).
53. Heaney, R. P., Recker, R. R., and Saville, P. D. Menopausal changes in calcium balance performance. *J. Lab. Clin. Med.* **92,** 953–963 (1978).
54. Heaney, R. P., Recker, R. R., and Saville, P. D. Menopausal changes in bone remodeling. *J. Lab. Clin. Med.* **92,** 953–963 (1978).
55. Seibel, M. J., Cosman, F., Shen, V., Gordon, S., Dempster, D. W., Ratcliffe, A., and Lindsay, R. Urinary hydroxypyridinium crosslinks of collagen as markers of bone resorption and estrogen efficacy in postmenopausal osteoporosis. *J. Bone Miner.* **9,** 881–889 (1993).
56. Delmas, P. D. Biochemical markers for the assessment of bone turnover. *In* "*Osteoporosis*" (B. L. Riggs and L. J. Melton III, eds.), pp. 319–350. Lippincott-Raven, Philadelphia, 1995.
57. Dempster, D. W., Shane, E. S., Horbert, W., Lindsay, R. A simple method for correlative light and scanning electron microscopy of human iliac crest bone biopsies: Qualitative observations in normal and osteoporotic subjects. *J. Bone and Mineral Res.* **1,** 15–21 (1986).
58. Jilka, R., Hangoc, G., Girasole, G., *et al.* Increased osteoclast development after estrogen loss: Mediation by interleukin-6. *Science* **257,** 88–91 (1992).
59. Pacifici, R., Brown, C., Puscheck, R., *et al.* Effect of surgical menopause and estrogen replacement on cytokine release from human blood mononuclear cells. *Proc. Natl. Acad. Sci. USA* **88,** 5134–5138 (1991).
60. Pacifici, R., Vannice, J. L., Rifas, L. *et al.* Monocytic secretion of interleukin-I receptor antagonist in normal and osteoporotic women: Effects of menopause and estrogen/progesterone therapy. *J. Clin. Endocrinol. Metab.* **77,** 1135–1141 (1993).
61. Raisz, L. G., Simmons, H. A. Effect of parathyroid hormone and cortisol on prostaglandins E_1 and E_2. *Endocrinology* **130,** 443–448 (1992).
62. Dempster, D. W. *In* "Osteoporosis", 2nd Edition (B. L. Riggs and L. J. Melton III, eds.), pp. 67–91. Lippincott-Raven Publishers, Philadelphia, 1995.
63. Girasole, G., Jilka, R., Passeri, G. *et al.* 17β-Estradiol inhibits interleukin-6 production by bone marrow-derived stromal cells and osteoblasts in vitro: A potential mechanism for the antiosteoporotic effect of estrogens. *J. Clin. Invest.* **89,** 883–891 (1992).
64. Melton, L. J., III, and Riggs, B. L. Epidemiology of age-related fractures. *In* "The Osteoporotic Syndrome" (L. V. Avioli, ed.), pp. 45–72. Grune & Stratton, New York, 1983.

65. Greendale, G. A., and Judd, H. L. The menopause: Health implications and clinical management. *J. Am. Geriatr. Soc.* **41,** 426–436 (1993).
66. Chang, R. J., and Judd, H. L. The ovary after menopause. *Clin. Obstet. Gynecol.* **24,** 181–191 (1981).
67. Lindsay, R., Coutts, J. R. T., and Hart, D. M. The effect of endogenous oestrogen on plasma and urinary calcium and phosphate in oophorectomized women. *Clin. Endocrinol.* **6,** 87–93 (1977).
68. Cauley, J. A., Gutai, J. P., Kuller, L. H., LeDonne, D., and Powell, J. G. The epidemiology of serum sex hormones in postmenopausal women. *Am. J. Epidemiol.* **129,** 1120–1131 (1989).
69. Greendale, G. A., Edelstein, S., and Barrett-Connor, E. Endogenous sex steroids and bone mineral density in older women and men: The Rancho Bernardo study. *J. Bone Miner.* **12,** 1833–1843 (1997).
70. Rozenberg, S., Ham, H., Bosson, D., Peretz, A., and Robyn, C. Age, steroids, and bone mineral content. *Maturitas* **12,** 137–143 (1990).
71. Van Betesteijn, E. C. H., van Laarhoven, J. P. R. M., Smals, A. G. H. Body weight and/or endogenous estradiol as determinants of cortical bone mass and bone loss in healthy early postmenopausal women. *Acta Endocrinol.* **127,** 226–230 (1992).
72. Spector, T. D., Thompson, P. W., Perry, L. A., McGarrigle, H. H., and Edwards, A. C. The relationship between sex steroids and bone mineral content in women soon after the menopause. *Clin. Endocrinol.* **34,** 37–41 (1991).
73. Cauley, J. A., Gutai, J. P., Kuller, L. H., and Powell, J. G. Reliability and interrelations among sex hormones in postmenopausal women. *Am. J. Epidemiol.* **133,** 50–57 (1991).
74. Heaney, R. P. Nutrition and risk for osteoporosis. *In* "Osteoporosis" (R. Marcus, D. Feldman, and J. Kelsey, eds.), pp. 483–509. Academic Press, San Diego, 1996.
75. Nilas, L., and Christiansen, C. Rates of bone loss in normal women: Evidence of accelerated trabecular bone loss after the menopause. *Eur. J. Clin. Invest.* **18,** 529–534 (1988).
76. Looker, A. C., Orwoll, E. S., Johnston, C. C., Lindsay, R., Wahner, H. W., Dunn, W. L., Calvo, M. S., Harris, T. B., and Heyse, S. P. Prevalence of low femoral bone density in older U.S. adults from NHANES III. *J. Bone Miner.* **12,** 1761–1768 (1997).
77. Riggs, B. L., Khosla, S., Melton, L. J., III. A unitary model for involutional osteoporosis: Estrogen deficiency causes both type I and type II osteoporosis in postmenopausal women and contributes to bone loss in aging men. *J. Bone Miner. Res.* **13,** 763–773 (1998).
78. Khosla, S., Atkinson, E. J., Melton, L. J., III, and Riggs, B. L. Effects of age and estrogen status on serum parathyroid hormone levels and biochemical markers of bone turnover in women: A population-based study. *J. Clin. Endocrinol. Metab.* **82**(5), 1522–1527 (1997).
79. Ooms, M. E., Lips, P., Roos, J. C., vander Vijgh, W. J. F., Popp-Snijders, C., and Bezemer, P. D. Vitamin D status and sex hormone binding globulin: Determinants of bone turnover and bone mineral density in elderly women. *J. Bone Miner. Res.* **10,** 1177–1187 (1995).
80. Kuller, L. H., Cauley, J. A., Lucas, L., Cummings, S., and Browner, W. S. Sex steroid hormones, bone mineral density, and risk of breast cancer. *Environ. Health Perspect.* **105,** 593–599 (1997).
81. Lindsay, R., Aitken, J. M., Anderson, J. B., Hart, D. M., MacDonald, E. B., and Clark, A. C. Long-term prevention of postmenopausal osteoporosis by oestrogen. *Lancet* **i,** 1038–1041 (1976).
82. Lindsay, R., Hart, D. M., Purdie, P., Ferguson, M. M., Clark, A. C., and Krasszewski, A. Comparative effects of oestrogen and a progestogen on bone loss in postmenopausal women. *Clin. Sci. Mol. Med.* **54,** 193–195 (1978).
83. Lindsay, R., Hart, D. M., Forrest, C., and Baird, C. Prevention of spinal osteoporosis in oophorectomized women. *Lancet* **ii,** 1151–1154 (1980).
84. Christiansen, C., and Rodbro, P. Does postmenopausal bone loss respond to estrogen replacement therapy independent of bone loss rate. *Calcif. Tissue Int.* **35,** 720–722 (1983).
85. Christiansen, C., Christiansen, M. S., and McNair, P. Prevention of early postmenopausal bone loss: Conducted 2 years study in 315 normal females. *Eur. J. Clin. Invest.* **10,** 273–279 (1980).
86. Davis, M. E., Lanzl, L. H., and Cox, A. B. Detection, prevention and retardation of postmenopausal osteoporosis. *Obstet. Gynecol.* **36,** 187–198 (1970).
87. Ettinger, B., Genant, H. K., and Cann, C. E. Long-term estrogen therapy prevents bone loss and fracture. *Ann. Intern. Med.* **102,** 319–324 (1985).
88. Horsman, A., Gallagher, J. C., Simpson, M., and Nordin, B. E. C. Prospective trial of estrogen and calcium in postmenopausal women. *Br. Med. J.* **2,** 789–792 (1977).
89. Lindsay, R., Hart, D. M., and Clark, D. M. The minimum effective dose of estrogen for prevention of postmenopausal bone loss. *Obstet. Gynecol.* **63,** 759–763 (1984).
90. Nachtigall, L. E., Nachtigall, R. H., and Nachtigall, R. D. Estrogen replacement therapy I: A 10-year prospective study in the relationship to osteoporosis. *Obstet. Gynecol.* **53,** 277 (1979).
91. Quigley, M. E. T., Martin, B. L., Burnier, A. M., and Brooks, P. Estrogen therapy arrests bone loss in elderly women. *Am. J. Obstet. Gynecol.* **156,** 1516–1523 (1987).
92. Recker, R. R., Saville, P. D., and Heaney, R. P. The effect of estrogens and calcium carbonate on bone loss in postmenopausal women. *Ann. Intern. Med.* **87,** 649–655 (1977).
93. Meema, S., Bunker, M. L., and Meema, H. E. Preventive effect of estrogen on postmenopausal bone loss. *Arch. Intern. Med.* **135,** 1436–1440 (1975).
94. Riis, B., Thomsen, K., Strom, V., and Christiansen, C. The effect of percutaneous estradiol and natural progesterone on postmenopausal bone loss. *Am. J. Obstet. Gynecol.* **156,** 61–65 (1987).
95. Jensen, G. F., Christiansen, C., and Transbol, I. Treatment of postmenopausal osteoporosis: A controlled therapeutic trial comparing oestrogen/gestagen, 1,25dihydroxyvitamin D_3 and calcium. *Clin. Endocrinol.* **16,** 515–524 (1982).
96. Ettinger, B., Genant, H. K., and Cann, C. E. Postmenopausal bone loss is prevented by treatment with low-dosage estrogen and calcium. *Ann. Intern. Med.* **106,** 40–45 (1987).
97. Finn-Hensen, M., Christiansen, C., and Transbol, I. Postmenopausal bone loss is prevented by treatment with low-dosage estrogen with calcium. *Obstet. Gynecol.* **60,** 493–496 (1982).
98. Horsman, A., James, M., and Francis, R. The effect of estrogen dose on postmenopausal bone loss. *N. Engl. J. Med.* **309,** 1405–1407 (1983).
99. Lafferty, F. N., and Helmuth, D. O. Postmenopausal estrogen replacement: The prevention of osteoporosis and systemic effects. *Maturitas* **7,** 147–159 (1985).
100. Munk-Jensen, N., Pors Nielsen, S., Obel, E. B., and Eriksen, P. B. Reversal of postmenopausal vertebral bone loss by oestrogen and progestogen: A double blind placebo controlled study. *Br. Med. J.* **296,** 1150–1152 (1988).
101. Al-Azzawi, F., Hart, D. M., and Lindsay, R. Long-term effect of oestrogen replacement therapy on bone mass as measured by dual photon absorptiometry. *Br. Med. J.* **294,** 1261–1262 (1987).

102. Lindsay, R., Hart, D. M., MacLean, A., Clark, A. C., Kraszewski, A., and Garwood, J. Bone response to termination of oestrogen treatment. *Lancet* **i,** 1325–1327 (1978).
103. Eiken, P., Nielsen, S. P., and Kolthoff, N. Effects on bone mass after eight years of hormonal replacement therapy. *Br. J. Obst. G.* **104,** 702–707 (1997).
104. Speroff, L., Rowan, J., Symons, J., Genant, H., Wilborn, for the CHART Study Group. The comparative effect on bone density, endometrium, and lipids of continuous hormones as replacement therapy (CHART Study). A randomized controlled trial. *JAMA* **276,** 1397–1403 (1996).
105. The Writing Group for the PEPI Trial. Effects of hormone therapy on bone mineral density. Results from the postmenopausal estrogen/progestin interventions (PEPI) trial. *JAMA* **276,** 1389–1396 (1996).
106. Naessen, T., Berglund, L., and Ulmsten, U. Bone loss in elderly women prevented by ultralow doses of parenteral 17β-estradiol. *Am. J. Obstet. Gynecol.* **177,** 115–119 (1997).
107. Genant, H. K., Lucas, J., Weiss, S., Akin, M., Emkey, R., McNaney-Flint, H., Downs, R., Mortola, J., Watts, N., Yang, H. M., Banav, N., Brennan, J. J., Nolan, J. C., for the Estratab/Osteoporosis Study Group. Low-dose esterified estrogen therapy. Effects on bone, plasma estradiol concentrations, endometrium, and lipid levels. *Arch. Intern. Med.* **157,** 2609–2615 (1997).
108. Prior, J. C., Vigna, Y. M., Wark, J. D., Eyre, D. R., Lentle, B. C., Li, D. K. B., Ebeling, P. R., and Atley, L. Premenopausal ovariectomy-related bone loss: A randomized, double-blind, one-year trial of conjugated estrogen or medroxyprogesterone acetate. *J. Bone Miner.* **12,** 1851–1863 (1997).
109. Orwoll, E. S., Bauer, D. C., Vogt, T. M., Fox, K. M., for the Study of Osteoporotic Fractures Research Group. Axial bone mass in older women. *Ann. Intern. Med.* **124,** 187–196 (1996).
110. Lindsay, R., Nieves, J. W., Formica, C., Henneman, E., Woelfert, L., Shen, V., Dempster, D. W., and Cosman, F. Parathyroid hormone increases vertebral bone mass and may reduce vertebral fracture incidence in estrogen treated postmenopausal women with osteoporosis. *Lancet* **350,** 550–555 (1997).
111. Genant, H. K., Cann, C. E., Ettinger, B., and Gordon, G. S. Quantitative computed tomography of vertebral spongiosa: A sensitive method for detecting early bone loss after oophorectomy. *Ann. Intern. Med.* **97,** 699–705 (1982).
112. Lufkin, E. G., Wahner, H. W., O'Fallon, W. M., *et al.* Treatment of postmenopausal osteoporosis with transdermal estrogen. *Ann. Intern. Med.* **117,** 1–9 (1992).
113. Savvas, M., Studd, J. W. W., Norman, S., Leather, A. T., and Garnett, T. J. Increase in bone mass after one year of percutaneous oestradiol and testosterone implants in postmenopausal women who have previously received long-term oestrogens. *Br. J. Obstet. Gynecol.* **99,** 757–760 (1992).
114. Stevenson, J. C., Cust, M. P., Gangar, K. F., Hillard, T. C., Lees, B., and Whithead, M. I. Effects of transdermal versus oral hormone replacement therapy on bone density in spine and proximal femur in postmenopausal women. *Lancet* **336,** 265–269 (1990).
115. Christiansen, C., and Riis, B. T. Beta-estradiol and continuous norethisterone: A unique treatment for established osteoporosis in elderly women. *J. Clin. Endocrinol. Metab.* **71,** 836–841 (1990).
116. Paganini-Hill, A., Chao, A., Ross, R. K., and Henderson, B. E. Exercise and other factors in the prevention of hip fracture: The Leisure World study. *Epidemiology* **2,** 16–25 (1991).
117. Christiansen, C., Christiansen, M. S., and Transbol, I. Bone mass in postmenopausal women after withdrawal of estrogen/gestagen replacement therapy. *Lancet* **i,** 459–461 (1981).
118. Horsman, A., Nordin, B. E., and Crilly, R. G. Effect on bone of withdrawal of oestrogen therapy. *Lancet* **ii,** 33 (1979).
119. Felson, D. T., Zhang, Y., Hannan, M. T., Kiel, D. P., Wilson, P. W., and Anderson, J. J. The effect of postmenopausal estrogen therapy on bone density in elderly women. *N. Engl. J. Med.* **329,** 1141–1146 (1993).
120. Paganini-Hill, A., Ross, R. K., Gerkins, V. R., Henderson, B. E., Arthur, M., and Mack, T. M. Menopausal estrogen therapy and hip fractures. *Ann. Intern. Med.* **95,** 28–31 (1981).
121. Hutchinson, T. A., Polansky, J. M., and Fienstein, A. R. Postmenopausal oestrogens protect against fracture of hip and distal radius. *Lancet* **ii,** 705–709 (1979).
122. Kreiger, N., Kelsey, J. L., and Holford, T. R. An epidemiological study of hip fracture in postmenopausal women. *Am. J. Epidemiol.* **116,** 141–148 (1982).
123. Weiss, N. S., Szekely, D. R., Dallas, R., English, M. S., Abraham, I., and Schweid, A. I. Endometrial cancer in relation to patterns of menopausal estrogen use. *JAMA* **242,** 261–264 (1979).
124. Burch, J. C., Byrd, B. F., and Vaughn, W. K. The effects of long-term estrogen on hysterectomized women. *Am. J. Obstet. Gynecol.* **118,** 778–782 (1974).
125. Kiel, D. P., Felson, D. T., and Anderson, J. J. Hip fracture and the use of estrogens in postmenopausal women. *N. Engl. J. Med.* **317,** 1169–1174 (1987).
126. Williams, A. R., Weiss, N. S., Ure, C., *et al.* Effect of weight, smoking, and estrogen use on the risk of hip and forearm fractures in post-menopausal women. *Obstet. Gynecol.* **60,** 695–699 (1982).
127. Cauley, J., Seeley, K., Ensrud, K., Ettinger, B., Black, D., and Cummings, S. R. Estrogen replacement therapy and fractures in older women. *Ann. Intern. Med.* **122,** 9–16 (1995).
128. Hulley, S., Grady, D., Bush, T., *et al.* Randomized trial of estrogen plus progestin for secondary prevention of coronary heart disease in postmenopausal women. *JAMA* **280,** 605–613 (1998).
129. Cummings, S. R., Black, D. M., Nevitt, M. C., *et al.* Appendicular bone density and age predict hip fracture in women. The Study of Osteoporotic Fractures Research Group. *JAMA* **263,** 665–668 (1990).
130. Henneman, P. H., and Wallach, S. A review of the prolonged use of estrogens and androgens in postmenopausal and senile osteoporosis. *Arch. Intern. Med.* **100,** 705–709 (1957).
131. Liberman, U. A., Weiss, S. R., Broll, J., Minne, H. W., Qyan, H., Bell, N. H., *et al.* Effect of oral alendronate on bone mineral density and the incidence of fractures in postmenopausal osteoporosis. *N. Engl. J. Med.* **333,** 1437–1433 (1995).
132. Marcus, R. Effects of hormone replacement therapies on bone mineral density (BMD) results from the postmenopausal estrogen and progestin interventions trial (PEPI). *J. Bone Miner. Res.* **10,** S197 (1995). [Abstract]
133. Villareal, D., Civitelli, R., Chines, A., and Avioli, L. Subclinical vitamin D deficiency in postmenopausal women with low vertebral bone mass. *J. Clin. Endocrinol.* **72,** 628–634 (1991).
134. Cheema, C., Grant, B. F., and Marcus, R. Effects of estrogen on circulating free and total 1,25dihydroxyvitamin D and on the parathyroid vitamin D axis in postmenopausal women. *J. Clin. Invest.* **83,** 537–542 (1989).
135. Nordin, B. E. C. Clinical significance and pathogenesis of osteoporosis. *Br. Med. J.* **i,** 571–576 (1971).
136. Heaney, R. P. A unified concept of osteoporosis. *Am. J. Med.* **39,** 377–380 (1965).
137. Nieves, J. W., Komar, L., Cosman, F., and Lindsay, R. Calcium potentiates the effect of estrogen and calcitonin on bone mass: Review and analysis. *Am. J. Clin. Nutr.* **67,** 18–24 (1998).
138. Dawson-Hughes, B., Dallal, G. E., Krall, G. E., *et al.* A controlled trial of the effect of calcium supplementation on bone den-

sity in postmenopausal women. *N. Engl. J. Med.* **323,** 878–883 (1990).

139. Chapuy, M. C., Arlot, M. E., Delmas, P. D., and Meunier, P. J. Effect of calcium and cholecalciferol treatment for three years on hip fractures in elderly women. *Br. Med. J.* **308,** 1081–1082 (1994).

140. Lindsay, R., and Tohme, J. Estrogen treatment of patients with established postmenopausal osteoporosis. *Obstet. Gynecol.* **76,** 290–295 (1990).

141. Lufkin, E. G., Wahner, H. W., O'Fallon, W. M., *et al.* Treatment of postmenopausal osteoporosis with transdermal estrogen. *Ann. Intern. Med.* **117,** 1–9 (1992).

CHAPTER 42

Selective Estrogen Receptor Modulators

ETHEL S. SIRIS Columbia University College of Physicians and Surgeons, and Toni Stabile Center for the Prevention and Treatment of Osteoporosis, Columbia-Presbyterian Medical Center, New York, New York 10032

DEBRA H. SCHUSSHEIM Department of Medicine, Columbia University College of Physicians and Surgeons, New York, New York 10032

DOUGLAS B. MUCHMORE Lilly Research Laboratories, Eli Lilly and Company, Indianapolis, Indiana 46285

INTRODUCTION

Selective estrogen receptor modulators (SERMs) constitute a group of chemical compounds that are distinct from estrogen. They bind and interact with estrogen receptors and possess estrogen agonist or antagonist properties at different target tissues. Their role in clinical medicine is evolving. Early SERMs, then generally called estrogen agonist–antagonist agents, included clomiphene, used in the treatment of infertility as an ovulation induction agent, and tamoxifen (and more recently toremifene), used in the management of breast cancer, especially estrogen receptor-positive cancers in postmenopausal women. However, the potential roles for SERMs have expanded to take greater advantage of their ability to offer postmenopausal women many of the benefits of hormone replacement therapy without many of the problems.

The ideal SERM would provide an estrogen-like effect at bone, preserving bone mass and reducing the risk of osteoporotic fracture. Additionally, it would lower the risk of coronary artery disease—the leading cause of death in women in the United States—through improvements in lipoprotein profiles, improved vascular endothelial function, and possibly other mechanisms. Unlike estrogen, however, the ideal SERM would exert no proliferative effect at the uterine endometrium, so that there would be no regular or irregular uterine bleeding. At least, there would be no increased risk and, at best, a lowering of risk of endometrial cancer. At the breast, the ideal SERM would not cause mastalgia, would not increase breast cancer risk, and would indeed lower the risk of estrogen receptor-positive breast cancers. Additionally, the ideal SERM would control effectively symptoms of menopause such as vaginal dryness and hot flashes as well as estrogen. Finally, it might be expected to provide a reduction in the risk of dementia in aging women, a possible effect of conventional hormone replacement therapy. Although the ideal SERM does not yet exist, several of these attractive properties are present in at least two members of this group, tamoxifen and raloxifene.

This chapter discusses our current understanding of the mechanism of action of SERMs and reviews the effects on the skeleton of tamoxifen and raloxifene, the two SERMS for which there are both preclinical and clinical data. Additionaly, the clinical effects of these two drugs on lipids, uterus, and breast, as well as their overall clinical safety and tolerability, are considered.

CONCEPT OF A SERM

The initial development of antiestrogens for use in the therapy of hormonally responsive breast cancers emerged from a recognition of their ability to compete with estradiol for binding to the estrogen receptor. With the exception of some 7α-alkylated steroids such as ICI 182, 780 and ICI 164, 384, which are "pure" antiestrogens, the chemically diverse group of synthetic compounds that have come to be studied in this area have possessed tissue-specific agonist and antagonist properties. Figure 1 depicts the chemical structures of several of these compounds, including the triphenylethylenes clomiphene and tamoxifen and the benzothiophene, raloxifene. Also shown are structures of three derivatives of tamoxifen, droloxifene, toremifene, and idoxifene. Not shown are the structures of other SERMS such as benzopyrans, ormeloxifene, and levormeloxifene.

MECHANISM OF ACTION OF SERMS

By definition, SERMs exert their biological effects through specific, high-affinity interactions with estrogen receptors. Advances in estrogen receptor biology have elucidated new levels of complexity in the systems that mediate estrogen effects. It is now possible to develop coherent explanations for the seemingly contradictory properties that allow SERMs to act as estrogen agonists in some tissues and as estrogen antagonists in others.

"Classical" Mechanism of Estrogen Action

The classical paradigm of estrogen action invokes high-affinity binding of estrogenic ligands to the estrogen receptor, resulting in conformational changes in the receptor that lead to receptor dimerization. The dimerized ligand-bound receptor then interacts with transcription factors (proteins) that enable the receptor to bind to and activate (or repress) transcription at DNA promoter sites containing the estrogen response element (ERE) consensus sequence [1]. This promoter activates the gene transcription of classical estrogen target genes such as vitellogen or progesterone receptor. These gene products are generally associated with reproductive tissues and their functions. It is now known that several distinct gene promoter sequences, including the AP-1 promoter [2], the retinoic acid receptor-$\alpha 1$ promoter [3], and the transforming grow factor-β (TGF-β) promoter [4], are activated by ligand-bound estrogen receptors. Differential activation of these various estrogen response pathways offers an attractive explanation for the mechanisms by which SERMs exert their simultaneous agonist and antagonist actions. To explore possible mechanisms of SERM action, raloxifene will serve as an example.

Antagonist Mechanism of SERMs

X-ray crystallographic evidence demonstrates that raloxifene binds in the same ligand-binding pocket of the estrogen receptor as estradiol. Critical hydroxyl groups of the two ligands coordinate to the same amino acids that are present in this pocket [5]. However, the basic side chain of receptor-bound reloxifene interferes with the location of the C-terminal α-helix of the estro-

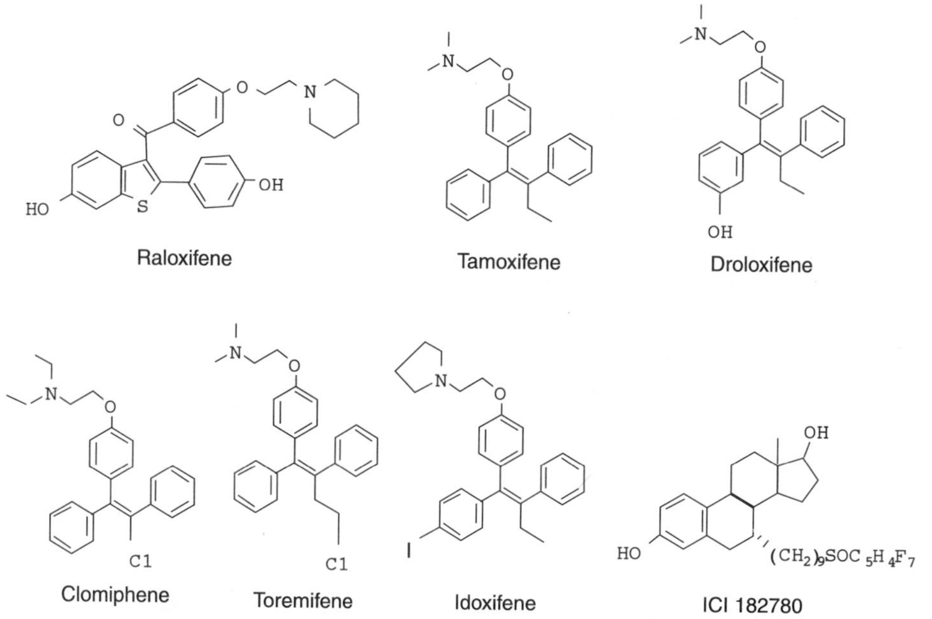

Raloxifene

Tamoxifene

Droloxifene

Clomiphene

Toremifene

Idoxifene

ICI 182780

FIGURE 1 Chemical structures of several SERMs as well as the pure antiestrogen ICI 182,780.

gen receptor, rotating this element of the receptor away from its usual location and guiding it to a position where it appears to block access to a portion of the receptor known as Activation Function-2 (AF-2). AF-2 is implicated in the transcriptional control of estrogen-responsive genes, and mutation of the estrogen receptor in this region can convert agonists to antagonists, and vice versa [6]. Blockade of the AF-2 region by the C-terminal α-helix of the receptor following raloxifene binding would thus be expected to interfere with the transcriptional control of estrogen responsive genes.

This inference from crystallographic studies regarding the role of the C-terminal α-helix of the estrogen receptor protein in mediating differential effects of agonists and antagonists has been confirmed in experiments that have subjected the C-terminal α-helix to mutational substitutions that modify the ability of the estrogen receptor to interact with agonists and antagonists in a fusion protein assay [7]. In this work, the assay depends on the ability of ligands to bind to and modify the function of a fusion protein that consists of a recombinase component and selected components of the estrogen receptor protein. Following ligand binding to the estrogen receptor portion of the fusion protein, the recombinase portion of the protein is activated to mediate a recombination event. This event is identified by a change in phenotype of yeast that has been engineered to signal the recombination by changing color of the colonies. This model is thus able to provide insight into early functional consequences of agonist and antagonist binding in a system that does not depend on gene transcription and the complex interactions of transcriptional helper proteins that may modify transcriptional activity. The model was then tested using fusion proteins containing different sequence fragments of the estrogen receptor.

The estrogen receptor has previously been subdivided into six domains (A–F), which correspond to different functional regions of the receptor. When agonists are bound to a fusion protein derived from a wild-type estrogen receptor sequence that includes the D, E, and F domains of the receptor, the recombinase is activated by both agonists and antagonists. This implies that both ligand binding and initial functional changes following ligand binding occur similarly for both antagonists and agonists. However, it proved possible to discriminate between agonist and antagonist activity by using fusion proteins that included deleted or mutated sequences of the estrogen receptor. For instance, deletion of the D "spacer" domain from the fusion protein caused activation by agonists but not by antagonists. Further, deletion of *both* D and F domains (leaving only the E domain) restored activation by antagonists. Further experiments aimed at mutating the F domain implicated the conformational positioning of this region of the receptor as critical in mediating differential effects of agonists and antagonists [7].

In addition to the key role played by the AF-2 region there is evidence that other portions of the ligand-binding domain (within the E domain of the receptor) are crucial in mediating the antagonist actions of raloxifene. Study of a mutant ER with substitution of tyrosine for the aspartate at residue 351 renders an agonist response to raloxifene [8]. Interestingly, this substitution has been observed in experimental conditions whereby tumors have become dependent on tamoxifen for growth [9]. Further, this key residue is involved in coordination to the basic side chain of raloxifene when it is bound by wild-type estrogen receptors [5].

It thus appears that the ability of selective antagonists such as raloxifene to block some estrogen actions depends on the conformation assumed by the C-terminal α-helix after the ligand is bound. By virtue of receptor-binding affinity comparable to that of estradiol, raloxifene competes for estrogen receptor occupancy and acts as a competitive antagonist in the classical estrogen pathway. This activity establishes an estrogen antagonist profile of action.

Another possible mechanism of SERM antagonist activity relates to the effect that SERMs may have on ligand-bound dimerized estrogen receptors. Tamoxifen has been shown to "destabilize" ER dimers, resulting in interference with estrogen-stimulated gene transcription in a yeast model system [10].

Agonist Mechanisms of SERMs

Additional evidence has demonstrated that the raloxifene-bound estrogen receptor is able to *activate* transcription of other, non-ERE-dependent gene pathways. One such alternate transcription target is TGF-β. TGF-β3 is stimulated by estrogen *in vivo* and has antiresorptive properties in bone [11]. It thus represents a candidate gene to explain estrogen action in bone. Because raloxifene has been demonstrated to have estrogen-like antiresorptive activity in bone [12], it was of interest to determine whether raloxifene would promote TGF-β3 transcription in the same way estrogen does. Using an *in vitro* transient transfection system, it was demonstrated that raloxifene, in the presence of estrogen receptors, could activate TGF-β3 transcription [4].

This investigation involved a panel of mutant estrogen receptors and established that agonist actions occurred even in estrogen receptor mutants that lack the DNA-binding domain that is necessary for the activation of transcription of ERE-dependent genes. As shown in Fig. 2, various mutant estrogen receptors were

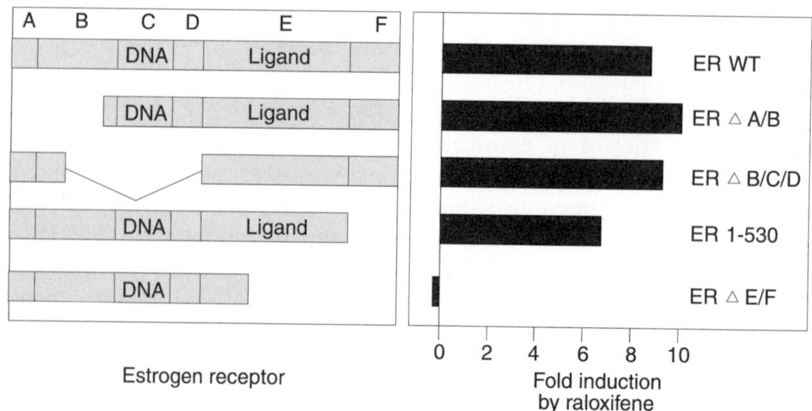

FIGURE 2 Estrogen receptor genomic material was cotransfected into host cells along with a reporter construct consisting of the TGF-β promoter placed ahead of the luciferase reporter gene. Activation of transcription by raloxifene, as determined by the induction of light production, is indicated by the horizontal bars on the right side of the figure. As shown in the first bar, cells cotransfected with the wild-type estrogen receptor demonstrated a greater than eightfold induction of activity of the reporter construct compared to control cells. Results using constructs that contained various mutant receptor sequences are shown in subsequent lines and indicate that the ligand-binding domain, but not the DNA-binding domain, of the estrogen receptor is required for raloxifene activation of TGF-β transcription. Reproduced from Yang *et al.* [4], with permission.

cotransfected along with a reporter construct consisting of the TGF-β promoter placed ahead of the luciferase reporter gene. Activation of transcription, as determined by the induction of light production, is indicated by the horizontal bars on the right side of Fig. 2. As shown in the first line of Fig. 2, cells cotransfected with the wild-type estrogen receptor demonstrated greater than eightfold induction of activity of the reporter construct compared to control cells. Results using constructs that contained various mutant receptor sequences are shown in subsequent lines. When the N-terminal portion of the estrogen receptor was deleted there was no change in transcription activation; this part of the gene sequence codes for the Activation Function-1 (AF-1) region of the receptor. AF-1 is believed to interact with helper proteins to facilitate gene transcription of certain target sequences. Similarly, elimination of the DNA-binding domain of the receptor had little effect. Deletion of the C-terminal portion of the receptor (the AF-2 region) had a modest impact on TGF-β3 promoter activity. However, when a deletion that interrupts ligand binding was used in the construct, transcription activation was eliminated. These results are consistent with the concept that raloxifene, acting by binding to the ligand-binding domain of the estrogen receptor, activates alternate gene pathways such as TGF-β3 through molecular mechanisms that are distinct from those involved in the actions of estradiol to activate "classical" estrogen target genes. Further, the fact that endogenous estrogen metabolites can activate these same pathways underscores the potential physiologic relevance of these alternate responses.

In addition to these non-ERE pathways there is evidence that different ERE-mediated pathways can respond differently to different ligands. Thus tamoxifen is as effective an agonist as estradiol in a CAT reporter system when the reporter is constructed using the β-globulin promoter, whereas it is ineffective when the reporter is constructed using a thymidylate kinase promoter. In contrast, raloxifene is nearly devoid of agonist activity with either promoter construct [13]. These results suggest that the promoter context may modulate the specificity of response to different ligands, offering additional mechanisms of SERM agonist specificity.

Alternative Pathways of Estrogen Action

Thus, it is clear that alternate pathways of estrogen action exist. These different pathways could offer attractive explanations for SERM action through the ligand-specific differential activation of different pathways. Studies have demonstrated not only that raloxifene could activate transcription through the TGF-β3 promoter, but that estradiol itself was without agonist activity in this system [4]. This indicated that various endogenous estrogenic substances may act through at least two distinct gene transcription pathways and that SERMs such as raloxifene may have agonist actions in some pathways while having antagonist actions in others. Fig-

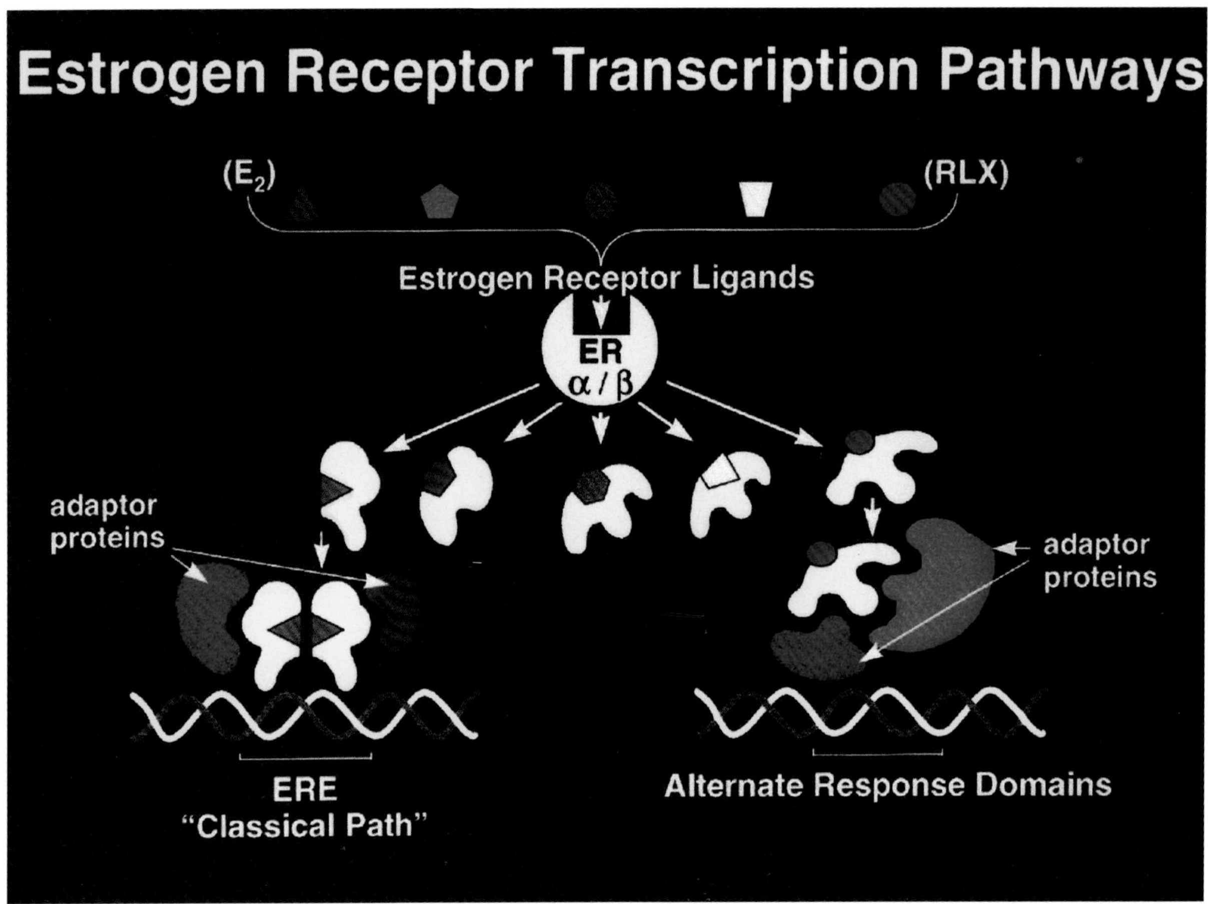

Figure 3 Dual pathways of estrogen action. Shown across the top are potential estrogen receptor ligands, which may include estradiol, estrogen metabolites, or SERMs. These ligands bind in the ligand-binding pocket of the estrogen receptor, resulting in ligand-specific conformations of the receptor. As indicated, different receptor isoforms (ERα or ERβ) may be available in the target tissue. The receptor conformation that results from interaction with estradiol leads to receptor dimerization, followed by binding to and activation of the DNA consensus sequence known as the estrogen response element (ERE), as seen on the left side of the diagram. This pathway is operative in reproductive tissues. SERMs may act as competitive antagonists of this pathway due to the inability of the SERM-bound receptor conformation to dimerize and activate ERE-dependent genes. Alternatively, receptor/ligand interactions may result in conformations that are able to activate alternate response pathways, as depicted on the right side of the figure. These pathways may be active in other estrogen responsive tissues, such as bone or vascular tissue. These alternative pathways and their ligand-specific sensitivities may explain the apparently contradictory ability of SERMs to have estrogen agonist effects in some tissues and estrogen antagonist effects in other tissues.

ure 3 presents a schematic representation of these alternative pathways of estrogen action. Shown across the top of Fig. 3 as colored geometric shapes are various potential estrogenic ligands. These all bind with high affinity to the ligand-binding domain of the estrogen receptor, which is shown as a circular shape near the center of Fig. 3. Implicit in this conceptualization is the ability of the various ligands to compete for binding occupancy in proportion to their equilibrium-binding constants and local concentrations.

After binding to the receptor, "classical" estrogen agonists then effect conformational change in the receptor, which allows two ligand-bound receptors to dimerize, interact with helper proteins, bind to the palindromic estrogen response element promoter sequence, and activate the transcription of specific target genes. However, other ligands induce a different three-dimensional conformational structure of the receptor that facilitates interaction with different helper proteins, resulting in the activation of transcription of alternate estrogen target gene sequences. As noted previously, several alternate estrogen response gene systems have been identified, including the TGF-β gene family [4], the AP-1 gene family [2], and the retinoic acid receptor gene family [3]. One may anticipate that different SERM ligands may have differential effects on transcription at these various alternate pathways. This has been demonstrated thus far for AP-1-mediated transcription vs ERE-mediated transcription [2]. An expected outcome of further investigations would be the identification of new SERMs with distinctive pharmacological profiles, pointing to the potential existence of new families of "designer estrogens."

Role of Other Accessory Factors

In addition to the possibility that different ligands may differentially activate different gene response pathways, there are other possible explanations for SERM profiles of activity. A number of transcription "helper" proteins that interact with the estrogen receptor have been identified, and these may function as coactivators or corepressors depending on the presence or absence of various ligands [14]. Studies have shown that mutant receptors lacking a functional AF-2 region are unable to discriminate between agonists and antagonists [15]. These mutant receptors are still responsive to coactivation by the helper protein known as glucocorticoid receptor interacting protein-1 (GRIP-1), and these authors hypothesize that the intact AF-2 region in the wild-type receptor acts as a "molecular switch" to activate or repress transcription, depending on the specific ligand that is bound [15].

Role of Estrogen Receptor Isoforms

Additional mechanisms of tissue selectivity of SERMs may also depend on the discovery of a novel estrogen receptor isoform known as ERβ [16]. ERβ has substantial sequence homology with ERα, but the presence of distinct isoforms of the estrogen receptor offers an additional potential mechanism for ligand-dependent tissue selectivity. For instance, the ability of raloxifene or other ligands such as estradiol or tamoxifen to stimulate transcription at a specific estrogen target sequence (the AP-1 promoter site) is highly dependent on the species of estrogen receptor used in the assay [2]. Thus, estradiol and tamoxifen are highly effective estrogen agonists at the AP-1 site when ERα is employed in a cotransfection assay in which an estrogen receptor (ERα or ERβ) and an AP-1 reporter construct are employed. In contrast, raloxifene and the antiestrogen ICI 164381 are nonstimulatory when ERα is the receptor isoform employed. Alternatively, when ERβ is used, estradiol is devoid of activity, but raloxifene and ICI 164381 are strongly stimulatory. Given that estrogen receptor isoform distribution varies from tissue to tissue [17,18] these results offer further potential explanations for differential tissue effects of SERMs.

Another possible mediator of selective actions of different ligands involves the recognized ability of ligand-bound estrogen receptors to form heterodimers in which a ligand–ERα complex can dimerize with a ligand–ERβ complex [19]. The biological significance of these heterodimers remains speculative, but these various results involving estrogen receptor isoforms further underscore the potential range of SERM specificities and the possibilities of developing new compounds with unique tissue-specific profiles of activity.

Summary of SERM Mechanisms

There are thus many potential explanations for the tissue selective actions of SERMs. These include differential effects of ligands on receptor conformation, leading to differential effects on gene transcription of several different gene families. The roles of different domains of the estrogen receptor and of different transcriptional helper proteins are only recently being elucidated. Further, ligand-specific modulation of the function of the estrogen receptor isoforms α and β, coupled with the emerging understanding of the tissue distribution of these receptor species, can explain the tissue selective estrogen agonist and antagonist action of estrogen receptor ligands in ways that are only now being unraveled. The extent to which these new insights will provide a basis for rational drug design to optimize tissue targeting of hormone agonist and/or antagonist activity is uncertain at present, but these new insights should provide a coherent basis for further investigations.

TAMOXIFEN

Tamoxifen is a nonsteroidal SERM compound initially produced in England in 1966 [20]. It was originally developed as an antifertility agent but, paradoxically, was found to induce ovulation in infertile women [21,22]. It was also found in animal studies that this agent had antitumor activity in carcinogen-induced rat mammary tumor models [23,24]. In 1971, the clinical efficacy of tamoxifen in women with metastatic breast cancer was reported [25]. At that time, tamoxifen was only one of numerous "antiestrogen" compounds being evaluated for the treatment of advanced breast cancer, but its distinct advantages were its high antitumor potency and its low side effect profile. In fact, tamoxifen seemed to have none of the troublesome side effects observed with high-dose estrogen therapy or androgen therapy that were standard treatments at that time.

In 1973, tamoxifen was approved in the United Kingdom for the treatment of breast cancer, with subsequent approval in the United States for the treatment of advanced disease in postmenopausal women in 1977. Since that time, additional approvals have been obtained for other applications of tamoxifen, including its use as the initial endocrine therapy for estrogen receptor (ER)-positive disseminated breast cancer in premenopausal women, for the treatment of metastatic breast cancer in men and, in 1998, for the prevention of breast cancer in healthy women at high risk. The Early Breast Cancer Trialists' Collaborative Group meta-analysis, published in 1992, strongly supported the case that adjuvant tamoxifen therapy prolongs both disease-free and overall survival 10 years after diagnosis [26].

Most of the approximately six million patient years of exposure to tamoxifen results from its use in the treatment of breast cancer. Because prolonged tamoxifen therapy is prescribed for many women and survival occurs for long periods after treatment, it became important to know whether the drug had effects on other organ systems, such as the skeleton.

Preclinical Studies on Bone

In 1986, an examination of tamoxifen on bone using an *in vitro* system demonstrated that tamoxifen inhibited parathyroid hormone-induced bone resorption in fetal rat long bones [27]. Subsequent reports of the effects of tamoxifen on skeletal mass in animals were contradictory. A reduction in bone mass, measured by femur ash weight and X-ray densitometry, in ovariectomized rats treated with tamoxifen compared with placebos was reported [28]. In contrast, tamoxifen was found to maintain bone mass in mature ovariectomized and young growing rats [29].

Reports on the effects of tamoxifen on bone remodeling were also conflicting. One study demonstrated that tamoxifen did not prevent calcitriol-stimulated bone resorption in rats *in vivo* [30]. However, another study of ovariectomized rats showed that tamoxifen acted as a potent inhibitor of bone resorption and prevented the increases in osteoclast number and resorbing surface length that were usually seen with ovarian hormone deficiency [31]. A number of later studies confirmed the antiresorptive effects of tamoxifen and supported the hypothesis that tamoxifen prevented skeletal alterations from ovarian hormone deficiency, possibly by acting as an estrogen agonist on bone [27,31a].

Clinical Studies on Bone

Although there was initially a concern that tamoxifen might accelerate postmenopausal bone loss in human subjects, several studies have reported protection against bone loss. The first clinical studies were performed in women receiving adjuvant tamoxifen for the treatment of early stage breast cancer. Dual-photon absorptiometry was used to study the effects of tamoxifen (10 mg twice daily) on bone mineral density (BMD) of the lumbar spine and radius and on biochemical measures of bone metabolism in 140 postmenopausal women with axillary node-negative breast cancer in a 2-year randomized, double-blind, placebo-controlled trial [32]. In the tamoxifen-treated group, the mean BMD of the lumbar spine increased by 0.61% per year, whereas in those given placebo it decreased by 1.00% per year ($p < 0.001$). There was no difference between the two groups in radial BMD. Serum osteocalcin and alkaline phosphatase concentrations, markers of bone turnover, decreased significantly in women given tamoxifen ($p < 0.001$ for both variables). Data published on the same cohort after 5 years of tamoxifen treatment showed that the effect of tamoxifen on the lumbar spine BMD persisted [33]. Serum indices of bone turnover were also significantly lower in tamoxifen-treated subjects after 5 years of follow-up. Other studies have reported similar findings [34,35].

In a study of tamoxifen effects on bone remodeling, transiliac bone biopsies were obtained from 41 women with breast cancer. Twenty-two of those women had been treated with tamoxifen for a minimum of 15 months and 19 had been untreated. A significantly lower tissue-based bone formation rate and a longer remodeling period were found in tamoxifen-treated women [36]. Mean and maximum resorption cavity depth were reduced in tamoxifen-treated patients compared with untreated patients. Calculated and directly measured indices of cancellous bone structure were similar in the two groups, although data indicated a trend toward greater connectivity of bone in tamoxifen-treated patients.

The effect of tamoxifen on BMD and bone metabolism has also been studied in postmenopausal women without breast cancer [37]. Fifty-seven subjects were randomized to receive either tamoxifen (20 mg/day) or placebo for 2 years. In women taking tamoxifen, the mean BMD of the lumbar spine increased by 1.4% whereas in women given placebo it declined by 0.7% ($p < 0.1$). The effect of tamoxifen was maximal after 1 year, with no further separation of the groups thereafter. There was no significant effect of tamoxifen on the proximal femur. Significant decreases in serum alkaline phosphatase and urinary excretion of hydroxyproline, *n*-telopeptides, and calcium occurred, results similar to those found in postmenopausal women with breast cancer.

The effect of tamoxifen on BMD in premenopausal women has also been evaluated. Two studies in premenopausal women, with and without breast cancer, have shown decreases in BMD at the radius, spine, and hip [38,39]. Tamoxifen was evaluated in a breast cancer chemoprevention trial involving 179 healthy premenopausal women randomized to 20 mg/day of the agent or to placebo [39]. BMD decreased progressively and significantly in the lumbar spine and the hip for women on tamoxifen but not for those on placebo. The mean annual loss in lumbar BMD per year over the 3-year study period in tamoxifen-treated patients who remained premenopausal throughout the study was 1.44% compared with a modest gain of 0.24% per year for women on placebo. In the same study, however, data from healthy postmenopausal women showed that tamoxifen had the opposite effect. Tamoxifen thus appeared to have estrogen-like properties in bone when used in the presence of low circulating estrogen levels, but antagonist effects when circulating estrogen levels were high. It has been proposed that the prevailing estrogen milieu is therefore important and may dictate tamoxifen's ultimate activity in bone. However, in a study of 38 postmenopausal women examining the effects of combination therapy with tamoxifen and estrogen, contradictory results emerged. In these subjects, tamoxifen alone led to an annual increase in BMD of the femur and spine by 2 and 1.5%, respectively, when compared with placebo [40]. The addition of hormone replacement therapy to tamoxifen resulted in a further 2% annual increase in BMD of the femur and no effect on spine BMD. Thus, further studies are needed to clarify this issue.

Preliminary data on the effects of tamoxifen on fracture risk in healthy pre- and postmenopausal women have been reported from the NSABP Breast Cancer Prevention Trial, involving over 13,000 women at high risk of developing breast cancer. After an average period of observation of 3.6 years, there was a 35% ($p = 0.013$) reduction in risk of fractures of the spine, hip, and wrist with tamoxifen compared with placebo [41].

Clinical Studies on Serum Lipids and Cardiovascular Events

Studies have shown that tamoxifen exerts a favorable effect on the lipid profile in postmenopausal women with early stage breast cancer [42]. In a 2-year, randomized, double-blind, placebo-controlled trial of therapy with tamoxifen (10 mg twice a day) in 140 postmenopausal women with a history of node-negative breast cancer, tamoxifen-treated women showed a significant decrease in fasting plasma levels of total cholesterol after 3 months. The mean decrease of 26 mg/dl with tamoxifen contrasted with a mean increase of 2 mg/dl with placebo. The decrease in total cholesterol seen in the tamoxifen-treated women persisted at 6 and 12 months. Estimated low-density lipoprotein (LDL) cholesterol levels were also decreased significantly in tamoxifen-treated women compared with placebo at 3, 6, and 12 months. At 3 months, the mean decrease for tamoxifen-treated women was 28 mg/dl compared with a mean increase of 2 mg/dl for placebo-treated women. During the first 12 months, plasma triglyceride levels increased, and small but significant decreases in high-density lipoprotein (HDL) cholesterol were observed for tamoxifen-treated women. However, ratios of total cholesterol to HDL cholesterol and of LDL to HDL cholesterol changed favorably.

The lipid profile changes observed with tamoxifen use may play a role in reducing mortality from coronary artery disease. Data from an adjuvant tamoxifen trial indicate that there may be a reduction in the incidence of fatal myocardial infarction in postmenopausal women receiving tamoxifen compared with controls [43]. A similar study showed a significant reduction in the incidence of hospital admissions for cardiac disease in postmenopausal women taking tamoxifen as adjuvant therapy when compared with controls [44].

Clinical Studies on the Uterus

A major concern of long-term tamoxifen use is uterine stimulation and the increased risk of endometrial cancer. The National Surgical Adjuvant Breast and Bowel Project, the largest randomized trial of adjuvant tamoxifen versus placebo, reported an absolute risk of tamoxifen-induced endometrial cancer of one to two cases annually per 1000 women treated and a relative risk of two to three times greater than that seen in women with breast cancer not treated with tamoxifen [45]. This study found that 15 of 1419 women randomized to receive 20 mg of tamoxifen daily for 5 years developed endometrial cancer, as did 8 of 1220 nonrandomized tamoxifen-treated patients. Two of 1424 women randomized to receive placebo, but who subsequently developed recurrent disease and were treated with tamoxifen, also developed endometrial cancer.

The cumulative incidence of endometrial cancers in all women treated with tamoxifen in the major adjuvant trials has been 0.9%, compared with 0.2% in the control groups [46]. It appears that the risk of endometrial cancer increases with the duration of tamoxifen use. Investigators have reported that women who receive tamoxifen for at least 5 years were at greater risk of developing endometrial carcinoma than those who received it for a shorter period of time [45,47].

Adverse Effects from Tamoxifen

The most frequent side effects associated with tamoxifen are hot flashes, especially in premenopausal women; mild nausea; vaginal bleeding or discharge; and fluid retention. Thromboembolic disease has been reported to occur infrequently with tamoxifen administration [48]. Data from adjuvant trials indicate a possible increase in, but low overall incidence of, thromboembolic disorders (1 to 3%) in tamoxifen users that is similar to the risk seen with hormone replacement therapy [45,46,49]. Some studies attribute this to a decline in the activity of antithrombin III with tamoxifen; however, other studies have failed to detect an association [50,51].

RALOXIFENE

Initial studies with raloxifene in the 1980s were directed at evaluating its potential in the management of patients with breast cancer. Preclinical studies validated its ability to inhibit the binding of estradiol to the estrogen receptor and to block the estradiol-dependent proliferation of MCF-7 breast cancer cells [52]. Later studies in rodents confirmed that raloxifene effects on carcinogen-induced tumors were similar to those with tamoxifen [53]. Very limited studies in women with advanced breast cancer who had recently ceased to respond to tamoxifen revealed no antitumor effect of raloxifene in this population [54]. The agent was not pursued further at that time as a cancer therapy, but subsequent recognition of its activity in bone and its potential utility as an alternative to estrogen as an osteoporosis therapy led to its rebirth. In particular, preclinical data suggested that raloxifene fulfilled the SERM profile of inhibiting bone loss, lowering cholesterol, and causing no stimulation of breast or uterine tissue. These findings led to a series of human studies evaluating the safety and efficacy of raloxifene in postmenopausal women in the prevention and treatment of osteoporosis. As of this writing, the agent has been approved in a number of countries for the prevention of osteoporosis, and phase III trials are near completion to evaluate the efficacy and safety of raloxifene in the treatment of established osteoporosis.

Preclinical Studies on Bone

Preclinical studies have evaluated the effects of raloxifene on bone mass, quality, and architecture in ovariectomized rats in experiments extending over 12 months. Raloxifene was found to be comparable to both estrogen and tamoxifen [12] in the prevention of cancellous bone loss as assessed by bone densitometry [12,55] and histomorphometric volume analysis [56]. Studies revealed that 17 α-ethynyl estradiol was approximately 25 times more potent than raloxifene in preserving bone mineral density in the ovariectomized rat [55]. Also in the ovariectomized rat model, raloxifene has been shown to reduce urinary collagen cross-links and serum osteocalcin to sham-operated levels comparable to those seen with estrogen [57].

Histomorphometric analyses in the rat tibia indicated that both estrogen and raloxifene inhibited the increases in osteoclast number, eroded perimeter, trabecular separation, and bone turnover that arise soon after ovariectomy, although estrogen substantially reduced the cancellous bone formation rate whereas raloxifene did not [58]. In other studies, however, the addition of raloxifene after significant bone loss had been established led to similar reductions in both bone resorption and bone formation. Biomechanical strength after ovariectomy in rats was studied in the lumbar vertebrae and neck and diaphysis of the femur; raloxifene and estrogen were similar in maintaining mechanical integrity and strength in this model [59]. Raloxifene has also been shown to prevent the bone loss that occurs in female rats treated with an LH-RH agonist [60].

Clinical Studies on Bone

Effects of raloxifene, 200 or 600 mg per day, versus conjugated estrogens, 0.625 mg per day, and placebo on markers of bone turnover were evaluated in 251 healthy postmenopausal women treated in a randomized, double-blind trial over 8 weeks. Significant reductions in serum alkaline phosphatase, urinary pyridinoline, and urinary calcium were found with both doses of raloxifene and estrogen compared to placebo, and the magnitude of the changes was similar with the three active treatments [61]. However, a study comparing conjugated estrogens (0.625 mg) with 60 mg of raloxifene showed that while estrogen suppressed serum levels of insulin-like growth factors, the 60-mg raloxifene dose did not to the same degree [62].

Bone remodeling in early postmenopausal women receiving cyclic hormone replacement therapy, 60 mg raloxifene or no treatment was evaluated in a study using calcium tracer kinetic methods with a constant diet and metabolic balance conditions [63]. Subjects were studied at baseline and at 4 and 31 weeks to allow an assessment of both early and late changes in remodeling. Both estrogen and raloxifene produced significant positive calcium balance shifts and significant reductions in bone resorption at both time points, but the suppressant effect of estrogen on resorption was greater than raloxifene at 31 weeks. There was no change in bone formation by either agent at 4 weeks, but at 31 weeks estrogen but not raloxifene reduced formation. At the 31 week point, therefore, the suppression of remodeling was greater for estrogen than raloxifene, although the remodeling balance was the same for both agents. The authors point out that the lack of suppression of formation by raloxifene at 31 weeks is consistent with the studies in ovariectomized rats in which estrogen but not raloxifene suppressed cancellous bone-forming activity [58] and the failure of raloxifene to suppress some serum markers of bone formation in postmenopausal women [62].

The effects of raloxifene at doses of 30, 60, or 150 mg daily or daily placebo for 24 months were evaluated in 601 postmenopausal women with baseline lumbar spine bone mineral density T scores ranging from 2.5 SD below to 2.0 SD above the mean value of young normal women [64]. As shown in Fig. 4, each of the doses of raloxifene produced small but significant increases in bone mineral density of the lumbar spine, total hip, and total body whereas placebo use led to a small decrease in bone density. The differences in bone density between raloxifene (60 mg) and placebo at 24 months were 2.4% at the lumbar spine, 2.4% at the total hip, and 2.0% for the total body ($p < 0.001$ for all comparisons). At the total body and the total hip the magnitude of these changes was roughly similar to that seen with both conjugated estrogen and 5 mg of alendronate in the prevention of menopausal bone loss [16], but was about 50% less than that seen at the lumbar spine [16]. The raloxifene trial differed from the alen-

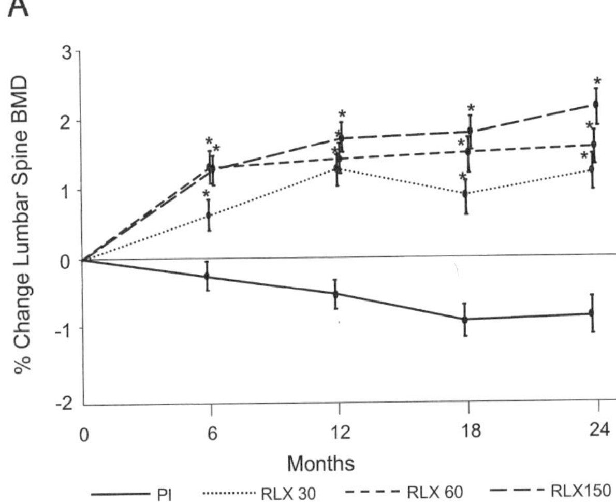

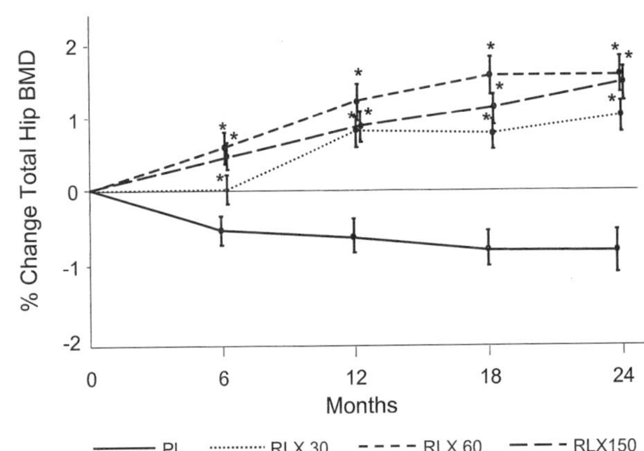

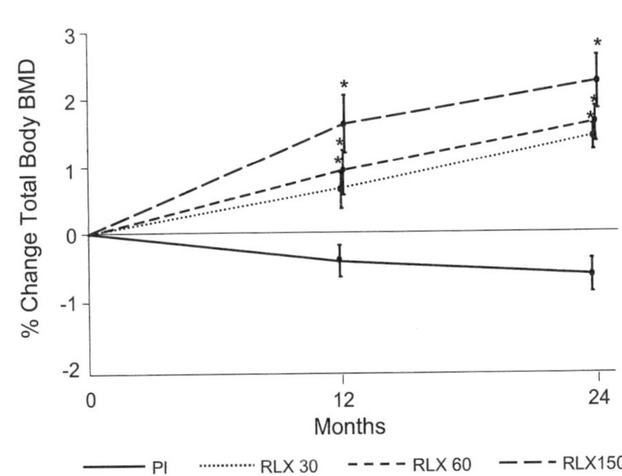

Figure 4 Effects of placebo and raloxifene at doses of 30, 60, and 150 mg on BMD of the spine (a), total hip (b), and total body (c) during a 24-month-long controlled clinical trial in postmenopausal women with initial T scores ranging from −2.5 to 2.0 SD. Significant increases in BMD compared to placebo were seen with all raloxifene doses at all postbaseline time points shown $*p < 0.029$. Reproduced with permission from Delmas *et al.* [64].

dronate study in the magnitude of the degree of bone loss in the placebo groups, so the direct comparison of data must be made with caution.

In this same study, all doses of raloxifene led to statistically significant decreases in three markers of bone turnover, serum bone-specific alkaline phosphatase, and osteocalcin and urinary C-telopeptide of type 1 collagen (data on the latter two biomarkers are shown in Fig. 5); at month 24 the 60-mg dose was associated with decreases in the median values of the three markers by 15, 23, and 34%, respectively, which represented a decrease from mean baseline values typical of postmenopausal women to values similar to those of premenopausal women [65].

A 6-month prevention study involving 51 older postmenopausal women (18 years postmenopause) compared 60 mg of raloxifene with 0.625 mg of conjugated estrogens and placebo with respect to changes in bone mineral density at the lumbar spine and hip [62]. There were significant increases above baseline at the lumbar spine for both estrogen and raloxifene, but 6 months of raloxifene yielded a significantly lower percentage increase than estrogen (1.3% vs 3.2%, $p = 0.029$). At the femoral neck, raloxifene patients had a significant increase in bone density (2.8%) vs a nonsignificant increase for estrogen patients (1.6%), but these changes did not differ significantly from each other in this small study.

To date there has been only one completed study reporting the effects of raloxifene in older postmenopausal women with established osteoporosis (143 women with a mean age of 68 years and at least one prevalent vertebral fracture) who were treated for 1 year with placebo or one of two doses of raloxifene in a randomized blinded design [66]. In this study, all patients received supplements of calcium (750 mg) and vitamin D (400 U) daily. Small but significant increases in bone density were seen at the 1-year time point at the total proximal femur and ultra distal radius with 60 mg raloxifene and at the ultradistal radius with 120 mg raloxifene, each compared with placebo. Both 60 and 120 mg of raloxifene led to significant decreases (compared to placebo) in median values for serum bone-specific alkaline phosphatase (44 and 38%) and osteocalcin (32 and 32%) and urinary C-telopeptide of type 1 collagen (54 and 49%).

More recently, 2-year interim analysis results from a large prospective randomized, placebo-controlled, double-blind clinical trial comparing two doses of raloxifene (60 and 120 mg per day) to placebo in a cohort of 7705 postmenopausal women with prevalent osteoporosis were reported to show a 44% reduction in percentage of women experiencing incident vertebral fracture [67]. Raloxifene reduced the percentage of women in this study experiencing two or more incident fractures by 61%. All subjects in the trial received daily calcium (500 mg) and vitamin D (400–600 IU) supplementation. The bone mineral density changes seen in the spine and hip in this study were similar to those seen in the raloxifene osteoporosis prevention trials, with a 2–3% increase compared to the control group.

Clinical Studies on Serum Lipids and Coagulation Factors

Measurement of serum lipids has been an additional assessment in two studies in which the effects of raloxi-

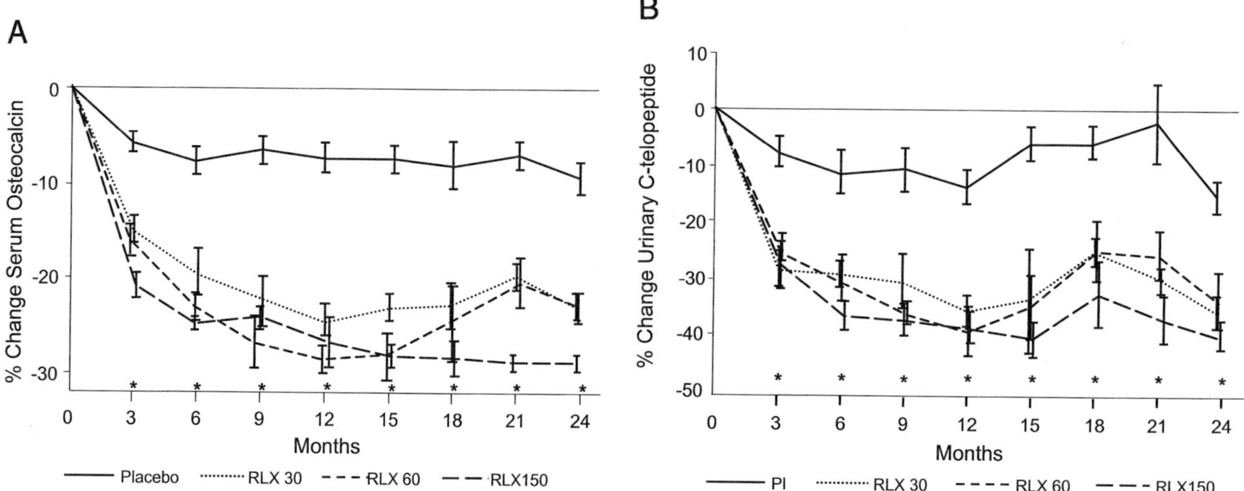

FIGURE 5 These data describe changes in bone turnover markers, serum osteocalcin (a) and urinary C-telopeptide (b), in the study described in Fig. 4. All doses of raloxifene significantly reduced these markers at all time points as shown. *All $p < 0.05$ vs placebo. Reproduced with permission from Delmas *et al.* [64].

fene on bone mineral density were examined in postmenopausal women [61,64]. In a short-term study of 251 postmenopausal women treated with 200 or 600 mg raloxifene daily for 8 weeks [61], serum LDL cholesterol was found to be reduced by 9.5 and 12.6%, respectively, by the two raloxifene doses, compared to baseline; there was no increase in HDL with either dose.

Subsequently, these data were confirmed by results of the osteoporosis prevention study described earlier with 601 postmenopausal women receiving either 60 or 120 mg of raloxifene or placebo daily for 2 years. Significant median percentage decreases from baseline were found at 2 years for total cholesterol (6.4 and 9.7%) and LDL (10.1 and 14.1%); there was no significant increase in HDL nor was there an increase in triglycerides [64] as may be seen with estrogen.

In a study comparing the effects of raloxifene and estrogen on serum lipids and coagulation factors [68], 390 healthy postmenopausal women were randomized to placebo, hormone replacement therapy (HRT) with conjugated estrogen (0.625 mg) and medroxyprogesterone acetate (2.5 mg), or raloxifene (60 or 120 mg), all taken daily for 6 months. A series of serum lipids and coagulation factors were measured at baseline and at 3 and 6 months. Compared with placebo, both raloxifene doses significantly reduced LDL cholesterol by 12%, a result similar to the significant reduction of 14% seen with HRT. HRT significantly increased HDL (11%), but raloxifene had no effect; however, raloxifene raised HDL subfraction 2 cholesterol significantly by 15–17%, contrasted with a significant 33% increase with HRT. Raloxifene but not HRT significantly lowered fibrinogen by 12–14%, and HRT increased triglycerides by 20% and decreased plasminogen activator inhibitor-1 by 29% whereas raloxifene had no effect on these levels. The pattern of raloxifene-induced effects had a greater resemblance to patterns seen with tamoxifen than estrogen, and as noted earlier, patients with breast cancer receiving tamoxifen have a lower risk of fatal myocardial infarction [43]. It has been proposed that these favorable effects of raloxifene upon several of these biochemical markers may be associated with some protection against cardiovascular disease, but further studies are required to determine if this is the case.

Clinical Studies on the Uterus

Studies evaluating uterine safety with raloxifene have included evaluations of endometrial thickness utilizing transvaginal ultrasound and endometrial biopsies performed in healthy postmenopausal women as well as in women participating in clinical trials for the prevention or treatment of osteoporosis. There were no changes in endometrial thickness with 60 or 150 mg of raloxifene compared with placebo in studies with nearly 1000 women [69]; 150 mg raloxifene daily for 1 year had the same lack of endometrial stimulation in another study in which the comparator was hormone replacement therapy; estrogen use in that study produced significant increases in endometrial thickness and uterine volume [70]. Endometrial biopsies after 8 weeks of raloxifene, 200 to 600 mg per day, revealed no endometrial proliferation [71]. In the osteoporosis prevention study described earlier, 2 years of raloxifene at doses of 30, 60, or 150 mg daily did not differ from placebo in terms of endometrial thickness [64]; the same absence of uterine stimulation was found in the 1-year study of raloxifene (60 or 120 mg) versus placebo in postmenopausal women with osteoporosis [66]. These data support the preclinical finding that raloxifene has estrogen antagonist effects at the uterus, unlike tamoxifen with its partial agonist effect at the endometrium.

Clinical Studies of the Breast

Raloxifene use was not associated with mastalgia in osteoporosis patients receiving 60 or 120 mg per day for a year [66]. In addition, preliminary safety analyses of breast cancer incidence in the more than 7000 women enrolled in osteoporosis clinical trials with raloxifene revealed that with a median exposure of 28 months of treatment there was a marked reduction of about 50% in the incidence of estrogen receptor-positive breast cancers in raloxifene-treated women [72,73]. The risk reduction in breast cancer seen to date with raloxifene in an osteoporosis population is similar to that seen with tamoxifen over a somewhat longer period of observation (42 months on average) in normal women at high risk for breast cancer [41]. Further studies are clearly needed to determine what the long-term effects of both raloxifene and tamoxifen will be with regard to possible breast cancer risk reduction.

Adverse Effects from Raloxifene

Raloxifene use is associated with an increase in the frequency but not severity of hot flashes in women who experience them and with muscle cramps (6–7% of women in the clinical trials to date) [74]. A three-to fourfold increase in the relative risk of venous thromboembolic disease was seen with raloxifene [74], a finding comparable to what has been reported with both postmenopausal estrogen [75–77] and tamoxifen [48,49].

References

1. Clark, J. H., Schrader, W. T., and O'Malley, B. W., "Textbook of Endocrinology" (J. D. Wilson and D. W. Foster, eds.), pp. 35–90. Saunders, New York, 1992.
2. Paech, K., Webb, P., Kuiper, G. G. J. M., Nilsson, S., Gustafsson, J., Kushner, P., and Scanlan, T. S. Differential ligand activation of estrogen receptors ERα and ERβ at AP1 sites. *Science* **277,** 1508–1510 (1997).
3. Elgort, M. G., Zou, A., Marschke, K. B., and Allegretto, E. A. Estrogen and estrogen receptor antagonists stimulate transcription from the human retinoic acid receptor-alpha 1 promoter via a novel sequence. *Mol. Endocrinol.* **10,** 477–487 (1996).
4. Yang, N. N., Venugopalan, M., Hardikar, S., and Glasebrook, A. Indentification of an estrogen response element activated by metabolites of 17β estradiol and raloxifene. *Science* **273,** 1222–1225 (1996).
5. Brzozowski, A. M., Pike, A. C., Dauter, Z., Hubbard, R. E., Bonn, T., Engstrom, O., Ohman, L., Greene, G. L., Gustafsson, J. A., and Carlquist, M. Molecular basis of agonism and antagonism in the oestrogen receptor. *Nature* **389,** 753–758 (1997).
6. Montano, M. M., Ekena, K., Krueger, K. D., Keller, A. L., and Katzenellenbogen, B. S. Human estrogen receptor ligand activity inversion mutants: receptors that interpret antiestrogens as estrogens and estrogens as antiestrogens and discriminate among different antiestrogens. *Mol. Endocrinol.* **10,** 230–242 (1996).
7. Nichols, M., Rientjes, J. M., and Stewart, A. F. Different positioning of the ligand binding domain helix 12 and the F domain of the estrogen receptor accounts for functional differences between agonists and antagonists. *EMBO J.* **17,** 765–773 (1998).
8. Levenson, A. S., and Jordan, V. C. The key to the antiestrogenic mechanism of raloxifene is amino acid 351 (aspartate) in the estrogen receptor. *Cancer Res.* **58,** 1872–1875 (1998).
9. Levenson, A. S., Catherino, W. H., and Jordan, V. C. Estrogenic activity is increased for an antiestrogen by a natural mutation of the estrogen receptor. *J. Steroid Biochem. Mol. Biol.* **60,** 261–268 (1997).
10. Wang, H., Peters, G. A., Zeng, X., Tang, M., Ip, W., and Khan, S. A. Yeast two-hybrid system demonstrates that estrogen receptor dimerization is ligand-dependent *in vitro. J. Biol. Chem.* **40,** 23322–23329 (1995).
11. Yang, N. N., Bryant, H. U., Hardikar, S., Sato, M., Galvin, R. J., Glasebrook, A. L., and Termine, J. D. Estrogen and raloxifene stimulate transforming growth factor-beta 3 gene expression in rat bone: a potential mechanism for estrogen- or ralozifene-mediated bone maintenance. *Endocrinology* **137,** 2075–2084 (1996).
12. Black, L. J., Sato, M., Rowley, E. R., Magee, D. E., Bekele, A., Williams, D. C., Cullinan, G. J., Bendele, R., Kauffman, R. F., Bensch, W. R., Frolik, C. A., Termine, J. D., and Bryant, H. U. Raloxifene (LY139481 HCl) prevents bone loss and reduces serum cholesterol without causing uterine hypertrophy in ovariectomized rats. *J. Clin. Invest.* **93,** 63–69 (1994).
13. Watanabe, T., Inoue, S., Ogawa, S., Ishii, Y., Hiroi, H., Ikeda, K., Orimo, A., and Muramatsu, M. Agonistic effect of tamoxifen is dependent on cell type, ERE promoter context, and estrogen receptor subtype: functional difference between estrogen receptors alpha and beta. *Biochem. Biophys. Res. Commun.* **236,** 140–145 (1997).
14. Shibata, H., Spencer, T. E., Onate, S. A., Jenster, G., Tsai, S. Y., Tsai, M.-J., and O'Malley, B. W. Role of co-activators and co-repressors in the mechanism of steroid/thyroid receptor action. *Recent Prog. Horm. Res.* **52,** 141–165 (1997).
15. Norris, J. D., Fan, D., Stallcup, M. R., and McDonnell, D. P. Enhancement of estrogen receptor transcriptional activity by the coactivator GRIP-1 highlights the role of activation function 2 in determining estrogen receptor pharmacology. *J. Biol. Chem.* **273,** 6679–6688 (1998).
16. Kuiper, G. G., and Gustafsson, J. A. The novel estrogen receptor-beta subtype: potential role in the cell- and promoter-specific actions of estrogens and anti-estrogens. *FEBS Lett* **410,** 87–90 (1997).
17. Couse, J. F., Lindzey, J., Grandien, K., Gustafsson, J., and Korach, K. Tissue distribution and quantitative analysis of estrogen receptor-α (ERα) and estrogen receptor-β (ERβ) messenger ribonucleic acid in the wild-type and ERα-knockout mouse. *Endocrinology* **139,** 4613–4621 (1997).
18. Kuiper, G. G., Carlsson, B., Grandien, K., Enmark, E., Haggblad, J., Nilsson, S., and Gustafsson, J. A. Comparison of the ligand binding specificity and transcript tissue distribution of estrogen receptors alpha and beta. *Endocrinology* **138,** 863–870 (1997).
19. Pace, P., Taylor, J., Suntharalingam, S., Coombes, R. C., and Ali, S. Human estrogen receptor beta binds DNA in a manner similar to and dimerizes with estrogen receptor alpha. *J. Biol. Chem.* **272,** 25832–25838 (1997).
20. Harper, M. J. K., and Walpole, A. L. Contrasting endocrine activities of *cis* and *trans* isomers in a series of substitutes triphenyethylenes. *Nature* **212,** 87 (1966).
21. Klopper, A., and Hall, M. New synthetic agent for the induction of ovulation: Preliminary trial in women. *Br. Med. J.* **2,** 152–154 (1971).
22. Williamson, J. G., and Ellis, J. D. The induction of ovulation by tamoxifen. *J. Obstet. Gynaecol. Br. Commonwealth* **80,** 844–847 (1973).
23. Jordan, V. C. Antitumor activity of the antiestrogen ICI 46,474 (tamoxifen) in the dimethylbenzanthracene (DMBA)-induced rat mammary carcinoma model. *J. Steroid Biochem.* **5,** 354 (1974).
24. Nicholson, R. I., and Golder, M. P. The effect of synthetic antioestrogens on the growth and biochemistry of rat mammary tumours. *Eur. J. Cancer* **11,** 571–579 (1975).
25. Cole, M. P., Jones, C. T. A., and Todd, I. D. H. A new antioestrogen agent in late breast cancer: An early clinical appraisal of ICI 46,474. *Br. J. Cancer* **25,** 270–275.
26. Early Breast Cancer Trialists' Collaborative Group. Systemic treatment of early breast cancer by hormonal, cytotoxic immunotherapy. *Lancet* **339,** 1–15, 71–85 (1992).
27. Stewart, P. H., and Stern, P. H. Effects of the antiestrogens tamoxifen and clomiphene on bone resorption in vitro. *Endocrinology* **118,** 125–131 (1986).
28. Feldmann, S., Minne, H. W., Parvizi, S., Pfeifer, M., Lempert, U. G., Bauss, F., and Ziegler, R., *Bone Miner.* **7,** 245–254 (1989).
29. Turner, R. T., Wakley, G. K., Hannon, K. S., and Bell, N. H. Tamoxifen prevents the skeletal effects of ovarian hormone deficiency in rats. *J. Bone Miner. Res.* **2,** 449–456 (1987).
30. Goulding, A., Gold, E., and Fisher, L. Effects of clomiphene and tamoxifen in vivo on the bone resorbing effects of parathyroid hormone and of high oral doses of calcitriol ($1,25(OH)_2D_3$) in rats with intact ovarian function consuming low calcium diet. *Bone Miner.* **8,** 185–193 (1990).
31. Turner, R. T., Wakley, G. K., Hannon, K. S., Bell, N. H. Tamoxifen onhibits osteoclast-mediated resorption of trabecular bone in ovarian hormone-deficient rats. *Endocrinology* **122,** 1146–1150 (1988).

31a. Arnett, T. R., Lindsay, R., and Dempster, D. W. Effect of oestrogen and antioestrogens on osteoclast activity in vitro (abstract). *J. Bone Miner. Res.* **1**(Suppl.), 99 (1986). [Abstract]

32. Love, R. R., Mazess, R. B., Barden, H. S., Epstein, S., Newcomb, P. A., Jordan, V. C., Carbone, P. P., and Demets, D. L. Effects of tamoxifen on bone mineral density in postmenopausal women with breast cancer. *N. Engl. J. Med.* **326,** 852–856 (1992).
33. Love, R. R., Barden, H. S., Mazess, R. B., Epstein, S., and Chappell, R. J. Effect of tamoxifen on lumbar spine bone mineral density in postmenopausal women after 5 years. *Arch. Intern. Med.* **154,** 2585–2588 (1994).
34. Ward, R. L., Morgan, G., Dalley, D., and Kelly, P. J. Tamoxifen reduces bone turnover and prevents lumbar spine and proximal femoral bone loss in early postmenopausal women. *Bone Miner.* **22,** 87–94 (1993).
35. Kristensen, B., Ejlertsen, B., Dalgaard, P., Larsen, L., Holmegaard, S. N., Transbol, I., and Mouridsen, H. T. Tamoxifen and bone metabolism in postmenopausal low-risk breast cancer patients: a randomized study. *J. Clin. Oncol.* **12,** 992–997 (1994).
36. Wright, C. D., Garrahan, N. J., Stanton, M., Gazet, J. C., Mansell, R. E., and Compston, J. E. Effect of long term tamoxifen therapy on cancellous bone remodeling and structure in women with breast cancer. *J. Bone Miner. Res.* **9,** 153–159 (1994).
37. Grey, A. B., Stapleton, J. P., Evans, M. C., Tatnell, M. A., Ames, R. W., and Reid, I. R. The effect of the antiestrogen tamoxifen on bone mineral density in normal late postmenopausal women. *Am. J. Med.* **99,** 636–641 (1995).
38. Gotfredson, A., Christiansen, C., and Palshof, T. The effect of tamoxifen on bone mineral content in premenopausal women with breast cancer. *Cancer* **53,** 853–857 (1984).
39. Powles, T. J., Hickish, T., Kanis, J. A., Tidy, A., and Ashley, S. Effect of tamoxifen on bone mineral density measured by dual energy x-ray absorptiometry in healthy premenopausal and postmenopausal women. *J. Clin. Oncol.* **14,** 78–84 (1996).
40. Chang, J., Powles, T. J., Ashley, S. E., Gregory, R. K., Tidy, V. A., Treleaven, J. G., and Singh, R. The effect of tamoxifen and hormone replacement therapy on serum cholesterol, bone mineral density and coagulation factors in healthy postmenopausal women participating in a randomized, controlled tamoxifen prevention study. *Ann. Oncol.* **7,** 671–675 (1996).
41. Wickerham, D. L., Costantino, J. C., Fisher, B., *et al.* The initial results from NSABP Protocol P-1: A clinical trial to determine the worth of tamoxifen for preventing breast cancer in women at increased risk. *In* "Proceedings of the American Society of Clinical Oncology 34th Annual Meeting," Plenary Session, 1998. [Abstract #3A]
42. Love, R. R., Newcomb, P. A., Wiebe, D. A., Surawicz, T. S., Jordan, V. C., Carbone, P. P., and Demets, D. L. Effects of tamoxifen therapy on the lipid and lipoprotein levels in postmenopausal patients with node negative breast cancer. *J. Natl. Cancer Inst.* **82,** 1327–1332 (1990).
43. McDonald, C. C., and Stewart, H. J. Fatal myocardial infarction in the Scottish adjuvant tamoxifen trial. *Br. Med. J.* **303,** 435–437 (1991).
44. Rutqvist, L. E., and Mattson, A. Cardiac and thromboembolic morbidity among postmenopausal women with early stage breast cancer in a randomized trial of adjuvant tamoxifen. *J. Natl. Cancer Inst.* **85,** 1398–1406 (1993).
45. Fisher, B., Costantino, J. P., Redmond, C. K., *et al.* Endometrial cancer in tamoxifen-treated breast cancer patients: Findings from the National Surgical Adjuvant Breast and Bowel Project (NSABP) B-14. *J. Natl. Cancer Inst.* **86,** 527–537 (1994).
46. Jaiyesimi, I. A., Buzdar, A. U., Decker, D. A., and Hortobagyi, G. N. Use of tamoxifen for breast cancer: twenty eight years later. *J. Clin. Oncol.* **13,** 513–529 (1995).
47. van Leeuwen, F. E., Benraadt, J., Coebergh, J. W., *et al.* Risk of endometrial cancer after tamoxifen treatment of breast cancer. *Lancet* **343,** 448–452 (1994).
48. Lipton, A., Harvey, H. A., and Hamilton, R. W. Venous thrombosis as a side effect of tamoxifen treatment. *Cancer Treat. Rep.* **68,** 887–889 (1984).
49. Fornander, T., Rutqvist, L. E., Cedermark, D., *et al.* Adjuvant tamoxifen in early stage breast cancer: effects on intercurrent morbidity and mortality. *J. Clin. Oncol.* **9,** 1740–1748 (1991).
50. Enck, R. E., and Rios, C. M. Tamoxifen treatment of metastatic breast cancer and antithrombin III levels. *Cancer* **53,** 2607–2609 (1984).
51. Auger, M. J., and Mackie, M. J. Effects of tamoxifen in blood coagulation. *Cancer* **61,** 1316–1319 (1988).
52. Wakeling, A. E., Valcaccia, B., Newboult, E., and Green, L. R. Non-steroidal anti-estrogens: Receptor binding and biological response in rat uterus, rat mammary carcinoma and human breast cancer cells. *J. Steroid Biochem.* **20,** 111–120 (1984).
53. Clemens, J. A., Bennett, D. R., Black, L. J., and Jones, C. D. Effects of a new anti-estrogen, keoxifene (LY 156758), on growth of carcinogen-induced mammary tumors and on LH and prolactin levels. *Life Sci.* **32,** 2869–2875 (1983).
54. Buzdar, A. U., Marcus, C., Holmes, F., Hug, V., and Hortobagyi, G. Phase II evaluation of LY 156758 in metastatic breast cancer. *Oncology* **45,** 344–345 (1988).
55. Sato, M., Kim, J., Short, L. L., Slemenda, C. W., and Bryant, H. U. Longitudinal and cross sectional analysis of raloxifene effects on the tibiae from ovariectomized aged rats. *J. Pharmacol. Exp. Ther.* **272,** 1252–1259 (1995).
56. Evans, G. L., Bryant, H. U., Magee, D. E., and Turner, R. T. Raloxifene inhibits bone turnover and prevents further cancellous bone loss in adult ovariectomized rats with established osteopenia. *Endocrinology* **137,** 4139–4144 (1996).
57. Frolik, C. A., Bryant, H. U., Black, E. C., Magee, D. E., and Chandrasekhar, S. Time-dependent changes in biochemical bone markers and serum cholesterol in ovariectomized rats: effects of raloxifene HCl, tamoxifen, estrogen and alendronate. *Bone* **18,** 621–627 (1996).
58. Evans, G. L., Bryant, H. U., Magee, D., Sato, M., and Turner, R. T. The effects of raloxifene on tibia histomorphometry in ovariectomized rats. *Endocrinology* **134,** 2282–2288 (1994).
59. Turner, C. H., Sato, M., and Bryant, H. U. Raloxifene preserves bone strength and bone mass in ovariectomized rats. *Endocrinology* **135,** 2001–2005 (1994).
60. Bryant, H. U., Cole, H. W., Rowley, E. R., *et al.* Raloxifene and LY117015 prevent bone loss induced by an LH-RH agonist without estrogen-like stimulation of the uterus. *In* "10th ICE I." p 572, 1996.
61. Draper, M. W., Flowers, D. E., Huster, W. J., Neild, J. A., Harper, K. D., and Arnaud, C. A controlled trial of raloxifene (LY139481) HCl: impact on bone turnover and serum lipid profile in healthy postmenopausal women. *J. Bone Miner. Res.* **11,** 835–842 (1996).
62. Gunness, M., Prestwood, K., Lu, Y., *et al.* Histomorphometric, bone marker and bone mineral density response to raloxifene HCl and Premarin in postmenopausal women. *In* "79th annual meeting of the Endocrine Society," p. 67, 1997.
63. Heaney, R. P., and Draper, M. W. Raloxifene and estrogen: comparative bone remodeling kinetics. *J. Clin. Endocrinol. Metab.* **82,** 3425–3429 (1997).
64. Delmas, P. D., Bjarnason, N. H., Mitlak, B. H., Ravoux, A.-C., Shah, A. S., Huster, W. H., Draper, M., and Christiansen, C. Effects of raloxifene on bone mineral density, serum cholesterol concentrations, and uterine endometrium in postmenopausal women. *N. Engl. J. Med.* **337,** 1641–1647 (1997).
65. Hosking, D., Chilvers, C., Christiansen, C., Ravn, P., Wasnich, R., Ross, P., McClung, M., Balske, A., Thompson, D., Daley, M., and Yates, A. J. Prevention of bone loss with alendronate in

postmenopausal women under 60 years of age. *N. Engl. J. Med.* **338,** 485–492 (1998).
66. Lufkin, E. G., Whitaker, M. D., Argueta, R., Caplan, R. H., Nikelsen, T., and Riggs, B. L. Raloxifene treatment of postmenopausal osteoporosis. *J. Bone Miner. Res.* **12,** S150 (1997).
67. Ettinger, B., Black, D., Cummings, S., Genant, H., Gluer, C., Lips, P., Knickerbocker, R., Eckert, S., Nickelsen, T., and Mitlak, B., *Osteopor. Int.* **8**(Suppl. 3), 11 (1998). [Abstract]
68. Walsh, B. W., Kuller, L. H., Wild, R. A., Paul, S., Farmer, M., Lawrence, J. B., Shah, A. S., and Anderson, P. W. Effects of raloxifene on serum lipids and coagulation factors in healthy postmenopausal women. *JAMA* **279,** 1445–1451 (1998).
69. Huster, W., Shah, A., Cohen, F., *et al.* Effect of raloxifene on the endometrium in healthy postmenopausal women. *In* "The North American Menopause Society 8th Annual Meeting." Boston, MA, 1997.
70. Scheele, W., Symanowski, S. M., Neale, S., *et al.* Raloxifene does not cause stimulatory effects on the uterus in healthy postmenopausal women. *In* "79th Annual Meeting of the Endocrine Society." p. 498, 1997.
71. Boss, S. M., Huster, W. J., Neild, J. A., Glant, M., Eisenhut, C. C., and Draper, M. Effects of raloxifene hydrochloride on the endometrium of postmenopausal women. *Am. J. Obstet. Gynecol.* **177,** 1458–1464 (1997).
72. Jordan, V. C., Glusman, J. E., Eckert, S., Lippman, M., Powles, T., Costa, A., Morrow, M., and Norton, L. Incident primary breast cancers are reduced by raloxifene: integrated data from multicenter, double-blind, randomized trials in 12,000 postmenopausal women. *In* "Proceedings of the American Society of Clinical Oncology 34th Annual Meeting," 1998. [Abstract 466]
73. Cummings, S. R., Norton, L., Eckert, S., Grady, D., Cauley, J., Knickerbocker, R., Black, D. M., Nickelsen, T., Glusman, J., and Krueger, K. Raloxifene reduces the risk of breast cancer and may decrease the risk of uterine cancer in post-menopausal women. Two year findings from the Multiple Outcomes of Raloxifene Evaluation (MORE). *In* "Proceedings of the American Society of Clinical Oncology 34th Annual Meeting," 1998. [Abstract 3]
74. Eli Lilly and Company, "Raloxifene Prescribing Information." Indianapolis, IN.
75. Daly, E., Vessey, M. P., Hawkins, M. M., Carson, J. L., Gough, P., and Marsh, S. Risk of venous thromboembolism in users of hormone replacement therapy. *Lancet* **348,** 977–980 (1996).
76. Jick, H., Derby, L. E., Myers, M. W., Vasilakis, C., and Newton, K. M. Risk of hospital admission for idiopathic venous thromboembolism among users of postmenopausal oestrogens. *Lancet* **348,** 981–983 (1996).
77. Grodstein, F., Stampfer, M. J., Goldhaber, S. Z., Manson, J. E., Colditz, G. A., Speizer, F. E., Willett, W. C., and Hennekens, C. H. Prospective study of exogenous hormones and risk of pulmonary embolism in women. *Lancet* **348,** 983–987 (1996).

Androgens

ERIC ORWOLL Oregon Health Sciences University, Endocrinology and Metabolism, Portland VA Medical Center, Portland, Oregon 97207

Androgens have myriad actions on the skeleton throughout life. During adolescence, those effects clearly promote skeletal growth and the accumulation of mineral mass, and for many years there has been hope that these anabolic effects will be useful in the prevention and therapy of metabolic bone disease in later life. In fact, the essential nature of the effects of androgens in bone remains uncertain, and the clinical usefulness of androgens is clearly defined in only a few situations. Nevertheless, there is an increasing interest in how the actions of androgens are integrated into the broad scheme of bone metabolism and how those effects can be adapted for prevention and therapy.

MECHANISMS OF ANDROGEN ACTION IN BONE: THE ANDROGEN RECEPTOR

Colvard *et al.* [1] first reported specific androgen-binding sites and androgen receptor RNA in human osteoblast-like cells derived from both male and female patients. Androgen and estrogen receptor concentrations were approximately the same, and the authors speculated that androgens and estrogens each play important roles in skeletal physiology in both sexes. Other reports confirmed the presence of androgen-binding sites and androgen receptor RNA in osteoblastic cells of human and animal origin [2–7]. The binding affinity of the androgen receptor found in osteoblastic cells ($K_D = 1\text{–}3 \times 10^{-10}$) is typical of that found in other classically androgen-responsive tissues, and exposure to androgen results in translocation of the receptor into the nucleus, presumably as a function of high-affinity DNA binding [3,4] Testosterone and dihydrotestosterone (DHT) appear to have similar binding affinities [2,6]. The number of specific androgen-binding sites in osteoblasts (1000–3000 sites/cell) is in a range associated with androgenic effects in other tissues. Androgen binding is specific, without significant competition by estrogen, progesterone, or dexamethasone. The character of androgen receptor RNA is similar to that in prostate and other tissues [8], as is the size of the androgen receptor protein when analyzed by Western blotting (~110 kDa) [6]. All these data are consistent with the precept that androgen effects in osteoblasts are at least in part exerted via a receptor-mediated process typical of the steroid hormone superfamily.

The regulation of the androgen receptor in osteoblasts is not well characterized, but it may be upregulated autologously by up to two- to three-fold [7]. A positive effect of androgen on androgen receptor gene transcription has been reported in osteoblastic cells, further suggesting that androgens may positively affect the responsiveness of osteoblasts to androgenic stimulation [9]. These are interesting observations, as the promoter for the androgen receptor contains no obvious androgen response elements, suggesting the effect of androgens on the androgen receptor may be via nonandrogen receptor-mediated mechanisms (e.g., via AP-1 pathways) [10]. Whether the androgen receptor in osteoblasts exists in several forms [11], whether it undergoes processing similar to that described in other tissues (phosphorylation, turnover, etc.) [12], or whether it can mediate nongenomic effects [13] is not yet known.

Androgen receptors are also present in other cells in the bone microenvironment. Mizuno *et al.* [14] described the presence of androgen receptor immunoreactivity in mouse osteoclast-like multinuclear cells. Estrogen receptors have been reported to be present in osteoclast-like giant cells [15], suggesting that sex steroids may act directly on these cells to modulate bone resorption. In addition, marrow-derived stromal cells have been shown to contain both androgen and estrogen receptors [16] and to be responsive to sex steroids during the regulation of osteoclastogenesis. Because androgens are so important in bone at the time of puberty, it is not surprising that androgen receptors are also present in epiphyseal chondrocytes [17]. The presence of androgen receptors in a variety of cell types important for bone remodeling reinforces the importance of androgens in these processes and illustrates the complexity of their effects.

Finally, the description of specific binding sites for weaker androgens (dehydroepiandrosterone, DHEA) [18] raises the possibility that DHEA or similar compounds may have direct effects in bone. In fact, Bodine *et al.* [19] showed that DHEA caused a rapid alteration in c-*fos* and c-*jun* expression in human osteoblastic cells, an action that was independent of the effects of more classical androgens (DHT, testosterone, androstenedione). This disparity was present, despite the fact that all caused significant increases in transforming growth factor β (TGF-β) activity.

METABOLISM OF ANDROGENS IN BONE: AROMATASE AND 5α-REDUCTASE ACTIVITIES

Testosterone is the major circulating androgen in both sexes, but there is abundant evidence in a variety of tissues that the eventual cellular effects of testosterone may be the result not only of direct action but also of the effects of testosterone metabolites formed in tissues as the result of local enzyme activities. The most important of these are estradiol (formed by the aromatization of testosterone) and dihydrotestosterone (the result of 5α reduction of testosterone).

There is evidence that both aromatase and 5α-reductase are present in bone [6,20,21]. Interestingly, Turner *et al.* [22] found that periosteal cells do not have detectable 5α-reductase activity, raising the possibility that the enzyme may be functional in only selected skeletal compartments. From a clinical perspective, the possible importance of this enzymatic pathway is suggested by the presence of skeletal abnormalities in patients with 5α-reductase deficiency [23]. These data point to a possible role for 5α-reduction in the regulation of androgen action in bone, but the importance of the enzyme and whether it is present uniformly in cells involved in bone modeling/remodeling remain uncertain.

The microsomal enzyme aromatase cytochrome P450 is essential for the formation of estrogens from androgen precursors. It is an enzyme that is well known to be regulated in a very pronounced tissue-specific manner [24]. Aromatase activity has been reported in bone, both from mixed cell populations derived from both sexes [25–27] and from osteoblastic cell lines [6,28,29]. Aromatase in bone can result not only in the formation of estradiol, but also the weaker estrogen, estrone, from its adrenal precursors androstenedione and dehydroepiandrosterone [25]. In addition to aromatase itself, osteoblasts contain enzymes that are able to interconvert estradiol and estrone (estradiol-17β hydroxysteroid dehydrogenase) and to hydrolyse estrone sulfate to estrone (estrone sulfatase) [28]. The clinical impact of aromatase activity has been suggested by the reports of women [30] and men [31] with enzyme deficiencies who presented with a phenotype that included an obvious delay in bone age. The presentation of men with aromatase deficiency is very similar to that of a man with estrogen receptor deficiency, namely lack of epiphyseal closure, tall stature, and osteopenia [32], suggesting that aromatase (and estrogen action) play a substantial role in male skeletal physiology. Despite these indications that some of the effects of androgens in bone may be mediated by aromatase activity and estrogen, there is convincing evidence that some (if not most) of the impact of androgens in the skeleton is direct. For instance, both *in vivo* and *in vitro* systems reveal the effects of the nonaromatizable androgen DHT to be essentially the same as those of testosterone (*vida infra*).

EFFECTS OF ANDROGENS ON THE CELLULAR BIOLOGY OF BONE

Androgens have direct effects on osteoblast function. Kasperk *et al.* [33] demonstrated that androgens increase the proliferation of osteoblast-like cells in primary cultures (murine and human) and in a transformed human osteoblastic cell line (TE-85) by 100–300%. Testosterone and nonaromatizable androgens (DHT and fluoxymesterone) are equally effective, an observation made by other investigators [2,34]. Testosterone and DHT have also been reported to cause an increase in creatine kinase activity and [^{3}H] thymidine incorporation into DNA in rat diaphyseal bone [35]. Moreover, androgen treatment appears to increase the proportion of cells expressing alkaline phosphatase activity, possibly representing a shift toward a more differentiated phenotype. These findings have been interpreted to indicate a positive effect of androgens on osteoblastic numbers and differentiation.

The actions of androgens in the osteoblast certainly must be considered in the context of a very complex endocrine, paracrine, and autocrine environment. In fact, androgens do interact with other well-known modulators of osteoblast function. DHT increases the expression of TGF-β mRNA in human osteoblast primary cultures [36] and hence androgens may accelerate osteoblast differentiation via this mechanism. Similar results were reported using a human clonal cell system [2]. Other growth factor systems may also be influenced by androgens. Conditioned media from DHT-treated primary osteoblast cultures is mitogenic, and DHT pretreatment increases the mitogenic response to fibroblast growth factor and to insulin-like growth factor II (IGF-II) [36]. In part, this may be due to slight increases in IGF-II binding in DHT-treated cells [36]. IGF-I and IGF-II levels in osteoblast conditioned media are not affected by androgen treatment [36,37].

In addition to growth factors, androgens appear to affect other major regulators of skeletal metabolism. In the human clonal osteoblast-like cell line SaOS-2, testosterone and DHT specifically inhibit the cAMP response elicited by the parathyroid hormone or the parathyroid hormone-related protein, possibly via an effect on the parathyroid hormone receptor–G_S–adenylate cyclase complex [38–40]. The production of prostaglandin E_2 (PGE_2), another important regulator of bone metabolism, is also affected by androgens, as both DHT and testosterone reduce PGE_2 production in calvarial organ cultures exposed to stimulation with parathyroid hormone or interleukin-1 [41]. The effects of androgens on parathyroid hormone action and PGE_2 production suggest that androgens could act to modulate (reduce) bone turnover in response to these agents. Similarly, androgens have been shown to have potent inhibitory effects on the production of interleukin-6 by stromal cells and the subsequent stimulation of osteoclastogenesis by marrow osteoclast precursors [16]. Interestingly, adrenal androgens (androstenediol, androstenedione, dehydroepiandrosterone) have similar inhibitory activities on interleukin-6 production by stroma [16]. The interaction between androgen action and interleukin-6 production may at least in part explain the marked increase in bone remodeling and resorption that follows orchiectomy. In this way, the effects of androgens seem to be very similar to those of estrogen, which inhibit osteoclastogenesis via mechanisms that also involve interleukin-6 inhibition.

Studies of the effects of androgens on other osteoblastic functions are less consistent. Whereas in some experiments androgens have promoted collagen synthesis in osteoblasts [2,34] there has been no effect in other reports [41,42]. The proliferative response to androgens has been reported to be blunted in calvarial cells [34], but the stimulatory effect of androgen on creatine kinase activity and [^{3}H] thymidine incorporation into DNA in long bone diaphysis was dependent on adequate vitamin D nutrition [35]. The divergence of these results may, to some extent, reflect differences in model systems.

ANDROGEN EFFECTS ON BONE: ANIMAL STUDIES

The effects of androgens on bone remodeling have been examined fairly extensively in animal models. Much of this work has been in species (rodents) not perfectly suited to reflect human bone metabolism, and certainly the field remains incompletely explored. Nevertheless, the animal models do provide valuable insights into the effects of androgens at organ and cellular levels.

Growing Male Animals

In most mammals there is a marked gender difference in skeletal morphology. The mechanisms responsible for these differences are complex and involve both androgenic and estrogenic actions. Estrogens are particularly important for the regulation of epiphyseal function and act to reduce the rate of longitudinal growth via influences on chondrocyte proliferation and action, as well as on the timing of epiphyseal closure [43]. Androgens appear to have somewhat opposite effects and tend to promote long bone growth, chondrocyte maturation, and metaphyseal ossification. Androgen deficiency retards those processes [44]. Nevertheless, excess concentrations of androgen will accelerate aging of the growth plate and reduce growth potential [45], possibly via conversion to estrogens.

The most dramatic effect of androgens during growth is on bone size. Male animals have larger bones and particularly thicker cortices than females [43,46]. The effects of androgens on this aspect of skeletal maturation can, to some extent, be assessed by observing the results of androgen withdrawal. In most studies, orchiectomy in young rats results in a reduction in cortical bone mass within 2–4 weeks. The reduction in cortical bone mass appears to result in part from a reduction in the periosteal bone formation rate induced by gonadectomy in males [47,48]. This response is distinctly different than that induced by oophorectomy, which results in an increase in periosteal apposition in the period immediately after surgery (Fig. 1). This divergent trend in the periosteal response to castration in male and female animals abolishes the sexual dimorphism usually present in radial bone growth. Although castration in the male tends to slow growth and weight gain, the effects on cortical bone histomorphometry are present in pair-fed rats and in groups in which there was no difference in growth rates [47,48], indicating that the skeletal effects are not merely the indirect result of changes in body size or composition. A lack of significant change in bone density following castration suggests that there is not a major impact of androgen deficiency on cortical porosity. Endosteal bone formation does not seem to be affected by orchiectomy [47]. Whereas estrogens appear to increase endosteal bone apposition, androgens probably have little effect at that site [43,46].

Cancellous bone mass is also reduced in castrate young male rats. Tibial metaphyseal bone volume and

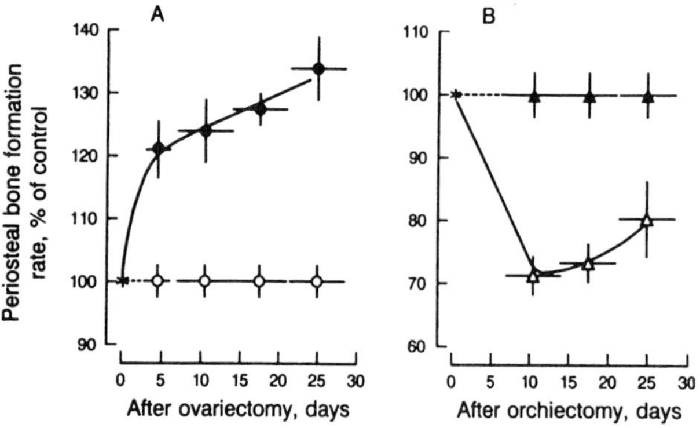

FIGURE 1 (A) The effect of ovariectomy (OVX) on periosteal bone formation rate. The mean ± SE (vertical bar) and tetracycline-labeling period (horizontal line) for intact controls (○) and OVX (●) rats are shown as a function of time after OVX. $p < 0.01$ for all OVX time points compared to intact controls. (B) The effect of orchiectomy (ORX) on periosteal bone formation rate. The mean ± SE and tetracycline-labeling period for intact controls (▲) and ORX (△) are shown as a function of time after ORX. $p < 0.01$ for all ORX time points compared to the same labeling period in intact controls. From Turner *et al.* [48].

vertebral bone mineral density are clearly reduced [47,49,50], an effect that is seen rapidly following castration [47]. An important issue that remains unresolved is whether the bone deficit is a result of actual loss of bone mass following castration or whether the differences between castrate and control animals result from a failure of castrate animals to accrue bone normally. Nevertheless, bone changes following orchiectomy occur in the presence of an increase in skeletal blood flow [51,52], osteoclast numbers and surface [47], serum and urine calcium levels [47], and increased serum tartrate-resistant acid phosphatase activity [53]. In sum, trabecular bone mass, as well as cortical mass, is clearly dependent on adequate androgen action in the growing male animal, but the specific mechanisms that mediate that effect are not well delineated.

These data in growing animals suggest that androgen deficiency during human childhood/adolescence would result in reduced bone size, cortical mass, and cancellous density. The effects are probably the result of a combination of deficiencies in both androgen and estrogen action. It is particularly important to understand and anticipate the results of hypogonadism during this period, as peak bone mass is considered a primary determinant of fracture risk later in life.

Mature Male Animals

In mature rats, androgen withdrawal also results in osteopenia. At a time when longitudinal growth has slowed markedly, pronounced differences between intact and castrate animals appeared in cortical bone ash weight per unit length, cross-sectional area, thickness, and bone mineral density [54–59]. Periosteal bone accretion is reduced [60] and endocortical bone loss is accelerated in the orchiectomized animals [61,62]. As might be expected in light of these changes in bone size, the maximum compressive load is decreased in cortical bone, although when corrected for cortical mass there is no evidence of an abnormality in bone strength [62]. In addition to changes in bone size, increased intracortical resorption cavities are reported to result from orchiectomy [63]. Cancellous bone volume is reduced rapidly after castration as well [60,63] and osteopenia becomes quite pronounced with time [58]. This bone loss appears to result in part from increases in bone resorption, as it is associated with increased resorption cavities, osteoclasts, and blood flow [55,60,63]. Interestingly, this initial phase of increased bone remodeling activity appears to subside somewhat with time [55,64], and by 4 months there is some evidence of a depression in bone turnover rates in some skeletal areas [55].

As a potential model for the effects of hypogonadism in humans, animal models therefore suggest an early phase of high bone turnover bone loss following orchidectomy, followed by a later reduction in remodeling rates. How long bone loss continues, and at what rate, is unclear. Both cortical and trabecular compartments are affected. The remodeling imbalance responsible for the loss of bone mass appears complex, as there are changes in rates of both bone formation and resorption and patterns that vary from one skeletal compartment to another.

The Female Animal

Of course androgens are present in females as well as males and may affect bone metabolism. Some evidence to support that concept includes the fact that flutamide (a specific androgen receptor antagonist) is capable of evoking osteopenia in intact (estrogenized) female rats [65]. This obviously suggests that androgens provide crucial support to bone mass independent of estrogens. Of interest, the character of the bone loss induced by flutamide suggested that estrogen prevents bone resorption whereas androgens stimulate bone formation. Dehydroepiandrosterone treatment has divergent effects (in both cortical and cancellous compartments) in intact and castrate female rats [66], perhaps reflecting an interaction or synergism between sex steroids and their effects on bone. These androgenic effects probably have counterparts in bone physiology in young women.

The Model of Androgen Resistance

The testicular-feminized (TFM, androgen receptor deficient) male rat provides an interesting model for the study of the unique effects of androgens in bone. In these rats, androgens are presumed to be incapable of action, but estrogen and androstenedione concentrations are considerably higher than in normal males [49,67]. Clear differences also exist between TFM and normal male rats in serum levels of calcium and phosphorus (increased), IGF-1 (decreased), and osteocalcin (increased). Results of bone mass measures suggest that TFM rats have reduced longitudinal and radial growth rates, but that cancellous volume and density are similar to those of normal rats. In selected sites, measures of bone mass and remodeling were intermediate between normal male and female values. This model clearly indicates that androgens play an independent role in normal bone growth and metabolism, but the model is complex and not easily dissected.

EFFECTS OF ANDROGENS ON THE SKELETON IN MEN

Puberty

Adolescence is associated with profound increases in bone mass in both sexes. Both axial and appendicular bone mass increase [68,69] with the addition of almost half of the total adult skeleton during this brief time. In boys, the rapid increase in indices of bone formation and skeletal mass during this period is closely linked to the pubertal stage [70,71] (Fig. 2) and to testosterone levels [70–73]. These data would suggest that testicular androgen secretion plays a role in the genesis of the adolescent increase in bone mass. In addition, however, the increase in adrenal androgens that occurs in the prepubertal period (adrenarche) [74] may also affect bone mass. Longitudinal bone growth (via epiphyseal action) has been reported to accelerate during adrenarche [75]. Bone mass accretion certainly occurs before sexual development begins [76] and could be influenced by the actions of adrenal androgens.

The overall result is a male skeleton that is larger in most dimensions, thus conferring a considerable biomechanical advantage. The total body mineral content is 25–30% greater in men [77]. Both the diameter and the cortical thickness (and hence the total mass and mineral content) of long bones are greater in men [78,79]. Vertebral size is also larger in men, even when other elements of body size (height, weight) are controlled [80]. These gender differences in bone size are not matched by differences in the essential composition of bone, as the

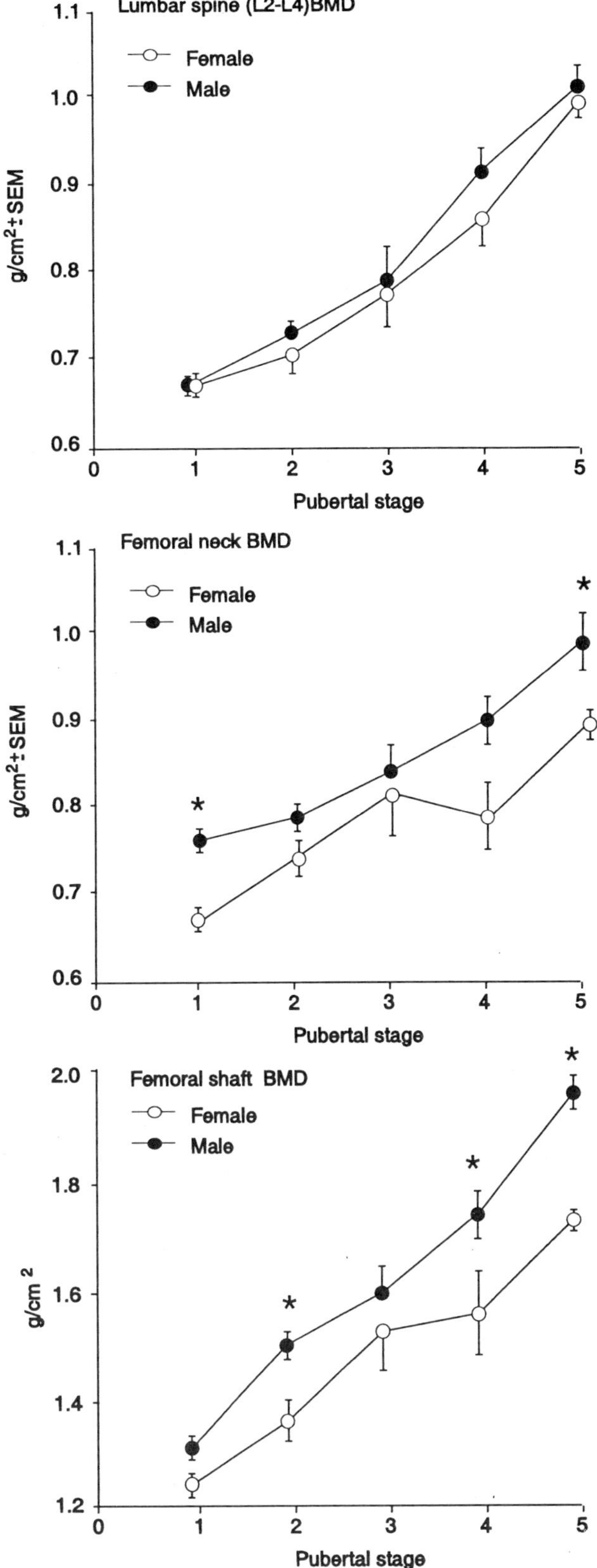

FIGURE 2 Relationship between BMD at the levels of the lumbar spine (L2–L4), femoral neck, and femoral shaft and pubertal stages in female and male subjects. *$p < 0.05$. From Bonjour *et al.* [71]; © The Endocrine Society.

true volumetric density of the bone in men and women is essentially the same [81].

That these pubertal changes in the male skeleton are related to androgen action is strongly suggested by several kinds of evidence. Genetic males with complete androgen resistance have a skeletal mass similar to that of women [82]. Moreover, the presence of androgen insufficiency, e.g., in patients with isolated gonadotrophin deficiency, results in abnormally low bone mass even when corrected for bone age [83]. Treatment of these patients with testosterone before epiphyseal closure results in a rapid increase in bone mass [84–86]. Finally, the short-term administration of testosterone to prepubertal boys quickly causes an increase in calcium retention and incorporation into bone [87] (Fig. 3).

Not only is androgen action essential for normal bone mass development, but the actual timing of the onset of puberty is fundamentally important as well. It is known that constitutionally delayed puberty can result in somewhat greater adult height [88], but bone mass is reduced in these patients even at the conclusion of sexual maturation [89]. In delayed puberty, bone density is also reduced, even when adjusted for bone age [90]. Constitutional delayed puberty is a common condition, and this reduction in peak adult bone mass may have important implications for eventual osteoporosis and fracture risk. More evidence for the importance of the timing of puberty comes from experience with the therapy of hypogonadal men who have not yet undergone puberty. In these patients there is a brisk increase in bone mass in response to testosterone therapy, but the final bone mass developed is impaired [84]. A similar response is seen in boys with constitutional pubertal delay treated with testosterone [90].

All these findings support a crucial role of androgen action during puberty in the development of adult bone mass in the male, probably as a result of both direct and indirect actions at the skeletal level. Because androgens are probably so important in the development of peak bone mass, there is great potential for the use of androgens as therapeutic agents during this period of life.

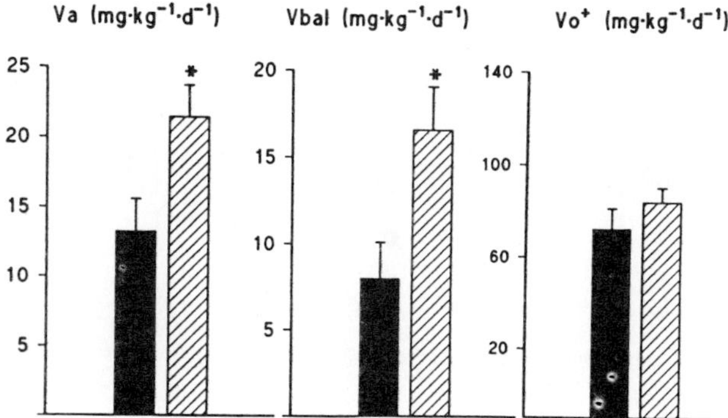

FIGURE 3 Changes in Va (dietary calcium absorption), Vbal (net calcium retention), and vo$^+$ (rate of bone accretion) in prepubertal children treated with testosterone (n = 6). solid bars, before testosterone; hatched bars, after testosterone. $*p < 0.05$. From Mauras *et al.* [87]. Reprinted with permission of the publisher via Copyright Clearance Center, Inc.

Estrogens vs Androgens in Puberty

The dynamic interplay between androgens and estrogens at the skeletal level during puberty is not well understood, but is probably quite important. That estrogen is essential for the development of peak bone mass in men has been highlighted by reports of young men with estrogen deficiency. Smith *et al.* [32] described a patient with an abnormality in the structure of the estrogen receptor (thus rendering him functionally estrogen deficient) who had a delayed bone age, tall stature, and profound osteopenia. A man with estrogen deficiency resulting from an aromatase deficiency was also noted to have a very similar phenotype [31]. The common abnormalities in bone age and stature in these two patients are to be expected as estrogens are essential for the normal closure of growth plates, even in men. The aberrations noted in bone mass are more difficult to understand, particularly since they exist in the face of testosterone levels that are actually higher (even strikingly higher) than in normal men. In one man with aromatase deficiency, estrogen treatment was noted to close the open epiphyses and result in an increase in bone mass. Whether the increase in bone mass resulted from the accumulation of mineral at the growth plates or was the result of a general skeletal effect of estrogen is unknown, but is of fundamental importance in the understanding of the respective roles of androgen and estrogen. If in fact the estrogen therapy resulted in an increase in bone mass unrelated to epiphyseal closure, estrogen would assume a more pivotal role in skeletal maturation in men and would shift therapeutic attention (e.g., in hypogonadal adolescents) to ensure the adequacy of estrogen as well as androgen action.

Adulthood: The Model of Hypogonadism

After peak bone mass is achieved during adolescence, androgens continue to be vitally important in the maintenance of bone health. Abnormal gonadal function is well known to incur risk for bone loss, and a wide variety of causes of gonadal failure result in osteopenia [59]. Hypogonadism is present in a substantial portion of men evaluated for metabolic bone disease [91], and hip fracture occurs more commonly in the presence of hypogonadism [92]. Both cortical and trabecular osteopenia is present, but cancellous bone loss seems most intense. Resulting changes in cancellous architecture are not well characterized, but in most reports there is evidence of reduced trabecular number [93,94]. In some series the degree of bone loss correlates with the level of serum testosterone [95,96], but is not a consistent finding. A threshold level of serum testosterone below which bone mass begins to decline, even in the absence of other skeletal stressors, has not been established. Finally, because hypogonadism in men is usually characterized by at least some degree of estrogen as well as androgen deficiency, a component of hypogonadal bone disease may be related to a lack of estrogen action. Although this issue is not well understood, it remains likely that androgen deficiency is a major determinant of the observed changes in bone metabolism (*vida supra*).

Androgen insufficiency may be an important component of several other forms of metabolic bone disease as well. For instance, in subjects treated with glucocorticoids, testosterone levels can be reduced substantially [97] and may contribute to bone loss. Similar interactions may result in remodeling alterations in patients with renal insufficiency, alcoholism, chemotherapy, and so on [59].

The mechanisms by which androgen withdrawal leads to bone loss in men have only begun to be explored. In the most direct assessment of the events following the onset of hypogonadism, Stepan and Lachman [98] examined changes in bone mass and biochemical indices of remodeling in a group of men undergoing castration. In the 1–3 years these men were followed after orchidectomy, vertebral bone loss was rapid (~7% per year) and progressed in conjunction with clear evidence of an increase in bone turnover (Fig. 4). Similar changes occur after the institution of GnRH agonist therapy in adult men [99]. Thus in the early stages of hypogonadism there appears to be an increase in remodeling and bone resorption, just as is seen in animal models of gonadal insufficiency. This concept is supported by data indicating that androgen action is important in the suppression of cytokines active in the stimulation of osteoclastogenesis [16]. Still more information is needed concerning the histomorphometric character of acute androgen deficiency and the effects on specific skeletal compartments. For instance, it is unclear to what extent an androgen-dependent depression of bone formation accompanies the increase in bone resorption and whether abnormalities in cortical bone metabolism are as profound as those reported to occur in cancellous bone.

Commonly, the diagnosis of hypogonadism is made in the subacute or chronic phases of the disorder, and most evaluations of the nature of hypogonadal bone

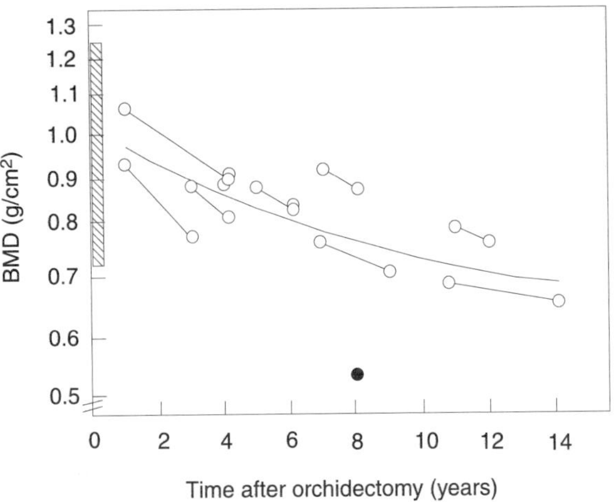

FIGURE 4 Scatter gram of lumbar spinal BMD as a function of time after orchidectomy in 12 men. In 8 patients the measurement was repeated after 1–3 years (O—O). The line is a regression (second order). Deletion of the repeated measurements made no significant difference to the regression. The hatched bar indicates the normal range in men 25–45 years of age for this laboratory. ●, value in a man who developed a hip fracture and died from its complications. From Stepan and Lachman [98]; © The Endocrine Society.

disease involve patients with long-standing reproductive disorders. In these patients the mechanisms responsible for osteopenia are particularly unclear and the histological pattern of the bone disorder is not well described. There are some small retrospective series available, and most other reports are uncontrolled and involve men in whom the hypogonadism was of varied causation and duration. For example, in a study of 13 men with long-standing hypogonadism, Francis and Peacock [94] found that bone remodeling and formation rates were reduced, and 1,25-dihydroxyvitamin D [$1,25(OH)_2D$] levels and intestinal calcium absorption were low in those with fracture. With testosterone therapy, $1,25(OH)_2D$ levels increased and there was a suggestion that indices of bone formation increased. Similarly, Delmas and Meunier [100] found decreased rates of formation in a small group of hypogonadal men, and formation was low in a single case report by Baran *et al.* [101], but vitamin D levels were not described. These contributions certainly raise the question of whether the osteopenia in patients with long-term androgen deficiency is to a major extent the result of a defect in bone formation. In contrast, Jackson *et al.* [102] described the histomorphometric character of chronically hypogonadal men without vitamin D deficiency and found no apparent defect in formation, but rather an increase in bone resorption. They suggested that earlier findings of a defect in bone formation were more the result of insufficient vitamin D action than of gonadal insufficiency. Actually, in all the available reports there is considerable subject heterogeneity, and the nature of remodeling is quite variable. In the face of this considerable patient diversity, inadequate controls, and the presence of other confounding medical conditions, no firm conclusions can be drawn concerning the remodeling defect induced by long-standing hypogonadism in men. If it is similar to that in postmenopausal women, one could expect the initial period of increased remodeling to be followed by one of relatively lower remodeling rates and slower rates of change in bone mass. Since the descriptions of osteoporosis by Fuller Albright half a century ago, a reduction in bone formation has been postulated to be a primary cause of hypogonadal bone disease. In fact, this precept remains essentially unproved.

Age-Related Declines in Androgen Levels: Contribution to Bone Loss in Men

The issue of the role of sex steroids in age-related bone loss has been considered in Chapter 15. Aging is associated with a clear decline in testicular and adrenal androgen levels in men [39,40] and there is considerable interest in the possibility that androgen replacement may attenuate that loss and reduce fracture rates in the elderly. Although there have been attempts to evaluate this hypothesis, most efforts have been indirect and less than conclusive. For instance, a variety of cross-sectional studies have examined the relationship between androgen levels and bone mass in older men. Some have suggested a significant association between androgen concentrations and bone mass [78,103–105], but others have not been able to substantiate an interaction between bone mass and either testosterone or adrenal androgens [106–109]. There continues to be much speculation about the role of the age-related decline in androgen levels in the development of bone loss in older men, and controversy surrounds the issue of whether androgen replacement is useful in the prevention of osteoporosis in older men.

Estrogens in Adult Men

The possibility that there is an important role for estrogens in the maintenance of adult bone mass in men must be considered. It is feasible that estrogens function in men to maintain bone mass, presumably in concert with the direct effects of androgens. Data suggest that estrogen levels are significantly associated with bone mass in elderly men [110] and that reduced estrogen levels may be related to the development of low bone mass in older men [111]. A fascinating series of male-to-female transsexuals indicate that in the presence of antiandrogen treatment or castration, estrogen treatment is capable of maintaining bone mass [112,113]. In fact, publications have suggested that serum concentrations of estrogens may be more closely related to bone mass in older men than androgens [114,115]. Despite the previous assumption that androgens provided the dominant gonadal steroid effect on bone in men, this new information demands that the role of estrogens, and interactions between sex steroids, be examined further. These controversies remain unresolved and clearly affect the question of the usefulness, and possible mechanisms of action, of androgen replacement therapy in older men with low bone mass.

INFLUENCE OF ANDROGENS ON BONE IN WOMEN

In premenopausal women, androgens apparently play an independent role in the determination of bone mass, and several studies have drawn attention to the role of androgens, in addition to estrogen and other factors, in the development of peak bone mass [116–119]. Both trabecular and cortical mass development are related to androgen levels. The fact that both testosterone and adrenal androgens (androstenedione) correlate with the achievement of peak density is reasonable given the important contribution of adrenal steroidogenesis to overall androgen activity in women.

The potential importance of androgens in the regulation of bone mass in young women is also illustrated by skeletal studies in patients with androgen excess. In hirsute, hyperandrogenic subjects with persistent menstruation bone mass is higher than in controls, whereas in hyperandrogenic women without menses bone mass is preserved despite low estrogen concentrations [117,120,121]. The tendency for weight to be increased in hyperandrogenic women was not found to explain the effects on bone mass. Once again, adrenal androgens were found to play an important role in the mediation of the androgen effect.

Androgens have been suggested to play an important role in skeletal metabolism in postmenopausal women as well. It is clear that androgen concentrations (particularly adrenal androgens) decline in the postmenopausal period [122] and it has been suggested that a fall in androgen action contributes to estrogen deficiency in the generation of postmenopausal bone loss. In fact, testosterone levels correlate with bone mass and rates of fall in bone density in perimenopausal women [123,124]. Although the available literature is not consistent, androgens have been implicated in the control of bone mass in the later postmenopausal period [75,125,126]. In this context, adrenal androgens (especially dehydroepiandrosterone) have been of particular interest. Finally, the use of small amounts of testosterone with estrogen replacement therapy in postmenopausal women has been reported to enhance the expected positive effects on bone density [127] and to cause changes in biochemical markers of bone remodeling that suggest reductions in osteoclastic activity with simultaneous increases in osteoblastic function [128]. In view of the complex interactions between androgens (testosterone and adrenal androgens) and estrogens potentially derived from them via aromatase activity, it is difficult to determine whether the putative associations between bone mass and androgens are the result of direct or indirect effects on bone. Also to be considered are changes in sex steroid-binding protein levels, weight, and body fat distribution [129] all of which may contribute to the relationship between sex steroid actions and postmenopausal bone metabolism.

ANDROGEN THERAPY: POTENTIALLY USEFUL ANDROGEN EFFECTS

Despite the relative paucity of research concerning androgen action in bone, there are several well-known effects, both direct and indirect, that may prove beneficial. An understanding of these actions was derived primarily from observations in animals or during human adolescence, but have the potential to be translated into therapeutic terms as well.

Growth-Promoting Effects

During adolescence, androgens appear to exert important effects on the skeleton. By the end of puberty, men have greater bone mass than women, a difference that is most marked in the cortical compartment (greater cortical diameter and thickness) [81,130,131]. Studies of the effects of testosterone on skeletal calcium accumulation during childhood strongly suggest that this is a direct effect [87]. In animals, orchidectomy reduces periosteal bone formation, an effect that is reversed with androgen therapy [48]. In genetic males with complete androgen insensitivity (androgen receptor dysfunction), the observation that skeletal size is similar to that in normal females strongly suggests that androgens play a major role [132].

However, there may also be indirect effects that account for a larger skeleton in men. For instance, before and through puberty boys have greater muscle and total body mass than girls, and the resultant increase in mechanical force exerted on the skeleton has been postulated to play a major role in the determination of bone mass [133,134]. Androgens may also affect the growth hormone/IGF-1 axis [135–137], which in turn may influence skeletal development. Finally, estrogen (derived from the aromatization of androgen) is very important for skeletal maturation [32] and may contribute to male skeletal development in ways that contribute to gender differences [132].

Because bone size and cortical thickness have profound effects on biomechanical strength and fracture resistance, these positive effects of androgens are of great potential use. The therapeutic impact of these actions may be most obvious during skeletal growth, e.g., in the therapy of pubertal forms of hypogonadism in boys. However, if the potential for androgen action on cortical thickness or bone size continues into adulthood, these effects could be useful in the prevention and therapy of common age-related disorders as well (especially osteoporosis). That androgens may continue to exert those actions is suggested by the observation that long bone dimensions continue to increase during adulthood, presumably due to periosteal bone accretion, and that this increase is more marked in men than in women [138].

Suppression of Bone Resorption

In a manner that seems very similar to that of estrogen, androgens seem to exert a moderating effect on cancellous osteoclastic bone resorption. Increases in osteoclastic activity follow quickly after castration in males [47,48,60] and appear to be prevented by nonaromatizable androgens [48]. *In vitro,* androgens prevent the increases in cytokine generation that, in large part, mediate osteoclastogenesis and resorption after gonadectomy in males [16]. Although there is considerable uncertainty about how the direct effects of androgens in bone cells are intertwined with the effects of estrogens derived from the aromatization of androgens, the effectiveness of nonaromatizable androgens in mediating these cellular effects points strongly to a primary androgen action.

Bone Formation

Androgens are the prototypical anabolic agents, and there has been considerable speculation that the effects of androgens in the skeleton may be in part the result of a stimulation of bone formation [139]. There are androgen receptors in osteoblasts [1,3] and evidence that androgens affect osteoblast activity [16,36,38,140]. During pubertal development, and in the periosteal space, there is considerable support for the contention that androgens enhance bone formation (vide supra). In addition to possible effects on bone growth, some have speculated that androgens may promote increased osteoblastic new bone formation in cancellous areas. However, peak cancellous bone density is similar in males and females, and in most studies the benefits of androgen administration on trabecular bone mass have been modest. Certainly there is little substantial evidence of a major anabolic effect. However, some reports suggest the possibility of impressive gains in bone density during androgen therapy of hypogonadal men. In view of the clear effects of androgens to reduce the increased rate of bone remodeling (and the rates of both resorption and formation) induced by castration, it is difficult to design experiments that directly examine the influence of androgens on bone formation in isolation. Thus the issue remains unresolved. If, in fact, androgens have positive effects on trabecular bone accumulation, there would be obvious therapeutic potential.

Androgens and 1GF-I

Androgens may exert many of their complex effects on bone metabolism via actions on cytokines and growth factors in the skeletal microenvironment. In addition, systemic levels of some of these substances are modulated by androgens (perhaps via conversion to estrogens) [141] and may also affect bone health. 1GF-I has potent actions on bone, and serum levels are increased by androgens [142]. If circulating 1GF-I levels have positive effects on bone (see other chapters), the increase stimulated by androgens may be beneficial.

Androgens and Muscle Strength

Muscle strength has long been considered responsive to androgens, and recent objective data suggest that contention. Because strength has been associated with increased bone mass and a reduction in fall propensity, this effect of androgens could be useful in reducing fracture risk. Certainly there remain unresolved issues (the effects of androgens on strength in physiologic concentrations, the usefulness of androgens in improving strength in the elderly, etc.), but the potential benefits of androgens acting on the skeleton via an effect on muscle may be substantial.

ANDROGEN REPLACEMENT IN HYPOGONADAL ADULT MEN

Androgen therapy in hypogonadal men has been shown to affect bone mass positively, at least in most patient groups [59,84,86,143]. For instance, Katznelson *et al.* [144] reported an increase in spinal bone mineral density (BMD) of 5–6% in a group of adult men with hypogonadism treated with testosterone for 18 months, although there was an insignificant increase in radial BMD (Fig. 5). As in the experience reported by Katznelson *et al.* [144] the increase in density following testosterone replacement generally appears to be most apparent in cancellous bone (e.g., lumbar spine), although the literature is not particularly consistent in this regard. Most reports indicate that the increase in bone mass with testosterone therapy can be expected to be modest in the short term (up to 24 months), but Behre *et al.* [145] noted an increase in spinal trabecular BMD of >20% in the first year of testosterone therapy in a group of hypogonadal men and further increases thereafter (Fig. 6). The most marked increases were observed in those with the lowest testosterone levels before therapy. In men treated for at least 3 years, bone density was found to be at levels normally expected for their ages. Although the experience remains small, there is a suggestion that the response to therapy in older men with hypogonadism can be expected to be similar to that in younger adult patients [145,146].

The cellular mechanisms responsible for improvements in bone mass are unclear. As discussed earlier, in the early phases of androgen deficiency (e.g., following castration) there appears to be a phase of increased remodeling and resorption, so that therapy may be beneficial because of an inhibitory effect on osteoclastic activity. However, in most available clinical studies, treated patient populations have had well-established hypogonadism and were characterized by an array of remodeling states. In these subjects the cellular effects of androgen replacement are not well known. In some reports, testosterone therapy appeared to result in an increase in cancellous bone formation [94,101], but in other series there appeared to be no clear remodeling trend induced by therapy [84]. Several groups have reported that biochemical indices of remodeling decline in response to testosterone replacement [144,147], which is what might be predicted if sex steroid deficiency results in an increase in remodeling and bone loss on that basis. Interestingly, some reports also suggest that osteocalcin levels may increase with androgen therapy [146,148], perhaps signaling an increase in bone formation.

In addition to the generally positive effects of androgen replacement therapy in hypogonadal men, additional benefits may be gained from the increases that have been noted in strength and lean body mass in these patients [144,146,149,150]. Because lean body mass and strength have been correlated with bone mass and a reduced propensity to fall, they may further serve to promote bone health and to reduce fracture risk.

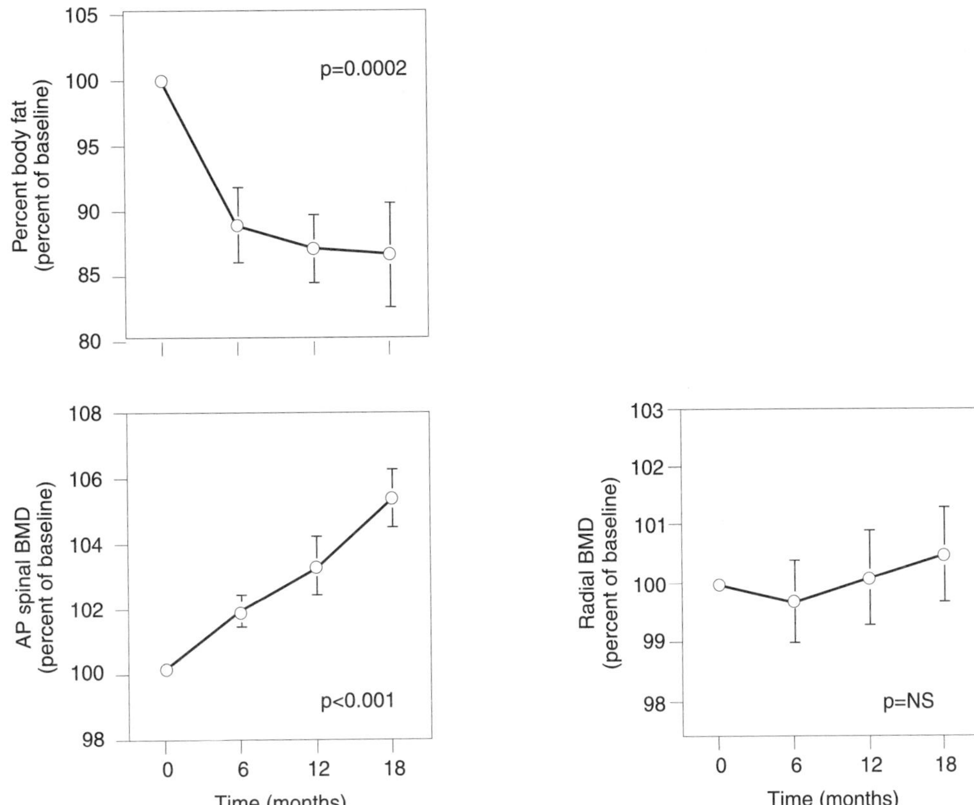

FIGURE 5 Changes in percentage body fat and BMD in hypogonadal men receiving testosterone replacement therapy. (a) Percentage body fat determined by bioelectric impedance analysis. (b) AP spinal BMD determined by dual-energy X-ray absorptiometry. (c) Radial BMD determined by single photon absorptiometry. Data are represented as the mean ± SEM percentage of the baseline. Statistical significance for analysis of the mean slope is shown in the bottom right-hand corner of each figure. From Katznelson *et al.* [144]; © The Endocrine Society.

Despite the generally positive tenor of most studies of the skeletal effects of testosterone replacement, in some patient groups, e.g., those with Kleinfelter's syndrome, the advantage associated with androgen therapy is questionable, as the available studies report very mixed results [151,152]. This may be because the level of androgen deficiency in Kleinfelter's (as in the case of some other causes of hypogonadism) is quite variable. These findings suggest the need to carefully consider the potential benefits of androgen replacement in each patient individually.

The most efficacious doses and routes of androgen administration for the prevention/therapy of bone loss in men remain uncertain. The specific testosterone levels necessary for an optimal effect have not been defined, but current practice is to attempt to ensure testosterone concentrations similar to those of normal young men. Moreover, whether the pulsatile pattern of testosterone exposure characteristic of intramuscular administration is more or less conducive to skeletal health than the more stable pattern produced by transdermal administration is unknown. In some studies, transdermal testosterone therapy appeared to be as effective as intramuscular administration in promoting bone mass [145]. Oral preparations of androgens are not appropriate in view of the higher incidence of adverse effects associated with their use.

Follow-Up of Treated Patients

The follow-up of hypogonadal men treated with testosterone, although not well codified, should certainly include careful monitoring for adverse effects. The risk of prostate disease in androgen-treated men is unknown, but regular prostate evaluations are necessary to ensure that any development of benign or malignant disease is detected early in its course. The development of erythrocytosis is not uncommon, particularly with intramuscular testosterone administration, and complete blood counts at 6- to 12-month intervals are useful to detect its appearance. Other problems that have been

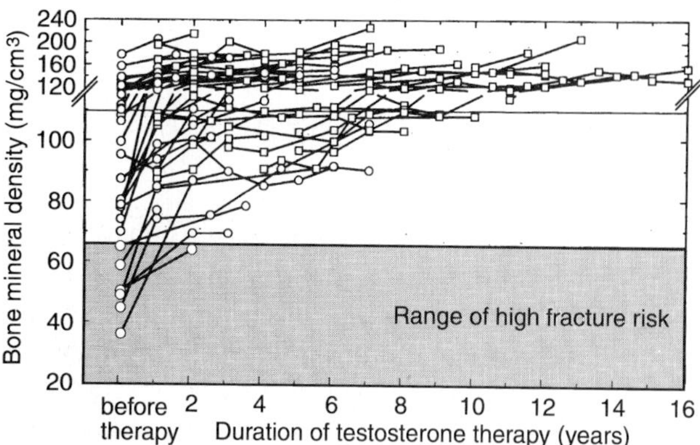

FIGURE 6 Increase in spinal BMD during long-term testosterone substitution therapy up to 16 years in 72 hypogonadal patients. Circles indicate hypogonadal patients with first quantitative computed tomography (QCT) measurement before institution of therapy, squares show those patients already receiving therapy at the first QCT. The dark shaded area indicates the range of high fracture risk, the unshaded area shows the range without significant fracture risk, and the light shaded area indicates the intermediate range where fractures may occur. From Behre *et al.* [145]; © The Endocrine Society.

postulated to be of concern in androgen-treated men are hyperlipidemia and sleep apnea [153].

In terms of skeletal disease, therapeutic success may be assessed via follow-up bone mass measures. In view of recent reports, increases in bone density can be anticipated in the average patient. Although the role of biochemical markers of remodeling is controversial, available data suggest that an adequate androgen effect should be accompanied by a fall in indices of bone resorption, an effect that should be especially useful if resorption markers are increased at baseline. Markers of bone formation may be more difficult to use at present in routine clinical situations, as some reports suggest increases follow therapy while others support a decline. The response may depend on the specific marker. Clearly, clinicians deciding on a follow-up strategy must be aware of the uncertainty currently inherent in the field and the vagaries of using the tools available (i.e., issues of measurement precision).

Unresolved Issues

Many additional unresolved issues concerning the role of androgen treatment in the prevention/therapy of osteoporosis in hypogonadal men remain, including

· The degree of hypogonadism (level of testosterone) at which adverse skeletal effects begin to occur is undefined, and hence it is difficult to decide upon the usefulness of therapy in many men with borderline levels of serum testosterone.

· Because hypogonadism in men results in deficiencies of estrogen as well as testosterone and because testosterone therapy results in increases in serum estrogen (as well as androgen) levels, the relative roles of estrogen vs testosterone in affecting skeletal health in hypogonadal men are unclear. It is unknown whether it is useful to assess estrogen concentrations in the diagnosis of hypogonadal bone disease in men or whether using estrogen levels to monitor the success of testosterone therapy is beneficial.

· In general, the available treatment studies are of relatively short duration, and it is unclear how long any increases in bone mass can be sustained and what eventual treatment effect can be expected.

· As of yet, the increase in bone mass that appears to accompany testosterone therapy is of uncertain usefulness in preventing fractures.

· Whether pretreatment age, duration of hypogonadism, degree of osteopenia, remodeling character, and associated medical conditions affect the therapeutic response is relatively unknown.

· Potential adverse effects of androgen therapy (e.g., prostate, lipid) are not well delineated.

ANDROGEN THERAPY IN EUGONADAL MEN

It has been hypothesized that androgens may have positive effects on bone formation and resorption (vida supra). The threshold level of androgens necessary to provide maximal skeletal benefits is unknown, and some have speculated that testosterone supplementation would benefit osteoporotic men even in the face of normal testosterone levels. The experience with this approach has been very limited, but Anderson *et al.* [154] found in an uncontrolled trial that testosterone supplementation was associated with an increase in bone density and a reduction in biochemical markers of remodeling in a group of osteoporotic, eugonadal men. This approach remains very much of uncertain benefit, and until its advantages are documented in controlled trials, it cannot be recommended. This is particularly true in view of the lack of knowledge concerning the potential adverse effects that may be associated with testosterone supplementation.

ANDROGEN REPLACEMENT IN ADOLESCENCE

Because adolescence is such a critically important pat of the process of attaining optimal peak bone mass, it is also especially vulnerable to disruption by alterations in gonadal function. Even constitutional pubertal delay is associated with a reduction in peak bone mass development, despite eventual full gonadal development [89,155]. The impairment in bone mass in adolescence with organic hypogonadism (hypogonadotropic hypogonadism) is similar to patients with this form of hypogonadism studied later in life, suggesting that the detrimental effect suffered in adolescence is the major cause of osteopenia [83]. In view of the major effects of androgens on the skeleton during growth (whether direct or indirect, as discussed earlier), the response to therapy of gonadal dysfunction during this time would be expected to be brisk. Although studies are few, this would appear to be the case [156]. Finkelstein *et al.* [84] reported that treatment of hypogonadal men with testosterone elicited the most robust skeletal response in those who were skeletally immature (open epiphyses) (Fig. 7). In young men considered to have constitutional delay of puberty, testosterone therapy results in a clear increase in bone mass, but whether this provides a solution to the problem of low peak bone mass in these patients is not yet known [90]. All this information suggests that the diagnosis of frank hypogonadism during childhood or adolescence carries with it the risk of impaired skeletal development and that there is an opportunity to improve bone mass with androgen therapy. In fact, from a skeletal perspective, it appears that therapy should be initiated before epiphyseal closure to maximize bone mass accumulation. Issues that are unresolved include whether bone mass can be normalized with therapy, the most appropriate doses and timing of therapy, and the source of the beneficial effects (androgen vs estrogen, growth factor stimulation, etc.).

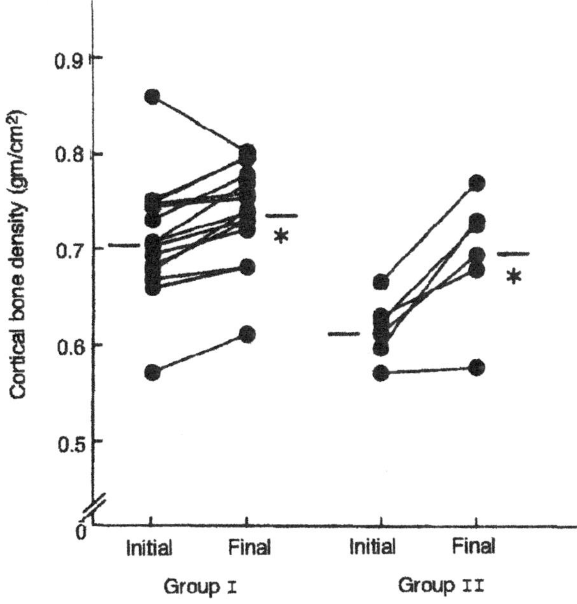

FIGURE 7 Cortical bone density before and after treatment of men with isolated GnRH deficiency who initially had fused epiphyses (group I) or who initially had open epiphyses (group II). Solid lines represent the mean cortical bone density, which increase significantly after treatment in both groups I and II ($p < 0.01$). Cortical bone density increased more in group II than in group I ($p < 0.05$). From Finkelstein *et al.* [84]; © The Endocrine Society.

ANDROGEN REPLACEMENT IN AGING MEN

Old age is associated with a panoply of physical changes in men, many of which have been speculated to be related, either directly or indirectly, to the decline in androgens that accompanies aging [157]. A few small trials of androgen administration in older men have suggested that there may be beneficial effects (increased strength and improved body composition) [146,150,158], and some reports, as of yet inconclusive, indicate that bone mass or biochemical indices of remodeling may improve [146,158]. Whether androgen replacement therapy can prevent or reverse bone loss in aging men is of enormous importance, but it remains uncertain. Until more definitive data are available concerning both advantages and disadvantages, testosterone replacement should not be utilized in elderly patients unless there is convincing evidence for androgen deficiency. This decision is difficult in many older men who have symptoms that can be associated with androgen deficiency but which are also common in the aged regardless of gonadal status (weakness, loss of libido or sexual ability, etc.). The identification of hypogonadism in this group is made especially challenging by the expected decline in androgen levels with age and the dirth of data concerning the levels (threshold concentrations) that are associated with adverse effects on bone.

ANDROGEN THERAPY IN SECONDARY FORMS OF METABOLIC BONE DISEASE

A variety of system illnesses and medications are associated with lowered testosterone levels [39], and it has been postulated that relative hypogonadism may contribute to the bone loss that also accompanies many of these conditions. For instance, renal insufficiency, glucocorticoid excess, posttransplantation, malnutrition, and alcoholism are all associated with osteopenia and with low testosterone concentrations. Although there is little experience with testosterone supplementation in these patients, there may be advantages to skeletal health as well as to other tissues (muscle, red cells, etc.). In a randomized study of crossover design, Reid *et al.* [159] reported that testosterone therapy apparently improved bone density (and body composition) in a small group of men receiving glucocorticoids (Fig. 8). Similarly, testosterone therapy apparently improved forearm bone mass in a small group of men with hemochromatosis (treated simultaneously with venesection) [143]. The number of patients affected by conditions associated with low testosterone levels is potentially quite large, and more information is needed to understand the role of androgen replacement in the prevention/therapy of concomitant bone loss.

ANDROGEN THERAPY IN WOMEN

In premenopausal women, androgens apparently play an independent role in the determination of bone mass, and several studies have drawn attention to the role of androgens, in addition to estrogen and other factors, in the development of peak bone mass [116–119]. Both trabecular and cortical mass development are related to androgen levels. The fact that both testosterone and adrenal androgens (androstenedione) correlate with the achievement of peak density is reasonable given the important contribution of adrenal steroidogenesis to overall androgen activity in women.

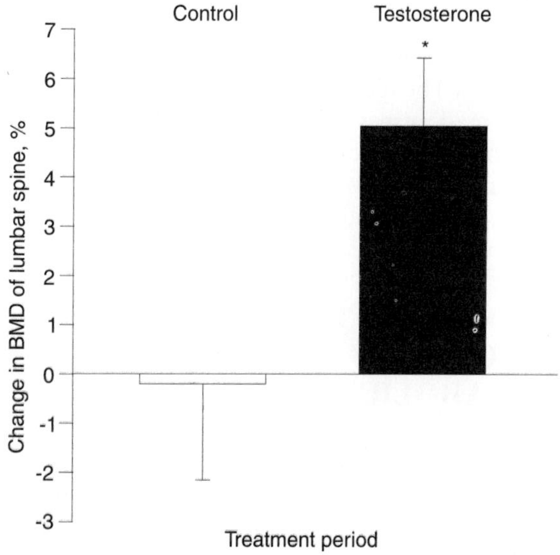

FIGURE 8 Rate of change in BMD of lumber spine during control or testosterone treatment periods (each of 6 months duration) in men receiving glucocorticoid therapy. Data are given as the mean ± SEM. There was a significant difference between groups ($p = 0.05$). The asterisk indicates a significant difference from 0 ($p = 0.005$). From Reid *et al.* [159].

In view of the relationships between androgens and bone mass in women, and the generally held belief that androgens might provide a unique benefit via a putative anabolic effect, there have been a variety of attempts to assess the usefulness of androgenic agents in women. Unfortunately, these benefits remain uncertain. Most commonly, orally administered androgens (e.g., stanozalol and nandrolone) or androgenic progestins (e.g., norethistrone) have been used in comparison with other treatments or placebo. In some of these trials, the effects of androgen therapy have been striking, with increases of forearm and vertebral bone mineral density of more than 20% in 2 years [160–164]. Unfortunately, most of these trials were not of randomized or controlled design, and/or the effects were not different from those of estrogen. In reports that included stricter control groups, the beneficial effects of androgens were much more modest (<5% increase in bone mineral density over 1–2 years) [165–169]. In one of the more convincing demonstrations of the potentially useful effects of androgens, Davis *et al.* [127] reported that the addition of testosterone to estrogen replacement in postmenopausal women has a salutary effect on lumbar spine and proximal femoral bone density [127] (Fig. 9).

Whether the benefits associated with androgen therapy in postmenopausal women are the result of "anabolic" actions remains unclear. Although experiments in adult rats utilizing similar anabolic steroids suggest an increase in periosteal bone formation, bone mineral density, and bone strength in cortical areas (compared with both intact and ovariectomized controls), there was no enhancement of trabecular bone mass (over intact controls). A distinction between clearly anabolic actions versus short-lived effects on bone resorption (remodeling transient) or indirect effects mediated by increased body weight or muscle mass is also not conclusively apparent in the clinical studies available. Biochemical markers of bone formation (osteocalcin, alkaline phosphatase) have not provided clearly supportive evidence of increased osteoblastic function, either in animal or in human studies [166,169–171].

In sum, clinical data in support of a clinical useful anabolic effect of androgenic steroids are tantalizing, but are by no means conclusive. Whether there are advantages of androgenic agents (or the combination of estrogen plus androgen) over estrogen replacement alone or over newer, specific antiresorptive approaches (potent bisphosphonates) is certainly not clear. In addition, potentially important adverse effects of androgens in postmenopausal women (hirsutism/virilization, lipid effects, and so forth) must be considered when assessing the usefulness of these therapies. At present, it is prema-

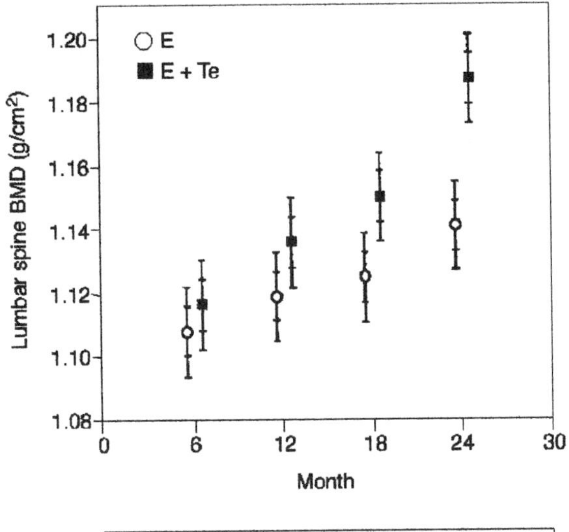

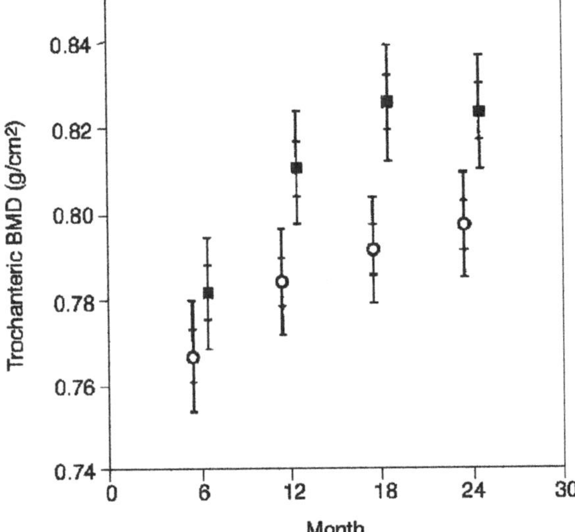

FIGURE 9 Effects of hormonal implants, either estradiol alone (E) or estradiol plus testosterone (E + T), on bone mineral density (g/cm^2): lumbar spine and femoral trochanter. Error bars represent SEM. From Davis *et al.* [127]. Reprinted with permission from Elsevier Science.

ture to choose androgen therapy as the primary approach in postmenopausal osteoporosis.

THERAPY WITH OTHER ANDROGENS

Several androgenic compounds may have effects on bone mass, and of most current interest are adrenal androgens. DHEA has become widely available as a supplement and has been the source of considerable recent debate. DHEA levels fall dramatically with aging in both sexes [157] and because DHEA can act as a precursor for both androgens and estrogens, there is some reason to expect that its administration may affect bone metabolism and bone mass. A variety of attempts have been made to link those changes with alterations in bone mass associated with age [106], but the information available to date is both inconclusive and incomplete. Labrie *et al.* [172] reported that cutaneous DHEA therapy in postmenopausal women was associated with an increase in spinal bone density, with reductions in some markers of bone remodeling (but increases in others) [172]. Similar studies are available in animals. There remains no long-term, well-controlled trials of DHEA supplementation in any coherent subject group, and until that information is available, no confident recommendations can be made. Of concern, there are also no available data concerning the potential risks associated with long-term therapy.

RESEARCH DIRECTIONS

The skeleton is an androgen responsive tissue, and theoretically there are a number of mechanisms by which androgen action may be important for skeletal health in both men and women. Clinical studies show that androgen therapy provides benefit, for the prevention and therapy of bone loss in hypogonadal men, and added gain may result from increases in muscle strength, particularly in older men at risk for falls. Nevertheless, the potential usefulness of androgen therapy, even in men, remains unclear. Major issues to be clarified include the appropriate criteria for patient selection, specifics of dosing and drug delivery, the nature of short- and long-term adverse effects, and the impact of therapy on fracture rates. Some of these issues can be clarified only with large-scale intervention trials. Androgens may have usefulness in women as well, but adverse effects loom as a more difficult problem. In both men and women, a greater understanding of the molecular mechanisms of androgen action in the skeleton may provide means to harness the beneficial effects of androgens without the disadvantages, for instance by the development of compounds with tissue-specific actions.

References

1. Colvard, D. S., *et al.* Identification of androgen receptors in normal human osteoblast-like cells. *Proc. Natl. Acad. Sci. USA* **86,** 854–857 (1989).
2. Benz, D. J., *et al.* High-affinity androgen binding and androgenic regulation of a $_1$(I)-procollagen and transforming growth factor-B steady state messenger ribonucleic acid levels in human osteoblast-like osteosarcoma cells. *Endocrinology* **128,** 2723–2730 (1991).

3. Orwoll, E. S., *et al.* Androgen receptors in osteoblast-like cell lines. *Calcif. Tissue Int.* **49,** 182–187 (1991).
4. Zhuang, Y. H. Subcellular location of androgen receptor in rat prostate, seminal vesicle and human osteosarcoma MG-63 cells. *J. Steroid Biochem. Molec. Biol.* **41,** 693–696 (1992).
5. Liesegang, P., *et al.* Human osteoblast-like cells contain specific saturable, high-affinity glucocorticoid, androgen, estrogen and 1a,25-dihydroxycholecalciferol receptors. *J. Androl.* **15,** 194–199 (1994).
6. Nakano, Y. The receptor, metabolism and effects of androgen in osteoblastic MC3T3 E1 cells. *Bone Miner.* **26,** 245–259 (1994).
7. Takeuchi, M., *et al.* Androgens directly stimulate mineralization and increase androgen receptors in human osteoblast-like osteosarcoma cells. *Biochem. Biophys. Res. Commun.* **204,** 905–911 (1994).
8. Chang, C., *et al.* Structural analysis of complementary DNA and amino acid sequences of human and rat androgen receptors. *Proc. Natl. Acad. Sci. USA* **85,** 7211–7215 (1988).
9. Wiren, K. M., *et al.* Transcriptional up-regulation of the human androgen receptor by androgen in bone cells. *Endocrinology* **138,** 2291–2300 (1997).
10. Kallio, P. J., *et al.* Androgen receptor-mediated transcriptional regulation in the absence of direct interaction with a specific DNA element. *Mol. Endocrinol.* **9,** 1017–1028 (1995).
11. Wilson, C. M., and McPhaul, M. J. A and B forms of the androgen receptor are present in human genital skin fibroblasts. *Proc. Natl. Acad. Sci. USA* **91,** 1234–1238 (1994).
12. Kemppainen, J. A., *et al.* Androgen receptor phosphorylation, turnover, nuclear transport, and transcriptional activation. *J. Biol. Chem.* **267,** 968–974 (1992).
13. Schumacher, M. Rapid membrane effects of steroid hormones: an emerging concept in neuroendocrinology. *Trends Neurosci.* **13,** 359–362 (1990).
14. Mizuno, Y., *et al.* Immunocytochemical identification of androgen receptor in mouse osteoclast-like multinucleated cells. *Calcif. Tissue Int.* **54,** 325–326 (1994).
15. Oursler, M. J., *et al.* Avian osteoclasts as estrogen target cells. *Proc. Natl. Acad. Sci. USA* **88,** 6613–6617 (1991).
16. Bellido, T., Jilka, R. J., Boyce, B. F., Girasole, G., Broxmeyer, H., Dalrymple, A., Murry, R., and Manolagas, S. C. Regulation of interleukin-6, osteoclastogenesis and bone mass by androgens: the role of the androgen receptor. *J. Clin. Invest.* **95,** 2886–2895 (1995).
17. Carracosa, A., *et al.* Biological effects of androgens and identification of specific dihydrotestosterone-binding sites in cultured human fetal epiphyseal chondrocytes. *J. Clin. Endocrinol. Metab.* **70,** 134–140 (1990).
18. Meikle, A. W., *et al.* The presence of a dehydroepiandrosterone-specific receptor binding complex in murine T cells. *J. Steroid Biochem. Mol. Biol.* **42,** 293–304 (1992).
19. Bodine, P. V. N., *et al.* Regulation of c-fos expression and TGF-B production by gonadal and adrenal androgens in normal human osteoblastic cells. *J. Steroid Biochem. Mol. Biol.* **52,** 149–158 (1995).
20. Schweikert, H. U., *et al.* Testosterone metabolism in human bone. *Acta Endocrinol.* **95,** 258–264 (1980).
21. Vittek, J., *et al.* The metabolism of 7a-^{3}H-testosterone by rat mandibular bone. *Endocrinology* **94,** 325–329 (1974).
22. Turner, R. T., *et al.* Failure of isolated rat tibial periosteal cells to 5a reduce testosterone to 5a-dihydrotestosterone. *J. Bone Miner. Res.* **5,** 775–779 (1990).
23. Fisher, L., *et al.* Clinical, endocrinological and enzymatic characterization of two patients with 5a-reductase deficiency: evidence that a single enzyme is responsible for the 5a-reduction of cortisol and testosterone. *J. Clin. Endocrinol. Metab.* **47,** 653–664 (1978).
24. Simpson, E. R., *et al.* Aromatase cytochrome P450, the enzyme responsible for estrogen biosynthesis. *Endocr. Rev.* **15,** 342–355 (1994).
25. Nawata, H., *et al.* Aromatase in bone cell: Association with osteoporosis in postmenopausal women. *J. Steroid Biochem. Mol. Biol.* **53,** 165–174 (1995).
26. Schweikert, H.-U., *et al.* Estrogen formation from androstenedione in human bone. *Clin. Endocrinol.* **43,** 37–42 (1995).
27. Yeh, J., *et al.* Expression of aromatase P450 in marrow from men and postmenopausal women. *In* "The Endocrine Society 77th Annual Meeting, Washington, DC." The Endocrine Society, 1995.
28. Purohit, A., *et al.* Estrogen synthesis by osteoblast cell lines. *Endocrinology* **131,** 2027–2029 (1992).
29. Tanaka, S., *et al.* Aromatase activity in human osteoblast-like osteosarcoma cell. *Calcif. Tissue Int.* **52,** 107–109 (1993).
30. Conte, F. A., *et al.* A syndrome of female pseudohermaphrodism, hypergonadotropic hypogonadism, and multicystic ovaries associated with missense mutations in the gene encoding aromatase (P450arom). *J. Clin. Endocrinol. Metab.* **78,** 1287–1292 (1994).
31. Morishima, A., *et al.* Aromatase deficiency in male and female siblings caused by a novel mutation and the physiological role of estrogens. *J. Clin. Endocrinol. Metab.* **80,** 3689–3698 (1995).
32. Smith, E. P., *et al.* Estrogen resistance caused by a mutation in the estrogen-receptor gene in a man. *N. Engl. J. Med.* **331,** 1056–1061 (1994).
33. Kasperk, C. H., *et al.* Androgens directly stimulate proliferation of bone cells in vitro. *Endocrinology* **124(3),** 1576–1578 (1989).
34. Gray, C., *et al.* Interaction of androgen and 1,25-dihydroxyvitamin D3: effects on normal rat bone cells. *J. Bone Miner. Res.* **7,** 41–46 (1992).
35. Somjen, D., *et al.* Direct and sex-specific stimulation by sex steroids of creatine kinase activity and DNA synthesis in rat bone. *Proc. Natl. Acad. Sci. USA* **86,** 3361–3365 (1989).
36. Kasperk, C., *et al.* Studies of the mechanism by which androgens enhance mitogenesis and differentiation in bone cells. *J. Clin. Endocrinol. Metab.* **71,** 1322–1329 (1990).
37. Canalis, E., *et al.* Regulation of insulin-like growth factor-II production in bone cultures. *Endocrinology* **129,** 2457–2462 (1991).
38. Fukayama, S., and Tashjian, H. J. Direct modulation by androgens of the response of human bone cells (SaOS-2) to human parathyroid hormone (PTH) and PTH-related protein. *Endocrinology* **125,** 1789–1794 (1989).
39. Gray, A., *et al.* Age, disease and changing sex hormone levels in middle-aged men: results of the Massachusetts male aging study. *J. Clin. Endocrinol. Metab.* **73,** 1016–1025 (1991).
40. Vermeulen, A. Androgens in the aging male. *J. Clin. Endocrinol. Metab.* **73,** 221–224 (1991).
41. Pilbeam, C. C., and Raisz, L. G. Effects of androgens on parathyroid hormone and interleukin-1-stimulated prostaglandin production in cultured neonatal mouse calvariae. *J. Bone Miner. Res.* **5,** 1183–1188 (1990).
42. Canalis, E., and Raisz, L. G. Effect of sex steroids on bone collagen synthesis *in vitro. Calcif. Tissue Res.* **25,** 105–110 (1978).
43. Turner, R. T., *et al.* Skeletal effects of estrogen. *Endocr. Rev.* **15,** 129–154 (1994).
44. Lebovitz, H. E., and Eisenbarth, G. S. Hormonal regulation of cartilage growth and metabolism. *Vitam. Horm. (NY)* **33,** 575–648 (1975).
45. Iannotti, J. P. Growth plate physiology and pathology. *Orthop. Clin. North Am.* **21,** 1–17 (1990).

46. Kasra, M., and Grynpas, M. D. The effects of androgens on the mechanical properties of primate bone. *Bone* **17,** 265–270 (1995).
47. Turner, R. T., *et al.* Differential effects of gonadal function in bone histomorphometry in male and female rats. *J. Bone Miner. Res.* **4,** 557–563 (1989).
48. Turner, R. T., *et al.* Differential effects of androgens on cortical bone histomorphometry in gonadectomized male and female rats. *J. Orthopaed. Res.* **8,** 612–617 (1990).
49. Vanderschueren, D., *et al.* Androgen resistance and deficiency have difference effects on the growing skeleton of the rat. *Calcif. Tissue Int.* 198–203 (1994).
50. Rosen, H. N., *et al.* Bone density is normal in male rats treated with finasteride. *Endocrinology* **136,** 1381–1387 (1995).
51. Schoutens, A., *et al.* Growth and bone haemodynamic responses to castration in male rats. Reversibility by testosterone. *Acta Endocrinol,* **107,** 428–432 (1984).
52. Kapitola, J., *et al.* Blood flow and mineral content of the tibia of female and male rats: Changes following castration and/or administration of estradiol or testosterone. *Bone* **16,** 69–72 (1995).
53. Ongphiphadhanakul, B., *et al.* Excessive L-thyroxine therapy decreases femoral bone mineral densities in the male rat: Effect of hypogonadism and calcitonin. *J. Bone Miner. Res.* **7,** 1227–1231 (1992).
54. Deleted in proof.
55. Verhas, M., and Schoutens, A. The effect of orchidectomy on bone metabolism in aging rats. *Calcif. Tissue Int.* **39,** 74–77 (1986).
56. Danielsen, C. C., *et al.* Long-term effect of orchidectomy on cortical bone from rat femur: Bone mass and mechanical properties. *Calcif. Tissue Int.* **50,** 169–174 (1992).
57. Vanderschueren, D., *et al.* Bone and mineral metabolism in the adult guinea pig: Long-term effects of estrogen and androgen deficiency. *J. Bone Miner. Res.* **7,** 1407–1415 (1992).
58. Vanderschueren, D., *et al.* Bone and mineral metabolism in aged male rats: short and long term effects of androgen deficiency. *Endocrinology* **130,** 2906–2916 (1992).
59. Orwoll, E. S. and Klein, R. F. Osteoporosis in men. *Endocr. Rev.* **16,** 87–116 (1995).
60. Gunness, M., and Orwoll, E. S. Early induction of alterations in cancellous and cortical bone histology after orchiectomy in mature rats. *J. Bone Miner. Res.* **10,** 1735–1744 (1995).
61. Vanderschueren, D., *et al.* Bone and mineral metabolism in the androgen-resistant (testicular feminized) male rat. *J. Bone Miner. Res.* **8,** 801–809 (1993).
62. Danielsen, C. C., *et al.* Long-term effect of orchidectomy on cortical bone from rat femur: bone mass and mechanical properties. *Calcif. Tissue Int.* **50,** 169–174 (1992).
63. Wink, C. S., and Felts, W. J. L. Effects of castration on the bone structure of male rats: a model of osteoporosis. *Calcif. Tissue Int.* **32,** 77–82 (1980).
64. Vanderschueren, D., *et al.* Time-related increase of biochemical markers of bone turnover in androgen-deficient male rats. *Bone Miner.* **26,** 123–131 (1994).
65. Goulding, A., and Gold, E. Flutamide-mediated androgen blockade evokes osteopenia in the female rat. *J. Bone Miner. Res.* **8,** 763–769 (1993).
66. Turner, R. T., *et al.* Dehydroepiandrosterone reduces cancellous bone osteopenia in ovariectomized rats. *Am. J. Physiol.* **258,** E673–E677 (1990).
67. Vanderschueren, D., *et al.* The aged male rat as a model for human osteoporosis: Evaluation by nondestructive measurements and biomechanical testing. *Calcif. Tissue Int.* **53,** 342–347 (1993).
68. Gilsanz, V., *et al.* Vertebral bone density in children: Effect of puberty. *Radiology* **166,** 847–850 (1988).
69. Lu, P. W., *et al.* Bone mineral density of total body, spine, and femoral neck in children and young adults: A cross-sectional and longitudinal study. *J. Bone Miner. Res.* **9,** 1451–1458 (1994).
70. Krabbe, S., *et al.* Effect of puberty on rates of bone growth and mineralisation. *Arch. Dis. Child.* **54,** 950–953 (1979).
71. Bonjour, J.-P., *et al.* Critical years and stages of puberty for spinal and femoral bone mass accumulation during adolescence. *J. Clin. Endocrinol. Metab.* **73,** 555–563 (1991).
72. Krabbe, S., *et al.* Longitudinal study of calcium metabolism in male puberty. *Poediatr. Scand.* **73,** 750–755 (1984).
73. Riis, B. J., *et al.* Bone turnover in male puberty: A longitudinal study. *Calcif. Tissue Int.* **37,** 213–217 (1985).
74. Odell, W. D. Puberty. *In* "Endocrinology" (L. J. DeGroot ed.). Saunders, Philadelphia, 1989.
75. Parker, L. N. Osteoporosis. *In* "Adrenal Androgens in Clinical Medicine," pp. 352–365. Academic, San Diego, 1989.
76. Slemenda, C. W., *et al.* Influences on skeletal mineralization in children and adolescents: evidence for varying effects of sexual maturation and physical activity. *J. Pediatr.* **125,** 201–207 (1994).
77. Rico, H., *et al.* Sex differences in the acquisition of total bone mineral mass peak assessed through dual-energy x-ray absorptiometry. *Calcif. Tissue Int.* **51,** 251–254 (1992).
78. Kelly, P. J., *et al.* Sex differences in peak adult bone mineral density. *J. Bone Miner. Res.* **5,** 1169–1175 (1990).
79. Fehily, A. M., *et al.* Factors affecting bone density in young adults. *Am. J. Clin. Nutr.* **56,** 579–586 (1992).
80. Gilsanz, V., *et al.* Gender differences in vertebral sizes in adults: biomechanical implications. *Radiology* **190,** 678–682 (1994).
81. Bonjour, J.-P., *et al.* Peak bone mass. *Osteopor. Int.* **1,** 7–13 (1994).
82. Munoz-Torres, M., *et al.* Bone mass in androgen-insensitivity syndrome: Response to hormonal replacement therapy. *Calcif. Tissue Int.* **57,** 94–96 (1995).
83. Finkelstein, J. S., *et al.* Osteoporosis in men with idiopathic hypogonadotropic hypogonadism. *Ann. Intern. Med.* **106,** 354–361 (1987).
84. Finkelstein, J. S., *et al.* Increase in bone density during treatment of men with idiopathic hypogonadotropic hypogonadism. *J. Clin. Endocrinol. Metab.* **69,** 776–783 (1989).
85. Arisaka, O., and Arisaka, M. Effect of testosterone on radial bone mineral density in adolescent male hypogonadism. *Acta Paediatr. Scand.* **80,** 378–380 (1991).
86. Devogelaer, J. P., *et al.* Low bone mass in hypogonadal males. Effect of testosterone substitution therapy, a densitometric study. *Maturitas* **15,** 17–23 (1992).
87. Mauras, N., *et al.* Calcium and protein kinetics in prepubertal boys. *J. Clin. Invest.* **93,** 1014–1019 (1994).
88. Uriarte, M. M., *et al.* The effect of pubertal delay on adult height in men with isolated hypogonadotropic hypogonadism. *J. Clin. Endocrinol. Metab.* **74,** 436–440 (1992).
89. Finkelstein, J. S., *et al.* Osteopenia in men with a history of delayed puberty. *N. Engl. J. Med.* **326,** 600–604 (1992).
90. Bertelloni, S., *et al.* Short-term effect of testosterone treatment on reduced bone density in boys with constitutional delay of puberty. *J. Bone Miner. Res.* **10,** 1488–1495 (1995).
91. Kelepouris, N., *et al.* Severe osteoporosis in men. *Ann. Intern. Med.* **123,** 452–460 (1995).
92. Stanley, H. L., *et al.* Does hypogonadism contribute to the occurrence of a minimal trauma hip fracture in elderly men? *JAGS* **39,** 766–771 (1991).
93. Jackson, J. A., and Kleerekoper, M. Bone histomorphometry in hypogonadal and eugonadal men with spinal osteoporosis. *J. Clin. Endocrinol. Metab.* **65,** 53–58 (1987).

94. Francis, R. M., and Peacock, M. Osteoporosis in hypogonadal men: role of decreased plasma 1,25-dihydroxyvitamin D, calcium malabsorption, and low bone formation. *Bone* **7,** 261–268 (1986).
95. Foresta, C., *et al.* Testosterone and bone loss in Klinefelter's syndrome. *Horm. Metab. Res.* **15,** 56–67 (1983).
96. Horowitz, M., *et al.* Osteoporosis and Klinefelter's syndrome. *Clin. Endocrinol. (Oxford)* **36,** 113–118 (1992).
97. Reid, I. R., *et al.* Plasma testosterone concentrations in asthmatic men treated with glucocorticoids. *Br. Med. J.* **291,** 574 (1985).
98. Stepan, J. J., and Lachman, M. Castrated men with bone loss: effect of calcitonin treatment on biochemical indices of bone remodeling. *J. Clin. Endocrinol. Metab.* **69,** 523–527 (1989).
99. Goldray, D., *et al.* Decreased bone density in elderly men treated with the gonadotropin-releasing hormone agonist decapeptyl (D-Trp^6-GnRH). *J. Clin. Endocrinol. Metab.* **76,** 288–290 (1993).
100. Delmas, P., and Meunier, P. J. L'osteoporose au cours du syndrome de Klinefelter. Donnees histologiques osseuses quantitatives dans cinq cas. Relation avec la carence hormonale. *Nouv. Presse Med.* **10,** 687 (1981).
101. Baran, D. T., *et al.* Effect of testosterone therapy on bone formation in an osteoporotic hypogonadal male. *Calcif. Tissue Res.* **26,** 103–106 (1978).
102. Jackson, J. A., *et al.* Bone histomorphometry in hypogonadal and eugonadal men with spinal osteoporosis. *J. Clin. Endocrinol. Metab.* **65,** 53–58 (1987).
103. McElduff, A., *et al.* Forearm mineral content in normal men: Relationship to weight, height, and plasma testosterone concentrations. *Bone* **9,** 281–283 (1988).
104. Murphy, S., *et al.* Sex hormones and bone mineral density in elderly men. *Bone Miner.* **20,** 133–140 (1993).
105. Rudman, D., *et al.* Relations of endogenous anabolic hormones and physical activity to bone mineral density and lean body mass in elderly men. *Clin. Endocrinol.* **40,** 653–661 (1994).
106. Barrett-Connor, E., *et al.* A prospective study of dehydroepiandrosterone sulfate (DHEAS) and bone mineral density in older men and women. *Am. J. Epidemiol.* **137,** 201–206 (1993).
107. Drinka, P. J., *et al.* Lack of association between free testosterone and bone density separate from age in elderly males. *Calcif. Tissue Int.* **52,** 67–69 (1993).
108. Meier, D. E., *et al.* Marked decline in trabecular bone mineral content in healthy men with age: lack of association with sex steroid levels. *J. Am. Geriatr. Soc.* **35,** 189–197 (1987).
109. Wishart, J. M., *et al.* Effect of age on bone density and bone turnover in men. *Endocrinol.* **42,** 141–146 (1995).
110. Slemenda, C. W., *et al.* Sex steroids, bone mass and bone loss in older men: Estrogens or androgens? (abst). *In* "Seventeenth Annual Meeting of the American Society for Bone and Mineral Research, Baltimore, MD." Blackwell Science, New York, 1995. [Abstract]
111. Bernecker, P. M., *et al.* Decreased estrogen levels in male patients with primary osteoporosis (abst). *In* "Seventeenth Annual Meeting of the American Society for Bone and Mineral Research, Baltimore, MD." Blackwell Science, New York, 1995. [Abstract]
112. Lips, P., *et al.* The effect of cross-gender hormonal treatment on bone metabolism in male-to-female transsexuals. *J. Bone Miner. Res.* **4,** 657–662 (1989).
113. Van Kesteren, P., *et al.* The effect of one-year cross-sex hormonal treatment on bone metabolism and serum insulin-like growth factor-1 in transsexuals. *J. Clin. Endocrinol. Metab.* **81,** 2227–2232 (1996).
114. Greendale, G. A., *et al.* Endogenous sex steroids and bone mineral density in older women and men: The rancho bernardo study. *J. Bone Miner. Res.* **12,** 1833–1843 (1997).
115. Slemenda, C. W., *et al.* Sex steroids and bone mass in older men. Positive associations with serum estrogens and negative associations with androgens. *J. Clin. Invest.* **100,** 1755–1759 (1997).
116. Buchanan, J. R., *et al.* Determinants of peak trabecular bone density in women: The role of androgens, estrogen, and exercise. *J. Bone Miner. Res.* **3,** 673–680 (1988).
117. Buchanan, J. R., *et al.* Effect of excess endogenous androgens on bone density in young women. *J. Clin. Endocrinol. Metab.* **67,** 937–943 (1988).
118. Daniel, M. Cigarette smoking, steroid hormones, and bone mineral density in young women. *Calcif. Tissue Int.* **50,** 300–305 (1992).
119. Leuenberger, P. K., *et al.* Determination of peak trabecular bone density: interplay of dietary fiber, carbohydrate, and androgens. *Am. J. Clin. Nutr.* **50,** 955–961 (1989).
120. Dixon, J. E., *et al.* Bone mass in hirsute women with androgen excess. *Endocrinol.* **30,** 271–277 (1989).
121. Prezelj, J., and Kocijancic, A. Bone mineral density in hyperandrogenic amenorrhoea. *Calcif. Tissue Int.* **52,** 422–424 (1993).
122. Ohta, H., *et al.* Which is more osteoporosis-inducing, menopause or oophorectomy? *Bone Miner.* **19,** 273–285 (1992).
123. Slemenda, C., *et al.* Sex steroids and bone mass. *Am. Soc. Clin. Invest.* **80,** 1261–1269 (1987).
124. Steinberg, K. K., *et al.* Sex steroids and bone density in premenopausal and perimenopausal women. *J. Clin. Endocrinol. Metab.* **69,** 533–539 (1989).
125. Gasperino, J. Androgenic regulation of bone mass in women. *Clin. Orthop. Rel. Res.* **311,** 278–286 (1995).
126. Vanderschueren, D., and Bouillon, R. Androgens and bone. *Calcif. Tissue Int.* **56,** 341–346 (1995).
127. Davis, S. R., *et al.* Testosterone enhances estradiol's effects on postmenopausal bone density and sexuality. *Maturitas* **21,** 227–236 (1995).
128. Raisz, L. G., *et al.* Comparison of the effects of estrogen alone and estrogen plus androgen on biochemical markers of bone formation and resorption in postmenopausal women. *J. Clin. Endocrinol. Metab.* **81,** 37–43 (1996).
129. Heiss, C. J., *et al.* Associations of body fat distribution, circulating sex hormones, and bone density in postmenopausal women. *J. Clin. Endocrinol. Metab.* **80,** 1591–1596 (1995).
130. Deleted in proof.
131. Martin, B. Aging and strength of bone as a structural material. *Calcif. Tissue Int.* **53**(Suppl. 1), S34–S40 (1993).
132. Vanderschueren, D. Androgens and their role in skeletal homeostasis. *Horm. Res.* **46,** 95–98 (1996).
133. Gilsanz, V., *et al.* Differential effect of gender on the sizes of the bones in the axial and appendicular skeletons. *J. Clin. Endocrinol. Metab.* **82,** 1603–1607 (1997).
134. van der Meulen, M. C. H., Ashford, M. W., Kiratli, B. J., Bachrach, L. K., and Carter, D. R. Determinants of femoral geometry and structure during adolescent growth. *J. Orthop. Res.* **14,** 22–29 (1996).
135. Keenan, B. S., *et al.* Androgen-stimulated pubertal growth: The effects of testosterone and dihydrotestosterone on growth hormone and insulin-like growth factor-I in the treatment of short stature and delayed puberty. *J. Clin. Endocrinol. Metab.* **76,** 996–1001 (1993).
136. Benbassat, C. A., *et al.* Circulating levels of insulin-like growth factor (IGF) binding protein 1 in aging men: Relationships to insulin, glucose, IGF, and dehydroepiandrosterone sulfate levels and anthropometric measures. *J. Clin. Endocrinol. Metab.* **82,** 1482–1491 (1997).

137. Tai-Pang, I., *et al.* Do androgens regulate growth hormone-building protein in adult men? *J. Clin. Endocrinol. Metab.* **80,** 1278–1282 (1995).
138. Ruff, C. B., and Hayes, W. C. Sex differences in age-related remodeling of the femur and tibia. *J. Orthoped. Res.* **6,** 886–896 (1988).
139. Orwoll, E. S. Androgens as anabolic agents for bone. *Trends Endocrinol. Metab.* **7,** 77–84 (1996).
140. Weinstein, R. S., Jilka, R. L., Parfitt, A. M., and Manolagas, S. C. The effects of androgen deficiency on murine bone remodeling and bone mineral density are mediated via cells of the osteoblastic lineage. *Endocrinology* **138,** 4013–4021 (1997).
141. Weissberger, A. J., and Ho, K. K. Y. Activation of the somatotropic axis by testosterone in adult males: evidence for the role of aromatization. *J. Clin. Endocrinol. Metab.* **76,** 1407–1412 (1993).
142. Mauras, N. R., Blizzard, R. M., Link, K., Johnson, M. L., Rogol, A. D., and Velduis, J. D. Augmentation of growth hormone secretion during puberty: evidence for a pulse amplitude-modulated phenomenon. *J. Clin. Endocrinol. Metab.* **64,** 596–601 (1987).
143. Diamond, T., *et al.* Effects of testosterone and venesection on spinal and peripheral bone mineral in six hypogonadal men with hemochromatosis. *J. Bone Miner. Res.* **6,** 39–43 (1991).
144. Katznelson, L., *et al.* Increase in bone density and lean body mass during testosterone administration in men with acquired hypogonadism. *J. Clin. Endocrinol. Metab.* **81,** 4358–4365 (1996).
145. Behre, H. M., *et al.* Long-term effect of testosterone therapy on bone mineral density in hypogonadal men. *J. Clin. Endocrinol. Metab.* **82,** 2386–2390 (1997).
146. Morley, J. E., *et al.* Effects of testosterone replacement therapy in old hypogonadal males: A preliminary study. *J. Am. Geriatr. Soc.* **41,** 149–152 (1993).
147. Wang, C., *et al.* Sublingual testosterone replacement improves muscle mass and strength, decreases bone resorption, and increases bone formation markers in hypogonadal men—A clinical research center study. *J. Clin. Endocrinol. Metab.* **81,** 3654–3662 (1996).
148. Guo, C.-Y., *et al.* Treatment of isolated hypogonadotropic hypogonadism effect on bone mineral density and bone turnover. *J. Clin. Endocrinol. Metab.* **82,** 658–665 (1997).
149. Wang, C., *et al.* Testosterone replacement therapy improves mood in hypogonadal men—A clinical research center study. *J. Clin. Endocrinol. Metab.* **81,** 3578–3583 (1996).
150. Sih, R., *et al.* Testosterone replacement in older hypogonadal men: a 12-month randomized controlled trial. *J. Clin. Endocrinol. Metab.* **82,** 1661–1667 (1997).
151. Kubler, A., *et al.* The influence of testosterone substitution on bone mineral density in patients with Klinefelter's syndrome. *Exp. Clin. Endocrinol.* **100,** 129–132 (1992).
152. Wong, F. H. W., *et al.* Loss of bone mass in patients with Klinefelter's syndrome despite sufficient testosterone replacement. *Osteopor. Int.* **7,** 281–287 (1993).
153. Swerdloff, R. S., and Wang, C. Androgen deficiency and aging in men. *West. J. Med.* **159,** 579–585 (1993).
154. Anderson, F. H., Francis, R. M., Peaston, R. T., and Wastell, H. J. Androgen supplementation in eugonadal men with osteoporosis: effects of six months' treatment on markers of bone formation and resorption. *J. Bone Miner. Res.* **12,** 472–478 (1997).
155. Finkelstein, J. S., Klibanski, A., and Neer, R. M. A longitudinal evaluation of bone mineral density in adult men with histories of delayed puberty. *J. Clin. Endocrinol. Metab.* **81,** 1152–1155 (1996).
156. Arisaka, O., *et al.* Effect of testosterone on bone density and bone metabolism in adolescent male hypogonadism. *Metabolism* **44,** 419–423 (1995).
157. Lamberts, S. W. J., van den Beld, A. W., and van der Lely, A. The endocrinology of aging. *Science* **278,** 419–424 (1997).
158. Tenover, J. S. Effects of testosterone supplementation in the aging male. *J. Clin. Endocrinol. Metab.* **75,** 1092–1098 (1992).
159. Reid, I. R., Wattie, D. J., Evans, M. C., and Stapleton, J. P. Testosterone therapy in glucocorticoid-treated men. *Arch. Intern. Med.* **156,** 1173–1177 (1996).
160. Need, A. G., *et al.* Comparison of calcium, calcitriol, ovarian hormones and nandrolone in the treatment of osteoporosis. *Maturitas* **8,** 275–280 (1986).
161. Need, A. G., *et al.* Effect of nandrolone therapy on forearm bone mineral content in osteoporosis. *Clin. Orthoped. Rel. Res.* **225,** 273–278 (1987).
162. Need, A. G., *et al.* Effects of nandrolone decanoate and antiresorptive therapy on vertebral density in osteoporotic postmenopausal women. *Arch. Intern. Med.* **149,** 57–60 (1989).
163. Need, A. G., *et al.* Cross-over study of fat-corrected forearm mineral content during nandrolone decanoate therapy for osteoporosis. *Bone* **10,** 3–6 (1989).
164. Berkenhager, J. C., *et al.* Can nandrolone add to the effect of hormonal replacement therapy in postmenopausal osteoporosis? *Bone Miner.* **18,** 251–265 (1992).
165. Chesnut, C. H. I., *et al.* Stanozolol in postmenopausal osteoporosis: Therapeutic efficacy and possible mechanisms of action. *Metabolism* **32,** 571–580 (1983).
166. Johansen, J. S., *et al.* Treatment of postmenopausal osteoporosis: is the anabolic steroid nandrolone decanoate a candidate? *Bone Miner.* **6,** 77–86 (1989).
167. Need, A. G., *et al.* Double-blind placebo-controlled trial of treatment of osteoporosis with the anabolic nandrolone decanoate. *Osteopor. Int.* **Suppl. 1,** S218–S222 (1993).
168. Passeri, M., *et al.* Effects of nandrolone decanoate on bone mass in established osteoporosis. *Maturitas* **17,** 211–219 (1993).
169. Lyritis, G. P., *et al.* Effect of nandrolone decanoate and 1-a-hydroxycalciferol on patients with vertebral osteoporotic collapse. A double-blind clinical trial. *Bone Miner.* **27,** 209–217 (1994).
170. Nordin, B. E. C., *et al.* New approaches to the problems of osteoporosis. *Clin. Orthoped. Rel. Res.* **200,** 181–197 (1985).
171. Aerssens, J., *et al.* Mechanical properties, bone mineral content, and bone composition (collagen, osteocalcin, IGF-1) of the rat femur: Influence of ovariectomy and nandrolone decanoate (anabolic steroid) treatment. *Calcif. Tissue Int.* **53,** 269–277 (1993).
172. Labrie, F., *et al.* Effect of 12-month dehydroepiandrosterone replacement therapy on bone, vagina, and endometrium in postmenopausal women. *J. Clin. Endocrinol. Metab.* **82,** 3498–3505 (1997).

Bisphosphonates

SOCRATES E. PAPAPOULOS Department of Endocrinology and Metabolic Diseases, Leiden University Medical Center, The Netherlands

INTRODUCTION

Geminal bisphosphonates are synthetic compounds, analogs of natural pyrophosphosphate in which the oxygen has been replaced by a carbon (Fig. 1). This modification renders bisphosphonates resistant to biological degradation and suitable for clinical use. The first bisphosphonate (etidronate) was synthesized in the past century by German chemists studying the reactions of phosphoric acid with other chemical entities and the stability of the P–C–P bond was first described (1). Because of their ability to inhibit crystallization and to complex metals in solution, bisphosphonates were used in numerous industrial applications long before their potential in the treatment of bone diseases was recognized. Examples include the oil and gas industry and the manufacturing of soaps, detergents, fertilizers, cosmetics, water softeners and toothpastes. In the 1960s, after the recognition of the role of pyrophosphosphate as a natural inhibitor of biomineralization, bisphosphonates were tested for their ability to inhibit calcification because pyrophosphate was hydrolyzable *in vivo.* During these experiments bisphosphonates were shown to inhibit bone resorption, an observation that initiated their development as treatments for skeletal disorders. Today a number of bisphosphonates have been approved for human use whereas others are being clinically developed. Their current therapeutic indications include osteoporosis, Paget's disease, malignancy-associated hypercalcemia, and skeletal complications from breast cancer and multiple myeloma (2–10). This chapter focuses on pharmacological issues relevant to the clinical application of bisphosphonates and to their use in the management of osteoporosis. This is the most common bone disease in the elderly and it is this area in which bisphosphonate use, although raising some controversy in the past, has proved to be one of the most clinically rewarding applications.

CHEMISTRY AND PHARMACOLOGY

All geminal bisphosphonates have two additional side chains, R1 and R2, respectively, allowing numerous substitutions and the development of a variety of analogs with different potencies and pharmacological properties. R1, together with the P–C–P part of the molecule, is responsible for the affinity of bisphosphonates for calcium crystals: This is why this region is sometimes collectively referred to as the "bone hook." The affinity of bisphosphonates for crystal surfaces is increased if R1 is a hydroxyl or an amino group because of the tridentate binding of this configuration to active sites of the calcium crystals (11). Most of the currently used bisphosphonates have a hydroxyl group (Table I). Binding to mineralized matrix is independent of the rest of the structure, and hydroxybisphosphonates with markedly different antiresorptive potencies have generally the same affinity for hydroxyapatite (12–16). The bone hook of the molecule mainly determines the physicochemical properties of the bisphosphonates, the most important being the inhibition of the growth of calcium crystals, an action that is probably responsible for their intrinsic property to inhibit the mineralization of bone. All bisphosphonates given at high doses can inhibit calcification and induce mineralization defects. This action is, however, clinically relevant only for etidronate given at high doses. The newer bisphosphonates have a much larger therapeutic window, and doses that suppress bone resorption effectively do not affect the mineralization of newly formed bone.

The effect of bisphosphonates on bone resorption is determined primarily by the structure of the R2 side chain of the molecule, which is also referred to as the "bioactive moeity." Small modifications in this part of the molecule may result in marked changes in antire-

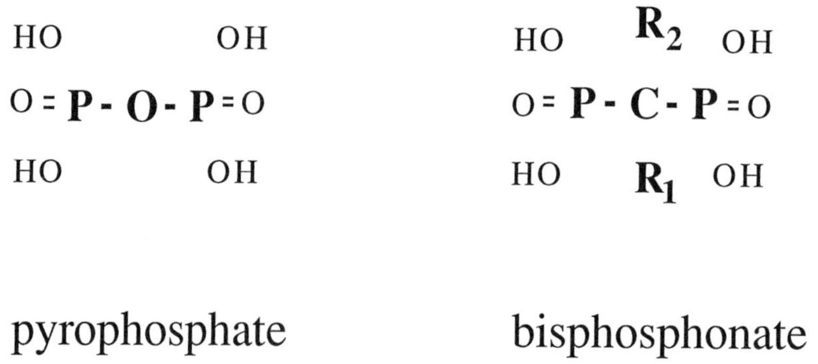

HO OH
O = P - O - P = O
HO OH

pyrophosphate

HO R_2 OH
O = P - C - P = O
HO R_1 OH

bisphosphonate

FIGURE 1 Chemical structure of pyrophosphate and geminal bisphosphonates.

sorptive potencies. Although no clear structure–activity relations have been established, it has been shown that a nitrogen functionality in an alkyl chain or a ring structure at R2 increases the potency of the bisphosphonates and their specificity for bone resorption. Nearly all of the newer potent bisphosphonates have a nitrogen function and are collectively named nitrogen-containing bisphosphonates. Studies, however, have demonstrated that the entire bisphosphonate molecule is involved in the cellular mechanism of antiresorptive action (17).

The mechanism of antiresorptive action of bisphosphonates has been a subject of intensive research for many years, but their molecular mechanism of action remained unknown until recently (4,18). A number of studies had already demonstrated that not all bisphosphonates share the same mechanism of action and that differences exist between nitrogen- and nonnitrogen-containing compounds. At the tissue level, bisphosphonates reduce bone turnover by decreasing the activation of new bone remodeling units. At the cellular level they suppress osteoclast-mediated bone resorption by inhibiting the activity of mature osteoclasts as well as the formation of osteoclasts from hematopoietic precursors that originate in the bone marrow. The former action may be due to a direct injury of the osteoclasts, shown for earlier developed bisphosphonates, or to an alteration of their cellular structure leading to loss of activity and/or earlier apoptosis, shown for nitrogen-containing bisphosphonates. The latter action can be direct through an effect on osteoclast precursors or indirect through stimulation of the production of an osteoclast-inhibiting factor by osteogenic cells (19,19a); these events occur at the bone surface rather than at the bone marrow compartment and lead to decreased formation of osteoclasts (20).

The relative contribution of these mechanisms to the antiresorptive action of bisphosphonates *in vivo* is not known and may not be the same for every individual compound.

Marked differences in antiresorptive potencies of bisphosphonates with only small modifications of the structure suggested a receptor-mediated action. However, no such receptor has been identified and no known second messengers have been found to be affected by bisphosphonates *in vitro.* Studies with macrophages showed that nitrogen-containing bisphosphonates, not ctidronate or clodronate, inhibit the prenylation of small GTP-binding proteins, such as *ras,* that are vital for a number of cellular functions, leading to increased apoptosis of these cells (21). It was suggested that a similar mechanism may be responsible for the effect of bisphosphonates on bone resorption. For the prenylation of these proteins, intermediates of the biosynthetic mevalonate pathway, such as geranylgeranyl pyrophosphate

TABLE I Bisphosphonates in Clinical Practice or in Development

1. 4-Amino-1-hydroxybutylidene bisphosphonic acid; Alendronate
2. Dichloromethylene bisphosphonic acid; Clodronate
3. 3-(1-Pyrrolidinyl)-1-hydroxypropylidene bisphosphonic acid; EB-1089
4. 1-Hydroxyethylidene bisphosphonic acid; Etidronate
5. 3-Methylpentylamino-1-hydroxypropylidene bisphosphonic acid; Ibandronate
6. Cycloheptylamino-methylene bisphosphonic acid; Incadronate
7. 6-Amino-1-hydroxyexilidene bisphosphonic acid; Neridronate
8. 3-Dimethylamino-1-hydroxypropylidene bisphosphonic acid; Olpadronate
9. 3-Amino-1-hydroxypropylidene bisphosphonic acid; Pamidronate
10. 2-(3-Pyridinyl)-1-hydroxyethylidene bisphosphonic acid; Risedronate
11. Chloro-4-phenylthiomethylene bisphosphonic acid; Tiludronate
12. 1-Hydroxy-2-(1H-imidazole-1-yl) ethylidene bisphosphonic acid; Zoledronate.

and farnesyl pyrophosphate, are essential. In long bone cultures *in vitro,* it was found that the formation of geranylgeranyl pyrophosphate is suppressed by bisphosphonate treatment (22). Taken together, these findings led to the conclusion that enzymes of the mevalonate pathway are the potential molecular targets of nitrogen-containing bisphosphonates, an area that is being explored intensively by various research groups.

Bisphosphonates share a number of pharmacological properties: low intestinal absorption, rapid elimination from the circulation, selective uptake by the skeleton, lack of circulating metabolites, renal excretion, and long skeletal retention. Differences also exist in their pharmacological and toxicological profiles as well as in their mechanism of action. It is, therefore, important that the specific properties of every individual bisphosphonate be determined and that results obtained with one bisphosphonate not be extrapolated readily to the whole class.

The absorption of bisphosphonates, which ranges between 0.5 and 5% of the orally administered dose, takes place primarily in the upper gastrointestinal tract and occurs probably along the intestinal cells (paracellularly) rather than across the cells (trancellularly) (23). Absorption decreases further in the presence of food or calcium, which binds the bisphosphonate. It is therefore mandatory to give oral bisphosphonate in the fasting state 30 min to 1 hr before meals with water only and never with milk. In the circulation, bisphosphonates are bound to plasma proteins, are cleared rapidly, and are taken up selectively by the skeleton. About 50% of the given dose concentrates in bone. Skeletal uptake depends on the rate of bone turnover, on the availability of active sites, and on the structure of the bisphosphonate; hydroxybisphosphonates show increased fractional retention compared to compounds with other substitutions at R1 (e.g., clodronate). For all bisphosphonates studied so far, no circulating metabolites have been identified and the rest of the administered dose is excreted by the kidney. Evidence shows that a renal tubular secretory mechanism may be involved in the elimination of at least some bisphosphonate. Impaired renal function reduces bisphosphonate excretion, leading to higher accumulation in the skeleton. Caution is, therefore, needed in their use in patients with renal failure inasmuch as clinical studies in such patients are sparse. Bisphosphonates are retained in the skeleton for a long time and their terminal half-life ranges from a few months to several years, depending on the species (24–27). It should be noted, however, that bisphosphonates affect a bone surface-related process and the active compound is that presented to this surface, whereas the bisphosphonate that is embedded in bone is biologically inert. Small quantities are probably released with continuing bone remodeling, but their metabolic fate has not been established.

Extensive studies in animals and humans have shown that the initial action of bisphosphonates is the suppression of bone resorption. Suppression of the rate of bone resorption depends further on the dose and the route of administration of the bisphosphonate as well as on the nature of the skeletal disease (28). After intravenous administration, the earliest change is detected after 24–48 hr. This contrasts with the more rapid action of calcitonin, which has led some investigators to recommend the combined use of calcitonin, and bisphosphonate when patients with life-threatening hypercalcemia are being treated. Suppression of bone resorption is followed by a second, slower decrease in the rate of bone formation due to the coupling of these two processes. Three to 6 months after the start of treatment, a new equilibrium between bone resorption and bone formation is reached at a lower level of bone turnover. During this period of dissociation of bone resorption from bone formation there is a transient increase in calcium balance and in calcium retention in the skeleton. In patients with increased bone turnover treated with high doses of potent bisphosphonates this early rapid suppression of bone resorption with the still unchanged bone formation rate may decrease serum calcium calcium concentrations with a compensatory increase in parathyroid hormone (PTH) secretion.

Pharmacodynamic and pharmacokinetic observations in animal and human models with different rates of bone turnover have led to two principal clinical uses of bisphosphonates. First, in conditions with excessive bone resorption, short-term courses with high doses are preferred; the limiting factor is the toxicological profile of the bisphosphonate. Examples include malignancy-associated hypercalcemia and Paget's disease of bone. Second, in conditions in which bone resorption is not increased excessively or there is an imbalance between bone resorption and bone formation, as in most patients with osteoporosis, lower doses given for longer periods constitute the preferred approach. An issue that can create some confusion among treating clinicians is the assumption that the total dose of bisphosphonate delivered to the skeleton will determine the final biological response. Studies in patients with high rates of bone turnover, such as Paget's disease, have shown that this is not true and that the magnitude of suppression of bone resorption depends largely on the amount of bisphosphonate presented to the bone surface at any particular time. If the same dose is divided over a long period, the final result will be different and the response will be incomplete. The possible implications of these pharmacodynamic principles have not yet been explored adequately in patients with osteoporosis.

BISPHOSPHONATES IN OSTEOPOROSIS

In osteoporosis there is an imbalance between bone resorption and bone formation leading to bone loss with every remodeling cycle. When this is accompanied by an increase in the activation of new bone remodeling units, more bone will be lost over the same period. In addition, this will affect the structure of the trabeculae leading to thinning and perforations with a subsequent increased risk for breaking. These form the rationale for the use of bisphosphonates, and other antiresorptive agents, in the treatment of osteoporosis. However, certain precautions needed to be taken as the doses used in the treatment of diseases with excessive bone resorption are not appropriate for the treatment of osteoporosis. Initial animal studies provided the necessary information (29). It was shown that the suppression of bone resorption during daily treatment with bisphosphonate (pamidronate) was dose dependent, reaching a plateau that was also dose dependent (Fig. 2). Of particular importance was the observation that this plateau was sustained despite the continuing administration of the bisphosphonate, which implied (1) that bone resorption can be suppressed mildly by daily treatment with low-dose bisphosphonate and (2) that the accumulation of the drug in the skeleton was not accompanied by a cumulative effect on bone metabolism. There was, thus, no evidence for the excessive suppression of bone remodeling, an undesirable effect that may reduce the ability of the skeleton to repair fatigue damage in osteoporotic patients. This pattern of response has now been confirmed repeatedly in long-term studies with nitrogen-containing bisphosphonates such as alendronate, ibandronate, pamidronate, and risedronate. Biochemical parameters of bone turnover were shown to decrease to the average of the premenopausal range (30).

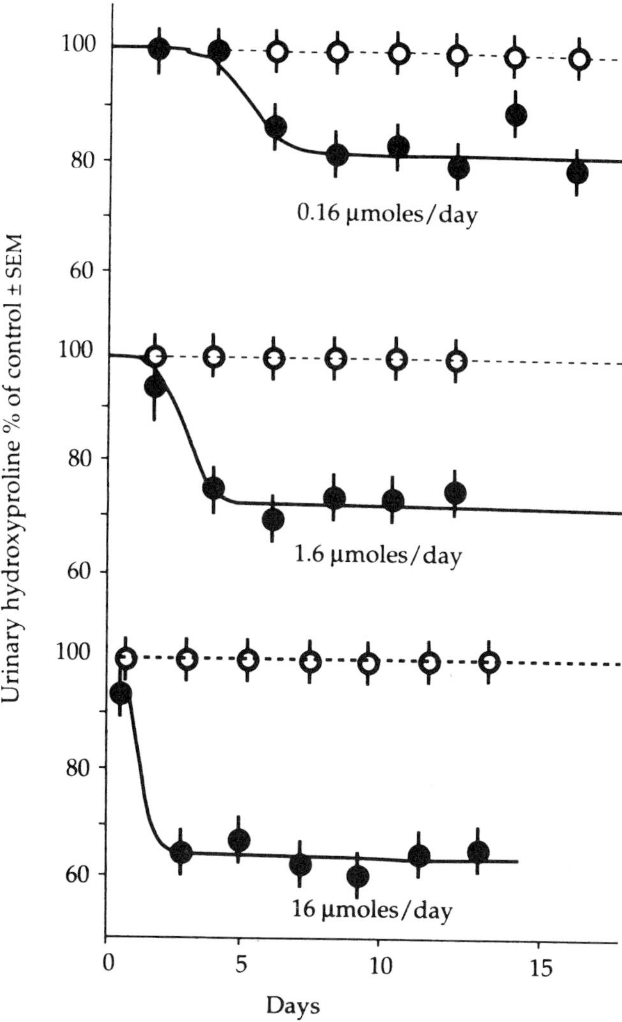

FIGURE 2 Changes in urinary hydroxyproline excretion in rats treated with daily injections of three different doses of pamidronate (●) or vehicle (○). From Reitsma *et al.* (29), with permission.

All bisphosphonates, independently of mode or route of administration, have been shown to significantly increase bone mineral density predominantly of trabecular bone. Studies with etidronate given intermittently (400 mg/day for 2 weeks every 3 months) showed that the initial increase in bone mineral density (BMD) is followed by a plateau, as would be expected by an antiresorptive therapy that reduces the bone remodeling space (31). However, open and controlled studies with daily oral administration of nitrogen-containing bisphosphonates, alendronate and pamidronate, showed that this increase, which occurred at all skeletal sites, is not confined to the first 2 years of treatment but that it continues thereafter significantly for up to 5 years, albeit at a lower rate (32–34). The reason for this further increase in BMD is not apparent and various explanations have been proposed (35). These include a possible anabolic effect of treatment due to small increases in circulating PTH or to a direct effect of the bisphosphonates on osteogenic cells or a readjustment of bone mass homeostasis. Of particular interest is the hypothesis that this is due to a higher degree of mineralization of bone due to the lower rate of bone turnover. This is supported by microradiographic studies of bone biopsies from rats treated with alendronate, but such evidence in humans is not yet available (36).

ANTIFRACTURE EFFICACY OF BISPHOSPHONATE TREATMENT

The aim of any pharmacological intervention in osteoporosis is the decrease in incident fractures in patients who have not yet sustained an osteoporotic fracture or of the progression of the disease in patients with prevalent fractures. Studies in various animal models with nitrogen-containing bisphosphonates showed that they preserve bone quality and improve the biomechanical properties of bone. Data on fracture prevention by bisphosphonates in humans are available with cyclical etidronate and alendronate. In two studies, cyclical etidronate appeared to be effective and reduced the incidence of vertebral fractures in patients with severe osteoporosis (37–39). The lower incidence of vertebral fractures was reported to be sustained for up to 7 years of treatment (40). However, an overall effectiveness of this regimen in reducing the incidence of new spinal fractures has not been shown under controlled conditions. There are no prospective data on the effect of cyclical etidronate on the incidence of nonvertebral fractures. An observational postmarketing survey suggested, however, that this may be the case (41).

Alendronate is the most extensively studied pharmacological agent in osteoporosis under (randomized controlled trial) (RCT) conditions. When given in different doses to postmenopausal women with osteoporosis, 20% of whom had prevalent fractures, it reduced significantly (by about 50%) the incidence of new vertebral deformities after 3 years (42). Pooling the data for all doses used, which was preplanned, was required to demonstrate this effect. The overall antifracture effectiveness of alendronate was supported further by a meta analysis of five RCTs (43). Its efficacy, however, was demonstrated in a study designed specifically to address this issue (fracture intervention trial, FIT). In this study, postmenopausal women with a mean age of 71 years, at least one prevalent vertebral fracture, and femoral neck BMD less than 2 SD of the mean of healthy premenopausal women were randomized to receive 5 mg/day alendronate or placebo for 3 years (44). All women also received 500 mg/day calcium. The dose of alendronate was increased to 10 mg/day after the second year, as in parallel trials this dose was shown to have optimal effects on BMD. New fractures occurred in 145/965 (15%) women in the placebo group and in 78/981 (8%) women in the alendronate-treated group. Active treatment also reduced the risk of multiple vertebral fractures and of wrist fractures significantly. Moreover, this was the first study to demonstrate a significant reduction in the incidence of new hip fractures (by 50%) in calcium and vitamin D-replete free-living women with osteoporosis. In the second arm of the FIT, more than 4000 women aged between 55 and 80 years with low femoral neck BMD but no prevalent vertebral fractures were treated with placebo or alendronate for 4 years. Five milligrams per day of alendronate was given the first 2 years and 10 mg/days the following 2 years. A full report of this study has not been published yet, but preliminary results showed that in women with a BMD T score of less than 2.5, alendronate reduced the incidence of new vertebral fractures by 52% and that of clinical fractures by 31%. Finally, in a multinational study (FOSIT), 1908 postmenopausal women with osteoporosis aged between 39 and 84 years were treated with placebo or 10 mg/day alendronate for 1 year (45). The incidence of nonvertebral fractures, which were captured as adverse events, was reduced significantly by 47% (19 patients on alendronate versus 37 patients on placebo). Thus, data obtained so far with alendronate in RCTs involving large numbers of osteoporotic women showed consistently significant and clinically relevant reductions in the incidence of new osteoporotic fractures. Information about the antifracture efficacy of other bisphosphonates is not yet available. Phase III studies with risedronate have been completed and results are expected in the near future.

An important issue that emerged from these studies is the relation between changes in BMD and reduction in the incidence of fractures. Although greater gains in BMD were generally associated with a higher reduction in fracture risk in the alendronate studies, the modest increases in BMD cannot fully explain the magnitude of the decrease in fracture incidence. By reducing the depth of the resorption cavities and by decreasing the rate of bone turnover, it may be that bisphosphonates decrease the risk of perforation of the trabeculae by the osteoclasts. These hypotheses need, however, to be explored further.

There is no information from controlled studies about the efficacy of bisphosphonates in men with osteoporosis. Preliminary data suggest, however, that they are also efficacious in this indication. Interesting, very promising data about the use of bisphosphonates (mainly pamidronate) have been reported in children with various forms of osteoporosis, including osteogenesis imperfecta (46,47). Such findings are outside the scope of this chapter but help evaluate the long-term safety of treatment as the growing skeleton is extremely sensitive to agents that may affect bone metabolism adversely.

GLUCOCORTICOID-INDUCED OSTEOPOROSIS

The first controlled study of bisphosphonate treatment in the prevention of glucocorticoid-induced bone loss was reported already in 1988 (48). Oral pamidronate (150 mg/day) was shown to prevent bone loss at both trabecular and cortical sites in glucocorticoid-treated patients after 1 year. Following this report there has been a remarkable paucity of controlled studies with bisphosphonates in this important clinical indication. Only several small nonrandomized studies with cyclical etidronate were reported (49,50). Controlled studies with cyclical etidronate and alendronate recently appeared in the literature, leading to approval of these treatments in various countries worldwide. Adachi *et al.* (51) conducted a randomized placebo-controlled study of the efficacy of cyclical etidronate in preventing bone loss in men and women who had recently (less than 3 months) started treatment with high doses of glucocorticoids for various indications. After 52 weeks there were significant differences in BMD of the spine and the trochanter between placebo and etidronate-treated groups (3.7 and 4.1%, respectively). No significant changes in the BMD of the femoral neck and the radius were noted. Of the postmenopausal women in the study, 1/31 treated with etidronate versus 7/32 treated with placebo had new vertebral fractures after 1 year, suggesting antifracture efficacy. Similar results for BMD were reported in a study of identical design by Roux and colleagues (52). In a larger placebo-controlled study of women and men treated for various periods with glucocorticoids, Saag *et al.* (53) showed that 5 or 10 mg/day alendronate significantly prevented bone loss at all skeletal sites after 48 weeks. Of the postmenopausal women in the study, 6/135 (4.4%) treated with alendronate versus 7/54 (13%) treated with placebo developed new vertebral fractures. Fracture incidence in both the etidronate and the alendronate studies was based on semiquantitative assessment of the X rays. The alendronate results indicate that it is efficacious in the prevention and treatment of glucocorticoid-induced osteoporosis.

These studies demonstrated the efficacy of bisphosphonates in the prevention and treatment of the most important cause of secondary osteoporosis, particularly in older women with increased risk of fractures. On the basis of these results and the current lack of reliable data about the relationship between BMD and fracture risk in glucocorticoid-treated patients, the possibility of offering bisphosphonates to elderly women about to start treatment with high doses of steroids should be considered carefully. Another important area of secondary osteoporosis in which the use of bisphosphonates is currently actively explored is posttransplantation osteoporosis, which can be particularly severe, especially in patients undergoing liver or heart transplantations.

SAFETY AND TOLERABILITY

Potential side effects of bisphosphonate treatment should be distinguished between those occurring at the bone tissue level and those due to general toxicity. Because of the long retention of the bisphosphonates in the skeleton and their property to inhibit the growth of calcium crystals *in vitro,* establishing skeletal safety forms a very important part of the development of these compounds as treatments for osteoporosis. In early studies, high doses of etidronate and clodronate induced fractures in dogs after 1 year (54). This was not the case with alendronate given to dogs for 3 years at a dose five times higher than the therapeutic dose (55). In addition, alendronate did not interfere with the normal healing and callus formation of experimentally induced fractures in dogs (56). Impairment of normal mineralization has been observed in animals and humans given high doses of etidronate. However, with the intermittent regimen used in the treatment of osteoporosis, no clinically significant osteomalacia has been reported (57–59). There are only anectodal reports of histologically confirmed osteomalacia with cyclical etidronate treatment (60,61). Bone biopsies of patients with osteoporosis treated with 5 or 10 mg/day alendronate for up to 3 years showed, compared to placebo, the expected decrease in the rate of bone turnover with no evidence of a mineralization defect (62–64). No impairment of mineralization during the treatment of osteoporotic patients with pamidronate (150 mg/day) for 2 years in a placebo-controlled trial or for 5 years in open studies has been encountered (unpublished observations). The same was also the case in patients with rheumatoid arthritis treated with pamidronate (300 mg/day) or placebo for 3 years (65). Furthermore, long-term pamidronate treatment did not affect the rapid mobilization of calcium from the skeleton or the responsiveness of the parathyroid glands to acutely induced hypocalcemia (66); this is in contrast to the findings during treatment with estrogens that were reported to decrease the sensitivity of the parathyroid glands to stimulation by EDTA-induced hypocalcemia (67). A related important issue is the reversibility of the effect of bisphosphonates on bone turnover and BMD after the discontinuation of treatment. There is agreement among studies that bone turnover, assessed biochemically, increases toward pretreatment values within 1 year of stopping treatment. This reemphasizes the lack of cumulative effects on bone metabolism. Reports on changes in BMD after stopping treatment did not provide consistent results. In short-term studies of postmenopausal women treated with tiludronate and alendronate, respectively, Reginster *et al.* (68) and Rossini *et al.* (69), reported no bone loss 6 months after stopping bisphosphonate treatment. In a small number of patients treated for at least 5 years (mean 6.5 years) with oral pamidronate, no change was found in spine or femoral neck BMD 2 years after the discontinuation of treatment, and despite the reactivation of bone metabolism (70). In contrast, in larger studies of alendronate in younger postmenopausal women, a progressive decrease in BMD followed treatment arrest at a rate similar to that of the placebo group (63). Thus there was no accelerated bone loss as occurs after stopping estrogens. It is not clear whether the initial rate of bone turnover, the length of treatment, or the dose of the bisphosphonate is responsible for these differences.

The overall safety profile of the bisphosphonates is excellent, provided that the general as well as the individual properties of the compounds are taken into consideration. When bisphosphonates are infused rapidly at high doses, they may form complexes with calcium in the circulation, which can be nephrotoxic. They should always be administered by slow infusion. Very potent bisphosphonates may be given, however, as bolus injections, an approach currently evaluated in phase III studies with intravenous ibandronate. In some patients treated for the first time with high doses of nitrogen-containing bisphosphonates, there is an increase in body temperature within the first 3 days of treatment that is associated with flu-like symptoms. This effect is transient, reverses within a few days without specific treatment and does not generally occur on the continuation of treatment or reexposure to the drug. The clinical and biochemical changes are those of an acute-phase reaction and it has been reported to be mediated by interleukin 6 and tumor necrosis factor-α (71,72). This response is not observed during the treatment of patients with osteoporosis with nitrogen-containing bisphosphonates, probably because of the much lower doses used.

Mild gastrointestinal (GI) complaints have been reported with the use of all bisphosphonates. Aminobisphonates, however, given orally can induce more severe GI side effects such as nausea, heartburn, and vomiting (73). A few cases with severe oesophagitis have been reported with oral pamidronate and alendronate in patients with osteoporosis (74,75). In all clinical trials involving a few thousand patients, alendronate given in doses between 5 and 20 mg/day had an incidence of GI side effects similar to that of the placebo-treated groups. In clinical trials, however, patients are carefully selected and followed. In daily practice, conditions may not be the same and there are some concerns about the GI effects of this bisphosphonate. In the FOSIT study, in which no careful selection of patients was done, the incidence of symptoms such as abdominal pain, dyspepsia, dysphagia, nausea, and vomiting was identical between the group receiving 10 mg/day alendronate and the group receiving placebo. Preliminary data from observations in a large number of general practices in the Netherlands suggest that about 10% of patients given alendronate will show GI intolerance in daily practice. This incidence is very similar to the one observed in controlled studies. Primary GI intolerance to aminobisphosphonates occurs usually within the first 4 weeks of treatment. Patients should be informed about this possibility and, in case of severe symptoms, treatment should be stopped. After reviewing with the patient the way the bisphosphonate was taken (with a full glass of water and not reclining after that), treatment can be reinstituted after 3 to 4 weeks. In case of reappearance of symptoms, treatment should be stopped. With oral pamidronate, GI effects appear to be dose related. In a placebo-controlled study of patients with osteoporosis, the incidence of GI side effects with 150 mg/day was low and distributed equally between pamidronate- and placebo-treated patients. In patients with rheumatoid arthritis, 300 mg/day pamidronate was associated with GI effects in 28% of the patients compared to 8% in placebo-treated patients. Daily doses higher than 300 mg/day induce GI side effects of varying severity in up to 50% of patients. Data on the GI toxicity of other nitrogen-containing bisphosphonates are not yet available from large controlled studies. The mechanism underlying this effect, as well as whether amino or nitrogen groups are primarily responsible, is not yet known.

SUMMARY

The evidence reviewed in this chapter underscores the important place of bisphosphonates in the treatment of osteoporosis. This is particularly true for alendronate which was shown to be efficacious in a number of randomized controlled studies. Of particular relevance to the scope of this book is that bisphosphonates were shown to be equally effective in younger as well as elderly postmenopausal women up to the age of 85 years (the highest age included in trials). Results of antifracture efficacy of other bisphosphonates given orally continuously (risedronate, pamidronate) or intravenously intermittently (ibandronate, pamidronate) are awaited, which will help position the whole class of these pharmacological agents in the management of osteoporosis.

References

1. Blomen, L. J. M. J. History of the bisphosphonates: discovery and history of the non-medical uses of bisphosphonates. *In* "Bisphosphonate on Bones" (O. L. M. Bijvoet, H. A. Fleisch, R. E. Canfield, and R. G. G. Russell, eds), pp 111–124. Elsevier, Amsterdam, 1995.
2. Geddes, A. D., D'Souza, S. M., Ebetino, F. H., and Ibbotson, K. J. Bisphosphonates: Structure-activity relationships and therapeutic implications. *In* "Bone and Mineral Research" (J. N. M. Heersche and J. A. Kanis, eds.), Vol. 8, pp. 265–306. Elsevier Science, Amsterdam, 1994.
3. Fleisch, H. Bisphosphonates: mechanism of action. *Endocr. Rev.* **19,** 80–100 (1998).
4. Fleisch, H. Bisphosphonates in bone disease. *In* "From the Laboratory to the Patient," 3rd Ed. The Parthenon Publishing Group, New York, 1997.

5. Fleisch, H. Bisphosphonates. Pharmacology and use in the treatment of tumour induced hypercalcaemic and metastatic bone disease. *Drugs* **42,** 919–944 (1991).
6. Yates, A. J., and Rodan, G. A. Alendronate and osteoporosis. *Drug Discov. Today* **3,** 69–78 (1998).
7. Rodan, G. A. Mechanism of action of bisphosnates. *Annu. Rev. Pharmacol. Toxicol.* **38,** 375–388 (1998).
8. Rogers, M. J., Watts, D. J., and Russell, R. G. G. Overview of bisphosphonates. *Cancer* (Suppl.) **80,** 1652–1660 (1997).
9. Papapoulos, S. E. Paget's disease of bone: clinical, diagnostic and therapeutic aspects. *Bailliere's Clin. Endocrinol. Metab.* **11,** 117–143 (1997).
10. Papapoulos, S. E. Bisphosphonates: pharmacology and use in the treatment of osteoporosis. *In* "Osteoporosis" (R. Marcus, D. Feldman, and J. Kelsey, eds.), pp 1209–1234, Raven Press, New York, 1996.
11. Benedict, J. J. The physical chemistry of the diphosphonates—Its relationship to their structural activity. *In* "Diphosphonates and Bone" (A. Donath and B. Courvoisier, eds.), pp 1–19, Symposium CEMO IV, Nyon Switzerland, Editions Medicine st Hygiene, Geneva, 1982.
12. van Beek, E., Hoekstra, M., van de Ruit, M., Löwik, C., and Papapoulos, S. Structural requirements for bisphosphonate actions in vitro. *J. Bone Miner. Res.* **12,** 1875–1882 (1994).
13. Sato, M., Grasser, W., Endo, N., Akins, R., Simmons, H., Thompson, D. D., and Rodan, G. A. Bisphosphonate action: Alendronate localization in rat bone and effects on osteoclast ultrastructure. *J. Clin. Invest.* **88,** 2095–2105 (1991).
14. Jung, A., Bisaz, S., and Fleisch, H. The binding of pyrophosphate and two diphosphonates on hydroxyapatite crystals. *Calcif. Tissue Res.* **11,** 269–280 (1973).
15. Sunberg, R., Ebetino, F. H., Mosher, C. T., and Roof, C. F. Designing drugs for stronger bones. *Chemtech* **21,** 304–309 (1991).
16. Sinoda, H., Adamek, G., Felix, R., Fleisch, H., Schenk, R., and Hagan, P. Structure-activity relationships of various bisphosphonates. *Calcif. Tissue Int.* **35,** 87–99 (1983).
17. van Beek, E., Löwik, C., Que, I., and Papapoulos, S. Dissociation of binding and antiresorptive properties of hydroxybisphosphonates by substitution of the hydroxyl with an amino group. *J. Bone Miner. Res.* **11,** 1492–1497 (1996).
18. Rodan, G. A., and Fleisch, H. Bisphosphonates: mechanisms of action. *J. Clin. Invest.* **97,** 2692–2696 (1996).
19. Shahni, M., Guenther, H., Fleisch, H., and Martin, T. J. Bisphosphonates act on bone resorption through mediation of osteoblasts. *J. Clin. Invest.* **91,** 2004–2011 (1993).
19a. Vitte, C., Fleisch, H., and Guenther, H. L. Bisphosphonates induce osteoblasts to secrete an inhibitor of osteoclast-mediated resorption. *Endocrinology* **137,** 2324–2333 (1996).
20. van Beek, E., Löwik, C. W. G. M., and Papapoulos, S. E. Effect of alendronate on the osteoclastogenic potential of bone marrow cells in mice. *Bone* **20,** 335–340 (1997).
21. Luckman, S. P., Huges, D. E., Coxon, F. P., Russell, R. G. G., and Rogers, M. J. Nitrogen-containing bisphosphonates inhibit the mevalonate pathway and prevent post-translational prenylation of GTP-binding proteins, including ras. *J. Bone Miner. Res.* **13,** 581–589 (1998).
22. van Beek, E., Löwik, C., van der Pluijm, G., and Papapoulos, S. The role of geranylgeranylation in bone resorption and its suppression by bisphosphonates in fetal bone explants in vitro; a clue to the mechanism of action of nitrogen-containing bisphosphonates. *J. Bone Miner. Res.* (1999).
23. Twiss, I. M., de Water, R., van Hartigh, J., Sparidans, R., Ramp-Koopmanschap, W., Bril, H., Wijdeveld, M., and Vermeij, P. Cytotoxic effects of pamidronate on monolayers of human intestinal epithelial (Caco-2) cells and its epithelial transport. *J. Pharma. Sci.* **83,** 699–703 (1994).
24. Mönkkönen, J., Koponen, H. M., and Yitalo, P. Comparison of the distribution of three bisphosphonates in mice. *Pharmacol. Toxicol.* **66,** 294–298 (1990).
25. Kastings, G. B., and Francis, M. D. Retention of etidronate in human, dog and rat. *J. Bone Miner. Res.* **7,** 513–522 (1992).
26. Lin, J. H., Duggan, D. E., Chen, I. W., and Ellsworth, R. L. Physiological desposition of alendronate, a potent anti-osteolytic bisphosphonate in laboratory animals. *Drugs Metab. Disp.* **19,** 926–932 (1991).
27. Kanis, J. A., Gerts, B. J., Singer, F., and Ortolani, S. Rationale for the use of alendronate in osteoporosis. *Osteopor. Int.* **5,** 1–13 (1995).
28. Papapoulos, S. E. Pharmacodynamics of bisphosphonates in man: Implications for treatment. *In* "Bisphosphonates on Bones" (O. L. M. Bijvoet, H. Fleisch, R. E. Canfield, and R. G. G. Russell, eds), pp. 231–245. Elsevier Science, Amsterdam, 1995.
29. Reitsma, P. H., Bijvoet, O. L. M., Verlinden-Ooms, H., and Wee van der Plas, L. J. A. Kinetic studies of bone and mineral metabolism during treatment with (3-amino-1-hydroxypropylidene)-1,1-bisphosphonate (APD) in rats. *Calcif. Tissue Int.* **32,** 145–157 (1980).
30. Garnero, P., Shih, W. J., Gineyts, E., Karpf, D. B., and Delmas, P. D. Comparison of new biochemical markers of bone turnover in postmenopausal osteoporotic women in response to alendronate treatment. *J. Clin. Endocrinol. Metab.* **79,** 1693–1700 (1994).
31. Heaney, R. P. The bone remodeling transient: Implications for the interpretation of clinical studies of bone mass changes. *J. Bone Miner. Res.* **9,** 1515–1523 (1994).
32. Valkema, R., Vismans, F.-J. F. E., Papapoulos, S. E., Pauwels, E. K. J., and Bijvoet, O. L. M. Maintained improvement in calcium balance and in bone mineral content in patients with osteoporosis treated with the bisphosphonate APD. *Bone Miner.* **5,** 183–192 (1989).
33. Liberman, U. A., Weiss, S. R., Bröll, J., *et al.* Effect of oral alendronate on bone mineral density and the incidence of fractures in postmenopausal osteoporosis. *N. Engl. J. Med.* **99,** 144–152 (1995).
34. Favus, M., Emkey, R., Leite, M., Devogelaer, J. P., Rodriguez, J., Peverly, C., Kauf, A., and Santora, A. Five-year treatment of osteoporosis in postmenopausal women with oral alendronate: effects on bone mass and turnover and safety. *J. Bone Miner. Res.* **12**(Suppl.) S150 (1997).
35. Rodan, G. A. Bone mass homeostasis and bisphosphonate action. *Bone* **20,** 1–4 (1997).
36. Meunier, P. J., and Boivin, G. Bone mineral density reflects bone mass but also the degree of mineralization of bone: therapeutic implications. *Bone* **21,** 373–377 (1997).
37. Storm, T., Thamsborg, G., Steiniche, T., Genant, H. K., and Sorensen, O. H. Effect of intermittent cyclical etidronate therapy on bone mass and fracture rate in women with postmenopausal osteoporosis. *N. Engl. J. Med.* **322,** 1265–1271 (1990).
38. Watts, N. B., Harris, S. T., Genant, H. K., *et al.* Intermittent cyclical etidronate treatment of postmenopausal osteoporosis. *N. Engl. J. Med.* **323,** 73–79 (1990).
39. Harris, S. T., Watts, N. B., Jackson, R. D., *et al.* Four-year study of intermittent cyclic etidronate treatment of postmenopausal osteoporosis: Three years of blinded therapy followed by one year of open therapy. *Am. J. Med.* **95,** 557–567 (1993).
40. Miller, P. D., Watts, N. B., Licata, A. A., *et al.* Cyclical etidronate in the treatment of postmenopausal osteoporosis: Efficacy and safety after seven years of treatment. *Am. J. Med.* **103,** 468–476 (1997).

41. van Staa, T. P., Abenheim, L., and Cooper, C. Use of cyclical etidronate and prevention of non-vertebral fractures. *Br. J. Rheumatol.* **37,** 87–94 (1998).
42. Liberman, U. A., Weiss, S. R., Bröll, J., *et al.* Effect of oral alendronate on bone mineral density and the incidence of fractures in postmenopausal osteoporosis. *N. Engl. J. Med.* **333,** 1437–1443 (1995).
43. Karpf, D. B., Shapiro, D. R., Seeman, E., *et al.* Prevention of non-vertebral fractures by alendronate: a meta analysis. *JAMA* **227,** 1159–1164 (1997).
44. Black, D. M., Cummings, S. R., Karpf, D. B., *et al.* Randomised trial of the effect of alendronate on risk of fractures in women with existing vertebral fractures. *Lancet* **348,** 1535–1541 (1996).
45. Pols, H. A. P. A multinational, placebo-controlled study of alendronate in postmenopausal women with osteoporosis; results from the FOSIT study. *J. Bone Miner. Res.* **12**(Suppl.) S172 (1997).
46. Brumsen, C., Hamdy, N. A. T., and Papapoulos, S. E. Long-term effects of bisphosphonates on the growing skeleton; studies of young patients with severe osteoporosis. *Medicine* **76,** 266–283 (1997).
47. Glorieux, F. H., Bishop, N. J., Plotkin, H., Chabot, G., Lanogu, G., and Travers, R. Cyclic administration of pamidronate in children with severe osteogenesis imperfecta. *N. Engl. J. Med.* **339,** 947–952 (1998).
48. Reid, I. R., King, A. R., Alexander, C. J., and Ibbeertson, H. K. Prevention of steroid induced osteoporosis with (3-amino-1-hydroxypropylidene)-1,1-bisphosphonate (APD). *Lancet* **i,** 143–146 (1988).
49. Struys, A., Snelder, A. A., and Mulder, H. Cyclical etidronate reverses bone loss of the spine and the proximal femur in patients with established corticosteroid-induced osteoporosis. *Am. J. Med.* **99,** 235–242 (1995).
50. Diamont, T., McGuigan, L., Barbagallo, S., and Bryant, C. Cyclical etidronate plus ergocalciferol prevents glucocorticoid-induced bone loss in postmenopausal women. *Am. J. Med.* **98,** 459–463 (1995).
51. Adachi, J. D., Bensen, W. G., Brown, J., *et al.* Intermittent etidronate therapy to prevent corticosteroid-induced bone loss. *N. Engl. J. Med.* **337,** 382–387 (1997).
52. Roux, C., Oriente, P., Laan, R., *et al.* Randomised trial of effect of cyclical etidronate in the prevention of corticosteroid-induced bone loss. *J. Clin. Endocrinol. Metab.* **83,** 1128–1143 (1998).
53. Saag, K. G., Emkey, R., Schnitzer, T. J., *et al.* Alendronate in the prevention and treatment of glucocorticoid-induced osteoporosis. *N. Engl. J. Med.* **339,** 292–299 (1998).
54. Flora, L., Hassing, G. S., Parfitt, A. M., and Villanueva, A. R. Comparative skeletal effects of two bisphosphonates in dogs. *Metab. Bone Dis. Rel. Res.* **2,** 389–407 (1980).
55. Balena, R., Markatos, A., Seedor, J. G., *et al.* Long-term safety of the aminobisphosphonate alendronate in adult dogs II. histomorphometric analysis of the L5 vertebrae. *J. Pharmacol. Exp. Ther.* **276,** 277–283 (1996).
56. Peter, C. P., Cook, W. O., Nunamaker, D. M., Provost, M. T., Seedor, J. G., and Rodan, G. A. Effect of alendronate on fracture healing and bone remodeling in dogs. *J. Orthop. Res.* **14,** 74–79 (1996).
57. Ott, S. M., Woodson, G. C., Huffer, W. E., Miller, P. D., and Watts, N. B. Bone histomorphometric changes after cyclic therapy with phosphate and etidronate disodium in women with postmenopausal osteoporosis. *J. Clin. Endocrinol. Metab.* **78,** 968–972 (1994).
58. Storm, T., Steiniche,T., Thamsborg, G., and Melsen, F. Changes in bone histomorphometry after long-term treatment with intermittent cyclic etidronate for postmenopausal osteoporosis. *J. Bone Miner. Res.* **8,** 199–208 (1993).
59. Axelrod, D. W., and Teitelbaum, S. L. Results of long-term cyclical etidronate therapy: Bone histomorphometric and clinical correlates. *J. Bone Miner. Res.* **9**(Suppl.) S136 (1994).
60. Thomas, T., Lafage, M. H., and Alexandre, C. Atypical osteomalacia after 2 year etidronate intermittent cyclic administration in osteoporosis. *J. Rheumatol.* **22,** 2183–2185 (1995).
61. Wimalawansa, S. J. Combined therapy with estrogen and etidronate has an additive effect on bone mineral density in the hip and the vertebrae: four year randomized study. *Am. J. Med.* **99,** 36–42 (1995).
62. Chavassieux, P. M., Arlot, M. E., Reda, C., Wel, L., Yates, A. J., and Meunier, P. J. Histomorphometric assessment of the long-term effects of alendronate on bone quality and remodeling in patients with osteoporosis. *J. Clin. Invest,* **100,** 1475–1480 (1997).
63. McGlung, M., Clemmensen, B., Daifotis, A., *et al.* Alendronate prevents postmenopausal bone loss in women with osteoporosis. *Ann. Int. Med.* **128,** 253–261 (1998).
64. Bone, H. G., Downs, R. W., Jr., Tucci, J. R., *et al.* Dose response relationships for alendronate treatment in osteoporotic elderly women. *J. Clin. Endocrinol. Metab.* **82,** 265–274 (1997).
65. Eggelmeijer, F., Papapoulos, S. E., van Passen, H. C., Dijkmans, B. A. C., Valkema, R., Westedt, M. L., Landman, J. O., Pauwels, E. K. J., and Breedveld, F. C. Increased bone mass with pamidronate treatment in rheumatoid arthritis; results of a three-year randomized, double blind trial. *Arthritis Rheum.* **39,** 396–402 (1996).
66. Landman, J. O., Schweitzer, D. H., Frölich, M., Hamdy, N. A. T., and Papapoulos, S. E. Recovery of serum calcium concentrations following acute hypocalcemia in patients with osteoporosis on long-term oral therapy with the bisphosphonate pamidronate. *J. Clin. Endocrinol. Metab.* **80,** 524–528 (1995).
67. Cosman, F., Nieves, J., Horton, J., Shen, V., and Lindsay, R. Effects of estrogen on the response to edetic acid infusion in postmenopausal osteoporotic women. *J. Clin. Endocrinol. Metab.* **78,** 939–943 (1994).
68. Reginster, J. Y., Lecart, M. P., Deroisy, R., *et al.* Prevention of postmenopausal bone loss by tiludronate. *Lancet* **2,** 3465–3468 (1989).
69. Rossini, M., Gatti, D., Zamberlan, N., Braga, V., Dorrizi, R., and Adami, S. Long-term effects of treatment course with oral alendronate of postmenopausal osteoporosis. *J. Bone Miner. Res.* **11,** 1833–1837 (1994).
70. Landman, J. O., Hamdy, N. A. T., Pauwels, E. K. J., and Papapoulos, S. E. Skeletal metabolism in patients with osteoporosis after discontination of long-term treatment with oral pamidronate. *J. Clin. Endocrinol. Metab.* **80,** 3465–3468 (1995).
71. Schweitzer, D. H., Oostendorp-vd Ruit, M., van der Pluijm, G., Löwik, C. W. G. M., and Papapoulos, S. E. Interleukin-6 and the acute phase response during treatment of patients with Paget's disease with the nitrogen-containing bisphosphonate dimethyl-amino-hydroxypropylidene bisphosphonate. *J. Bone Miner. Res.* **10,** 956–962 (1995).
72. Sauty, A., Pecherstorfer, M., Zimmer-Roth, I., Fioroni, P., Juillerat, L., Markert, M., Ludwig, H., Leuenberger, P., Burckhardt, P., and Thiebaud, D. Interleukin-6 and tumor Necrosis factor α levels after bisphosphonate treatment in vitro and in patients with malignancy. *Bone* **18,** 133–139 (1996).
73. Adami, S., and Zamberlan, N. Adverse effects of bisphosphonates. A comparative review. *Drug Safety* **14,** 158–170 (1996).
74. Lufkin, E. G., Argueta, R., Whitaker, M. D, Cameron, A. L., Wong, V. H., Egan, K. S., O'Fallon, W. M., and Riggs, B. L. Pamidronate: an unrecognized problem in gastrointestinal tolerability. *Osteopor. Int.* **4,** 320–322 (1994).
75. De Groen, P. C., Lubbe, D. F., Hirsch, L. J., *et al.* Esophagitis associated with the use of alendronate. *N. Engl. J. Med.* **335,** 1016–1021 (1996).

Calcitonin

CATHERINE E. WAUD AND JOHN L. STOCK
Endocrinology Division, University of Massachusetts Memorial Health Care and the Department of Medicine, University of Massachusetts Medical School, Worcester, Massachusetts 01605

INTRODUCTION

Calcitonin was named for its ability to regulate the "tone" of serum calcium and has been used in the treatment of disorders characterized by increased bone resorption [1]. In 1964 the thyroid was determined to be the source of calcitonin [2]. During fetal development the fourth pharyngeal pouch divides into two portions. The dorsal and ventral portions develop into the superior parathyroid and the ultimobrachial body, respectively. The ultimobrachial body joins the lateral wing of the thyroid and develops into parafollicular C-cells, which are the source of calcitonin. They eventually migrate into the thyroid proper and become indistinguishable from thyroid tissue itself [3].

Structure of Calcitonin Gene Products

The amino-terminal disulfide bone ring closure between the two cystine residues at positions 1 and 7 of this 32 amino acid peptide is important for its biological activity [4,5]. The calcitonin structure is well conserved during evolution. Seven of the first nine residues of calcitonin are common to all species, but there is variability in the rest of the molecule [5]. Most of the variation seen between species is found within the central portion where modifications account for the potency and duration of action of calcitonin. The more flexible the midportion (i.e., fewer side chains), the greater the number of conformational positions at the receptor binding site and the greater the potency [6]. Fish calcitonins, including salmon and eel calcitonin, are approximately 50 times more potent in mammals than human calcitonin [5].

The calcitonin gene has been localized to chromosome 11 [7]. Calcitonin is one cleavage product of a much larger protein. Alternate splicing of the precursor protein can result in other calcitonin-related peptides. Six exons encode three major peptides: calcitonin, katacalcin, and the calcitonin gene-related peptide (CGRP) [8]. The primary RNA transcript of the calcitonin gene is processed in a tissue-specific manner to produce calcitonin, katacalcin, or CGRP [9].

Katacalcin is a 21 amino acid protein flanking calcitonin on the carboxy terminus of the precursor protein [10]. Katacalcin is biologically active and can lower the serum calcium level almost as effectively as calcitonin. Katacalcin potentiates the effect of calcitonin by fivefold, suggesting that katacalcin and calcitonin may work through different receptors [11]. Katacalcin is localized in normal C cells of the thyroid. Like calcitonin, katacalcin levels appear to be higher in men than in women. Elevated levels are also found in medullary thyroid carcinoma [10].

CGRP is a 37 amino acid protein that is produced from the alternate processing of RNA transcript of the calcitonin gene [12]. Calcitonin and CGRP have identical 5′ sequences but nonhomologous 3′ sequences [8]. Because the concentration of CGRP is fivefold higher than calcitonin, it has been postulated that CGRP may be the major circulating product of the calcitonin gene [9]. CGRP can be extracted from medullary thyroid carcinoma tissue and has been found to be a potent vasodilator in both animals and humans [13,14]. CGRP is distributed throughout the central nervous system, especially in the hypothalamus [8], and may play a role in vascular control and in neuromodulation [9,12]. It has also been found in cardiovascular tissue where it may serve as a vasodilator [12]. Unlike calcitonin and katacalcin, CGRP levels are similar in men and women and do not decline with age [9].

The Calcitonin Receptor

The calcitonin receptor is a member of the G-protein subfamily of receptors that includes the PTH, GHRH,

VIP, and secretin receptors [12]. The binding of calcitonin to its receptor is followed by the production of cytoplasmic cyclic adenosine monophosphate and increased cytosolic calcium levels in the osteoclast which lead to the inhibition of osteoclast activity [15]. Calcitonin receptors have been found in osteoclasts and other organs, including the central nervous system [16,17]. There are at least two forms of the human calcitonin receptor [12]. The different isoforms may have variable expression in different tissues and may account for the different effects of calcitonin.

Calcitonin Action

Calcitonin has been shown to inhibit bone resorption directly [18], unlike PTH, which requires the presence of osteoblasts for its effect on the osteoclast [19]. The effects of calcitonin on isolated osteoclasts include the gradual slowing of cell motility, decreased pseudopodial protrusion and retraction, decreased margin ruffling, decreased cell migration, and reduction of the cell surface to 60% of the original cell area [15].

Although the major effect of calcitonin is to inhibit bone resorption, calcitonin may also enhance osteoblastic bone formation *in vitro* and *in vivo* [20]. Calcitonin receptors have been found on a variety of osteoblast-like cell lines, suggesting that the effect of calcitonin may be in part anabolic [20,21]. Calcitonin also increases renal 1-α-hydroxylase activity [17].

Calcitonin Secretion and Metabolism

Calcitonin has rapid antihypercalcemic action, is secreted in response to elevations in serum calcium concentration, and has a half-life of minutes. Gastrin and other gut hormones have been shown to stimulate calcitonin secretion [12]. The kidney is the main site of metabolism and little calcitonin can be detected in urine [22]. Although the major effect of calcitonin is to inhibit bone resorption, effects in liver, kidney, central nervous system, and gastrointestinal tract have been described [17].

EFFECTS OF AGING AND HORMONAL STATUS ON CALCITONIN

Except in medullary cancer of the thyroid, circulating calcitonin concentrations are low, particularly in women [23]. With the development of sensitive and reliable radioimmunoassay techniques, calcitonin has been detected in normal human circulation [23,24]. Calcitonin levels are higher in fetuses and during childhood growth spurts, adolescence, pregnancy, and lactation when bone resorption is increased [15,24,25]. Although it has been shown that estrogen and progesterone increase calcitonin secretion [26], the levels of calcitonin are not directly correlated with levels of estrogen [23]. Evidence from some studies support the hypothesis that the major function of calcitonin is to prevent the excess or unwanted bone resorption during times of skeletal stress [21,27]. This antiresorptive effect has been exploited in the investigation and use of calcitonin for the prevention and treatment of postmenopausal osteoporosis.

Calcitonin levels are higher in men than in women and decrease with age [28]. These differences are more dramatic with provocative testing [23,28] (Fig. 1). It was postulated that aging leads to the decreased secretory capacity of C cells or the diminished response of C cells to calcium stimulus [28] and that women may have lower calcitonin secretion [29] and calcitonin reserves than men [23]. However, another study did not find an age-related decrease in plasma calcitonin levels or a calcitonin secretory response to calcitonin infusion [29]. Taggert *et al.* showed that, although there was no difference in basal calcitonin levels between postmenopausal women with osteoporosis and normal controls, women with osteoporosis had a blunted response to calcium infusion [30]. The interstudy differences found may be explained by the type of calcitonin that is predominant in young and elderly women. Bucht *et al.* [30a] demonstrated that elderly women had predominantly high molecular weight calcitonin with low or undetectable levels of monomeric calcitonin. Young women had both the high molecular weight calcitonin as well as higher levels of the monomeric calcitonin.

Age-related decreases in calcitonin may be related to low vitamin D levels as vitamin D receptors have been found on parathyroid C cells. Impaired calcitonin secretion in elderly vitamin D-deficient subjects was nearly normalized by vitamin D administration [30b].

Several studies have suggested that estrogen's inhibition of bone resorption may be related to its effect on calcitonin secretion [23,27,31,32]. Stevenson *et al.* [27] showed that basal calcitonin concentrations in early menopause were increased by estrogen replacement therapy. Another study failed to find differences in calcitonin concentrations in postmenopausal women before and after treatment with estrogen, but did show that stimulated calcitonin concentrations were higher after estrogen treatment [32]. The estrogen deficiency of menopause may also accelerate the age-related decline of calcitonin secretion, thus increasing the sensitivity of the skeleton to bone-resorbing hormones [31]. Calcitonin levels rise with natural or synthetic estrogen replacement therapy, suggesting that the effect of estrogen on

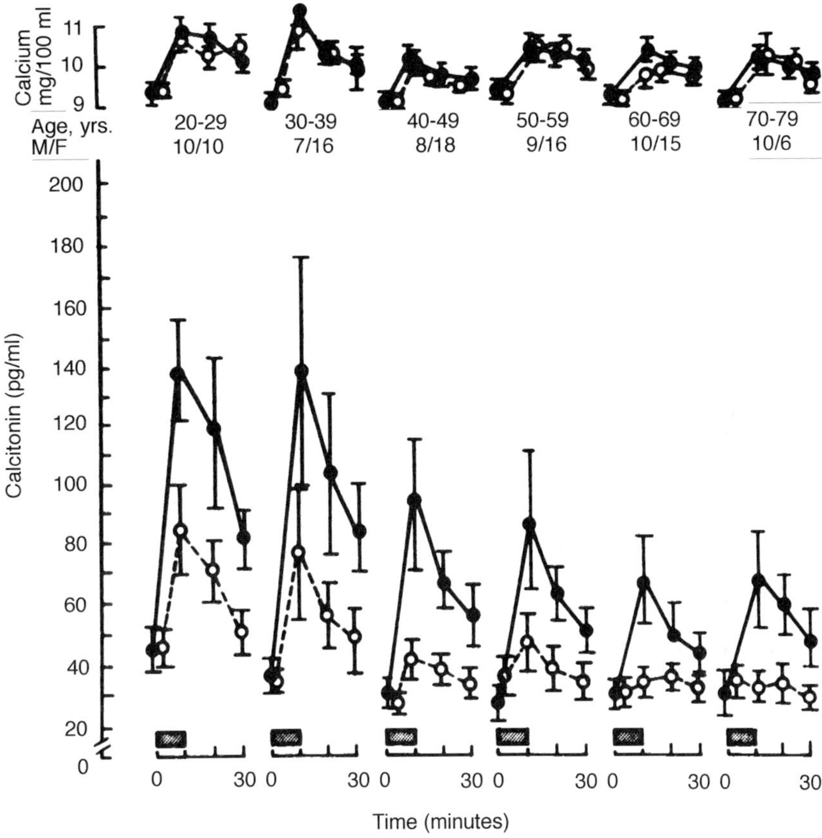

FIGURE 1 Influence of age and sex on plasma calcitonin in humans at baseline and with a 10-min infusion of calcium. ●, men; ○, women. From Deftos *et al.* [28].

bone density may be related in part to calcitonin secretion [27,31]. Hormone replacement therapy increases the size or numbers of C cells, and estrogen deficiency is associated with a decreased C cell mass [31]. *In vitro,* estrogen and progesterone increase calcitonin secretion in a dose-dependent manner. Because this effect is not inhibited by tamoxifen, the estrogen receptor may not be involved [26].

EFFICACY OF CALCITONIN IN THE PREVENTION AND TREATMENT OF POSTMENOPAUSAL OSTEOPOROSIS

Calcitonin has been used in the treatment of diseases characterized by increased osteoclastic bone resorption, including Paget's disease, osteoporosis, and hypercalcemia of malignancy [20]. Although numerous studies have investigated the effectiveness of calcitonin in the prevention and treatment of postmenopausal osteoporosis, many are limited by a lack of randomization or placebo controls, small number of subjects, short duration, varying preparations, different routes of administration, and different study endpoints. These factors make it difficult to compare studies. Concomitant medications, such as calcium, vitamin D, and estrogen, have also complicated interpretation of these studies. Bone mineral content (BMC) or bone mineral density (BMD) and biochemical markers of bone resorption have been used as short-term end points. However, these end points may not be correlated with bone strength or actual fracture risk. Further studies of actual fracture incidence are needed.

Parenteral Calcitonin

In 1985 the FDA approved salmon calcitonin for the treatment of postmenopausal osteoporosis. Salmon calcitonin has several advantages over human calcitonin. It is easy to synthesize on a large scale [5] and is the most potent of the natural calcitonins [16].

PREVENTION OF POSTMENOPAUSAL OSTEOPOROSIS

Bone Mineral Density There are few studies that assess the effect of parenteral salmon calcitonin for the prevention of postmenopausal bone loss. In a 2-year randomized study, MacIntyre *et al.* [33] allotted 70 early postmenopausal women to one of four treatment groups: placebo, calcitonin by subcutaneous injection (20 IU thrice weekly), estrogen and progesterone, and estrogen and progesterone in combination with calcitonin. Intermittent calcitonin was as effective as estrogen at maintaining vertebral BMC. No additional effect was seen when estrogen and calcitonin were combined. Drawbacks of this study include small numbers and an unusually high loss of BMC in the placebo group (10.2%). Mazzuoli *et al.* [34] demonstrated that patients who received intramuscular calcitonin (100 IU every other day) beginning 7 days after ovariectomy showed no change in BMC of the distal radius after 6 or 12 months of treatment. Patients who started calcitonin treatment 6 months after ovariectomy showed a significant decrease in BMC in the first 6 months, but no further decrease in the second 6 months, coinciding with calcitonin administration. These studies suggest that parenteral calcitonin treatment begun soon after menopause can delay bone loss associated with estrogen deficiency.

Bone Markers Serum concentrations of alkaline phosphatase activity and urinary hydroxyproline excretion were decreased in women treated with calcitonin alone or in combination with hormone replacement therapy [33,34]. There were no differences between treatment and control patients in the serum concentrations of the bone formation marker osteocalcin [34].

TREATMENT OF POSTMENOPAUSAL BONE LOSS

Bone Mineral Density Gennari *et al.* [35] studied 82 women with two or more vertebral fractures randomized to calcium only, calcium and daily calcitonin [100 IU], or calcium and alternate day calcitonin [100 IU] given by intramuscular or subcutaneous injection. Confounding this study was a high drop out rate with only 45 women completing the 1-year study (15 in each group). The control group lost significant BMC both at the hip and at the lumbar spine. The calcitonin-treated groups demonstrated significant increases in BMC in a dose-dependent manner at both sites after 1 year. Gruber *et al.* [36] randomized 45 women with atraumatic vertebral fractures and low total body calcium levels (TBC) to receive placebo or calcitonin (100 IU daily) by intramuscular or subcutaneous injection. At the end of 26 months, the calcitonin-treated group demonstrated a significant increase in TBC from baseline compared to a decrease in the placebo group. The effect of calcitonin on TBC appeared to diminish after 18 months, suggesting tolerance to the calcitonin treatment. There was no change in bone mass of the radius in either group. In a 12-month, double-blind, multicenter trial, Mazzuoli *et al.* [37] randomized postmenopausal women with one or more vertebral fractures to either intramuscular calcitonin (100 IU every other day) or placebo. The BMC of the distal forearm increased significantly in the treatment group and decreased significantly in the control group. Civitelli *et al.* investigated the relationship between bone turnover, defined by whole body retention of 99m Tc-methylene disphosphonate, and response to calcitonin treatment. Intermittent low-dose calcitonin by subcutaneous injection (50 IU every other day) increased vertebral BMC 22% in women with high turnover osteoporosis, but did not change in vertebral BMC in osteoporotic women with normal turnover. At the femur, there was a significant decrease in BMC in the group with normal turnover whereas the high turnover group did not lose or gain BMC during the 12 months of treatment [38].

Bone Markers In several studies, parenteral administration of calcitonin was associated with a reduction in urinary hydroxyproline excretion [35,37], but did not affect serum concentrations of alkaline phosphatase activity [35]. In the study by Civitelli *et al.* [38], women with high turnover osteoporosis demonstrated a greater decrease in serum concentrations of osteocalcin and urinary hydroxyproline excretion in response to calcitonin treatment than those women with normal turnover osteoporosis.

Fracture Prevention In 32 postmenopausal women with one or more vertebral fractures, treatment with intermittent intramuscular calcitonin (100 IU daily for 10 days each month) resulted in a 60% reduction in the incidence of new vertebral fractures. During the same period there was a 35–45% increase in new fractures in the 28 women in the control group [39,40]. These findings paralleled increases in axial bone mass and total body bone mineral content [40]. In a retrospective study, the relative risk of hip fracture was 0.69 in 2086 women who had been treated with parenteral calcitonin compared to 3532 age-matched controls [41].

Cost, inconvenience, and side effects have limited the use of parenteral calcitonin. Calcitonin administered by either subcutaneous or intramuscular routes is associated with nausea, vomiting, anorexia, diarrhea, abdominal pain, flushing, skin rashes, and inflammation at the injection site. Gastrointestinal complaints or hot flashes are seen in about 10–30% of women receiving parenteral calcitonin [42]. The side effects may subside with time, but they are often the reason for the discontinuation of calcitonin treatment. Potential allergic reactions to parenteral calcitonin mandate skin testing prior to starting therapy. The inconvenience of the injectable form, especially in elderly patients, may also be a limiting factor.

Nasal Calcitonin

PREVENTION OF POSTMENOPAUSAL BONE LOSS

Bone Mineral Density Nasal salmon calcitonin has many advantages over parenteral calcitonin. It is easier to administer, has fewer side effects, and is less expensive. The rate of absorption of nasal calcitonin is variable and is lower than the parenteral form. Estimates of the bioavailability of nasal calcitonin have ranged from 20 to 40% of the parenteral form [43–45]. In a short-term, double-blind study, Combe *et al.* compared the efficacy of nasal calcitonin to subcutaneous calcitonin. Patients with recent vertebral crush fractures were treated with either nasal calcitonin (200 IU daily) or subcutaneous calcitonin (50 IU daily). Both methods of administration were equivalent in decreasing the pain within 30 days and 50% of the patients had decreased pain within the first 10 days. There was no difference in markers of bone resorption in either group [46]. Reginster *et al.* [45] found no differences between the effects of nasal or intramuscular calcitonin on calcium, phosphorus, or parathyroid hormone levels.

The efficacy of nasal salmon calcitonin for the prevention of vertebral postmenopausal bone loss has been demonstrated in both short-term [47,48] and long-term [49–54] studies. Most studies have used daily dosing, but intermittent dosing has been evaluated as well. Lyritis *et al.* [48] compared nasal calcitonin (100 IU daily) to a placebo nasal spray in a double-blind, placebo-controlled study of early postmenopausal women. At the end of 1 year there was a significant increase in BMC of the spine and the proximal forearm in the treatment group compared to a loss of BMC in the placebo group. Gennari *et al.* [47] compared nasal calcitonin (200 IU every other day) to placebo in early postmenopausal women. At the end of 1 year, in the women treated with nasal calcitonin, there was a 3.3% increase in vertebral BMC, whereas there was a 3.5% decrease in BMC in the women treated with placebo. This beneficial effect was also seen in ovariectomized women who were treated with nasal calcitonin (200 IU daily) as either a continuous or a cyclic (3 months on, 1 month off) regimen within 30 days of bilateral ovariectomy. After 1 year of treatment, both the intermittent and the continuous calcitonin regimens were successful in preventing the rapid bone loss seen after ovariectomy [53]. The efficacy of nasal calcitonin in preventing postmenopausal bone loss has also been seen in longer studies. Reginster *et al.* [49,51,54] followed women for up to 5 years. Two hundred and fifty-one women who were within 72 months of menopause were randomized to three treatment groups: placebo, 50 IU nasal calcitonin, or 200 IU nasal calcitonin given 5 days per week. At the end of 2 years, lumbar spine BMD was decreased in the placebo group (6.28%), was increased minimally in the 50 IU nasal calcitonin group (0.82%), and was increased significantly in the 200 IU nasal calcitonin group (2.03%) [49]. In another study, 287 women within 3 years of menopause were assigned randomly to either a calcium-only group or a calcium plus nasal calcitonin group (50 IU 5 days per week). At the end of 3 years, of the 186 women who completed the study, there was an increase in lumbar BMD of 1.8% in the treatment group compared to a 5.8% decrease in the control group [54]. Long-term use of the nasal calcitonin was well tolerated and there was no evidence for the loss of effectiveness or tolerance in the women treated with nasal calcitonin. One hundred of these 186 women continued on a second protocol for an additional 2 years. Although the control group continued to lose lumbar BMD, the treatment group showed no change for the remainder of the study. Nasal calcitonin was well tolerated by the women at the end of the 5 years [51]. Overgaard *et al.* also showed that nasal calcitonin (100 IU daily) in early menopause prevented lumbar bone loss. However, unlike the previous studies, BMC at the distal forearm was measured and decreased about the same amount (2% per year) in the treatment and control groups. Thus, although spinal bone loss may be prevented by nasal calcitonin, there is no effect on peripheral bone loss in early menopause [52]. Another 2-year, randomized double-blind, placebo-controlled trial failed to show any efficacy of various doses of nasal calcitonin in 134 early postmenopausal women. Women within 3 years of menopause were randomized to daily calcium or calcium plus nasal calcitonin (100, 200, or 400 IU daily). After 24 months there was no significant difference in BMD of the lumbar spine or BMC of the distal forearm in patients receiving nasal calcitonin compared to control patients [50].

Bone Markers The effect of nasal calcitonin on biochemical markers of bone metabolism in healthy early postmenopausal women is variable. Serum markers of bone turnover decreased in several short-term studies [47,53]. However, several long-term studies showed no change [5,49,51,52].

In conclusion, there is some evidence that nasal calcitonin prevents vertebral bone loss in postmenopausal women. However, data are not conclusive for the distal radius and no data are available for prevention of loss at the hip.

TREATMENT OF POSTMENOPAUSAL OSTEOPOROSIS

Bone Mineral Density Thamsborg *et al.* [55] randomized 62 postmenopausal women with a history of Colles' fracture to either placebo or nasal calcitonin

(200 IU daily). There was no significant difference in lumbar spine, distal forearm, or femoral neck BMD between the placebo and nasal calcitonin groups after 2 years. Overgaard *et al.* [56] treated 37 women with a history of wrist fracture with nasal calcitonin (200 IU daily). At the end of 1 year, BMC of the distal forearm and lumbar spine did not change significantly in the calcitonin group, but decreased in the placebo group. In a study of 23 postmenopausal women with high turnover osteoporosis and vertebral fractures, Kapetanos *et al.* [57] demonstrated a 6.2% increase in lumbar spine BMD and an 8.7% increase in femoral neck BMD after 12 months of nasal calcitonin (100 IU twice daily). In a larger study of 208 postmenopausal women with osteoporosis, Overgaard *et al.* [44] randomized women to placebo or nasal calcitonin (50, 100, or 200 IU daily). In all groups, including placebo, the lumbar BMD increased over the 2-year treatment period and the effect was greatest in the 200 IU/day nasal calcitonin group. There was no significant effect on BMD of the distal forearm. Ellerington *et al.* [58] randomized 117 postmenopausal women with osteoporosis to receive placebo or nasal calcitonin (200 IU daily or thrice weekly) and followed BMD of the lumbar spine and hip. There were small increases in vertebral and hip BMD compared to controls in the subgroup of women treated with nasal calcitonin who were more than 5 years postmenopausal. The early postmenopausal women (less than 5 years) treated with nasal calcitonin experienced bone loss. The largest study to date enrolled 1175 women at 42 centers in the United States. In contrast to many of the studies already reviewed, this is a large, multicenter, double-blind, placebo-controlled trial that will likely yield definitive results regarding the efficacy of nasal calcitonin. Women were randomized to receive placebo or nasal calcitonin (100, 200, or 400 IU daily) for 5 years and interim results at 3 years have been reported [59]. Of the 1175 patients enrolled, 648 women were still receiving treatment after 3 years and there was no difference in the discontinuation rates between groups. After 1 year, lumbar spine BMD was increased significantly in all treatment groups compared to placebo (Fig. 2). Lumbar spine BMD in the 200 and 400 IU/day nasal calcitonin groups was not significantly different from placebo at 3 years, but was significantly increased from baseline. There was no significant difference in BMD changes at the hip between control and treatment groups. All subjects were treated with higher calcium (1000 mg) and vitamin D (400 IU) supplements, which may explain why no difference was seen compared to placebo.

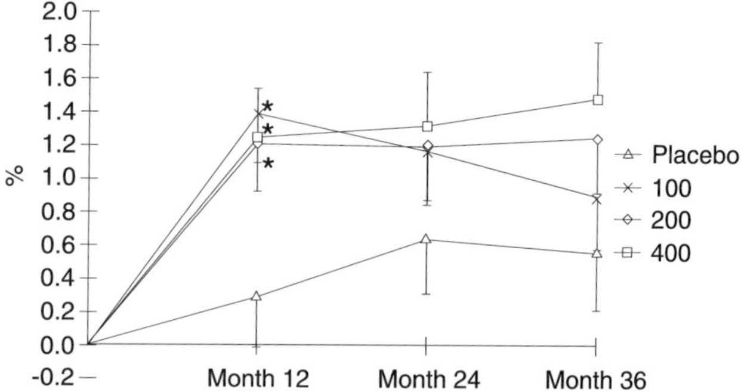

FIGURE 2 A significant increase in BMD at lumber spine compared to placebo is seen in postmenopausal women with established osteoporosis treated with nasal salmon calcitonin (200 IU daily) at 12 months. The changes are increased significantly compared to baseline at 3 years in all treatment groups. $^*p < 0.05$ by ANOVA. From Stock *et al.* [59].

Bone Markers The effects of nasal calcitonin treatment on biochemical markers of bone turnover in postmenopausal osteoporosis have been variable. Kraenzlin *et al.* showed that in 10 early menopausal women with high-turnover osteoporosis, nasal calcitonin (100 IU twice daily) rapidly decreased several markers of bone resorption, with maximum effect by 8 weeks of treatment. After 8 weeks there was a plateau in the response of resorption markers despite continued calcitonin treatment. After cessation of treatment, all markers returned to baseline [60]. Ellerington *et al.* [58] found no significant changes in bone markers in postmenopausal osteoporotic women treated with nasal calcitonin (200 IU daily or thrice weekly) for 2 years. Overgaard *et al.* [44] demonstrated a decrease in the urinary excretion of the cross-linked C-telopeptide of type I collagen after 9 months of nasal calcitonin treatment (50, 100, or 200 IU daily) in women previously described with established postmenopausal osteoporosis. Women with the least BMD response and those who had sustained fractures demonstrated less inhibition of bone resorption as measured by this bone marker. In the 3-year interim analysis of the 5-year multicenter nasal calcitonin trial, urinary excretion of the bone resorption marker cross-linked N-telopeptide of type I collagen was decreased compared to baseline in all nasal calcitonin treatment groups (100, 200, or 400 IU daily), but was reduced significantly compared to placebo only in the 400 IU/day group [59]. Serum concentrations of bone-specific alkaline phosphatase were decreased in the 400 IU/day calcitonin group at 1, 2, and 3 years [59].

Fracture Prevention Although numerous studies have investigated the effects of calcitonin treatment on BMD and bone markers, very few studies have used fracture incidence as an end point. Large numbers of patients and long-term studies are required to assess effects on fracture rates. In a 2-year study, Overgaard *et al.* [61] was able to assess fracture rates by pooling data from several treatment groups and then comparing the pooled group to a placebo group. The vertebral fracture rate in women treated with nasal salmon calcitonin was decreased to about one-third of that seen in the placebo group. However, this was a small study with a total of 12 new vertebral fractures in all groups. In the 3-year interim analysis of the large multicenter study in progress, individual doses of nasal calcitonin were compared to placebo. New vertebral fractures were decreased in the 100 IU/day group by 16.2%, in the 200 IU/day group by 37.4%, and in the 400 IU/day group by 16.0% compared to the placebo group, but only in the 200 IU/day group did the reduction reach significance [59] (Table I).

Combination Therapy

Many studies have investigated the efficacy of calcitonin administrated by parenteral or nasal routes, in combination with other regimens including phosphate [62], growth hormone [63,64], vitamin D [65], estrogen [33,66], anabolic steroids [67,68], PTH [69], and growth hormone [63,64,70,71]. These studies are of short duration and have included small numbers of patients with no definite conclusions.

Studies of calcitonin efficacy have not been limited to older patients with postmenopausal osteoporosis. Calcitonin has been effective in decreasing bone loss in patients with corticosteroid-induced osteoporosis, including patients with chronic obstructive pulmonary disease [72], sarcoidosis [72], liver transplantation [73], steroid-dependent asthma [72,74], and polymyalgia rheumatica [75]. Calcitonin may also be effective in preventing bone loss in young patients with thalassemia [76].

TABLE I New Vertebral Fractures in Postmenopausal Women with Established Osteoporosis Treated with Nasal Salmon Calcitonin or Placebo[a]

	Placebo	100 IU	200 IU	400 IU
No. patients with at least one new fracture/No. patients at risk	50/253	40/253	33/270	42/261
Relative risk to placebo (% reduction)		0.838 (16.2%)	0.626 (37.4%)	0.840 (16.0%)
p		0.404	0.037	0.403

[a] From Stock *et al.* [59].

Other Routes of Administration

Oral calcitonin is digested quickly by gastric enzymes. In one study of women with a history of hip fractures, rectal calcitonin was not effective [77]. Intrapulmonary aerosolized calcitonin closely approximated or exceeded the biological effect of injected calcitonin, but no data on efficacy were presented [78].

Analgesic Effect of Calcitonin

The analgesic effect of calcitonin has been demonstrated in patients with disorders characterized by increased bone resorption (osteoporotic vertebral fractures, Paget's disease) as well as in nonendocrine disorders (metastatic bone pain, posthysterectomy pain, pancreatitis, thalassemia) [21,76].

Lyritis *et al.* [79] demonstrated a significant reduction in bone pain in patients who were hospitalized for painful vertebral fractures that were less than 4 days old. The patients were randomized to either placebo or calcitonin (100 IU daily) by intramuscular injection. Calcitonin treatment resulted in a significant decline in pain scores and use of rescue analgesics. There was a significant reduction in pain associated with sitting, standing, and walking in the treatment group [79]. Patients with longstanding painful vertebral fractures also experienced a reduction in back pain [80]. Pun and Chan [81] demonstrated a similar effect on pain reduction with the use of nasal calcitonin. Eighteen patients with 1–4 acute, painful osteoporotic vertebral fractures were randomized to either a placebo nasal spray or nasal calcitonin (100 IU twice daily) for 4 weeks. Although there was decline in pain with time in patients in both groups, only in the treated group was there a significant reduction in pain compared with baseline as assessed by the overall use of analgesic medications and pain scores (Fig. 3).

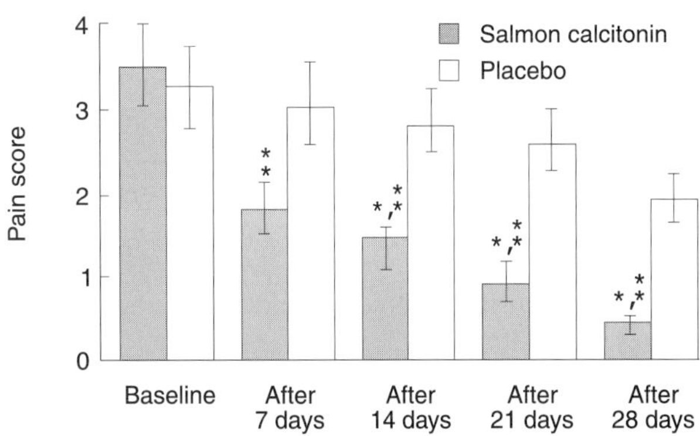

FIGURE 3 Treatment with nasal salmon calcitonin (100 IU twice daily) significantly decreases pain scores in patients with acute vertebral fractures. $*p \leq 0.05$ compared to placebo. $**p \leq 0.05$ compared to baseline. From Pun and Chan [81].

In a double-blind study of 100 patients with acute osteoporotic vertebral fracture, Lyritis *et al.* [82] demonstrated a reduction in pain scores, rescue analgesic use, and an improvement in mobility in the calcitonin-treated group. Calcitonin treatment and earlier mobilization resulted in lower urinary hydroxyproline excretion. As seen with parenteral calcitonin, the analgesic effect of nasal calcitonin is not limited to the first few weeks of treatment [83] and nasal calcitonin is as efficacious as parenteral calcitonin for the treatment of pain [46].

Although the etiology of the analgesic effect of calcitonin has not yet been elucidated, several hypotheses have been proposed. Epidural and subarachnoid injections of calcitonin result in analgesia [84], suggesting the presence of a calcitonin receptor in the central nervous system (CNS) that may be involved with pain perception [21]. Calcitonin may also enhance serotoninergic transmission in the CNS [42] and is associated with increasing circulating β-endorphins [84].

SUMMARY

Calcitonin, a 32 amino peptide synthesized in the parafollicular C-cells of the thyroid, is found in lower concentrations in women than in men and decreases with aging. Although estrogen deficiency affects calcitonin levels, the role of endogenous calcitonin in the pathophysiology of postmenopausal osteoporosis has yet to be determined.

Pharmacologic treatment with salmon calcitonin appears to delay lumbar vertebral bone loss in postmenopausal women. In women with established osteoporosis, calcitonin treatment increases vertebral BMD slightly and decreases the risk of new vertebral fractures. The possible analgesic effect of calcitonin may be an added benefit in the treatment of osteoporotic fractures. The duration of calcitonin efficacy and its effectiveness on the hip have not been determined. Calcitonin antibodies, down-regulation of receptors, and secondary hyperparathyroidism have all been proposed to contribute to the development of calcitonin resistance [85,86]. It has been suggested that the cyclic use of calcitonin may be as efficacious as continuous treatment and may reduce the risk of resistance and antibody formation [53]. Intermittent use may also have the added advantages of cost reduction and improvement in compliance.

Nasal calcitonin has been shown to be as safe and effective as parenteral calcitonin in preventing and treating postmenopausal bone loss with few of the problems associated with parenteral calcitonin. It has minimal side effects such as rhinorhhea and nasal mucosal irritation. Therefore, it has supplanted parenteral calcitonin in the management of postmenopausal osteoporosis. Although patients report short-term side effects with parenteral (64–75%) and nasal (32%) formulations, calcitonin has been used for up to 16 years without any serious or long-term side effects [43].

It is reasonable to consider the use of a safe, natural hormone, with antiresorptive effect on bone, that is deficient in postmenopausal and aging women. Although nasal calcitonin is one of the options for the treatment of postmenopausal bone loss, more extensive long-term data on the efficacy of both chronic and intermittent nasal calcitonin on vertebral and hip BMD and fracture rate are necessary before the role of nasal calcitonin, compared to estrogen replacement or bisphosphonates, can be fully defined for the prevention and treatment of postmenopausal osteoporosis.

References

1. Copp, D., Cameron, E., Cheney, B., Davidson, A., and Henze K. Evidence for calcitonin—a new hormone from the parathyroid that lowers blood calcium. *Endocrinology* **70,** 638–649 (1962).
2. Foster, G., Baghdiantz, A., Kumar M., Slack, E., Soliman, H., and MacIntyre, I. Thyroid origin of calcitonin. *Nature* **202,** 1303–1305 (1964).
3. Pearse, A., and Carvalheira, A. Cytochemical evidence for an ultimobranchial origin of rodent thyroid C cells. *Nature* **214,** 929–930 (1967).
4. McSheehy, P., Farina, C., Airaghi, R., Allievi, E., Banfi, S., Bertolini, D., Ferni, G., Frattola, D., Oneta, S., Pinza, M., Sorini, C., Valente, M., and Volontieri, A. Pharmacologic evaluation of the calcitonin analogue SB 205614 in models of osteoclastic bone resorption in vitro and in vivo: Comparison with salmon calcitonin and elcatonin. *Bone* **16,** 435–444 (1995).
5. Carstens, J., and Feinblatt, J. Future horizons for calcitonin: A U.S. perspective. *Calcif. Tissue Int.* **49** (Suppl. 2), S2–S6 (1991).
6. Epand, R., and Epand, R. Conformational flexibility and biological activity of salmon calcitonin. *Biochemistry* **25,** 1964–1968 (1986).
7. Hoppener, J., Steenbergh, P., Zandberg, J., Bakker, E., Pearson, P., Geurts van Kessel, A., Jansz, H., and Lips, C. Localization of the polymorphic human calcitonin gene on chromosome 11. *Hum. Genet.* **66,** 309–312 (1984).
8. Amara, S., Jonas, V., Rosenfeld, M., Ong, E., and Evans, R. Alternative RNA processing in calcitonin gene expression generates mRNAs encoding different polypeptide products. *Nature* **298,** 240–244 (1982).
9. Girgis, S., Stevenson, J., Lynch, C., Self, C., MacDonald, D., Bevis, P., Wimalawansa, S. Calcitonin gene-related peptide: Potent vasodilator and major product of calcitonin gene. *Lancet* 14–16 (1995).
10. Hillyard, C., Abeyasekera, G., Craig, R., Myers, C., Stevenson, J., and MacIntyre, I. Katacalcin: A new plasma calcium-lowering hormone. *Lancet* 846–848 (1983).
11. MacIntyre, I., Hillyard, C., Murphy, P., Reynolds, J., Gaines Das, R., and Craig, R. A second plasma calcium-lowering peptide from the human calcitonin precursor. *Nature* **300,** 460–462 (1982).
12. Martin, T., Findlay, D., and Moseley, J. Peptide hormones acting on bone. *In* "Osteoporosis" (R. Marcus, D. Feldman, and J. Kelsey, eds.), pp. 185–199. Academic Press, San Diego, 1996.

13. Brain, S., Williams, T., Tippins, J., Morris, H., and MacIntyre, I. Calcitonin gene-related peptide is a potent vasodilator. *Nature* **313,** 54–56 (1985).
14. Struthers, A., Brown, M., MacDonald, D., Beacham, J., Stevenson, J., Morris, H., and MacIntyre, I. Human calcitonin gene related peptide: A potent endogenous vasodilator in man. *Clin. Sci.* **70,** 389–393 (1986).
15. Zaidi, M., Datta, H., Moonga, B., and MacIntyre, I. Evidence that the action of calcitonin on rat osteoclasts is mediated by two G proteins acting via separate post-receptor pathways. *J. Endocrinol.* **126,** 473–481 (1990).
16. Avioli, L. Salmon calcitonin nasal spray. *Endocrine* **5,** 115–127 (1996).
17. Azria, M. 25 years of salmon calcitonin: From synthesis to therapeutic use. *Calcif. Tissue Int.* **57,** 405–408 (1995).
18. Martin, T., Robinson, C., and MacIntyre, I. The mode of action of thyrocalcitonin. *Lancet* 900–902 (1966).
19. Chambers, T., Athanasou N., and Fuller, K. Effect of parathyroid hormone and calcitonin on the cytoplasmic spreading of isolated osteoclasts. *J. Endocrinol.* **102,** 281–286 (1984).
20. Wallach, S., Farley, J., Baylink, D., and Brenner-Gati, L. Effects of calcitonin on bone quality and osteoblastic function. *Calcif. Tissue Int.* **52,** 335–339 (1993).
21. Deleted in proof.
22. Deftos, L. Calcitonin. *In* "Primer on the Metabolic Bone Disease Disorders of Mineral Metabolism" (M. J. Favus, ed.), 3rd Ed., pp. 82–87. Lippincott–Raven, Philadelphia, 1993.
23. Parthemore, J., and Deftos, L. Calcitonin secretion in normal human subjects. *J. Clin. Endocrinol. Metab.* **47,** 184–188 (1978).
24. Stevenson, J., Hillyard, C., MacIntyre, I., Cooper, H., and Whitehead, M. A physiological role for calcitonin: Protection of the maternal skeleton. *Lancet* 769–770 (1979).
25. Samaan N., Anderson, G., and Adam-Mayne, M. Immunoreactive calcitonin in the mother, neonate, child and adult. *Am. J. Obstet. Gynecol.* **121,** 622–625 (1975).
26. Greenberg, C., Kukreja, S., Bowser, E., Hargis, G., Henderson, W., and Williams, G. Effects of estradiol and progesterone on calcitonin secretion. *Endocrinology* **118,** 2594–2598 (1986).
27. Stevenson, J., Hillyard, C., Abevasekera, G., Phang, K., and MacIntyre, I. Calcitonin and the calcium-regulating hormones in postmenopausal women: Effect of oestrogens. *Lancet* 693–695 (1981).
28. Deftos, L., Weisman, M., Williams, G., Karpf, D., Frumar, A., Davidson, B., Parthemore, J., and Judd, H. Influence of age and sex on plasma calcitonin in human beings. *N. Eng. J. Med.* **302,** 1351–1353 (1980).
29. Tiegs, R., Body, J., Barta, J., and Heath, H. Secretion and metabolism of monomeric human calcitonin: Effects of age, sex, and thyroid damage. *J. Bone Miner. Res.* **1,** 339–349 (1986).
30. Taggart, H., Ivey, J., Sisom, K., Chesnut, C., Baylink, D., Huber, M., and Roos, B. Deficient calcitonin response to calcium stimulation in postmenopausal osteoporosis? *Lancet* 475–477 (1982).
30a. Bucht, E., Rong, H., Sjoberg, H.-E., Sjostedt, U., Granberg, B., and Torring, O., *Calcif. Tissue Int.* **56,** 32–37 (1995).
30b. Quesada, J., Mateo, A., Jans, I., Rodriguez, M., and Bouillon, R., *J. Bone Miner. Res.* **9,** 53–57 (1994).
31. Stevenson, J., Abeyasekera, G., Hillyard, C., Phang, K., MacIntyre, E., Campbell, S., Lane G., Townsend, P., Young, O., and Whitehead, M. Regulation of calcium-regulating hormones by exogenous sex steroids in early postmenopause. *Eur. J. Clin. Invest.* **13,** 481–487 (1983).
32. Morimoto, S., Tsuji, M., Okada, Y., Onishi, T., and Kumahara, Y. The effect of oestrogens on human calcitonin secretion after calcium infusion in elderly female subjects. *Clin. Endocrinol.* **13,** 135–143 (1980).
33. MacIntyre, I., Stevenson, J., Whitehead, M., Wimalawansa, S., Banks, L., and Healy, M. Calcitonin for prevention of postmenopausal bone loss. *Lancet* 900–902 (1988).
34. Mazzuoli, G., Tabolli, S., Bigi, F., Valtorta, C., Minisola, S., Diacinti, D., Scarnecchia, L., Bianchi, G., Piolini, M., and Dell'Acqua, S. Effects of salmon calcitonin on the bone loss induced by ovariectomy. *Calcif. Tissue Int.* **47,** 209–214 (1990).
35. Gennari, C., Chierichetti, S., Bigazzi, S., Fusi, L., Connelli, S., Ferrara R., and Zacchei, F. Comparative effects on bone mineral content of calcium and calcium plus salmon calcitonin given in two different regimens in postmenopausal osteoporosis. *Curr. Ther. Res.* **38,** 455–464 (1985).
36. Gruber, H., Ivey, J., Baylink, D., Matthews, M., Nelp, W., Sisom, K., Chestnut, C. Long-term calcitonin therapy in postmenopausal osteoporosis. *Metabolism* **33,** 295–303 (1984).
37. Mazzuoli, G., Passeri, M., Gennari, C., Minisola, S., Antonelli, R., Valtorta, C., Palummeri, E., Cervellin, G., Gonneli, S., and Francini, G. Effects of salmon calcitonin in postmenopausal osteoporosis: A controlled double-blind clinical study. *Calcif. Tissue Int.* **38,** 3–8 (1986).
38. Civitelli, R., Gonnelli, S., Zacchei, F., Bigazzi, S., Vattimo, A., Avioli, L., and Gennari, C. Bone turnover in postmenopausal osteoporosis: Effect of calcitonin treatment. *J. Clin. Invest.* **82,** 1268–1274 (1988).
39. Rico, H., Hernandez, E., Revilla, M., and Gomez-Castresana, F. Salmon calcitonin reduces vertebral fracture rate in postmenopausal crush fracture syndrome. *Bone Miner.* **16,** 131–138 (1992).
40. Rico, H., Revilla, M., Hernandez, E., Villa, L., and Alvarez de Buergo, M. Total and regional bone mineral content and fracture rate in postmenopausal osteoporosis treated with salmon calcitonin: A prospective study. *Calcif. Tissue Int.* **56,** 181–185 (1995).
41. Kanis, J. Johnell, O., Gullberg, B., Allander, E., Dilsen, G., Gennari, C., Lopes Vaz, A., Lyritis, G., Mazzuoli, G., Miravet, L., Passeri, M., Perez Cano, R., Rapado, A., and Ribot, C. Evidence for efficacy of drugs affecting bone metabolism in preventing hip fracture. *Br. Med. J.* **305,** 1124–1128 (1992).
42. Bannwarth, B., Schaeverbeke, T., and Dehais, J. Calcitonin and osteoporosis fact and fiction. *Rev. Rhum.* [*Engl. Ed*] **62,** 3–6 (1995).
43. Wimalawansa, S. Long- and short-term side effects and safety of calcitonin in man: A prospective study. *Calcif. Tissue Int.* **52,** 90–93 (1993).
44. Overgaard, K., and Christiansen, C. A new biochemical marker of bone resorption for follow-up on treatment with nasal salmon calcitonin. *Calcif. Tissue Int.* **59,** 12–16 (1996).
45. Reginster, J., Denis, D., Albert, A., and Franchimont, P. Assessment of the biological effectiveness of nasal synthetic salmon calcitonin (SSCT) by comparison with intramuscular (i.m.) or placebo injection in normal subjects. *Bone Miner.* **2,** 133–140 (1987).
46. Combe, B., Cohen, C., and Aubin F. Equivalence of nasal spray and subcutaneous formulations of salmon calcitonin. *Calcif. Tissue Int.* **61,** 10–15 (1997).
47. Gennari, C., Agnusdei, D., Montagnani, M., Gonnelli, S., and Civitelli, R. An effective regimen of intranasal salmon calcitonin in early postmenopausal bone loss. *Calcif. Tissue Int.* **50,** 381–383 (1992).
48. Lyritis, G., Magiasis, B., and Tsakalakos, N. Prevention of bone loss in early nonsurgical and nonosteoporotic high turnover patients with salmon calcitonin: The role of biochemical bone markers in monitoring high turnover patients under calcitonin treatment. *Calcif. Tissue Int.* **56,** 38–41 (1995).

49. Reginster, J., Deroisy, R., Lecart, M., Sarlet, N., Zegels, B., Jupsin, I., Belgium, L., de Longueville, M., and Franchimont, P. A double-blind, placebo-controlled, dose-finding trial of intermittent nasal salmon calcitonin for prevention of postmenopausal lumbar spine bone loss. *Am. J. Med.* **98,** 452–458 (1995).
50. Overgaard, K. Effect of intranasal salmon calcitonin therapy on bone mass and bone turnover in early postmenopausal women: A dose-response study. *Calcif. Tissue Int.* **55,** 82–86 (1994).
51. Reginster, J., Meurmans, L., Deroisy, R., Jupsin, I., Biquet, I., Albert, A., and Franchimont, P. A 5-year controlled randomized study of prevention of postmenopausal trabecular bone loss with nasal salmon calcitonin and calcium. *Eur. J. Clin. Invest.* **24,** 565–569 (1994).
52. Overgaard, K., Riis, B., Christiansen, C., and Hansen, M. Effect of salcatonin given intranasally on early postmenopausal bone loss. *Br. Med. J.* **299,** 477–499 (1989).
53. Fioretti, P., Gambacciani, M., Taponeco, F., Melis, G., Capelli, N., and Spinetti, A. Effects of continuous and cyclic nasal calcitonin administration in ovariectomized women. *Maturitas,* **15,** 225–232 (1992).
54. Reginster, J., Denis, D., Deroisy, R., Lecart, M., DeLongueville, M., Zegels, B., Sarlet, N., Noirfalisse, P., and Franchimont, P., Long-term (3 years) prevention of trabecular postmenopausal bone loss with low-dose intermittent nasal salmon calcitonin. *J. Bone Miner. Res.* **9,** 69–73 (1994).
55. Thamsborg, G., Jensen, J., Kollerup, G., Hauge, E., Melsen, F., and Sorensen, O. Effect of nasal salmon calcitonin on bone remodeling and bone mass in postmenopausal osteoporosis. *Bone* **18,** 207–212 (1996).
56. Overgaard, K., Riis, B., Christiansen, C., Podenphant, J., and Johansen, J. Nasal calcitonin for treatment of established osteoporosis. *Clin. Endocrinol.* **30,** 435–442 (1989).
57. Kapetanos, G., Symeonides, P., Dimitriou, C., Karakatsanis, K., and Potoupnis, M. A double blind study of intranasal calcitonin for established postmenopausal osteoporosis. *Acta Orthop. Scand.* **68**(Suppl. 275), 108–111 (1997).
58. Ellerington, M., Hillard, T., Whitcroft, S., Marsh, M., Lees, B., Banks, L., Whitehead, M., and Stevenson, J. Intranasal salmon calcitonin for the prevention and treatment of postmenopausal osteoporosis. *Calcif. Tissue Int.* **59,** 6–11 (1996).
59. Stock, J., Avioli, L., Baylink, D., Chestnut, C., Genant, H., Maricic, J., Silverman, S., Schaffer, A., and Feinblatt, J. P.R.O.O.F: prevention of recurrence of osteoporotic fractures. *J. Bone Miner. Res.* **12,** S149 (1997).
60. Kraenzlin, M., Seibel, M., Trechsel, U., Boerlin, V., Azria, M., Kraenzlin, C., and Haas, H. The effect of intranasal salmon calcitonin on postmenopausal bone turnover as assessed by biochemical markers: Evidence of maximal effect after 8 weeks of continuous treatment. *Calcif. Tissue Int.* **58,** 216–220 (1996).
61. Overgaard, K., Hansen, M., Jensen, S., and Christiansen, C. Effect of salcatonin given intranasally on bone mass and fracture rates in established osteoporosis: A dose-response study. *Br. Med. J.* **305,** 556–561 (1992).
62. Kuntz, D., Marie, P., Berthel, M., and Caulin, F. Treatment of post-menopausal osteoporosis with phosphate and intermittent calcitonin. *Int. J. Clin. Pharm. Res.* **6,** 157–162 (1986).
63. Holloway, L., Kohlmeier, L., Kent, K., and Marcus, R. Skeletal Effects of cyclic recombinant human growth hormone and salmon calcitonin in osteopenic postmenopausal women. *J. Clin. Endocrinol. Metab.* **82,** 1111–1117 (1997).
64. Gonnelli, S., Cepollaro, C., Montomoli, M., Gennari, L., Montagnani, A., Palmieri, R., and Gennari, C. Treatment of post-menopausal osteoporosis with recombinant human growth hormone and salmon calcitonin: A placebo controlled study. *Clin. Endocrinol.* **46,** 55–61 (1997).
65. Palmieri, G., Pitcock, J., Brown, P., Karas, J., and Roen, L. Effect of calcitonin and vitamin D in osteoporosis. *Calcif. Tissue Int.* **45,** 137–141 (1989).
66. Meschia, M., Brincat, M., Barbacini, P., Crossignani, P. G., and Albisetti, W. A clinical trial on the effects of a combination of elcatonin (carbocalcitonin) and conjugated estrogens on vertebral bone mass in early postmenopausal women. *Calcif. Tissue Int.* **53,** 17–20 (1993).
67. Cantatore, F., Loperfido, M., Mancini, L., and Carrozzo, M. Effect of calcitonin or the anabolic steroid decadurabolin on serum B2 microglobulin in osteoporotic postmenopausal women. *J. Rheum.* **19,** 1753–1755 (1992).
68. Szucs, J., Horvath, C., Kollin, E., Szathmari, M., and Hollo, I. Three-year calcitonin combination therapy for postmenopausal osteoporosis with crush fractures of the spine. *Calcif. Tissue Int.* **50,** 7–10 (1992).
69. Hesch, R., Busch, U., Prokop, M., Delling, G., and Rittinghaus, E. Increase of vertebral density by combination therapy with pulsatile 1-38hPTH and sequential addition of calcitonin nasal spray in osteoporotic patients. *Calcif. Tissue Int.* **44,** 176–180 (1989).
70. Aloia, J., Vaswani, A., Kapoor, A., Yek, J., and Cohn, S. Treatment of osteoporosis with calcitonin, with and without growth hormone. *Metabolism* **34,** 124-129 (1985).
71. Aloia, J., Vaswani, A., Meunier, P., Edouard, C., Arlot, M., Yeh, J., and Cohn, S. Coherence treatment of postmenopausal osteoporosis with growth hormone and calcitonin. *Calcif. Tissue Int.* **40,** 253–259 (1987).
72. Adachi, J. Corticosteroid-induced osteoporosis. *Am. J. Med. Sci.* **313,** 41–49 (1997).
73. Valerno, M., Loinaz, C., Larrodera, L., Leon, M., Moreno, E., and Hawkins, F. Calcitonin and bisphosphonates treatment in bone loss after liver transplantation. *Calcif. Tissue Int.* **57,** 15–19 (1995).
74. Luengo, M., Pons, F., Martinez de Osaba, M., and Picado, C. Prevention of further bone mass loss by nasal calcitonin in patients on long term glucocorticoid therapy for asthma: A two year follow up study. *Thorax* **49,** 1099–1102 (1994).
75. Adachi, J., Bensen, W., Bell, M., Bianchi, F., Cividino, A., Craig, G., Sturtridge, W., Sebaldt, R., Steele, M., Gordon, M., Themeles, E., Tugwell, P., Roberts, R., and Gent, M. Salmon calcitonin nasal spray in the prevention of corticosteroid-induced osteoporosis. *Br. J. Rheum.* **36,** 255–259 (1997).
76. Canatan, D., Akar, N., and Arcasoy, A. Effects of calcitonin therapy on osteoporosis in patients with thalassemia. *Arta Haematol.* **93,** 20–24 (1995).
77. Kollerup, G., Hermann, A., Brixen, K., Lindblad, B., Mosekilde, L., and Sorensen, O. Effects of Salmon calcitonin suppositories on bone mass and turnover in established osteoporosis. *Calcif. Tissue Int.* **54,** 12–15 (1994).
78. Deftos, L., Nolan, J., Seely, B., Clopton, P., Cote, G., Whitham, C., Florek, L., Christensen, T., and Hill, M. Intrapulmonary drug delivery of bone-active peptides: Bioactivity of inhales calcitonin approximates injected calcitonin. *J. Bone Miner. Res.* **11,** S95 (1996).
79. Lyritis, G., Tsakalakos, N., Magiasis, B., Karachalios, T., Yiatzides, A., and Tsekoura, M. Analgesic effect of salmon calcitonin in osteoporotic vertebral fractures: A double-blind placebo-controlled clinical study. *Calcif. Tissue Int.* **49,** 369–372 (1991).
80. Wallach, S., Cohn, S., Atkins, H., Ellis, K., Kohberger, R., Aloia, J., and Zanzi, I. Effect of salmon calcitonin on skeletal mass in osteoporosis. *Curr. Ther. Res.* **22,** 556–572 (1977).

81. Pun, K., and Chan, L. Analgesic Effect of intranasal salmon calcitonin in the treatment of osteoporotic vertebral fractures. *Clin. Ther.* **11,** 205–209 (1989).
82. Lyritis, G., Paspati, I., Karachalios, T., Iaokimidis, D., and Skarantavos, G. Pain relief from nasal salmon calcitonin in osteoporotic vertebral crush fractures. *Acta Orthop. Scand.* **68**(Suppl. 275), 112–114 (1997).
83. Tolino, A., Romano, L., Ronsini, S., Riccio, S., and Montemagno, U. Treatment of postmenopausal osteoporosis with salmon calcitonin nasal spray: Evaluation by bone mineral content and biochemical patterns. *Int. J. Clin. Pharm. Ther. Tox.* **31,** 358–360 (1993).
84. Avioli, L. Osteoporosis syndromes: Patient selection for calcitonin therapy. *Geriatrics* **47,** 58–67 (1992).
85. Sibilia, V., and Netti, C. Current therapies and future directions in osteoporosis management. *Pharmacol. Res.* **34,** 237–245 (1996).
86. Gennari, C., Agnusdei, D., and Camporeale, A. long term treatment with calcitonin in osteoporosis. *Horm. Metab. Res.* **25,** 484–485 (1993).

CHAPTER 46

Parathyroid Hormone

A. B. HODSMAN, L. J. FRAHER, AND P. H. WATSON
Department of Medicine and the Lawson Research Institute, St. Joseph's Health Centre, and the University of Western Ontario, London, Ontario, Canada N6A 4V2

INTRODUCTION

In all but the most recent textbooks of physiology, parathyroid hormone (PTH) as released in a pulsatile fashion by the parathyroid gland *in vivo* regulates serum calcium levels and the rate of bone remodeling turnover and is thought of as a bone-resorbing hormone. Although bone resorption is a prominent histological event seen in bone sections obtained from patients suffering from pathological secretion of PTH, osteoclasts do not present PTH receptors, and the enhanced bone resorption accompanying pathological PTH secretion appears to require the presence of osteoblasts [1,2]. Furthermore, patients with primary hyperparathyroidism are not automatically at risk for trabecular bone loss, despite evidence for increased bone turnover [3,4]. Presumably these individuals retain efficient coupling of bone formation and resorption during the remodeling cycle carried out by bone multicellular units (BMUs).

The anabolic properties of exogenously injected PTH (or, more concisely, bovine parathyroid gland extracts) were first reported in a series of serendipitous findings dating back to 1931 [5,6] in both human and animal situations. Some 45 years later, Reeve and colleagues, citing circumstantial evidence in both clinical hyperparathyroid states and animal data, used a synthetic human PTH(1-34) animo-terminal fragment to treat a small group of elderly individuals with osteoporosis [7,8]. They reported a dramatic histological improvement in bone turnover and structural trabecular growth.

Solid-state synthesis of peptides is expensive. During the next 20 years the supply of clinical drug remained limited. However, the small number of clinical trials evaluating the potential of exogenous PTH therapy to treat osteoporosis consistently demonstrated a beneficial anabolic effect [9–28]. Although the introduction of clinical axial bone densitometry facilitated clinical research greatly, the commercial development of PTH awaited the technologic advances needed for the inexpensive large-scale manufacture of peptides by fermentation. Indeed, the first report of a commercial dose-finding, 12-month controlled clinical trial evaluating the efficacy of hPTH(1-84) on bone mineral density (BMD) against a placebo drug is available only in abstract format [A randomised controlled multicentre study of 1-84 h PTH for treatment of postmenopausal osteoporosis Lindsay, R., Hodsman, A., Genant, H., Bolognese, M., Ettinger, M., for the PTH working group, *Bone* **23** (Suppl), S175 (1998).]

ADVANTAGES OF ANABOLIC AGENTS FOR REVERSAL OF OSTEOPOROSIS

There are strong epidemiologic associations between BMD measurements at either central (lumbar spine) or appendicular sites (femoral neck, distal radius, os calcis) and the current or future risk for osteoporotic fractures [29–31]. Current estimates suggest a twofold increase in the risk of fracture for every 1.0 standard deviation below average age- and sex-adjusted BMD, increasing dramatically if there is a preexisting fragility fracture in an individual with a low BMD [29,31]. To date, relatively small increments in BMD reported in published placebo-controlled clinical trials (of about 0.5 SD within the age-matched population variation) translate into an incident fracture reduction of approximately 50% within 2–4 years of starting such therapy [32].

There are currently two therapeutic strategies to treat osteoporosis. These strategies are illustrated in Fig. 1. For the purposes of Fig. 1, a fracture threshold has been indicated, but the gradient of risk is continuous (as it is for many biological variables such as blood pressure and cholesterol in ischemic vascular disease). The most

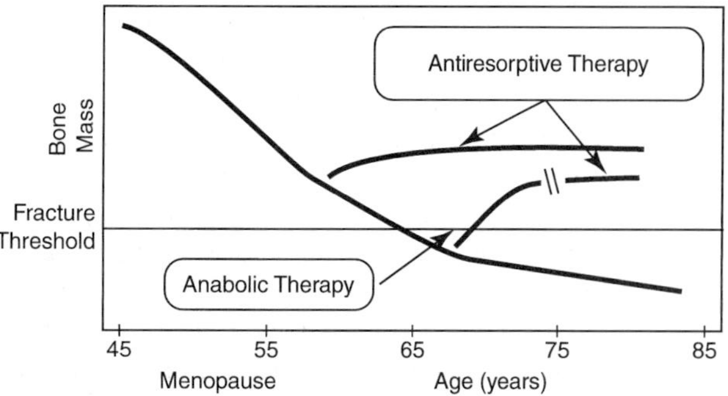

FIGURE 1 The relative efficacy of different strategies to maintain bone mass. (a) Antiresorptive strategy. Various agents (e.g., estrogens, bisphosphonates, calcitonin) will arrest ongoing age-related and postmenopausal bone loss. Reductions in bone resorption and turnover are observed, and gains in skeletal bone mass may occur due to the reduced bone resorption and perhaps to a reversal of the remodeling deficit. (b) Anabolic therapy. Agents such as PTH and sodium fluoride directly stimulate osteoblastic activity to increase bone mass, despite concurrent increases in bone turnover (i.e., there is an increase in both bone formation and resorption). The rapid increase in bone mass should accelerate the reduction in future fracture risk more effectively than the use of antiresorptive agents alone.

important role for an anabolic agent in bone would be the rapid induction of "new" bone formation in the skeleton to rapidly reduce the risk of fragility fractures. It is against this background that the role of PTH therapy is discussed.

Antiresorptive Agents

This approach relies on the inhibition of osteoclastic activity during the BMU remodeling activity, allowing osteoblastic function to continue unimpeded. The meticulously controlled clinical trials of the bisphosphonate alendronate have defined the benefits of this strategy; in the published fracture intervention trial (FIT), alendronate was given to elderly women (mean age 71 years, with at least one preexisting vertebral fracture) for approximately 3 years. During this time lumbar spine BMD measured by dual-energy X-ray absorptiometry (DEXA) increased by 6.2% (approximately 2% per year). New vertebral fracture rates fell by 47% ($p < 0.001$) and by 49% at the hip ($p < 0.05$) [32]. Similarly, evidence suggests that another antiresorptive agent, estrogen, reduces osteoporosis-related fractures by up to 50% [33–37]; one short-term controlled clinical trial supports epidemiologic or case-controlled data. In this study, elderly women (aged 66 years) with preexisting vertebral fractures were treated for 1 year with estrogen. Compared to placebo therapy, treated patients gained 5% in lumbar BMD ($p = 0.007$) and experienced 50% fewer vertebral fractures ($p = 0.04$) [35]. Thus, a gain in BMD at an axial measurement site (e.g., 4–8% at the lumbar spine) may reduce incident fractures by approximately 40–50%. Detailed reports of antiresorptive therapies are reviewed in other chapters of this publication.

Anabolic Agents

Two principal agents have been shown to stimulate osteoblast function within bone: sodium fluoride and analogues of PTH. Sodium fluoride and its slow-release formulations are discussed elsewhere in this publication. The landmark publication of Riggs *et al.* in 1982 suggested that plain sodium fluoride reduced vertebral fracture rates significantly [38]. The subsequent placebo-controlled trial demonstrated a rapid and linear gain in lumbar spine BMD of 9% per year over 4 years [39]. However, this result provided no evidence for a reduction in incident fractures [39]. Because the fluoride dose in this trial might have been toxic and adversely affected the matrix "quality" of newly formed bone, the lower dosed, "slow-release" fluoride formulation reported by Pak *et al.* [40] is an important study. In this randomized trial, fluoride-treated patients gained BMD in the lumbar spine of 4% per year and experienced a 64% reduction in incident vertebral fractures.

By whatever outcome measure used, PTH analogues have been shown to be anabolic, resulting in comparable gains in bone mass by comparison with fluoride. These gains are considerably more rapid than those seen with antiresorptive agents. However, fluoride therapy has not supported the dictate that gains in BMD translate into lower fracture rates. Because there are as yet no controlled trials reporting incident fractures in patients treated with PTH analogues, it is necessary to evaluate the potential mechanisms by which PTH has seemingly paradoxical anabolic effects, focusing on preclinical data in osteopenic animal models, as well as the available clinical evidence.

POTENTIAL MECHANISMS OF ANABOLIC ACTION

The physiological action of PTH is to maintain the ambient concentration of ionized calcium in blood by (a) influencing calcium reabsorption from the glomerular filtrate of kidney tubule cells and (b) indirectly enhancing calcium absorption from the gut by increasing the activity of the renal vitamin D-1-hydroxylase, which produces $1\alpha,25(OH)_2D_3$ [41,42]. PTH also initiates a series of events that result in the release of skeletal calcium by osteoclasts.

In 1931, Pehue *et al.* described the case history of an 8-year-old Parisian child who had succumbed to anemia due to the obliteration of his marrow space by bone; he was subsequently discovered to have had hypertrophic parathyroids [5]. Subsequently, in contrast to the findings in primary hyperparathyroidism, Selye [6] suggested that PTH could have a potent anabolic effect. Selye was able to mimic the clinical situation described by Pehue *et al.* He injected 14- to 30-day-old albino male rats daily with 5 IU of the recently available Eli Lilly parathyroid extract for 30 days. The result was the production of osteopetrotic bone with no suggestion of osteoclastic bone resorption at these low doses of parathyroid extract. Numerous investigators have since confirmed the anabolic action of PTH (used as either the 1-84 holohormone or various amino-terminal analogues). This anabolic effect of multiple intermittent doses of PTH rather than the bone catabolic effect of continuous exposure to the hormone has been coined the *PTH paradox* [43].

Both PTH(1-84) and PTH(1-34) act through dual-signaling pathways in target cells. In osteoblasts the type 1 PTH/PTHRP receptor is coupled to both the adenylate cyclase-activating G protein, Gs, and the phospholipase C-activating Gq protein. PTH requires the first two amino acids and some part of the amino acid 25–34 region to activate Gs, but only the 28–32 portion to activate Gq [44]. PTH fragments such as (1-desamino) hPTH(1-34), hPTH(8-84), or hPTH(28-48), which stimulate membrane-bound protein kinase C (PKC), but not adenylate cyclase in isolated osteoblasts, do not stimulate bone formation in the oophorectomized rat model of osteoporosis. However, hPTH(1-31) amide, which stimulates the adenylate cyclase pathway as effectively as hPTH(1-34) or hPTH(1-84), but not the PKC pathway, is capable of stimulating the growth of both trabecular and cortical bone in the same animal model [45,46]. Administration of analogues of cAMP as well as other agents such as forskolin, which directly activates the adenylate cyclase, mimic many of the effects of PTH on osteoblasts in culture, thus strongly suggesting that the bone anabolic properties of PTH are associated with its ability to activate the cAMP–protein kinase A pathway.

The exact cellular mechanisms and principal mediators of the action of PTH on osteoblasts have not been fully elucidated, but it is likely to result from a combination of activating growth factors available in the immediate bone marrow environment, as well as recruiting new populations of preosteoblasts from marrow stromal cells. In terms of the former there is strong evidence that PTH stimulates both insulin-like growth factor (IGF) and transforming growth factor-β (TGF-β) systems [47,48]. The insulin-like growth factor regulatory system comprises (1) two growth factors (IGF-I and IGF-II); (2) two receptors, the type I recognizing IGF-I, IGF-II, and insulin and the type 2 being a high-affinity receptor for IGF-II preferentially; (3) six binding proteins that can act as carrier proteins (circulating factors), delivery systems to the receptors (modulators of bioactivity), and shields from proteolytic enzymes (enhancing bioavailability); and (4) IGF-binding, protein-specific proteases (which release free IGFs for target cell binding). Following binding to the PTH receptor on osteoblasts and the generation of cAMP, these cells produce more IGF-II, IGFBP -1,-4,-5, and the IGFBP-3 and IGFBP-5 proteases [48]. PTH also directly stimulates the synthesis of TGF-β by mature osteoblasts [49]. It appears that IGF-I, IGF-II, and TGF-β, which have been secreted previously by osteoblasts, are bound to the collagen matrix of bone where they reside as a sort of growth factor bank. During cycles of bone remodeling, when PTH induces osteoclastic bone resorption, these factors are released into the immediate environment where they can act on resident osteoblasts [49]. The anabolic effect of PTH also results in the appearance of multistacked active osteoblasts at sites of bone formation. The origin of these cells is not certain. They might be osteoprogenitor cells from marrow precursors, PTH responsive postmitotic cells that have been recruited to the site by chemotaxis, or bone lining cells that have been induced to reenter proliferative cycles and pile up [50,51].

ANIMAL MODELS OF PTH EFFECTS ON BONE METABOLISM

Detailed investigation of the anabolic action of PTH requires a suitable animal model. The ovariectomized (OVX) mature rat develops osteopenia rapidly, which is characterized by a significant decrease in both cancellous bone mineral and bone mass and a marked increase in osteoblast and osteoclast activity typical of increased bone turnover [52–58]. The OVX rat has been accepted widely as a model for human postmenopausal osteoporosis because it closely parallels the early, rapid phase of bone loss characteristic of postmenopausal human bone loss [52,59]. The osteopenia of OVX rats shares many characteristics in common with the bone manifestations of perimenopausal bone loss, including increases in both bone resorption and activation frequency, with a relative deficiency in bone formation leading to a negative modeling balance [52,53,56,57,60].

The OVX rat has been used extensively as a model for the *in vivo* anabolic action of intermittent treatment with PTH [52,54,57,60–64]. Studies by the Kalu laboratory [57] have shown that hPTH(1–34) treatment of mature, OVX rats prevents the 50% reduction in trabecular bone volume following OVX and enhances bone volume to a level threefold that of sham-operated controls. PTH also reverses preexisting bone loss induced by OVX [52,60–62,64]. Meng and colleagues [65] have shown that the increase in the bone formation rate after intermittent therapy with PTH is primarily due to an increase in both total mineralization surface and the mineral apposition rate that occurs in the first week after the initiation of treatment [65]. Measurement of bone mineral density in PTH-treated rats has also shown positive increments in femur [66], vertebrae [66,67], and tibia [66,68,69], confirming histological data. All of these studies show a PTH-induced increase in bone formation chiefly by the induction of osteoblast function. Thus intermittent PTH therapy increases osteoblastic bone formation via increased activation frequency, resulting in positive bone balance [62].

Another important consideration is the quality of the bone produced by PTH therapy. Data from the rat have shown that PTH works primarily by increasing trabecular thickness, not number [60,70–72]. An assessment of trabecular connectivity demonstrates that PTH produces well-connected trabecular bone of normal three-dimensional architecture when used in combination with estrogen as an antiresorptive agent [64,71,73], but not when used on its own [71]. One last point to bear in mind is the biomechanical strength of PTH-induced bone formation, as nothing is gained if the newly formed bone does not provide the strength and support to protect against fractures. Numerous studies of load-to-failure rates in vertebral bodies, femoral shafts, and femoral necks have shown that bone from PTH-treated OVX rats performs consistently better than that from sham-operated controls [65,66,72–76]. This pattern held true even in a primarily cortical bone site (femoral shaft) [65] and correlated well with observations of increased tabecular thickness and bone mineral density [65,72].

Much effort has been applied to the problem of either augmenting the bone formation induced by PTH therapy or maintaining the gains of bone following the cessation of PTH therapy with an antiresorptive agent. Bisphosphonates are the antiresorptives of choice for a variety of reasons, but most notably because of their efficacy in achieving gains in bone mineral density in osteoporotic patients. Residronate has been evaluated carefully to determine if concurrent therapy is additive to the anabolic effect of PTH in the osteopenic rat model. These studies have shown that combination therapy with residronate and PTH provides no further advantage over PTH alone in the mature ovariectomized rat when vertebral bone mass and strength [76] and femoral neck strength [75] are assessed. Similar results were obtained with aged ovariectomized rats after evaluation of the first lumbar vertebra and proximal tibia by histomorphometry [77]. There has been some concern that PTH therapy may affect cortical bone width and strength adversely, but studies with PTH alone or residronate cotherapy show no effects of PTH on cortical bone in the ovariectomized rat and no advantage to residronate cotherapy [78–80].

However, studies with other bisphosphonates suggest that these compounds can blunt the anabolic effect of PTH on bone formation rates in cancellous bone of the ovariectomized rat. This has been found for pamidronate [81], tiludronate [82], and YM-175 [83]. Thus *concurrent* therapy of bisphosphonates and PTH does not appear to confer therapeutic advantages. However, *maintenance* of bone mass following cessation of PTH therapy may be achieved successfully by bisphosphonates [84].

CLINICAL EXPERIENCE OF PTH THERAPY IN OSTEOPOROTIC SUBJECTS

Although the clinical literature on the use of PTH peptides to treat osteoporosis dates back to 1976, it must be noted that published clinical protocols have been very heterogeneous, generally of short duration, experimental in design, and largely lacking appropriate randomized control groups. However, these studies have formed the scientific basis to explore the anabolic effects of PTH and related analogues in animal models of osteoporosis as referred to earlier. Subsequently, controlled randomized clinical trials have been initiated at phase II–III levels, but these studies are in progress. This chapter reviews the published clinical literature of PTH peptides to date. Most studies have utilized hPTH(1–34); however, the purity and specific activity of this peptide cannot be relied upon in the older literature. Using the highly purified synthetic hPTH(1–34) peptide, reported doses of 500 units should be equivalent to approximately 40 μg or 9.7 nmol of pure peptide.

Clinical Studies

Table I summarizes the available published studies [7–19,21,22,25–28,85–88]. Some 200 subjects (167 women and 33 men) have been treated in a heterogeneous series of protocols for periods varying between 6 and 36 months. In general, most subjects have been over 60 years of age with a diagnosis of osteoporosis. As can be seen in Table I, very few studies have employed a randomized design with acceptable controls. Most have used concomitant medications, either calcitriol or an

TABLE I Clinical Protocols Used in PTH Studies

Author[a] (year)	Age (years)[b]	Gender ♀:♂[c]	PTH dose	Study duration (months)	Concommitant therapy	Controls
Reeve *et al.* [7] (1976)[1]	N/A	4:0	"500" units	6	None	None
Reeve *et al.* [85] (1976)[1]	N/A	4:0	"500–2000" units	1–6	None	None
Reeve *et al.* [8] (1980)[2]	61	16:5	"500" units	6–24	None	None
Hesp *et al.* [9] (1981)	53–77	?	"500" units	12	None	None
Reeve *et al.* [10] (1981)[2]	61	18:5	"500" units	6	None	Four patients untreated
Slovik *et al.* [11] (1981)	50–70	5:1	450–750 units	1	None	None
Slovik *et al.* [12] (1986)	50	0:8	400–500 units	12	Calcitriol	None
Reeve *et al.* [13] (1987)[2]	64	12:1	1000–1500 units, 7-day cycles	12	Calcitriol	None
Neer *et al.* [14] (1987)	65	16:8	400–500 units either daily or in 6 week cycles	18–24	Calcitriol	Seven women on Ca or calcitriol
Hesch *et al.* [15] (1989)	50	2:6	750 units hPTH(1–38), 70-day cycles	14	Calcitonin	Five women on other treatments
Reeve *et al.* [16] (1990)[2]	64	11:1	500 units	12	Estrogen or androgen	Twelve patients on fluoride
Hodsman and Fraher [17] (1990)[3]	70	17:3	400 units PTH (1–38), 14-day cycles	6	Calcitonin	None
Reeve *et al.* [18] (1991)[2]	64	11:1	500 units	12	Estrogen or androgen	None
Hodsman *et al.* [19] (1991)[3]	70	17:3	400 units PTH (1–38), 14-day cycles	6	Calcitonin	None
Neer *et al.* [20] (1991)	N/A	15:0	400–500 units	12–24	Calcitriol	Fifteen women on Ca
Bradbeer *et al.* [21] (1992)[2]	64	11:0	450–750 units	6–12	Estrogen or androgen	None
Hodsman *et al.* [22] (1993)[4]	66	20:0	800 units, 28-day cycles	3	Calcitonin	None
Reeve *et al.* (1993)[2]	64	11:1	500 units	12	Estrogen or androgen	None
Finkelstein *et al.* [25] (1994)	30	20:0	500 units daily	6	Calcium and naferelin	Twenty woman on Naferelin
Sone *et al.* [26] (1995)	80	14:2	20 units daily	6	None	None
Hodsman *et al.* [27] (1997)[4]	67	39:0	800 units, 28-day cycles	24	Calcitonin	None
Lindsay *et al.* [28] (1997)	60	17:0	400 units daily	36	Estrogen	Seventeen on Estrogen

[a] Superscript by author indicates published data from the same study cohort.
[b] Arithmetic means.
[c] Numbers do not include "controls" who did not receive PT.

antiresorptive agent, and most have used calcium supplements.

The PTH peptide has usually been the hPTH(1–34) fragment, although three reports employed hPTH(1–38) [15,17,19], given in daily doses of 400 to 800 units. Most dose regimens have used daily subcutaneous injections, but the drug has been used in repeating cycles varying from 7 to 28 days [13,17,27] or from 6 to 10 weeks [14,15]. The only randomized, placebo-controlled trial is a 1-year dose-finding study using daily injections of hPTH(1–84), so far published only in abstract form [89].

Many unknown issues are raised by the use of PTH peptides as a prospective treatment for osteoporosis, although evidence to date highlights only the potential benefits. These clinical issues are discussed under the headings by which regulatory agencies currently examine data for the treatment of osteoporosis.

Fractures

There are no randomized controlled clinical trials that demonstrate the efficacy of PTH peptides to reduce the incidence of osteoporosis-related fractures. Although this outcome is clearly an imperative before accepting the efficacy of PTH as a useful treatment for osteoporosis, two studies have reported incident vertebral fractures during therapy with hPTH(1–34) [27,28], albeit that no true control groups were included for comparison. Hodsman *et al.* [27] reported a vertebral fracture incidence of 4.5/100 patient years in a group of elderly patients with preexisting vertebral fractures and receiving eight 28-day cycles of hPTH(1–34) over 2 years. Lindsay *et al.* [28] reported an incidence of 2.5/100 patient years in a comparable group of patients receiving daily hPTH(1–34) injections over 3 years. Because both studies enrolled high-risk female patients with an average of more than two preexisting vertebral fractures, an average age of over 60 years, and comparable BMD measurements, they document fracture incidences in a high-risk population. A reasonable historical comparison can be made with the "placebo" (calcium supplemented) arm of the fracture intervention trials, in whom new vertebral fracture incidence rates were documented at 10/100 patient years in a cohort of women with only one prevalent osteoporosis-related vertebral fracture followed for 3 years [32].

Whereas data for incident vertebral fractures in women with osteoporosis and prevalent vertebral fractures suggest a clinically important protective effect by PTH against further vertebral fracturing, it must be emphasized that these results have yet to be evaluated in appropriately controlled randomized clinical trials that incorporate concurrent controls.

Bone Mass Measurements

Figure 2 plots changes in BMD measurements in reported studies in which responses to PTH treatment have been followed by DEXA of the lumbar spine [20,27,89,90]. Other studies using quantitative computerized tomography (QCT) show even greater increments of 25–100% over baseline [12,15,16]. The striking

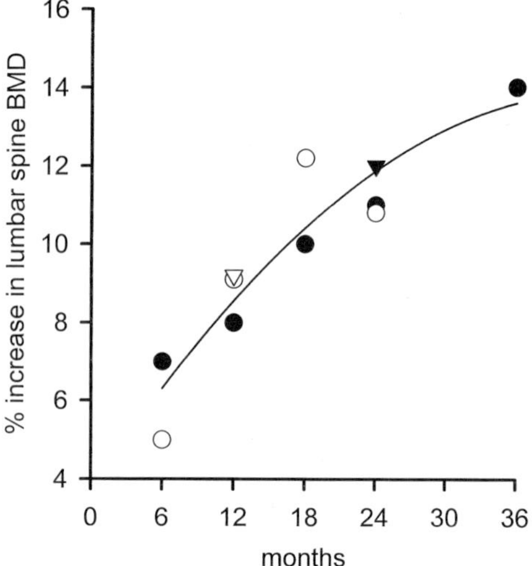

FIGURE 2 Composite changes in lumbar spine BMD measured by dual-energy X-ray absorptiometry during up to 3 years of therapy with PTH. The plot shows the average reported changes in BMD across time. Individual points represent mean data for separate publications (○, Hodsman *et al.* [27]; ●, Lindsay *et al.* [28]; △, Rittmaster *et al.* [89]; ▲, Near *et al.* [20]).

findings in Fig. 2 are that the skeletal gains in bone mass are remarkably consistent over time, even though the therapeutic protocols were dissimilar (see Table I). Changes in lumbar spine BMD average 8–9% during the first year and a further 3% after the second year. The second observation to be made suggests that the anabolic effects of PTH may plateau after the second year of therapy, independent of concomitant medication. This raises an important question as to the optimal use and duration of PTH therapy. Most importantly, does the use of PTH ultimately confer skeletal resistance to the drug and do we know enough about such a mechanism?

Figures 3 and 4 describe specific changes in BMD at both the lumbar spine and other measurement sites published by Hodsman *et al.* [27] and Lindsay *et al.* [28]. Both studies clearly document increments in spine BMD of 10–12% over 2–3 years of PTH(1–34) therapy. After 2 years of cycling PTH therapy, Hodsman *et al.* [27] found a small increase in femoral neck BMD (Fig. 3). However, Lindsay *et al.* [28] found significant increments in both femoral neck and total body calcium measurements (Fig. 4).

Extended data on appendicular BMD changes during PTH treatment are limited. There is a widespread belief that PTH results in decreased BMD at appendicular sites, mainly attributed to Neer *et al.* [20], who have reported a transient (but nonprogressive) reduction in distal radial BMD of 5.7% during the first year of PTH therapy. Hesp *et al.* [9] were unable to document an

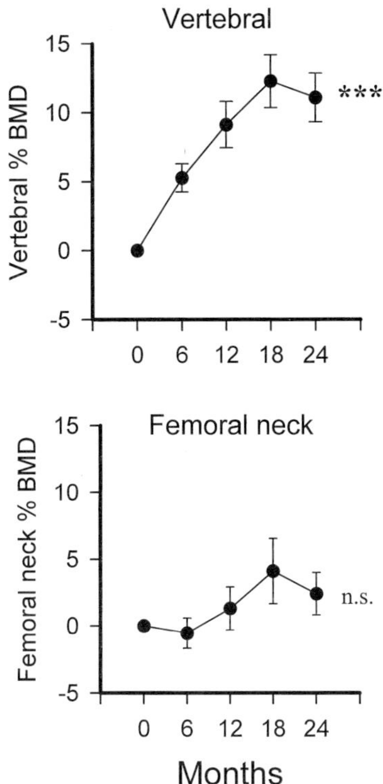

FIGURE 3 Changes in bone mineral density following treatment with 28-day cycles of hPTH(1-34), 800 IU/day, repeating every 3 months. $***p < 0.001$. Modified from Hodsman, A. B., Fraher, L. J., Watson, P. H., Ostbye, T., Stitt, L. W., Adachi, J. D., Taves, D. H., and Drost, D. (1997). *J. Clin. Endocrin. Metab.* **82,** 620–628; © The Endocrine Society.

improvement in external calcium balance in patients with osteoporosis treated with hPTH(1–34) daily for 12 months, whereas Slovik *et al.* [11] came to a similar conclusion after short-term (1 month) treatment. This has led to the hypothesis that anabolic agents used to treat osteoporosis may improve trabecular bone mass at the expense of diminishing cortical bone mass. Further evidence for this hypothesis has been supplied from the literature of fluoride therapy, in which patients who gained significant amounts of bone mass in the lumbar spine lost significant bone mass at the distal radius site [91,92].

Many reports have found no significant changes (neither improved nor decreased) in distal radius or femoral neck BMD over extended periods of PTH therapy [12,13,15,16,25,27,28,88]. Changes in BMD over the femoral neck have averaged 2–3% in two prospective studies (Fig. 3 and 4) [27,28] and 8% in total body bone mineral (Fig. 4) [28]. In the detailed multisite bone mass measurements reported by Lindsay *et al.* [28], significant gains in bone mass were found at all measured skeletal sites over a study period of 3 years (Fig. 4) [28].

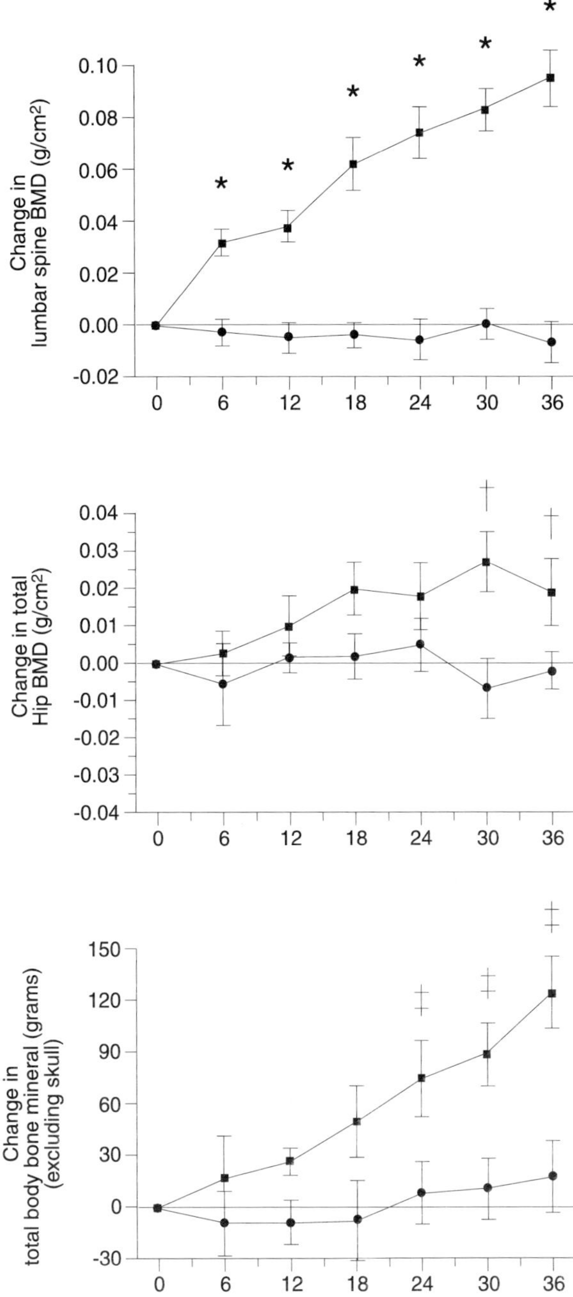

FIGURE 4 Changes in bone mineral density following hPTH(1-34), 400 IU/day. Data show two groups of patients: one treated with estrogen alone (●) and the other treated with estrogen plus PTH (■). $*p < 0.001$ vs estrogen; $^{\dagger}p < 0.05$ vs estrogen; $^{\ddagger}p < 0.02$ vs estrogen. Modified from Lindsay *et al.* [28], *Lancet* **350,** 550–555, by The Lancet, Ltd, 1997.

At the current time, evidence suggests that PTH therapy rapidly improves spinal bone mass without convincing evidence for a deleterious effect on the appendicular skeleton. Further exploration of any effects of PTH on the appendicular skeleton or on any beneficial effects of the improved axial skeletal mass on fracture rates requires that appropriate controlled clinical trials be conducted to answer this question.

Histology

As described in earlier sections, changes in bone histology can be detected in animal experiments very early on in the course of PTH therapy. Similar changes have been recorded in clinical studies [22].

After only 28 days of hPTH(1–34)injections, changes in both formation and resorption surfaces were increased two to five times those measured in a control panel of osteoporotic bone biopsies [22]. Similar findings were observed for bone formation rates and the activation frequency of bone remodeling; there was no evidence for impaired mineralization as measured by mineral apposition rates and trabecular architecture was apparently normal [22]. Reeve and co-workers [8,13,18,21,88] have reported changes in bone histomorphometry after 6 to 12 months of daily PTH therapy. Using each patient as an internal control, significant increases in trabecular area, trabecular width, and mean trabecular osteon wall thickness of between 5 and 25% over baseline measurements were documented [18,21]. Although the earlier study by Reeve and colleagues demonstrated increased trabecular osteoid surfaces (from 23.3 to 35.2%) and resorption surfaces (from 3.9 to 6.2%) [8], their later study demonstrated that if anything, these same parameters tended to decrease with time [88]. Although little kinetic data (based on *in vivo* tetracycline labels) are available from Reeve and co-workers, available evidence suggests that long-term PTH therapy (i.e., of more than 6 to 12 months duration) favors a positive osteon remodeling balance and normal bone architecture, but that the dramatic short-term histological evidence for increased bone turnover is not sustained over time.

Calcium Balance Studies

Prior to 1980, there were few methods to document changes in bone mass in response to any agent. Bone biopsies yield important information, but the measured parameters are not precise (typical CV ± 20%) [93]. Therefore, early studies relied on classical dietary calcium balance studies and radioisotopic techniques of assessing skeletal calcium accretion to determine the extent to which new therapies for osteoporosis improved skeletal "bone mass." The methodology of the following reports is not easy to follow, but the cited references provide a source for such documentation. Moreover, the reader should appreciate that the cited clinical protocols vary widely with respect to dose of PTH, duration of therapy, and concurrent medication (see Table I). Given these limitations, the results indicate enough consistency to describe the results in general terms.

In the initial report by Reeve *et al.* [7], four patients treated with PTH (500 units/day) demonstrated an improved dietary calcium balance averaging 7.3 mmol/day. Net diet absorption of ^{47}Ca averaged 3.4 mmol/day. Measured accretion of ^{47}Ca by the skeleton averaged 6.3 mmol/day. These data seemed to confirm that the observed improvements in bone histology were indeed due to an anabolic effect of the injected hPTH(1–34). A subsequent report on the short-term changes (less than 1 month) measured in the same subjects defined dose-dependent effects, with calcium balance improving over doses of 500 to 1000 units hPTH(1–34) per day, but deteriorating at doses of 1500 units/day [86]. In a small group of four patients treated with 450–750 units hPTH(1–34) over 1 month reported by Slovik *et al.* [11], a similar dose dependency was observed, with positive dietary calcium balance (2.2 mmol/day) seen only at the lower doses of PTH.

In summary, kinetic calcium data demonstrate trends toward positive dietary calcium balances during a variety of therapeutic PTH protocols. These techniques have not been as sensitive to changes in bone mass by dual-energy absorptiometric measurements, but they comprise the only existing evidence that prolonged PTH treatment does not result in consistent total body calcium depletion. However, two reports suggest that higher doses of PTH (>1000 units/day) may be deleterious to total body calcium balance [11,85].

Biochemical Markers of Bone Metabolism

It is beyond the scope of this chapter to discuss the development of biochemical markers of bone turnover in metabolic bone diseases. Their advantage for research purposes is principally the provision of noninvasive indicators of the balance between bone resorption and bone turnover [94–96]. In this section, discussion of biochemical markers of bone resorption will be restricted to urinary hydroxyproline and the collagen cross-linked peptides. Markers of bone formation will focus on total serum alkaline phosphatase and osteocalcin.

Because PTH is regarded as a hormone with potent bone-resorbing properties, leading to concomitant increases in urinary calcium excretion, other markers of bone resorption are of great importance. Reeve *et al.*

[13,18] reported a 26% increase in hydroxyproline excretion (OH-Pro) in patients treated with daily PTH [8], but either no change or a 100% fall in urinary OH-Pro in a small group of 12 patients who were treated with estrogen or androgen as concurrent antiresorptive therapy. When using a "high" dose of PTH (800 units/day), Hodsman *et al.* [22] reported a 53% increase in urine OH-Pro after 1 month of treatment with no significant changes in urine pyridinoline excretion. Finkelstein *et al.* [25] reported increases of both OH-Pro and pyridinoline excretion of approximately 125% in acutely hypoestrogenemic younger women after 6 months of PTH therapy. In longer term studies (24–36 months), both Hodsman *et al.* [27] and Lindsay *et al.* [28] reported an initial sharp increase in urinary N-telopeptide excretion during the first 6 months of hPTH(1–34) therapy followed by a gradual return toward baseline. Because these changes are associated with an apparent plateau in the gains in BMD, they raise the issue again that the skeleton may become refractory to PTH over 2–3 years, even though the treatment protocols and dosing were not comparable between the two studies.

It is not surprising that PTH increases collagen breakdown and subsequent excretion of its components as there is ample evidence for increased bone turnover during anabolic therapy (which involves concurrent bone resorption). However, the results reported by Reeve *et al.* [13,18] are at the lowest end of the spectrum, those of Lindsay *et al.* [28] are somewhere in the middle, and those of Finkelstein *et al.* [25] are at the highest end. A common link among these three studies is the use of concurrent estrogen replacement in elderly women with osteoporosis by Reeve *et al.* [13,18] and Lindsay *et al.* [28], together with the therapeutic induction of acute estrogen deficiency (as treatment for endometriosis with naferelin) by Finkelstein *et al.* [25]. This provides evidence for the potential benefits of combining antiresorptive agents with PTH therapy in an attempt to maximize gains in bone mass achieved by PTH alone.

Despite rather variable changes in markers of bone resorption, indices of bone formation have shown consistent increments. In response to exogenous PTH therapy, serum total alkaline phosphatase (tAP) levels increased from 15 to 104% [7,8,15,17,22,25,27,28] and average 40% over time. In the three studies reporting changes in serum osteocalcin (OC), both short [17,22]- and long [27,28]-term PTH treatment resulted in increments of 60 to 160%. Increases in tAP and/or OC have been seen only inconsistently during other anabolic treatments, specifically fluoride therapy [91,92], whereas acute, abrupt, and sustained reductions in both resorption and formation markers are seen with antiresorptive therapy (e.g., estrogen replacement or alendronate [95,96].

In summary, the reported measurements of biochemical markers for bone resorption and formation support the rapid onset of skeletal activation and bone turnover in response to PTH as reported histologically by Hodsman *et al.* [22]. Increments in bone formation markers are consistent and of considerable magnitude, in keeping with direct osteoblastic stimulation and bone anabolism [27,28]. Increments in bone resorption markers are less consistent, but appear to be less pronounced during concomitant therapy with estrogen. Because declines in biochemical markers of bone turnover after 2–3 years of therapy appear to be consistent, these markers may sustantiate the premise that skeletal resistance to the anabolic effects of PTH peptides might occur during the first 3 years of therapy.

Effects on Serum and Urinary Calcium

When given by continuous intravenous infusion, intravenous bolus, or subcutaneous injection, the biological effects of PTH are not the same. For example, continuous infusion of hPTH(1–34) caused marked bone resorption in the rat [97]. When infused into osteoporotic subjects, Hodsman *et al.* [22] reported that a given dose of hPTH(1–34) caused significantly larger increments in total serum calcium over 24 hr than the same dose given by a single subcutaneous injection. The PTH infusion led to a significant fall in biochemical markers of bone formation, suggesting, if anything, that continuous intravenous infusion of PTH is "antianabolic" [22]. Similar findings in osteoporotic subjects were reported by Cosman *et al.* [98], albeit that concurrent estrogen therapy might have mitigated the catabolic effects of PTH infusion.

Increments in serum calcium following subcutaneous PTH injection are delayed and do no peak until 4–8 hr postdosing [22,99], but they are generally within the normal physiological range. Because the clearance of injected PTH is so rapid, no obvious safety concern has arisen after over 20 years of PTH therapy; significant persistent hypercalcemia is unlikely to result from daily PTH injections. Nonetheless, short-term increments in serum $1{,}25(OH)_2D_3$ have been reported after subcutaneous hPTH(1–34) [17,100], together with increased fractional absorption of dietary calcium [17] and hypercalciuria [22,99]. However, of the two studies reporting long-term biochemical changes in response to hPTH(1–34) injections, neither sustained increments in serum $1{,}25(OH)_2D_3$ nor hypercalciuria persist within these elderly patients with osteoporosis [27,28].

ANALYSIS OF CONCURRENT THERAPIES USED WITH PTH PROTOCOLS

During the past 20 years, PTH therapy has been used in a heterogeneous fashion as a single agent, with or without nutritional calcium and vitamin D supplements [7–10,85,100]; with calcitriol [12,14,20]; with estrogen or androgen as a concurrent antiresorptive agent [16,18,21,88,101]; and in several cyclical protocols with or without antiresorptive agents [13,15,17,19,22,27]. The *concept* for the cyclical use of PTH should be distinguished from its direct anabolic effects on the skeleton. Because PTH also activates bone remodeling, cyclical protocols have attempted to exploit the ADFR hypothesis (A, activate remodeling; D, depress resorption in the activated bone modelling units; F, allow for a treatment-free period of bone formation; R, repeat the treatment cycle). In fact, none of the cyclical protocols can be considered as true ADFR protocols and should be regarded as hybrid anabolic protocols.

Despite the heterogeneity of these protocols, the overall results of therapy have been remarkably consistent: an increase in trabecular bone (as measured by BMD or histomorphometrically), with somewhat smaller changes in bone mass in the appendicular skeleton. All reported studies had small samples of treated subjects and thus a low power to dissect the interactions of concurrent therapies. Only the brief report by Neer *et al.* [20] used a true control group of patients treated with no other bone-active agents except nutritional calcium supplements. However, some guarded conclusions can be made.

1. The earliest studies by Reeve and co-workers, using daily PTH injections but without concurrent therapy, unequivocally show increased trabecular bone mass (histological outcome) and increased skeleton accretion (^{47}Ca kinetics), with a small trend toward an overall positive calcium balance (classical diet balance techniques). Given the poor precision of dietary calcium balance techniques, (CV $\pm$ 2.1 mmol/day [86]), the reported changes in calcium balance ranged from -3.7 to 2.2 mmol/day [11,13,18]. Much larger samples would be required to answer the question of whether PTH therapy, given alone, is beneficial or injurious to the skeleton as a whole? Current clinical trials in progress will answer this question more economically using total body bone mass measurements obtained by dual-energy X-ray absorptiometry.

2. The studies by Neer and co-workers combined concurrent calcitriol with daily PTH injection therapy [11,12,14,20]. This strategy was adopted because the earlier dietary calcium balance studies of Reeve and co-workers demonstrated minimal adaptations of dietary calcium absorption despite obvious histomorphometric restoration of trabecular bone and increased urinary Ca excretion. Because exogenous PTH does increase serum 1,25(OH)$_2$D levels [17,99] and is associated with increased fractional ^{45}Ca absorption, the need for the addition of calcitriol therapy remains unproven. The changes in lumbar BMD reported by Neer and co-workers are comparable to other studies but theirs is the one group to report significant losses of BMD at the radius in a controlled clinical trial (15 patients on calcium, 15 patients on PTH + calcitriol 0.25 μg/day, over 2 years) [20]. The control group lost 1.7% and the experimental group lost 5.7% in radial BMD—all in the first year of treatment. The greater and abrupt loss of appendicular bone mass in the experimental group might indicate a permanent loss to cortical bone, but an alternative explanation includes the possibility of a "transient" effect consistent with increased intracortical modeling.

3. The concurrent use of antiresorptive agents, specifically estrogen, is attractive. If estrogen can selectively blunt the resorptive action of PTH on bone without deleterious inhibition of its anabolic effects, this combination would be ideal. The experimental literature is confusing. Cosman *et al.* [98] infused PTH over 20 hr (approximately 800 units to each of 17 estrogen-treated and 15 estrogen-deficient postmenopausal women with osteoporosis). The estrogen-deficient women had a significantly higher excretion of bone resorption markers (urinary OH-Pro and deoxypyridinoline), suggesting a protective effect of estrogen on resorption. However, in a similar experiment, Tsai *et al.* [102] infused 400 units/day for 3 days to three groups of subjects, premenopausal and postmenopausal women with and without osteoporosis. They found no differences in serum calcium or urinary OH-Pro excretion and concluded that estrogen did not have such a protective effect. Using an alternative approach of calcium deprivation to induce endogenous 2° hyperparathyroidism, the same group reached similar conclusions [104]. Marcus *et al.* [104] gave acute (20 min) infusions of graded doses of PTH to 15 postmenopausal women before and after starting estrogen replacement, and no differences were found in serum 1,25(OH)$_2$D increments or urinary cAMP excretion as a result of estrogen therapy. They concluded that the renal–endocrine axis was not affected by estrogen deficiency. The flaw in these arguments is the fact that clinical responses to PTH infusion favor bone catabolism, whereas intermittent injections favor anabolism [22].

In the study by Reeve *et al.* [18], daily PTH injections and concurrent estrogen therapy were combined in nine women. By comparison with historical controls (women treated with PTH alone) [8], calcium balance studies were improved significantly; cotreatment with estrogen actually led to a 12% decrease in urinary calcium [18] rather than the 14% increase seen historically [8]. The 3-year study by Lindsay's group comparing estrogen-treated patients with and without daily PTH injection is now complete [28]. To date there are no controlled factorial studies to test the estrogen effect independently of PTH; therefore the protective effect of estrogen remains speculative.

No clinical studies combining bisphosphonates with PTH have been reported to date. As discussed earlier, data for bisphosphonate interactions with PTH in animal models are also unclear, with contradictory evidence that the *concurrent* use of bisphosphonates may blunt the anabolic agents of PTH. This is an important issue. Given the increase in skeletal bone remodeling induced by an activation drug such as PTH (at the BMU level), it is likely that the remodeling space within all skeletal bone envelopes will be enlarged as a transient state [105]. The enlarged remodeling space could be exploited by antiresorptive drugs as *maintenance* therapy after discontinuing PTH. This hypothesis has not been fully tested experimentally.

However, Rittmaster *et al.* [89] have presented preliminary clinical data in a group of 77 patients with osteoporosis previously treated for 1 year with one of three doses of hPTH(1–84) or placebo. These patients were subsequently treated with oral alendronate (10 mg daily). After 12 months, BMD increased further in patients previously treated with PTH in both the lumbar spine (approximately 6%) and the femoral neck (approximately 3%). These increments were no larger than those seen in previously placebo-treated patients (7 and 3%, respectively). In a subgroup of 30 patients, total body calcium measurements by DEXA also increased during 12 months of alendronate therapy (approximately 3%), but there was no difference between patients treated previously with hPTH(1–84) or placebo. In contrast, Hodsman *et al.* [107] treated a similar group of osteoporotic women, treated previously with cyclical hPTH(1–34), using 28-day cycles of oral clodronate (400 mg/day), repeating every 3 months. As can be seen in Fig. 5, cyclical clodronate failed to prevent small declines in bone mass over the 2-year observation period. Thus, at this junction, there is no evidence to confirm or refute the hypothesis that the potentially increased size of the remodeling space induced by PTH therapy can be exploited by sequential bisphosphonate therapy. The role of bisphosphonates in maintaining gains in bone mass induced by PTH awaits further study.

Cyclical therapy with PTH is of interest in so far that it might provide insights as to how the hormone might ultimately be given in the most economical fashion,

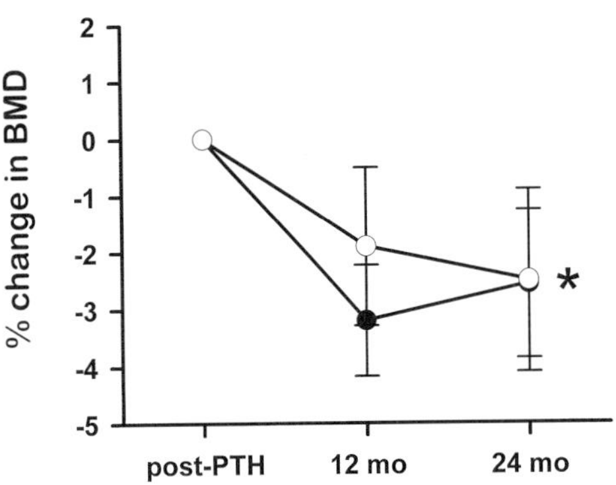

FIGURE 5 Maintenance therapy with 28-day cycles of clodronate, 400 mg/day, repeating every 3 months. Modified from Hodsman *et al.* [108]; these patients had previously received 28-day cycles of PTH therapy as described by Hodsman *et al.* [27]. $^{*}p < 0.05$ compared to post-PTH values.

but the literature to date adds little that is not already known about the actions of PTH. Hesch and Hodsman have combined cyclical PTH(1–34) and PTH(1–38) with concomitant or sequential cycles of calcitonin [15,17,19,22,27]. There is little evidence that the antiresorptive action of calcitonin provides any additional clinical benefit. Short cycles of PTH (400–500 units/day) for less than 14 days provide little evidence of skeletal activation of bone turnover or anabolism [13,17,19], although biochemical responses are detectable within this time frame. However, 28-day cycles of high-dose PTH (800 units daily) appear to provide a strong stimulus for the activation of bone turnover [22] and anabolic effects on bone mass [22,27]. The reported changes in lumbar spine BMD, with small increments in femoral neck BMD with 28-day cycles of high-dose PTH, may provide an alternative approach to harnessing the anabolic effects of PTH, but there are no controlled trials comparing cycles of PTH therapy with daily injections.

PHARMACOKINETICS OF PTH ADMINISTRATION

Since all therapeutic protocols have reported the response of the skeleton to daily subcutaneous injections, this section focuses on the pharmacodynamic responses to PTH when given by this route.

In a small study involving four healthy young subjects, Kent *et al.* [108] reported that after subcutaneous administration of 1250 units hPTH(1–34) (100 μg, 20nmol), the time to reach maximum plasma concentration, T_{max} was approximately 15 min, with immunoreactive PTH concentrations decaying to baseline after 180–240 min. Two additional reports in estrogen-treated postmenopausal osteoporotic subjects and in both young and untreated postmenopausal subjects [99,109] provided very similar data, i.e., peak immunoreactive increments in serum hPTH(1–34) levels at 20–30 min postinjection, increasing 10- to 15-fold over baseline (depending on injected dose), and decaying within a $T_{1/2}$ of about 75 min.

The only detailed pharmacodynamic study published for other PTH peptides is a dose-finding single subcutaneous injection report on hPTH(1–84). Schwietert *et al.* [110] reported minimal changes in total serum calcium in response to single injections of up to 5 μg hPTH(1–84)/kg (approximately 0.5 nmol/kg). However, with this peptide, absorption appeared to provide a double peak in C_{max}, with an early peak occurring <20 min postinjection and a second peak appearing 1.5–2 hr later. This pharmacokinetic profile occurred at all doses of hPTH(1–84) and appears to be different from that observed after hPTH(1–34) dosing.

It is therefore quite possible that different PTH peptides have different biological properties on bone metabolism together with different safety profiles.

IMMUNOLOGICAL RESPONSES TO EXOGENOUS PTH

Of the available reports in which antibody formation was deliberately sought, 8 out of 75 patients apparently developed anti-hPTH(1–34) antibodies in low titers [7,13,15,18,27]. Four patients discontinued hPTH(1–34) therapy because of generalized urticarial reactions or local irritation at the injection site [7,8]. Although an 11% incidence of anti-PTH(1–34) antibodies may seem high, it is likely that these early reports reflect impurities in the hPTH(1–34) formulations that were used; native hPTH(1–34) is a naturally occurring peptide and should not be immunogenic. Whether the newer PTH analogues possess this drawback awaits further clinical testing.

SIDE EFFECTS DURING PTH THERAPY

From Table I, it can be seen that close to 200 patients with osteoporosis have been treated with PTH. Of these, no deaths have been reported. As discussed earlier, 4 patients probably experienced sufficiently severe immunological responses to hPTH(1–34) to discontinue therapy. Eight patients may have demonstrated immunological reactions to an (impure) hPTH(1–34) product and/or local irritation at the injection site. Several patients developed mild nausea and arthralgia in one study [25]. Mild hypercalcemia and hypercalciuria have been observed, but neither have resulted in documented clinical consequences and no increased incidence of renal calculus formation has been reported to date. Hodsman *et al.* [27] have raised an issue about the long-term safety of PTH on renal function. In this report, 39 patients were treated with cyclical high dose PTH (800 units per day for four 28 day cycles/year over 2 years). This patient group experienced a significant 10% increase in serum creatinine (albeit within the normal range of age-related serum creatinine). Thus, PTH-induced hypercalciuria might conceivably affect renal function.

SUMMARY

To date, the 25-year clinical experience of PTH therapy indicates that this is an important anabolic agent with the potential to reverse osteoporosis. Very few safety concerns have been raised over treatment periods of 2–3 years. The introduction of PTH peptides/analogues holds promise for a new class of agents that might reduce fractures in osteoporotic individuals. However, there are many outstanding questions raised by the published literature; the order in which the authors listed them in no way reflects their order of importance.

1. The safety prolife of PTH peptides remains to be established. Although ongoing, long-term, placebo-controlled trials will establish this, a small minority of patients develop sustained hypercalcemia and hypercalciuria, and there is at least one report of declining renal function over time [27].

2. Although PTH holds the promise of rapid increments in skeletal bone mass in osteoporotic subjects, several unanswered questions arise; (a) Is this benefit accompanied by corresponding reductions in fracture risk? Definitive data exist for the antiresorptive bisphosphonate class of drugs (particularly alendronate), but are conflicting for the anabolic drug sodium fluoride. Fracture data after PTH therapy are very limited. (b) Are the anabolic benefits to the skeleton restricted to the trabecular envelope? Do patients lose cortical bone as suggested by the radial bone mass data reported by Neer *et al.* [20]? This important question is crucial but other data regarding the radius, total body calcium balance [28], and total body bone mineral density [28] suggest that the effect of PTH treatment is most potent at trabecular sites but is not detrimental to cortical bone. Again, we await the appropriate conduct of controlled clinical trials.

3. Given that PTH therapy induces rapid gains in bone mass (assessed by BMD measurement), can these gains be translated into sustainable bone mass? Animal data suggest that concomitant or sequential

bisphosphonate therapy either blunts the skeletal response to PTH or blunts subsequent therapy with the peptide [82,83,112], although this is not an invariable finding [79]. To date, the only clinical studies suggest that concurrent estrogen therapy and daily PTH injections result in significant increments in total body BMD, as well as increments at axial sites [28]. As presented in abstract form, sequential therapy with alendronate following 1-year therapy with daily hPTH(1–84) injections resulted in marked gains in both axial and appendicular bone mass [89]. This approach may suggest a role for antiresorptive therapy as a sequential regimen in the overall management of osteoporosis rather than concomitant therapy.

4. Is concurrent medication necessary during PTH therapy? Most studies have utilized a variety of agents (including calcium, vitamin D or calcitriol, calcitonin, and estrogen). While the published data employing such strategies are not convincing, factorially designed clinical trials have not been done.

5. Will cycles of PTH injections prove to be as effective as continued daily dosing? This question has a significant impact on cost and compliance impact.

6. Does the skeleton develop some form of resistance to continued PTH therapy? If so, does interval rechallenge work? Does rechallenge after antiresorptive therapy work?

7. Will analogues of PTH be better anabolic agents than hPTH(1–34) or hPTH(1–84)?

References

1. Parfitt, A. M. The actions of parathyroid hormone on bone: relation to bone remodeling and turnover, calcium homeostasis, and metabolic bone disease. Part 3 or 4 parts: PTH and osteoblasts, the relationship between bone turnover and bone loss, and the state of the bones in primary hyperparathyroidism. *Metabolism* **25,** 1033 (1976).
2. McSheehy, P. M., and Chambers, T. J. Osteoblastic cells mediate osteoclastic responsiveness to parathyroid hormone. *Endocrinology* **118,** 824–828 (1986).
3. Grey, A. B., Evans, M. C., Stapleton, J. P., and Reid, I. R. Body weight and bone mineral density in postmenopausal women with primary hyperparathyroidism. *Ann. Intern. Med.* **121,** 745–749 (1994).
4. Parisien, M., Cosman, F., Mellish, R. W. E., Schnitzer, M., Nieves, J., Silverberg, S. J., Shane, E., Kimmel, D., Recker, R. R., Bilezikian, J. P., Lindsay, R., and Dempster, D. W. Bone structure in postmenopausal hyperparathyroid, osteoporotic, and normal women. *J. Bone Miner. Res.* **10,** 1393–1399 (1995).
5. Pehu, M., Policard, A., and Dufort, A. L'Osteoporose ou maladie des os marmoreens. *La Press Med.* **53,** 999 (1931).
6. Selye, H. On the stimulation of new bone formation with parathyroid extract and irradiated ergosterol. *Endocrinology* **16,** 547–558 (1932).
7. Reeve, J., Hesp, R., Williams, D., Klenerman, L., Zanelli, J. M., Darby, A. J., Tregear, G. W., Parsons, J. A., and Hume, R. Anabolic effect of low doses of a fragment of human parathyroid hormone on the skeleton in postmenopausal osteoporosis. *Lancet* **1,** 1035–1038 (1976).
8. Reeve, J., Meunier, P. J., Parsons, J. A., Bernat, M., Bijvoet, O. L. M., Courpron, P., Edouard, C., Klenerman, L., Neer, R. M., Renier, J. C., Slovik, D., Vismans, F. J. F. E., and Potts, J. T. J. Anabolic effect of human parathyroid hormone fragment on trabecular bone in involutional osteoporosis: a multicentre trial. *Br. Med. J.* 1340–1344 (1980).
9. Hesp, R., Hulme, P., Williams, D., and Reeve, J. The relationship between changes in femoral bone density and calcium balance in patients with involutional osteoporosis treated with human parathyroid hormone fragment (hPTH 1-34). *Metab. Bone Dis. Rel. Res.* **2,** 331–334 (1981).
10. Reeve, J., Arlot, M., Bernat, M., Charhon, S., Edouard, C., Slovik, D., Vismans, F. J. F. E., and Meunier, P. J. Calcium-47 kinetic measurements of bone turnover compared to bone histomorphometry in osteoporosis: the influence of human parathyroid (hPTH 1-34) therapy. *Metab. Bone Dis. Rel. Res.* **3,** 23–30 (1981).
11. Slovik, D. M., Neer, R. M., and Potts, J. T. J. Short-term effects of synthetic human parathyroid hormone-(1–34) administration on bone mineral metabolism in osteoporotic patients. *J. Clin. Invest.* **68,** 1261–1271 (1981).
12. Slovik, D. M., Rosenthal, D. I., Doppelt, S., Potts, J. T. J., Daly, M. A., Campbell, J. A., and Neer, R. M. Restoration of spinal bone in osteoporotic men by treatment with human parathyroid hormone (1-34) and 1,25-dihydroxyvitamin D. *J. Bone Min. Res.* **1,** 377–381 (1986).
13. Reeve, J., Arlot, M., Price, T. R., Edouard, C., Hesp, R., Hulme, P., Ashley, J. P., Zanelli, J. M., Green, J. R., Tellez, M., Katz, D., Spinks, T. J., and Meunier, P. J. Periodic courses of human 1-34 parathyroid peptide alternating with calcitriol paradoxically reduce bone remodelling in spinal osteoporosis. *Eur. J. Clin. Invest.* **17,** 421–428 (1987).
14. Neer, R. M., Slovik, D., Doppelt, S., Daly, M., Rosenthal, D., LO, C., and Potts, J. The use of parathyroid hormone plus 1,25-dihydroxyvitamin D to increase trabecular bone in osteoporotic men and postmenopausal women. *In* "Osteoporosis 1987" (C. Christiansen, J. S. Johansen, and B. J., Riis, eds.), pp. 929–835. Osteopress Aps, Kobenhavn, Denmark, 1987.
15. Hesch, R. D., Busch, U., Prokop, M., Delling, G., and Rittinghaus, E. F. Increase of vertebral density by combination therapy with pulsatile 1-38 hPTH and sequential addition of calcitonin nasal spray in osteoporotic patients. *Calcif. Tissue Int.* **44,** 176–180 (1989).
16. Reeve, J., Davies, U. M., Hesp, R., McNally, E., and Katz, D. Treatment of osteoporosis with human parathyroid peptide and observations on the effect of sodium fluoride. *Br. Med. J.* **301,** 314–318 (1990).
17. Hodsman, A. B., and Fraher, L. J. Biochemical responses to sequential human parathyroid hormone (1-38) and calcitonin in osteoporotic patients. *Bone Miner.* **9,** 137–152 (1990).
18. Reeve, J., Bradbeer, J. N., Arlot, M., Davies, U. M., Green, J. R., Hampton, L., Edouard, C., Hesp, R., Hulme, P., Ashby, J. P., Zanelli, J. M., and Meunier, P. J. hPTH 1-34 treatment of osteoporosis with added hormone replacement therapy: biochemical, kinetic and histological responses. *Osteopor. Int.* **1,** 162–170 (1991).
19. Hodsman, A. B., Steer, B. M., Fraher, L. J., and Drost, D. J. Bone densitometric and histomorphometric responses to sequential

human parathyroid hormone (1-38) and salmon calcitonin in osteoporotic patients. *Bone Miner.* **14,** 67–83 (1991).
20. Neer, R., Slovik, D., Daly, M., LO, C., Potts, J., and Nussbaum, S. Treatment of post-menopausal osteoporosis with daily parathyroid hormone plus calcitriol. *In* "Osteoporosis" (C. Christiansen and K. Overgaard, eds.). Osteopress APS, Copenhagen, 1991.
21. Bradbeer, J. N., Arlot, M. E., Meunier, P. J., and Reeve, J. Treatment of osteoporosis with parathyroid peptide (hPTH 1-34) and oestrogen: Increase in volumetric density of iliac cancellous bone may depend on reduced trabecular spacing as well as increased thickness of packets of newly formed bone. *Clin. Endocrinol. (Oxf.)* **37,** 282–289 (1992).
22. Hodsman, A. B., Fraher, L. J., Ostbye, T., Adachi, J. D., and Steer, B. M. An evaluation of several biochemical markers for bone formation and resorption in a protocol utilizing cyclical parathyroid hormone and calcitonin therapy for osteoporosis. *J. Clin. Invest.* **91,** 1138–1148 (1993).
23. Bikle, D. D., and Rasmussen, H. The ionic control of 1,25-dihydroxyvitamin D3 production in isolated chick renal tubules. *J. Clin. Invest.* **55,** 292 (1975).
24. Pierides, A. M., Edwards, W. G., Cullum, U. X., *et al.* Hemodialysis encephalopathy with osteomalacic fractures and muscle weakness. *Kidney Intl.* **18,** 115–124 (1980).
25. Finkelstein, J. S., Klibanski, A., Schaefer, E. H., Hornstein, M. D., Schiff, I., and Neer, R. M. Parathyroid hormone for the prevention of bone loss induced by estrogen deficiency. *N. Engl. J. Med.* **331**, 1618–1623 (1994).
26. Sone, T., Fukunaga, M., Ono, S., and Nishiyama, T. A small dose of human parathyroid hormone (1-34) increased bone mass in the lumbar vertebrae in patients with senile osteoporosis. *Min. Electrol. Metab.* **21,** 232–235 (1995).
27. Hodsman, A. B., Fraher, L. J., Watson, P. H., Ostbye, T., Stitt, L. W., Adachi, J. D., Taves, D. H., and Drost, D. A randomized controlled trial to compare the efficacy of cyclical parathyroid hormone versus cyclical parathyroid hormone and sequential calcitonin to improve bone mass in postmenopausal women with osteoporosis. *J. Clin. Endocrinol. Metab.* **82,** 620–628 (1997).
28. Lindsay, R., Nieves, J., Formica, C., Henneman, E., Woelfert, L., Shen, V., and Dempster, D. Randomised controlled study of effect of parathyroid hormone on vertebral bone mass and fracture incidence among postmenopausal women on oestrogen with osteoporosis. *Lancet* **350,** 550–555 (1997).
29. Ross, P. D., Davis, J. W., Epstein, R. S., and Wasnich, R. D. Pre-existing fractures and bone mass predict vertebral fracture incidence in women. *Ann. Int. Med.* **114,** 919–923 (1991).
30. Cummings, S. R., Black, D. M., Nevitt, M. C., Browner, W., Cauley, J., Ensrud, K., Genant, H. K., Palermo, L., Scott, J., and Vogt, T. M. Bone density at various sites for prediction of hip fractures. *Lancet* **341,** 72–75 (1993).
31. Marshall, D., Johnell, O., and Wedel, H. Meta-analysis of how well measures of bone mineral density predict occurrence of osteoporotic fractures. *Br. Med. J.* **312,** 1254–1259 (1996).
32. Black, D. M., Cummings, S. R., Karpf, D. B., Cauley, J. A., Thompson, D. E., Nevitt, M. C., Bauer, D. C., Genant, H. K., Haskell, W. L., Marcus, R., Ott, S. M., Torner, J. C., Quandt, S. A., Reiss, T. F., and Ensrud, K. E. Randomised trial of effect of alendronate on risk of fracture in women with existing vertebral fractures. *Lancet* **348,** 1535–1541 (1997).
33. Kiel, D. P., Felson, D. T., Anderson, J. J., Wilson, P. W. F., and Moskowitz, M. A. Hip fracture and the use of estrogens in postmenopausal women. *N. Engl. J. Med.* **317**(19), 1169–1174 (1987).
34. Naessen, T., Persson, I., Adami, H., Bergstrom, R., and Bergkvist, L. Hormone replacement therapy and the risk for first hip fracture. *Ann. Int. Med.* **113,** 95–103 (1990).
35. Lufkin, E. G., Wahner, H. W., O'Fallon, W. M., Hodgson, S. F., Kotowicz, M. A., Lane, A. W., Judd, H. L., Caplan, R. H., and Riggs, B. L. Treatment of postmenopausal osteoporosis with transdermal estrogen. *Ann. Int. Med.* **117,** 1–9 (1992).
36. Eiken, P., Kolthoff, N., and Pors Neilsen, S. Effect of 10 years' hormone replacement therapy on bone mineral content in postmenopausal women. *Bone* **19,** 191S–193S (1996).
37. Maxim, P., Ettinger, B., and Spitalny, G. M. Fracture protection provided by long-term estrogen treatment. *Osteopor. Int.* **5,** 23–29 (1995).
38. Riggs, B. L., Seeman, E., Hodgson, S. F., Taves, D. R., and O'Fallon, W. M. Effects of the fluoride/calcium regimen on vertebral fracture occurrence in postmenopausal osteoporosis. *N. Engl. J. Med.* **306,** 446–450 (1982).
39. Kleerekoper, M., Peterson, E. L., Nelson, D. A., Phillips, E., Schork, M. A., Tilley, B. C., and Parfitt, A. M. A randomized trial of sodium fluoride as a treatment for postmenopausal osteoporosis. *Osteopor. Int.* **1,** 155–161 (1991).
40. Pak, C. Y. C., Sakhaee, K., Adams-Huet, B., Piziak, V., Peterson, R. D., and Poindexter, J. R. Treatment of postmenopausal osteoporosis with slow-release sodium fluoride—Final report of a randomized control group. *Ann. Intern. Med.* **123**(6), 401–408 (1995).
41. Bilezikian, J. P., Marcus, R., and Levine, M. A., "The Parathyroids." Raven Press, New York, 1994.
42. Brabant, G., Prank, K., and Schofl, C., *Trends Endocrinol. Metab.* **3,** 183–190 (1992).
43. Morley, P., Whitfield, J. F., and Willick, G. E. Anabolic effects of parathyroid hormone on bone. *Trends Endocrinol. Metab.* **8,** 225–231 (1997).
44. Whitfield, J. F., Morley, P., Langille, R., and Willick, G. E. Adenyl ceclase-activating anabolic agents: parathyroid hormone and protaglandins E. *In* "Anabolic Treatments for Osteoporosis" (J. E. Whitfield and P. Morley, eds.), pp. 109–145. CRC Press, Boca Raton, FL, 1998.
45. Rixon, R. H., Whitfield, J. F., Gagnon, L., Isaacs, R. J., Maclean, S., Chackravarthy, B., Durkin, J. P., Neugebauer, W., Ross, V., Sung, W., and Willick, G. E. Parathyroid hormone fragments may stimulate bone growth in ovariectomized rats by activating adenylate cyclase. *J. Bone Miner. Res.* **9,** 1179–1189 (1994).
46. Whitfield, J. F., Morley, P., Willick, G. E., Ross, V., Barbier, J.-R., Isaacs, R. J., and Ohannessian-Barry, L. Stimulation of growth of femoral trabecular bone in ovariectomized rats by the novel parathyroid hormone fragment, hPTH(1-31), (Ostabolin). *Calcif. Tissue Int.* **58,** 81–87 (1996).
47. Dempster, D. W., Cosman, F., Parisien, M., Shen, V., and Lindsay, R. Anabolic actions of parathyroid hormone on bone. *Endoc. Rev.* **14,** 690–709 (1993).
48. Johansson, A., and Rosen, C. J. The insulin-like growth factors: potential anabolic agents for the skeleton. *In* "Anabolic Treatments for Osteoporosis" (J. E. Whitfield and P. Morley, eds.), pp. 185–205. CRC Press, Boca Raton, FL, 1998.
49. Canalis, E. Skeletal growth factors. *In* "Osteoporosis" (R. Marcus, D. Feldman, and J. Kelsey, eds.), pp. 266–238. Academic Press, San Diego, 1996.
50. Dobnig, H., and Turner, R. T. Evidence that intermittent treatment with parathyroid hormone increases bone formation in adult rats. *Endocrinology* **136,** 3624–3638 (1995).
51. Watson, P. H., Lazowski, D. A., Han, V. K. M., Fraher, L. J., Steer, B. M., and Hodsman, A. B. Parathyroid hormone restores bone mass and enhances osteoblast insulin-like growth factor-1 gene expression in ovariectomized rats. *Bone* **16,** 1–9 (1995).
52. Liu, C. C., Kalu, D. N., Salerno, E., Echon, R., Hollis, B. W., and Ray, M. Preexisting bone loss associated with ovariectomy

in rats is reversed by parathyroid hormone. *J. Bone Miner. Res.* **6,** 1071–1080 (1991).

53. Frost, H. M., and Jee, W. S. S. On the rat model of human osteopenias and osteoporoses. *Bone Miner.* **18,** 227–236 (1992).
54. Hori, M., Uzawa, T., Morita, K., Noda, T., Takahashi, H., and Inoue, J. Effect of human parathyroid hormone (PTH(1-34)) on experimental osteopenia of rats induced by ovariectomy. *Bone Miner.* **3,** 193–199 (1988).
55. Hock, J. M., Gera, I., Fonesca, J., and Raisz, L. G. Human parathyroid hormone (1-34) increases rat bone mass in ovariectomized and orchidectomized rats. *Endocrinology* **122,** 2899–2904 (1988).
56. Wronski, T. J., Dann, L. M., Scott, K. S., and Cintrón, M. Long-term effects of ovariectomy and aging on the rat skeleton. *Calcif. Tissue. Int.* **45,** 360–366 (1989).
57. Liu, C. C., and Kalu, D. N. Human parathyroid hormone-(1-34) prevents bone loss and augments bone formation in sexually mature ovariectomized rats. *J. Bone Miner. Res.* **5,** 973–982 (1990).
58. Wronski, T. J., Yen, C.-F., Burton, K. W., Mehta, R. C., Newman, P. S., Soltis, E. E., and DeLucca, P. P. Skeletal effects of calcitonin in ovariectomized rats. *Endocrinology* **129,** 2246–2250 (1991).
59. Kalu, D. N. The ovariectomized rat model of postmenopausal bone loss. *Bone Miner,* **15,** 175–192 (1991).
60. Kimmel, D. B., Bozzato, R. P., Kronis, K. A., Coble, T., Sindrey, D., Kwong, P., and Recker, R. R. The effect of recombinant human (1-84) or synthetic human (1-34) parathyroid hormone on the skeleton of adult osteopenic ovariectomized rats. *Endocrinology* **132(4),** 1577–1584 (1993).
61. Shen, V., Dempster, D. W., Mellish, R. W. E., Birchman, R., Horbert, W., and Lindsay, R. Effects of combined and separate intermittent administration of low-dose human parathyroid hormone fragment (1-34) and 17β-estradiol on bone histomorphometry in ovariectomized rats with established osteopenia. *Calcif. Tissue Int.* **50,** 214–220 (1992).
62. Wronski, T. J., Yen, C.-F., and Dann, L. M. Parathyroid hormone is more effective than estrogen or bisphosphonates for restoration of lost bone mass in ovariectomized rats. *Endocrinology* **132,** 823–831 (1993).
63. Jerome, C. P. Anabolic effect of high doses of human parathyroid hormone (1-38) in mature intact female rats. *J. Bone Miner. Res.* **9,** 933–942 (1994).
64. Tada, K., Yamanuro, T., Okumura, H., Kasai, R., and Takahashi, H. Restoration of axial and appendicular bone volumes by hPTH (1-34) in parathyroidectomized and osteopenic rats. *Bone* **11,** 163–169 (1990).
65. Meng, X. W., Liang, X. G., Birchman, R., Wu, D. D., Dempster, D. W., Lindsay, R., and Shen, V. Temporal expression of the anabolic action of PTH in cancellous bone of ovariectomized rats. *J. Bone Miner. Res.* **11,** 421–429 (1996).
66. Mosekilde, L., Danielsen, C. C., and Gasser, J. The effect on vertebral bone mass and strength of long term treatment with antiresorptive agents (estrogen and calcitonin), human parathyroid hormone-(1-38), and combination therapy, assessed in aged ovariectomized rats. *Endocrinology* **134,** 2126–2134 (1994).
67. Wronski, T. J., Cintrón, M., and Dann, L. M. Temporal relationship between bone loss and increased bone turnover in ovariectomized rats. *Calcif. Tissue Int.* **43,** 179–183 (1988).
68. McMurtry, C. T., Schranck, F. W., Walkenhorst, D. A., Murphy, W. A., Kocher, D. B., Teitelbaum, S. L., Rupich, R. C., and Whyte, M. P. Significant developmental elevation in serum parathyroid hormone levels in a large kindred with familial benign (Hypocalciuric) hypercalcemia. *Am. J. Med.* **93,** 247–258 (1992).
69. Gunness-Hey, M., and Hock, J. M. Loss of the anabolic effect of parathyroid hormone on bone after discontinuation of hormone in rats. *Bone* **10,** 447–452 (1989).
70. Lane, N. E., Thompson, J. M., Strewler, G. J., and Kinney, J. H. Intermittent treatment with human parathyroid hormone (hPTH[1-34]) increased trabecular bone volume but not connectivity in osteopenic rats. *J. Bone Miner. Res.* **10,** 1470–1477 (1995).
71. Shen, V., Dempster, D. W., Birchman, R., Xu, R., and Lindsay, R. Loss of cancellous bone mass and connectivity in ovariectomized rats can be restored by combined treatment with parathyroid hormone and estradiol. *J. Clin. Invest.* **91,** 2479–2487 (1993).
72. Li, M., Mosekilde, L., Sogaard, C. H., Thomsen, J. S., and Wronski, T. J. Parathyroid hormone monotherapy and cotherapy with antiresorptive agents restore vertebral bone mass and strength in aged ovariectomized rats. *Bone* **16,** 629–635 (1995).
73. Shen, V., Birchman, R., Xu, R., Otter, M., Wu, D., Lindsay, R., and Dempster, D. W. Effects of reciprocal treatment with estrogen and estrogen plus parathyroid hormone on bone structure and strength in ovariectomized rats. *J. Clin. Invest.* **96,** 2331–2338 (1995).
74. Mosekilde, L., Danielsen, C. C., Sogaard, C. H., McOsker, J. E., and Wronski, T. J. The anabolic effects of parathyroid hormone on cortical bone mass, dimensions and strength—assessed in a sexually mature, ovariectomized rat model. *Bone* **16,** 223–230 (1995).
75. Sogaard, C. H., Wronski, T. J., McOsker, J. E., and Mosekilde, L. The positive effect of parathyroid hormone on femoral neck bone strength in ovariectomized rats is more pronounced than that of estrogen or bisphosphonates. *Endocrinology* **134,** 650–657 (1994).
76. Mosekilde, L., Sogaard, C. H., McOsker, J. E., and Wronski, T. J. PTH has a more pronounced effect on vertebral bone mass and biomechanical competence than antiresorptive agents (estrogen and bisphosphonate)—assessed in sexually mature, ovariectomized rats. *Bone* **15,** 401–408 (1994).
77. Qi, H., Li, M., and Wronski, T. J. A comparison of the anabolic effects of parathyroid hormone at skeletal sites with moderate and severe osteopenia in aged ovariectomized rats. *J. Bone Miner. Res.* **10,** 948–955 (1995).
78. Wronski, T. J., and Yen, C.-F. Anabolic effects of parathyroid hormone on cortical bone in ovariectomized rats. *Bone* **15,** 51–58 (1994).
79. Baumann, B. D., and Wronski, T. J. Response of cortical bone to antiresorptive agents and parathyroid hormone in aged ovariectomized rats. *Bone* **16,** 247–253 (1995).
80. Mosekilde, L., Danielsen, C. C., Sogaard, C. H., McOsker, J. E., and Wronski, T. J. The anabolic effects of parathyroid hormone on cortical bone mass, dimensions and strength—assessed in a sexually mature, ovariectomized rat model. *Bone* **16,** 223–230 (1995).
81. Cheng, P. T., Chan, C., and Muller, K. Cyclical treatment of osteopenic ovariectomized adult rats with PTH(1-34) and pamidronate. *J. Bone Miner. Res.* **10,** 119–126 (1995).
82. Delmas, P. D., Vergnaud, P., Arlot, M. E., Pastoureau, P., Meunier, P. J., and Nilssen, M. H. L. The anabolic effect of human PTH (1-34) on bone formation is blunted when bone resorption is inhibited by bisphosphonate tiludronate—Is activated resorption a prerequisite for the in vivo effect of PTH on formation in a remodelling system? *Bone* **16(6),** 603–610 (1995).
83. Mashiba, T., Tanizawa, T., Takano, Y., Takahashi, H. E., Mori, S., and Norimatsu, H. A histomorphometric study on effects of single and concurrent intermittent administration of human

PTH(1-34) and bisphosphonate cimadronate on tibial metaphysis in ovariectomized rats. *Bone* **17,** 273S–278S (1997).
84. Takano, Y., Tanizawa, T., Mashiba, T., Endo, N., Nishida, S., and Takahashi, H. E. Maintaining bone mass by bisphosphonate incadronate disodium (YM175) sequential treatment after discontinuation of intermittent human parathyroid hormone (1-34) administration in ovariectomized rats. *J. Bone Miner. Res.* **11,** 169–177 (1996).
85. Reeve, J., Tregear, G. W., and Parsons, J. A. Preliminary trial of low doses of human parathyroid hormone 1-34 peptide in treatment of osteoporosis. *Clin. Endocrinol.* **21,** 469–477 (1976).
86. Lee, D. B. N., Drautbar, N., and Kleeman, C. R. Disorders of phosphorous metabolism. *In* "Disorders of Meneral Metabolism" (F. Bronner, and J. W. Coburn, eds.), pp. 283. Academic Press, New York, 1981.
87. Maloney, N. A., Ott, S. M., Alfrey, A. C., Mill, N. L., Coburn, J. W., and Sherrard, D. J. Histological quantitation of aluminum in iliac bone from patients with renal failure. *J. Lab. Clin. Med.* **99,** 206–216 (1982).
88. Reeve, J., Arlot, M. E., Bradbeer, J. N., Hesp, R., Mcally, E., Meunier, P. J., and Zanelli, J. M. Human parathyroid peptide treatment of vertebral osteoporosis. *Osteopor. Int.* S199–S203 (1993).
89. Rittmaster, R. J., Bolognese, M., Ettinger, B., Hanley, D., Hodsman, A. B., Kendler, D. L., and Rosen, C. J. Treatment of osteoporosis with parathyroid hormone followed by alendronate. *Bone* **23** (Suppl), S517 (1998). [Abstract]
90. Gregg, E. W., Kriska, A. M., Salamone, L. M., Roberts, M. M., Anderson, S. J., Ferrell, R. E., Kuller, L. H., and Cauley, J. A. The epidemiology of quantitative ultrasound: A review of the relationships with bone mass, osteoporosis and fracture risk. *Osteopor. Int.* **7,** 89–99 (1997).
91. Riggs, B. L., Hodgson, S. F., O'Fallon, W. M., Chao, E. Y. S., Wahner, H. W., Muhs, J. M., Cedel, S. L., and Melton, L., III, Effect of fluoride treatment on the fracture rate in postmenopausal women with osteoporosis. *N. Engl. J. Med.* **322,** 802–809 (1990).
92. Hodsman, A. B., and Drost, D. J. The response of vertebral bone mineral density during the treatment of osteoporosis with sodium fluoride. *J. Clin. Endocrinol. Metab.* **69,** 932–938 (1989).
93. Chavassieux, P. M., Arlot, M. E., and Meunier, P. J. Intersample variation in bone histomorphometry: comparison between parameter values measured on two contiguous transiliac bone biopsies. *Calcif. Tissue Int.* **37,** 345–350 (1985).
94. Delmas, P. D., Schlemmer, A., Gineyts, E., Riis, B., and Christiansen, C. Urinary excretion of pyridinoline crosslinks correlates with bone turnover measured on iliac crest biopsy in patients with vertebral osteoporosis. *J. Bone Miner. Res.* **6,** 639–644 (1991).
95. Riis, B. J., Overgaard, K., and Christiansen, C. Biochemical markers of bone turnover to monitor the bone response to postmenopausal hormone replacement therapy. *Osteopor. Int.* **5,** 276–280 (1995).
96. Garnero, P., Shih, W. J., Gineyts, E., Karpf, D. B., and Delmas, P. D. Comparison of new biochemical markers of bone turnover in late postmenopausal osteoporotic women in response to alendronate treatment. *J. Clin. Endocrinol. Metab.* **79(6),** 1693–1700 (1994).
97. Tam, C. S., Heersche, J. N. M., Murray, T. M., and Parsons, J. A. Parathyroid hormone stimulates the bone apposition rate independently of its resorptive action: differential effects of intermittent and continuous administration. *Endocrinology* **110,** 506–512 (1981).
98. Cosman, F., Shen, V., Xie, F., Seibel, M., Ratcliffe, A., and Lindsay, R. Estrogen protection against bone resorbing effects of parathyroid hormone infusion. *Ann, Int. Med.* **118,** 337–343 (1993).
99. Lindsay, R., Nieves, J., Henneman, E., Shen, V., and Cosman, F. Subcutaneous administration of the amino-terminal fragment of human parathyroid hormone-(1-34): kinetics and biochemical response to estrogenized osteoporotic patients. *J. Clin. Endocrinol. Metab.* **77,** 1535–1539 (1993).
100. Reeve, J., Arlot, M., Bernat, M., Edouard, C., Hesp, R., Slovik, D., Vismans, F. J. F. E., and Meunier, P. J. Treatment of osteoporosis with human parathyroid fragment 1-34: a positive final tissue balance in trabecular bone. *Metab. Bone. Dis. Rel. Res.* **2,** 355–360 (1980).
101. Lindsay, R., Cosman, F., Nieves, J., Dempster, D. W., and Shen, V. A controlled clinical trial of the effects of 1-34hPTH in estrogen treated osteoporotic women. *J. Bone Miner. Res.* **8,** S130 (1995). [Abstract]
102. Tsai, K.-S., Ebeling, P. R., and Riggs, B. L. Bone responsiveness to parathyroid hormone in normal and osteoporotic postmenopausal women. *J. Clin. Endocrinol. Metab.* **69,** 1024–1027 (1989).
103. Ebeling, P. R., Jones, J. D., Burritt, M. F., Duerson, C. R., Lane, A. W., Hassager, C., Kumar, R., and Riggs, B. L. Skeletal responsiveness to endogenous parathyroid hormone in postmenopausal osteoporosis. *J. Clin. Endocrinol. Metab.* **75,** 1033–1038 (1992).
104. Marcus, R., Villa, M. L., Cheema, M., Cheema, C., Newhall, K., and Holloway, L. Effects of conjugated estrogen on the calcitriol response to parathyroid hormone in postmenopausal women. *J. Clin. Endocrinol. Metab.* **74,** 413–418 (1992).
105. Parfitt, A. M. Morphologic basis of bone mineral measurements: Transient and steady state effects of treatment in osteoporosis. *Miner. Electrol. Metab.* **4,** 273–287 (1980).
106. Hodsman, A. B., Fraher, L. J., and Watson, P. H. Parathyroid hormone: The clinical experience and prospects. *In* "Anabollic Treatments for Osteoporosis" (J. E. Whitfield, and P. Morley, eds.). CRC Press, Boca Raton, FL, 1997.
107. Hodsman, A. B., Fraher, L., and Adachi, J. A clinical trial of cyclical clodronate as maintenance therapy following withdrawal of parathyroid hormone, in the treatment of post-menopausal osteoporosis. *J. Bone Miner. Res.* **10,** S200 (1995). [Abstract]
108. Kent, G. N., Loveridge, N., Reeve, J., and Zanelli, J. M. Pharmacokinetics of synthetic human parathyroid hormone 1-34 in man measured by cytochemical bioassay and radioimmunoassay. *Clin. Sci.* **68,** 171–177 (1985).
109. Fraher, L. J., Hodsman, A. B., Steer, B. M., and Freeman, A. A comparison of the pharmacokinetics of subcutaneous parathyroid hormone in healthy young and elderly osteoporotic subjects. *J. Bone Miner. Res.* **8,** S253 (1993). [Abstract]
110. Schweitert, H. R., Groen, E. W. J., Sollie, F. A. E., and Jonkman, J. H. G. Single-dose subcutaneous administration of recombinant human parathyroid hormone [rhPTH(1-80)] in healthy postmenopausal volunteers. *Clin. Pharmacol. Therap.* **61,** 360–376 (1997).
111. Mashiba, T., Tanizawa, T., Takano, Y., Takahashi, H. E., Mori, S., and Norimatsu, H. A histomorphometric study on effects of single and concurrent intermittent administration of human PTH(1-34) and bisphosphonate cimadronate on tibial metaphysis in ovariectomized rats. *Bone* **17,** 273S–278S (1995).

CHAPTER 47

Growth Hormone and Insulin-like Growth Factor I as Therapeutic Modalities for Age-Related Osteoporosis

LEAH RAE DONAHUE AND CLIFFORD J. ROSEN
The Jackson Laboratory, Bar Harbor Maine, and the Maine Center for Osteoporosis Research and Education, Bangor Maine 04401

INTRODUCTION

Aging in humans is associated with a heightened risk for osteoporotic fractures [1]. In part, this can be attributed to a higher frequency of falling in older individuals [2]. However, an age-related decline in bone mineral density and a marked increase in bone turnover [3] accompany aging. These factors all contribute to enhanced skeletal fragility and fracture. Aging is also accompanied by major perturbations in other organ systems. In the elderly, lean body mass is reduced markedly, and body fat is increased as well as redistributed [4]. As total muscle mass declines, motor function also deteriorates, increasing the likelihood of falling. The musculoskeletal atrophy of aging heightens the risk of fracture and enhances the likelihood of subsequent disability [4].

Coincident with a rather dramatic age-associated decline in bone mineral density (BMD) is a pronounced dampening of growth hormone (GH) secretion [5]. This process has been labeled the "sommatopause" [5,6]. Through complex deconvolution analysis it has been established that GH secretory pulses decline in magnitude and frequency with aging [5]. This is almost certainly related to a reduction in endogenous GH releasing stimuli and an increase in somatostatin secretion [5]. These changes in GH secretion result in a marked decline in circulating insulin-like growth factor I (IGF-I), insulin-like growth factor binding proteins (IGFBP)-3, and IGFBP-5 [7]. Because IGF-I is a potent growth-promoting factor for muscle cells as well as osteoblasts, investigators have speculated that the "sommatopause" is responsible for the musculoskeletal atrophy of aging [6]. Although this thesis has never been proven, age-related changes in body composition parallel the declining production of IGF-I and its regulatory components. So if musculoskeletal deterioration during aging can be halted or reversed by restoring growth hormone or IGF-I, then the potential for savings in terms of both health care dollars and quality of remaining life could be immense.

Since the seminal work of Rudman and colleagues in the 1980s, and the coincident availability of recombinant GH and IGF-I, investigators have earnestly examined how elements of the GH/IGF axis might be manipulated to enhance skeletal and muscle function [8,9]. This chapter reviews how various therapeutic approaches working through the GH/IGF axis could increase serum IGF-I in the elderly and how such a rise might translate into higher bone mass, less fractures, and better functional outcomes in the high-risk osteoporotic patient.

IGF-I AND ITS REGULATORY COMPONENTS

IGF-I is a ubiquitous polypeptide that plays a major role in promoting cell growth and differentiation in various tissues [10–12]. IGF-I is also essential for longitudinal growth, stimulating both the proliferation and the differentiation of chondrocytes. In the adult skeleton, IGF-I is an important coupling factor, which can stimulate proliferation and differentiation of osteoblasts as well as recruitment of osteoclasts [10–12]. The skeleton is also a major reservoir for both IGF-I and IGF-II, as these peptide are constantly being synthesized and bound to hydroxyapatite and IGFBPs [10–12].

The circulation is a major depot for IGF-I. Multiple tissues contribute to the total IGF-I concentration in blood. However, IGF-I does not circulate free in serum. It is bound to a family of six IGF-specific, high-affinity, insulin-like growth factor binding proteins [12]. Only IGFBP-3, the largest and most abundant IGFBP, is fully saturated with IGF-I and IGF-II [12]. Liver is the major factory for IGF-I production and hepatic synthesis is principally under the control of growth hormone. However, kidney and bone also contribute to the circulating pool. Each tissue has the capacity to synthesize and export IGF-I, but regulation of expression at the site of origin is controlled by tissue-specific hormones, as well as paracrine and autocrine factors. Even though circulating IGF-I concentrations reflect the total amount of IGF-I in the body, the relative proportion of IGF-I in a single tissue may differ from the proportion of IGF-I in serum. Moreover, the presence of stimulatory or inhibitory IGFBPs within a given organ system can alter IGF bioactivity dramatically, even though IGF-I concentrations parallel those found in the serum.

Several factors regulate the absolute concentration of IGF-I in the circulation. Growth hormone remains the principal regulator of serum IGF-I and IGFBP-3 [13]. Growth hormone-deficient (GHD) states are associated with low levels of serum IGF-I, whereas acromegaly (or gigantism), a disorder of increased GH secretion, is characterized by high serum levels of IGF-I. However, disorders of insulin, thyroxine, testosterone, or parathyroid hormone production can all have subtle influences on circulating IGF-I levels [12,13]. Also, both endogenous and exogenous estradiol can affect serum and skeletal IGF-I concentrations in women [12,13].

By far the most important cofactor that controls IGF-I synthesis in the liver is nutritional status. Protein calorie undernutrition leads to inhibition of hepatic IGF-I production as well as synthesis of several inhibitory IGFBPs [9,12,13]. The most dramatic example of this is noted in children with suboptimal nutrient intake who manifest growth retardation that almost certainly is a function of impaired hepatic IGF-I production despite enhanced growth hormone release [12]. Similarly, in the aging elder, protein-calorie malnutrition can lead to reduced serum IGF-I and peripheral resistance to endogenous GH. Acute and chronic illnesses can also suppress hepatic IGF-I production. Numerous studies show that serum IGF-I represents the sum of several perturbations in the GH/IGF-I axis, and therefore any causal relationship between skeletal or serum IGF-I concentrations and osteoporosis in the elderly must be interpreted with caution [14].

Age is another factor that influences circulating levels of IGF-I. After age 50, serum IGF-I levels decline in both men and women, although males consistently have higher levels throughout the later decades of life [15,16]. Multiple factors contribute to this age-associated decline. First, growth hormone secretion is reduced, primarily because somatostatinergic tone is increased [5]. However, other factors also suppress GH secretion. These include declining testosterone levels, increased adiposity (possibly mediated through leptin), aberrant sleep patterns, and reduced exercise patterns [5,17]. Second, as noted earlier, protein depletion is very common in the elderly and can affect serum IGF-I profoundly. Finally, there may be some peripheral resistance to endogenous and exogenous pulses of GH that occurs with advanced age [6].

In summary, aging is associated with marked alterations in GH secretion and IGF-I production. Some of these changes are related to environmental factors, whereas others may be genetically or hormonally programmed. Irrespective of etiology, low serum IGF-I and low bone mineral density are both common features in older individuals [14]. Whether these two phenotypes are causally related still remains to be determined.

IGF-I AND AGE-RELATED OSTEOPOROSIS

Age-related bone loss is a major cause of osteoporotic fractures in the elderly, yet the pathogenesis of this syndrome is not totally clear [18]. It is known that bone resorption increases with advancing age [3,18,19]. This may be related to reduced calcium and vitamin D intake leading to secondary hyperparathyroidism and increased calcium mobilization from the skeleton [18–21]. In addition, elderly women who lose bone rapidly also demonstrate some uncoupling in the remodeling cycle, as bone formation rates do not match the rapidity of bone resorption [20,21]. Evidence suggests that osteoblast resistance to IGF-I occurs in bone cells harvested from the elderly [22]. This resistance, coupled with evidence that there is reduced recruitment of osteoblast progenitors, suggests that age-related bone loss is magnified by defective osteoblastogenesis.

Because the skeletal and circulating IGF regulatory systems are so important in maintaining the differentiated osteoblastic phenotype, much attention has focused on reduced IGF-I as an etiologic factor in age-related osteoporosis. Several studies have shown an age-associated reduction in circulating IGF-I due to reduced GH secretion [5,17]. As noted earlier, changes in GH secretion with age are related to several factors, but the end result is a dampening of GH pulses and amplitudes. Cross-sectional studies have also established that serum IGF-I and bone density at several skeletal sites in older postmenopausal women are correlated [23–25]. Also, Kurland *et al.* [26] have noted a strong relationship between serum IGF-I and BMD in middle-aged men with severe idiopathic osteoporosis. Low levels of IGF-I in men with this syndrome are also related to reduced bone formation by histomorphometry, suggesting that there may be a causal relationship between IGF-I and bone turnover in this group of osteoporotic individuals [26].

Boonen *et al.* [25] noted that cortical and trabecular IGF-I concentrations in the human femoral neck decline by more than one-third from the age of 23 to 92 years. These findings, along with an earlier study by Nicholas and co-workers, confirm that skeletal IGF-I is reduced markedly in the elderly and that this decline is similar to the age-associated drop in serum IGF-I [5,17,27,28]. These findings do not prove that low IGF-I levels cause reduced bone mineral density but rather that aging is accompanied by a reduction in both IGF-I and bone mass.

In addition to a global reduction in serum and skeletal IGF-I, there may be other perturbations in the IGF regulatory system that could contribute to impaired bone formation in the elderly. In particular, there are likely to be alterations in the production and breakdown of inhibitory and stimulatory IGFBPs [29]. Several roles for the IGFBPs and their related proteases have emerged from *in vitro* studies utilizing various osteoblast-derived cell lines. These include sequestering IGFs to inhibit their biological activity, prolonging the half-life of IGFs, and enhancing the biological response of target tissues to IGFs by targeting the peptides to particular cell types or by fixing them in adjacent compartments [13,30–34]. Alterations in the IGFBPs could impact bone remodeling and accentuate age-related bone loss. Of particular interest is IGFBP-5, one of the IGFBPs that potentiates IGF action [34,35]. IGFBP-5 is specific for IGF-I and IGF-II but is able to associate directly with the osteoblast surface to stimulate mitogenesis in the absence of either peptide [34–36]. IGFBP-5 is present in the extracellular matrix and may facilitate storage of IGFs by complexing with IGFs and then binding to hydroxyapatite [34–36]; IGFs would then be available to participate in bone remodeling, possibly by stimulating nearby osteoblasts during bone formation [31,35–37]. Regulation of inhibitory and stimulatory skeletal IGFBPs may be a key process in bone remodeling and may be disorded in the elderly [38]. For example, in contrast to stimulatory IGFBP-5 is IGFBP-4, a binding protein that acts to inhibit IGF actions by sequestering IGFs and preventing association with IGF receptors [12,38]. IGFBP-5 declines with age and may contribute to reduced osteoblastic activity, whereas IGFBP-4 is increased markedly in the serum of elderly individuals and is highest among those who sustain a hip fracture [38,39]. Furthermore, IGFBP-4 concentrations correlate closely with PTH and both rise with age [39,40]. Finally, IGFBP-3, a major circulating binding protein that can be either inhibitory or stimulatory, is produced by osteoblasts and is regulated by growth hormone [9,10,12]. Serum IGFBP-3 also declines with age and may contribute to changes in bone turnover in the elderly [7,41,42].

Thus, a scenario could be constructed whereby elderly individuals with reduced serum and skeletal IGF-I, IGFBP-3, and IGFBP-5 concentrations who are also calcium deficient develop secondary hyperparathyroidism. This leads to a marked increase in bone resorption, but also enhanced synthesis of IGFBP-4 that prevents IGF-I-induced stimulation of bone formation. Uncoupling the remodeling unit in this manner could increase the risk of osteoporotic fractures markedly as bone loss becomes pronounced. This pathophysiologic scenario could have implications therapeutically, as replacement or pharmacologic administration of IGF-I, or GH, might restore the remodeling balance in the aged skeleton. Hence, a strong rationale for utilizing components of the GH/IGF axis as therapeutic options in the elderly with osteoporosis has been proposed. Table I summarizes the various manipulations that could result in increased serum IGF-I and thus serve as anabolic agents for age-related osteoporosis. It should be noted that this chapter examines only the role of the GH/IGF-I axis or its components as treatments for age-related osteoporosis. However, it must be pointed out that intermittent parathyroid hormone (PTH) administration increases skeletal IGF-I and may exerts its anabolic effects on bone via this mechanism [43]. Ironically, PTH therapy does not affect circulating IGF-I concentrations. Similarly, testosterone can stimulate the local production of IGF-I and may have a slight effect on increasing serum

TABLE I Agents That Could Potentially Enhance Tissue or Serum IGF-I and May Have Utility in Treating Age-Related Osteoporosis

Agent	↑ IGF-I[a]	Clinical trial[b]	Osteoporosis utility	Reference
rhIGF-I	++++	Yes	±?	[50–53]
rhGH	++++	Yes	−???	[8,9,48–53]
GHRH	++	Yes	???	[67]
GHRP[c]	++	Yes	??	[17,67]
Protein supplement	++	Yes	+?	[65]
Testosterone	+	Yes	+???	[74]
PTH	−	Yes	++	[43]
rhIGFBP-5	±	No	????	—
IGF/BP3	+++++	Yes	+???	[43,56]

[a] A plus sign represents the degree of increase in serum IGF-I or potential utility for treating osteoporosis. A minus sign means no effect was reported.

[b] Whether there are ongoing phase I, II, or III studies utilizing this approach to raise IGF-I in elderly individuals.

[c] A family of growth hormone-releasing peptides and nonpeptide that increase GH secretion independent of GHRH.

IGF-I in men [44,44a]. In adolescent men and women, testosterone also stimulates GH secretion, but data concerning the effects of androgens on serum IGF-I in the elderly are meager.

GH OR IGF-I AS THERAPEUTIC OPTIONS FOR OSTEOPOROSIS

Low bone mineral density as a result of chronic growth hormone deficiency (GHD) in adulthood can lead to osteoporotic fractures [45]. The U.S. FDA has approved the use of recombinant human GH (rhGH) for growth hormone deficiency in adults. In part, this indication was based on compelling data from the United States and Europe that rhGH treatment for GHD increases BMD at several skeletal sites after 2 years of treatment [46,47]. However, no studies have shown that rhGH can increase bone mass in the elderly to the extent noted in GHD, even though both skeletal and serum IGF-I levels are low initially and are increased by exogenous administration [47]. The reasons for this disparate response between young and old to rhGH or rhIGF-I are not entirely clear. Originally, Rudman *et al.* [8] reported a 1.6% increase in lumbar BMD following 6 months of rhGH treatment to elderly males with low serum IGF-I. A subsequent follow-up of that cohort failed to show a consistent effect from rhGH on spine, hip, or total body BMD [9]. Other short-term studies have also been unable to show a strong positive effect from rhGH treatment on bone mineral density, even though markers of bone turnover increase in the elderly [48–51]. Similarly, Holloway *et al.* [51] could not establish a benefit from rhGH treatment alone that was greater than treatment with the antiresorptive medication, calcitonin. Furthermore, MacLean *et al.* [52] reported that total body BMD decreased after 1 year of low-dose rhGH in elderly men and women who were classified as frail by indices of physical performance. Moreover, there was no correlation between serum IGF-I and measures of physical performance in that same cohort either at baseline or after treatment (D. P. Kiel, personal communication). It is even more notable that the results of these studies were negative despite consistent and significant increases of serum IGF-I into the young normal range. Taken together, these data would suggest that IGF-I deficiency was not the pathogenic factor in age-related osteoporosis or that other factors, including the IGFBPs, limit the bioactivity of IGF-I in the skeleton of older individuals. However, it should be noted that long-term studies with rhGH or rhIGF-I in elderly individuals have not gone beyond 24 months. Based on previous GH trials, it might take several years to see a beneficial effect from growth factor treatment, especially with respect to the aging skeleton [46,47].

The absence of an anabolic skeletal effect in the elderly has not deterred investigations with rhIGF-I and IGF-I/IGFBP-3 as antiosteoporotic treatments. Ebeling *et al.* [53] investigated several doses of rhIGF-I in younger postmenopausal women and found that bone turnover was stimulated and the lowest dose of rhIGF-I could increase bone formation more than resorption. Few side effects were noted with rhIGF-I at doses of 30 and 60 μg/kg/day [53]. More recently, Ghiron *et al.* [50] administered low-dose IGF-I (15 μg/kg/day b.i.d) to elderly women and found a selective increase in bone formation without changes in bone resorption. These data suggest that rhIGF-I in low doses may have an effect on bone turnover and potentially (although not measured in the Ghiron study) BMD. The findings by Ghiron *et al.* [50] are also consistent with short-term studies by Grinspoon and colleagues [54] in young fasting women. In those studies, much higher doses of rhIGF-I were well tolerated and produced an increase in bone formation that exceeded bone resorption. These effects were pronounced, considering those women exhibited a decline in serum IGF-I and a rise in IGFBP-1, another inhibitory IGF-binding protein [54].

Serum levels of IGFBP-3 are reduced in some osteoporotic patients, and because of the concern about hypoglycemia during rhIGF-I treatment, an alternative approach for using rhIGF-I in age-related osteoporosis has emerged [23,24,55]. IGF-I complexed to IGFBP-3 and administered daily as a soluble complex subcutaneously has been shown to increase serum IGF-I concentrations markedly in the young and elderly without serious adverse effects. Based on earlier animal studies, the IGF-I/IGFBP-3 complex can enhance bone formation and bone mass strongly [56]. Dose ranging studies using the IGF-I/IGFBP-3 complex (0.3–6.0 mg/kg) in young volunteers and healthy elderly adults have shown that this agent is safe and well tolerated (D. Rosen, personal communication). No episodes of hypoglycemia were noted, even at high doses of complex. Similarly, in a phase I trial, 7 consecutive days of rhIGF-I/IGFBP-3 at doses of 0.5–2.0 mg/kg/day by continuous subcutaneous infusion via a mini pump produced no serious side effects to healthy elders. Furthermore, procollagen peptide (a marker of bone formation) increased 50% over the 7-day period and remained elevated for an additional 7 days after discontinuation of treatment (D. Rosen, personal communication). Despite a concomitant rise in deoxypyridinoline with complex administration, this rise did not persist posttreatment. Thus, this form of IGF-I administration could have utility in patients with osteoporosis.

Future osteoporosis therapies could also center on manipulating IGFBPs or IGFBP proteases, some of which are specific for particular IGFBPs and operate in tissue-restricted environments (e.g., one skeletal IGFBP-4 protease works only at a very low pH) [57]. Bone cells in culture and human bone cells *in vivo* produce enzymes that stimulate the breakdown of several IGFBPs. These include nonspecific matrix metalloproteases and plasmin that will degrade more than one kind of IGFBP and IGFBP-specific proteases [57–59]. Because IGFBP-5 fragments have been shown to enhance the action of IGFs on bone cells, IGFBP-5 protease may be the regulatory agent in IGF/IGFBP-mediated bone differentiation [60]. In some physiological conditions, IGFBP-5 protease will also degrade IGFBP-3 and -4, and proteolysis of IGFBP-5 has been shown to be responsive to PTH and prostaglandin E_2 [61]. IGFBP-4 also has a specific protease that is induced by PTH and estrogen, effectively limiting the inhibitory capacity of IGFBP-4 in medium from osteoblastic cell culture [62]. Consequently, the induction of specific proteases to release or sequester IGFs via IGFBPs could be used therapeutically to manipulate the bioavailability of the IGFs. However, at the current time no human or animal studies have been undertaken.

GH/IGF-I AS SHORT-TERM TREATMENT OF CATABOLIC STATES ASSOCIATED WITH OSTEOPOROSIS

Hip fractures are the most feared complication of the osteoporosis syndrome [63]. This is due to the high mortality (upward of 20%) and the tremendous morbidity associated with this event [63]. Although hip fractures do not kill people directly, the baseline nutritional status of those who fracture, the trauma itself, the surgery required for repair, and the predisposing frailty associated with hip fracture lead to poor outcomes. Two independent groups have noted a dramatic drop in serum IGF-I in elders after a hip fracture [64,65]. These changes in IGF-I were accompanied by significant declines in femoral BMD and lean body mass 8 weeks after the fracture [65]. Even though some of the hip fracture subjects were malnourished or chronically sick prior to their fracture, these findings demonstrate that the injury and the resultant surgery strongly limit IGF-I production. Furthermore, this decline in IGF-I can be tied directly to increases in total body catabolism. No studies have shown yet that a low serum IGF-I is directly related to morbidity or mortality after a hip fracture. However, Bonjour *et al.* [65] established that baseline IGF-I after hip surgery was a surrogate marker for prolonged hospitalization postsurgical fixation. Because much of the annual cost for osteoporosis (i.e., 13 billion dollars in the United States) centers on hospitalization and rehabilitation after hip fractures, therapies utilizing the GH/IGF-I axis or its components make sound medical and economic sense [66].

Several therapeutic strategies have been initiated in order to reduce hospital stays and morbidity after a hip fracture. Bonjour *et al.* [65] demonstrated convincingly that 6 months of protein supplementation to elderly patients posthip fracture increases serum IGF-I by 75%, reduces bone loss by half, improves muscle strength, and shortens rehabilitation times. Growth hormone treatment has also been attempted in some elders post-hip fracture, but at the present time those trials have been somewhat inconclusive and safety has yet to be established.

Another approach under consideration in the elderly is the use of growth hormone-releasing hormone (GHRH) or GH-releasing peptide analogues to induce modest increases in serum IGF-I and to prevent protein breakdown. There are several advantages to the use of these agents. First, there are few side effects reported with their use in elderly individuals [67]. Second, the growth hormone/IGF-I axis remains intact. Third, the ease of administration (oral or subcutaneous) is appealing. Fourth, the rise in IGF-I with use of these agents is far lower than after treatment with GH or rhIGF-I [67]. Preliminary studies in elders suggest that both oral and subcutaneous forms of these secretagogues raise serum IGF-I only 40–60% above baseline [67]. Functional responses to these short-term therapies have yet to be reported. Finally, there is an ongoing 3-month placebo-controlled randomized phase II clinical trial of IGF-I/IGFBP-3 complex administered for 2 months to

24 elderly men and women who have sustained a hip fracture. Results of that study will be awaited with considerable interest [68].

DISADVANTAGES OF rhGH OR rhIGF-I TREATMENT FOR AGE-RELATED OSTEOPOROSIS

There are clear disadvantages to utilizing growth hormone or growth factors for the long-term treatment of age-related osteoporosis or the short-term sequelae resulting from hip fractures. Besides the lack of strong evidence that bone formation will be enhanced more than bone resorption in the elderly or that BMD will be increased dramatically, there are also acute side effects from recombinant rhGH and rhIGF-I treatment [8,9,48–53] (also see Table I). The most common short-term side effects are edema and water retention, clinically significant gynecomastia in men, carpal tunnel syndrome, and tachycardia/orthostasis (limited primarily to rhIGF-I). Hypoglycemia is noted only with high doses of rhIGF-I and then only under certain circumstances. These agents have to be given parenterally, and the cost of rhGH treatment for 1 year to GHD patients is already considered to be quite high.

There may also be long-term considerations that will limit enthusiasm for these treatments in the immediate future. Several lines of evidence raise concerns about such therapy. First, it should be noted that IGF-I and its receptors act as anti-apoptic agents [69]. Hence prolonged cell survival, which may seem appealing, also raises the question of whether these agents could promote neoplastic transformation or prolong malignant cell life. Second, a report from the Physician's Health Cohort suggested that the highest quartile of serum IGF-I was associated with a more than threefold greater risk of future prostate cancer [70]. Third, it is well known that IGF-I is a growth-promoting agent for MCF-7 breast cancer cells [69]. Tamoxifen, a potent antitumor agent, lowers serum IGF-I and may exert its effect on neoplastic tissue by working through inhibition of IGF-I synthesis [71]. Finally, in acromegaly, a chronic disorder associated with high circulating levels of IGF-I, colonic polyps are a very frequent finding. All these lines of circumstantial evidence raise concern about the long-term safety of growth hormone, IGF-I, or other growth factors in the treatment of chronic diseases such as osteoporosis.

SUMMARY

Work since the 1980s has produced some exciting and innovative approaches to understanding the relationship of IGF-I to the skeleton. The IGF regulatory system is ubiquitous, complex, and multifaceted. It is regulated by numerous hormonal and paracrine factors that control matrix deposition and bone mineral density. New evidence has emerged that there are also genetic determinants that affect total skeletal and serum IGF-I concentrations [72,73]. Aging results in a dramatic decline in IGF-I that may lead to accelerated bone loss and accentuate osteoporosis in the elderly population. Therapies aimed at replacing low levels of IGF-I or altering IGF bioactivity via rhGH, rhIGF-I, IGF-I/IGFBP-3, or IGFBPs have great potential as anabolic options for treating osteoporosis. However, there are significant limitations to these therapies that will have to be resolved before these agents will be approved for the augmentation or enhancement of the aging skeleton.

References

1. Hui, S. L., Slemenda, C. W., and Johnston, C. C. Age and bone mass as predictors of fracture in a prospective study. *J. Clin. Invest.* **81,** 1804–1809 (1988).
2. Greenspan, S. L., Myers, E. R., Maitland, L. A., Resnick, N. M., and Hayes, W. C. Fall severity and bone mineral density as risk factors for hip fracture in ambulatory elderly. *JAMA* **271,** 128–133 (1994).
3. Dresner-Pollak, R., Parker, R. A., Poku, M., Thompson, J., Seibel, M. J., and Greenspan, S. L. Biochemical markers of bone turnover reflect femoral bone loss in elderly women. *Calcif. Tissue Int.* **59,** 328–333 (1996).
4. Nevitt, M. C., Cummings, S. R., and Hudes, E. S. Risk factors for injurious falls: a prospective study. *J. Gerontol.* **56M,** 164–171 (1991).
5. Veldhuis, J. D., Iranmanesh, A., and Weltman, A. Elements in the pathophysiology of diminished GH secretion in aging humans. *Endocrine* **7,** 41–48 (1997).
6. Hoffman, A. R., Lieberman, S. A., Butterfield, G., Thompson, J., Hintz, R. R. L., Ceda, G. P., and Marcus, R. Functional consequences of the Somatopause and its treatment. *Endocrine* **7,** 73–76 (1997).
7. Rajaram, S., Baylink, D. J., and Mohan, S. IGFBPs in serum and other biological fluids. *Endoc. Rev.* **18,** 801–831 (1997).
8. Rudman, D., Feller, A. G., and Nelgrag, H. S. Effect of human GH in men over age 60. *N. Engl. J. Med.* **323,** 52–60 (1990).
9. Rudman, D., Feller, A. G., and Chohn, L. Effect of rhGH on body composition in elderly men. *Horm. Res.* **36,** 73–81 (1991).
10. Mohan, S., and Baylink, D. J. Autocrine and paracrine aspects of bone metabolism. *Growth Gen. Horm.* **6,** 1–9 (1990).
11. Bautista, C., Baylink, D. J., Mohan, S. Isolation of a novel IGF binding protein from human bone: a potential candidate for fixing IGF-II in human bone. *Biochem. Biophys. Res. Commun.* **176,** 756–763 (1991).
12. Jones, J., and Clemmons, D. R. IGFs and their binding proteins. *Endocrin. Rev.* **16,** 3–32 (1995).
13. Zapf, J., and Froesch, E. IGFs/somatomedins: structure, secretion, biological actions and physiological roles. *Horm. Res.* **24,** 121–130 (1986).
14. Rosen, C. J. Growth hormone, IGFs and the senescent skeleton. *J. Cell. Biochem.* **58,** 346–348 (1994).

15. Grogean, T., Vereault, D., Millard, P. S., and Rosen, C. J. A comparative analysis of methods to measure IGF-I in human serum. *Endocr. Metab.* **4,** 109–114 (1997).
16. Donahue, L. R., Hunter, S. J., Sherblom, A. P., and Rosen, C. J. Age-related changes in serum IGFBPs in women. *J. Clin. Endocrinol. Metab.* **71,** 575–579 (1990).
17. Rosen, C. J., and Conover, C. Growth insulin like growth factor-I axis in aging: a summary of an NIA sponsored symposium. *J. Clin. Endocrinol. Metab.* **82,** 3919–3922 (1997).
18. Kiel, D. P. The approach to osteoporosis in the elderly patient. *in* "Osteoporosis: Diagnostic and Therapeutic Principles" (CJ Rosen ed.) pp. 225–238. Human Press, Totowa, NJ (1996).
19. Garnero, P., Hausherr, E., Chapuy, M. C., Marcelli, C., *et al.* Markers of bone resorption predict hip fractures in elderly women: the EPIDOS prospective study. *J. Bone Miner. Res.* **11,** 1531–1538 (1996).
20. McKane, W., Khosla, S., Egan, K., and Riggs, B. L. Role of calcium intake in modulating age-related increases in PTH and bone resorption. *J. Clin. Endocrinol. Metab.* **81,** 1699–1703 (1996).
21. Kamel, S., Brazier, M., Picar, C., Boitte, F., Sarzason, L., Desmet, G., and Sebert, J. L. Urinary excretion of pyridinoline crosslinks measured by immunoassay and HPLC techniques in normal subjects and elderly patients with vitamin D deficiency. *Bone Miner.* **26,** 197–208 (1994).
22. Davis, P. Y., Frazier, C. R., Shapiro, J. R., and Fedarko, N. S. Age-related changes in effects of IGF-I on human osteoblast like cells. *Biochem. J.* **324,** 753–760 (1997).
23. Sugimoto, T., Nishiyama, K., Kuribayashi, F., and Chihara, K. Serum levels of IGF-I, IGFBP-2, and IGFBP-3 in osteoporotic patients with and without spine fractures. *J. Bone Miner. Res.* **12,** 1272–1279 (1997).
24. Romagnoli, E., Minisola, S., Carnevale, V., Rosso, R., Pacitti, M. T., Scarda, A., Scarnecchia, L., and Mazzuoli, G. Circulating levels of IGFBP-3 and IGF-I in perimenopausal women. *Osteopor. Int.* **4,** 305–308 (1994).
25. Boonen, S., Aerssens, J., Dequekeer, J., Nicholson, P., Chung, X., Lovert, G., Verhehe, G., and Bouillon, R. Age-associated declines in human femoral neck and cortical and trabecular content of IGF-I. *Calcif. Tissue Int.* **61,** 173–178 (1997).
26. Kurland, E. S., Rosen, C. J., Cosman, F., McMahon, D., Chan, F., Shane, E., Lindsay, R., Dempster, D., and Bilezikian, J. P. IGF-I in men with idiopathic osteoporosis. *J. Clin. Endocrinol. Metab.* **82,** 2799–2805 (1997).
27. Nicholas, V., Prewett, A., Beltica, P., Mohan, S., Finkelman, R., Baylink, D. J., and Farley, A. J. Age-related declines in IGF-I and TGF-beta in femoral cortical bone from men and women. *J. Clin. Endocrinol. Metab.* **78,** 1011–1016 (1994).
28. Boonen, S., Lesaffre, E., Dequeker, J., Aerssens, J., Nijs, J., Pelemans, W., and Bouillon, R. Relationship between baseline IGF-I and femoral neck bone density in women aged over 70 years. *J. Am. Ger. Soc.* **44,** 1301–1306 (1996).
29. Mohan, S. IGF-binding proteins in bone cell regulation. *Growth Regul.* **3,** 65–68 (1993).
30. Zapf, J., Schoenle, E., Jagars, G., Sand, I., Grunwald, J., and Froesch, E. R. Inhibition of the action of nonsuppressible IGF activity on isolated rat fat cells by binding to its carrier protein. *J. Clin. Invest.* **63,** 1077–1084 (1979).
31. Clemmons, D. R., Elgin, R. G., Han, V. K. M., Casella, S. J., D'Ercole, A. J. and Van Wyk, J. J. Cultured fibroblast monolayers secrete a protein that alters the cellular binding of somatomedin C/IFG I. *J. Clin. Invest.* **77,** 1548–1556 (1986).
32. Elgin, R. G., Busby, W. H. J., and Clemmons, D. R. An IGF binding protein enhances the biologic response to IGF-I. *Proc. Natl. Acad. Sci. USA* **84,** 3254–3258 (1987).
33. Blum, W. F., Jenne, E. W., Reppin, F., *et al.* IGF-I binding protein complex is a better mitogen than free IGF-I. *Endocrinology* **125,** 766–772 (1989).
34. Jones, J., Gockerman, A., Busby, J. W., *et al.* Extracellular matrix contains IGFBP-5: potentiation of the effects of IGF-I. *J. Cell Biol.* **121,** 679–687 (1993).
35. Andress, D. L., and Brinbaum, R. S. Human osteoblast-derived IGF binding protein-5 stimulates osteoblast mitogenesis and potentiates IGF action. *J. Biol. Chem.* **267,** 22467–22472 (1992).
36. Roghani, M., Hossenlopp, P., LePage, P., Ballard, A., and Binoux, M. Isolation from human CSF of a new IGFBP with selective affinity for IGF-II. *FEBS Lett.* **255,** 253–258 (1989).
37. Hayden, J., Mohan, S., and Baylink, D. J. The IGF system and the coupling of formation to resorption. *Bone* **17,** 93–98S (1995).
38. Mohan, S., and Baylink, D. J. Serum IGFBP-4 and IGFBP-5 in aging and age-associated diseases. *Endocrine* **7,** 87–91 (1997).
39. Rosen, C. J., Donahue, L. R., Hunter, S. J., *et al.* The 24/25 kDa serum IGFBP is increased in elderly women with hip and spine fractures. *J. Clin. Endocrinol. Metab.* **74,** 24–27 (1992).
40. Mohan, S., Farley, J. R., and Baylink, D. J. Age-related changes in IGFBP-4 and IGFBP-5 in human serum and bone: implications for bone loss with aging. *Progr. Growth Factor Res.* **6,** 465–473 (1995).
41. Gelato, M. C., and Frost, R. A. IGFBP-3 Functional and structural implications in aging and wasting syndromes. *Endocrine* **7,** 81–85 (1997).
42. Johansson, A., Forslund, A., Hambraeus, L., Blum, W., and Ljunghall, S. Growth hormone dependent IGFBP-3 is a major determinant of bone mineral density in healthy men. *J. Bone Miner. Res.* **9,** 915–921 (1993).
43. Rosen, C. J., Donahue, L. R., and Hunter, S. J. IGFs and bone: the osteoporosis connection. *Proc. Soc. Exp. Biol. Med.* **206,** 83–102 (1994).
44. Ho, K. Y., Evans, W. S., Blizzard, R., *et al.* Effects of sex and age on twenty four hour profiles of GH secretion in men. *J. Clin. Endocrinol. Metab.* **64,** 51–58 (1987).
44a. Hobbs, C. J., Plymate, S. R., Rosen, C. J., and Adler, R. A. Testosterone administration increases IGF-I in normal men. *J. Clin. Endocrinol. Metab.* **77,** 776–780 (1993).
45. Rosen, T., Hannsson, H., Granhed, H., Szucs, J., and Bengtsson, B. A. Reduced bone mineral content in adults with GHD. *Acta Endocrinol.* **129,** 201–206 (1993).
46. Beshyah, S. A., Kyd, P., Thomas, E., Fairny, A., and Johnston, D. G. The effects of prolonged GH replacement on bone turnover and bone mineral density in hypopituitary adults. *Clin. Endocrinol.* **42,** 249–254 (1995).
47. Marcus, R. Skeletal effects of GH and IGF-I in adults. *Endocrine* **7,** 53–55 (1997).
48. Papadakis, M. A., Grady, D., Black, D., Tremey, M. J., Goding, G. A. W., and Grunfeld, C. GH replacement in healthy older men improves body composition but not functional activity. *Ann. Int. Med.* **124,** 708–716 (1996).
49. Thompson, J. L., Butterfield, G. E., and Marcus, R. The effects of recombinant rhIGF-I and GH on body composition in elderly women. *J. Clin. Endocrinol. Metab.* **80,** 1845–1852 (1995).
50. Ghiron, L., Thompson, J., Halloway, L., Hintz, R. L., Butterfield, G., Hoffman, A., and Marcus, R. Effects of rhIGF-I and GH on bone turnover in elderly women. *J. Bone Miner. Res.* **10,** 1844–1877 (1995).
51. Holloway, L., Kohlmeier, L., Kent, K., and Marcus, R. Skeletal effects of cyclic recombinant human GH and salmon calcitonin in osteopenic postmenopausal women. *J. Clin. Endocrinol.* **82,** 1111–1117 (1997).

52. Maclean, D., Kiel, D. P., and Rosen, C. J. Low dose rhGH for frail elders stimulates bone turnover in a dose dependent manner. *J. Bone Miner. Res.* **10,** S1458 (1995).
53. Ebeling, P., Jones, J., O'Fallon, W., Janess, C., and Riggs, B. L. Short term effects of recombinant IGF-I on bone turnover in normal women. *J. Clin. Endocrinol. Metab.* **77,** 1384–1387 (1993).
54. Grinspoon, S. K., Baum, H. B. A., Peterson, S., and Klibanski, A. Effects of rhIGF-I administration on bone turnover during short-term fasting. *J. Clin. Invest.* **96,** 900–905 (1995).
55. Wuster, C., Blum, W., Sclemilch, S., Ranke, M., and Ziegler, R. Decreased serum IGFs and IGFBP-3 in osteoporosis. *J. Intern. Med.* **234,** 249–255 (1993).
56. Bagi, C. M., Brommage, R., DeLeon, L., Adams, S., Rosen, D., and Sommer, A. Benefit of systemically administered rhIGF-I/IGFBP-3 on cancellous bone in ovariectomized rats. *J. Bone Miner. Res.* **9,** 1301–1105 (1994).
57. Kanzaki, S., Hilliker, S., Baylink, D. J., and Mohan, S. Evidence that human bone cells in culture produce IGFBP-4 and IGFBP-5 proteases. *Endocrinology* **134,** 383–392 (1994).
58. Conover, C., and Kiefer, M. Regulation and biological effects of endogenous IGFBP-5 in human osteoblastic cells. *J. Clin. Endocrinol. Metab.* **76,** 1153–1159 (1993).
59. Fowlkes, J., Enghild, J., Suzuki, K., and Nagase, H. Matrix metalloproteinases degrade IGFBP-3 in dermal fibroblast cultures. *J. Biol. Chem.* **269,** 25742–25746 (1994).
60. Thraillkill, K., Quarles, L. D., Nagase, H., Suzuki, K., Serra, D., and Fowlkes, J. Characterization of IGFBP-5 degrading proteases produced throughout murine osteoblast differentiation. *Endocrinology* **136,** 3527–3533 (1995).
61. Hakeda, Y., Kawaguchi, H., Hurley, M., Pilbeam, C., Abreu, C., Linkhart, T., Mohan, S., Kumegawa, M., Raisz. Intact IGFBP-5 associates with bone matrix and the soluble fragments of IGFBP-5 accumulated in culture medium of neonatal mouse calvariae by PTH and prostaglandin E2 treatment. *J. Cell Physiol.* **166,** 370–379 (1996).
62. Kudo, Y., Iwashita, M., Itatsu, S., Iguchi, and Takeda, Y. Regulation of IGFBP-4 protease activity by estrogen and PTH in SaOS-2 cells: implications for the pathogenesis of postmenopausal osteoporosis. *J. Endocrinol.* **150,** 223–229 (1996).
63. Keene, G., Parker, M., and Pryor, G. Mortality and morbidity after hip fractures. *Br. Med. J.* **307,** 1248–1250 (1993).
64. Cook, F., Rosen, C. J., Vereault, D., Steffens, C., Kessenich, C. R., Greenspan, S., Ziegler, T. R., Watts, N. B., Mohan, S., and Baylink, D. J. Major changes in the circulatory IGF regulatory system after hip fracture surgery. *J. Bone Miner. Res.* **11,** S 327 (1996).
65. Bonjour, J. P., Schurch, M. A., Chevalley, T., Ammann, P., and Rizzoli, R. Protein intake, IGF-I and osteoporosis. *Osteopor. Int.* **7,** S36–S42 (1997).
66. Ray, N. F., Chan, J. K., Thamer, M., and Melton, L. J. Medical expenditures for the treatment of osteoporotic fractures in the U.S. in 1995: Report from the NOF. *J. Bone Miner. Res.* **12,** 24–35 (1997).
67. Khorram, O., Laughlin, G. A., and Yen, S. S. Endocrine and metabolic effects of long-term administration of growth releasing hormone 1-29 NH2 in age advanced men and women. *J. Clin. Endocrinol. Metab.* **82,** 1472–1479 (1997).
68. Geuseirs, P., Bouillon, R., Broos, P., Rosen, D. M., Adams, S., Sanders, M., Raus, J., Boorlu, S. *Bone* **23** 55:1037 (1998).
69. LeRoith, D., Parrizas, M., and Blakesley, V. A. IGF-I receptor and apoptosis. *Endocrine* **7,** 103–105 (1997).
70. Chan, J. M., Stampfer, M. J., Giovannucci, E., Gann, Ph., Wilkinson, P., Hennekens, C. H., and Pllack. Plasma IGF-1 and prostate cancer risk: A prospective study. *Science* **279,** 563–566 (1998).
71. Shewman, D. A., Stock, J. L., Rosen, C. J., Heiniluoma, K. M., Hogue, M. M., Morrison, A. M., Doyle, E. M., Ukena, T., Weale, G., and Baker, S. The effects of estrogen and tamoxifen on lipoprotein a and IGF-I in healthy postmenopausal women: A randomized placebo controlled trial. *Arter. Thromb.* **14,** 1586–1593 (1994).
72. Rosen, C. J., Kurland, E. S., Vereault, D., Adler, R. A., Rackoff, P. J., Craig, W. Y., Witte, S., Rogers, J., and Bilezikian, J. P. An association between serum IGF-I and a simple sequence repeat in the IFG-I gene. Implication for genetic studies of bone mineral density. *J. Clin. Endocrinol. Metab.* **83,** 2286–2290 (1998).
73. Rosen, C. J., Dimai, H. P., Vereault, D., Donahue, L. R., Beamer, W. G., Farley, J., Linkhart, S., Linkhart, T., Mohan, S., and Baylink, D. J. Circulating and skeletal IGF-I concentrations in two inbred strains of mice with different bone mineral densities. *Bone* **21,** 217–223 (1997).

CHAPTER 48

Fluoride Therapy of Established Osteoporosis

K.-H. WILLIAM LAU AND DAVID J. BAYLINK

Departments of Medicine and Biochemistry, Loma Linda University, and Mineral Metabolism Research Center, Jerry L. Pettis Memorial V. A. Medical Center, Loma Linda, California 92357

INTRODUCTION

One of the characteristics of aging is the age-dependent decrease in bone density (Fig. 1). When the bone density is reduced to a level that is below the putative "fracture threshold" [1], the risk for fragility fractures is increased and osteoporosis develops. If the patient has a bone density that is near the fracture threshold (i.e., has only a modest decrease in bone density), the preferred treatment would be a preventive therapy in which the patient is treated with an antiresorptive agent to essentially maintain bone mass by preventing further bone loss. There are several effective antiresorptive therapies, such as bisphosphonates, estrogens, and calcitonins. However, these antiresorptive therapies are not expected to cause large increases in bone density. Thus, if the patient has a bone density that is much below the fracture threshold (i.e., established osteoporosis), the patient would still be at high fracture risk even on an antiresorptive therapy. Ideally, such a patient needs a corrective therapy that is an osteogenic agent, which, in turn, increases bone formation and bone mass. To date, only two osteogenic agents have been shown to effectively stimulate bone formation and cause large increases in bone density in humans. These two agents are parathyroid hormone and fluoride. Of these two agents, fluoride is the only orally active and bone-specific agent that causes large increases in spinal bone density in patients [2–4]. Thus, fluoride is considered a potentially useful osteogenic therapy for osteoporosis.

This chapter reviews and discusses the clinical use of fluoride for established osteoporosis. Advantages and disadvantages of the fluoride therapy are addressed. Because a high benefit-to-risk profile of a drug is essential for efficacy of a therapy, the authors also propose a strategy to improve this profile of the fluoride therapy. In addition, information regarding the molecular mechanism of action of fluoride is considered to be a relevant issue and will also be discussed.

ANABOLIC ACTIONS OF FLUORIDE

Historical Background

Clinical observations in the 30s indicated that (1) prolonged industrial exposure to excessive fluoride led to skeletal fluorosis, characterized by osteosclerosis and calcification of ligaments and tendons [5], and (2) the severity of skeletal fluorosis correlated with the extent and duration of exposure to fluoride [6]. Based on these findings, Rich and co-workers [7–9] have proposed that low doses of fluoride may be used therapeutically in humans to increase bone formation and thereby strengthen the skeleton without severe osteosclerosis or other skeletal side effects.

Subsequent clinical use of fluoride in patients with osteoporosis has confirmed its usefulness to increase spinal bone density. Bone histomorphometric studies indicated that (a) the effect of fluoride to increase bone mass was due entirely to an increase in bone formation and not to a reduction in bone resorption and (b) the increase in bone formation was mediated through the stimulation of osteoblast proliferation [3,10]. Such results confirm that fluoride is an anabolic agent for bone cells and that osteogenic properties of fluoride are mediated primarily by an increase in osteoblast proliferation.

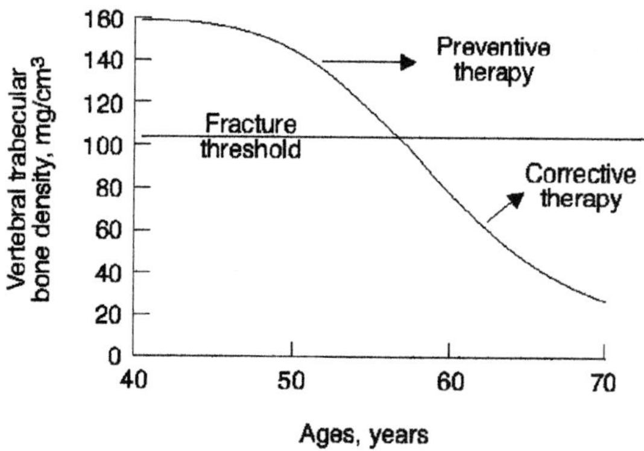

FIGURE 1 Schematic plot of the relationship between vertebral trabecular bone density and age. The fracture threshold line represents the putative spinal bone density value (i.e., 100 mg/cm^3, measured by QCT), above which the risk for osteoporotic spinal fractures is low and below which the risk for spinal fracture progressively increases. By definition, the risk of an osteoporotic spinal fracture can be reduced by preventing the spinal bone density from decreasing below the "fracture threshold" (as with preventive therapies). When the spinal bone density has already decreased to a value below the fracture threshold (i.e., established osteoporosis), corrective osteogenic therapy is required to restore the bone density deficit. Adapted from Libanati *et al.* [98], with permission.

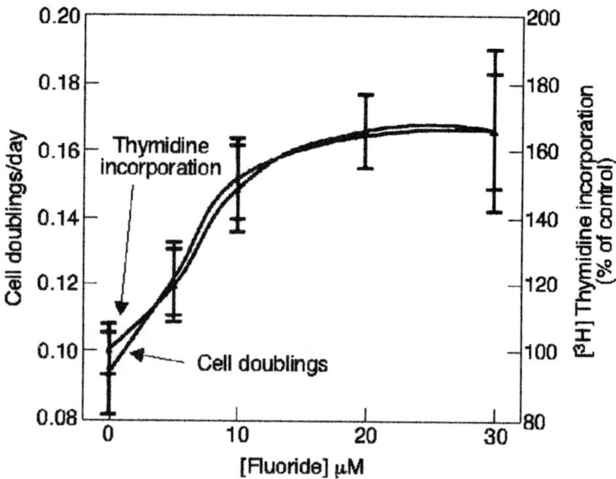

FIGURE 2 Fluoride increases human bone cell proliferation *in vitro.* Normal human bone cells were isolated from the trabecular bone of femoral head samples obtained during hip replacement surgery with collagenase digestion. Human bone cell proliferation was measured by [^{3}H]thymidine incorporation into DNA and by the number of cell population doublings per day. Each data point is the mean ± SEM of six replicates. Adapted from Wergedal *et al.* [14], with permission.

Fluoride Actions on Bone Cells

The demonstration by Farley *et al.* [11] in 1983 that fluoride stimulated the proliferation of primary chicken bone cells has provided the first conclusive evidence that fluoride acts directly on bone cells to exert its anabolic actions. The optimal stimulatory dose was approximately 10 μM, which is similar to the effective serum fluoride concentrations (i.e., basal level at 5–10 μM and peak level at 30 μM) in fluoride-treated patients [12], suggesting that *in vitro* bone cell mitogenic effect may be clinically relevant. The mitogenic action of fluoride was subsequently confirmed by a number of laboratories on bone cells of various species, including humans [13–22], as shown in Fig. 2, which illustrated that fluoride at clinically relevant concentrations (i.e., 5–15 μM) significantly increased DNA synthesis and the cell doubling in normal human bone cells. Thus, these bone cell mitogenic effects of fluoride are entirely compatible with the past bone histomorphometric findings of a fluoride-induced increase in osteoblast proliferation [3,10].

There is also evidence that fluoride, at mitogenic doses, acts directly on bone cells to stimulate several mature osteoblastic activities, i.e., synthesis of alkaline phosphatase [11,14,15,17,20,23], collagen [11,14,20,23], and osteocalcin [14,20,23]. Mitogenic doses of fluoride also increased transient calcium uptake [24,25] and sodium-dependent phosphate transport [22,26] in isolated bone cells *in vitro.* Thus, it is speculated that the stimulatory effects of fluoride on osteoblast proliferation and activity are responsible for the fluoride-dependent stimulation of bone formation. Consistent with the speculation that fluoride promotes the progression of proliferation and activation of osteoprogenitor cells leading to increased bone formation, fluoride at mitogenic doses stimulated the formation of bone nodule (an index of *de novo* bone formation) in rat bone cell monolayer cultures [13,16,27].

Characteristics of *in Vitro* Mitogenic Activity of Fluoride on Bone Cells

Studies of the *in vitro* bone cell mitogenic activity of fluoride have revealed seven unique and important characteristics, which are relevant to the molecular mechanism whereby fluoride promotes bone cell proliferation: (1) the mitogenic dose of fluoride is very low (i.e., 10–100 μM) and is at least two orders of magnitude lower than the doses of fluoride required for the effects on other biological systems (i.e., millimolar level) [28]. (2) Consistent with the *in vivo* observations that the osteogenic action of fluoride is skeletal tissue specific, the *in vitro* mitogenic activity of fluoride is also specific for cells of skeletal origin [11,14]. (3) The *in vitro* bone cell mitogenic activity of fluoride requires the presence of a bone cell growth factor, such as insulin-like growth factor (IGF)-I or transforming growth factor (TGF)β [21,29]. (4) Fluoride potentiates the mitogenic actions of bone cell growth factors, such as IGF-I, both *in vivo* [30] and *in vitro* [28]. (5) The *in vitro* bone cell mitogenic activity of fluoride is sensitive to changes in the concentrations of inorganic phosphate in culture medium [24,29]. (6) Fluoride acts primarily on osteoprogenitor cells and/or undifferentiated osteoblasts rather than the highly differentiated, mature osteoblasts [23,31,32]. (7) The bone cell mitogenic action of fluoride is associated with increases in the overall tyrosine phosphorylation status of several cellular proteins, including MAP kinase (MAPK) [22,28,33,34]. Thus, any model for the molecular mechanism of the bone cell mitogenic action of fluoride must account for these properties.

Proposed Molecular Mechanism of Fluoride on Bone Cell Proliferation

Several models of the mechanism of mitogenic action of fluoride have been proposed (Table I). Kawase and Suzuki [35] have postulated that fluoride (at millimolar concentrations) stimulates the proliferation of L-929 fibroblasts by activating protein kinase C (a protein serine kinase) through a heterotrimeric GTP-binding protein (G protein). Reed *et al.* [21] have suggested that the bone cell mitogenic activity of fluoride may be mediated through enhancing the cell sensitivity to TGFβ (a bone cell growth factor). Because fluoride treatment triggers a transient increase in the intracellular calcium level [24,25] that is associated with the cell proliferation process in many cell types, the involvement of a transient increase in intracellular calcium in the bone cell mitogenic activity of fluoride has been suggested [24,25]. On the basis of their findings that fluoride at the 15–50 mM level activated phospholipase D in human SaSO-2 osteosarcoma cells, Bourgoin *et al.* [36] have proposed that the bone cell mitogenic activity of fluoride may involve phospholipase D activation through a G protein. While each of these proposed mechanisms is intriguing and merits further investigation, none of these models can account for all of the aforementioned characteristics of the bone cell mitogenic action of fluoride, e.g., low (micromolar) effective doses of fluoride, the cell and tissue specificity of the mitogenic action of fluoride, and/or the absolute requirements of an appropriate growth factor.

TABLE I Proposed Mechanisms of Mitogenic Action of Fluoride

Proposed mechanism	Reference
Stimulation of protein kinase C through activation of G proteins	35
Modulation of cell sensitivity to transforming growth factor β	21
Acute transient increase in intracellular calcium	24, 25
Stimulation of phospholipase D through activation of G proteins	36
Inhibition of an osteoblastic fluoride-sensitive phosphotyrosine phosphatase	28, 37
Activation of protein tyrosine kinases through a Gi/o protein	22, 42, 43

The authors have proposed a molecular mechanism (shown in Fig. 3) of the bone cell mitogenic activity of fluoride that involves the stimulation of the MAPK mitogenic signal transduction pathway through inhibition of a fluoride-sensitive phosphotyrosine phosphatase (PTP) [37]. The MAPK signaling pathway has at least four tyrosine phosphorylation regulatory points: (1) the growth factor receptor, (2) rasGAP, (3) Raf, and (4) MAPK (identified in Fig. 3 as 1 to 4, respectively). The authors postulate that the dephosphorylation of one or more of these signaling proteins may be mediated by fluoride-sensitive PTPs and that fluoride inhibits the activity of one or more fluoride-sensitive PTPs in osteoblasts, causing an inhibition of tyrosine dephosphorylation of one or more of these four signaling proteins of the MAPK pathway. As a result, the overall tyrosine phosphorylation level of these signaling proteins rises, which leads to prolongation of the mitogenic signal initiated by a bone cell growth factor, resulting in the enhancement of the growth-factor mediated stimulation of proliferation and/or differentiation of osteoblasts.

This model is supported by a large body of strong, albeit circumstantial, evidence [37]. Moreover, this model is tenable and attractive because it accounts for each of the aforementioned seven characteristics of the bone cell mitogenic activity of fluoride. First, the inhibitory doses of fluoride for the fluoride-sensitive PTP in osteoblasts are in the same low micromolar dose range that stimulates bone cell proliferation and bone formation *in vitro* and *in vivo* [11,12]. Second, that the fluoride-sensitive PTP is unique to cells of skeletal origin is compatible with the *in vitro* and *in vivo* observations of the skeletal specificity of the mitogenic action of fluoride [11,14]. Third, while the fluoride-dependent inhibition of dephosphorylation of cellular phosphotyrosine proteins can increase their overall tyrosine phosphorylation level, it is effective only when the basal level of phosphorylation has been increased in response to activation of a protein tyrosine kinase (PTK). Thus, the optimal mitogenic action of fluoride would require the presence of a bone cell growth factor to increase the basal tyrosine phosphorylation of cellular proteins. Fourth, because the mitogenic actions of bone cell growth factors, such as IGF-I, are mediated through direct activation of the PTK activity of their corresponding receptor and because the mitogenic actions of fluoride are presumed to be mediated by an inhibition of phosphotyrosine dephosphorylation, it follows that fluoride should interact

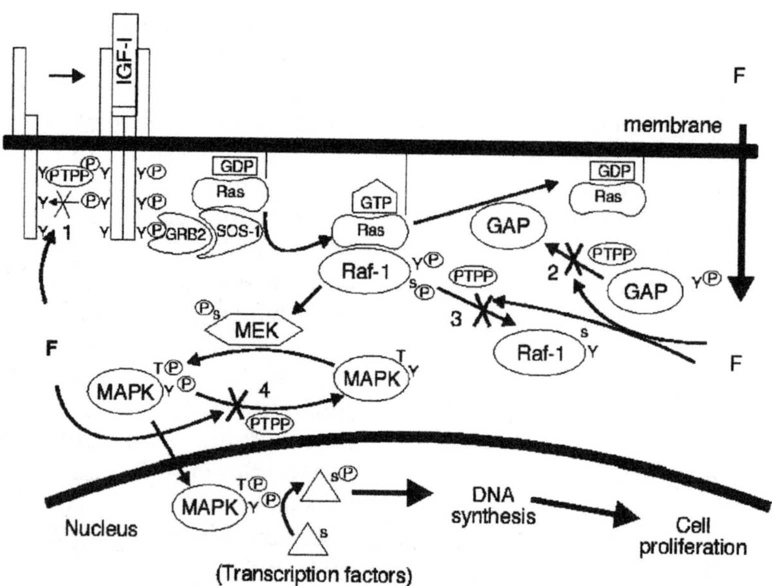

FIGURE 3 A proposed molecular mechanism for the mitogenic action of fluoride on bone cells. The model involves the stimulation of the MAP kinase (MAPK) mitogenic signal transduction pathway through inhibition of a fluoride-sensitive phosphotyrosine phosphatase (PTP). The MAPK signaling pathway is usually initiated with the binding of a growth factor (e.g., IGF-I) to its cell surface receptor, which triggers the autophosphorylation and activation of the intrinsic protein tyrosine kinase (PTK) activity of the receptor. The activated growth factor receptor recruits and phosphorylates docking proteins, such as Shc and/or Grb, which targets Sos to the membrane to mediate the exchange of GDP to GTP on Ras. The GTP-bound Ras is active, whereas the hydrolysis of the Ras-bound GTP to GDP inactivates the Ras, a process that is catalyzed by rasGAP. However, tyrosine phosphorylation of rasGAP prevents the binding of Ras to rasGAP, so that it blocks the GTP hydrolysis and maintains Ras in the GTP-bound activated form. The activated Ras mediates the tyrosine phosphorylation and activation of a protein serine kinase, Raf, which phosphorylates and activates MEK. The activated MEK phosphorylates MAPKs (also known as ERKs) at both a threonine and a tyrosine residue, resulting in activation of MAPKs, which, in turn, migrate into the nucleus to phosphorylate and activate a number of transcription factors, the actions of which collectively lead to increased gene expression, DNA synthesis, cell proliferation, and/or differentiation. Consequently, the mitogenic MAPK signal transduction pathway is stimulated when key members of this pathway are tyrosine phosphorylated, whereas tyrosine dephosphorylation of these signaling proteins results in an inhibition of the MAPK pathway and the consequent cell proliferation process. There are at least four tyrosine phosphorylation regulatory points: (1) the growth factor receptor, (2) rasGAP, (3) Raf, and (4) MAPK (identified as 1 to 4, respectively). This model postulates that the dephosphorylation of one or more of these signaling proteins may be mediated by fluoride-sensitive PTPs. Upon entering bone cells, fluoride inhibits the activity of one or more fluoride-sensitive PTPs, causing an inhibition of the tyrosine dephosphorylation of one or more of these four signaling proteins of the MAPK pathway. As a result, this leads to prolongation of the mitogenic signal initiated by a bone cell growth factor, resulting in the enhancement of the growth factor-mediated stimulation of the proliferation of osteoblasts. Reproduced from Libanati *et al.* [98], with permission.

with PTK-activating growth factors to promote bone cell proliferation and bone formation as it was reported both *in vivo* [30] and *in vitro* [28]. Fifth, fluoride can act, in coordination with divalent cations, as a transition state analogue of inorganic phosphate [38], which is a potent inhibitor of most, if not all, PTPs. Several known transition-state analogues of phosphate (e.g., vanadate, molybdate), at concentrations that inhibited the fluoride-sensitive PTP, also stimulated bone cell proliferation to the same extent as fluoride [28,39]. Thus, it is not surprising that the bone cell mitogenic activity of fluoride is sensitive to changes in phosphate concentration in culture medium [24,40]. Sixth, the osteoprogenitor cells (and less differentiated bone cells) produce more growth factors [23,41] and contain more of this fluoride-sensitive PTP [32] than the more differentiated osteoblasts. As predicted by the authors' model, previous *in vitro* studies show that the less differentiated osteoprogenitor cells are the preferred target cells for fluoride [23,31,32]. Finally, that the model involves the MAPK signal transduction pathway is consistent with the findings that fluoride increases the overall tyrosine phosphorylation level of MAPK and associated signaling proteins in bone cells [33,34].

Caverzasio and Bonjour [22,42,43] have shown that treatments with millimolar concentrations of fluoride in the presence of 10–50 μM aluminum also stimulated cell proliferation and increased the MAPK tyrosine phosphorylation level in rodent bone cells *in vitro*. However, there appeared to be an absolute requirement of aluminum ion, suggesting that the active ingredient may be the fluoroaluminate ion (AlF_4^-) rather than the free fluoride ion [42,43]. This bone cell mitogenic action of AlF_4^- was blocked by a PTK inhibitor, genistein [22], and pertussis toxin, a presumed specific inhibitor of Gi or Go proteins. Based on these findings, these investigators have proposed an alternative model, which also involves activation of MAPK. In contrast to the model shown in Fig. 3, their model postulates that the active species is AlF_4^- (rather than free fluoride ion), which acts directly on a specific Gi/o protein in bone cells, leading to the subsequent activation of one or more PTKs, which, in turn, are responsible for activation of the MAPK signal transduction pathway by phosphorylating key signaling proteins, including Shc and MAPK [43].

Although their data are, in general, compatible with their conclusions, their model fails to reconcile several important discrepancies, such as the cell/tissue specificity, the requirement of growth factor(s), or the sensitivity to phosphate concentration. More importantly, the effective doses of fluoride in their studies were at least an order of magnitude higher than the therapeutic serum fluoride level in patients [12] and were also higher than the effective fluoride doses in most previous *in vitro* studies [13–21,23,24]. The requirement of a high fluoride concentration raises serious questions about the clinical relevance of these findings with respect to the *in vivo* fluoride action on bone formation. In addition, it should be pointed out that AlF_4^- is not the fluoride ion. Because aluminum ion or AlF_4^- is a mitogen for many cell types [44–47], the authors cannot overlook the possibility that the apparent discrepancies observed between the laboratory of Bonjour and theirs may be due to the fact that what they described are related to the mechanism of AlF_4^-, while what the authors observed are relevant to the molecular mechanism of the fluoride ion. Consistent with this speculation, there are several significant differences between the responses to fluoride and those to aluminum and fluoride mixture. For example, fluoride increased the overall level of tyrosine phosphorylation and activity of $p44^{mapk}$ (Erk 1) in human bone cells [34], whereas the aluminum fluoride mixture increased the tyrosine phosphorylation level of $p42^{mapk}$ (Erk2) [43]. Nevertheless, much work, such as knocking out the appropriate PTPs, PTKs, and/or Gi/o gene, will be needed to definitively resolve the discrepancies between the two models.

In summary, there is a large body of evidence indicating that the molecular mechanism of bone cell mitogenic activity of fluoride involves a fluoride-dependent enhancement of the MAPK mitogenic signal transduction pathway. Regardless of whether the enhancement is due to an inhibition of a unique fluoride-sensitive PTP or a direct stimulation of PTKs through a Gi/o protein, these observations raise the possibility that one may increase bone cell proliferation by enhancing a key signal transduction pathway and, as such, these findings open up a new and exciting research area in which this key signal transduction pathway may be used as the screening target for discovery of new anabolic drugs for osteoporosis and related bone diseases.

FLUORIDE PHARMACOKINETICS

Good fluoride responders (those who show large increases in spinal bone density) are characterized by relatively high levels of serum fluoride, increased extrarenal clearance, and decreased renal fluoride clearance [48]. A positive correlation between the urinary fluoride level and the spinal bone mineral content was reported in good responders [49]. In addition, the fluoride-mediated increase in bone mineral content appeared to be associated with the age-related reduction in renal functions [50]. Accordingly, fluoride pharmacokinetics and bioavailability are important factors of skeletal response to the fluoride therapy. In addition to the dosage and body size of the patient, four additional factors would influence fluoride pharmacokinetics and bioavailability: (1) fluoride salts and forms, (2) gastrointestinal absorption, (3) tissue deposition, and (4) renal clearance.

Fluoride Salts and Forms

Two fluoride salts are currently available for human uses: sodium fluoride (NaF) and monofluorophosphate (MFP). Like NaF, MFP stimulates osteoblast proliferation and bone formation both *in vivo* [51] and *in vitro* [52]. However, MFP appears to have three important advantages over NaF: (1) NaF frequently causes gastric irritation due to gastric absorption and formation of hydrofluoric acid with hydrochloric acid in the stomach.

In contrast, MFP is not absorbed in the stomach, does not react with hydrochloric acid, and is hydrolyzed by alkaline phosphatase to release free fluoride ion for rapid absorption in the duodenum [52]. Accordingly, MFP has much less undesirable gastrointestinal side effects than NaF. (2) While the intestinal absorption of NaF is reduced significantly by calcium [53], dietary calcium has no effect on the intestinal absorption of MFP [54]. Thus, MFP can be taken simultaneously with calcium without concern of decreased absorption. (3) The bioavailability of fluoride ion for MFP salt was much higher than that for NaF salt [55–57]. These observations together raise the interesting possibility that MFP is a better fluoride salt for fluoride therapy than NaF.

In addition to plain NaF and MFP, both fluoride salts are also available in enteric-coated and sustained-release preparations. The enteric-coated (galenic) formulations would minimize gastrointestinal irritations. The sustained-release preparations enable a gradual release of fluoride ion, allowing the maintenance of the serum fluoride at the therapeutic level without sharp postabsorption peaks. This is illustrated in Fig. 4 in which a large postabsorption peak in the serum fluoride level was seen in patients with plain MFP therapy, but not in patients treated with a 12-h sustained-release form of MFP [58]. That therapies with sustained-release fluoride preparations avoid postabsorption peaks has been confirmed by others [59]. It is important to eliminate the postabsorption peaks because these peaks are not required for an osteogenic effect, but they could significantly increase the fluoride deposition in bone, which has a deleterious effect on bone quality.

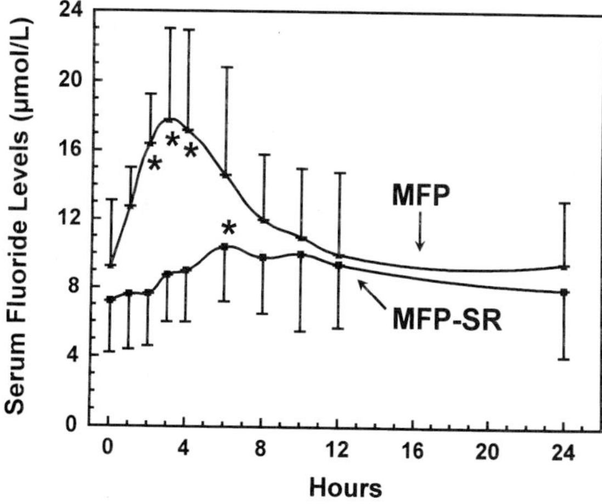

FIGURE 4 Serum fluoride levels (mean and SD) over 24 hr in six osteoporotic patients following a single 76-mg dose of either plain monofluorophosphate (MFP) or 12-hr slow-release MFP (MFP-SR). $*p < 0.05$. Reproduced from Resch *et al.* [58], with permission.

Fluoride Absorption

Upon oral administration, the ingested fluoride is absorbed rapidly and extensively from the gastrointestinal tract into the circulation, presumably through passive mechanisms [60,61]. While the majority of the fluoride is absorbed in the small intestine, mostly in the duodenum and jejunum [62], it is unique among the halides in that a significant amount of fluoride is also absorbed in the stomach [63]. While the rate of gastric fluoride absorption depends primarily on the pH, i.e., inversely proportional to the pH of the gastric contents [62,63], the efficiency of intestinal absorption of fluoride is influenced by three key factors: (1) the type of fluoride salt and the galenic formulation. For example, while several factors can reduce the intestinal absorption of NaF [53,64], these factors do not affect the absorption of fluoride from MFP [65]. (2) The type and amount of other ions in the intestine, such as Ca^{2+}, Mg^{2+}, Al^{3+}, other di- or trivalent cations, and Cl^- [66]. In this regard, di- and trivalent cations have been shown to reduce the rate and extent of the intestinal fluoride absorption, presumably due to the formation of poorly absorbed fluoride compounds, e.g., CaF_2 [66]. (3) The physiological and pathological state of patients, such as age, body acid–base equilibrium, gastric and urine pH, and renal functions [67]. Long-term balance studies in rats indicated that the net secretion of fluoride into the gastrointestinal tract (i.e., fecal excretion > dietary intake) could occur when plasma fluoride concentrations were high [63]. This raises the possibility that a small component of the absorbed fluoride can be resecreted into the gastrointestinal tract.

Tissue Distribution

In humans, the absorbed fluoride enters the circulation and is distributed primarily into two major compartments: (a) extracellular fluids and soft tissue, where it has a relatively short half-life of a few hours, and (b) hard tissues (bone, calcified cartilages, and teeth), where it has a much longer half-life of up to several years. The main deposition (or storage) site for the fluoride ion is the bone, where the fluoride ion is exchanged for hydroxyl groups in the hydroxyapaptite molecule to form fluoroapatite, which is biologically inert. However, fluoride ions are not distributed homogeneously in bone, but are deposited mostly in areas that are actively mineralizing (i.e., sites of bone formation) during fluoride treatment [68]. Thus, in addition to the serum concentration of fluoride (which is influenced by the dosage) and the exposure time (which is related to the treatment duration), the amount of fluoride deposited in bone is also determined by the bone formation rate. Fluoride deposited in the skeleton is removed by osteoclastic resorption during remodeling. Part of the released bone fluoride is probably recycled into new bone minerals, while the rest is excreted in the urine. Therefore, the fluoride content in bone would drop slowly, but progressively, once fluoride therapy is stopped [69]. This slow release appears to account for the relatively long half-life of fluoride in the bone.

Renal Clearance

After absorption into the circulation, serum fluoride is either deposited in bone or excreted. In humans, 75% of the total excreted fluoride is in the urine, 12–20% is in feces, and 5–13% is in sweat [70]. Fluoride is filtered freely in the kidney [71], and the amount of renal fluoride clearance depends on the filtered load (i.e., the glomerular filtration rate × blood fluoride concentration) and free water clearance: the greater the free water clearance, the greater the fluoride excretion [71]. However, because urinary pH is one of the key determinants of urinary fluoride clearance rate and because diet can influence urinary pH, vegetarian diets, which are alkaline, could lead to greater fluoride retention [72].

Some investigators have suggested that renal fluoride excretion may be used as a clinical index to predict the subsequent increase in bone density [49,73]. This suggestion was based on the direct correlation observed between urinary fluoride excretion and the increase in bone density in a group of osteoporotic patients with normal renal function [73]. However, it is possible that an increase in urinary fluoride may merely reflect a higher serum fluoride level in these patients, which itself determined the subsequent osteogenic response. This alternative interpretation would be consistent with the findings of another study in which there was a lower renal fluoride clearance and a greater extrarenal clearance in good responders [48]. It should, however, be emphasized that, inasmuch as the kidney is the major excretory route of fluoride, even a moderate impairment of renal function would predispose to excessive fluoride retention during fluoride therapy [74]. Increased fluoride retention would increase the risk of skeletal fluorosis. Therefore, fluoride should only be used as a therapy with caution or not at all in patients with renal insufficiency [75,76].

THERAPEUTIC SERUM LEVEL OF FLUORIDE

Three observations have led to the suggestion that the serum level of fluoride is the primary determinant of the skeletal response. First, *in vitro* studies indicate that the fluoride ion acts directly on osteoblast-line cells; thus, the circulating fluoride ion, rather than the bone matrix bound fluoride (in form of fluoroapatite), is probably the biologically active species. Second, the optimal *in vitro* osteogenic doses of fluoride were similar to the effective serum fluoride concentrations in fluoride-treated patients. Third, good fluoride responders showed a higher serum fluoride level than poor responders [48]. It has also been shown that the osteogenic response (increases in spinal bone density) correlated positively with the daily oral dose (Fig. 5), but not with treatment duration [77]. Because the serum fluoride concentration is primarily determined by the oral dose, these findings provide further indirect support for the premise that serum fluoride concentration is the major determinant of the skeletal response. Accordingly, the serum fluoride level is probably the most important index for monitoring the therapeutic dose.

Ideal Serum Fluoride Level

The optimum serum fluoride concentrations for osteogenic actions in humans have not been established convincingly because (1) there is a paucity of controlled data on dose–effect relationships and (2) commercial determinations of serum fluoride vary among laboratories, partly due to the fact that the standard curve is not linear such that measurements usually involve extrapolation. In 1970, Taves [78] proposed that fasting serum fluoride levels be maintained between 5 and 10 μM for an osteogenic response in humans. Although these proposed limits have been referred to frequently as the "therapeutic window" for fluoride therapy, this putative "window" was based solely on theoretical as-

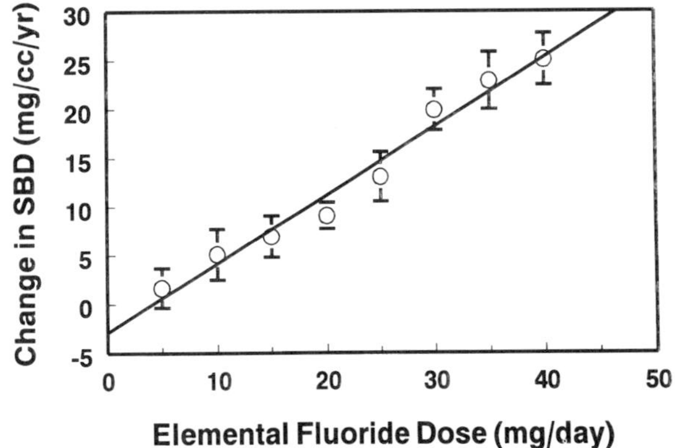

FIGURE 5 The daily dose of fluoride was related to the rate of change in spinal bone density in 41 osteoporotic patients receiving fluoride (range 15 to 43 mg/day) and calcium (1500 mg/day). Adapted from Dure-Smith *et al.* [77], with permission.

sumptions that have not been confirmed. However, there is circumstantial evidence arguing for these limits. Anecdotal data indicate that serum fluoride concentrations below 5 μM rarely produce a significant increase in bone formation in humans. Thus, it is reasonable to have this level as the minimal level. The determination of the upper limit is more difficult. *In vitro* studies disclose that the dose-dependent stimulation of human osteoblast proliferation and differentiation persists at fluoride concentrations of 10–30 μM (Fig. 2), but is linear only up to ~10 μM [14]. Although it is likely that a higher serum fluoride level will produce greater increases in bone formation in humans (Fig. 5), it is also conceivable that the greater increases in bone formation by higher fluoride doses would be offset by a greater incidence of harmful side effects. Thus, the optimal upper limit of fluoride dose should be one that yields the highest benefit-to-risk ratio. Unfortunately, information about the relationship between benefit-to-risk data and serum fluoride concentration is currently missing. However, it would seem reasonable that an appropriate fluoride dose should be one that yields a blood fluoride level that stays within the linear portion of the mitogenic dose–response curve, i.e., 10 μM. The rationale for recommending 5 to 10 μM as a safe and effective level is based on two additional observations: (1) a consistent stimulation of bone formation was observed in patients when fasting serum fluoride levels were maintained at 5–10 μM [12,79] and (2) no serious side effects were observed at a serum fluoride level of 5–10 μM. Until more information concerning the benefit-to-risk ratio of fluoride in humans becomes available, a morning predose serum fluoride concentration of 5–10 μM would seem to be a reasonable therapeutic serum concentration for adults with established osteoporosis.

Serum Fluoride Measurements

Because the putative "therapeutic window" of serum fluoride level is relatively narrow, regular monitoring of fasting serum fluoride concentrations is recommended highly in patients receiving fluoride therapy to detect abnormally high or subtherapeutic fluoride levels [12,71]. However, the timing of serum fluoride measurements is an important issue as the oral intake of fluoride frequently produces acute postabsorption peaks, which are usually three times the morning predose level. Thus, measurements during the postabsorption peak period could yield misleading information. Because it is reasoned that the morning predose level would most likely represent the steady-state serum fluoride level and as such would be an acceptable representation of the mean serum level throughout the 24-hr dosing period, the authors measure the serum fluoride concentration just before the morning fluoride dose [12].

Dosage and Regimen of Fluoride Therapy

Analyses of recent randomized, prospective, placebo-controlled studies appear to indicate that the dosage and the regimen of fluoride treatment each play an important role in determining therapeutic efficacy [80–84]. A study done at the Mayo Clinic, Rochester, Minnesota [80,82], and one at the Henry Ford Hospital, Detroit, Michigan [81], showed that postmenopausal women who were treated with 75 mg plain NaF/day (or 34 mg/day elemental fluoride) for 4 years did not significantly reduce the vertebral fracture rate compared to the placebo-treated subjects, despite a highly significant increase (35%) in spinal bone density. However, an extended analysis of the Mayo Clinic study revealed that a subgroup of 50 patients who had received lower fluoride doses (i.e., <75 mg/day) due to side effects and who had a smaller increase in spinal bone density (i.e., <17%) and a lower serum fluoride level (i.e., <8 μM) exhibited moderate but significant decreases in the spinal fracture rate [82]. Accordingly, it seems that higher doses of fluoride, while showing very rapid increases in bone density and larger increments in serum fluoride levels, did not reduce the spinal fracture rate, whereas lower doses of fluoride, which yielded lesser increments in serum fluoride levels and bone density, were therapeutically effective in reducing the fracture rate.

Two potential mechanisms may explain the lack of a beneficial effect on spinal fractures in patients treated with higher doses of fluoride. First, histomorphometric evaluation of transilial biopsy samples from the Mayo Clinic study showed clear evidence for osteomalacia, even though these patients had received daily supplementation of 1500 mg calcium carbonate during the study [85]. Accordingly, if higher serum fluoride concentrations produced a relatively large increase in bone formation, it follows that the higher the increment in serum fluoride level, the greater the demand for calcium, and the greater calcium demand may result in the development of osteomalacia in the patient. Conversely, patients with a smaller increase in bone formation would be expected to have a lesser tendency toward osteomalacia. Thus, it is possible that the lack of a significant reduction in the spinal fracture rate with higher fluoride doses may be attributed to the osteomalacia. The second potential explanation relates to the fact that higher fluoride doses result in an increased deposit of fluoride into bone mineral (due to higher serum fluoride concentrations), which can have a deleterious effect on bone quality and strength and which leads to the lack of a beneficial effect on fracture rate reduction. Nevertheless, these clinical studies clearly illustrate the importance of fluoride dosage on its clinical efficacy.

The usual daily dosage of fluoride for established osteoporosis is 20 to 30 mg of elemental fluoride [12]. This dose range is used to obtain a morning predose serum fluoride level between 5 and 10 μM. However, it should be emphasized that the required fluoride dose that would achieve optimum serum fluoride concentrations within the putative "therapeutic window" is influenced by age, intestinal and renal functions, and other clinical factors [50] and is likely to vary from one individual to another. As intestinal and renal functions decline, as in old age (most patients with established osteoporosis are in their seventh and eighth decades), serum fluoride concentrations would rise. Consequently, it may require some adjustments in the fluoride dosage in order to maintain serum fluoride concentration within the putative "therapeutic window."

The contention that dosage regimen and scheduling can also be an important factor in the fluoride therapy is demonstrated by the prospective, randomized, controlled study that was carried out by investigators at the University of Texas Southwestern Medical Center in Dallas, Texas [84,85]. In this study, postmenopausal osteoporotic women were treated for 4 years with an intermittent slow-release NaF [50 mg NaF/day (23 mg/day of elemental fluoride) and 800 mg/day calcium citrate supplementation] in a dosage regimen consisting of 14-month cycles (12 months receiving fluoride and 2 months off therapy). Unlike the Mayo Clinic study, patients in this study showed a marked decrease in spinal fracture rate accompanying a moderate increase in bone density. This study, however, differed from the Mayo Clinic study in four important aspects: (1) this study used a lower fluoride dose (23 mg/day vs 34 mg/day elemental fluoride); (2) the study employed a slow-release NaF preparation as opposed to plain NaF, (3) the patients were supplemented with calcium citrate, which is more soluble and readily absorbed than calcium carbonate [86], which was used in the other two studies; and (4) the treatment regimen contained a 2-month "off" fluoride period per year of treatment to reduce fluoride incorporation in bone minerals. It was speculated that the time "off" fluoride period together with the use of calcium citrate would facilitate the resolution of any potential osteomalacia that might have occurred during the therapy. Consistent with this speculation, there was no evidence for osteomalacia and secondary hyperparathyroidism in patients treated with the intermittent regimen [83,84]. Moreover, the "off" fluoride period could also reduce the amount of fluoride deposited in bone. Accordingly, the lack of osteomalacia and the reduced fluoride incorporation in bone may attribute to the significant reduction in the fracture rate. Consequently, these observations indicate that regimens containing moderate and cyclic doses of fluoride may have important advantages over continuous fluoride regimens for the treatment of established osteoporosis.

SKELETAL RESPONSE TO FLUORIDE THERAPY

The osteogenic actions of fluoride are characterized by increases in osteoblast proliferation and activity, bone formation, and bone mass. Accordingly, clinical responses to the fluoride therapy may be assessed by increases in serum bone formation biochemical markers, bone formation histomorphometric parameters, and bone density.

Biochemical Bone Formation Markers

Serum biochemical markers, such as skeletal alkaline phosphatase and osteocalcin, are useful in assessing bone formation in response to therapy in patients [87]. Accordingly, serial measurements of these bone formation markers are often used as an acute quantitative index of the skeletal response to fluoride [88,89]. Fluoride therapy significantly increases serum levels of skeletal alkaline phosphatase [87] and osteocalcin [89,90] within weeks in treated patients. Figure 6 shows that increases in skeletal alkaline phosphatase activity precede bone density gains and improvement of clinical symptoms (e.g., reducing back pain). Serum skeletal alkaline phosphatase also correlates to the fluoride-

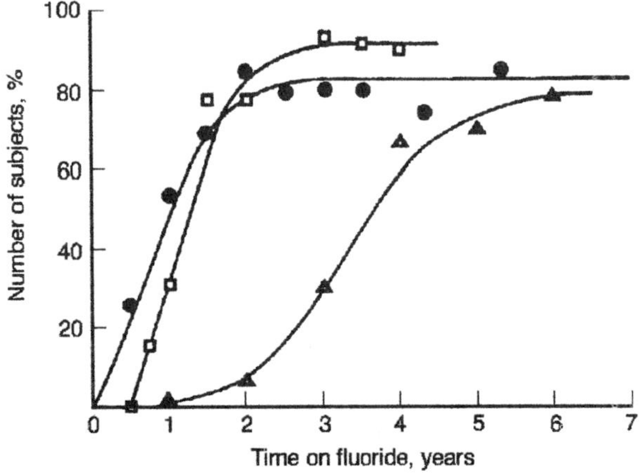

FIGURE 6 The time-dependent effects of fluoride therapy on serum skeletal alkaline phosphatase activity (●), decreased back pain (□), and thickened trabeculae on vertebral X rays, which reflect the increase spinal bone density (△) in osteoporotic patients. Reproduced from Farley *et al.* [88], with permission.

dependent increase in histomorphometric bone biopsy measures of bone formation [88]. Thus, serum bone formation markers, i.e., skeletal alkaline phosphatase activity, are useful early indicators of the osteogenic response to fluoride in humans.

Fluoride therapy can also cause osteomalacia. Increases in the serum level of skeletal alkaline phosphatase is associated frequently with osteomalacia. Hence, an increase in serum alkaline phosphatase activity may not allow the distinction between the two potential causes of a rise in this serum marker, namely increased bone formation or defective mineralization (osteomalacia). Other markers may be needed in assisting in distinguishing these two potential responses to the fluoride therapy. Accordingly, while the increase in serum alkaline phosphatase is associated with calcium deficiency and osteomalacia, there will also be changes in other markers typically associated with secondary hyperparathyroidism, such as a decrease in urine calcium, an increase in serum PTH, and an increase in urine bone resorption markers. In contrast, there should be no such changes in these markers accompanying the rise in serum alkaline phosphatase activity associated with increased bone formation. In vitamin D deficiency-associated osteomalacia, there is an increase in skeletal alkaline phosphatase but not an increase in serum procollagen peptides (another serum bone formation biochemical marker). Thus, one could measure serum procollagen peptide levels to assess the osteogenic action of fluoride or as a means of determining whether the increase in skeletal alkaline phosphatase indicates a mineralization defect.

Bone Histomorphometry

Bone histomorphometric studies in a number of animal models have clearly indicated that fluoride treatment increased the osteoid and bone formation histomorphometric parameters in cancellous bones [37,91–96] and increased the number of osteoblasts and osteoblast-covered surface [19,94,97]. These findings confirm that fluoride stimulates bone formation and indicate that the increase is due to a fluoride-mediated increase in osteoblast proliferation. Bone histomorphometric data of fluoride therapy in humans are almost exclusively derived from transilial biopsies. Fluoride therapy also caused large increases in osteoblast number without direct effects on bone resorption parameters in humans [3,10]. Hence, it is generally believed that the rise in the number of active osteoblasts stimulates bone formation, resulting in a subsequent overfilling of the resorption excavation cavity [Fig. 7], which, in turn, leads to an increase in trabecular bone volume with a thickening of trabeculae and an increase in osteoid volume [98]. This concept is strongly supported by bone histomorphometric data, which also indicate that the increase in osteoid volume is due, in large part, to an increase in osteoid surface and, to a lesser extent, to an increase in osteoid thickness [10,99–102].

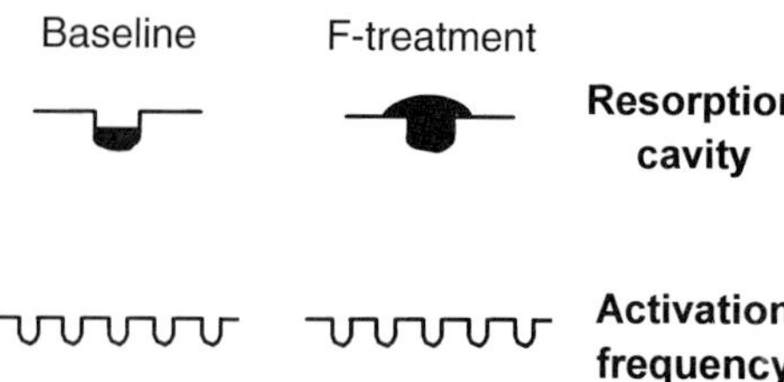

FIGURE 7 Model of the effect of fluoride on bone formation. In osteoporosis, the resorption cavities are underfilled due to impaired bone formation, increased bone resorption, or both. As a consequence, bone density decreases at a given site with each cycle of bone remodeling. Fluoride corrects this deficit by promoting an overfilling of the resorptive cavity (and thereby increasing wall thickness). The activation frequency (the number of active resorptive sites created per unit of bone surface/unit of time in a given unit of bone) is not affected significantly by fluoride. Reproduced from Libanati *et al.* [98], with permission.

There is also compelling histomorphometric evidence that fluoride therapy is often associated with a delay in mineralizing newly synthesized osteoid, as shown in Fig. 8, which indicates that there was a 14-fold increase in the mineralization lag time in fluoride-treated patients over that in placebo control subjects in the Mayo Clinic study [85]. This mineralization defect has been reported in humans [85,102–104] as well as in several animal species [95,105–107]. This defect may be related to the fluoride dose and availability of calcium to adequately mineralize the newly formed osteoid matrix [3,100,102,108]. Because the elderly patients have a reduced intestinal calcium absorption efficiency, the calcium insufficiency due to rapid and large increases

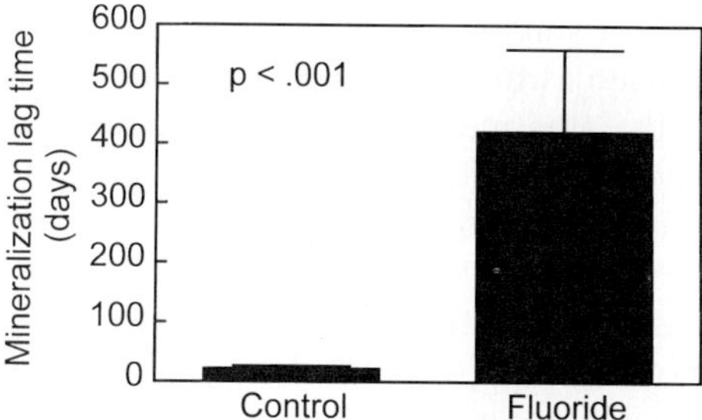

FIGURE 8 Effect of 4 years of fluoride therapy on the mineralization lag time in iliac crest biopsy samples from the Mayo Clinic prospective placebo-controlled clinical trial. The mineralization lag time is a specific measure of the degree of osteomalacia. Values represent mean ± SEM. This presents compelling bone histomorphometric evidence that fluoride treatment causes osteomalacia. Adapted from Lundy *et al.* [85], with permission.

in bone formation in response to fluoride therapy would probably be more pronounced in the elderly subjects. Thus, large and rapid increases in bone formation are more likely associated with the mineralization defect than smaller and slower increases.

While the fluoride-associated osteomalacia is probably related to the calcium deficiency, we cannot overlook the possibility that high fluoride incorporation into bone mineral may at least, in part, play a role in the mineralization defect through physicochemical interactions with bone minerals that directly retard the mineralization process per se. The fluoride-induced osteomalacia, along with high fluoride incorporation in bone mineral, could significantly impair the biomechanical properties of bone, which, in turn, could increase fracture risk. Accordingly, it may be speculated that the greater the incidence of osteomalacia, the greater the incidence of harmful skeletal side effects. If this speculation is confirmed, it is conceivable that the calcium deficiency-associated osteomalacia may have attributed, to some extent, to the lack of positive effects in some past fracture studies.

Bone Density

An important end point of the osteogenic effect of fluoride therapy is to increase bone density. Bone density at both axial and appendicular skeletal sites in humans can be measured with high precision and accuracy by noninvasive methods, viz. quantitative computed tomography (QCT) and dual-energy X-ray absorptiometry (DXA). Because fluoride increases bone density preferentially at axial trabecular skeletal sites more than that at appendicular cortical sites, the effects of fluoride on these two skeletal compartments will be addressed separately.

Axial Skeleton

Lateral lumbar spine X-ray analysis (Fig. 9) clearly shows that treatment of an osteoporotic patient with fluoride (30 mg elemental fluoride/day) and calcium carbonate (1500 mg/day) for 3.5 years led to an increase in bone density attended by a coarsening of vertebral trabeculae and an increased prominence of the vertebral end plates. This confirms the contention that fluoride therapy increases the trabecular bone mass of the axial skeleton in humans. Measurements of bone density by either DXA or QCT also show a marked increase in the axial trabecular (lumbar spine) bone density in fluoride-treated patients. Depending on the dosage and regimen, the observed annual increase in spinal bone density in fluoride-treated patients may vary between 4–10% (with DXA) and 20–30% (with QCT), respectively. A larger

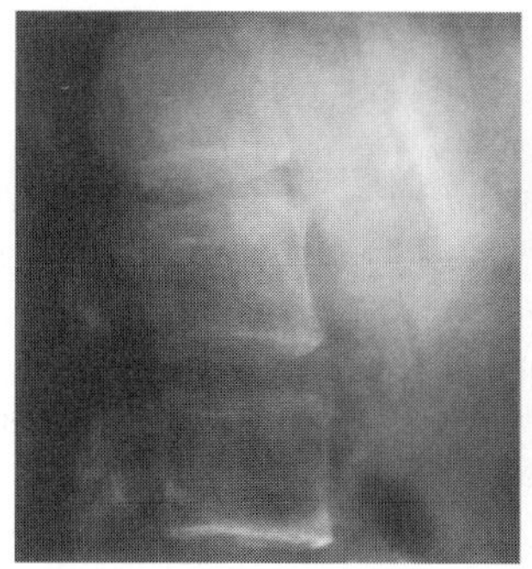
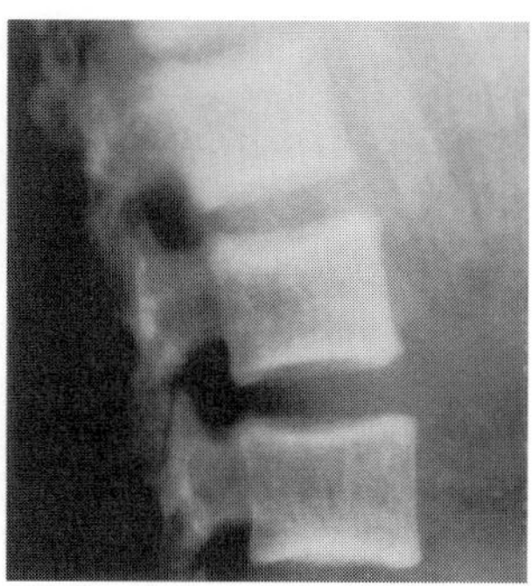

FIGURE 9 Lateral lumbar spinal X ray of a 60-year-old postmenopausal woman before (left) and after (right) 3.5 years of therapy with fluoride (30 mg elemental fluoride/day) and calcium carbonate (1500 mg/day). Note the remarkable increase in bone density of the trabeculae and the end plates. Reproduced from Libanati *et al.* [98], with permission.

percentage increase is seen with QCT, because QCT, unlike DXA, measures trabecular bones exclusively and because fluoride therapy increases trabecular bone mass preferentially.

The increase in spinal bone density in response to fluoride is progressive with treatment duration [4,80,109,110], as shown in Fig. 10, which shows that the increase in spinal bone density in postmenopausal osteoporotic women is proportional with time on therapy for at least 5 years. While the dose–response increase in spinal bone density has not been evaluated rigorously with prospective controlled studies, there seems to be a dose–response increase in spinal bone density between 5 and 40 mg/day of elemental fluoride

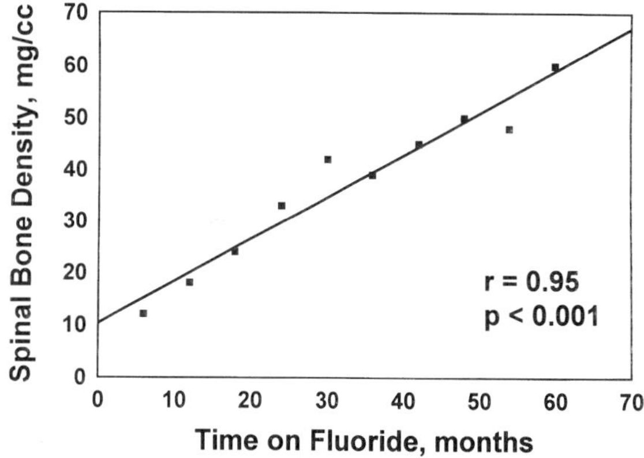

FIGURE 10 The fluoride-dependent increase in spinal bone density as measured by QCT as a function of time in 510 osteoporotic patients treated with fluoride (30 ± 8 mg elemental fluoride/day) and calcium carbonate (1500 mg/day) for up to 5 years. Note the apparent linear increase in spinal bone density with fluoride treatment time for up to 5 years. Reprinted with permission from Lau *et al.* (1998). Osteogenic actions of fluoride: its therapeutic use for established osteoporosis. In (J. F. Whitfield and P. Morley, Eds.) Anabolic treatments for osteoporosis. pp. 207–254. Copyright CRC Press, Boca Raton, Florida.

(Fig. 5). Thus, it is likely that the increase in spinal bone density in response to fluoride is proportional to the dosage and treatment duration. Conversely, the fluoride-induced increase in spinal bone density is unrelated to the severity of osteoporosis, the patient's age, or the cause of the disease [50,98]. Accordingly, patients may show increases in spinal trabecular bone density from a very low value (e.g., 20 mg/cc) to a value above the typical peak bone density of 100 mg/cc. Moreover, fluoride therapy is as effective in increasing spinal bone density in patients with glucocorticoid-induced osteoporosis as in those with postmenopausal osteoporosis [111].

It is intriguing to note that the gain in spinal bone density from the fluoride therapy is not maintained after the therapy is discontinued [112]. The rate of spinal bone loss after cessation of fluoride therapy is similar to the spinal bone gain rate during the therapy [112], raising the possibility that fluoride-treated osteoporotic patients who have an increase in spinal bone density during the fluoride therapy may also be at risk for bone loss after discontinuation of the therapy. Another intriguing aspect of the fluoride therapy is that not all patients would respond to fluoride therapy with an increase in spinal bone density. Twenty to 25% of the osteoporotic patients do not manifest an increase in spinal bone density in response to fluoride therapy and therefore are considered nonresponders [3,101,113]. The causes of the nonresponsiveness and the individual variability in response to fluoride therapy are unknown at this time. A better understanding of the molecular mechanism whereby fluoride exerts its osteogenic actions should shed light on the cause of the nonresponsiveness.

Appendicular Skeleton

Total body bone scintigrams indicate that increased bone formation is seen in both the axial and the appendicular skeleton after 11 months of fluoride therapy [114]. There is also radiological [115] and bone density [80,116,117] evidence that fluoride therapy increases new bone formation in several appendicular skeletal sites that contain a large amount of trabecular bones, such as knee, ankle, foot, hips, diaphysis of tibia, and femoral condyle. Accordingly, these observations provide compelling evidence that fluoride acts on both the axial and the appendicular skeleton, but preferably at the trabecular bone sites.

The magnitude of the increases on appendicular skeletal sites is much smaller than that seen on the axial trabecular skeleton (Fig. 11). Accordingly, even under the best circumstances, the increase in bone density of the appendicular skeleton appears to be of less clinical significance than the increase in axial bone density. However, it should be noted that the osteoporotic deficit

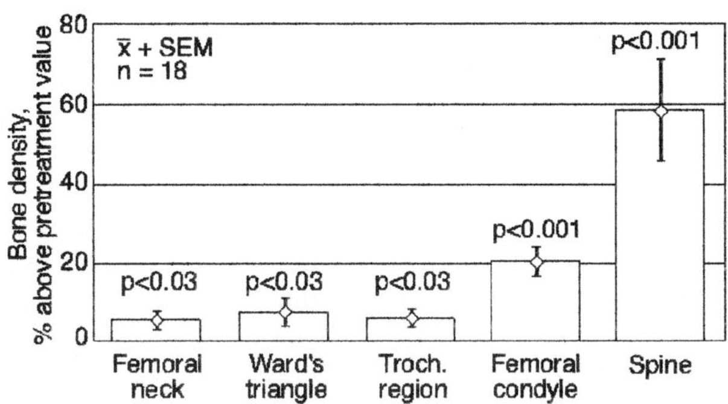

FIGURE 11 Site-specific increases in bone density in osteoporotic patients in response to fluoride therapy. Increases in bone density were measured by QCT in the spine and femoral condyle and by DXA in the hip. Note that only trabecular bone density was measured by QCT in the spine and femoral condyle, whereas cortical and trabecular bone density was measured by DXA in the hip. Thus, the different responses in the spine and hip are, in part, due to different measuring techniques. Bone density increases associated with fluoride therapy are typically larger in the spine than in the appendicular skeleton and are also typically larger in trabecular bone compared to cortical bone. Reproduced from Dure-Smith *et al.* [77], with permission.

at appendicular bone sites (i.e., hip) is also less severe than that at the spine. The relative differences in bone density changes between the appendicular and the axial skeleton could be, in part, the result of the lower inherent turnover of cortical bone compared to that of trabecular bone. An important issue, however, is whether the small increase in the hip bone density, which is usually seen with the fluoride therapy, would be sufficient to reduce hip fracture risks in osteoporotic patients. In this respect, there is currently no reliable evidence supporting the contention that fluoride may reduce hip fracture risks significantly.

The effect of fluoride on the appendicular skeleton appears to be enhanced by mechanical loading, as fluoride seems to increase bone density of weight-bearing bones preferentially over nonweight-bearing bones [114]. Mechanical loading increases the production of growth factors in bone cells and bones [118]. Accordingly, it has been speculated that the more significant increases in bone formation and bone density in weight-bearing bones are the result of a synergism between the growth factor released by bone cells during mechanical loading and mitogenic action of fluoride [119]. This potential synergy is consistent with the proposed mechanism of fluoride action, as the model (Fig. 3) predicts a synergistic interaction between the actions of bone growth factor and fluoride.

Another relevant issue to the fluoride therapy on peripheral bone density is that, in the placebo-controlled prospective study of the Mayo Clinic [80], there was a highly significant 7.7% per year decrease in forearm bone density in fluoride-treated patients, despite a marked increase in spinal bone density. It was interpreted by the investigators that the increase in trabecular spinal bone density occurs at the expense of the cortical bone of the peripheral skeleton. However, there was clear evidence for severe osteomalacia in the fluoride-treated patients in that study (Fig. 8), suggesting that these patients might have developed calcium deficiency. Accordingly, it is possible that the calcium deficiency and the accompanying secondary hyperparathyroidism associated with the fluoride therapy in these patients could be, to some extent, responsible for this peripheral cortical bone loss [85]. In this respect, in the placebo-controlled prospective study of the University of Texas Southwestern Medical Center, the fluoride-treated patients, who showed no evidence of osteomalacia and/or calcium deficiency, did not lose any bone mass at peripheral bone sites [83,84]. Therefore, these findings are consistent with the premise that the cortical bone loss at peripheral bone sites may be related to fluoride-induced calcium deficiency and secondary hyperparathyroidism.

SIDE EFFECTS OF FLUORIDE THERAPY

Fluoride therapy in humans has several significant side effects, such as gastrointestinal irritation, peripheral bone pain, calcium deficiency, stress fractures, and hip fractures.

Gastrointestinal Irritation

Free fluoride ion can be absorbed through the stomach and can react with gastric acids to form hydrofluoric acid, which is an irritant. Accordingly, when plain NaF was used to treat osteoporotic patients in the past, gastrointestinal irritation was a frequent side effect, i.e., >25% of patients who received the therapy would experience this side effect [71]. The severity of this side effect is dose related. The most common symptoms include epigastric pain, nausea, and vomiting, which can be treated effectively with antiacids or H_2 blockers or by decreasing the fluoride dose. In rare cases, patients who are treated with large doses of plain NaF can develop duodenal ulceration and bleeding, which requires temporary discontinuation of the therapy. However, with the recent use of new galenic-sustained release or enteric-coated formulations of fluoride, which avoid gastric absorption and interaction with gastric acids, the gastrointestinal irritation side effect is virtually eliminated.

Peripheral Bone Pain

In 10 to 40% of patients receiving fluoride therapy, severe pain may be developed at peripheral joints, such as knees, ankles, or feet [119,120]. The pain usually subsides within a few days when the therapy is discontinued. This side effect is also dose related and is less frequent in patients receiving relatively low daily doses (<20 mg of elemental fluoride), especially when the drug is given in a cyclic regimen [121].

The etiology of peripheral bone pain is a controversial issue. Some investigators suggest that the peripheral bone pain may be derived from stress fracture that occurs in some fluoride-treated patients [122–124]. The authors propose that the pain is related to a marked increase in bone formation locally by fluoride therapy [98,125,126], a phenomenon that is analogous to the bone pain experienced in rapidly growing children. This possibility is supported by three pieces of circumstantial evidence: (1) the total body bone scintigram demonstrates that increased uptake in the lower skeleton is diffuse and bilaterally symmetrical [114] and moreover that the pain is also frequently bilateral, which is rare for stress fractures. (2) Radiological changes indicative of new bone formation have been found in association with painful episodes in some patients [115]. (3) Pain diminishes with 2–3 days after discontinuation of fluoride therapy and returns with reinstitution of fluoride therapy. Based on these observations, the authors believe that the majority of the peripheral bone pain in the lower extremities during fluoride therapy is due to a local rapid increase in periosteal bone formation. Fluoride therapy can cause stress fracture [80,122–124], which can be painful, but the authors believe that stress fractures are only a minor contributing factor of the peripheral pain syndrome associated with fluoride therapy.

Calcium Deficiency

Calcium deficiency is a serious side effect because it could lead to secondary hyperparathyroidism, increased bone resorption, and perhaps also peripheral bone loss and osteomalacia [73,127]. Accordingly, early studies with fluoride therapy have included the daily supplementation of a large dose of calcium carbonate in the hope that this would ensure a sufficient amount of calcium available to prevent calcium deficiency and the accompanying secondary hyperparathyroidism and also to allow for adequate mineralization of the newly formed bone matrix to avoid osteomalacia. Unfortunately, despite the calcium supplementation, some elderly osteoporotic patients still developed osteomalacia and calcium deficiency [73,104,127], presumably because they have a reduced calcium absorption efficiency such that calcium supplementation alone is insufficient to overcome the calcium deficiency resulted from exuberant bone formation associated with the therapy.

In addition to causing secondary hyperparathyroidism and increased bone resorption and bone loss, calcium deficiency may also promote the deposition of fluoride in bone. It has been shown that there was a greater increase in fluoride deposited in bone in rats fed a low calcium diet than rats fed a normal calcium diet [128]. Similarly, osteomalacia can impair the healing of microdamage in the bone, thereby leading to an accumulation of microdamage in the skeleton. Thus, to avoid this possible complication of calcium deficiency, it is necessary to routinely monitor patients for signs of calcium deficiency, such as a low urine calcium, a high serum PTH, and a marked increase in bone formation [127]. Calcium deficiency and osteomalacia can be corrected easily by treatment with calcitriol [or $1\alpha(OH)D$] and calcium.

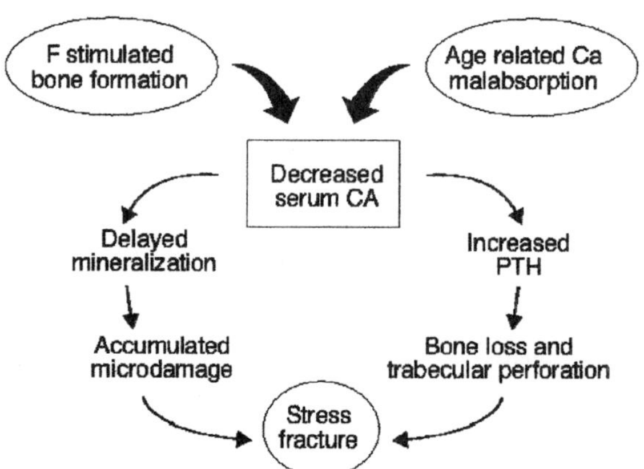

FIGURE 12 Proposed pathogenic mechanism(s) of stress fracture development in fluoride-treated osteoporotic patients. The fluoride-induced increase in bone formation in the presence of calcium malabsorption (such as occurs in elderly subjects) results in a state of secondary hyperparathyroidism, which, in turn, results in cortical bone resorption and cortical bone loss. The weakened bone develops microdamage for which healing is delayed because of the osteomalacia and, as a result, the patient is at risk for stress fractures. Reproduced from Libanati *et al.* [98], with permission.

Stress Fractures

Fluoride therapy appears to increase the prevalence of stress fractures in weight-bearing appendicular skeleton (primarily in the legs) [80]. Peripheral stress fractures occur almost exclusively in patients who have a low lumber spine density, i.e., patients with severe osteoporosis [129]. However, this can be considered a relatively benign complication because these fractures are predominantly incomplete fractures and because in all cases, the stress fractures healed after a transitory drug discontinuation [110,129].

The etiology of stress fractures is largely unknown. Because stress fractures are more likely to develop in patients who have severe osteoporosis and who show a rapid and large increase in serum skeletal alkaline phosphatase activity in response to fluoride, the authors postulate that the major underlying causes of stress fractures are (1) the rapid increase in bone formation in response to the therapy and (2) the resulting calcium deficiency. The authors speculate that the greater the fluoride-induced increase in bone formation, the greater the calcium deficit. This situation would be further exaggerated by the poor calcium absorption in elderly patients (Fig. 12). Accordingly, on the one hand, calcium deficiency causes the secondary hyperparathyroidism, which results in cortical bone loss, which, in turn, reduces the biomechanical strength of the bone. On the other hand, it also delays mineralization (i.e., osteomalacia), which impairs microdamage healing in the skeleton. Accumulation of microdamage and increased cortical bone loss, together, increase the risk of hip stress fractures and hip fractures, especially in those who already have a weakened skeleton. Therefore, this model further emphasizes the importance of assuring adequate calcium absorption in patients receiving fluoride therapy for established osteoporosis.

Another potential contributing factor to stress fractures is the improved ability of the fluoride-treated patients to engage in physical activity that results from the reduction of symptoms (e.g., back pain) due to therapy. Accordingly, in patients who respond to fluoride therapy with large increases in spinal bone density, there is decreased back pain, which allows the patient to engage in increased amounts of physical activity. This increase in physical activity, coupled with the calcium deficiency, may be responsible for the increased incidence of stress fractures, especially in patients with severe osteoporosis.

Hip Fractures

The most disturbing of all potential side effects of the fluoride therapy is the possibility that fluoride treatment may increase the incidence of hip fractures [130,131]. Theoretically, fluoride may cause hip fractures through three mechanisms: (1) fluoride-induced calcium deficiency; as discussed earlier, calcium deficiency can lead to significant peripheral cortical bone loss as a consequence of the accompanying secondary hyperparathyroidism. (2) Osteomalacia, which impairs healing of microdamages. Accumulation of a significant amount of unrepaired microdamages could lead to stress and hip fractures. (3) A high level of fluoride deposition in bone minerals, which can cause a deterioration in bone quality and strength, which, in turn, could increase the risk for hip stress fractures.

Because of the serious nature of hip fractures, a retrospective analysis was performed on more than 1000 patient-years of fluoride treatment by five international medical centers who have extensive experience in the use of fluoride therapy to evaluate the issue of fluoride-induced hip fractures [132]. This analysis indicated that hip fracture risk is increased in osteoporotic patients because of the bone deficit and that the risk was unaffected by fluoride therapy. Two additional studies also did not confirm the contention that fluoride causes hip fractures: (1) a study of more than 250 patients, followed for over a 5-year period, showed that fluoride did not increase the frequency of hip fractures [133]. (2) Studies with intermittent slow-release fluoride showed no increase in incidence of hip or stress fractures [83,84]. To add to the controversy, another study showed that the fluoridation of drinking water not only did not increase, but significantly reduced hip fracture incidence [134]. Moreover, although *experimentally* fluoride can reduce bone quality in osteofluorosis (where one might expect a high prevalence of bone fractures), one sees extra skeletal calcifications but not excessive bone fractures [109,110,126]. Much additional work is needed to resolve the issue whether fluoride therapy causes hip fractures.

EFFICACY OF FLUORIDE THERAPY

The efficacy of fluoride therapy of established osteoporosis may be evaluated according to its ability to (a) reduce symptoms, (b) improve bone strength and quality, and (c) reduce fracture rates.

Symptoms

A major symptom of osteoporosis is back pain. There is an abundance of evidence that fluoride therapy significantly reduces back pain [3,88,135]. This is an important benefit because it gives the patient feelings of increased strength and reduced morbidity. This also allows the patient to become more physically active and to participate in physical therapy and exercise programs. Thus, this improves the quality of life significantly.

Bone Quality and Strength

Fluoride therapy increases the incorporation of fluoride into bone mineral crystals in both humans and animals. A survey of past human studies wherein bone fluoride content data are available reveals that the amount of fluoride in bone ash is proportional to the total amount of fluoride taken by the patients (Fig. 13), indicating that the dosage and duration of the fluoride therapy may determine the amount of fluoride that is deposited in bone. Past studies in animal models have led to the general conclusion that deposition of a large amount of fluoride into bone mineral reduces bone quality and strength significantly [136]. Turner *et al.* [137] observed in rodents (and subsequently confirmed in rabbits) that deleterious effects of fluoride on cortical bone quality and strength are seen once the bone fluoride level reaches about 0.5% (i.e., 5000 to 10,000 ppm). Thus, these investigators have suggested that the bone fluoride level should be kept below 0.45% (i.e., putative "maximum safe level") to avoid harmful effects on bone quality and strength [137].

Evidence shows that deposition of a high level of fluoride in human bone also has a deleterious effect on bone quality and strength. Sogaard and co-workers [138] reported that there was a significant 45% reduction of trabecular bone strength and a 58% decrease in trabecular bone quality in 12 osteoporotic patients after 5 years of therapy with NaF (an accumulated oral dose of approximately 45 g), which led to an accumulation of bone fluoride of approximately 0.85%. Similarly, patients in the Mayo Clinic study [80,82] who received an accumulated fluoride dose of approximately 50 g elemental fluoride and deposited a bone fluoride level of approximately 0.95% showed increased peripheral fracture rates and had no beneficial effect on the spinal fracture rate reduction, despite a large increase in spinal bone den-

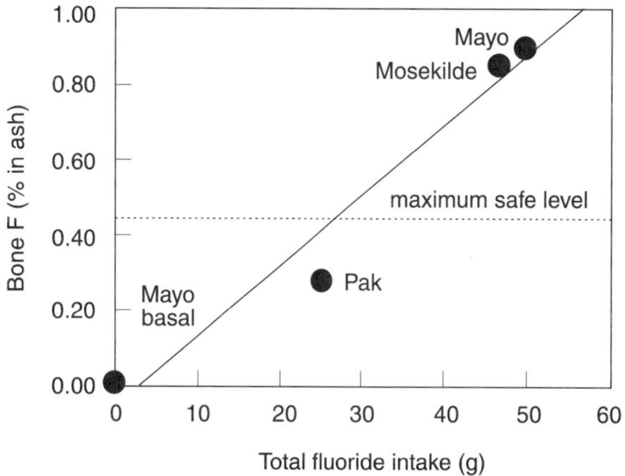

FIGURE 13 Relationship between total elemental fluoride taken orally in clinical trials and the corresponding subsequent bone fluoride concentrations. The total oral fluoride intake and bone fluoride concentrations are calculated from data obtained from Refs. 84, 85, and 138, respectively. The putative "maximum safe bone fluoride level" (0.45% in bone ash) was suggested by Turner *et al.* [137].

sity. Conversely, the fluoride-treated patients in the slow-release intermittent dosage study [83,84], wherein the bone fluoride level of the treated patients was less than 0.3%, exhibited an impressive reduction in spinal fracture rates without an increase in peripheral fracture rates.

A high level of bone fluoride deposition may act through three means to reduce bone strength and quality.

Fluoride Deposition Alters Physicochemical Properties of Bone Mineral Crystals

Fluoride treatment produces a number of significant changes in the bone mineral phase. Incorporation of fluoride in bone minerals leads to the substitution of fluoride for the hydroxyl group in apatite to form fluoroapatite crystals [139], which improves the apatite crystallinity of bone minerals, increases crystal size, and decreases the degree of lattice distortion [140]. Fluoride incorporation also increases the width and thickness of the mineral crystal without an effect on the crystal length [139]. These effects on bone minerals *in vivo* lead to a significant increase in bone mineral density (i.e., increased calcium content per unit dry bone weight) and microhardness in cortical bones [141,142], which may, in turn, diminish bone quality because the increased bone mineral density is expected to produce an increased compressive strength but a reduced bending strength. Thus, high levels of fluoride deposition can reduce bone strength in response to bendings.

Fluoride Incorporation May Produce Histologically Abnormal Bone

The fluoride ion does not diffuse in large amounts into preformed hydroxyapatite crystals in highly mineralized bone, but it is incorporated into fluoroapatite crystals during new bone mineralization. Thus, most of the fluoride is deposited in actively mineralizing areas of the bone [143]. Accordingly, fluoride treatment could produce distinct areas of high mineral density in cortical bones [140,141,143,144]. In addition to the hypermineralized areas, fluoride treatment also produces areas of undermineralized matrix. The cause for the hypomineralization could be partly due to calcium deficiency and the consequent mineralization defect brought on by the increased calcium demand to mineralize the new bone formed during the fluoride treatment [145]. The combination of hypermineralized and hypomineralized areas produces a picture of mottled bone with low mineral density (but well-organized matrix) and hypomineralized halos around mottled lacunae [68,146,147]. The increased variability of bone mineral content with areas of high and low mineral density may weaken the bone integrity and therefore could be an important contributor to decreased quality of the fluoride-treated bone [148].

Fluoride Causes Calcium Deficiency and Osteomalacia

In addition to an increased level of fluoride disposition, large doses of fluoride may cause calcium deficiency and osteomalacia. As discussed earlier, calcium deficiency and the accompanying secondary hyperparathyroidism would increase bone resorption and promote trabecular perforation, which, in turn, leads to the deterioration of trabecular microarchitecture and bone quality, resulting in a reduction in bone strength. Osteomalacia would impair the repair of microdamage, the accumulation of which will further corrupt the trabecular integrity, causing a significant reduction in bone strength and bone quality. Therefore, fluoride-induced calcium deficiency and osteomalacia, which can be associated with a high level of bone fluoride deposition, may be, in part, responsible for the reduced bone strength and quality.

Vertebral Fracture Rate

Past uncontrolled studies have suggested that a significant reduction in the vertebral fracture rate is frequently associated with increased spinal bone density in fluoride-treated osteoporotic patients [2,3,121,149–153] and that there appeared to be a strong inverse relationship between spinal bone density and vertebral fracture rate [1,153]. Accordingly, a past comparison evaluation between spinal bone density measured by QCT and spinal fracture rate has indicated that spinal bone density is a key determinant of vertebral fracture risks and also provided a putative "fracture threshold" of 100 mg/cm^3 for females and 132 mg/cm^3 for males [1]. Thus, it is reasonable to anticipate that patients who respond to fluoride therapy with an increase in spinal bone density would show a reduction in the vertebral fracture rate. Consistent with this speculation, a retrospective study [153] wherein 510 osteoporotic patients treated with an average daily dose of 30 mg elemental fluoride for 5 years showed a marked and progressive increase in spinal bone density and an exponential decrease in the vertebral fracture rate as a function of the increase in spinal bone density (Fig. 14). Also, the vertebral fracture rate in good responders to fluoride therapy (i.e., with a significant increase in vertebral trabecular bone density) was 76% less than that in poor responders (Fig. 15).

The view that fluoride therapy has a beneficial effect on vertebral fracture rates, however, is not accepted universally. Contrary to most uncontrolled studies, a

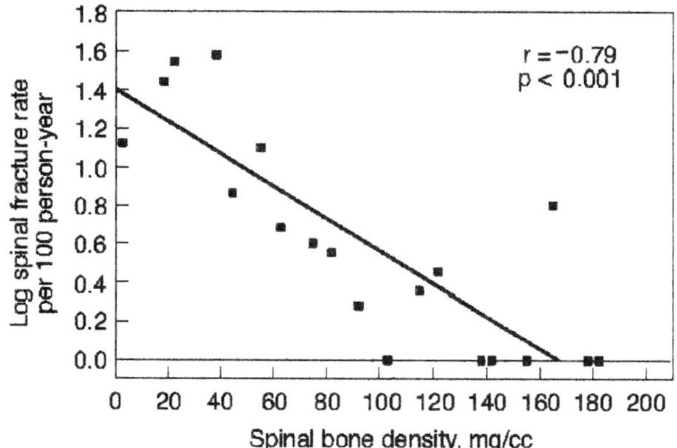

FIGURE 14 Relationship between spinal bone density during fluoride therapy and the spinal fracture rate in 510 patients. The spinal fracture rate decreases as a function of increasing bone density during fluoride therapy, suggesting that the bone accumulated during fluoride therapy has a positive impact on vertebral mechanical strength. Reproduced from Farley *et al.* [153], with permission.

placebo-controlled study indicated that fluoride therapy did not reduce the vertebral fracture rate significantly, despite an impressive increase in spinal bone density [116]. This issue is further confounded by results of several prospective, placebo-controlled studies that provided conflicting conclusions on the efficacy of fluoride therapy on the vertebral fracture rate in osteoporotic patients [80–84]. On the one hand, in the two NIH-sponsored clinical trials wherein patients were treated with a relatively high dose of plain NaF [80,81], therapy did not reduce vertebral fracture rates, even though the spinal bone density was increased greatly. On the other hand, patients in the clinical trial with an intermittent

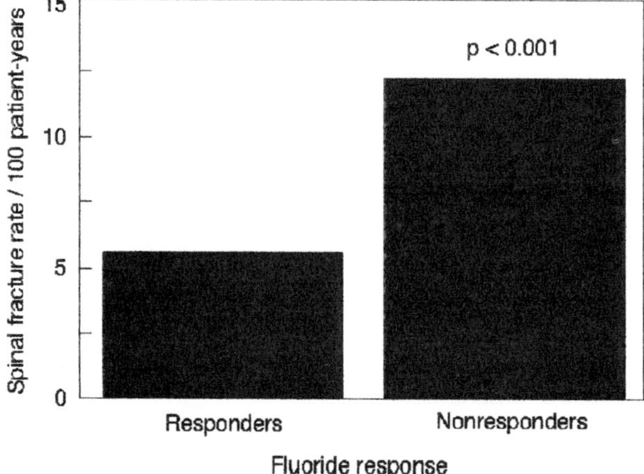

FIGURE 15 The spinal fracture incidence in osteoporotic patients who responded to fluoride therapy with a significant increase in spinal bone density (i.e., responders) compared to the spinal fracture incidence of those osteoporotic patients who failed to respond to fluoride (nonresponders). Reproduced from Farley *et al.* [153], with permission.

regimen of a low dose of slow-release NaF preparation showed only a moderate increase in spinal bone density but an impressive reduction in vertebral fracture rates [83,84]. To add to the controversy, the follow-up extended observation and reanalysis of the data of the Mayo Clinic's NIH-sponsored trial revealed that patients who had a relatively low serum fluoride level with a corresponding smaller increase in spinal bone density had unequivocally reduced spinal fracture rates [82]. In addition, Ringe *et al.* (154) have reported that a 3-year intermittent (3 months on fluoride, 1 month off fluoride) treatment with a low dose of MFP showed an impressive reduction in vertebral fractures and an improvement of back pain in male patients with idiopathic osteoporosis compared to the control group. Despite the fact that several additional placebo-controlled, prospective studies, including the FAVOS study [155], have been conducted, this controversy has not been resolved satisfactorily. Consequently, the issue concerning the efficacy of fluoride therapy with respect to the reduction of spinal fracture rate remains controversial [156,157]. Nevertheless, these prospective, controlled clinical trials have clearly demonstrated that, under optimal conditions, significant reductions in vertebral fracture rates can be achieved with fluoride therapy.

In order to define optimal conditions that would allow beneficial effects on vertebral fracture rates, it would be essential to understand the reason(s) for the contrasting effects of these clinical studies on spinal fracture rates. Theoretical assessments of skeleton responses from fluoride therapy suggest that there are at least three potential explanations for the different results of these fluoride clinical studies with respect to vertebral fracture rates.

LOSS OF TRABECULAR CONNECTIVITY AND NUMBER

Loss of trabecular connectivity and number is a characteristic of established osteoporosis. Thus, the issue as to whether fluoride therapy would promote trabecular connectivity and/or restore trabecular number is relevant to clinical efficacy with respect to vertebral fracture risk. There is currently no convincing evidence that fluoride therapy can restore trabecular number and connectivity [158]. If fluoride cannot increase the number and/or connectivity of trabeculae, then fluoride treatment which only increases the thickness and volume of remaining trabecular, alone may not be sufficient to reestablish the biomechanical integrity of the skeleton. Accordingly, while the thickened but less connected trabeculae in the fluoride-treated skeleton may increase the biomechanical strength compared to the osteoporotic trabeculae, the strength per unit of bone mass would still be less than that of normal skeleton. Consequently, the number and connectivity of the trabeculae existing in the patient before fluoride therapy could be a significant variable in determining the efficacy of the therapy on fracture risks. In other words, the more severe the disease, the less likely fluoride would be to completely correct the fracture risk. The fact that patients enrolled in the intermittent slow release NaF trial appeared to have less severe osteoporosis (i.e., higher basal spinal bone density) than those who participated in the two NIH-sponsored studies [80–84] may in part explain the observation of a significant reduction in spinal fracture risk in the intermittent slow release study but not in the two NIH-sponsored clinical trials. However, it should be noted that the authors' study of 510 patients, patients with severe osteoporosis, who had large increases in bone density in response to fluoride therapy, seemed to fall on the same line relating final bone density to fracture rate as those patients who had less severe osteoporosis and an increase in bone density in response to fluoride [153]. Therefore, it seems likely that the protective effect of fluoride depends to a considerable extent on the amount of new bone added, irrespective of the number of trabeculae. Based on these findings, the authors reason that even if fluoride therapy can only thicken trabeculae and thereby increase bone density above the fracture threshold, fluoride therapy could still improve the symptoms and morbidity of the patients and reduce fracture risks.

Calcium Deficiency and Osteomalacia

As indicated earlier, the fluoride-induced calcium deficiency and osteomalacia together may contribute to increases in vertebral fragility and fractures. In this respect, many patients in the Mayo Clinic study have clearly developed osteomalacia, which appeared to be related to calcium deficiency [85]. In contrast, there is no evidence that patients in the intermittent slow release study, who had received a lower dose of fluoride, developed this side effect or secondary hyperparathyroidism [83,84]. Therefore, the observed differences with respect to vertebral fracture risks may also be in part attributed to whether the patients developed calcium deficiency and/or osteomalacia.

Fluoride Deposition in Bone Mineral

As discussed earlier, a high level deposition of fluoride in bone mineral crystals can affect bone quality and strength adversely. Because the daily fluoride dose in the Mayo Clinic study was larger than that in the intermittent slow release regimen study and because, unlike the Mayo Clinic study, which was a continuous regimen, the intermittent slow release study contained a 2-month off fluoride period, the fluoride-treated patients in the Mayo Clinic study received a significantly larger total accumulated fluoride dose than those in the intermittent slow release study. Moreover, patients in the intermittent study by Pak *et al.* [83,84] were on a slow release fluoride, which produces an area under the serum fluoride curve much smaller than that with the acute release fluoride [58]. Accordingly, the amount of fluoride deposition in bone mineral in the fluoride-treated patients of the intermittent slow release study is correspondingly significantly lower than that found in the fluoride-treated patients of the Mayo Clinic study (Fig. 13). It is interesting to note that the bone fluoride level in the fluoride-treated patients of the Mayo Clinic study (i.e., 0.95%) was above, whereas that in the fluoride-treated patients of the intermittent study was below, the putative "maximum safe level" (i.e., 0.45%). Consequently, the difference in the bone fluoride level may, to some extent, account for different efficacy with respect to vertebral fracture risk in these two placebo-controlled prospective studies.

STRATEGIES TO IMPROVE FLUORIDE THERAPY

Table II summarizes the advantages and disadvantages of fluoride therapy. It is clear that fluoride therapy can have several side effects, as well as many significant advantages as an anabolic agent for the treatment of established osteoporosis. While most of the side effects of fluoride therapy appear to be manageable, two serious side effects, namely calcium deficiency and reduced bone quality and strength, significantly outweigh the advantages, thereby giving fluoride therapy an unfavorable benefit-to-risk profile. In order for the fluoride therapy to be an effective anabolic therapy for established osteoporosis, this benefit-to-risk profile must be improved. Accordingly, the authors propose a strategy to

TABLE II Advantages and Disadvantages of Fluoride Therapy of Established Osteoporosis[a]

Advantage	Disadvantage
1. Oral administration	1. Gastrointestinal irritation
2. Large increases in bone density	2. Peripheral bone pain
3. Increases bone formation in trabecular and cortical–endosteal bone sites	3. Calcium deficiency
4. No increase in bone resorption	4. Osteomalacia
5. Specific for bone	5. Stress fractures
6. Unique mechanism of action	6. Decreased bone material quality and strength

[a] Reprinted with permission from Lau *et al.* [37]. Copyright CRC Press, Boca Raton, Florida.

improve the benefit-to-risk profile of fluoride therapy (Table III). Because most of these undesirable side effects of fluoride therapy are caused by calcium deficiency and high fluoride deposition in bone minerals, the strategy focuses on (1) the prevention of calcium deficiency and (2) the reduction of fluoride deposition in bone. Because fluoride therapy does not promote trabecular connectivity and because a further loss of trabecular connectivity and number could have a detrimental effect on bone quality and strength, the authors further propose that combination therapy of fluoride with an antiresorption therapy may be necessary, especially when the patient has an elevated bone resorption rate.

Strategy to Avoid Calcium Deficiency

Calcium deficiency is an important potential consequence of fluoride therapy [127]. In the opinion of the authors, this could even have been a problem in the FAVOS study [155]. Calcium deficiency appears to be the cause of two significant side effects, i.e., osteomalacia and stress fractures. In this context, one certainly does not want to increase spinal bone density only to have the patient suffer a painful stress fracture. To avoid potential complications of calcium deficiency, the authors recommend that the fluoride-treated patient should be monitored regularly (e.g., every few months) for signs of calcium deficiency, such as low urine calcium, a high serum PTH, and a marked increase in bone formation [127]. Regular monitoring of signs of calcium deficiency could alert physicians to take necessary precautionary interventions. To prevent calcium deficiency, it would be necessary to provide the patient with sufficient amounts of calcium in a bioavailable form (e.g., calcium citrate). In older patients who may have insufficient intestinal calcium absorption, it may be necessary to give calcitriol in a dosage of 0.25–0.5 μg/day or 1α(OH)D in a dosage of 0.5–1.0 μg/day to enhance intestinal calcium absorption. The authors believe that these steps, when taken together, would minimize the occurrence of calcium deficiency and the associated side effects, such as secondary hyperparathyroidism, osteomalacia, and/or stress fractures.

TABLE III Proposed Strategy to Improve the Benefit-to-Risk Profile of Fluoride Therapy

Prevent calcium deficiency
- Regularly monitor signs of calcium deficiency
- Supplement with bioavailable calcium salt
- Increase intestinal calcium absorption with calcitriol or 1α(OH)D_3

Avoid a high fluoride deposition into bone mineral
- Use dose of fluoride to produce serum level of 5–10 μM
- Use slow-release preparations
- Use intermittent, cyclic regimen
- Avoid calcium deficiency

Add an antiresorption therapy if bone resorption is elevated

Strategy to Reduce Fluoride Deposition in Bone Mineral

Because poor bone quality and reduced bone strength appear to result in part from high fluoride deposition in bone minerals, it is important to minimize the amount of bone fluoride deposition. In this regard, based on fluoride measurements in bone ash and bone-breaking strength in the rat, Turner [136,137] concluded that the maximum safe amount of fluoride in bone ash was about 0.45%. Although the authors' study, in collaboration with Dr. Einhorn, found no deterioration in bone strength in rats with fluoride concentrations in the bone ranging up to 1% fluoride in the bone ash [159], the authors have accepted Dr. Turner's suggestion that the maximum safe level of fluoride is 0.45% in order to be conservative. Accordingly, it would be important to avoid the accumulation of bone fluoride level above this putative "maximum safe level."

One of the major determinants of fluoride deposition in bone ash is fluoride intake (Fig. 13). Accordingly, the issue of fluoride dosage becomes an important issue. The patient should be given a sufficient fluoride dose that would effectively increase bone density, but yet the dose should not be so high as to cause an excessive accumulation of fluoride in bone minerals. Figure 2 indicates that the *in vitro* mitogenic dose–response curve of fluoride is nonlinear in that there is no additional increase in mitogenic activity at doses above 10–15 μM. The authors believe that the fluoride dose should be on a linear portion of the mitogenic dose–response curve. They also speculate that when the blood fluoride level increases above a certain level (i.e., 10–15 μM), there would not be any greater increase in bone cell mitogenic activity, but it would increase the amount of bone fluoride deposition significantly. Regarding the latter issue, it has been shown that there is a proportionality between the serum fluoride level and the amount of fluoride deposited in bone [136,137]. For the reasons given earlier, the authors believe that the optimal blood fluoride level should be between 5 and 10 μM. Thus, patients should be given an appropriate fluoride dose that yields a blood fluoride level that is maintained between 5 and 10 μM for a desirable therapeutic result (i.e., an increased spinal bone density without a decreased bone strength).

As mentioned earlier, the amount of fluoride deposited in bone is directly proportional to the circulating fluoride concentration, i.e., the larger the area under the fluoride serum curve, the more fluoride will be deposited in bone. As shown in Fig. 4, the area under the curve of plain MFP was much greater than that of the slow-release formulation because of the postabsorptive serum fluoride peak. This postabsorptive peak of fluoride is undesirable as it is not essential for *in vivo* efficacy [83,84,89], but it would markedly increase the amount of bone fluoride deposition. Thus, it seems advisable to use slow-release fluoride preparations to limit fluoride deposition in bone minerals.

Another approach to reduce the bone deposition of fluoride without reducing the efficacy of fluoride therapy is to use cyclic therapy. It has been demonstrated previously in the rat that the mitogenic effect of fluoride on the osteoblast persists for weeks even after fluoride withdrawal [160]. Moreover, in humans (following the discontinuation of fluoride therapy), the half-life for the disappearance of the increase in bone formation, as measured by bone formation markers, was much slower than that for the disappearance of serum fluoride [58]. Thus, it is likely that a cyclic regimen would considerably reduce the amount of fluoride incorporation into bone without impairing the mitogenic effect. For instance, in Dr. Pak's cyclic fluoride study [83,84], in which patients received a daily dose of 23 mg elemental fluoride for 12 months during the 14-month cycle (i.e., 2 months off fluoride period), the patient probably would obtain the same increase in bone density as if the drug was given continuously for the entire 14 months. However, there would be significantly less (i.e., about 15%) fluoride incorporated in bone for the same amount of bone formation. Consistent with this idea, Fig. 13 shows that the amount of bone deposition in Dr. Pak's cyclic fluoride study was much lower than the two continuous fluoride therapies (i.e., studies of Mayo Clinic and Dr. Mosekilde). The benefits of slow-release cyclic fluoride preparation in the treatment of osteoporosis on vertebral fracture rates have been demonstrated convincingly by the studies of Pak [83,84] and Ringe [154,161]. Another study also indicates that intermittent slow-release NaF therapy produced normal bone histomorphometric parameters [162], in contrast to continuous fluoride therapy, where evidence of calcium deficiency and osteomalacia can be seen [85]. Accordingly, the use of cyclic therapy instead of continuous therapy would seem to be a logical approach.

Although the regimen used successfully by Dr. Pak contained a 2-month "off fluoride period" in a 14-month cycle, there is no compelling evidence that this regimen is the most appropriate regimen. Thus, additional work to determine the "optimum" cyclic regimen would be important. There is some data on this issue (described later) that can be used to formulate reasonable cycle times. Ideally, the optimum cyclic regimen would be one that contains the shortest possible fluoride treatment period with the longest possible "off fluoride period" without a sacrifice in therapeutic efficacy. In this respect, the optimum cyclic regimen would probably depend on the biological half-lives of serum fluoride level and the fluoride-induced bone formation. The half-life for the decrease in serum fluoride after the discontinuation of slow-release MFP was approximately 2 days and the half-life for serum osteocalcin (a marker of bone formation) after 6–12 months of fluoride therapy was 39 days [89]. It should be noted that the half-life of the fluoride-induced increase in serum osteocalcin is much longer than that of serum fluoride. This raises the possibility that fluoride therapy may be stopped for 1 month or longer after 6–12 months of fluoride therapy, during which time the serum fluoride level would return to the pretreatment level, but the bone formation rate would remain stimulated. A better understanding of appropriate rate constants between the persistence of osteogenic effects of fluoride and the duration of fluoride treatment would help in designing more optimized cyclic regimens. Consequently, several laboratories, including the authors, are in the process of determining the optimum cyclic regimen for fluoride therapy of established osteoporosis.

Finally, as discussed earlier, calcium deficiency, in addition to causing osteomalacia and stress fractures, can also enhance fluoride deposition in bone [128]. Therefore, it is important to avoid calcium deficiency during fluoride therapy. If these strategies are followed, it should be possible to minimize the fluoride deposition in bone without a significant loss in therapeutic efficacy.

Combination Therapy with an Antiresorptive Therapy

The bone resorption rate in the osteoporotic postmenopausal patient is frequently elevated above the premenopausal level. If the patient is treated with fluoride to increase bone formation when she also has an increased bone resorption, which increases the perforations of the trabeculae, this would not be an optimum therapeutic strategy. Accordingly, because fluoride acts predominantly at the axial trabecular bone sites, the realistic goal of fluoride therapy is to increase the bone density of the central skeleton with fluoride therapy and, at the same time, preserve the bone density of the peripheral skeleton with antiresorptive therapy. To achieve this objective, it seems reasonable to use combination therapy with an antiresorptive agent if the bone resorption rate of the patient is elevated above the postmenopausal level. In this regard, estrogens, bisphosphonates, or calcitonins should be considered. The goal is to decrease bone resorption with an estrogen or a bisphosphonate at the same time to increase the thickness of the remaining trabeculae by fluoride. In this context, the authors were initially concerned that because fluoride acts only at remodeling sites to increase wall thickness (Fig. 7) and does not stimulate bone formation on a neutral surface, the decrease in remodeling sites caused by an antiresorptive agent could impair the effect of fluoride to increase density. However, the authors have, in fact, shown significant increases in spinal bone density with the combination of estrogen and fluoride [163]. They were also able to show similar results at hip bone density. Consequently, under the conditions of the study, estrogen did not inhibit the effect of fluoride to increase bone density. Consistent with the contention that a combination therapy of fluoride and an antiresorptive agent has benefits, it has been shown that the combination therapy of fluoride and etidronate appears to be superior to the therapy of etidronate alone in increasing lumbar spine bone mineral mass and in preserving hip bone mass in corticosteroid-induced osteoporosis [164]. Therefore, the authors believe that the combination therapy of fluoride and an antiresorptive agent has a good rationale as a therapy of osteoporosis.

SUMMARY

It has been well recognized for decades that fluoride has both beneficial and detrimental effects on the skeleton. On the one hand, it is well documented that fluoride is a bone cell-specific, anabolic agent that effectively stimulates cancellous bone formation and increases spinal bone density, without an increase in bone resorption. On the other hand, studies have also demonstrated that fluoride may cause calcium deficiency and osteomalacia, which reduces the integrity of bone, and that high bone deposition of fluoride could greatly reduce the biomechanical properties and strength of the skeleton. These undesirable side effects, together, significantly reduce the benefit-to-risk profile of fluoride therapy and thereby diminish its therapeutic values. Accordingly, fluoride therapy of established osteoporosis has been a highly controversial issue [156,157]. However, at the present time fluoride is the only orally active, bone-specific, anabolic agent that increases bone formation and bone density at appropriate skeletal sites, i.e., trabecular and cortical–endosteal bone sites. Because there is a great need of an effective bone-specific anabolic agent for the treatment of established osteoporosis, a reasonable option for anabolic therapy would be to take advantage of the benefits (i.e., bone-specific anabolic actions) of fluoride and to somehow improve the therapy to minimize the adverse side effects of fluoride (i.e., calcium deficiency and high bone fluoride incorporation).

This chapter has proposed a set of strategies to improve the advantage-to-disadvantage profile of fluoride therapy. The strategies were intended to (1) avoid calcium deficiency and osteomalacia and (2) find a way to reduce the amount of fluoride deposited in bone minerals. If applied appropriately, these strategies, should increase bone density without producing osteomalacia and without increasing the bone fluoride concentration up to a level that would impair bone quality. In this regard, some of the concepts of the authors proposed strategy have been incorporated into studies of Dr. Pak [83,84], Dr. Ringe [154,161], and the authors group (153), which have provided convincing beneficial results with respect to the reduction in fracture rate.

Acknowledgments

This work was supported in part by research grants from the National Institutes of Health (DE08681) and the Veterans Administration.

References

1. Odvina, C. V., Wergedal, J. E., Libanati, C. R., Schulz, E. E., and Baylink, D. J. Relationship between trabecular body density and fractures: a quantitative definition of spinal osteoporosis. *Metabolism* **37,** 221–228 (1988).
2. Riggs, B. L., Hodgson, J. F., Hoffman, D. L., Kelly, P. J., Johnson K. A., and Taves, D. Treatment of primary osteoporosis with fluoride and calcium: clinical tolerance and fracture occurrence. *J. Am. Med. Assoc.* **243,** 446–449 (1980).
3. Briancon, D., and Meunier, P. J. Treatment of osteoporosis with fluoride, calcium, and vitamin D. *In* "The Orthopedic Clinics of North America" (H. M. Frost, ed.), Vol. 12, pp. 629–648. Saunders, Philadelphia, 1981.
4. Farley, S. M. G., Libanati, C. R., Mariano-Menez, M. R., Tudtud-Hans, L. A., Schulz, E. E., and Baylink, D. J. Fluoride therapy for osteoporosis promotes a progressive increase in spinal bone density. *J. Bone Miner. Res.* **5**(Suppl. 1), S37–S42 (1990).
5. Moller, P. F., and Gudjonsson, S. V. Massive fluorosis of bones and ligaments. *Acta Radiol. (Stockholm)* **13,** 269–272 (1932).
6. Roholm, K., "Fluorine Intoxication: A Clinical Hygienic Study." H. K. Lewis, Co. Ltd., London, 1937.
7. Rich, C., and Ensinck, J. Effect of sodium fluoride on calcium metabolism of human beings. *Nature* **191,** 184–185 (1961).
8. Rich, C., Ensinck, J., and Ivanovich, P. The effects of sodium fluoride on calcium metabolism of subjects with metabolic bone diseases. *J. Clin. Invest.* **43,** 545–556 (1964).
9. Rich, C., and Ivanovich, P. Response to sodium fluoride in severe primary osteoporosis. *Ann. Intern. Med.* **63,** 1069–1074 (1965).
10. Harrison, J. E., McNeill, K. G., Sturtridge, W. C., Bayley, T. A., Murray, T. M., Williams, C., Tam, C., and Fornasier, V. Three-year changes in bone mineral mass of osteoporotic patients based on neutron activation analysis of the central third of the skeleton. *J. Clin. Endocrinol. Metabol.* **52,** 751–758 (1981).

11. Farley, J. R., Wergedal, J. R., and Baylink, D. J. Fluoride directly stimulates proliferation and alkaline phosphatase activity of bone forming cells. *Science* **222,** 330–332 (1983).
12. Baylink, D. J. Serum fluoride levels. "Primers on the Metabolic Bone Diseases and Disorders of Mineral Metabolism" (M. J. Favus, ed.), 2nd Ed., pp. 262–263. Raven Press, New York, 1993.
13. Hall, B. K. Sodium fluoride as an initiator of osteogenesis from embryonic mesenchyme *in vitro. Bone* **8,** 111–116 (1987).
14. Wergedal, J. E., Lau, K.-H. W., and Baylink, D. J. Fluoride and bovine bone extract influence cell proliferation and phosphatase activities in human bone cell cultures. *Clin. Orthopaed. Rel. Res.* **233,** 274–282 (1988).
15. Khokher, M. A., and Dandona, P. Fluoride stimulates ^{3}H-thymidine incorporation and alkaline phosphatase production by human osteoblasts. *Metabolism* **39,** 1118–1121 (1990).
16. Bellows, C. G., Heersche, J. N. M., and Aubin, J. E. The effects of fluoride on osteoblast progenitors *in vitro. J. Bone Miner. Res.* **5**(Suppl. 1), S101–S105 (1990).
17. Lau, K.-H. W., Yoo, A., and Wang, S. P. Aluminum stimulates the proliferation and differentiation of osteoblasts in vitro by a mechanism that is different from fluoride. *Mol. Cell. Biochem.* **105,** 93–105 (1991).
18. Simmons, D. J., Seitz, P., Kidder, L., Klein, G. L., Waeltz, M., Gundberg, C. M., Tabuchi, C., Yang, C., and Zhang, R. W. Partial characterization of rat marrow stromal cells. *Calcif. Tissue Int.* **48,** 326–334 (1991).
19. Modrowski, D., Miravet, L., Feuga, M., Bannie, F., and Marie, P. J. Effect of fluoride on bone and bone cells in ovariectomized rats. *J. Bone Miner. Res.* **7,** 961–969 (1992).
20. Kassem, M., Mosekilde, L., and Eriksen, E. F. 1,25-Dihydroxyvitamin D_3 potentiates fluoride-stimulated collagen type I production in cultures on human bone marrow stromal osteoblast-like cells. *J. Bone Miner. Res.* **8,** 1453–1458 (1993).
21. Reed, B. Y., Zerwekh, J. E., Antich, P. P., and Pak, C. Y. C. Fluoride-stimulated [^{3}H]thymidine uptake in a human osteoblastic osteosarcoma cell line is dependent on transforming growth factor β. *J. Bone Miner. Res.* **8,** 19–25 (1993).
22. Burgener, D., Bonjour, J. P., and Caverzasio, J. Fluoride increases tyrosine kinase activity in osteoblast-like cells: regulatory role for the stimulation of cell proliferation and Pi transport across the plasma membrane. *J. Bone Miner. Res.* **10,** 164–171 (1995).
23. Kassem, M., Mosekilde, L., and Eriksen, E. F. Effects of fluoride on human bone cells in vitro: differences in responsiveness between stromal osteoblast precursors and mature osteoblasts. *Acta Endocrinol.* **130,** 381–386 (1994).
24. Farley, J. R., Hall, S. L., Herring, S., and Tanner, M. A. Fluoride increases net ^{45}Ca uptake by SaOS-2 cells: the effect is phosphate dependent. *Calcif. Tissue Int.* **53,** 187–192 (1993).
25. Zerwekh, J., Morris, A., Padalino, P., Gottschalk, F., and Pak, C. Y. C. Fluoride rapidly and transiently raises intracellular Ca in human osteoblasts. *J. Bone Miner. Res.* **5**(Suppl. 1), S131–S136 (1990).
26. Selz, T., Caverzasio, J., and Bonjour, J.-P. Fluoride selectively stimulates Na-dependent phosphate transport in osteoblast-like cells. *Am. J. Physiol.* **260,** E833–E838 (1991).
27. Bellows, C. G., Aubin, J. E., and Heersche, J. N. M. Differential effects of fluoride during initiation and progression of mineralization of osteoid nodules formed *in vitro. J. Bone Miner. Res.* **8,** 1357–1363 (1993).
28. Lau, K.-H. W., Farley, J. R., Freeman, T. K., and Baylink, D. J. A proposed mechanism of the mitogenic action of fluoride on bone cells: inhibition of the activity of an osteoblastic acid phosphatase. *Metabolism* **38,** 858–868 (1989).
29. Farley, J. R., Tarbaux, N., Hall, S., and Baylink, D. J. Evidence that fluoride-stimulated ^{3}[H]thymidine incorporation in embryonic chick calvarial cell cultures is dependent on the presence of a bone mitogen, sensitive to changes in the phosphate concentration, and modulated by systemic skeletal effectors. *Metabolism* **37,** 988–995 (1988).
30. Ammann, P., Rizzoli, R., Caverzasio, J., and Bonjour, J.-P. Fluoride potentiates the osteogenic effects of IGF-I in aged ovariectomized rats. *Bone* **22,** 39–43 (1998).
31. Bellows, C. G., Heersche, J. N. M., and Aubin, J. E. The effects of fluoride on osteoblast progenitors in vitro. *J. Bone Miner. Res.* **5**(Suppl. 1), S101–S105 (1990).
32. Farley, J. R., Tarbaux, N., Hall, S., and Baylink, D. J. Mitogenic action(s) of fluoride on osteoblast line cells: determinants of the response *in vitro. J. Bone Miner. Res.* **5**(Suppl. 1), S107–S113 (1990).
33. Thomas, A. B., Hashimoto, H., Baylink, D. J., and Lau, K.-H. W. Fluoride at mitogenic concentrations increases the steady state phosphotyrosyl phosphorylation level of cellular proteins in human bone cells. *J. Clin. Endocrinol. Metabol.* **81,** 2570–2578 (1996).
34. Wu, L.-W., Yoon, H. K., Baylink, D. J., Graves, L. M., and Lau, K.-H. W. Fluoride at mitogenic doses induces a sustained activation of $p44^{mapk}$, but not $p42^{mapk}$, in human TE85 osteosarcoma cells. *J. Clin. Endocrinol. Metabol.* **82,** 1126–1135 (1997).
35. Kawase, T., and Suzuki, A. Studies on the transmembrane migration of fluoride and its effects on proliferation of L-929 fibroblasts (L cells) *in vitro. Arch. Oral Biol.* **34,** 103–107 (1989).
36. Bourgoin, S. G., Harbour, D., and Poubelle, P. E. Role of protein kinase Cα, Arf, and cytoplasmic calcium transient in phospholipase D activation by sodium fluoride in osteoblast-like cells. *J. Bone Miner. Res.* **11,** 1655–1665 (1996).
37. Lau, K.-H. W., Åkesson, K., Libanati, C. R., and Baylink, D. J. Osteogenic actions of fluoride: its therapeutic use for established osteoporosis. *In* "Anabolic Treatments for Osteoporosis" (J. F. Whitfield and P. Morley, eds.), pp. 207–254. CRC Press, Boca Raton, FL, 1998.
38. Antonny, D., Bigay, J., and Chabre, M. A novel magnesium-dependent mechanism for the activation of transduction by fluoride. *FEBS Lett.* **268,** 277–280 (1990).
39. Lau, K.-H. W., Tanimoto, H., and Baylink, D. J. Vanadate stimulates bone cell proliferation and bone collagen synthesis *in vitro. Endocrinology* **123,** 2858–2867 (1988).
40. Lau, K.-H. W., and Baylink, D. J. Phosphotyrosyl protein phosphatases: potential regulators of cell proliferation and differentiation. *Crit. Rev. Oncogen.* **4,** 451–471 (1993).
41. Kasperk, C. H., Wergedal, J. E., Strong, D. D., Farley, J. R., Wangerin, K., Gropp, H., Ziegler, R., and Baylink, D. J. Human bone cell phenotypes differ depending on their skeletal site of origin. *J. Clin. Endocrinol. Metabol.* **80,** 2511–2517 (1995).
42. Caverzasio, J., Imai, T., Ammann, P., Burgener, D., and Bonjour, J.-P. Aluminum potentiates the effect of fluoride on tyrosine phosphorylation and osteoblast replication *in vitro* and bone mass *in vivo. J. Bone Miner. Res.* **11,** 46–55 (1996).
43. Caverzasio, J., Palmer, G., Suzuki, A., and Bonjour, J.-P. Mechanism of the mitogenic effect of fluoride on osteoblast-like cells: evidence for a G protein-dependent tyrosine phosphorylation process. *J. Bone Miner. Res.* **12,** 1975–1983 (1997).
44. Jones, T. R., Antonetti, D. L., and Reid, T. W. Aluminum ions stimulate mitosis in murine cells in tissue culture. *J. Cell. Biochem.* **30,** 31–39 (1986).
45. Smith, J. B. Aluminum ions stimulate DNA synthesis in quiescent cultures of swiss 3T3 cells. *J. Cell. Physiol.* **118,** 298–304 (1984).

46. Boyer, J. L., Waldo, G. L., Evans, T., Northup, J. K., Downes, C. P., and Harden, T. K. Modification of AlF_4^-- and receptor-stimulated phospholipase C activity by G-protein $\beta\gamma$ subunits. *J. Biol. Chem.* **264,** 13917–13922 (1989).
47. Paris, S., Chambard, J.-C., and Pouyssegur, J. Tyrosine kinase-activating growth factor potentiate thrombin- and AlF_4^- induced phosphoinositide breakdown in hamster fibroblasts. Evidence for positive cross-talk between the two mitogenic signaling pathways. *J. Biol. Chem.* **263,** 12893–12900 (1988).
48. Kraenzlin, M. E., Kraenzlin, C., Farley, S. M. G., Fitzsimmons, R. J., and Baylink, D. J. Fluoride pharmacokinetics in good and poor responders to fluoride therapy. *J. Bone Miner. Res.* **5**(Suppl. 1), S49–S52 (1990).
49. Duursma, S. A., Raymakers, J. A., de Raadt, M. E., Karsdorp, N. J. G. H., van Dijk, A., and Glerum, J. Urinary fluoride excretion in responders and nonresponders after fluoride therapy in osteoporosis. *J. Bone Miner. Res.* **5**(Suppl. 1), S43–S47 (1990).
50. Murray, T. M., Harrison, J. E., Bayley, T. A., Josse, R. G., Sturtridge, W. C., Chow, R., Budden, F., Laurier, L., Pritzker, K. P. H., Kandel, R., Vieth, R., Strauss, A., and Goodwin, S., Fluoride treatment of postmenopausal osteoporosis: age, renal function, and other clinical factors in osteogenic response. *J. Bone Miner. Res.* **5**(Suppl. 1), S27–S35 (1990).
51. Sebert, J. L., Richard, P., Mennecier, I., Bisset, J. P., and Loeb, G. Monofluorophosphate increases lumbar bone density in osteopenic patients: a double-masked randomized study. *Osteopor. Int.* **5,** 108–114 (1995).
52. Farley, J. R., Tarbaux, N. M., Lau, K.-H. W., and Baylink, D. J. Monofluorophosphate is hydrolyzed by alkaline phosphatase and mimics the actions of NaF on skeletal tissues *in vitro. Calcif. Tissue Int.* **40,** 35–42 (1987).
53. Jowsey, J., and Riggs, B. L. Effect of concurrent calcium ingestion on intestinal absorption of fluoride. *Metabolism* **27,** 971–974 (1978).
54. Ericsson, Y. Monofluorophosphate physiology: general considerations. *Caries Res.* **17**(Suppl. 1), 46–55 (1983).
55. Delmas, P. D., Dupuis, J., Duboeuf, F., Chapuy, M. C., and Meunier, P. J. Treatment of vertebral osteoporosis with disodium monofluorophosphate: comparison with sodium fluoride. *J. Bone Miner. Res.* **5**(Suppl. 1), S143–S147 (1990).
56. Rigalli, A., Morosano, M., and Puche, R. C. Bioavailability of fluoride administered as sodium fluoride or sodium monofluorophosphate to human volunteers. *Arzneimittel-Forschung* **46,** 531–533 (1996).
57. van Asten, P., Duursma, S. A., Glerum, J. H., Ververs, F. F., van Rijn, H. J., and van Dijk, A. Absolute bioavailability of fluoride from disodium monofluorophosphate and enteric-coated sodium fluoride tablets. *Eur. J. Clin. Pharmacol.* **50,** 321–326 (1996).
58. Resch, H., Libanati, C., Talbot, J., Tabuenca, M., Farley, S., Bettica, P., Tritthart, W., and Baylink, D. Pharmacokinetic profile of a new fluoride preparation: sustained-release monofluorophosphate. *Calcif. Tissue Int.* **54,** 7–11 (1994).
59. Erlacher, L., Templ, H., and Magometschnigg, D. A comparative bioavailability study on two new sustained-release formulations of disodiummonofluorophosphate versus a nonsustained-release formulation in healthy volunteers. *Calcif. Tissue Int.* **56,** 196–200 (1995).
60. Hodge, H. C., and Smith, F. A. Fluoride. *In* "Disorders of Mineral Metabolism" (F. Bronner and J. W. Coburn, eds.) Vol. 1, pp. 439–481. Academic Press, New York, 1981.
61. Cremer, H. D., and Bütner, W. Absorption of fluorides. *In* "Fluorides and Human Health," pp. 75–91. World Health Organization, Monograph Series, Geneva, 1970.
62. Whitford, G. M. Intake and metabolism of fluoride. *Adv. Dent. Res.* **8,** 5–14 (1994).
63. Whitford, G. M. Effects of plasma fluoride and dietary calcium concentrations on GI absorption and secretion of fluoride in the rat. *Calcif. Tissue Int.* **54,** 421–425 (1994).
64. Ekstrand, J., and Ehrnebo, M. Influences of milk products on fluoride bioavailability in man. *Eur. J. Clin. Pharmacol.* **16,** 211–215 (1979).
65. Duursma, S. A., Raymakers, J. A., Fakkeldij, T. M. V., and van Asten, P. Pharmacokinetics of monofluorophosphate. *Res. Clin. Forums* **15,** 21–31 (1993).
66. Richards, A., Kragstrup, J., and Nielsen-Kudsk, F. Pharmacokinetics of chronic fluoride ingestion in growing pigs. *J. Dent. Res.* **64,** 425–430 (1985).
67. Rao, G. S. Dietary intake and bioavailability of fluoride. *Annu. Rev. Nutri.* **4,** 115–136 (1984).
68. Boivin, G., Chavassieux, P., Chapuy, M. C., and Meunier, P. J. Skeletal fluorosis: histomorphometric analysis of bone changes and bone fluoride content in 29 patients. *Bone* **10,** 89–99 (1989).
69. Boivin, G., Chapuy, M. C., and Baud, C. A., and Meunier, P. J. Fluoride content in the human iliac bone, results in controls, patients with fluorosis, and osteoporotic patients treated with fluoride. *J. Bone Miner. Res.* **3,** 497–502 (1988).
70. Gabovich, R. D., and Ovrutsky, G. D. Fluorine in stomatology and hygiene. "NIH Publ. 78-785." National Institutes of Health, Bethesda, MD, 1977.
71. Pak, C. Y. C. Fluoride and osteoporosis. *Proc. Soc. Exp. Biol. Med.* **191,** 278–286 (1989).
72. Ekstrand, J., Ehrnebo, M., and Boreus, L. O. Fluoride bioavailability after intravenous and oral administration: importance of renal clearance and urine flow. *Clin. Pharmacol. Ther.* **23,** 329–337 (1978).
73. Duursma, S. A., Glerum, J. H., van Dijk, A., Bosch, R., Kerkhoff, H., van Putten, J., and Raymakers, J. A. Responders and nonresponders after fluoride therapy in osteoporosis. *Bone* **8,** 131–136 (1987).
74. Ekstrand, J., and Spak, C.-J. Fluoride pharmacokinetics: its implications in the fluoride treatment of osteoporosis. *J. Bone Miner. Res.* **5**(Suppl. 1), S53–S61 (1990).
75. Spencer, H., Kramer, L., Gatza, C., Norris, C., Wiatrowski, E., and Gandhi, V. C. Fluoride metabolism in patients with chronic renal failure. *Arch. Intern. Med.* **140,** 1331–1335 (1980).
76. Kanis, J. A., and Meunier, P. J. Should we use fluoride to treat osteoporosis? *Q. J. Med.,* **210,** 145–164 (1984).
77. Dure-Smith, B. A., Kraenzlin, M. E., Farley, S. M., Libanati, C. R., Schulz, E. E., and Baylink, D. J. Fluoride therapy for osteoporosis: a review of dose response, duration of treatment, and skeletal sites of action. *Calcif. Tissue Int.* **49**(Suppl.), S64–S72 (1991).
78. Taves, D. R. New approach to the treatment of bone disease with fluoride. *Fed. Proc.* **29,** 1185–1187 (1970).
79. van Kesteren, R. G., Duursma, S. A., Visser, W. J., van der Sluys, V., and Backer Dirks, O. Fluoride in serum and bone during treatment of osteoporosis with sodium fluoride, calcium, and vitamin D. *Metabol. Bone Dis. Rel. Res.* **4,** 31–37 (1982).
80. Riggs, B. L., Hodgson, S. F., O'Fallon, W. M., Chao, E. Y., Wahner, H. W., Muhs, J. M., Cedel, S. L., and Melton, L. J., III, Effect of fluoride treatment on the fracture rate in postmenopausal women with osteoporosis. *N. Engl. J. Med.* **322,** 802–809 (1990).
81. Kleerekoper, M., Peterson, E. L., Nelson, D. A., Phillips, E., Schork, M. A., Tilley, B. C., and Parfitt, A. M. A randomized trial of sodium fluoride as a treatment for postmenopausal osteoporosis. *Osteopor. Int.* **1,** 155–161 (1991).

82. Riggs, B. L., O'Fallon, W. M., Lane, A., Hodgson, S. F., Wahner, H. W., Muhs, J., Chao, E., and Melton, L. J., III. Clinical trial of fluoride therapy in postmenopausal osteoporotic women: extended observations and additional analysis. *J. Bone Miner. Res.* **9,** 265–275 (1994).
83. Pak, C. Y., C., Sakhaee, K., Piziak, V., Peterson, R. D., Breslau, N. A., Boyd, P., Poindexter, J. R., Herzog, J., Heard-Sakhaee, A., Haynes, S., Adams-Huet, B., and Reisch, J. S. Slow-release sodium fluoride in the management of postmenopausal osteoporosis. A randomized controlled trial. *Ann. Intern. Med.* **120,** 625–632 (1994).
84. Pak, C. Y. C., Sakhaee, K., Adams-Huet, B., Piziak, V., Peterson, R. D., and Poindexter, J. R. Treatment of postmenopausal osteoporosis with slow-release sodium fluoride. Final report of a randomized controlled trial. *Ann. Intern. Med.* **123,** 401–408 (1995).
85. Lundy, M. W., Stauffer, M., Wergedal, J. E., Baylink, D. J., Featherstone, J. D., Hodgson, S. F., and Riggs, B. L. Histomorphometric analysis of iliac crest bone biopsies in placebo-treated versus fluoride-treated subjects. *Osteopor. Int.* **5,** 115–129 (1995).
86. Pak, C. Y. C., Sakhaee, K., Parcel, C., Poindexter, J., Adams, B., Bahar, A., and Beckley, R. Fluoride bioavailability from slow-release sodium fluoride given with calcium citrate. *J. Bone Miner. Res.* **5,** 857–862 (1990).
87. Taylor, A. K., Lueken, S. A., Libanati, C. R., and Baylink, D. J. Biochemical markers of bone turnover for the clinical assessment of bone metabolism. *Rheum. Dis. Clin. North Am. Osteopor.* **20,** 589–607 (1994).
88. Farley, S. M. G., Wergedal, J. E., Smith, L. C., Lundy, M. W., Farley, J. R., and Baylink, D. J. Fluoride therapy for osteoporosis: characterization of the skeletal response by serial measurements of serum alkaline phosphatase activity. *Metabolism* **36,** 211–218 (1987).
89. Battman, A., Resch, H., Libanati, C. R., Ludy, D., Fischer, M., Farley, S., and Baylink, D. J. Serum fluoride and serum osteocalcin levels in response to a novel sustained release monofluorophosphate preparation, comparison with plain monofluorophosphate. *Osteopor. Int.* **7,** 48–51 (1997).
90. Dandona, P., Coumar, A., Gill, D. S., Bell, J., and Thomas, M. Sodium fluoride stimulates osteocalcin in normal subjects. *Clin. Endocrinol.* **29,** 437–441 (1988).
91. Chavassieux, P. Bone effects of fluoride in animal models in vivo. A review and a recent study. *J. Bone Miner. Res.* **5**(Suppl. 1), S95–S99 (1990).
92. Cheng, P.-T., and Bader, S. M. Effects of fluoride on rat cancellous bone. *Bone Miner.* **11,** 153–161 (1990).
93. Marie, P. J., and Hott, M. Short-term effects of fluoride and strontium on bone formation and resorption in mouse. *Metabolism* **35,** 547–571 (1986).
94. Kragstrup, J., Richards, A., and Fejerskov, O. Experimental osteofluorosis in the domestic pig: a histomorphometric study of vertebral trabecular bone. *J. Dent. Res.* **63,** 885–889 (1984).
95. Chavassieux, P., Pastoureau, P., Boivin, D., Chapuy, M. C., Delmas, P. D., and Meunier, P. J. Dose effects on ewe bone remodeling of short-term sodium fluoride administration—a histomorphometric and biochemical study. *Bone* **12,** 421–427 (1991).
96. Lundy, M. W., Farley, J. R., and Baylink, D. J. Characterization of a rapidly responding animal model for fluoride-stimulated bone formation. *Bone* **7,** 289–293 (1986).
97. Ream, L. J. The effect of short-term fluoride ingestion on bone formation and resorption in the rat femur. *Cell Tissue Res.* **221,** 421–430 (1981).
98. Libanati, C., Lau, K.-H. W., and Baylink, D. J. Fluoride therapy for osteoporosis. *In* "Osteoporosis" (R., Marcus, D., Feldman, and J., Kelsey, eds.), Chapt. 66, pp. 1259–1277. Academic Press, San Diego, 1996.
99. Kuntz, D., Marie, P., Naveau, B., Maziere, B., Tubiana, M., and Ryckewaert, A. Extended treatment of primary osteoporosis by sodium fluoride combined with 25-hydroxycholecalciferol. *Clin. Rheumatol.* **3,** 145–153 (1984).
100. Eriksen, E. F., Mosekilde, L., and Melsen, F. Effects of sodium fluoride, calcium, phosphate, and vitamin D_2 on trabecular bone balance and remodeling in osteoporosis. *Bone* **6,** 381–389 (1985).
101. Harrison, J. E., Bayley, T. A., Josse, R. G., Murray, T. M., Sturtridge, W., Williams, C., Goodwin, S., Tam, C., and Fornasier, V. The relationship between fluoride effects on bone histology and on bone mass in patients with postmenopausal osteoporosis. *Bone Miner.* **1,** 321–333 (1986).
102. Olah, A. J., Reutter, F. W., and Dambacher, M. A. Effects of combined therapy with sodium fluoride and high doses of vitamin D in osteoporosis. A histomorphometric study in the iliac crest. *In* "Fluoride and Bone" (B., Courvoisier, A., Donath, and C. A., Baud, eds.), pp. 242–253. Bern, Huber, 1978.
103. Baylink, D. J., and Bernstein, D. S. The effects of fluoride therapy on metabolic bone disease. *Clin. Orthop. Rel. Res.* **55,** 51–85 (1967).
104. Compston, J. E., Chadha, S., and Merrett, A. L. Osteomalacia developing during treatment of osteoporosis with sodium fluoride and vitamin D. *Br. Med. J.* **281,** 910–911 (1980).
105. Snow, G. R., and Anderson, C. Short-term chronic fluoride administration and trabecular bone remodeling in beagles: a pilot study. *Calcif. Tissue Int.* **38,** 217–221 (1986).
106. Spencer, G. R., el-Sayed, F. I., Kroening, G. H., Pell, K. L., Shoup, N., Adams, D. F., Franke, M., and Alexander, J. E. Effects of fluoride, calcium and phosphorus on porcine bone. *Am. J. Vet. Res.* **32,** 1751–1774 (1971).
107. Gedalia, I., Hodge, H. C., Anaise, J., White, W. E., and Menczel, J. The effect of sodium monofluorophosphate and sodium fluoride on bone immobilization in rats. *Calcif. Tissue Res.* **5,** 146–152 (1970).
108. Jowsey, J., Riggs, B. L., Kelly, P. J., and Hoffmann, D. L. Effect of combined therapy with sodium fluoride, vitamin D and calcium in osteoporosis. *Am. J. Med.* **53,** 43–49 (1972).
109. Kleerekoper, M., and Balena, R. Fluorides and osteoporosis. *Annu. Rev. Nutri.* **11,** 309–324 (1991).
110. Kleerekoper, M. Fluorides and the skeleton. *Crit. Rev. Clin. Lab. Sci.* **33,** 139–161 (1996).
111. Rizzoli, R., Chevalley, T., Slosman, D. O., and Bonjour, J.-P. Sodium monofluorophosphate increases vertebral bone mineral density in patients with corticosteroid-induced osteoporosis. *Osteopor. Int.* **5,** 39–46 (1995).
112. Talbot, J. R., Fischer, M. M., Farley, S. M., Libanati, C., Farley, J., Tabuenca, A., and Baylink, D. J. The increase in spinal bone density that occurs in response to fluoride therapy for osteoporosis is not maintained after the therapy is discontinued. *Osteopor. Int.* **6,** 442–447 (1996).
113. Budden, F. H., Bayley, T. A., Harrison, J. E., Josse, R. G., Murray, T. M., Sturtridge, W. C., Kandel, R., Vieth, R., Strauss, A. L., and Goodwin, S. The effect of fluoride on bone histology depends on adequate fluoride absorption and retention. *J. Bone Miner. Res.* **3,** 127–132 (1988).
114. Schulz, E. E., Libanati, C. R., Farley, S. M., Kirk, G. A., and Baylink, D. J. Skeletal scintigraphic changes in osteoporosis treated with sodium fluoride: concise communication. *J. Nuclear Med.* **25,** 651–655 (1984).
115. Schulz, E. E., Engstrom, H., Sauser, D. D., and Baylink, D. J. Osteoporosis: radiographic detection of fluoride-induced extra-axial bone formation. *Radiology* **159,** 457–462 (1986).

116. Resch, H., Libanati, C., Farley, S., Bettica, P., Schulz, E., and Baylink, D. J. Evidence that fluoride therapy increases trabecular bone density in a peripheral skeletal site. *J. Clin. Endocrinol. Metabol.* **76,** 1622–1624 (1993).
117. Dambacher, M. A., Ittner, J., and Ruegsegger, P. Long-term fluoride therapy of postmenopausal osteoporosis. *Bone* **7,** 199–205, (1986).
118. Rawlinson, S. C., Mohan, S., Baylink, D. J., and Lanyon, L. E. Exogenous prostacyclin but not prostaglandin E2 produces similar responses in both G6PD activity and RNA production as mechanical loading, and increases IGF-II release, in adult cancellous bone in culture. *Calcif. Tissue Int.* **53,** 324–329 (1993).
119. Farley, S. M., Libanati, C. R., Schulz, E. E., Kirk, G. A., and Baylink, D. J. Fluoride stimulates bone formation in the peripheral skeleton, particularly at weight bearing sites. *Clin. Res.* **32,** 394A (1984). [Abstract]
120. Riggs, B. Treatment of osteoporosis with sodium fluoride: an appraisal. *In* "Bone and Mineral Research" (W. A., Peck, ed.), pp. 366–393. Elsevier, Amsterdam, 1983.
121. Pak, C. Y. C., Sakhaee, K., Zerwekh, J. E., Parcel, C., Peterson, R., and Johnson, K. Safe and effective treatment of osteoporosis with intermittent slow-release sodium fluoride: argumentation of vertebral bone mass and inhibition of fractures. *J. Clin. Endocrinol. Metabol.* **68,** 150–159 (1989).
122. O'Duffy, J. D., Wahner, H. W., O'Fallon, W. M., Johnson, K. A., Muhs, J. M., Beabout, J. W., Hodgson, S. F., and Riggs, B. L. Mechanism of acute lower extremity pain syndrome in fluoride-treated osteoporotic patients. *Am. J. Med.* **80,** 561–566 (1986).
123. Schnitzler, C. M., and Solomon, L. Trabecular stress fractures during fluoride therapy for osteoporosis. *Skel. Radiol.* **14,** 276–279 (1985).
124. Bayley, T. A., Harrison, J. E., Murray, T. M., Josse, R. G., Sturtridge, W., Pritsker, K. P., Strauss, A., Vieth, R., and Goodwin, S. Fluoride induced fractures: relation to osteogenic effect. *J. Bone Miner. Res.* **5**(Suppl. 1), S217–S222 (1990).
125. Gruber, H. E., and Baylink, D. J. The effects of fluoride on bone. *Clin. Orthop. Rel. Res.* **267,** 264–277 (1991).
126. Kleerekoper, M., and Mendlovic, D. B. Sodium fluoride therapy of postmenopausal osteoporosis. *Endocr. Rev.* **14,** 312–323 (1993).
127. Dure-Smith, B. A., Farley, S. M., Linkhart, S. G., Farley, J. R., and Baylink, D. J. Calcium deficiency in fluoride treated osteoporotic patients despite calcium supplementation. *J. Clin. Endocrinol. Metab.* **81,** 269–275 (1996).
128. Beary, D. The effects of fluoride and low Ca on the physical properties of the rat femur. *Anat. Rec.* **164,** 305–316 (1969).
129. Devogelaer, J. P., and Nagant de Deuxchaisnes, C. Fluoride therapy of type I osteoporosis. *Clin. Rheumatol.* **14**(Suppl. 3), 26–31 (1995).
130. Hedlund, L. R., and Gallagher, J. C. Increased incidence of hip fracture in osteoporotic women treated with sodium fluoride. *J. Bone Miner. Res.* **4,** 223–225 (1989).
131. Gutteridge, D. H., Price, R. I., Kent, G. N., Prince, R. L., and Michell, P. A. Spontaneous hip fractures in fluoride-treated patients: potential causative factors. *J. Bone Miner. Res.* **5**(Suppl. 1), 205–212 (1990).
132. Riggs, B. L., Baylink, D. J., Kleerekoper, M., Lane, J. M., Melton, L. J., and Meunier, P. J. Incidence of hip fractures in osteoporotic women treated with sodium fluoride. *J. Bone Miner. Res.* **2,** 123–126 (1987).
133. Farrerons, J., Rodriguez de la Serna, A., Guanabens, N., Armadans, L., Lopez-Navidad, A., Yoldi, B., Renau, A., and Vaque, J. Sodium fluoride treatment is a major protector against vertebral and nonvertebral fractures when compared with other common treatments of osteoporosis: a longitudinal, observational study. *Calcif. Tissue Int.* **60,** 250–254 (1997).
134. Lehmann, R., Wapniarz, M., Hofmann, B., Pieper, B., Haubitz, I., and Allolio, B. Drinking water fluoridation: bone mineral density and hip fracture incidence. *Bone* **22,** 273–278 (1998).
135. Bernstein, D. S., and Cohen, P. Use of sodium fluoride in the treatment of osteoporosis. *J. Clin. Endocrinol.* **27,** 197–210 (1967).
136. Turner, C. H., Akhter, M. P., and Heaney, R. P. The effects of fluoridated water on bone strength. *J. Orthop. Res.* **10,** 581–587 (1992).
137. Turner, C. H., Hasegawa, K., Zhang, W., Wilson, M., Li, Y., and Dunipace, A. J. Fluoride reduces bone strength in older rats. *J. Dent. Res.* **78,** 1475–1481 (1995).
138. Sogaard, C. H., Mosekilde, L., Richards, A., and Mosekilde, L. Marked decrease in trabecular bone quality after five years of sodium fluoride therapy—assessed by biomechanical testing of iliac crest bone biopsies in osteoporotic patients. *Bone* **15,** 393–399 (1994).
139. Eanes, E. D., and Reddi, A. H. The effect of fluoride on bone mineral apatite. *Metab. Bone Dis.* **2,** 3–11 (1979).
140. Singer, L., Armstrong, W. D., Zipkin, I., and Frazier, P. D. Chemical composition and structure of fluorotic bone. *Clin. Orthop. Rel. Res.* **99,** 303–312 (1974).
141. Franke, J., Runge, H., Grau, P., Fengler, F., Wanka, C., and Rempel, H. Physical properties of fluorosis bone. *Acta Orthop. Scand.* **47,** 20–27 (1976).
142. Yamamoto, K., Wergedal, J. E., and Baylink, D. J. Increased bone microhardness in fluoride treated rats. *Calcif. Tissue Res.* **15,** 45–54 (1974).
143. Grynpas, M. D. Fluoride effects on bone crystals. *J. Bone Miner. Res.* **5,** S169–S175 (1990).
144. Lundy, M. W., Russell, J. E., Avery, J., Wergedal, J. E., and Baylink, D. J. Effect of sodium fluoride on bone density in chickens. *Calcif. Tissue Int.* **50,** 420–426 (1992).
145. Wiers, B. H., Francis, M. D., Hovanick, K., Ritchie, C. K., and Baylink, D. J. Theoretical physical chemical studies of the cause of fluoride-induced osteomalacia. *J. Bone Miner. Res.* **5**(Suppl. 1), S63–570 (1990).
146. Baylink, D. J., and Bernstein, D. S. The effects of fluoride therapy on metabolic bone disease. *Clin. Orthop. Rel. Res.* **55,** 51–85 (1967).
147. Fratzl, P., Roschger, P., Eschberger, J., Abendroth, B., and Klaushofer, K. Abnormal bone mineralization after fluoride treatment in osteoporosis: a small-angle X-ray scattering study. *J. Bone Miner. Res.* **9,** 1541–1549 (1994).
148. Carter, D. R., and Beaupre, G. S. Effects of fluoride treatment on bone strength. *J. Bone Miner. Res.* **5**(Suppl. 1), S177–S184 (1990).
149. Riggs, B. L., Seeman, E., Hodgson, S. F., Taves, D. R., and O'Fallon, W. M. Effect of fluoride/calcium regimen on vertebral fracture occurrence in postmenopausal osteoporosis: comparison with conventional therapy. *N. Engl. J. Med.* **306,** 446–450 (1982).
150. Lane, J. M., Healey, J. H., Schwartz, E., Vigorita, V. J., Schneider, R., Einhorn, T. A., Suda, M., and Robbins, W. C. Treatment of osteoporosis with sodium fluoride and calcium: effects on vertebral fracture incidence and bone histomorphometry. *Orthop. Clin. North Am.* **15,** 728–745 (1984).
151. Mamelle, N., Meunier, P. J., Dusan, R., Guillaume, M., Martin, J. L., Gaucher, A., Prost, A., Zeigler, G., and Netter, P. Risk benefit of sodium fluoride treatment in primary vertebral osteoporosis. *Lancet* **2,** 361–365 (1988).
152. Heaney, R. P., Baylink, D. J., Johnson, C. C., Melton, L. J., III, Meunier, P. J., Murray, T. M., and Nagant de Deuxchaisnes, C.

Fluoride therapy for the vertebral crush fracture syndrome (a status report). *Ann. Intern. Med.* **111,** 687–680 (1989).
153. Farley, S. M., Wergedal, J. E., Farley, J. R., Javier, G. N., Schulz, E. E., Talbot, J. R., Libanati, C. R., Lindegren, L., Bock, M., Goette, M. M., Mohan, S. S., Kimball-Johnson, P., Perkel, V. S., Cruise, R. J., and Baylink, D. J. Spinal fractures during fluoride therapy for osteoporosis: relationship to spinal bone density. *Osteopor. Int.* **2,** 213–218 (1992).
154. Ringe, J. D., Dorst, A., Kipshoven, C., Rovati, L. C., and Setnikar, I. Avoidance of vertebral fractures in men with idiopathic osteoporosis by a three year therapy with calcium and low-dose intermittent monofluorophosphate. *Osteopor. Int.* **8,** 47–52 (1998).
155. Meunier, P. J., Sebert, J.-L., Reginster, J.-Y., Briancon, D., Appelboom, T., Netter, P., Loeb, G., Rouillon, A., Barry, S., Evreux, J.-C., Avouac, B., Marchandise, X., and the FAVO Study Group, Fluoride salts are no better at preventing new vertebral fractures than calcium-vitamin D in postmenopausal osteoporosis: the FAVO Study. *Osteopor. Int.* **8,** 4–12 (1998).
156. Pak, C. Y. C., Zerwekh, J. E., Antich, P. P., Bell, N. H., and Singer, F. R. Slow-release sodium fluoride in osteoporosis. *J. Bone Miner. Res.* **11,** 561–564 (1996).
157. Kleerekoper, M. Fluoride: the verdict is in, but the controversy lingers. *J. Bone Miner. Res.* **11,** 565–567 (1996).
158. Zerwekh, J. E., Hagler, H. K., Sakhaee, K., Gottschalk, F., Peterson, R. D., and Pak, C. Y. C. Effect of slow-release sodium fluoride on cancellous bone histology and connectivity in osteoporosis. *Bone* **15,** 691–699 (1994).
159. Einhorn, T., Wakley, G., Linkhart, S., Rush, E., Maloney, S., Faierman, E., and Baylink, D. Incorporation of sodium fluoride into cortical bone does not impair the mechanical properties of the appendicular skeleton in rats. *Calcif. Tissue Int.* **51,** 127–131 (1992).
160. Chavassieux, P., Boivin, G., Serre, C. M., and Meunier, P. J. Fluoride increases rat osteoblast function and population after in vivo administration but not after in vitro exposure. *Bone* **14,** 721–725 (1993).
161. Ringe, J., Kipshoven, C., Rovati, L., and Setnikar, I. Therapy of idiopathic male osteoporosis: a 3-year study with Ca and low dose intermittent monofluorophosphate. *In* "Osteoporosis" (S. E., Papapoulos, ed.), pp. 383–390. Elsevier, Amsterdam (1996).
162. Schnitzler, C. M., Wing, J. R., Raal, F. J., van der Merwe, M. T., Mesquita, J. M., Gear, K. A., Robson, H. J., and Shires, R. Fewer bone histomorphometric abnormalities with intermittent than with continuous slow-release sodium fluoride therapy. *Osteopor. Int.* **7,** 376–389 (1997).
163. Libanati, C. R., and Baylink, D. J. Fluoride and estrogen combination therapy for osteoporosis. *J. Bone Miner. Res.* **8**(Suppl. 1), S335 (1993). [Abstract]
164. Lems, W. F., Jacobs, J. W., Bijlsma, J. W., van Veen, G. J., Houben, H. H., Haanen, H. C., Gerrits, M. I., and van Rijn, H. J. Is addition of sodium fluoride to cyclical etidronate beneficial in the treatment of corticosteroid induced osteoporosis? *Ann. Rheum. Dis.* **56,** 357–363 (1997).

CHAPTER 49

Vitamin D

MURRAY J. FAVUS The University of Chicago Pritzker School of Medicine, Chicago, Illinois 60637

INTRODUCTION

Changes in the skeleton with aging may become clinically manifest as bone loss, increased bone fragility, and fracture. A rational approach to the prevention of progressive bone loss and fracture depends on a detailed understanding of the physiology of bone turnover and the age-related changes in bone formation and resorption and calcium balance. As vitamin D is known to play an important role in normal skeletal growth and development and in the prevention of rickets in children and osteomalacia in adults, considerable interest has focused on understanding vitamin D biologic actions on bone. Extensive clinical and animal studies support the concept that vitamin D deficiency and altered vitamin D metabolism contribute to bone loss and fracture in aging. Vitamin D deficiency in the elderly and the effects of vitamin D repletion are discussed in detail in Chapter 17. This chapter reviews the evidence for age-related alterations in vitamin D metabolism and the efficacy of vitamin D, vitamin D metabolites, and analogues in preventing fractures. A major action of vitamin D is to increase the efficiency of intestinal Ca absorption. As Ca intake and the effects of aging on Ca balance are discussed in detail in Chapters 3 and 40, this chapter considers Ca intake only as it may influence vitamin D metabolism and intestinal Ca absorption.

EVIDENCE FOR ALTERED VITAMIN D METABOLISM IN AGING

Normal Control of Intestinal Ca Absorption and Vitamin D

Dietary Ca absorption is incomplete, and the efficiency of Ca absorption is correlated inversely with Ca intake [1,2]. The relationship between Ca intake and absorption depends on the level of Ca intake, with a greater efficiency of absorption during low intakes and a less efficient but linear relationship at luminal Ca concentrations greater than 1.5 m*M* [3]. Dietary Ca is absorbed by both passive diffusion and a vitamin D-dependent cellular active transport process [4,5]. The latter is responsible for the highly efficient transport of Ca during low intakes, while passive diffusional mechanisms, driven by concentration, electrical, and osmotic gradients [5], dominate at higher levels of luminal Ca. In response to a low Ca diet, Ca absorption becomes more efficient through an increase in the number of transporters (V_{max}) with no change in the affinity of the transport system for Ca [3,5].

The intestinal Ca active transport process is dependent on adequate vitamin D, and therefore vitamin D deficiency will be most evident during low levels of dietary Ca intake. At higher intakes of Ca, when luminal Ca concentrations are greater than 1.5 m*M,* diffusional, vitamin D-independent Ca transport mechanisms predominate.

The naturally occurring vitamin D_3[1] and the synthetic vitamin D_2 are biologically inert and require sequential hydroxylation at the C-25 position in the liver and at the C-1 position in the kidney to confer full biologic activity [6]. The cellular actions of vitamin D occur through binding of the steroid to the intracellular vitamin D receptor (VDR), which is a member of the steroid hormone superfamily of trans-activating transcription factors [7]. The dihydroxylated form of vitamin D, 1,25-dihydroxyvitamin D [$1,25(OH)_2D$], is considered to be the hormonal form of the vitamin based on its high specific binding affinity for the VDR compared to vitamin D_2 and D_3 and the hepatic 25-hydroxyvitamin D

[1]Vitamin D without a subscript is a generic term that refers to vitamin D in general. Specific forms of vitamin D include vitamin D_3 (cholecalciferol) and the synthetic vitamin D_2 (ergocalciferol). Both are metabolized to their 25-hydroxyvitamin D and $1,25(OH)_2D$ forms. $1,25(OH)_2D_3$ is also known as calcitriol, and the two terms may be used interchangeably.

(25OHD) metabolites and its greater potency in exerting known biologic actions of vitamin D such as stimulation of intestinal Ca transport [7]. Thus, sufficient amounts of $1,25(OH)_2D$ must be synthesized for optimal stimulation of the Ca active transport process, as during low intake of Ca.

Renal proximal tubule synthesis of $1,25(OH)_2D$ is tightly regulated to meet skeletal requirements. Increases in 25-hydroxyvitamin D-1α-hydroxylase (1-OHase) activity, $1,25(OH)_2D$ production, and circulating $1,25(OH)_2D$ levels occur during growth, pregnancy, lactation, or when dietary Ca intake is low or inadequate to meet body Ca requirements. Under these conditions, Ca needs are met through the increased efficiency of intestinal Ca active transport. 1-OHase activity is stimulated by parathyroid hormone (PTH) as during low Ca intake [8] and during low phosphate diet (LPD) [9]. Insulin-like growth factor-I (IGF-I) [10,11] also has direct stimulatory actions on the 1-OHase, whereas calcitonin [12] and estrogen [13] may regulate 1-OHase activity through direct or indirect mechanisms.

Serum $1,25(OH)_2D$ Levels and Intestinal Ca Absorption in Aging

There is a weak positive correlation between serum $1,25(OH)_2D$ levels and rates of intestinal Ca absorption [14] due in part to the wide range of serum $1,25(OH)_2D$ levels, which may vary fourfold within the general population of men and women. Also, rates of intestinal Ca absorption may vary twofold independent of dietary Ca intake. Thus, ambient serum $1,25(OH)_2D$ levels are poor predictors of intestinal Ca absorption rates.

Several studies have reported an age-related decline in serum $1,25(OH)_2D$ levels that is most evident after age 65 [14–18]. Others have reported either no decline with age [19–23] or increasing levels until age 65 and then a decline thereafter [24,25]. $1,25(OH)_2D$ production rates have not been measured *in vivo* in aging individuals; however, the lack of decline in vitamin D-binding protein (DBP) with age and a decrease in calculated free $1,25(OH)_2D$ levels beginning about 10 years after menopause [26] support the concept that $1,25(OH)_2D$ production decreases with aging. Estrogen status may influence DBP concentration, and therefore DBP levels may vary independent of age. Measurements of total $1,25(OH)_2D$ and DBP and calculation of free $1,25(OH)_2D$ indicate that the latter levels are independent of menopausal (estrogen) status [27,28]. The tendency for metabolic clearance of $1,25(OH)_2D$ to decrease from early to later adult years in otherwise healthy women [25] may contribute to the stability or increase in serum $1,25(OH)_2D$ with age. Changes in serum 25OHD concentrations may occur in elderly subjects poorly repleted with vitamin D. The levels of serum 25OHD in elderly subjects in the United States may be lower than once thought [29], but the impact of these lower levels on serum $1,25(OH)_2D$ levels and calcium absorption is not yet known.

Several studies have explored the mechanism of the age-related decrease in serum $1,25(OH)_2D$ levels by measuring serum $1,25(OH)_2D$ levels in response to the intravenous administration of PTH (Table I). Using infusions of PTH, which is a major stimulus and regulator of the renal 1-OHase, $1,25(OH)_2D$ synthetic capacity was tested in young adults, older subjects, and patients with osteoporosis. Baseline serum $1,25(OH)_2D$ levels were lower in osteoporotic women compared to age-matched controls in two studies [30,31], whereas Tsai *et al.* [32] found that elderly women (mean age 78 years) had the same baseline serum levels of $1,25(OH)_2D$ in the presence and absence of a hip fracture. The response to PTH also varied among the studies. Riggs *et al.* [31] and Sorensen *et al.* [30] found that PTH infusion increased serum $1,25(OH)_2D$ levels in age-matched postmenopausal women with and without osteoporosis. In contrast, Silverberg *et al.* [33] found an impaired rise in serum $1,25(OH)_2D$ in response to PTH in women with postmenopausal osteoporosis compared to age-matched women without osteoporosis. Tsai *et al.* [32] also found the response to PTH was blunted in elderly subjects with or without osteoporosis (presence of a hip fracture). Slovik *et al.* [34] administered PTH to healthy young adults (mean age 29 years) and postmenopausal women with osteoporosis (age 58 years) and found a twofold increase in serum $1,25(OH)_2D$ levels in the young adults and no rise in serum levels in the osteoporotic women. While the serum $1,25(OH)_2D$ levels were clearly different between the two groups, one cannot determine whether the defect in secretory response to PTH was due to the effect of age or osteoporosis. Some of the differences in results among these studies may be due to the dose of PTH and the length of the PTH infusion. However, these studies support an age-related decline in baseline $1,25(OH)_2D$ levels (Fig. 1) and strongly suggest that aging with or without osteoporosis may be associated with impaired PTH stimulation of the renal 1-OHase. These results agree with studies in rats, in which there is a clear age-related defect in 1-OHase activity and response to PTH.

Like serum $1,25(OH)_2D$ levels, intestinal Ca absorption has also been reported to decline or remain stable with aging. The seeming discrepancy in the observations may be due in part to the different techniques employed in measuring Ca absorption. Measurement of net Ca absorption by external Ca balance [1,35], jejunal perfusion [3], and radioisotopic Ca absorption tests [1,36,37]

TABLE I Regulation of 1,25(OH)2D Serum Levels by Parathyroid Hormone Stimulation Tests

Subjects[a]	No. per group	Age (years)	Serum baseline[b]	1,25(OH)2D (pg/ml) incremental increase[b]	Reference
Young	6	29	49 ± 10	45 ± 25	Slovik *et al.* [34]
Osteoporosis	5	58	42 ± 9	0	
Postmenopausal	10	67	53 ± 8	19 ± 5	Riggs *et al.* [31]
Postmenopausal + osteoporosis	12	67	31 ± 4	20 ± 6	
Osteoporosis	9	69	19 ± 3	16 ± 7	Sorensen *et al.* [30]
Nonosteoporosis	9	69	35 ± 3	15 ± 8	
Premenopausal	10	37	37 ± 7	64 ± 13	Tsai *et al.* [32]
Postmenopausal	8	61	34 ± 5	40 ± 11	
Elderly	10	78	20 ± 6	25 ± 3	
Elderly + hip fracture	8	78	21 ± 3	13 ± 3	

[a] Osteoporosis diagnosed by fracture.
[b] Values are mean ± SEM.

reveal a decline in absorption after menopause. In contrast, calculated true Ca absorption (fractional Ca absorption × dietary Ca) measured by either a stable isotope (^{42}Ca) or double Ca radioisotopes (^{45}Ca, ^{47}Ca) shows no decline with age [22,25].

Age-Related Loss of Intestinal Adaptation to Dietary Ca Restriction

HUMAN STUDIES

As the vitamin D-dependent component of total Ca absorption is active mainly during dietary Ca restriction and because women at all ages tend to ingest diets low in Ca (see Chapter 40), estimates of vitamin D-dependent Ca transport in aging may be more meaningful. There is considerable evidence that adaptation of the Ca active transport process to low Ca intake is diminished or lost in aging men and women [3,35,38]. Such data has been obtained using external Ca balance or perfusion of the jejunum and ileum with solutions of varying Ca concentrations (Fig. 2). Thus, aging prevents the usual physiologic adaptation or increase in net Ca absorption during a low Ca diet (LCD). These procedures for measuring Ca absorption, while time-consuming and less frequently employed in recent years, nevertheless provide a quantitative measure of the absolute amount of Ca absorbed and are not sensitive to the variabilities of dilution of Ca in the intestinal lumen and binding of Ca to luminal contents as may occur with the use of small amounts of stable isotopes or radioisotopes of Ca. The loss of intestinal adaptation during LCD in older men and women occurs despite the development of negative Ca balance and bone loss. Thus, with aging, there appears to be a loss of the usual signal that stimulates renal 1,25(OH)$_2$D synthesis in the presence of a low Ca diet, elevated PTH, and negative Ca balance. These observations argue against the concept that Ca absorption and 1,25(OH)$_2$D are lower in older subjects because they require less Ca. In young adults, ingestion of a low Ca diet for 1–2 weeks is sufficient to increase serum 1,25(OH)$_2$D levels and Ca active transport [3]. The loss of adaptation to LCD may be demonstrated in men and women as early as the fifth decade [3,35]. Length of exposure to LCD is also not limiting, as measurements of Ca balance in older males ingesting a low Ca diet found no evidence of an increase in net Ca absorption even after 1 year of dietary Ca restriction [35,38].

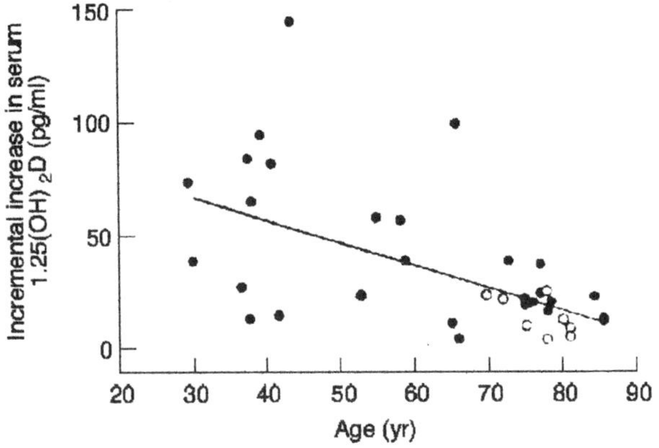

FIGURE 1 Relationship between incremental increase in serum 1,25(OH)$_2$D$_3$ levels following bovine parathyroid hormone 1-34 infusion and age in normal subjects (●) and patients with hip fracture (○). From Tsai *et al.* [32]. Reproduced from **The Journal of Clinical Investigation, 1984, vol. 73, 1668–1672,** by copyright permission of The American Society for Clinical Investigation.

There is some evidence for an intestinal resistance to 1,25(OH)$_2$D$_3$ in aging humans that may contribute to the reduction in intestinal Ca absorption. Ebeling *et al.* [21] found an age-related decline in VDR levels in duodenal mucosal biopsy specimens from 35 women.

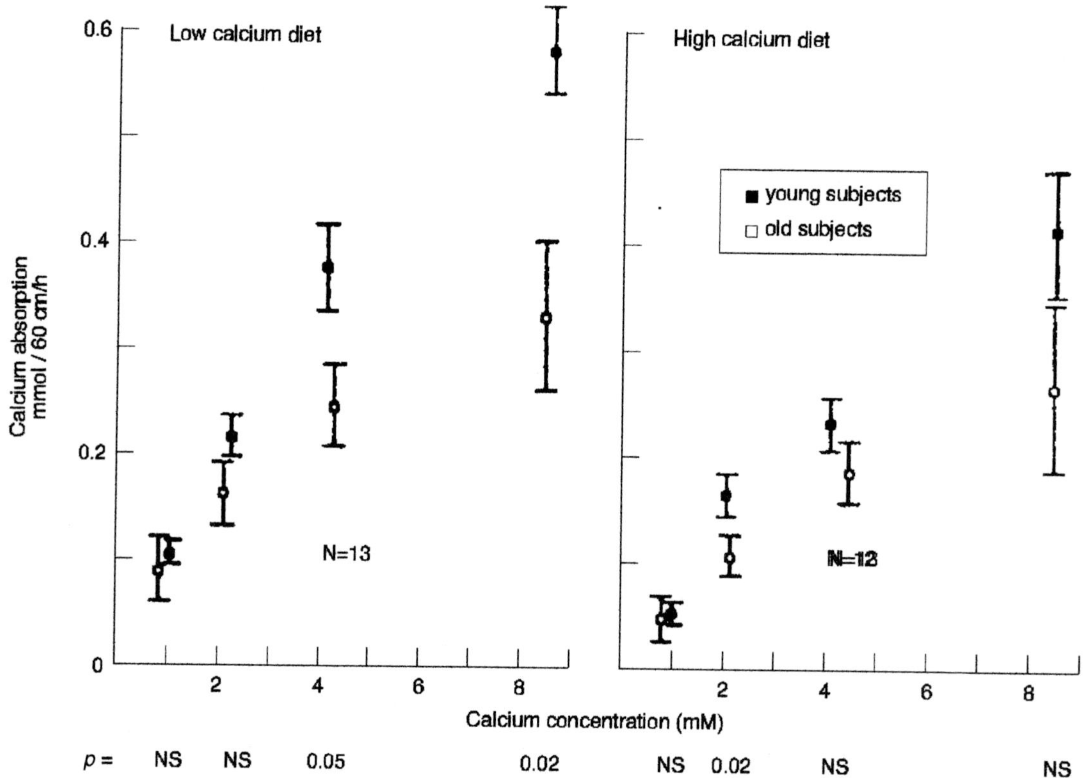

FIGURE 2 Effect of age on Ca absorption by triple lumen perfusion technique. Values are mean ± SEM for seven young and six old subjects studied during a low Ca diet and six subjects in each group during high Ca intake. From Ireland and Fordtron [3]. Reproduced from **The Journal of Clinical Investigation, 1973, vol. 52, 1680–1685,** by copyright permission of The American Society for Clinical Investigation.

In these women, fractional Ca absorption did not decline with age, although serum PTH and $1,25(OH)_2D_3$ levels increased, suggesting an age-related resistance to $1,25(OH)_2D_3$. Thus, with aging, both reduced $1,25(OH)_2D_3$ production and decreased target tissue response to $1,25(OH)_2D_3$ contribute to the decline in Ca absorption and to the loss of adaptation to low Ca intakes.

REGULATION OF $1,25(OH)_2D_3$ SYNTHESIS

Studies in aging rats fed LCD clearly show that they develop a negative Ca balance due to the loss of an increase in 1-OHase activity, serum $1,25(OH)_2D$ levels, and small intestinal Ca active transport [39,40]. Intestinal VDR content is lower in aging rats [41]. However, the time course and magnitude of the responses of the Ca active transport system to $1,25(OH)_2D_3$ are no different in young and old rats [42], suggesting that resistance to the actions of $1,25(OH)_2D_3$ may not be the major factor in the loss of adaptation.

The nature of the age-related defective production of $1,25(OH)_2D_3$ has been studied extensively in adult and aging rats. The loss of renal proximal tubule 1-OHase stimulation during LCD is not overcome by either endogenous or exogenous PTH [43,44]. Further, a low phosphorus diet (LPD), which stimulates 1-OHase activity by a mechanism that is independent of PTH [45], is also ineffective in stimulating 1-OHase in adult (4-month-old) and aging (24-month-old) rats [46]. The age-dependent loss of 1-OHase activity has been thought to result from a decrease in renal function with age and therefore would be irreversible. However, in recent studies, IGF-I administration reversed the failure of 1-OHase activity to increase in adult and aging rats fed either LPD or LCD and restored enzyme activity and serum $1,25(OH)_2D_3$ levels to or toward the levels found in young rats fed the same diets [46]. IGF-I administration did not increase 1-OHase activity in young rats fed either LCD or LPD, and the dose of IGF-I alone was insufficient to increase enzyme activity in young or older rats fed a normal Ca and P diet. Thus, the actions of IGF-I to stimulate 1-OHase activity and the decline in serum growth hormone and IGF-I levels with age [47] suggest that the age-related loss of 1-OHase activity may be due in part to a reduction in IGF-I production.

Actions of Vitamin D on Bone

There is extensive evidence that $1,25(OH)_2D_3$ stimulates both bone formation and bone resorption; however, the mechanisms of such actions remain unclear.

As osteoblastic cells contain the VDR, the actions of $1,25(OH)_2D_3$ on bone formation likely result from a direct stimulatory action of the steroid hormone on osteoblast differentiation and osteoblastic synthetic functions. Specifically, $1,25(OH)_2D_3$ increases bone matrix production through the expression of several osteoblast genes, including alkaline phosphatase, osteocalcin, osteopontin, and type I collagen [48,49]. $1,25(OH)_2D_3$ also stimulates the secretion of transforming growth factor-β [50] and IGF-I binding protein and suppresses IGF-I [51]. $1,25(OH)_2D_3$ also promotes the progression of immature, proliferating osteoblasts through maturation stages to form mature, nondividing osteoblasts [52]. The effects on osteoblastic differentiation and matrix synthesis may be the mechanisms through which vitamin D promotes normal skeletal development. Prevention of rickets may also depend on these actions on osteoblasts; however, the demonstration of healing of rachitic lesions in children with hereditary vitamin D-dependent rickets with intravenous calcium [53] argues for a major effect of vitamin D to be on intestinal mineral transport.

Osteoclastic bone resorption is also stimulated by $1,25(OH)_2D_3$; however, this may be an indirect effect as the mature osteoclast does not contain the VDR. Evidence shows that $1,25(OH)_2D_3$ can induce the differentiation of immature osteoclastic precursor cells to differentiate into bone-resorbing cells [54]. Thus, $1,25(OH)_2D_3$ stimulation of osteoclastic bone resorption may result from an indirect stimulation of mature osteoclasts via the osteoblasts.

There is very limited experimental evidence for a change in $1,25(OH)_2D_3$ action on bone cells with aging; however, the age-related decline in bone cell VDR content in rats [41] may create a resistance of bone cells to $1,25(OH)_2D_3$ action similar to that suggested for intestine.

VITAMIN D EFFICACY IN THE TREATMENT OF OSTEOPOROSIS

Vitamin D (D_2 and D_3) in physiologic replacement and pharmacologic doses has been used to correct vitamin D depletion in the elderly and to prevent vitamin D deficiency at all ages (see discussion by Gloth in Chapter 17). Because the age-related defect in $1,25(OH)_2D_3$ synthesis contributes to the decline in intestinal Ca absorption and perhaps to defective osteoblast function in the elderly, clinical trials of vitamin D_2, D_3, $1,25(OH)_2D_3$, and the synthetic analogue 1α-hydroxyvitamin D_3 have been conducted in postmenopausal women and in elderly men and women with osteoporosis. Since the late 1970s, over 50 such studies have been conducted using vitamin D or metabolites as treatment for osteoporosis. This discussion has selected for analysis only randomized, prospective trials with adequate blinding of treatment assignment in which vitamin D or an analogue either alone or in combination with calcium supplementation, was compared with a placebo, no intervention, or calcium supplements. Further, studies using fracture rates of the hip, vertebrae, or appendicular skeleton as the primary end point have been the focus of this chapter. While several additional studies used change in bone density as the primary end point, they are not included in the detailed review, as the effect of treatment on bone density becomes important only after the intervention has shown efficacy in reducing fracture rates.

Reduction in Hip Fracture

Chapuy *et al.* [55] randomly assigned 3270 elderly French women to either 800 IU vitamin D and 500 mg supplemental Ca or double placebo (Table II). At 3 years of follow-up, treatment effect was significant in reducing the appearance of new hip fractures (odds ratio of 0.68, with 99% confidence interval of 0.53 to 0.93) [56]. The effects of therapy were evident by 18 months of treatment, at which time hip fractures were 43% lower than placebo-treated controls (Fig. 3). In contrast, Lips *et al.* [57] randomized 2578 elderly men and women to either 400 IU vitamin D_3 or placebo and observed no decrease in rates of hip fracture in the treated compared to placebo after 3 years. Thus, one of two studies supports the efficacy of vitamin D and Ca supplement in reducing hip fracture. The lack of efficacy in the Lips trial may have been due to the lack of calcium supple-

TABLE II Effect of Vitamin D_3 Therapy on Hip Fracture

Year	Subjects	N	Mean age (years)	Rx[a]	Follow-up (years)	Odds ratio	Reference
1992	Elderly	3270	84 ± 6	D_3 + Ca vs PL	1.5 3.0	0.72 (0.49 to 1.06) 0.68 (0.50 to 0.93)	Chapuy *et al.* [55]
1996	Elderly	2578	80 ± 6	D_3 vs PL	3.0	1.21 (0.73 to 2.02)	Lips *et al.* [57]

[a] PL, placebo; Ca, Ca supplement. Entry criteria for subjects is indicated.
[b] 99% confidence intervals are shown in parentheses, as calculated by Gillespie *et al.* [56].

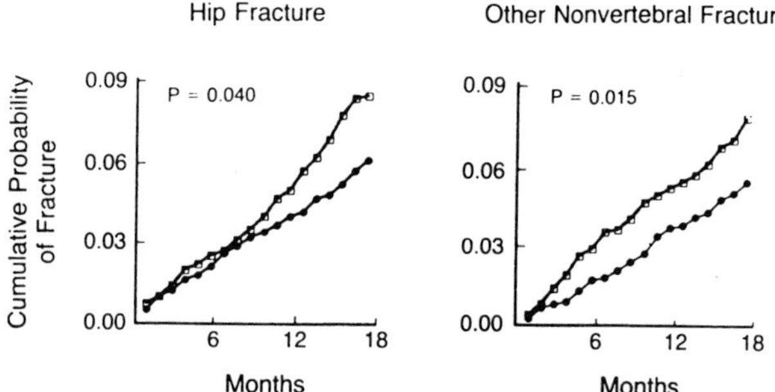

FIGURE 3 Proportion of postmenopausal women in the experimental groups (calcitriol; Ca only) who did not develop new vertebral fractures during the 3-year study. In comparison of the treatment groups: $*p < 0.01$; $**p < 0.001$. Reprinted from Chapuy *et al.* [55], with permission.

mentation or to the lower dose of vitamin D (400 IU vs 800 IU). Because the population studied by Chapuy *et al.* [55] had, on average, low to low-normal serum 25-hydroxyvitamin D levels, the results may be applicable only to subjects with marginal vitamin D stores. Whether such therapy will be effective in a population with relatively normal serum 25-hydroxyvitamin D levels such as in the United States where selected foods are fortified with vitamin D and where vitamin supplements are widely used will require additional randomized trials.

There are no randomized clinical trials in which calcitriol or 1α-hydroxyvitamin D_3 have been tested for efficacy in the reduction of hip fracture.

New Vertebral Fractures

Six randomized controlled trials have compared $1,25(OH)_2D_3$ or 1α-hydroxyvitamin D_3 with either Ca supplementation or placebo in women with established osteoporosis (Table III). Over 1 to 3 years of follow-up, the appearance of new vertebral fractures decreased significantly in three studies and was unchanged in the other three. At least part of the difference in outcomes may be related to the dose of $1,25(OH)_2D_3$ used. The studies by Aloia *et al.* [58], Gallagher and Riggs [59], and Ott and Chestnut [60] used a similar protocol, which called for $1,25(OH)_2D_3$ to be started at 0.5 μg per day and then increased until hypercalciuria or hypercalcemia developed. Calcium intake varied among the three studies and was restricted to varying degrees depending on the appearance of hypercalciuria and hypercalcemia. As a result, Aloia *et al.* [58] used a higher dose than the other two sites (0.8 μg per day vs. 0.6 and 0.4 μg per day). None of the three studies resulted in a reduction in the vertebral fracture rate; however, there was a trend for reduction in new fractures in the Aloia study, which used the higher dose.

Tilyard *et al.* [61] randomized 622 New Zealand women with established osteoporosis (all had at least one vertebral fracture) to either 0.5 μg/day $1,25(OH)_2D_3$ or 1000 mg/day Ca (Table III). By the third year of treatment (Fig. 4), the difference in fracture rates between the two groups was highly significant (odds ratio of 0.28, with 99% confidence interval of 0.13 to 0.58) [56]. However, the significant differences reached during the second and third years resulted from a threefold increase in new vertebral fractures in the Ca-treated group, whereas the fracture rate in the calcitriol-treated group was unchanged. The increase in fracture rate among those receiving Ca supplements is unusual in that Ca supplements have been used in placebo groups in several prospective studies without increases in fracture rates. High drop-out rates during the first year may have changed the composition of the control group such that it became excessively enriched with women experiencing an acceleration in fracture rates. Therefore, this study must be interpreted with caution, as the results do not clearly support an efficacious action of calcitriol

TABLE III Effect of Vitamin D or Analogue Therapy on Appearance of New Vertebral Deformity or Fracture

Year	Subjects[a]	N[b]	Rx[c]	Control	Follow-up (years)	Results	Reference
1988	Vert fx	27	1,25D	Placebo	2.0	No difference in fx rates	Aloia *et al.* [58]
1989	Vert fx	62	1,25D	Placebo	1.0	Fx rates decreased	Gallagher *et al.* [70]
1989	Vert fx	72	1,25D	Placebo	2.0	No difference in fx rates	Ott and Chestnut [60]
1990	Vert fx	40	1,25D	Placebo	2.0	No difference in fx rates	Gallagher and Riggs [59]
1992	Vert fx	432	1,25D	Ca	3.0	Fewer fxs in Rx group	Tilyard *et al.* [61]
1994	Fx	74	1αD +Ca	PL +Ca	1.0	Fx rates decreased	Orimo *et al.* [62]

[a] Entry criteria for subjects are indicated.
[b] Number completing the study.
[c] 1,25D, calcitriol; Ca, calcium supplements; $1\alpha D_3$, 1α-hydroyxvitamin D_3.

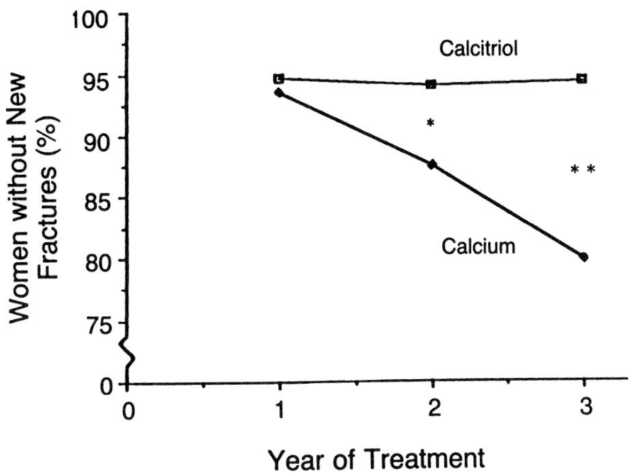

FIGURE 4 Cumulative probability of hip fracture and other appendicular fractures in the placebo group (□) and the group treated with vitamin D_3 and Ca supplement (●). Estimated by life table method and based on the length of time to first fracture. Reprinted from Tilyard *et al.* [61], with permission. Copyright 1992 Massachusetts Medical Society. All rights reserved.

in the prevention of new vertebral fractures in women with established osteoporosis.

In a smaller study of 74 Japanese women with osteoporosis, Orimo *et al.* [62] reported that bone density of the lumbar spine and proximal femur tended to increase and new vertebral fractures tended to decrease over 1 year of treatment with 1α-hydroxyvitamin D_3 (Table III). However, the smaller number of subjects that completed the trial limits the power of the study to conclude that the vitamin D analogue is effective in reducing the rate of new vertebral fractures.

There have been no randomized studies of vitamin D_2 or D_3 vs placebo or Ca supplementation on the rates of vertebral fracture.

Effect on Appendicular Fracture Rates

Two studies designed to assess the effects of therapy on hip fracture also measured other nonvertebral fractures (Table IV). In the study by Chupay *et al.* [55], 18 months of therapy reduced nonvertebral fracture rates by 32% compared to placebo (Fig. 3). Lips *et al.* [57] found no reduction in appendicular fractures at 3.5 years of follow-up using 400 IU vitamin D_3 daily vs placebo. Therefore, these two studies suggest that the dose of vitamin D_3 must be at least 800 IU per day and that Ca supplements should be part of the management plan to reduce appendicular fracture rates. However, other factors, such as the underlying level of vitamin D depletion, may have influenced the outcomes of these trials. Thus, the very limited data are insufficient to reach a conclusion as to the efficacy of vitamin D with or without Ca supplementation on appendicular fractures in the elderly.

Adverse Effects of Therapy

$1,25(OH)_2D_3$ has a narrow dose–response range [63]. Doses of 0.25 μg and below have no consistent effect on intestinal Ca absorption. Doses between 02.5 and 0.75 μg per day increase intestinal Ca absorption and urine Ca excretion. Hypercalciuria and hypercalcemia become more frequent and approach 100% as doses increase above 0.75 μg per day. Trials of $1,25(OH)_2D_3$ on fracture rates have used between 0.25 and 1.0 μg per day in subjects who were largely vitamin D replete and with normal serum and urine Ca. In the largest trial of calcitriol [61], 0.25 μg twice daily caused hypercalcemia in only 2 of 314 women (0.6%) sufficient to discontinue therapy, and hypercalciuria was greater than 300 mg/24 hr in only 16% (vs 7% in the Ca-treated controls). No significant decline in renal function was detected in a subset of the treated group, and one woman in a subset of 120 who underwent renal ultrasonography was found to have nephrocalcinosis. No subject developed clinical symptoms of stone formation or passage. In studies using doses of calcitriol in the range of 0.25 to 1.0 μg per day, bone density of the lumbar spine [58,64], total body [65], and distal radius [58] increased in some studies and not in others [66,60]. No information is available on the effects of calcitriol on proximal femur bone density. At the commonly used doses, $1,25(OH)_2D_3$ suppresses bone turnover as indicated by reduction in the levels of bone biochemical markers [67,68]. Therefore, decreased bone turnover is one mechanism whereby $1,25(OH)_2D_3$ may improve

TABLE IV Effect of Vitamin D or Calcitriol Therapy on Appendicular Fracture Rates

Year	Subjects	*N*	Rx[a]	Control	Follow-up (years)	Results	Reference
1992	Elderly	3270	D+Ca	Placebo	1.5	Fx rates decreased	Chapuy *et al.* [55]
1992	Vert fx	432	1,25D	Ca	3.0	Fx rates decreased	Tilyard *et al.* [61]
1996	Elderly	2578	D	Placebo	4.0	Fx rates unchanged	Lips *et al.* [57]

[a] D, vitamin D_3; Ca, Ca supplement.

bone mass and decreases vertebral fracture rates. Bone biochemical markers are also consistent with direct effects of $1,25(OH)_2D_3$ on osteoblast function, as serum osteocalcin increases during $1,25(OH)_2D_3$ therapy as a result of a direct stimulation of osteocalcin gene expression [69]. It appears that at higher doses (2.0 μg and above), calcitriol may stimulate osteoclast-mediated bone resorption, resulting in the appearance or worsening of hypercalciuria and hypercalcemia [69].

SUMMARY

There is abundant evidence that as men and women age, they develop a negative Ca balance and bone loss. Defective synthesis and decreased circulation of $1,25(OH)_2D_3$ may contribute to the bone loss through the reduction of basal intestinal Ca absorption and loss of the physiologic adaptive increase in Ca absorption during low Ca intake. In addition, decreased osteoblast synthetic function in aging may result in part from reduced $1,25(OH)_2D_3$ action. Despite these observations, the use of $1,25(OH)_2D_3$ and its analogue 1α-hydroxyvitamin D_3 in clinical trials has failed to clearly demonstrate efficacy in reducing fracture rates and improving bone mass. Additional basic information on bone cell function in aging and the effects of $1,25(OH)_2D_3$ are required along with further clinical studies to determine whether these biologically active vitamin D metabolites and analogues are useful in fracture prevention.

References

1. Heaney, R. P., Recker, R. R., Stegman, M. R., and Moy, A. J. Calcium absorption in women: Relationships to calcium intake, estrogen status, and age. *J. Bone Miner. Res.* **4,** 469–475 (1989).
2. Heaney, R. P., Weaver, C. M., and Fitzsimmons, M. L. The influence of calcium load on absorption fraction. *J. Bone. Miner. Res.* **11,** 1135–1138 (1990).
3. Ireland, P., and Fordtran, J. S. Effect of dietary calcium and age on jejunal calcium absorption in humans studied by intestinal perfusion. *J. Clin. Invest.* **52,** 2672–2681 (1973).
4. Favus, M. J., Walling, M. E., and Kimberg, D. V. Effects of 1,25-dihydroxycholecalciferol on intestinal calcium transport in cortisone-treated rats. *J. Clin. Invest.* **52,** 1680–1685 (1973).
5. Favus, M. J. Factors that influence absorption and secretion of calcium in the small intestine and colon. *Am. J. Physiol.* **248,** G147–G157 (1985).
6. Horst, R. L., and Reinhardt, T. A. Vitamin D metabolism. *In* "Vitamin D" (D. Feldman, F. H. Glorieux, and J. W. Pike, eds.), pp. 13–31. Academic Press, San Diego, 1997.
7. Pike, J. W. The vitamin D receptor and its gene. *In* "Vitamin D" (D. Feldman, F. H. Glorieux, and J. W. Pike, eds.), pp. 105–125. Academic Press, San Diego, 1997.
8. Garabedian, M., Holick, M. F., DeLuca, H. F., and Boyle, I. T. Control of 25-hydroxycholecalciferol metabolism by parathyroid glands. *Proc. Natl. Acad. Sci. USA* **69,** 1673–1676 (1972).
9. Tanaka, Y., and DeLuca, H. F. The control of 25-hydroxyvitamin D metabolism by inorganic phosphate. *Arch. Biochem. Biophys.* **154,** 566–574 (1973).
10. Nesbitt, T., and Drezner, M. K. Insulin-like growth factor-I regulation of renal 25-hydroxyvitamin D-1-hydroxylase activity. *Endocrinology* **132,** 133–138 (1993).
11. Condamine, L., Vztovsnik, F., Friedlander, G., Menaa, C., and Garabedian, M. Local action of phosphate depletion and insulin-like growth factor 1 on in vitro production of 1,25-dihydroxyvitamin D by cultured mammalian kidney cells. *J. Clin. Invest.* **94,** 1673–1679 (1994).
12. Horiuchi, N., Takahashi, H., Matsumoto, T., Shimazawa, E., Suda, T., and Ogata, E. Salmon calcitonin-induced stimulation of 1-alpha, 25-dihydroxycholecalciferol synthesis in rats involving a mechanism independent of cAMP. *Biochem. J.* **184,** 269–275 (1979).
13. Castillo, L., Tanaka, Y., DeLuca, H. F., and Sunde, M. L. The stimulation of 25-hydroxyvitamin D_3-1alpha-hydroxylase by estrogen. *Arch. Biochem. Biophys.* **179,** 211–217 (1977).
14. Gallagher, J. C., Riggs, B. L., Eisman, J., Hamstra, A., Arnaud, S., and DeLuca, H. F. Intestinal calcium absorption and serum vitamin D metabolites in normal subjects and osteoporotic patients. Effect of age and dietary calcium. *J. Clin. Invest.* **64,** 729–736 (1979).
15. Quesada, J. M., Coopmans, W., Ruiz, B., Aljama, P., Jans, I., and Bouillon, R. Influence of vitamin-D on parathyroid function in the elderly. *J. Clin. Endocrinol. Metab.* **75,** 494–501 (1992).
16. Clemens, T. L., Zhou, X., Myles, M., Endres, D., and Lindsay, R. Serum vitamin D_2 and vitamin D_3 metabolite concentrations and absorption of vitamin D_2 in elderly subjects. *J. Clin. Endocrinol. Metab.* **63,** 656–660 (1986).
17. Dandona, P., Menon, R. K., Shenoy, R., Houlder, S., Thomas, M., and Mallinson, W. J. W. Low 1,25-dihydroxyvitamin D, secondary hyperparathyroidism, and normal osteocalcin in elderly subjects. *J. Clin. Endocrinol. Metab.* **63,** 459–462 (1986).
18. Fujisawa, Y., Kida, K., and Matsuda, H. Role of change in vitamin D metabolism with age in calcium and phosphorus metabolism in normal human subjects. *J. Clin. Endocrinol. Metab.* **59,** 719–726 (1998).
19. Lund, B., and Sorensen, O. H. Measurement of 25-hydroxyvitamin D in serum and its relation to sunshine, age, and vitamin D. *Scand. J. Clin. Lab. Invest.* **39,** 23–30 (1979).
20. Orwoll, E. S., and Meier, D. E. Alterations in calcium, vitamin D, and parathyroid hormone physiology in normal men with aging: Relationship to the development of senile osteoporosis. *J. Clin. Endocrinol. Metab.* **63,** 1262–1269 (1986).
21. Ebeling, P. R., Sandgren, M. E., Dimagno, E. P., Lane, A. W., DeLuca, H. F., and Riggs, B. L. Evidence of an age-related decrease in intestinal responsiveness to vitamin D: Relationship between serum 1,25-dihydroxyvitamin D_3 and intestinal vitamin D receptor concentration in normal women. *J. Clin. Endocrinol. Metab.* **75,** 176–182 (1992).
22. Ebeling, P. R., Yergey, A. L., Vieira, N. E., Burritt, M. F., O'Fallon, W. M., Kumar, R., and Riggs, B. L. Influence of age on effects of endogenous 1,25-dihydroxyvitamin D on calcium absorption in normal women. *Calcif. Tissue Int.* **55,** 330–334 (1994).
23. Sherman, S. S., Hollis, B. W., and Tobin, J. D. Vitamin D status and related parameters in a healthy population: The effects of age, sex and season. *J. Clin. Endocrinol. Metab.* **71,** 405–413 (1990).
24. Epstein, S., Bryce, G., Hinman, J. W., Miller, O. N., Riggs, B. L., Hui, S. L., and Johnston, C. C. J. The influence of age on bone mineral regulation hormones. *Bone,* **7,** 421–425 (1986).

25. Eastell, R., Yergey, A. L., Vieira, N. E., Cedel, S. L., Kumar, R., and Riggs, B. L. Interrelationship among vitamin D metabolism, true calcium absorption, parathyroid function, and age in women: Evidence of an age-related intestinal resistance to 1,25-dihydroxyvitamin D action. *J. Bone Miner. Res.* **6,** 125–132 (1991).
26. Prince, R. L., Dick, I., Devine, A., Price, R., Gutteridge, D. H., Kerr, D., Criddle, A., Garcia-Webb, P., and St. John, A. The effects of menopause and age on calcitropic hormones: A cross-sectional study of 655 healthy women aged 35 to 90. *J. Bone Miner. Res.* **10,** 835–842 (1995).
27. Prince, R. L., Dick, I., Garcia-Webb, P., and Retallack, R. W. The effects of the menopause on calcitriol and parathyroid hormone: Responses to a low dietary calcium stress test. *J. Clin. Endocrinol. Metab.* **70,** 1119–1123 (1990).
28. Falch, J. A., Oftebro, H., and Hang, E. Early postmenopausal bone loss is not associated with a decrease in circulating levels of 25-hydroxyvitamin D, 1,25-dihydroxyvitamin D, or vitamin D-binding protein. *J. Clin. Endocrinol. Metab.* **64,** 836–841 (1987).
29. Thomas, M. K., Lloyd-Jones, D. M., Thadhani, R. I., Shaw, A. C., Deraska, D. J., Kitch, B. T., Vamakas, E. C., Dick, I. M., Prince, R. L., and Finkelstein, J. S. Hypovitaminosis D in medical inpatients. *N. Engl. J. Med.* **338,** 777–783 (1998).
30. Sorensen, O. H., Lumholtz, B., Lund, B., Hjelmstrand, I. L., Mosekilde, L., Melsen, F., Bishop, J. E., and Norman, A. W. Acute effects of parathyroid hormone on vitamin D metabolism in patients with the bone loss of aging. *J. Clin. Endocrinol. Metab.* **54,** 1258–1261 (1982).
31. Riggs, B. L., Hamstra, A., and DeLuca, H. F. Assessment of 25-hydroxyvitamin D 1α-hydroxylase reserve in postmenopausal osteoporosis by administration of parathyroid extract. *J. Clin. Endocrinol. Metab.* **53,** 833–835 (1981).
32. Tsai, K. S., Heath, H., III., Kumar, R., and Riggs, B. L. Impaired vitamin D metabolism with aging in women. Possible role in pathogenesis of senile osteoporosis. *J. Clin. Invest.* **73,** 1668–1672 (1984).
33. Silverberg, S. J., Shane, E., DeLaCruz, L., Segre, G. V., Clemens, T. L., and Bilezikian, J. P. Abnormalities in parathyroid hormone secretion and 1,25-dihydroxyvitamin D_3 formation in women with osteoporosis. *N. Engl. J. Med.* **320,** 277–281 (1989).
34. Slovik, D. M., Adams, J. S., Neer, R. M., Holick, M. F., and Potts, J. T., Jr. Deficient production of 1,25-dihydroxyvitamin D in elderly osteoporotic patients. *N. Engl. J. Med.* **305,** 372–374 (1981).
35. Malm, O. J. Calcium requirement and adaptation in adult man. *Scand. J. Clin. Lab. Invest.* **10**(Suppl.36), 108–199 (1958).
36. Avioli, L. V., McDonald, J. E. and Lee, S. W. The influence of age on the intestinal absorption of ^{47}Ca in women and its relation to ^{47}Ca absorption in postmenopausal osteoporosis. *J. Clin. Invest.* **44,** 1960–1967 (1965).
37. Bullamore, J. R., Gallagher, J. C., Wilkinson, R., Nordin, B. E. C., and Marshall, D. H. Effect of age on calcium absorption. *Lancet,* **2,** 535–537 (1970).
38. Nicolaysen, R. The absorption of calcium as a function of the body saturation with calcium. *Acta Physiol. Scand.* **5,** 201–209 (1943).
39. Armbrecht, H. J., Forte, L. R., and Halloran, B. P. Effect of age and dietary calcium on renal 25(OH)D metabolism, serum 1,25(OH)$_2$D, and PTH. *Am. J. Physiol.* **246,** E266–E270 (1984).
40. Armbrecht, H. J., Gross, C. J., and Zenser, T. V. Effect of dietary calcium and phosphorus restriction on calcium and phosphorus balance in young and old rats. *Arch. Biochem. Biophys.* **210,** 179–185 (1981).
41. Horst, R. L., Goff, J. P., and Reinhardt, T. A. Advancing age results in reduction of intestinal and bone 1,25-dihydroxyvitamin D receptor. *Endocrinology* **126,** 1053–1057 (1990).
42. Lee, D. B. N., Walling, M. W., Levine, B. S., Gafter, U., Silis, V., Hodsman, A., and Coburn, J. W. Intestinal and metabolic effect of 1,25-dihydroxyvitamin D_3 in normal adult rat. *Am. J. Physiol.* **240,** G75–G78 (1981).
43. Armbrecht, H. J., Wongsurawat, N., and Paschal, R. E. Effect of age on renal responsiveness to parathyroid hormone and calcitonin in rats. *J. Endocrinol.* **114,** 173–178 (1987).
44. Friedlander, J., Janulis, M., Tembe, V., Ro, H. K., Wong, M. S., and Favus, M. J. Loss of parathyroid hormone-stimulated 1,25-dihydroxyvitamin D_3 production in aging does not involve protein kinase A or C pathways. *J. Bone Miner. Res.* **9,** 339–345 (1994).
45. Hughes, M. R., Brumbaugh, P. F., Haussler, M. R., Wergedal, J. E., and Baylink, D. J. Regulation of serum 1,25-dihydroxyvitamin D_3 by calcium and phosphate in the rat. *Science* **190,** 578–579 (1975).
46. Wong, M. S., Sriussadaporn, S., Tembe, V., and Favus, M. J. Insulin-like growth factor I increases renal 1,25(OH)$_2$D$_3$ biosynthesis during low-P diet in adult rats. *Am. J. Physiol.* **272,** F698–F703 (1997).
47. Zadik, Z., Chalew, S. A., McCarter, R. J., Meistas, M., and Kowarski, A. A. The influence of age on the 24-hour integrated concentration of growth hormone in normal individuals. *J. Clin. Endocrinol. Metab.* **60,** 513–516 (1985).
48. Demay, M. B., Kierman, M. S., DeLuca, H. F., and Kronenberg, H. M. Characterization of 1,25-dihydroxyvitamin D_3 receptor interactions with target sequence in the rat osteocalcin gene. *Mol. Endocrinol.* **6,** 557–562 (1992).
49. Fraser, J. D., and Price, P. A. Induction of matrix Gla protein synthesis during prolonged 1,25-dihydroxyvitamin D_3 treatment of osteosarcoma cells. *Calcif. Tissue Int.* **46,** 270–279 (1990).
50. Finkelman, R. D., Linkhart, T. A., Mohan, S., Lau, K. H., Baylink, D. J., and Bell, N. H. Vitamin D deficiency causes a selective reduction in deposition of transforming growth factor β in rat bone: Possible mechanism for impaired osteoinduction. *Proc. Natl. Acad. Sci. USA* **88,** 3657–3660 (1991).
51. Scharla, S. H., Strong, D. D., Mohan, S., Baylink, D. J., and Linkhart, T. A. 1,25-Dihydroxyvitamin D_3 differentially regulates the production of insulin-like growth factor-1 (IGF-1) and IGF binding protein-4 in mouse osteoblasts. *Endocrinology* **129,** 3139–3146 (1991).
52. Aubin, J. E., and Heersche, J. N. M. Vitamin D and osteoblasts. *In* "Vitamin D" (D. Feldman, F. H. Glorieux, and J. W. Pike, eds.), pp. 313–328. Academic Press, San Diego, 1997.
53. Chou, S., Hannah, S. S., Lowe, K. E., Norman, A. W., and Henry, H. L. Tissue-specific regulation by vitamin D status of nuclear and mitochondrial gene expression in kidney and intestine. *Endocrinology* **136,** 5520–5526 (1995).
54. Suda, T., and Takahashi, N. Vitamin D and osteoclastogenesis. *In* "Vitamin D" (D. Feldman, F. H. Glorieux, and J. W. Pike, eds.), pp. 329–340. Academic Press, San Diego, 1997.
55. Chapuy, M. C., Arlot, M. E., Duboeuf, F., Brun, J., Crouzet, B., Arnaud, S., Delmas, P. D., and Meunier, P. J. Vitamin D_3 and calcium to prevent hip fractures in elderly women. *N. Engl. J. Med.* **327,** 1637–1642 (1992).
56. Gillespie, W. J., Henry, D. A., O'Connell, D. L., and Robertson, J. Vitamin D and vitamin D analogues in the prevention of fractures in involutional and post-menopausal osteoporosis. *In* "Musculoskeletal Injuries Module of the Cochrane Database of Systemic Reviews" (W. J. Gillespie, R. Madhok, G. D. Murray, C. M. Robinson, and M. F. Swiontkowski, eds.). Cochrane Collaboration, Oxford, 1997.
57. Lips, P., Graafmans, W. C., Ooms, M. E., Bezemer, P. D., and Bouter, L. M. Vitamin D supplementation and fracture incidence

in elderly persons. A randomized, placebo-controlled clinical trial. *Ann. Intern. Med.* **124,** 400–406 (1996).

58. Aloia, J. F., Vaswani, A., Yeh, J. K., Ellis, K., Yasumura, A., and Cohn, S. H. Calcitriol in the treatment of postmenopausal osteoporosis. *Am. J. Med.* **84,** 401–408 (1988).
59. Gallagher, J. C., and Riggs, B. L. Action of 1,25-dihydroxyvitamin D on calcium balance and bone turnover and its effect on vertebral fracture rate. *Metabolism* **39**(Suppl.1), 30–34 (1990).
60. Ott, S. M., and Chestnut, C. H., III. Calcitriol treatment is not effective in postmenopausal osteoporosis. *Ann. Intern. Med.* **110,** 267–274 (1989).
61. Tilyard, M. W., Spears, G. F. S., Thomson, J., and Dovey, S. Treatment of postmenopausal osteoporosis with calcitriol or calcium. *N. Engl. J. Med.* **326,** 357–362 (1992).
62. Orimo, H., Shiraki, M., Hayashi, Y., Hoshino, T., Onaya, T., Miyazaki, S., Kurosawa, H., Nakamura, T., and Ogawa, N. Effects of 1-hydroxyvitamin D_3 on lumbar bone mineral density and vertebral fractures in patients with postmenopausal osteoporosis. *Calcif. Tissue Res.* **54,** 370–376 (1994).
63. Klein, R. G., Arnaud, S. B., Gallagher, J. C., DeLuca, H. F., and Riggs, B. L. Intestinal calcium absorption in exogenous hypercortisolism. *J. Clin. Invest.* **60,** 253–259 (1977).
64. Arthur, R. S., Piraino, B., Candib, D., Cooperstein, L., Chen, T., West, C., and Puschett, J. Effect of low-dose calcitriol and calcium therapy on bone histomorphometry and urinary calcium excretion in osteoporotic women. *Miner. Electrolyte Metab.* **16,** 385–390 (1990).
65. Gallagher, J. C., and Goldgar, D. Treatment of postmenopausal osteoporosis with high doses of synthetic calcitriol. A randomized controlled study. *Ann. Intern. Med.* **113,** 649–655 (1990).
66. Falch, J. A., Odegaard, O. R., Finnanger, M., and Matheson, I. Postmenopausal osteoporosis: No effect of three years treatment with 1,25-dihydroxycholecalciferol. *Acta Med. Scand.* **221,** 199–204 (1987).
67. Riggs, B. L., and Nelson, K. I. Effect of long term treatment with calcitriol on calcium absorption and mineral metabolism in postmenopausal osteoporosis. *J. Clin. Endocrinol. Metab.* **61,** 457–461 (1985).
68. Gallagher, J. C., Jerpbak, C. M., Jee, W. S. S., Johnson, K. A., DeLuca, H. F., and Riggs, B. L. 1,25-Dihydroxyvitamin D_3: Short- and long-term effects on bone and calcium metabolism in patients with postmenopausal osteoporosis. *Proc. Natl. Acad. Sci. USA* **79,** 3325–3329 (1982).
69. Zerwekh, J. E., Sakahee, K., and Pak, C. Y. C. Short-term 1,25-dihydroxyvitamin D3 administration raises serum osteocalcin in patients with postmenopausal osteoporosis. *J. Clin. Endocrinol. Metab.* **60,** 615–617 (1985).
70. Gallagher, J. C., Riggs, B. L., Recker, R. R., and Goldgar, D. The effect of calcitriol on patients with postmenopausal osteoporosis with special reference to fracture frequency. *Proc. Soc. Exp. Biol. Med.* **191,** 287–291 (1989).

Index

A

C

D

E

F

G

H

I

J

K

P

T

ISBN 0-12-098655-8